CONTEMPORARY PERSPECTIVES IN HEARING ASSESSMENT

FRANK E. MUSIEK

Dartmouth-Hitchcock Medical Center

WILLIAM F. RINTELMANN

Professor Emeritus, Wayne State University School of Medicine

ALLYN AND BACON

Boston • London • Toronto • Sydney • Tokyo • Singapore

Executive Editor: Stephen D. Dragin
Editorial Assistant: Bridget McSweeney
Senior Editorial-Production Administrator: Joe Sweeney
Editorial-Production Service: Walsh & Associates, Inc.
Composition Buyer: Linda Cox
Manufacturing Buyer: Dave Repetto
Cover Administrator: Jennifer Hart

Library of Congress Cataloging-in-Publication Data

Musiek, Frank E.
    Contemporary perspectives in hearing assessment / Frank E. Musiek,
William F. Rintelmann.
        p.   cm.
    Includes bibliographical references and index.
    ISBN 0-205-27457-9
    1. Audiometry.   I. Rintelmann, William F.   II. Title.
RF294.M87   1999
617.8'075—dc21   98-55568
                                                                        CIP

Printed in the United States of America

10 9 8 7 6 5 4 3 2   03 02 01 00

Contents

PREFACE

Contemporary Perspectives in Hearing Assessment represents an update of *Hearing Assessment*, 2nd edition, published in 1991. Both the 1991 and the earlier 1979 editions of this text have been well received in the field of audiology. The primary purpose of this book is to serve as a text for graduate-level audiology courses concerned with the assessment of the peripheral and central auditory systems. It should also be a useful reference for practicing audiologists, otolaryngologists, and other clinicians and scientists who are concerned with the assessment of hearing in its normal and disordered states.

This new text, while retaining the informative and important basic chapters dealing with fundamental concepts of clinical audiology, also provides new data on the more complex and sometimes controversial assessment procedures critical to the practice of contemporary audiology. Comprehensive explanations of various aspects of diagnostic audiology are brought to the reader by contributors who are well-recognized authorities in their areas of specialization.

While the clinical procedures of some topics (e.g., pure-tone audiometry, clinical masking, etc.) have changed little in the past decade, other topics (evoked potentials, otoacoustic emissions, etc.) have continued to evolve and expand largely due to the scientific emphasis placed on these topics. As a consequence, the scope and magnitude of some chapters are proportionately greater than others.

The coverage of classic behavioral site-of-lesion tests has been omitted to provide necessary space for topics that are more relevant as we approach the millennium. Though information on classic behavioral site-of-lesion tests remains historically important, it is beyond the scope of this text to review these tests. Those interested in a review of this aspect of audiology are referred to *Hearing Assessment*, 2nd edition.

A unique aspect of this text is the accompanying compact disc (CD) that has been prepared by Richard Wilson. The purpose of this CD is to provide graduate students an opportunity to have some experience with acoustic stimuli that might not be readily available. Hence, students will have a chance to better comprehend certain clinical concepts that may not be well understood by textual explanation alone.

The editors are indebted to each of the authors for providing comprehensive and up-to-date coverage of their assigned topics. Also, we wish to thank Patty Cantlin for providing secretarial assistance connected with this book, and Kathy Whittier for her editorial assistance. Finally, we appreciate the support of our wives, Sheila and Sandy, for their patience and understanding during the time this book was in progress.

FRANK E. MUSIEK, Ph.D.

Dr. Musiek is presently Professor of Otolaryngology in the Department of Surgery as well as Professor of Neurology in the Department of Medicine at the Dartmouth Medical School. He is also Director of Audiology at the Dartmouth-Hitchcock Medical Center in Lebanon, New Hampshire. He has published over 120 articles and book chapters in audiology and related fields. He is co-editor of the book *Central Auditory Assessment: Foundations in Clinical Correlates*, as well as co-author of the books *Neuroaudiology: Case Studies, Central Auditory Processing Disorders: New Perspectives*, and *The Efferent Auditory System*. Dr. Musiek has also edited a monograph entitled "Contemporary Issues in Audiology." He is the Hitchcock Foundation Henry Heyl Award winner for Excellence in Clinical Research. He was selected as the "Baylor College of Medicine James Jerger Lecturer for 1996."

WILLIAM F. RINTELMANN, Ph.D.

After a 35-year career serving on the faculties of several universities, Dr. Rintelmann retired in 1995 as Professor and Chairman, Department of Audiology, Wayne State University School of Medicine. His publications include over 80 articles and book chapters on various topics of clinical audiology. He is also co-editor of *Principles of Speech Audiometry* (1983) and editor of *Hearing Assessment* (1979) and (1991). He is a Fellow of the American Speech-Language-Hearing Association, member and past Executive Board member of the American Auditory Society, and member of the American Academy of Audiology. He received the "Career Award in Hearing" in 1997 from the American Academy of Audiology.

CONTRIBUTORS

Jane A. Baran, Ph.D.
University of Massachusetts
Department of Communication Disorders
Amherst, MA 01003-0410

Christopher D. Bauch, Ph.D.
Mayo Clinic
Section Of Audiology
Rochester, MN 55905

Fred H. Bess, Ph.D.
Vanderbilt University Medical Center
Vanderbilt Bill Wilkerson Center for Otolaryngology
 and Communication Sciences
Department of Hearing and Speech Sciences
Nashville, TN 37212-2197

Allan Diefendorf, Ph.D.
Indiana University School of Medicine
Department of Audiology and Speech-Language
 Pathology
Indianapolis, IN 46202

John D. Durrant, Ph.D.
University of Pittsburgh
Center for Audiology, UPMC
Otolaryngology & Communication
Pittsburgh, PA 15213

John A. Ferraro, Ph.D.
University of Kansas Medical Center
Hearing and Speech Center
Kansas City, KS 66160-7605

Theodore J. Glattke, Ph.D.
University of Arizona
Department of Speech and Hearing Sciences
Tucson, AZ 85721

Judith S. Gravel, Ph.D.
Albert Einstein College of Medicine
Department of Audiology
Bronx, NY 10461

James W. Hall III, Ph.D.
Vanderbilt University
Balance and Hearing Center
Nashville, TN 37212-3102

Andrea Hedley-Williams, M.S.
Vanderbilt University Medical Center
Vanderbilt Bill Wilkerson Center for Otolaryngology
 and Communication Sciences
Department of Hearing and Speech Sciences
Nashville, TN 37212-2197

Linda J. Hood, Ph.D.
LSU Medical Center
Kresge Hearing Research Laboratory of the South
New Orleans, LA 70112

Lisa L. Hunter, Ph.D.
University of Minnesota
Department of Otolaryngology
Minneapolis, MN 55455-0301

Gary P. Jacobson, Ph.D.
Henry Ford Hospital
Division of Audiology
Detroit, MI 48202-2689

Wei Wei Lee, M.D.
Department of Otolaryngology
Albert Einstein College of Medicine
Bronx, NY 10461

Michael J. Lichtenstein, M.D.
Audie L. Murphy Memorial Veterans Hospital
Division of Geriatrics and Gerontology
Geriatrics Research Education and Clinical Center
San Antonio, TX

Brenda L. Lonsbury-Martin, Ph.D.
University of Miami School of Medicine
Department of Otolaryngology (805)
Miami, FL 33101

Robert H. Margolis, Ph.D.
University of Minnesota
Department of Otolaryngology
Minneapolis, MN 55455-0301

Glen K. Martin, Ph.D.
University of Miami School of Medicine
Department of Otolaryngology (805)
Miami, FL 33101

Frank E. Musiek, Ph.D.
Dartmouth Hitchcock Medical Center
Sections of Otolaryngology and Neurology
Lebanon, NH 03756

William F. Rintelmann, Ph.D.
Professor Emeritus, Wayne State University
    School of Medicine
Department of Audiology
35407 North 59th Street
Cave Creek, AZ 85331-9159

Martin S. Robinette, Ph.D.
Mayo Arrowhead Primary Care Center
Glendale, AZ 85308

Jay W. Sanders, Ph.D.
Vanderbilt University
Division of Hearing and Speech Sciences
Nashville, TN 37240

Sabina A. Schwan, M.A.
Comprehensive Audiology, Inc.
Grosse Pointe, MI 48230

Thomas H. Simpson, Ph.D., CCC-A
Wayne State University
Department of Audiology and Speech-Language
    Pathology
Detroit, MI 48202

Anne L. Strouse, Ph.D.
VA Medical Center
Audiology (126)
Mountain Home, TN 37684

Fred F. Telischi, M.D.
University of Miami
Department of Otolaryngology
Miami, FL 33101

Robert G. Turner, Ph.D.
LSU Medical Center
Communication Disorders
New Orleans, LA 70112-2262

Bruce A. Weber, Ph.D.
Duke University Medical Center (retired)
Department of Audiology
Durham, NC 27710

Laura Ann Wilber, Ph.D.
Northwestern University
Audiology Department
Evanston, IL 60208-3550

Richard H. Wilson, Ph.D.
VA Medical Center
Audiology (126)
Mountain Home, TN 37684

CHAPTER 1

PURE-TONE AUDIOMETRY: AIR AND BONE CONDUCTION

LAURA ANN WILBER

INITIAL CONCEPTS

Pure-tone audiometry (air and bone conduction) should serve as the base for audiologic evaluation. After completing a history and obtaining pure-tone audiometric thresholds, one should have at least preliminary answers to the basic questions: (1) Does this person have a hearing loss? (2) Is this hearing loss likely to be correctable by medicine or surgery? (3) Is this hearing loss likely to interfere with communication? Although other procedures are necessary to refine these answers and to determine the probable site of the pathology, the basic picture should be clear after completion of pure-tone air and bone conduction.

Since we recognize that pure-tone audiometry is the base for the rest of our audiologic testing and evaluation, it is somewhat surprising to realize that the procedure did not exist until the latter part of the nineteenth century. In addition, normative threshold values for pure-tone audiometers did not exist officially in this country until 1951 with the publication of the American Standards Association Document: "Audiometers for General Diagnostic Purposes". Z24.5 (ASA, 1951).

Pure-tone audiometry as we know it today probably began after the presentation in 1919 by C. C. Bunch and L. W. Dean (Bunch, 1943) of the "Pitch Range Audiometer" before the American Otologic Society. By 1922 Fowler and Wegel had developed the Western Electric 1A audiometer, which was the first commercially available vacuum tube audiometer existent in the United States (Bunch, 1943). Further, a standard procedure for pure-tone threshold testing was not officially established until 1978 (ANSI, 1978).

WHISPER TESTS

Physicians and others did test hearing, however, before the audiometer became commercially available. One of the first threshold tests of hearing probably was the "whisper" test. As recently as 1996, a report appeared that suggested that clinicians (general practice physicians) should employ the test (Eeckhof, de Bock, de Laat, Dap, Schaapveld, & Springer, 1996). Whisper tests and tests using spoken voice will be discussed in detail in Chapter 2 on Speech Audiometry. To summarize, the procedure is used to try to determine whether the patient has normal hearing. Generally, the examiner uses either spoken voice or whispered voice at a specified distance from the patient and determines whether the patient responds appropriately or not to a question or command. The obvious problem with this type of procedure is that it is difficult to determine the level of one's voice or whisper. This author has measured "whispers" from 20 dB to 65 dB sound pressure level (SPL) at 3 feet, depending on the talker. It also is not possible to determine which ear is responding to the whisper or spoken voice. Despite its inadequacies, we still receive forms from the government or insurance companies asking for results of "SV" (spoken voice) and "WV" (whispered voice).

As concern about the need for surgery or medical treatment of middle ear pathology became more prevalent, as well as the ability to carry out such treatment, it was realized that it was necessary to determine the extent of the hearing loss and to differentiate hearing loss caused by problems in the external/middle ear versus those in the inner ear.

TUNING FORK TESTS

Probably the earliest technique used to differentiate conductive and sensorineural hearing losses is still in use today. Tuning fork tests were used to determine whether the patient had "normal" hearing at several frequencies, and they also enabled the physician to predict the probability of middle ear pathology. Tuning fork tests, which may have been used first simply to indicate more accurately whether the patient heard sounds equally well at different pitches, became critical in evaluating the possibility of a conductive component. Certain tuning fork tests are still commonly used today by otologists, some audiologists, and others as a quick method of assessing the probability of conductive pathology. Although most audiologists probably do not routinely use tuning fork tests, they still need to be sufficiently familiar with them to discuss patient test findings, including tuning fork results, with otologists or neurologists. In addition, tuning fork tests can be used as a "quick and dirty test" to compare to one's bone conduction results.

To administer the test, the examiner first strikes the tuning fork usually on his or her own arm or leg or some other object so that it emits a sound. The strength with which the tuning fork is struck, as well as the material with which the tuning fork is made, will control the intensity of the sound from the fork as well as the length of time it takes for the tone to decay. We have found differences in intensity greater than 30 dB between fork presentations depending upon the striking strength and the metal with which the tuning fork was made. Thus, hearing sensitivity with the tuning fork becomes difficult to quantify. It is possible for experienced examiners to use tuning forks to estimate air-conduction thresholds by determining the difference in seconds between the length of time the patient and the examiner heard the tone. This may be done at various test frequencies. The tuning fork is held in front of the pinna, or its shank is placed on the forehead or the mastoid process depending on the specific test. It also is possible to use masking when testing with forks. Most commonly, the Baranay noise box is used for tuning fork masking. The basic problem of the Baranay noise box is that its frequency response does not produce adequate masking especially for high frequencies (see Chapter 3).

Table 1.1 describes five basic tuning fork tests in use today. The Schwabach has been used for air conduction as well as bone conduction, although it is commonly considered a measure of bone conduction. In this test one must rely on the examiner's ability to consistently strike the fork. The Schwabach and Rinne help determine whether the sensorineural system is normal. The difference between the tuning fork and audiometric tests is that the tuning fork air-bone difference normally is classified as present or absent (except with very experienced examiners who may be able to say whether the difference is small, moderate, or large), whereas the audiometer allows one to quantify the air-bone gap fairly precisely in decibels.

The Bing and Weber tests can be done using a bone vibrator and an audiometer in place of a tuning fork. The Gellè can be accomplished by changing air pressure in the ear canal with the probe from an acoustic immittance device and using the probe tone for the air-conduction Gellè. One may use a bone vibrator (or tuning fork) plus the air pressure change created by the acoustic immittance device for the bone-conducted Gellè.

In the hands of a careful and experienced examiner, tuning fork tests can provide a great deal of information about

TABLE 1.1   Tuning fork tests.

TEST	DEFINITIONS AND PROCEDURES
Schwabach	Place the tuning fork on the mastoid and determine the difference in seconds that the tone is heard by the examiner and the patient. If it is heard for a longer time by the patient, it is a prolonged Schwabach and one assumes conductive hearing loss. If it is heard for a shorter time by the patient, it is a shortened Schwabach and one assumes a sensorineural hearing loss.
Rinne	Determine if the patient hears the tone longer by air conduction (AC) or bone conduction (BC). If the patient hears the tone for a longer time by BC than AC, the Rinne is negative and suggests a conductive (or mixed) lesion.
Bing	Occlude the ear. If the tone appears louder when the ear is occluded this indicates normal hearing or a sensorineural hearing loss. If the tone does *not* get louder, this indicates a conductive hearing loss.
Weber	Place the tuning fork in the center of the forehead. If the patient hears the tone in the poorer ear this indicates a conductive component, whereas, if it is heard in the better ear the loss is probably sensorineural. This test is usually done only with frequencies 256 Hz to 1024 Hz. (*Note:* The tone *may* lateralize to the ear with the greatest cochlear reserve [best bone conduction] regardless of the conductive component).
Gellè	Increase the air pressure in the auditory canal. In stapes fixation the increase of air pressure usually does not affect, or decreases, the loudness for bone conduction, but it does decrease loudness for air conduction. Normally in other conductive pathology air conduction thresholds will also be decreased.

Based in part on work reported by Tonndorf (1964).

the probability, and even degree, of conductive pathology. However, they do not provide numerical threshold data. One can only determine relative intensities for air and bone thresholds. The results can be reported and compared from one examiner to another but only in a gross sense. With experience, one may be able to delineate those who have normal hearing from those with mild, moderate, or severe-profound losses with or without conductive pathology. Unfortunately, these tests are more susceptible to error than audiometric tests. For example, the Weber will normally lateralize *either* to the ear with the better cochlear reserve *or* to the ear with the greater conductive component. However, for no obvious reason it may lateralize to an ear with poorer cochlear reserve or a lesser conductive component. The reason for this occurrence might be that the contour of the skull causes the tone to reach the cochlea quicker for one ear than the other (phase advance). We have seen instances in which the Weber, done audiometrically or with tuning forks, lateralizes to one ear at one frequency and to the other at another frequency. In addition, we have found instances in which the placement (i.e., forehead vs. dental) of the tuning fork or bone vibrator will affect the tonal lateralization.

Most tuning fork tests can be easily influenced by the manner in which the patient is questioned. For example, while doing the Bing, if one asks the patient after the ear is occluded if the tone appears to be louder than before, one is more likely to get an affirmative response than if one simply asks the patient to tell what, if anything, happened to the tone when the ear was occluded. The latter is the more acceptable question since it is less likely to influence the response of the patient. Many patients in their desire to be cooperative are all too willing to respond in whatever way they believe the examiner expects or wishes. Similarly, when administering the Weber, it is best to simply ask where the patient hears the tone (rather than in which ear it is heard).

Thus, with tuning fork tests one can determine whether the patient hears better at one frequency than another, whether hearing is essentially normal or not, and whether there is probable conductive pathology. Tuning fork tests can be done at any frequency for which one has a tuning fork, but generally they are done at 256 or 512 Hz. One is extremely unlikely to obtain positive Bing or Gellè results at frequencies above 512 Hz. Useful information may be obtained with the Schwabach or Rinne at higher frequencies, although it usually is somewhat more difficult to obtain reliable lateralization or air-bone differences with forks above 1024 Hz. Probably the 512 Hz fork is the most commonly used, although it is not quite as likely to produce a positive Bing as is the 256 Hz fork. Finally, it is generally best to draw conclusions with tuning fork tests only if one has tested two or more frequencies with at least two procedures.

METHODS OF THRESHOLD MEASUREMENT

As suggested above, with the advent of the pure-tone audiometer, it became possible to determine the threshold of hearing for the patient. For a discussion of the audiometer and procedures for calibration, refer to Chapter 17. The audiometer can be used for speech testing and for special auditory tests but in this chapter we will discuss the use of the audiometer only as a device for obtaining pure-tone thresholds for hearing.

CONCEPT OF THRESHOLD

The concept of threshold of hearing is both simple and complex. Clinicians (especially otolaryngologists and audiologists) tend to use one type of definition, whereas psychoacousticians use another that is slightly different. The American National Standards Institute defines the threshold of hearing and the threshold of audibility (ANSI, S1.1, 1994; ANSI S3.20, 1995). These documents define threshold: "For a given listener and specified signal, the minimum (a) sound pressure level (b) force level that is capable of evoking an auditory sensation in a specified fraction of the trials" (ANSI, 1994, p. 36; ANSI, 1995, p. 19). The definition goes on to say that the characteristics of the test signal, of the procedure, and so on should be defined.

The obvious problem is what is meant by "evoking an auditory sensation." Strictly speaking, in most audiologic testing, the threshold of audibility probably is not attained. In most audiologic test procedures a compromise is made between determining the faintest level at which an auditory sensation can be evoked and the level at which the examinee will *respond* to the presence of an auditory stimulus using available audiometric test equipment in a reasonable length of time. It is clear that the procedure that one uses to measure "threshold" will determine to a large extent the value that will be obtained as threshold.

The level at which the examinee responds will be affected by whether: (1) the test stimulus is presented in 1 dB steps (or any fraction thereof) or in 5 dB steps; (2) the signal appears in the presence of a defined noise or in "quiet"; (3) the patient must indicate whether he or she believed a signal has occurred after a specific clue (such as a light flash) or with no clue; (4) the criterion for definition of threshold is the level at which the examinee responds 50% of the time, more than 50% of the time, or some other specified percentage; and (5) it is done by an examiner or a computer system. These are, of course, only a few of the variables that might affect the outcome of threshold measurement.

The working definition of "threshold of hearing" for the clinician should probably be the faintest level at which the patient will respond consistently (at least 50% of the time) to the presence of a specific auditory signal using a specified technique. Some of these techniques will be discussed later. However, both ANSI terminology documents note that threshold may be defined as "the lowest input level at which responses occur in at least 50% of a series of ascending trials" (ANSI, 1995, p. 10). It should be noted that the American Speech-Language-Hearing Association (ASHA) has developed a recommended procedure (ASHA, 1977) and the American National Standards Institute (ANSI) and the International Standards Organization (ISO) have produced standards for pure-tone audiometric test procedures (ANSI, 1978, 1992; ISO, 1982, 1984). However, even when one of these standard procedures is used, one should realize that one may not obtain a "true auditory threshold" for the examinee.

PSYCHOPHYSICAL PROCEDURES

It is important to decide on the psychophysical procedure that will be used in determining threshold of hearing for pure tones by individuals. The contribution made by the psychoacousticians to our understanding of why the patient responds as he or she does and which procedures are most likely to elicit the most sensitive and reliable data cannot be underestimated.

Before deciding which psychophysical method one wishes to use, one must first consider the reasons for which the measurements are being made. For example, some questions might be whether the person will respond to sound, in what way the person will respond, to determine whether the person has a hearing loss or not in a gross sense, to determine the person's specific hearing level for compensation purposes, or to determine the probabilities of the person having conductive pathology. Second, one must consider the nature of the specific stimulus that one plans to use: in this case, pure tones or tonal stimuli of varying intensities and durations. Third, one must consider the person being tested. For example, it would be inappropriate to expect an infant to operate a switch or even to raise its hand in response to the tone (see Chapter 10). The method used, therefore, must be appropriate to the person, to the stimuli, and most of all, to answer the measurement question.

Stevens (1958, 1960) described seven procedures for determining *absolute threshold.* The absolute threshold was defined by ANSI S3.20 as the "minimum stimulus that evokes a response (about 50% of the time) in a specified fraction of trials" (ANSI, 1995, p. 13). Earlier Stevens defined absolute threshold as "the value that divides the continuum of stimuli into two classes—those to which the organism reacts and those to which it does not" (Stevens, 1960, p. 33). Stevens' procedures are: (1) single stimuli, (2) counting, (3) forced choice, (4) adjustment, (5) limits, (6) tracking, and (7) staircase. Although he pointed out that it was not possible to define absolute threshold absolutely

since it shifts in time, he did describe procedures that might be used to try to determine the threshold of hearing for a given subject at a given point in time.

All of the above methods have been used alone, in combination, or in modified form to attempt to determine the subject/patient's threshold of hearing. Depending on the procedure, the stimulus (in this case a pure tone) is on either continuously or during discrete time intervals.

In the *single stimuli method* the tone is on or off at a particular intensity level and the examinee is asked to indicate whether the tone is present. If he or she believes that it is present, he or she may indicate yes by saying so, by pushing a button, by raising his or her hand, and so on. If the examinee does not believe that it is present, he or she will do nothing. Threshold is defined as the level at which the stimulus is correctly perceived as present 50% of the time. One may use another requirement such as 75% of the time, but generally in clinical usage 50% is considered the threshold point.

If, instead of randomly presenting the stimulus at various intensities, it is varied in a systematic procedure from levels above and below the threshold, it is called a *method of limits*. This may be done using a continuous tone as originally described, or discrete tone bursts. The subject is instructed to indicate when he or she "just hears" the tone. A modification of this procedure is used in most clinical situations, as will be described in more detail later in this chapter under *conventional procedures*. In the latter case, referred to as *modified method of limits*, the stimulus is increased in specified intensity intervals until the examinee indicates that he or she has heard it. The tone is then attenuated by a specified amount and again increased in discrete steps until the subject indicates that the tone is present.

The modified method of limits is not very different from the *staircase procedure* in which the intensity levels are also discrete and fixed. The response at a particular level during one trial will determine the level of the next trial. Specifically, if the stimulus did not elicit a response, the intensity is increased by a fixed amount, whereas if a response was elicited it is decreased by a fixed step interval. In the procedures described above the examinee knows that a signal will occur, but he or she usually does not know *when*. In the *forced choice method* the examinee knows when the stimulus *may* have been presented, but he or she does not necessarily know *if* it was. In this procedure during a fixed time interval, which is usually defined by a light clue, the subject is required to indicate whether the stimulus was present. In a variation of this, the subject knows both that the tone was present and that it occurred during one of a series of time intervals (usually no more than four). In the latter case a signal such as a light flash is given, and the subject indicates in which discrete time interval the stimulus occurred. The forced choice procedure was originally used with research subjects, but it easily is adaptable to most clinical situations with cooperating alert patients. Robinson and Watson (1972) indicated that the optimal time interval for a single interval procedure is between one and three seconds. They further reported that in the multiple interval procedure the time between successive observations is usually about half a second.

One more variant on the above procedures is the *counting method*. This was used at one time in classrooms when many children were tested simultaneously. A series of tones was presented through headsets to each of the children and they were asked to indicate how many tones they heard during the time interval. In this case, the tones were attenuated in discrete steps, so by comparing the number of tones perceived by the child against the number given, one could decide the faintest level at which the child heard. The problem was that the child might lose count or copy from a neighbor. The procedure also has been used with some telephone tests of hearing. Another variant used today with difficult to test patients is to give 1 to 3 stimuli at a given intensity level. The patient is asked to indicate how many were heard. This often produces more reliable, if not more sensitive, threshold data.

Besides procedures that use discrete stimulus presentations, some methods use *constant stimuli*. In these procedures the stimulus is always present and the question is how faint it may be and still be perceived as audible by the examinee. In one procedure, the *method of adjustment*, the examinee controls an attenuator and adjusts the intensity of the tone until it is "just audible" (or in some cases, until it is "just inaudible"). The level to which the examinee adjusts the intensity is defined as threshold.

In another procedure, the *method of limits* described above using discrete stimuli, the stimuli may also be constantly on but systematically varied by the examiner. The examinee indicates when the tone is just audible, as it is increased and decreased in a specified range.

A variation on the continuous stimuli method of limits procedure is called *tracking* (more commonly called the "Bekesy" procedure). It was described by Bekesy (1947) and by Oldfield (1949). In this procedure the examinee presses a button or activates a switch for as long as he or she hears the tone and releases the button, or deactivates the switch when the tone disappears. The stimulus intensity is automatically increased or decreased depending on the subject's action. It should be noted that in the original design described by Bekesy, the stimulus frequency was changed automatically at the same time the intensity was increasing and decreasing.

With persons who have hearing losses, it usually is easier to determine threshold of hearing when the pure-tone frequency is fixed. This is because the time constants of the frequency change are such that the subject may not have reached threshold at one frequency before the next frequency is presented. If there is a dramatic difference in threshold (i.e., sharp slope) from one frequency to another, this often will not be reflected in the continuously varying frequency procedure.

Although all of the methods described above may be used with a clinical population, each procedure may not be equally effective for each individual. For example, the single interval forced choice procedure in which a stimulus may or may not occur during a fixed time interval normally produces very reliable and sensitive threshold data for research subjects. However, for *some* patients an uncertain time interval is thought to be of help clinically since it avoids predisposing the patient whose hearing level is unknown from responding when there is no stimulus. For example, it is not uncommon for both children and adults to establish their own rhythmic pattern of indicating the presence of a stimulus regardless of whether one was introduced. If the examinee is told that a signal may or may not occur in a given time interval, some patients will respond positively in each time interval. If this occurs, the clinician should either use a method of rewarding the patient only for a correct response, or use another forced choice procedure, in which several time intervals occur and the patient is asked in which interval the stimulus occurred. Again, some patients will either invariably pick a specific interval (e.g., number two) or will become more concerned with guessing an interval than listening for a tone. The distinction may be that generally the research subject appears to interpret the important question as being whether he or she can respond correctly to the presence of a stimulus, while the patient with a hearing loss may respond in a completely different manner simply because his or her goal is to define a level at which he or she can respond rather than his or her ability to accomplish the task. If it is clear that the patient will not easily break a pattern response when a forced choice technique is used, it may be necessary to vary time intervals, or to use another procedure.

As suggested above when obtaining patient thresholds, the time interval between stimulus presentations for an alert cooperating person is generally between one and three seconds. However, when the patient begins to respond at short time intervals, such as once every two seconds regardless of the time of stimulus presentation, the time period between signal presentations may be expanded to five or ten seconds. Finally, in clinical testing, one will find some patients who appear to need several seconds before they are able to respond to the presented stimulus. We have seen some patients who were consistently able to respond to the presence of a sound but who required a five- to ten-second time interval between the end of the stimulus and the time when they were able to produce a response. This *may* suggest the presence of some neurologic dysfunction.

In psychoacoustic signal detection experiments, when using forced choice procedures, it is common to establish a specific criterion level for the patient. The subject may be asked, for example, to respond when he or she is 90% sure that a stimulus has occurred during a given time interval. When a strict criterion is employed, one expects that the response will require a greater intensity than it will if the subject is asked to respond if he or she thinks that he or she has a 10% probability of correctly identifying the stimulus. In the latter instance he or she is likely to guess much more often and the level at which he or she responds will be fainter. Generally, the purpose of these experiments is not simply to define the level at which the subject can detect a signal but to determine probabilities of signal detection. Some experiments are designed to determine not only the listener's ability to discriminate the presence of a signal embedded in noise, but also his or her ability to adapt a particular strategy for responding to the presence of the stimulus. The display of data generated from these experiments generally is called a *receiver operating characteristic (ROC) curve*. This function relates the probability of a response being given when the signal is, in fact, absent. Egan, Greenberg, and Schulman (1961) showed that there could be considerable difference in the probability curves that were generated depending upon whether the subject was instructed to be strict, medium, or lax in making a decision. Again, it is probably evident that there are many variations which can occur on this theme.

The outcome of these experiments (or any threshold measurement procedure) can be affected in other ways, such as indicating to the examinee that he or she will be rewarded financially or in some other way if he achieves a particular percent correct criterion. If the subject is punished either by a mild electric shock or even by a signal light indicating a wrong answer, then the correct response percentage also will change. Some variations on these behavior modification techniques can be used effectively with patients. For example, in testing young children it usually is helpful to smile and nod one's head enthusiastically when the child correctly responds to the presence of a tone. One also may frown or look dejected when the child responds when the sound is absent. (This author does *not* recommend or condone the use of electric shock for children or in fact *any* persons as a reinforcer or as a punisher for incorrect response.)

In psychoacoustic experiments it also has been shown that one can dramatically affect the results by giving the subject false feedback information. If one gives a light signal indicating the response was false when it was not, this can confuse the subject and will change the level at which he or she responds to the presence of the stimulus. One should thus be careful not to give a patient false visual information. For example, if the clinician frowns in response to something occurring in the examining room at the same time that the patient is responding correctly to the presentation of a tone, this will confuse the patient and may result in false threshold estimations.

It should be remembered that signal detection theory, which has helped so much to delineate psychophysical test procedure experiments and has provided a means to study the effect of variables, is actually a mathematical model designed to determine whether an electrical signal has occurred in the presence of noise. Originally these experiments were developed in electrical engineering (Tanner & Sorkin, 1972). Mathematical concepts may be used with human beings by asking that the human respond in the ways described above, but one should remember that it is infinitely easier to accurately detect the presence or absence of a signal in the presence of noise on an oscilloscope or with a computer than in a human's auditory system. The results from the machine are not so likely to be contaminated by human problems such as fatigue, desire to be rewarded, desire to confuse or confound the examiner, or the constant change that appears to occur in a human's true auditory receptive ability.

Finally, criterion levels may be defined much more easily for electronic equipment than humans. Every clinician is likely to have been confronted at one time or another with a patient who had been instructed very carefully to respond as soon as a tone was heard, but who did not respond consistently after repeated instructions and reinstructions. Just as the clinician becomes convinced that this patient has the largest threshold variation ever reported, the patient suddenly says, "Oh! You meant I should tell you *every time* I heard that itty bitty noise. Well, why didn't you tell me that's what you wanted me to do?" At this point the psychoacoustician generally has a distinct advantage over the clinician in that the former can walk out of the room and let the computer continue the testing.

CONVENTIONAL PROCEDURES

The majority of hearing tests for children and adults will be administered using so-called "conventional" procedures. For years the term "conventional" procedure was used with no clear definition of what it meant. In recent years, most often it referred to manual audiometry using the modified Hughson-Westlake technique (Carhart & Jerger, 1959), which is essentially an ascending technique using a modified method of limits procedure. In this procedure the patient/subject (examinee) is asked to indicate when he or she hears the tone either by raising his or her hand or finger or by pushing a button. The level of the tone is increased or decreased depending on the response (see Figure 1.1).

Briefly, with the manual procedure the examiner first familiarizes the examinee with the test tone by producing the stimulus at a presumed supra-threshold level or by gradually increasing the tone's intensity until the examinee responds. Then the tone is presented in short bursts of one to two seconds with silent intervals of varying length between tone presentations. The tone presentations are decreased in intensity until the examinee ceases to respond

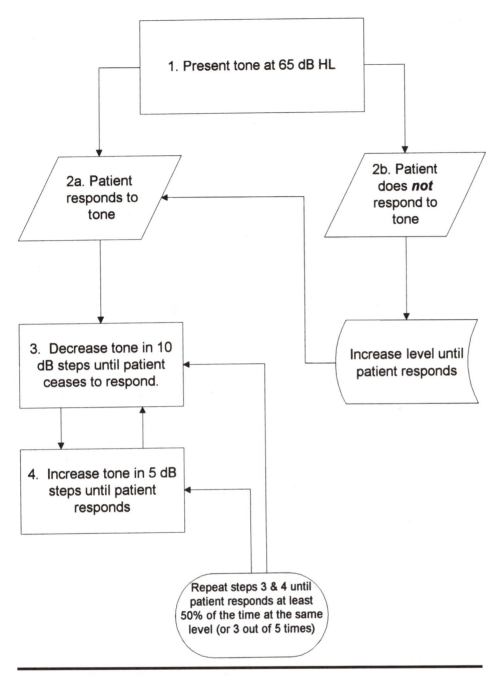

FIGURE 1.1 Flow chart for audiometric testing.

when it is presented. At that point, the intensity of the tone is increased. If the examinee responds when the tone is presented, the tone is lowered in intensity by 10 dB, and then it is increased in 5 dB steps until the examinee again responds. This ascending procedure is repeated until the examinee responds at least 50% of the time at a given level. Since most audiometer attenuators operate in 5 dB steps, in practice this level normally is achieved when one obtains two out of three or three out of five correct responses at a given intensity. A detailed description of the manual pure-tone audiometry procedure is described in *Asha* (ASHA, 1977) and in the ANSI standard S3.21 (ANSI, 1978). Working Group 3 (TC43/WG3) of ISO also developed an international standard for pure-tone testing (ISO, 1984). This Working Group has developed a series of standard procedure documents. The first standard defined procedures to use in industrial testing using automatic and manual threshold testing (ISO, 1982). The initial draft proposal of the manual procedure by the Group differed from the Hughson-Westlake method and was called a *bracketing procedure.* It more closely approximates an automatic procedure. As proposed, after familiarization, the tone is increased in specified steps and then decreased in specified steps. The faintest level at which the examinee responds to the tone on three ascending passes and on three descending passes is averaged to determine the threshold for hearing at a given frequency. The ascending technique described above was added as an alternate test procedure and is now considered equivalent to the bracketing procedure. In fact, a systematic study was carried out by Arlinger (1979) to see if there was a substantial difference in the threshold values obtained with the two techniques outlined above. The results indicated that both procedures yielded similar thresholds.

In any event, it is no longer sufficient for an examiner to say a "conventional" procedure was used. It is important to define specifically the procedure or to state that the ASHA 1977, ANSI 1978, or ISO 1984 procedure was used. *All of the above* standards and recommendations require that the examiner note on the audiogram (or report) if deviations from the described procedure were used. It is recognized that certain patients cannot be tested using any of the specific manual audiometric techniques described above and that special techniques must be used in these cases. In the latter instances, it is especially important to describe in detail the technique that was used.

Another "conventional" procedure for pure-tone testing is automatic (self-recording) audiometry. It is outside the limits of this chapter to discuss the procedures for Bekesy audiometry as it was used for diagnostic purposes, but automatic machines often are used to determine audiometric thresholds. In this procedure the examinee normally is asked to push a button when the tone is heard and to release the button when the tone fades away. The machine automatically decreases and increases the intensity of the tone as the button is pushed and released. An X-Y plotter may be attached to the attenuator output so that one may obtain a graphic representation of the examinee's response while increasing and decreasing the intensity of the sound. The midpoint of the ascending and descending patterns (Reger, 1952) or some other specific trace point is used to define the threshold level. It has been shown that the point on the tracing that one chooses to call "threshold" can affect the correlation of these results with manual techniques (Harbert & Young, 1966). The problem of comparing manual to automatic thresholds has been discussed in detail by Rintelmann (1975) especially as applied to industrial hearing conservation procedures.

A second automatic technique is a preprogrammed computerized method that essentially has replaced the Bekesy technique, especially in industrial applications (see Chapter 16). In one computerized procedure, the examinee presses a button if he or she thinks a sound has occurred. If the sound did occur, the program calls for a fainter stimulus to be emitted at a discrete level. Attenuation may continue in discrete steps until the subject does not respond, at which time the intensity is increased. This may mirror the modified Hughson-Westlake technique described above. With the exception that this procedure may be done with single tone bursts and discrete interval steps, it also is very much like the automatic procedure described above. In another preprogrammed computerized technique a tonal signal is presented at a predetermined intensity level. A light flashes and the subject responds by pushing a button to indicate whether he or she believes a tone presentation occurred or not. At certain randomly prescribed intervals the light will flash, but no tone will be presented. Again, the subject must indicate whether he or she believes a tone occurred. The faintest level at which the subject correctly identifies a specified percentage of tonal stimuli is labeled threshold. These procedures use the forced choice technique discussed above. There are many variations on the above procedures. Currently an ANSI working group is trying to develop a standard for computerized audiometry. The current ISO standard simply states that test results with a computerized system should yield thresholds that are the same as with the manual procedure (ISO, 1984).

No matter which of the techniques outlined above are used, it is clear that the examinee may respond at whatever supra-threshold level he or she desires or he or she may fail to respond at all, even when the tone is audible. The examinee's concept of "hearing the tone" will influence the results obtained. It is important that the examiner instruct the examinee in a manner likely to elicit the faintest response levels. For example, one may say: "Be sure to push the button *as soon as* you hear the tone and let the button go *as soon as* it goes away. Remember, I want to find the *very faintest* level at which you can hear this tone." One may tell the examinee to respond as soon as he or she hears the tone no matter how quiet it is, that it is all right to guess, and that the subject should indicate even if he or she only *thinks* he or she hears the tone. If too many false positive responses occur, one must reinstruct the examinee.

Various techniques can be used for children or older persons who have difficulty in responding consistently to the stimulus. Patients who have tinnitus, regardless of age, often have difficulty, especially at high frequencies. Others have short attention spans. Others may forget the stimulus for which they are listening, or the response that is expected. In these instances one may ask the patient to count the number of beeps (giving varying numbers of tonal stimuli usually 1 to 4, at a given intensity level) or to point to the ear in which he or she hears the sound. Assuming the patient can count or can point, these procedures should yield reliable threshold results. If the examinee wishes to deceive the examiner, it is quite possible that he or she will respond only at supra-threshold levels. It is beyond the scope of this chapter to discuss ways in which this can be detected or the procedures to overcome it (see Chapter 14), but one must always remember that it is possible that at a given time the examinee may not be responding at the faintest level at which he or she can hear.

Green (1972) described somewhat facetiously the "finger" test in which he discusses the height or way the finger is raised. In many instances one truly can determine how close to threshold one is by noting the alacrity and height to which the examinee raises his finger or hand. Although this particular observation is not always foolproof, the careful clinician will try to observe the examinee's behavior in order to gain more information about the examinee's probable reception of sound.

One 2-year-old child whom we tested refused to raise his hand consistently, but he did say "no" firmly each time the tone was presented. It is the clinician's job to encourage, to cajole, and occasionally even to bully the examinee into responding as closely as possible to his or her threshold of audibility.

The conventional procedures described above have as their advantage that they are highly repeatable. It is not yet clear by how much the results of any of these "conventional" techniques will vary from the "true threshold of audibility" for a given examinee; but for practical purposes, these techniques will enable one to determine with a high degree of confidence whether the examinee has normal hearing or a mild, moderate, severe, or profound hearing loss.

HISTORY

Before beginning the actual test procedure it is important to establish rapport with the patient and to learn something about that patient. Both of these can be accomplished while taking a history. A skillful clinician often can determine the probable hearing level (how loud does one have to speak to be understood), the possible cause of the problem (specific answers to questions), and the probable rehabilitative needs (chief complaint) while taking the history. This also affords the clinician an opportunity to establish a relaxed atmosphere in which the patient feels that his or her concerns are of paramount importance to the clinician.

Table 1.2 presents an outline of the areas that should be covered. One should always be able to modify the questions asked depending on the answers. In some cases one will wish to probe for more information (if, for example, the patient reports that other family members have hearing losses), and in some cases specific areas need not be covered (birth history in the case of most adults). It is important to listen to the answers and to the way in which they are given. If the clinician starts thinking about the next question, he or she may miss an important part of an answer. If the patient volunteers information that the clini-

TABLE 1.2   Primary components of a case history.

I. Identifying Information
  A. Name, address, date of birth, current date, referral source
  B. Occupation (include schooling level for children)
II. Chief Complaint—or Reason for Referral
III. Previous Evaluations
  A. Hearing
  B. Other medical (ENT, neurologic, pediatric, etc.)
  C. Other non-medical (speech, language, psychological, etc.)
IV. History
  A. Birth (includes pre-, peri-, and postnatal)*
  B. Developmental*
  C. Medical (diseases, injuries, and medical concerns)
  D. Familial (relatives with known or suspected hearing loss)
V. Current Complaints
  A. Hearing difficulty (where, under what conditions)
    1. Normal response to sound (speech, music, environmental)
    2. Able to use telephone (which ear)
    3. Stable or progressive loss (how long)
    4. One or both ears
  B. Other specific complaints related to ears
    1. Tinnitus (description of sound—ringing, buzzing, hissing, etc., and time frame)
    2. Vertigo (spinning, unsteadiness, etc.)
    3. Ear infections
    4. Ear surgery
VI. Current (recent) Medical
  A. Disease (Systemic illness, e.g., diabetes, renal, etc.)
  B. Head injuries
  C. Noise exposure
  D. Medication
    1. Ototoxic
    2. Other
VII. Rehabilitation History
  A. Hearing aids
  B. Aural rehabilitation
  C. Speech-language pathology*
  D. Remedial reading*
  E. Other

*Usually only asked with pediatric or infant populations

cian had planned to ask later, that should be noted and the questions not asked again.

Probably the single most important question revolves around the chief complaint (Why are you here today?). This concern should help direct subsequent questioning and testing. It should also, inasmuch as possible, be answered to the patient's satisfaction at the end of the test session. Referring to this question during the test session also reassures the patient that the clinician is really trying to gain the information necessary to help him or her.

It behooves the audiologist to address the history even if one already has been obtained during the session by a physician. Sometimes patients remember answers after the questions have been asked more than once. Sometimes they are more willing to be frank with the audiologist than the physician (and sometimes, vice versa). Although it may not be necessary to repeat all of the questions, at least one should determine the chief complaint, communication problems, and eliminate major causal factors.

PROCEDURES FOR CONVENTIONAL PURE-TONE AUDIOMETRY

After one has obtained a history, one should choose an appropriate method of measurement and basic stimuli. Remember it is important to determine not only the amount of hearing loss but something of its nature. The most basic procedures for determining gross site of lesion (i.e., conductive or sensorineural) are the air and bone conduction tests. In this chapter each will be discussed separately, but it is important to remember that both must be administered to obtain the basic diagnostic information. It also is important to recognize that in addition to pure-tone tests one will normally also administer acoustic immittance (Chapters 4 and 5) and speech tests (Chapter 2) to determine whether the loss is conductive or sensorineural. More subtle diagnostic information will be obtained using other physiologic and psychologic test procedure (see Chapters 6, 7, 8, and 13).

AIR-CONDUCTION TESTS

When obtaining behavioral air-conduction thresholds, one is measuring a response to sound passed through the entire auditory pathway. However, when observing an infant, one may be misled into thinking that a child "hears" when in fact the sound may be received only at a subcortical level. In most instances, the requirement of a specific voluntary action increases the probability that the patient has "heard" in the psychological sense (see Chapters 10, 11, and 15). Thus, one may believe with *some* degree of assurance that if the examinee responds to pure-tone stimuli at normal threshold levels the basic auditory system is reasonably intact from the external ear to the auditory cortex. However, ability to respond to pure-tones does *not* imply that the auditory system is completely undamaged. It will be shown in other chapters (2 and 13) that in some retrocochlear lesions the subject may be able to respond to pure tones at normal threshold levels but may not be able to handle speech stimuli or complex tonal stimuli in a normal manner. Despite this problem, if the examinee makes consistent *voluntary* responses to sound stimuli, those sounds probably have reached the auditory cortex. With

pure-tone testing, one is generally concerned with determining whether the patient has a peripheral hearing loss; that is, a loss at the level of the cochlea, middle, or external ear. Although in many instances damage to the VIIIth nerve also will result in a pure tone hearing loss, its significance will not be discussed here.

Responses to pure tones at normal (or above normal) hearing levels only mean the examinee hears a sound at these normal intensity levels. A response at a normal intensity level does not indicate that the tone necessarily is received or perceived in a normal manner, that is, it may be distorted or it may have no tonal quality at all. It is thus important to try to determine *what* the examinee hears as well as how faint a tone the subject can respond to. This usually can be learned by careful questioning at some time during the test session.

Air conduction tests are administered either using earphones, in the sound field using loudspeakers, or as mentioned earlier using tuning forks. In the next paragraphs we will be concerned with pure tone air-conduction testing using earphones or loudspeakers.

Earphone Testing

At present there are ANSI standards for earphones that are placed on the pinna (supra-aural) and for those that go into the ear (insert receivers), but there are no official standards for those that are enclosed in circumaural cushions or enclosures (that is, cushions that encircle the pinna as opposed to supra-aural cushions that rest on the pinna) (ANSI, 1996; Zwislocki, Kruger, Miller, Niemoeller, Shaw, & Studebaker, 1988), so it will be assumed here that supra-aural or insert earphones are used. Interim values for circumaural cushions are given in the appendix to ANSI S3.6-1996 (ANSI, 1996). A discussion of the importance of this distinction is given in Chapter 17 on calibration.

Whether an earphone is placed on, in, or over an ear, it is important that the diaphragm be placed opposite the opening to the ear canal. When the earphone is placed on *or* in the ear, hair or anything else that can block the opening to the ear canal should be moved away. It behooves the clinician to visually inspect the ear canal to make sure there is no cotton, excessive cerumen, or other object in the external ear. Sometimes persons who are in pain will put cotton in the ear canal and forget that it is there, which, of course, will create or add to a hearing loss. If possible, the ear should be cleared of cerumen. If cerumen extends out into the canal, it may block the opening of the insert receiver. However, if the cerumen is not impacted and totally occluding the ear canal, blocking the receiver, or touching the eardrum, it appears to have little, if any, effect on hearing thresholds. If threshold testing does reveal a conductive hearing loss and there appears to be cerumen, it should be removed by a competent person and the test should be repeated after the cerumen has been removed. It is a mistake to fail to repeat the test after cerumen removal, even if a conductive loss was found. By repeating the test one can determine whether the cerumen contributed to the initial test results.

Testing should be done in a room that is quiet enough to avoid masking by the noise in the room. The maximum sound pressure level (SPL) that may exist in a room in order to obtain thresholds as low as "0" dB hearing level (HL) are given in ANSI S3.1 (ANSI, 1991) and are shown in Table 1.3. Note that the values are lower for covered ears (earphones over both ears) than uncovered. If one is doing bone-conduction or sound field testing (see below), one must use the *uncovered* values as criterion values for room noise.

The covered values presume the use of supra-aural cushions. Although it is possible to obtain fainter and possibly more reliable thresholds in the presence of room noise using circumaural cushions (Villchur, 1970) or insert receivers (Wilber, Kruger, & Killion, 1988), the fact is that these effects have not yet been incorporated into the standards. This is expected in the next version of S 3.1, currently in draft stage.

In the case of supra-aural earphones, one should be sure that the earphone fits snugly over the ear and that the headband is adjusted appropriately. The earphones must be placed tightly over the ears or there will be a low-frequency transmission loss (such as evidenced in open ear mold fittings) that will be reflected in the measured thresholds. Occasionally one will find a patient whose head is too large for conventional headsets. In this instance, one may use two headsets with the earphone from one headset on one ear and the other earphone from the same headset on the upper part of the head and vice versa. Whether the head is large or small, it is infinitely better to use earphones with a headband than to try to hold the earphone in place. The

examiner's hand is unlikely to maintain consistent pressure against the pinna. A few manufacturers have provided earphone headbands for children, although they are difficult to find. We know of no commercially available headbands for infants. It will behoove the clinician to have available at least one headset that is the appropriate size for children, otherwise the insufficient pressure exerted by the band holding the phone in place may allow escape of sound, creating the presence of an erroneous low-frequency hearing loss and possibly slippage so that the high frequencies also may be in error.

In addition, when testing with supra-aural earphones, it is important to be sure that the pinna or ear canal does not collapse. In some instances when earphones are placed on the ear (especially with geriatric patients), the ear canal or the pinna may collapse to occlude the external auditory meatus. This will not be visibly apparent since current earphones are not transparent. One can get some notion of this possibility by pushing on the pinna with one's fingers prior to putting on the earphones and observing whether the opening into the canal appears to collapse. If one finds an apparent conductive loss with a normal tympanogram or positive acoustic reflex, one should suspect the possibility of an occluded ear canal. If a collapsing canal is suspected, one must use other procedures, such as sound field testing, insert receivers, or some method of keeping the canal propped open. The use of insert receivers will obviate this problem. When using insert receivers, however, one must be careful to insert them into the ear canal firmly and hold them in place until the foam tip has adjusted to the canal shape.

The patient should be seated in the examining room in a comfortable chair. Some clinicians prefer to have the patient facing the window between the examining room and the test area so that they can monitor facial expressions and bodily changes more readily—as well as maintain a type of contact with the patient that usually enhances rapport. When facing the patient, it also is possible to use facial expression to encourage responses. Others prefer to have the patient facing away so that he or she will not be influenced by any motions of the examiner and so that the patient will not spend time trying to "read" the examiner. This author normally uses the first approach but is careful not to allow the patient to see changes in posture or movement that would indicate when the signal is being activated.

When obtaining pure-tone air-conduction thresholds, one generally begins with a 1000 Hz tone. Although there is no compelling reason for starting at 1000 Hz (human sensitivity is slightly better at 2000 Hz, for example), some early studies by Harris (1945) and by Dadson and King (1952) indicated that test-retest reliability was slightly better at 1000 (or 1024) Hz than at the other frequencies tested. Perhaps for that reason, 1000 Hz is the recommended

TABLE 1.3 Acceptable ambient noise levels.

FREQUENCY (Hz)	UNDER EARPHONES ONLY (IN dB SPL)	SOUND FIELD OR BONE CONDUCTION (IN dB SUPL)
125	34.0	28.0
250	22.5	18.5
500	19.5	14.5
1000	26.5	14.0
2000	28.0	8.5
4000	34.5	9.0
8000	43.5	20.5

Acceptable noise levels (in dB SPL for octave bands) in audiometric test rooms when testing is expected to reach "0" dB HL (ANSI, 1991).

starting point in both the ANSI and ISO standard procedures. After establishing a threshold at that frequency using procedures described above and shown in Figure 1.1, one proceeds to the next highest octave frequency and so on through 8000 Hz, and then one establishes threshold for the lower frequencies of 250 and 500 Hz. If there is a difference of 20 dB or more between threshold values for adjacent octaves, one should test the intra-octave frequency. (For example, if the value for 1000 Hz is 25 dB and the value for 2000 Hz is 50 dB one should test 1500 Hz). When testing children or others whose attention span is very short or who are difficult to test, one may wish to first obtain threshold values at 500 and 2000 Hz for each ear. Following those four thresholds one may try testing the remaining frequencies. By finding thresholds for a high and low frequency, one can gain a basic impression of the examinee's response to sound. While the information from two frequencies is not sufficient to make a full comment on the examinee's hearing, these frequencies will enable one to make some statement regarding the probable hearing level of the patient and his or her probable communication problems. One should indicate which frequency was used initially if it was not 1000 Hz.

Before testing the second ear, one should retest the threshold at 1000 Hz to obtain an estimate of test-retest reliability. If agreement is ±10 dB, continue testing the next ear. If the agreement is poorer than ±10 dB, one must determine the cause of the poor test-retest agreement. Reinstructing the patient may solve the problem. In some cases it will be clear that the patient has "caught on" to the task, and his or her second responses are more accurate.

Although it is not within the scope of this chapter to discuss speech audiometry (see Chapter 2), we have found it helpful to use the speech recognition threshold (SRT) results as guidelines for pure tone test expectations especially in the case of young children. If the 1000 Hz threshold is considerably different than that obtained for speech, it is appropriate to test a frequency other than 1000 Hz to see if the second pure tone threshold is more compatible with the SRT. It should be expected that one of the frequencies of 500, 1000, or 2000 will be within ±5 to 10 dB of the SRT. Occasionally the SRT may be better than the thresholds for any of these three frequencies. However, if no pure-tone threshold is within ±5 dB of the SRT, one should suspect that the pure tone threshold results are inaccurate. The reason for the inaccuracy may be that speech is more familiar and probably more interesting than pure tones or it may indicate a functional overlay (see Chapter 14).

It is important to be sure that one is testing through the earphones (not through speakers when the earphones are on) and that the appropriate earphones are used. It helps to ask the patient to raise the hand on the side where he or she hears the sound (or to point to the ear with the sound).

However, often if all thresholds are obtained in this manner, they may be slightly poorer than thresholds obtained by simply asking the examinee to respond by raising his or her hand or pushing a response button when he or she hears a tone. It is difficult for many people to determine in which ear the sound is being heard at or very near their auditory threshold. In addition, the sound does not always have the same tonal quality near threshold that it does at supra-threshold levels. In any case, at some time during the test it is appropriate to ask the patient *where* he or she hears the sound to make sure that one has not inadvertently reversed the earphones.

When testing via earphone, one should expect the possibility of crossover if the air-conduction threshold is poorer than 40 dB HL. If the air-conduction threshold is 40 dB poorer than the bone-conduction threshold of the contralateral ear, crossover may occur but since one normally tests air conduction in both ears before testing by bone conduction, initially one cannot be sure of the bone-conduction threshold levels. Therefore, if responses occur at levels greater than 40 dB HL, one should consider using masking. The necessity of, and procedures for masking are discussed in detail in Chapter 3.

Sometimes it is difficult to teach young children to respond to the presence of the tone rather than to the presence of the masking noise. However, many children as young as 2 to 3 years of age can be taught this difference and will respond appropriately even when masking is used. A much more difficult problem is convincing the 2-year-old to use earphones. Many children in the 18- to 30-month-old range do not like to have anything on their heads and object strenuously when earphones are placed on them. Some children can be persuaded to wear the "hat" or "astronaut headphones," others cannot be so persuaded. This usually is not a problem for children below 1 year of age, but it is difficult to find appropriate headbands for babies. In this case, the insert receiver is the most viable alternative. When the child totally refuses earphones or they will not fit, sound field testing may be used.

Sound Field Testing Using Frequency Modulated Signals (Warble Tones) and Narrowband Noises

If the patient cannot be tested by earphones, it may be necessary to use sound field testing in order to obtain an indication of the levels at which the patient hears the tones. It is not possible to use pure tones in the sound field in an audiometric test booth (or regular room) because of standing waves. These create an impossible calibration situation and in addition require the examinee's head to be held in a rigid position. Pure tones probably can be used in an anechoic chamber, provided one has carefully padded all reflecting surfaces, including the chair in which the patient sits, in order to avoid any possibility of reflected sound.

Normally, however, one will be using an audiometric test booth and thus pure tones should not be used. As an alternative, one may use frequency modulated signals (commonly referred to as *warble tones*) or narrow bands of noise. The current audiometer standard describes the appropriate acoustic characteristics of both frequency modulated tones and narrowband noise (ANSI, 1996). The standard also gives the reference equivalent threshold sound pressure level (RETSPL) for sound field testing in either binaural (0° azimuth) or monaural (at 0°, 45°, and 90° azimuths) conditions.

When doing sound field testing, it is necessary to make sure that there is no object between the loudspeaker and the ear of the patient. It also is important to try to eliminate reflecting surfaces in the sound room (Stream & Dirks, 1974). The advantage of warble tone over narrow bands of noise was pointed out by Orchik and Rintelmann (1978) and Stephens and Rintelmann (1978). The latter study showed that for patients with flat hearing losses, warble tones and narrow bands of noise yield equivalent thresholds; however, if the patient has a high frequency loss because of the spread of the noise band, one will not get an accurate representation of the loss. That is, since a narrow band of noise as produced by current commercial audiometers has a spectrum that encompasses adjacent frequency bands at some point (6 to 20 dB fainter in most cases), the individual may respond to the noise from the adjacent frequency band rather than the test band. Since the purpose of testing is to determine the nature and degree of loss, it appears clear that warble tones are preferable to narrowband noise.

It probably is not important to use warble tones or narrow bands of noise under earphones, since most children who will wear earphones will respond equally well to warble tones or pure tones (Robinson & Vaughan, 1976).

As mentioned earlier, one of the disadvantages of sound field testing is that one cannot tell with which ear the patient is responding. When testing in the sound field, it is important to place the examinee in the location at which the intensity of the sound was measured. One way to do this is to suspend a weight on a string in the test chamber at a precise distance from the loudspeaker(s). The weight can be lowered to touch either the center of the patient's head (if necessary) or the microphone when calibrating. The examiner is again urged to use earphones whenever possible, since this will more accurately allow one to determine threshold values for each ear separately. As long as one realizes the limitations of sound field testing, it appears to be an acceptable procedure for tonal (although not pure tone) testing. See Chapter 10 for further discussion.

One can assume monaural testing only if there is a large difference between ears, or if the non-test ear is properly masked or occluded. Finally, comparisons of sound field

and specific earphone RETSPLs are given in Annex A of ANSI S3.6 (ANSI, 1996).

BONE-CONDUCTION TESTS

Bone-Conduction Theories

Before Bekesy's experiments, there was a question as to whether the auditory pathway for bone conduction was the same as for air conduction. Based on his work (Bekesy, 1932, 1960), it was recognized that the pathway is the same once sound reaches the cochlea. After that, investigators became concerned with determining how sound was conducted by bone conduction. Probably the most lucid explanation of bone-conduction hearing was presented by Tonndorf (1966).

Tonndorf described three modes of bone conduction as being: (1) energy radiated into the external canal (sometimes known as osseotympanic) in which vibratory sound from the osseous portion of the canal is conducted into the external auditory meatus and thence through the tympanic membrane using the normal air-conduction pathway; (2) acceleration of the temporal bone (also known as inertial bone conduction) caused by both the inertial response of the ossicular chain (probably especially at the footplate of the stapes) and the inner ear fluids; and (3) distortional vibrations of the temporal bone (also known as compressional bone conduction) that set up the traveling wave within the cochlea.

The normal ear probably makes use of all three modes in receiving the bone-conducted signal. However, the patient with a conductive lesion cannot (Tonndorf, 1964). If the problem is in the external ear, the first mode will be affected, since even if sound radiates into the external canal it will not be carried through the tympanic membrane. The inertial and compressional aspects will probably not be affected by external ear pathology. But, if the patient has an ossicular fixation or ossicular discontinuity, he or she will lose modes (1) and (2) to a greater or lesser extent depending on where the ossicular abnormality occurs, and will be left only with the third, or compressional, bone-conduction pathway. Note also that the relationship between frontal bone and mastoid bone conduction threshold will vary depending on the presence and site of a conductive lesion. The fact that the "Carhart notch" (average bone conduction loss of 5 dB at 500 Hz, 10 dB at 1000 Hz, 15 dB at 2000 Hz, and 5 dB at 4000 Hz) found in cases of otosclerosis disappears after successful stapes surgery is one indication that the apparent hearing loss by bone conduction is an artifact. It probably reflects only a loss of the inertial and osseotympanic components of bone conduction that are restored when the ossicular chain is repaired.

Although it is true that one may never determine "true" cochlear reserve using conventional bone-conduction tests, one may obtain reliable estimates of it. Certainly, one will have an indication of whether there is a difference between the air-conduction and bone-conduction thresholds (air-bone gap), which is indicative of conductive pathology and of the amount of gain in hearing that may be expected following successful middle ear surgery.

Note also that it is not possible for true bone-conduction thresholds to be poorer than true air-conduction thresholds. Since air-conduction values reflect the sum of the loss of hearing in the external and middle ear and that of the inner ear (measured by bone conduction), it is obvious that true air-conduction thresholds must always be the same or poorer than bone-conduction thresholds. Because of various testing artifacts (poor calibration, thick skull, unusual amount of fatty tissue on the mastoid, abnormal impedance at the ear drum, normal subject variation, etc.), one may occasionally obtain values in which bone-conduction thresholds *appear* to be poorer than air-conduction thresholds.

Bone-Conduction Test Procedures

The most commonly used procedure for bone-conduction testing is mastoid placement. Two other techniques, frontal bone placement and the sensorineural acuity level (SAL) procedure, also have been used. The latter test rarely is used today because of the improvement of techniques of conventional bone-conduction testing, masking, and calibration.

It is interesting to realize that we have only had threshold values for bone conduction since 1966 when Lybarger published the HAIC (Hearing Aid Industry Conference) bone-conduction norms (Lybarger, 1966). These values were first incorporated into the Appendix of the ANSI Standard for Artificial Headbone Calibration in 1972 and revised in 1981 and 1992 (ANSI, 1972, 1992). The present audiometer standard (ANSI, S3.6–1996) includes the expected threshold values for frontal and mastoid bone conduction placement. Specifications for a mechanical coupler (artificial mastoid or headbone) for calibrating bone vibrators used in audiometry has been published (ANSI S3.13–1987). See Chapter 17 for further discussion of calibration.

A second problem, masking, still exists, but it is not as significant as it once was, since our understanding of masking techniques has improved and since the use of narrow-band and effective masking has become more routine (see Chapter 3). Finally, advances have been made in bone vibrators (i.e., those with more mass and more reliable electronic circuitry, such as the Radioear B-71 and B-72) in the last few years that enable us to obtain even more reliable and sensitive threshold data today. The procedures described below for testing via bone conduction differ in detail but not in purpose. The basic problems mentioned above that preclude actual measurement of precise cochlear reserve exist in each method.

Mastoid Bone Conduction.   Mastoid placement is used most often because it seems convenient, it is traditional, and it requires slightly less power to measure threshold with mastoid placement than frontal bone placement, but generally other differences are not significant (Dirks, 1964a; Dirks & Malmquist, 1969). Please note that although one may correctly calibrate to compensate for the intensity difference between mastoid and frontal bone placement, the characteristics of current vibrators do not allow one to drive the vibrators at equally high hearing levels because of distortion possibilities. The improvement in sensitivity with mastoid placement thus will enable the examiner to measure a wider range of hearing levels. This latter reason *may* be why most audiologists prefer to use mastoid placement. However, there is evidence that the current vibrators, such as the Radioear B-72 (Dirks & Kamm, 1975) have greatly reduced the previous distortion problem.

In the United States bone-conduction testing traditionally has been carried out by holding the vibrator in place on the mastoid process with a headband. Although we pay lip service to the fact that this should have a static force of approximately 5.4 newtons (N) (ANSI, 1996), in fact, the force is generally closer to 400 grams (Dirks, 1964b). Studies by Konig (1957) indicated that higher static pressures resulted in slightly more reliable thresholds. However, there is a point beyond which the patient will not allow the examiner to increase pressure. We have found, for example, that when using a pressure of 1000 grams, even research subjects have difficulty in tolerating the physical pressure. There is a definite indentation on the head where the vibrator was located when testing is completed. A static force of 500 grams does not appear to be unduly uncomfortable for the majority of patients and is a practical if not ideal pressure.

Unfortunately, current commercially available headbands for vibrators do not allow one to regulate and monitor static pressure. This becomes an even more difficult problem with the smaller heads of children. In the latter case pressures may not reach static force values of 250 grams. It should be mentioned that the solution in testing is *not* one of holding the vibrator by hand. Pressure will not be constant with this method either, and one may dampen the stimulus output from the vibrator.

In addition to the static pressure, the positioning of the vibrator on the mastoid process also will affect the bone-conduction threshold results. With the larger hearing-aid type of vibrator, (i.e., Radioear B-70A) placement does not always make a great deal of difference since this vibrator covers a large area of the mastoid. However, with the round tipped vibrators currently recommended by ANSI (e.g., B-71) placement may make a considerable difference (ANSI, 1996). To help control reliability, the clinician is advised to place the vibrator on the mastoid process, turn on the tone, and move the vibrator from place to place, asking the examinee at which place the tone appears to be the loudest. This place will sometimes vary from one frequency to another, so to avoid changing placement for each frequency, one may use a specific frequency such as 500 Hz. It is, of course, difficult for young children and for some adults to indicate verbally at which place the tone appears loudest. In these cases, one must simply find a convenient place on the mastoid for placement. Further, one must always be sure that the vibrator does not touch the pinna and that as much of the hair as possible is pushed away from under the vibrator. Obviously, eyeglasses with temples that extend behind the pinna also must be removed.

In the United States, the ear ipsilateral to the vibrator is left unoccluded and an earphone is placed on the contralateral ear for the purpose of masking. This is advisable since the currently used threshold values were obtained using an open ear ipsilateral to the vibrator and contralateral masking (ANSI, 1996). This was done since covering both ears could cause an occlusion effect in cases other than bilateral conductive loss, and because the fact of "0" dB intra-aural attenuation for bone conduction means that masking must be used whenever there is an air-bone gap. If the contralateral ear is covered with a masking earphone, an occlusion effect will result unless the ear has a conductive hearing loss or masking is used. The occlusion effect will result in a false impression of bone-conduction sensitivity since it elevates low frequency thresholds (Dirks & Swindeman, 1967; Goldstein & Hayes, 1965; Huizing, 1960). This phenomenon may be reduced by using insert receivers for masking. Some clinicians prefer to obtain unmasked bone-conduction thresholds first and then repeat the test using appropriate masking if there is an air-bone gap of 5 to 10 dB at more than two frequencies. If there is no difference between the air-conducted and bone-conducted thresholds, there is no reason to mask. As mentioned above, normative threshold values for bone conduction were obtained using masked threshold data, since it was assumed that in most instances masking would be used and since it was realized that contralateral masking would affect slightly the obtained thresholds.

Whether the earphone is used contralaterally or ipsilaterally, one must provide enough masking to the contralateral ear to overcome the occlusion effect that will occur in the low frequencies. This effect can be as great as 25 dB at 500 Hz (Feldman, Grimes, & Shur, 1971). It should be emphasized, however, that the occlusion effect is highly variable and thus cannot easily be subtracted in the case of conductive loss ears (Dirks & Swindeman, 1967; Feldman et al., 1971). Normally an effective masking level of 30 dB will be enough to override the occlusion effect and to allow one to obtain accurate bone conduction thresholds (Whittle, 1965). An explanation of this as well as other procedures for masking are given in detail in Chapter 3.

After the vibrator is in place and the pressure is judged, or measured, to be correct the procedure for testing bone conduction is essentially the same as for air conduction (see Figure 1.1). Audiologists commonly use the ASHA (1977) or ANSI (1978, 1992) approved modified Hughson-Westlake technique (Carhart & Jerger, 1959) described above, including familiarizing the patient with the test tone. The patient is asked to respond when the tone is heard. The patient may need to be given additional instructions when masking is introduced. Bone conduction testing may be done using automatic or manual audiometry assuming appropriate calibration was performed.

As pointed out earlier, the only advantage of mastoid placement is that it will enable one to obtain slightly more sensitive threshold values than will frontal placement. It may, however, lull the clinician into believing that the side with the bone vibrator is the side being tested.

Frontal Bone.   Frontal bone placement probably is more defensible as a technique than mastoid placement, since it has been shown to be somewhat more reliable than mastoid placement (Dirks, 1964b; Studebaker, 1962), and since other possible contaminating factors mentioned below will not exist; however, it appears to be less popular with most clinicians. In this technique one must always use masking since both cochlea are stimulated. Without masking it is not possible to know which ear was tested. In this technique the vibrator is placed in the center of the forehead and one rarely has to worry about hair between the skin and the vibrator and never about touching the pinna. It generally is easier to obtain a static pressure that approximates 5.4 N with currently available headbands using frontal placement (Dirks, 1964b).

The procedure for obtaining threshold is the same as for air conduction or bone conduction with mastoid placement except that one must *always* use masking in the contralateral ear. The results obtained are assumed to be from the unmasked ear.

After thresholds are obtained for one ear, masking is changed to the contralateral ear. In the United States the test ear generally is unoccluded. If both ears are occluded, one must account for the occlusion effect. However, as mentioned above, the ear with a conductive loss will have little or no occlusion effect, while the normal ear or ear with a sensorineural loss will have an occlusion effect. Since one may not know in advance whether a conductive lesion exists, it is difficult to know whether to subtract the occlusion effect. Therefore, it seems more sensible not to cover the test ear. It should be mentioned again that insert receivers can minimize the occlusion effect, but they will not necessarily eliminate it.

SAL.   The third technique, *sensorineural acuity level (SAL)*, was developed by Jerger and Tillman (1960) at a time when it was critical for the surgeon to know as precisely as possible the acuity level of the sensorineural mechanism and when calibration and masking techniques were less precise. In the SAL technique, white noise masking is introduced into the bone vibrator, which is placed on the forehead while hearing is tested by air conduction. Air-conduction thresholds are obtained with and without masking. The shift that occurs when masking is presented is called the *SAL shift* and is compared to the average shift obtained under the same conditions for a group of normal-hearing subjects. The difference between the expected (local norms) and obtained shifts is the SAL threshold.

Problems with the SAL are: (1) Both ears are occluded, (2) some patients with sensorineural hearing loss have an abnormally large threshold shift with masking, and (3) difficulty in determining normative shifts. A useful application of the SAL, although not widely recognized, is in assessment of pseudohypacusis (see Chapter 14).

The three test procedures discussed above all have one common deficit. They cannot allow one to truly measure the cochlear reserve, since the normal ear uses modes of bone conduction that the ear with a conductive component cannot. Thus, these procedures will all underestimate the true level of the cochlear reserve to greater or lesser extents. Nonetheless, they all point to the probability of the presence or absence of conductive pathology. Finally, each of the three measures when properly used predict with high accuracy the expected post-operative air-conduction threshold. Since it always is important to know not only whether conductive pathology exists but what may be expected for post-operative hearing levels, the latter is most helpful. Clearly, when the pathology has a serious morbidity probability, the expected post-operative hearing levels are of little importance, but with pathologies not expected to cause serious illness or death (such as otosclerosis) it is very important to be able to predict with high probability the post-operative hearing levels.

Extended High-Frequency Audiometry

Another procedure that can be used with either air conduction or bone conduction, depending on instrumentation, is *extended high-frequency audiometry*. In this procedure one tests the hearing in the frequency range *above* 8000 Hz. High-frequency audiometry purportedly can reveal sensorineural hearing losses related to ototoxicity (Dreschler, van der Hulst, Tange, & Urbanus, 1985; Fausti, Larson, Noffsinger, Wilson, Phillips, & Fowler, 1994; Goldstein, Shulman, & Kisiel, 1987; Rappaport, Fausti, Schechter, & Frey, 1986; van der Hulst, Dreschler, & Urbanus, 1988), noise exposure (Gauz, Smith, & Hinkle, 1986; Goldstein et al., 1987), or other pathologies (Gauz et al., 1986; Goldstein et al., 1987; Rahko & Karma, 1986) before the hearing loss is evident in frequencies at or below 8000 Hz.

Various investigators (Frank & Dreisbach, 1991; Gauz, Smith, & Hinkle, 1986; Green, Kidd, & Stevens, 1987; Matthews, Lee, Mills, & Dubno, 1997; Okstad, Laukli, & Mair, 1988; Stelmachowicz, Beauchaine, Kalberer, Langer, & Jesteadt, 1988) have looked at the variability of the air and bone systems and found them to be comparable in variability to other systems with only somewhat larger standard deviations in the higher frequencies. For example, Green and colleagues (1987) reported the standard deviations for their younger subjects as 2.5 dB in the 8 to 14 Hz range and 4.5 dB in the range above that. There also have been some attempts to establish normative threshold data for high-frequency test procedures. Part of the problem relates to the fact that even more than at lower frequencies, age will influence the determination of a normal range of hearing (Matthews et al., 1997). At the present time both ANSI and ISO have established working groups to look at high-frequency audiometry both in terms of test equipment and in terms of possible normative data. Interim normative values for high-frequency thresholds for two types of earphones are given in the appendix to the audiometer standard (ANSI, 1996).

The specific test procedure to be used varies with instrumentation. In one case a probe tube is placed down the ear canal. In another, high-fidelity circumaural earphones are used. In the third approach, a large bone vibrator is used to transduce the signal. It is probable that most clinicians will use circumaural earphones for extended high-frequency testing. Since there are no official standards for this procedure yet, the reader is advised to use the ANSI interim values and proceed with caution. In theory the idea of extended high-frequency audiometry is excellent, but in practice there still appear to be some problems (calibration, normative data) that may preclude its routine use at this time. It should, however, prove quite useful (with the above cautions) when tracking hearing acuity change over time with patients who are exposed to noise or to ototoxic medications.

THE UNRESPONSIVE OR DIFFICULT TO TEST

The psychophysical procedures described earlier and the conventional procedures outlined above clearly require the cooperation of the subject/patient since the examinee must respond by word, by hand signal, or by manipulation of buttons or attenuators to indicate whether the stimulus is or is not heard. Although it is relatively easy to test the cooperating adult who wishes to know the faintest level at which he or she can hear, for the young child or patient who does not wish to respond, the procedure is not so simple. It is difficult to test the uncooperative individual who wishes to make the clinician believe that his or her hearing is much worse (or better) than it is (see Chapter 14). It also is difficult to test an individual who is unable to communicate verbally with the clinician because of the lack of a verbal language system or because he or she uses a different language than the clinician. In the latter instance, gestures may be used effectively to describe what is wanted. Finally, it will be especially tedious to attempt to test the patient who appears not to notice or care whether the sounds that enter his or her environment are present or absent.

Despite the difficulty, it is important to try to test the unresponsive or difficult-to-test individual using behavioral techniques. Although the electrophysiologic procedures (described in detail in Chapters 4–8) can give a great deal of information about the organism's ability to receive sound, the perception, or definition and usefulness, of the reception can best be assessed with behavioral techniques. If electrophysiologic tests indicate that the child or nonresponsive adult does not receive sound (at the level of the cochlea or higher), it probably is not necessary to do behavioral testing, but if sound *is* received by the child's auditory system, it is important to know if it is usable. (It should be noted, however, that this author has obtained behavioral thresholds on individuals who reportedly had no response to various electrophysiologic procedures.)

The difficult-to-test individual is considered to be one who because of maturation level, mental level, emotional well being, or attitude is unable or unwilling to cooperate with the examiner using conventional test procedures. It must be remembered that this individual may be quite testable using special test procedures. However, in some instances it will be impossible to establish rapport and cooperation sufficient to allow one to determine the threshold of hearing or even an approximation thereof. In these instances, one may need to use the electrophysiologic procedures described in Chapters 4 through 8. Also see Chapters 10 and 11 for assessing hearing in the pediatric population via both electrophysiologic and behavioral techniques. Note that many of the procedures described for children may also be used for the adult who is difficult to test. Finally, refer to Chapter 12 for discussion of hearing problems related to aging.

VARIABLES AND PROBLEMS THAT INFLUENCE MEASUREMENT

Throughout this chapter some of the problems that may affect threshold measurements in a clinical population have been discussed. In addition to the currently insoluble problem of whether true auditory thresholds *can* be obtained from human subjects, there are specific factors that should be re-emphasized.

First, with supra-aural earphone placement it is imperative that the diaphragm of the earphone be opposite the opening of the ear canal, that the canal not collapse, and that there is no air leak between the cushion and the ear. If

the earphone is off to one side of the canal, if the canal collapses, if headband pressure is insufficient, and so on, one will not obtain accurate measurement of the examinee's hearing threshold. It takes a little more time to make sure that the hair is not in front of the ear and that the earphone is properly placed, but without these precautions the measurement results may be meaningless.

Second, with insert receivers it is important to make sure the ear is clear of obstructions, including cerumen that might block the end of the receiver. It also is important to make sure that the receiver is placed firmly and deeply into the ear canal and that its surrounding foam has time to expand to fill the canal.

Third, positioning the patient in the sound field must be done carefully. As pointed out, it is important that when one uses two loudspeakers in a sound field, each ear should be an equal distance from the face of the loudspeaker. It probably is best to use 0° azimuth for sound field testing, although 45° and 90° may be used for monaural testing. (In special procedures such as hearing aid evaluations, one may wish speakers to be at 0° and 180° azimuth relative to the listener's face.) Loudspeaker calibrations must be made at the place where one expects the listener's head to be. If the subject's head is not at the spot where the microphone was placed, one will get an inaccurate representation of his or her threshold. In addition, if there is anything between the patient's ear and the loudspeaker (e.g., a parent's hand, the examiner's body, or any other object), one may obtain erroneous thresholds. As far as is possible, the head of the listener should be in the same plane as the loudspeaker. It may be difficult to move the speakers or patient up and down to compensate for the difference in height of the listener, but if this is feasible it should be done.

Fourth, bone vibrator placement must be carefully controlled. As mentioned earlier, the spot on the mastoid on which the vibrator is placed will change the threshold test results to some extent. The change can be as great as 10 dB. It is most important that the vibrator not touch the pinna. In addition, the pressure with which the vibrator is affixed to the mastoid process should be controlled, since this will change the threshold test result as well as the reliability of the threshold measurements.

Fifth, extended high-frequency audiometry can be used with circumaural earphones or a special bone vibrator to assess hearing above 8 kHz—especially if monitoring possible changes in hearing for a given individual—but it should be interpreted with caution when trying to determine precise hearing threshold levels.

Sixth, besides proper use of test equipment, the attention and cooperation of the patient will influence threshold measurements. If the examinee is not interested in the stimulus, does not care to play games, or is trying to simulate a hearing loss, the results will not be accurate. In the case of young children and some adults, it may be necessary to interrupt the test procedure from time to time to reinstruct them and to reestablish rapport. If there is something else that is interesting in the sound room, such as toys, flashing lights, or other visual stimuli, children may become distracted and not pay attention. If the patient is frightened, concerned, or distrusts the examiner, threshold measurements are likely to be inaccurate. Many persons begin to lose attention when one approaches threshold and may need to be revived again (sometimes just giving a louder stimulus will renew attention).

In some instances when testing children, as well as others who are unresponsive or difficult to test, one will obtain consistent play responses at supra-threshold levels and inconsistent responses as threshold is approached. This is probably because the patient's attention begins to wander since tones are not inherently interesting and so he or she must constantly be brought back to the task. Fatigue can affect the results for all patients. If the patient is tired or sleepy or if it is nap time for the child, the results will not be as accurate or as close to true threshold as might otherwise be obtained. In short, any physical, mental, or emotional factor that affects the human can affect his or her ability to respond to pure tones. This is true even if the examinee is concerned about the level at which he or she hears and wishes to cooperate. Despite these comments, it should be pointed out that with patience it is possible to reliably test patients who are so sick that they are on gurneys, who are in intensive care units, or who throw tantrums when they first enter the test room.

It is possible that the type of psychophysical test procedure will influence results. However, there appear to be no systematic investigations that clearly delineate the dB difference that might result from one procedure versus another. Clearly it has been shown that the modified Hughson-Westlake procedure will yield reliable results— but whether it consistently yields the most sensitive thresholds has not been demonstrated yet.

In addition, environmental physical factors also may influence test results. Temperature and ventilation must be appropriately controlled. In one test room that it was necessary to use, the temperature often reached or even exceeded 90°. Under those conditions some children yielded threshold test results that were as much as 15 dB poorer than they were at other times when the room was more comfortable. The precise effect that temperature, humidity, or ventilation will have on a subject will, of course, vary from one person to another and even from one time to another. Thus, the clinician is well advised to try to obtain the most comfortable, pleasant atmosphere possible in order to enhance the probability of obtaining reliable and accurate threshold measurements.

Finally, one should realize when trying to obtain threshold for pure tones or other tonal stimuli, that one must be sure of the calibration of one's equipment, of the ability

and willingness of the patient to respond, of the condition of the test environment, and of the interest and competence of the examiner. Failure to control any of these variables may prevent one from obtaining accurate and reliable measurements of the patient's threshold of hearing for pure tones. However, lest one doubt the possibility of ever obtaining worthwhile pure tone air- and bone-conduction threshold measurements, if the examiner remembers the reason for the test and attends to the procedures for controlling appropriate variables, reliable and accurate audiometric threshold data can and will be obtained.

REFERENCES

American National Standards Institute. (1972). *American National Standard for an Artificial Headbone for the Calibration of Audiometer Bone Vibrators* (ANSI S3.13). New York: Author.

American National Standards Institute. (1978). *Manual Pure-Tone Threshold Audiometry* (ANSI S3.21-1978, R1992). New York: Author.

American National Standards Institute. (1987). *American National Standard Specification for a Mechanical Coupler for Measurement of Bone Vibrators* (ANSI S3.13-1987). New York: Author.

American National Standards Institute. (1991). *American National Standard Maximum for Permissible Ambient Noise Levels for Audiometric Test Rooms* (ANSI S3.1-1991). New York: Author.

American National Standards Institute. (1992). *American National Standard Reference Equivalent Zero for the Calibration of Pure-Tone Bone Conduction Audiometers* (ANSI S3.43-1992). New York: Author.

American National Standards Institute. (1994). *American National Standard Acoustical Terminology* (ANSI S1.1-1994). New York: Author.

American National Standards Institute. (1995). *American National Standard Psychoacoustical Terminology* (ANSI S3.20-1995). New York: Author.

American National Standards Institute. (1996). *American National Standard Specifications for Audiometers* (ANSI S3.6-1996). New York: Author.

American Speech-Language-Hearing Association. (1977). Guidelines for manual pure-tone threshold audiometry. *Asha*, *19*, 236–240.

American Standards Association. (1951). *Audiometers for General Diagnostic Purposes* (Z24.5). New York: Author.

Arlinger, S. D. (1979). Comparison of ascending and bracketing methods in pure tone audiometry. *Scandinavian Audiology*, *8*, 247–254.

Bekesy, G. v. (1932). Zur theorie des horens bei der schallaufnahme durch knochenleitung. *Annal. Physik.*, *13*, 111–136.

Bekesy, G. v. (1947). A new audiometer. *Acta Oto-Laryngologica Stockholm*, *35*, 411–422.

Bekesy, G. v. (1960). *Experiments in Hearing*. New York: McGraw-Hill.

Bunch, C. C. (1943). *Clinical Audiometry*. St. Louis: C. V. Mosby.

Carhart, R., & Jerger, J. J. (1959). Preferred method for clinical determination of pure-tone thresholds. *Journal of Speech and Hearing Disorders, 24*, 330–345.

Dadson, R. S., & King, J. H., (1952). A determination of the normal threshold of hearing and its relation to the standardization of audiometers. *Journal of Laryngology and Otolaryngology, 66*, 366–378.

Dirks, D. (1964a). Factors related to bone conduction reliability. *Archives of Otolaryngology, 79*, 551–558.

Dirks, D. (1964b). Bone-conduction measurements. *Archives of Otolaryngology, 79*, 594–599.

Dirks, D. D., & Kamm, C., (1975). Bone vibrator measurements: Physical characteristics and behavioral thresholds. *Journal of Speech and Hearing Research, 18*, 242–260.

Dirks, D., & Malmquist, C. M. (1969). Comparison of frontal and mastoid bone-conduction thresholds in various conductive lesions. *Journal of Speech and Hearing Research, 12*, 725–746.

Dirks, D. D., & Swindeman, J. G. (1967). The variability of occluded and unoccluded bone-conduction thresholds. *Journal of Speech and Hearing Research, 10*, 232–249.

Dreschler, W. A., van der Hulst, R. J., Tange, R. A., & Urbanus, N. A. (1985). The role of high-frequency audiometry in early detection of ototoxicity. *Audiology, 24* (6), 387–395.

Eekhof, J. A., de Bock, G. H., de Laat, J. A., Dap, R., Schaapveld K., & Springer, M. P. (1996). The whispered voice: The best test for screening for hearing impairment in general practice? *British Journal of General Practice, 46,* 473–474.

Egan, J. P., Greenberg, C. Z., & Schulman, A. I. (1961). Interval of time uncertainty in auditory detection. *Journal of the Acoustical Society of America, 33*, 771–778.

Fausti, S. A., Larson, V. D., Noffsinger, D., Wilson, R. H., Phillips, D. S., & Fowler, C. G. (1994). High-frequency audiometric monitoring strategies for early detection of ototoxicity. *Ear and Hearing, 15* (3), 232–239.

Feldman, A. (1961). Problems in the measurement of bone conduction. *Journal of Speech and Hearing Disorders, 26,* 39–44.

Feldman, A. S., Grimes, C. T., & Shur, I. B. (1971). *Studies of the Occlusion Effect.* New York: SUNY Upstate Medical Center.

Frank, T., & Dreisbach, L. E. (1991). Repeatability of high-frequency thresholds. *Ear and Hearing, 12,* 294–295.

Gauz, M. T., Smith, M. M., & Hinkle, R. R. (1986). The simplified HF E-800 high-frequency audiometer: Clinical applications. *Journal of Audiological Research, 26* (2), 121–134.

Goldstein, B., Shulman, A., & Kisiel, D. (1987). Electrical high-frequency audiometry. Preliminary medical audiologic experience. *Audiology, 26* (6), 321–31.

Goldstein, D. P., & Hayes, C. S. (1965). The occlusion effect in bone-conduction hearing. *Journal of Speech and Hearing Research, 8*, 137–148.

Green, D. M., Kidd, G. Jr., & Stevens, K. N. (1987). High-frequency audiometric assessment of a young adult population. *Journal of the Acoustical Society of America, 81* (2), 485–94.

Green, D. S. (1972). Pure tone air conduction thresholds. In J. Katz (Ed.), *Handbook of Clinical Audiology.* Baltimore: Williams and Wilkins.

Harbert, F., & Young, I. M. (1966). Amplitude of Bekesy tracings with different attenuation rates. *Journal of the Acoustical Society of America, 39*, 914–919.

Harris, J. D. (1945). Group audiometry. *Journal of the Acoustical Society of America, 17*, 73–76.

Huizing, E. (1960). Bone conduction, the influence of the middle ear. *Acta-Otolaryngologica, 155*-Sup, 1–99.

International Standards Organization. (1982). *Acoustics—Pure Tone Air Conduction Threshold Audiometry for Hearing Conservation Purposes* (ISO/DIS 6189.2). Geneva: Author.

International Standards Organization. (1984). *Acoustics—Pure-Tone Audiometric Test Methods* (ISO/DIS 8253). Geneva: Author.

Jerger, J., & Tillman, T. W. (1960). A new method for the clinical determination of sensorineural acuity level (SAL). *Archives of Otolaryngology, 71*, 948–955.

König, E. (1957).*Variations in Bone Conduction as Related to the Force of Pressure Exerted on the Vibrator.* Chicago: Beltone Translations.

Lybarger, S. (1966). Interim bone conduction thresholds for audiometry. *Journal of Speech and Hearing Research, 9*, 483–487.

Matthews, L. J., Lee, F-S., Mills, J. H., & Dubno, J. (1997). Extended high-frequency thresholds in older adults. *Journal of Speech-Language-Hearing Research, 40*, 208–214.

Okstad, S., Laukli, E., & Mair, I. W. (1988). High-frequency audiometry: Comparison of electric bone-conduction and air-conduction thresholds. *Audiology, 27* (1), 17–26.

Oldfield, R. C. (1949). Continuous recoding of sensory thresholds and other psychophysical variables. *Nature, 164*, 581.

Orchik, D. J., & Rintelmann, W. F. (1978). Comparison of pure-tone, warble-tone and narrow-band noise thresholds of young normal-hearing children. *Journal of the American Audiological Society, 3*, 214–220.

Rahko, T., & Karma, P. (1986). New clinical finding in vestibular neuritis: High-frequency audiometry hearing loss in the affected ear. *Laryngoscope, 96* (2), 198–199.

Rappaport, B. Z., Fausti, S. A., Schechter, M. A., & Frey, R. H. (1986). A prospective study of high-frequency auditory function in patients receiving oral neomycin. *Scandinavian Audiology, 15* (2), 67–71.

Reger, S. N. (1952). A clinical and research version of the Bekesy audiometer. *Laryngoscope, 62*, 1333–1351.

Rintelmann, W. F. (1975). Manual and automatic audiometry. In J. B. Olishifski & E. R. Harford (Eds.), *Industrial Noise and Hearing Conservation.* Chicago: National Safety Council.

Robinson, D. E., & Watson, C. S. (1972). Psychophysical methods in modern psychoacoustics. In J. Tobias (Ed.), *Foundations of Modern Auditory Theory.* New York: Academic Press.

Robinson, D. O., & Vaughan, C. R. (1976). Relative efficiency of warble-tone and conventional pure-tone testing with children. *Journal of the American Audiological Society, 1*, 252–257.

Rudmose, W. (1962). *Pressure vs. Free Field Thresholds at Low Frequencies.* Copenhagen: Fourth International Congress Acoustics.

Shaw, G. M., Jardine, C. A., & Fridjhon, P. (1996). A pilot investigation of high-frequency audiometry in obscure auditory dysfunction (OAD) patients. *British Journal of Audiology, 30* (4), 233–237.

Stelmachowicz, P. G., Beauchaine, K. A., Kalberer, A., Langer, T., & Jesteadt, W. (1988). The reliability of auditory thresholds in the 8 to 20 kHz range using a prototype audiometer. *Journal of the Acoustical Society of America, 83* (4), 1528–1535.

Stephens, M. M., & Rintelmann, W. F. (1978). Influence of audiometric configuration on pure-tone, warble-tone and narrow band noise thresholds for adults with sensorineural hearing losses. *Journal of the American Audiological Society, 3,* 221–226.

Stevens, S. S. (1958). Problems and methods of psychophysics. *Psychological Bulletin, 55,* 177–196.

Stevens, S. S. (1960). Mathematics, measurement and psychophysics. In S. S. Stevens (Ed.), *Handbook of Experimental Psychology.* New York: John Wiley & Sons.

Stream, R. W., & Dirks, D. D. (1974). Effect of loudspeaker position on differences between earphone and free-field thresholds (MAP and MAF). *Journal of Speech and Hearing Research, 17,* 549–568.

Studebaker, G. A. (1962). Placement of vibrator in bone-conduction testing. *Journal of Speech and Hearing Research, 5,* 321–331.

Tanner, W. P., Jr., & Sorkin, R. D. (1972). The theory of signal detectability. In J. Tobias (Ed.), *Foundations of Modern Auditory Theory.* New York: Academic Press.

Tonndorf, J. (1964). Animal experiments in bone conduction: Clinical conclusions. *Annals of Otology, Rhinology and Laryngology, 73,* 659–679.

Tonndorf, J. (1966). Bone conduction—studies in experimental animals. *Acta-Otolaryngologica, 213*-Sup, 132.

van der Hulst, R. J., Dreschler, W. A., & Urbanus, N. A. (1988). High frequency audiometry in prospective clinical research of ototoxicity due to platinum derivatives. *Annals of Otology, Rhinology and Laryngology, 97* (2 Pt. 1), 133–137.

Villchur, E., (1970). Audiometer earphone mounting to improve intersubject and cushion-fit reliability. *Journal of the Acoustical Society of America, 48,* 1387–1396.

Whittle, L. S., (1965). A determination of the normal threshold of hearing by bone conduction. *Journal of Sound Vibrations, 2,* 227–248.

Wilber, L. A., Kruger, B. A., & Killion, M. C. (1988). Reference threshold levels for the ER-3A insert earphone. *Journal of the Acoustical Society of America, 83,* 669–676.

Zwislocki, J., Kruger, B., Miller, J. D., Niemoeller, A. F., Shaw, E. A., & Studebaker, G. (1988). Earphones in audiometry. *Journal of the Acoustical Society of America, 83,* 1688–1689.

CHAPTER 2

AUDITORY MEASURES
WITH SPEECH SIGNALS

RICHARD H. WILSON
ANNE L. STROUSE

The most important sounds transduced by the ear are sounds that compose speech signals. Speech signals are important because speech is the medium through which language-based communications are transmitted. The importance of the relation between speech signals and hearing was recognized over a century ago by Oscar Wolf who considered speech "the most perfect method of testing the hearing power, inasmuch as it embodies the most delicate shades in the pitch, intensity, and character of sound" (Gruber, 1891, p. 131). This chapter concentrates on the language, concepts, and variables associated with a variety of speech signals used to evaluate the auditory system. An instructive adjunct to the chapter is an audio compact disc that contains examples of many of the speech signals that are available for use in audiology clinics and research laboratories (see Appendix A for a detailed listing). Tracks #1 through #32 contain speech materials discussed in this chapter. Tracks #33 through #40 contain materials discussed in Chapters 10 and 13. The last track (#41) is a presentation made by Dr. Raymond Carhart during a dedication at Northwestern University (March 28, 1973). The first half of the presentation is on Channel 1 with the second half on Channel 2. Dr. Carhart was introduced by Dr. Tom Tillman, who briefly recounted the highlights of Dr. Carhart's career. The lecture is a reminiscence of the audiology program at Northwestern between 1941 and 1973 with mention made of the academic and scholarly philosophy behind the program, of the broad research topics of the thirty-year span, and of many of the students who matriculated through the doctoral program. Finally, the paucity in this chapter of a detailed historical perspective of speech audiometry is not meant to minimize the significance of early contributions. Previous annotations that are readily available provide a complete historical component (see Feldmann, 1960; Konkle & Rintelmann, 1983; Martin, 1997; Mendel & Danhauer, 1997; Olsen & Matkin, 1991; Tillman & Olsen, 1973).

Speech audiometry incorporates both *sensitivity* and *acuity* measures (Ward, 1964). Sensitivity measures are threshold measures that typically are referred to as the *speech-recognition threshold (SRT)* (ANSI, 1996, p. 4) and the *speech-detection threshold (SDT)*. Acuity measures are supra-threshold measures that typically are referred to as the speech-recognition score, word-recognition performance, or some combination thereof. The difference between threshold and supra-threshold measures is also related to the designation of the independent and dependent variables. With threshold measures we define the decibel hearing level (dB HL) (dependent variable) at which a certain percent correct recognition performance (typically 50% correct) (independent variable) is achieved. The independent and dependent variables are reversed with supra-threshold measures in which we define the percent correct recognition performance (dependent variable) that is achieved at certain decibel hearing levels (independent variable).

PSYCHOMETRIC FUNCTION

Threshold and supra-threshold data both represent points on a psychometric function, which is a graphic plot that relates some aspect of patient performance (output) to a stimulus dimension (input). With speech audiometry, the aspect of patient performance usually is percent correct detection, recognition, or identification and the stimulus dimension is the presentation level of the signal. Typically, patient performance is plotted on the ordinate (*y*-axis). The level of the signal, which usually is expressed in terms of *decibels sound-pressure level (dB SPL), decibels hearing level (dB HL)* (ANSI, 1996), or in terms of decibels *signal-to-noise (S/N) ratio*, is plotted on the abscissa (*x*-axis). Signal-to-noise ratio is a linear relation on the dB scale that involves subtracting the level of the signal from the level of the noise. For example, if an 80 dB HL signal is presented in 72 dB HL of background noise, the S/N ratio would be 8 dB. Likewise, a 70 dB SPL signal presented in 75 dB SPL of noise would produce a –5 dB S/N ratio.

Figure 2.1 illustrates detection (circles) and recognition (triangles) psychometric functions for the W-1 spondaic words spoken by Hirsh (Hirsh, Davis, Silverman, Reynolds, Eldert, & Benson, 1952); 24 listeners with normal hearing participated in the study (Cambron, Wilson, & Shanks, 1991). The lines through both sets of data are the

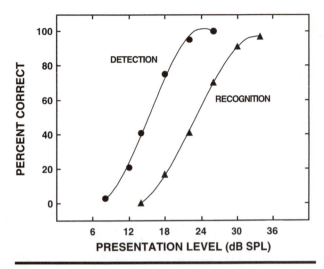

FIGURE 2.1 Detection (circles) and recognition (triangles) psychometric functions (n = 24) for the W-1 spondaic words spoken by Hirsh. (Adapted from Cambron et al., 1991)

the 20% and 80% correct points. For simplicity's sake and because the slope on this part of the curvilinear function approaches linearity, the slope of the function can be expressed simply as $\Delta y / \Delta x$. Over the 20% to 80% correct range, the slopes of the functions in Figure 2.1 are different, with the function for detection being steeper (8.0%/dB) than the function for recognition (6.5%/dB). These slopes, which are not as steep as slopes typically associated with functions for spondaic words, may be influenced by the method used to generate them. Consider the functions in both panels of Figure 2.2, in which individual functions *A, B, C, D,* and *E* (dashed lines) are averaged with the mean functions depicted with solid lines and circles. The functions of the mean data in both panels of Figure 2.2 (circles) were obtained by averaging the percent correct performance of subjects *A–E* at selected presentation levels (i.e., averaging the *y* datum points at each *x* point). Functions

best-fit, third-degree polynomials. (Equations for orthogonal polynomials are useful because the goodness of fit can be described and because any point on the function [in terms of either the *x*-axis or *y*-axis] can be calculated with ease and precision; additionally, the first derivative of a polynomial defines the slope function. Appendix B contains a brief discussion of polynomials.) The data in Figure 2.1, which are functions for the mean percent correct data points (ordinate) versus presentation level in dB SPL (abscissa), are instructive in a couple of ways. First, the detection and recognition functions are separated by 7.2 dB at 20% correct to 8.9 dB at 80% correct, with detection requiring less energy for comparable performance. The thresholds (50% points) are at 15.3 dB SPL (detection) and 23.2 dB SPL (recognition), which demonstrate a 7.9 dB difference between the two response tasks. Because the detection task is easier than the recognition task, the detection task requires less energy (sound-pressure level) than the recognition task to achieve the same performance criteria. Generally, the difficulty of the listening condition or test material determines the spot or location in the *x*-axis domain of the psychometric function.

Second, the *slopes* of the psychometric functions in Figure 2.1 merit discussion. With word-recognition data, the slope of the function is expressed as the percent correct per decibel (%/dB), meaning how much the percent correct recognition changes with each increment in the decibel presentation level. Although (mean) psychometric functions for word-recognition are usually sigmoidal or S-shaped, for simplification, the slope is calculated on what is termed the linear portion of the function, which usually is between

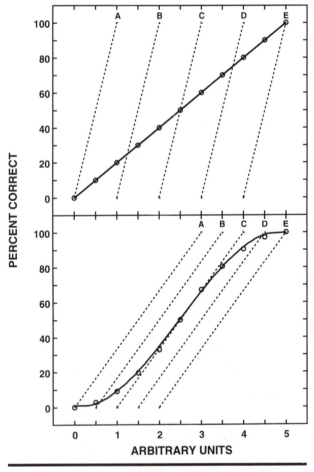

FIGURE 2.2 Schematized psychometric functions for individuals *(A–E)* and for the mean data (open symbols) calculated by averaging the percent correct *(y)* at each arbitrary unit *(x).* (Adapted from Wilson & Margolis, 1983)

averaged in this manner are the best predictors of subject performance at a given signal level, but the functions are influenced substantially by intersubject variability, as can be seen by comparing the data in the two panels of Figure 2.2. There is an inverse relation between intersubject variability and the slope of a function. Large intersubject variability decreases (flattens) the slope of the mean function (upper panel), whereas small intersubject variability increases (steepens) the slope of the mean function (lower panel). Although the mean functions in Figure 2.2 represent performance of the groups, the mean functions do not represent performance by any member of the groups. Function C in each panel is more representative of the performance by each member of the group, especially in terms of the slope of the function. The mean C functions in both panels were obtained by averaging the presentation levels of subjects A–E at selected percent correct points (i.e., averaging the x data points at each y point). The mean C functions, which are means of the individual functions, best predict the slope of individual functions. The majority of data presented throughout this chapter will be in terms of psychometric functions compiled using one of these two methods.

As was demonstrated in Figure 2.2, intersubject variability has a substantial influence on the slope of the mean psychometric function. The type of test material also has a substantial influence on the slope of a psychometric function. Past accounts indicate that the easier the word-recognition material, the steeper the slope of the function. For example, the psychometric function for digit materials is steeper than the function for spondaic words; likewise, the function for spondaic words is steeper than the function for monosyllabic words. In both of these comparisons, for a variety of reasons, listening to and repeating the former material is an easier task than listening to and repeating the latter material. The explanation of the easier the material, the steeper the slope of the function, however, is only superficially correct. The mechanism underlying the slope of a function is the homogeneity (similarity) of the experimental subjects and of the experimental items that compose the listening condition or test materials.

In the above example of digits, spondaic words, and monosyllabic words, then, the conclusion can be reached that digit materials are more homogenous than the spondaic words and that spondaic words are more homogenous than monosyllabic words. Empirically these relations were investigated under the hypothesis that the more homogeneous the psychometric functions for the individual words of a word list, the steeper the slope of the mean psychometric function for those words (Wilson & Strouse, in review). Two sets of monosyllabic word materials (PB-50s recorded by Rush Hughes and CID W-22s recorded by Hirsh) were selected for study because the slope of the W-22 function is

somewhat steeper than the slope of the PB-50 function (Heckendorf, Wiley, & Wilson, 1997). Twelve subjects with normal hearing participated. Representative findings are illustrated in Figure 2.3 with the psychometric functions for the individual subjects in the upper panels and the psychometric functions for the individual words in the lower panels; the mean data are depicted with symbols. The List 3, W-22 data are in the left panels and the List 8, PB-50 data are in the right panels (List 4, W-22 data and List 9, PB-50 data were obtained but are not shown here). Several relations are apparent in the figure. First, the slope of the mean function for the W-22s (2.8%/dB) is steeper than the slope of the mean function for the PB-50s (1.4%/dB). Second, the intersubject variability gauged by the spread of the functions in the top panels is less than the interword variability gauged by the spread of the functions in the corresponding bottom panels. Third, comparing the spread of functions in the bottom panels of Figure 2.3, the interword variability of the W-22s is substantially less than the interword variability of the PB-50s. That is, the psychometric functions for the W-22 words are more homogeneous than the psychometric functions for the PB-50 words, thereby supporting the hypothesis that the more homogeneous the individual functions, the steeper the slope of the mean function.

The data in Figure 2.4 represent the final step in the dissection of the mean psychometric function for word recognition. The data are from two words on List 3 of the W-22s, *are* (top panel) and *add* (bottom panel). In the figure, the filled symbols represent the mean data for each word with the thin straight lines representing the data of each of the 12 subjects. With most subjects, the recognition scores go from 0% correct to 100% correct in one 8 dB presentation increment (if a smaller step size had been used, then steeper functions for the individual subjects would have been obtained). The data from one subject in each panel, however, vacillates (dashed lines) and one subject in the top panel always scored 100% correct (triangles). The data in Figure 2.4 indicate how different the individual subject responses are to different words and support the notion that the more homogeneous the components of a mean function, the steeper the slope of that mean function. This concept applies to the mean function of each subject (stimulus differences) and to mean functions of a group of subjects (stimulus differences and subject differences).

The issues of intersubject variability and interstimulus variability are compounded when subjects with hearing impairment are evaluated. With respect to word-recognition ability, the population with hearing loss is less homogeneous than the population with normal hearing. Further, the interstimulus or interword variability probably is exaggerated when subjected to the variety of auditory limitations imposed on a group of listeners with hearing loss.

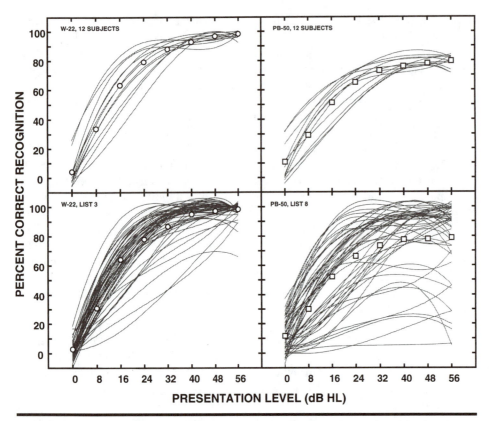

FIGURE 2.3 Psychometric functions for the individual subjects (n = 12) and for the individual words (n = 50) obtained for List 3, W-22 (Hirsh recording, left panels) and for List 8, PB-50 (Rush Hughes recording, right panels). The open symbols in each panel epresent the mean data. (Adapted from Wilson & Strouse, in review)

For these reasons, psychometric functions for subjects with hearing impairment (1) are displaced to higher presentation levels than functions for listeners with normal hearing and (2) have slopes that are more gradual (by as much as a factor of two or more) than the slopes of functions for the same materials from subjects with normal hearing.

FACTORS AFFECTING SPEECH RECOGNITION AND IDENTIFICATION

The ability of a listener to understand speech is affected many factors including the presentation level of the material, the presentation and response modes, the characteristics of the speech materials, and characteristics of the listener including language experiences and status of the auditory system.

Calibration of Speech Signals

Speech audiometry materials recorded on compact disc (or other recorded media) must have a reference tone recorded on one track (Wilson, Preece, & Thornton, 1990). The level of speech signals is defined in ANSI S3.6-1996 as:

> The level of the rms sound pressure of a 1000 Hz signal adjusted so that the deflection of the volume level indicator produced by the 1000 Hz signal is equal to the average peak deflection produced by the speech signal. The level indicated by the monitoring meter for a preliminary carrier phrase may be taken as the level indication of the speech material immediately following when the material is delivered in a natural manner at the same communication level as the carrier phrase. (p. 13)

For system calibration, the 1000 Hz calibration tone is set to 0 dB on the monitoring meter of the audiometer. With older audiometers the monitoring meter was a vu meter (ANSI, 16.5-1954), but the current ANSI specification for audiometers (S3.6-1996) defines the monitoring meter (dB meter) as one that has a 3 dB maximum and a −20 dB minimum with a response time that reaches the 0 dB point in 350 ms (±10% or 35 ms) with no more than 1.5% overshoot (p. 13). For vu meters the ballistic standards are a little more strict, namely, read 0 vu in 300

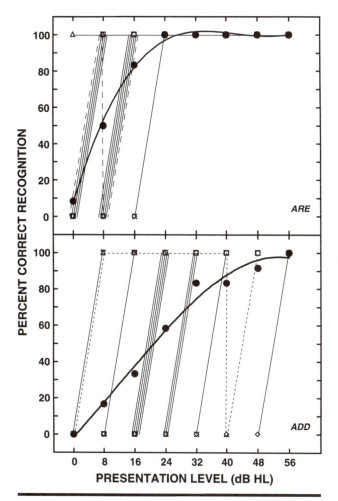

FIGURE 2.4   Psychometric functions for two words on List 3 of the W-22s, *are* (top panel) and *add* (bottom panel). The thin straight lines represent the data of each of the 12 subjects and the filled symbols indicate mean data. (Adapted from Wilson & Strouse, in review)

ms (±10%) with 1 to 1.5 vu overshoot (ANSI, 16.5-1954). The levels of speech stimuli whose sustained peak energy is maintained for <300–350 ms (e.g., monosyllabic words) cannot be measured accurately because these brief durations are less than the ballistic time constants of vu or dB meters. For this reason, some recorded materials with short durations do not reflect the level of the calibration tone. [Track 1 of the audio CD on both the left and right channels contains a 30 s, 1000 Hz calibration tone that is preceded by a 300 ms, 1000 Hz tone that can be used to check the ballistic characteristics of a monitoring (vu or dB) meter. Courtesy of the Auditory Research Laboratory, Mountain Home, Tennessee.]

Earphone.   The standard reference sound-pressure level for speech is defined in ANSI S3.6-1996 as 12.5 dB above

the 1000 Hz standard for a given transducer. Thus, if the standard sound-pressure level for a given earphone (insert or supra-aural) at 1000 Hz were 7.5 dB, then the standard reference level for speech through that earphone would be 20 dB SPL.

Sound Field.   Certain audiologic procedures, like functional gain on hearing aids and the evaluation of young children, require a free-field (i.e., an anechoic chamber) or sound-field (i.e., a sound-treated booth) environment. In the sound field, loudspeakers serve as the transducers with *azimuth* used to describe the relation between the head of the subject (ears) and the sound source. In Figure 2.5 the head of the subject is pointed at loudspeaker *A* and is denoted as the 0° azimuth. Adjacent to the right ear is the 90° azimuth (loudspeaker *B*), behind the head is the 180° azimuth (loudspeaker *C*), and adjacent to the left ear is the 270° azimuth (loudspeaker *D*). Our ability to hear in a sound field changes as a function of the azimuth of the stimulus source. The data in Figure 2.6 illustrate this point. In the figure, the listener has the left ear open and the right ear occluded with a foam insert and a muff. The *near ear* refers to the ear closer to the sound source, whereas the *far ear* refers to the ear farther from the sound source. In the example in Figure 2.6, about 4 dB less energy is required to reach threshold at the three near-ear azimuths

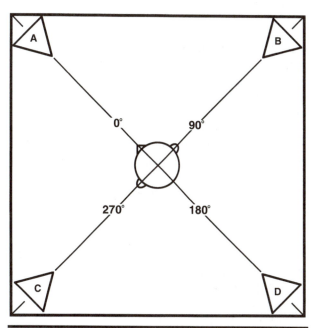

FIGURE 2.5   A schematic representation of the orientation of the head in a sound-field environment that illustrates the azimuth locations (in degrees) with respect to the face of the listener. The triangles with letters *A–D* represent loudspeaker locations.

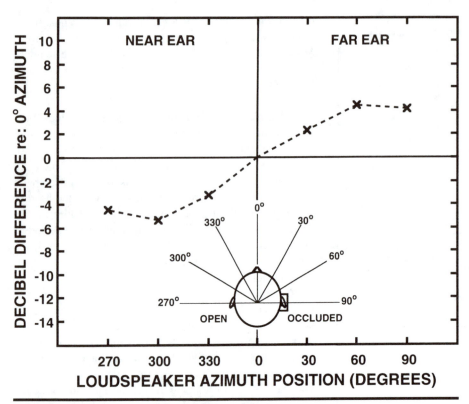

FIGURE 2.6 A schematic that represents the changes in the speech thresholds that occur for the left ear of a listener with the right ear occluded as the sound source rotates from the near-ear locations (270° to 330°), through the 0° azimuth that serves as the reference threshold, to the far-ear locations (30° to 90°). (Adapted from Wilson & Margolis, 1983)

(270°, 300°, and 330°) than at the 0° azimuth. In contrast, as the signal source moves to a far-ear location (30°, 60°, and 90° in this example), the left ear is in the acoustic shadow of the head and about 4 dB more energy is required to reach threshold than at the 0° azimuth. The acoustic shadow of the head (termed the *head-shadow effect*) acts like a low-pass filter imposing level, spectral, and phase changes on the signal as the signal crosses the head. Thus in this example, there is about an 8 dB difference between signal (speech) levels from near-ear and far-ear sources. In sound field, speech is calibrated minimally at 1 m for binaural listening to 14.5 dB SPL (0° azimuth) and for monaural listening to 16.5, 12.5, and 11.0 dB SPL for 0°, 45°, and 90° azimuths, respectively (ANSI, 1996, p. 23; also see Breakey & Davis, 1949; Dirks, Stream, & Wilson, 1972; Tillman, Johnson, & Olsen, 1966).

Presentation Level

A recent survey of audiological practices indicated that the majority of audiologists continue to use a variety of methods to select a single presentation level for word-recognition tests (Martin, Woodrick-Armstrong, & Champlin, 1994).

Seventy-five percent of audiologists reported that they administer word-recognition tests at a single presentation level, the most common of which was 40 dB above the speech-recognition threshold (SRT) or above the pure-tone average. This reference system is termed *sensation level (SL)* and in the above example would be expressed as 40 dB SL. In the same survey, approximately 20% of respondents reported using a *most comfortable listening (MCL) level* for word-recognition testing. Even a smaller percentage reported that testing was performed at a specified hearing level (e.g., 50 dB HL), or by obtaining word-recognition scores at several hearing levels to determine a segment of the psychometric function and/or maximum performance.

When the SRT or pure-tone average is used as the reference, most clinicians present word lists at 25 to 40 dB SL (25 dB SL corresponds to the beginning of the plateau at which normal hearing subjects attain scores of 90% or better on most word-recognition tests; 40 dB SL represents a comfortable listening level for most normal hearing persons). Adding a fixed sensation level to the SRT, however, will not always result in a valid maximum word-recognition score, especially for patients with sensorineural hearing loss. The level at which maximum scores are obtained differs substantially among patients. As will be discussed in a subsequent section, the level needed to yield a maximum word-recognition score also depends on such variables as type of test material (and recording) and the speaker. The use of MCL for speech as the presentation level for word-recognition testing is also not recommended since in most cases this level will not result in maximum performance. For the majority of patients, the level required for maximum word-recognition performance is higher than the MCL (Ullrich & Grimm, 1976).

Although use of a single presentation level for estimates of word-recognition ability remains popular in clinical practice, the use of a single level is not supported by data, especially for subjects with sensorineural hearing loss. As a result, many audiologists recommend evaluating word-recognition abilities at multiple levels, which defines a portion of the psychometric function and ensures that the test is being administered at a level at which maximum performance can be obtained (Boothroyd, 1968; Edgerton & Danhauer, 1979). *At a minimum*, word-recognition tests should be presented at two hearing levels (between 50 and 90 dB HL). The first set of words are presented at 50 dB HL or 15 dB above the three-frequency pure-tone average, whichever is the higher level. Word-recognition performance at or near 50 dB HL gives an indication of the need of the patient for amplification through his or her ability to understand normal conversational speech in quiet. Scores should then be obtained in 10 or 20 dB steps until the patient gets ≥80% correct or in the opinion of the audiologist the patient will not achieve 80% correct at any presentation level. It is not uncommon, therefore, to evaluate word-recognition at two or three hearing levels, especially with cases in which word-recognition ability at a high level (e.g., 90 dB HL) routinely is obtained. The use of this approach is especially valuable for differentiating between cochlear and retrocochlear pathology, which will be discussed in detail later in this chapter.

Presentation Mode

Most often in the clinical setting the speech stimulus is a word presented either in isolation or preceded by a carrier phrase (e.g., "Say the word . . ."). Some clinical settings employ other types of stimuli like speech sounds used with young children, nonsense syllables, and sentences. The speech materials are presented to the patient at calibrated decibel hearing levels (ANSI, 1996) with the source of the materials being either monitored-live voice (MLV) or from a recording. With the MLV technique the audiologist says the materials naturally and monitors the level of the words on a vu (or dB) meter. The problem with the MLV technique is that each time a

word is spoken, even by the same speaker, it has different acoustic characteristics. As Kruel, Bell, and Nixon (1969) succinctly stated, "tests ought not to be thought of as the written lists of words but as recordings of these words" (p. 289). Thus, for standardization and reliability purposes, recorded materials (typically from a compact disc) are the preferred presentation mode (Brandy, 1966). The differences between test materials recorded by different speakers will be considered in detail later in this chapter. Recordings from a compact disc are calibrated by adjusting the vu meter to 0 vu using the 1000 Hz calibration tone that is on one track of the compact disc. Regardless of the presentation mode, the vu (or dB) meter must have ballistic characteristics that conform to the appropriate ANSI standard for vu meters (ANSI, C16.5-1954) or dB meters. [Note 1 vu = 1 dB only for a sinusoid (IEEE, 1993).]

The data in this chapter described for speech recognition and identification were collected using air-conducted signals via insert or supra-aural earphones. At times, however, it may be necessary to obtain speech-recognition data via bone conduction. In such cases, the speech signal is transduced by a bone vibrator placed on the mastoid bone, or occasionally on the frontal bone at the midline of the forehead. Bone-conducted speech testing may be useful in evaluating patients for whom it is difficult to elicit reliable responses to pure-tone signals. It can also assist in confirming the presence and extent of an air-bone gap. The application of bone-conduction speech testing is limited by the frequency response and output limitations of the bone-conduction vibrator.

Response Mode

The response mode required of the patient takes one of several forms including *detection*, *recognition*, and *identification*. With the detection response, the patient only has to respond when the signal is present, that is, the patient only has to identify the presence of the signal and does not have to define any characteristics of the signal. The most common detection task in audiology is pure-tone audiometry. Speech signals, however, may be used with a detection response mode. In the earlier literature, *speech awareness* and *threshold of audibility* were synonymous with detection.

With the recognition response, the patient not only has to be aware of the signal but has to define characteristics of the signal. Verbally repeating words in an open-set paradigm is the most common example of a recognition task. With word tests, the patient repeats the stimulus word. With sentence materials, the patient repeats or shadows the sentence. An alternative to the verbal response is the written response on a prepared scoresheet. Written responses are less prone to scoring errors than are verbal responses, especially with inexperienced audiologists (Nelson & Chaiklin, 1970). The written response technique, which is too time-consuming to justify use in the routine clinical setting, is also useful with certain nonverbal patients (e.g., laryngectomy patients). Until the early 1980s, the term *speech discrimination* was used instead of word recognition. As in other disciplines, *discrimination* is now reserved for paradigms in which patients make comparative judgments about two or more signals.

The identification response is a special case of the recognition response. Whereas the recognition response is an open-set response in that the patient has no a priori knowledge of what the target stimulus will be, the identification response is a closed-set response in that the patient responds by pointing to one of (usually) four to six alternatives displayed visually. As illustrated in Figure 2.7, the

alternatives may be depicted as either pictures (top panel) or words (bottom panel). The response mode has a substantial influence on the performance that is achieved by the patient. The data in Figure 2.8 (Wilson & Antablin, 1982) are from 24 young adults with normal hearing who responded in three ways to the *Picture Identification Task* materials (Wilson & Antablin, 1980), including one recognition mode (oral recall) and two identification modes (pointing to words or pictures). The materials were presented in 70 dB SPL speech-spectrum noise and the subjects were not required to respond to each stimuli (i.e., it was not a forced-choice paradigm). As expected, the differences between the recognition (open set) and the identification (closed set) functions were 35 to 45% (9–12 dB) with identification requiring less energy. Because the subjects were not required to respond to stimuli, the identification functions approached 0% correct recognition. Had the subjects been required to respond to each stimulus, the lowest percent correct identification would have been 25% correct. Interestingly, the 8% (2 dB) difference between the two identification functions was significant. Why the difference between the data from the word and picture response modes? The authors contended that interpreting pictures required more cognitive processing than interpreting the words.

Scoring of the response can take one of several forms. With word tests, the target word can be scored as a unit or as components of the unit. For example, with a consonant-vowel-consonant (CVC) monosyllabic word, the whole

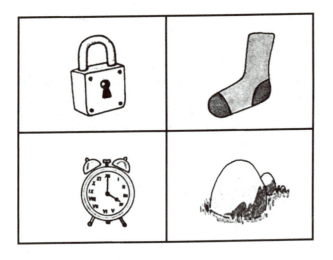

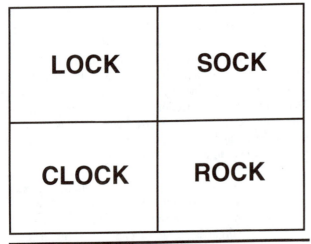

FIGURE 2.7 Example response foils for a word-identification task involving pictures (top panel) and words (bottom panel). (Adapted from Wilson & Antablin, 1980)

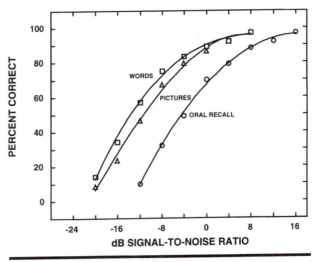

FIGURE 2.8 Psychometric functions (n = 24) for two closed-set, word-identification tasks (words = squares and pictures = triangles) and an open-set, word-recognition task (oral recall = circles). The stimulus materials were the same for the three response tasks. (Adapted from Wilson & Antablin, 1982)

word may be scored as correct or incorrect, which gives one tally/word, or the two consonants and the vowel may be scored individually, which gives three tallies/word (Boothroyd, 1968). More traditionally, the word is scored as a unit. Likewise, with sentences, scoring may be based on the entire sentence or upon selected target words within the sentence.

Redundancy and Uncertainty in Spoken Speech/Word Recognition

To the individual with normal hearing, spoken language contains more information or cues than are necessary to understand the content of the message. Simplistically, our language structure has *extrinsic redundancies* that involve information from phonemes to syntax, whereas listeners have *intrinsic* language *redundancies* that are based on their experience with the language (Miller, 1951). The more extrinsic and intrinsic redundancies the communication has, the easier the message is to comprehend. As illustrated in Figure 2.9 from Miller, Heise, and Lichten (1951), the comprehension of digit material is much easier than the comprehension of words in sentences. This is mainly because the listener has a very limited response choice with digits (almost a closed set), whereas the response choice with words in sentences is somewhat broader. The comprehension of words in sentences (Figure 2.9, circles) is easier than the comprehension of the same words in isolation (triangles) because the non-target words in the sentences contain cues (redundancies) that are not available with the words in isolation. For the same reasons, nonsense

syllables are more difficult to comprehend than words in isolation. Of major importance with intrinsic redundancies is how familiar the listener is with the words of the spoken language. As shown in Figure 2.10, Rosenzweig and Postman (1957) demonstrated that there was an inverse relation between the word threshold (in terms of the number of trials required to comprehend the word) and the frequency of use of the word. The more often a word is used, the easier that word is to understand.

The combination of extrinsic and intrinsic redundancies makes spoken language easily understood, even when both redundancies are somewhat reduced. In circumstances in which either the extrinsic or intrinsic redundancies are completely eliminated, however, comprehension of the message is eliminated. The following are extreme examples of these two conditions. First, if the extrinsic redundancies of a message are reduced by presenting the message at a level below the threshold of the listener, then there is no comprehension, even though the full complement of intrinsic redundancies is available. Second, when a listener with normal hearing encounters a foreign language for the first time, the listener usually does not understand anything that is spoken. Although the foreign language contains the full complement of extrinsic redundancies, the intrinsic redundancies of the listener are totally lacking, thereby reducing language comprehension to zero. As will be discussed in the Degraded Speech Tests section of this chapter, the extrinsic redundancies in spoken language can be reduced selectively in a number of ways involving physically altering the speech signal by masking, filtering, distorting, and so on. Additionally, hearing loss (which is an audibility,

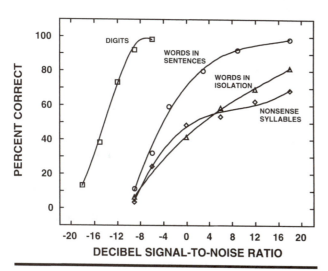

FIGURE 2.9 Psychometric functions obtained for digits (squares), words in sentences (circles), words in isolation (triangles), and nonsense syllables (diamonds). (Adapted from Miller et al., 1951, Figures 1 and 3)

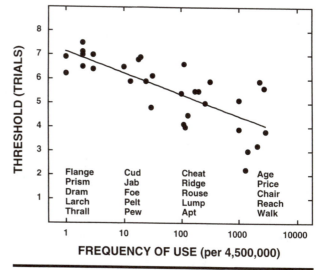

FIGURE 2.10 Thresholds for selected words based on their frequency of usage. (Adapted from Rosenzweig & Postman, 1957, Table 1 and Figure 1)

filtering, distorting mechanism) is a major culprit in reducing the extrinsic redundancies of spoken language. Intrinsic redundancies likewise can be reduced by a variety of causes that range from limited exposure to language to a physical insult to the language centers of the brain caused by trauma or a vascular episode.

Collectively, the processes that reduce extrinsic and intrinsic redundancies create *uncertainty* with the listener. The more uncertain the individual is about the listening condition, the poorer the performance. To demonstrate this effect, Green (1961) created frequency uncertainty with pure tones. When the listeners did not know from trial to trial what the pure-tone frequency was, thresholds required about 3 dB more energy than did the threshold when the pure-tone frequency was the same from trial to trial. Similar effects have been shown in the temporal domain in which the time of signal onset was the uncertainty variable (Egan, Greenberg, & Schulman, 1961; Green & Weber, 1980). With speech stimuli, signal uncertainty can be introduced in a number of ways (Pollack, 1959). For example, changing the speaker from trial to trial reduces performance in comparison to the same speaker on each trial (Creelman, 1957; Kirk, Pisoni, & Miyamoto, 1997; Mullennix, Pisoni, & Martin, 1989). Likewise, if the level of the speech presentation is different from trial to trial, then uncertainty is created in the task of the listener.

Finally, since redundancy, uncertainty, and many of the related concepts in language are rooted in the psychology literature it seems appropriate to mention the literature that has evolved in the past decade dealing with the theories of and variables associated with *spoken word recognition* (Frauenfelder & Tyler, 1987). The early work in experimental psychology with word recognition was restricted to written word recognition. As more and more studies deal with spoken word recognition, it is becoming apparent that the theories and concepts that apply to written word recognition do not necessarily apply to spoken word recognition.

Masking

As with pure-tone signals, speech signals presented in one ear at levels high enough to cross over to the opposite ear require that masking be used in the nontest ear. Both threshold and supra-threshold speech testing can require masking the nontest ear with either broadband or speech-spectrum noise. The rules for masking speech signals, which are dependent upon the type of transducer (i.e., insert or supra-aural earphone), are presented in Chapter 3. [Track 2 of the audio CD contains a 30 s sample of broadband (white) noise (left channel) and a 30 s sample of speech-spectrum noise (right channel). Courtesy of the Auditory Research Laboratory, Mountain Home, Tennessee.]

THRESHOLD MEASURES

In speech audiometry, threshold usually is defined as the point on a psychometric function at which 50% correct responses occur with spondaic word test materials. As the response criterion changes, the point on the function changes (e.g., two out of three correct responses corresponds to the 67% correct point on the function). Historically, our modern-day use of speech thresholds can be traced to three investigations. (For a review of other historical reports, see Wilson & Margolis, 1983.) First, Hughson and Thompson (1942) reported a three-year study in which "speech reception thresholds" were established with sentence materials (Fletcher & Steinberg, 1929) presented by monitored live voice. The subjects, who had a variety of hearing impairments, were required to repeat the sentences verbatim. A bracketing technique was used to define threshold in decibels "below which the subject can no longer repeat at least two thirds of the sentences correctly" (p. 531). Second, Hudgins, Hawkins, Karlin, and Stevens (1947), who were working at the Harvard Psycho-Acoustic Laboratory (PAL) during World War II, introduced the spondaic word as the speech signal to measure "the loss of hearing for speech." Four criteria were satisfied with the spondaic words "(1) familiarity, (2) phonetic dissimilarity, (3) normal sampling of English speech sounds, and (4) homogeneity with respect to basic audibility" (p. 58). Hudgins and colleagues devised two lists of 42 spondaic words each; a carrier phrase (e.g., "Number one . . .", etc.) preceded each word. Two versions of the spondaic words were recorded on vinyl disc with a 1000 Hz calibration tone. PAL Auditory Test No. 9 pre-attenuated the words such that successive groups of six words were recorded 4 dB below the level of the previous set, which provided a 24 dB range across the 42 words. PAL Auditory Test No. 14 had the spondaic words recorded at the same level.

Following World War II, the spondaic word materials and a simple question sentence test (PAL Auditory Test No. 12) were used in the Aural Rehabilitation program at Deshon General Hospital to establish thresholds for speech signals (Hirsh, 1947). Third, Hirsh and colleagues (1952), working at the Central Institute for the Deaf (CID) under contracts from the then Veterans Administration (VA) and Navy, reduced the list of 84 spondaic words to 36 words by eliminating the easiest and most difficult words. Based on psychometric functions obtained on the 36 words, ±2 dB adjustments were made to some of the words to make them more homogeneous with respect to audibility. These 36 spondaic words were recorded as the CID W-1 lists. A second version, the CID W-2 lists, were recorded with each subsequent set of 3 words recorded 3 dB below the level of the previous set. These 36 spondaic words continue in use as the standard material with which to establish thresholds for speech. [Track 3 of the audio CD is a recording of 12 of the spondaic words spoken by a female speaker (left channel) and by Hirsh (right channel). Courtesy of the Auditory Research Laboratory, Mountain Home, Tennessee; G. Donald Causey, VA Medical Center, Washington, D.C.; and Technisonic Studios, Inc., St. Louis, Missouri.]

Stimulus Materials

Spondaic Words. The psychometric function for the 36 W-1 spondaic words is relatively steep, 8%/dB (Hirsh et al., 1952). Two characteristics contribute to this steepness. First, there are only 36 words, which constitutes an approximate "closed set" of test materials. Second, if the patient correctly recognizes one of the two syllables, then the whole word should be correctly recognized; there are of course exceptions, e.g., *hothouse* and *hotdog*. If the spondaic words were equivalent with respect to threshold, then the recognition threshold for each word would be the same. Many studies demonstrate that the thresholds and slopes of the psychometric functions associated with each of the 36 spondaic words are different, even on a group of listeners with normal hearing (Beattie, Edgerton, & Svihovec, 1975; Bowling & Elpern, 1961; Cambron et al., 1991; Conn, Dancer, & Ventry, 1975; Curry & Cox, 1966; Young, Dudley, & Gunter, 1982). Table 2.1 lists the 50% correct thresholds (dB SPL) and slopes of the psychometric functions (%/dB) for each of the 36 W-1 spondaic words spoken by Tillman that were obtained from 20 young adults with normal hearing (from Young et al., 1982). The mean threshold was 18.7 dB SPL but the thresholds varied 6.4 dB from 15.2 dB SPL (*hotdog*) to 21.6 dB SPL (*greyhound*). Using ±1 standard deviation, 26 words were described as homogeneous with respect to threshold. Even greater variability was observed with the slope data.

The mean slope was 10%/dB, but the range was from 6.1%/dB (*farewell*) to 20.6%/dB (*schoolboy*), a 14.5%/dB range. Using ±1 standard deviation to define the slope variability, 22 words were described as homogeneous. Young and colleagues observed that only 15 spondaic words were homogeneous in terms of both threshold and slope of the psychometric function. Clinically, it is important that each spondaic word used as a stimulus item can be perceived at essentially the same level, since the measure of interest is the level necessary for a 50% correct response (Bilger, Matthies, Meyer, & Griffiths, in press). It would be ideal to use a homogeneous set of test words, as we are able with pure-tone signals, to increase the precision with which the SRT can be established.

Another example of the variability associated with the spondaic word materials is illustrated in Figure 2.11 in which thresholds for each of the 36 W-1 spondaic words are plotted for two speakers, a male speaker (Hirsh) on the ordinate and a female speaker (VA compact disc) on the abscissa. The diagonal line in this bivariate plot represents

TABLE 2.1   The thresholds (dB SPL) and slopes of the psychometric functions (%/dB) for each of the W-1 spondaic words spoken by Tillman. Twenty young adults with normal hearing were studied. (From Young et al., 1982)

SPONDAIC WORD	THRESHOLD (dB SPL)	SLOPE (%/dB)
airplane	17.1	17.3
armchair	17.0	8.0
baseball	17.4	11.3
birthday	18.8	6.9
cowboy	17.5	13.7
daybreak	20.3	8.8
doormat	19.9	12.5
drawbridge	18.3	12.0
duckpond	18.7	7.5
eardrum	18.1	8.3
farewell	20.3	6.1
grandson	19.9	10.2
greyhound	21.6	11.3
hardware	17.5	13.7
headlight	18.7	7.5
horseshoe	17.6	13.8
hotdog	15.2	10.3
hothouse	17.2	13.8
iceberg	16.5	16.3
inkwell	18.5	8.2
mousetrap	20.1	8.8
mushroom	19.9	7.9
northwest	18.9	11.3
oatmeal	21.2	12.0
padlock	19.4	11.5
pancake	20.0	7.8
playground	18.1	11.5
railroad	18.9	8.5
schoolboy	20.1	20.6
sidewalk	19.6	10.8
stairway	18.2	7.8
sunset	21.3	11.3
toothbrush	19.7	11.5
whitewash	16.4	9.0
woodwork	19.2	11.5
workshop	17.6	10.0

equal thresholds. The data are from 22 young adults with normal hearing (Cambron et al., 1991). Although the mean thresholds (filled symbol) are ±0.5 dB, the dispersion of the other datum points in the figure indicates substantial (1) interword threshold variability that is greater for the female speaker (8.8 dB) than for the male speaker (6.4 dB) and (2) interspeaker threshold variability. The thresholds for the words spoken by the female speaker ranged from 18.4 dB SPL (*hotdog*) to 27.2 dB SPL (*daybreak*), whereas the thresholds for the words spoken by the male speaker ranged from 19.7 dB SPL (*workshop*) to 24.6 dB SPL (*oatmeal*). The smaller threshold range for the words spoken

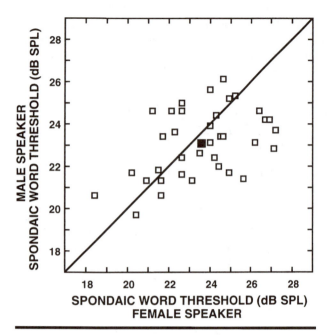

FIGURE 2.11   A bivariate plot of the spondaic-word thresholds spoken by a male speaker (Hirsh) (ordinate) and the VA female speaker (abscissa). The filled symbol represents the mean data. (Adapted from Cambron et al., 1991)

by the male speaker was to be expected because the levels of some of the spondaic words were amplified 2 dB, attenuated 2 dB, or unaltered before the final recordings were made in order to make the thresholds of the words more homogeneous (Hirsh et al., 1952). The levels of the spondaic words spoken by the female speaker were only equated by equal peak deflections on a vu meter. The interspeaker threshold variability associated with each spondaic word ranged from 4.3 dB for *grandson* (27.1 dB SPL female speaker; 22.8 dB SPL male speaker) to –3.4 dB for *mushroom* (21.2 dB SPL female speaker; 24.6 dB SPL male speaker). Remember that this variability is based on data from young adults with normal hearing. This variability will be compounded when the materials are evaluated on patients with hearing loss.

Sentences.   Although utilized clinically less frequently than spondaic words, sentence materials have also been shown to be efficient for determining thresholds for speech (Dubno, Dirks, & Morgan, 1984; Hagerman, 1982). Sentences have the advantage that the slope of the psychometric function is steeper than for single words (Plomp, 1986). The two most widely used sentence tests designed specifically for obtaining thresholds for speech include *Speech Reception Threshold Testing Using Sentence Stimuli* (Plomp & Mimpen, 1979) and the *Hearing In Noise Test (HINT)* (Nilsson, Soli, & Sullivan, 1994). Both tests are designed

to determine threshold with sentence materials either in quiet or in the presence of noise using an adaptive psychophysical procedure. In this technique, the first sentence is presented below threshold and is increased by 2 dB steps until the sentence is correctly repeated. Subsequent sentences are presented once each, with the presentation level dependent upon the accuracy of the preceding response. Presentation levels are decreased 2 dB after a correct response and increased 2 dB after an incorrect response. To be scored as correct, the listener must correctly repeat the entire sentence. Simple, meaningful sentences are used as stimuli. The Plomp and Mimpen materials consist of 10 lists of 13 Dutch sentences. Each sentence contains 8 or 9 syllables and is read by a female speaker (e.g., translated from Dutch, *My neighbor bought a new car*). The test has been shown to be highly reliable for clinical use in listeners with normal hearing and with different degrees of sensorineural hearing loss. Data are available for speech thresholds measured in quiet as well as in noise.

Nilsson and colleagues (1994) developed the *Hearing In Noise Test (HINT)*, which is composed of 250 sentences, derived from British sentences and rewritten in American English. The sentences are 6 to 8 syllables in length and include both monosyllabic and polysyllabic words (e.g., *The boy fell from the window*). The task of the listener in the adaptive test paradigm is to repeat the entire sentence. Each sentence is scored as correct or incorrect with minor exceptions made for article substitutions and verb tense. The reliability and sensitivity of the test have been established and normative data for both quiet and noise conditions are available (Nilsson, Soli, & Sumida, 1995). [Track 4 of the audio CD contains 10 examples of HINT sentences (left channel) presented in a background of noise (right channel). Sentences 1, 3, 4, 7, 8, and 9 are examples of items that also are included in the children's version of the HINT (HINT-C). Courtesy of Michael Nilsson and Sigfrid Soli, House Ear Institute, Los Angeles, California.]

Protocols for Estimating Thresholds for Speech

Typically the speech-recognition threshold (SRT) measured with spondaic words is defined as the decibel hearing level at which 50% of the words are recognized correctly. Similarly, the speech-detection threshold (SDT) measured with spondaic words is defined as the decibel hearing level at which 50% of the words are detected. Although there is no ANSI standard that defines a protocol to establish thresholds for speech, ASHA has put forth a guideline (1979) and a revised guideline (1988) with suggested protocols for establishing SRTs. The need for such a standard was clearly enunciated by Tillman and Olsen (1973), who observed that a systematic procedure ". . . confines all clinicians to the same operational definition of threshold, and thus reduces variability in estimates of the speech reception threshold produced by variations in this definition" (pp. 45–46). Basically, there are three protocols, which are derived from the classical method of limits, used to establish thresholds for speech—*bracketing*, *ascending or descending*, and *adaptive*. Although each of the three procedures involves ascending and descending signal presentation levels, the procedures differ in the rules governing signal presentation, test termination, and threshold computation. When spondaic words are used with any of the threshold protocols, the patient should be familiarized with the words either by having the patient read the words and repeat them verbally, or by having the patient listen to the words presented at a comfortable listening level and repeat them verbally. Familiarity with the spondaic words is an important factor in determining degree of intelligibility in that better performance is achieved when the listener knows the stimulus material for which he is listening, that is, when uncertainty is reduced (Conn et al., 1975; Tillman & Jerger, 1959).

Bracketing Psychophysical Procedure. The so-called bracketing procedure used to establish speech-recognition thresholds is basically the modified Hughson-Westlake procedure (Carhart & Jerger, 1959) that is used in pure-tone testing except that spondaic words serve as the stimuli. The procedure involves presentation of a spondaic word 30 to 40 dB above the estimated threshold. The estimated threshold can be from the pure-tone thresholds, from the history and observations of the patient, or from both. During the initial descent, one word is presented at each 10 to 15 dB decrement. When one word is missed, the presentation level is incremented 10 dB and a word is presented at that level and each of 5 dB decrements until a word is missed. This 10 dB up and 5 dB down procedure is continued until the threshold criterion is met. The stopping rule for a threshold (defined as 50% correct) is two of four words correctly repeated at a given presentation level. If other threshold criteria are used—for example, two of three words correct at a given level—then a notation should be made of the threshold criterion. Although this procedure is one of "bracketing," the level of threshold is determined from the descending portion of the track. To establish threshold from the ascending portion of the track, the above procedure can be reversed.

Ascending/Descending Psychophysical Procedure. In pursuit of a systematic, standardized protocol, Tillman and Olsen (1973) suggested a threshold procedure that was modeled after PAL Auditory Test No. 9 and CID Auditory Test W-2, both of which attached a decibel value to each spondaic word, 0.67 dB (6 words/4 dB) and 1.0 dB (3 words/3 dB), respectively. In addition to each word being assigned a decibel value, this threshold procedure, which is described in this section and embraced by ASHA

(1979, 1988), has the following features: (1) spondaic words that are familiar to the listener, (2) a descending level approach to threshold (ascending can be used as well), and (3) threshold defined as the 50% correct point. Four steps are involved in establishing the speech-recognition threshold (SRT) with this technique.

Step 1: Familiarize the patient with the 36 spondaic words presenting the words to the patient at a comfortable listening level and having the patient repeat the words. Words that the patient misses during familiarization should not be used in the test protocol.

Step 2: An initial presentation level for the test protocol is estimated by presenting one spondaic word at each 10 dB decrement starting 30 to 40 dB above the estimated threshold, which can be estimated from the pure-tone audiogram. When one word is missed at a given level, a second word is presented at the same level. The test protocol is initiated 10 dB above the level at which two words are missed.

Step 3: The test protocol, which involves the presentation of two spondaic words at each 2 dB decrement, has both a starting and stopping rule. The starting rule is satisfied when five of the first six words are repeated correctly. The stopping rule (termination of the test protocol) is satisfied when five of six words are incorrect. (Other combinations of words and presentation decrements can be used.)

Step 4: The Spearman-Kärber formula (Finney, 1952), which is derived in the subsequent section, is used to compute the 50% point. With this formula, the number of correct responses is subtracted from the initial presentation level that was estimated in Step 2. A correction factor of one is added to the difference to compensate for the extra word included at the initial presentation level (different correction factors are used with other combinations of number of words and presentation decrements). The sum is the threshold in decibels hearing level.

The Spearman-Kärber formula was described independently in the English literature (Spearman, 1908) and in the German literature (Kärber, 1931). A paper by Wilson, Morgan, and Dirks (1973) observed that it was this statistical procedure that was actually involved in the PAL Auditory Test No. 9 and CID W-2 speech threshold techniques. The formula is as follows:

$$T_{50\%} = i + \tfrac{1}{2}d - d(r)/n \qquad (2.1)$$

in which $T_{50\%}$ is the speech-recognition threshold defined as the 50% correct point, i is the initial (or highest) presentation level, d is the decrement (or increment) size in decibels, r is the number of correct responses, and n is the number of words presented at each presentation level. When $d = n$, formula 2.1 can be reduced to

$$T_{50\%} = i + \tfrac{1}{2}d - r \qquad (2.2)$$

Formula 2.2 is the one used in Step 4 above to compute the SRT.

Two examples of the SRT procedure are provided on the SRT worksheets shown in Figure 2.12. First, on the left panel a 2 dB step protocol with 2 words/step was used. The initial presentation level was 40 dB HL and nine responses were correct. Substituting in formula 2.2 the following is derived

$$T_{50\%} = 40 + \tfrac{1}{2}(2) - 9$$

$$T_{50\%} = 32 \text{ dB HL}$$

Second, on the right panel a 5 dB step protocol with 5 words/step was used. The initial presentation level was 85 dB HL and eight responses were correct. Again, substituting in formula 2.2, the following threshold is derived

$$T_{50\%} = 85 + \tfrac{1}{2}(5) - 8$$

$$T_{50\%} = 79.5 \text{ dB HL}$$

Finally, for an example in which the step size and number of words per step is unequal, the following serves as an example. Given $i = 72$ dB SPL, $d = 3$ dB steps, $r = 12$ correct, and $n = 5$ words/step, then substituting in formula 1 the following threshold is derived

$$T_{50\%} = 72 + \tfrac{1}{2}(3) - 3(12)/5$$

$$T_{50\%} = 72 + 1.5 - 7.2$$

$$T_{50\%} = 66.3 \text{ dB SPL}$$

Although discussion of the Spearman-Kärber formula in this section was restricted to the descending SRT procedure, the Spearman-Kärber formula can be applied to data obtained from an ascending SRT procedure and to a variety of other data from which the 50% point needs to be derived.

Adaptive Psychophysical Procedure. An alternate method for measuring speech thresholds is by adaptive testing, in which the signal presentation level is dependent upon the responses of the listener to the previously presented signal or signals (ANSI, 1995). The signal level may be under the direct control of the listener or may be adjusted by the examiner. Adaptive techniques take many forms, ranging in complexity from the simple adaptive technique that has a single observation interval to the two-interval, forced-choice (2IFC) procedures. With the simple adaptive technique in a word-recognition task, the listener repeats the word or sentence presented in the observation interval. The 2IFC procedure, which is more complicated, is used in psychoacoustic experiments involving detection tasks. With the 2IFC adaptive technique in a speech-detection task,

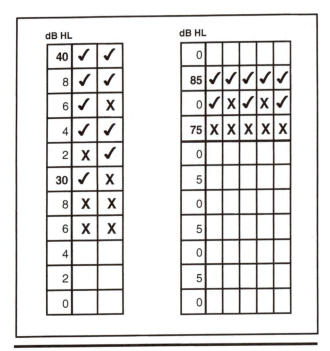

FIGURE 2.12 Examples of SRT worksheets for the 2 dB (left) and 5 dB (right) test intervals.

there are two observation intervals in each trial (usually defined by lights) with only one interval containing the signal presentation. The listener knows that on each trial a signal will be presented either in the first or second observation interval. The listener is required to indicate the interval in each trial in which the signal occurred (i.e., the listener is forced to respond, even if nothing was heard in either interval). Consequently, 2IFC procedures avoid the influence of response criteria that is common with the ascending/descending threshold procedures.

Both the simple and more complicated adaptive procedures employ the same operating rules. For example, both use a small step size (usually 2 dB) and a strategy that places most of the signal presentations in close proximity to a specified point on the psychometric function. The target point on the psychometric function is determined by the rules governing the track (Levitt, 1971). For example, if the target point is 70.7% correct, then the two-down, one-up rule is used in which the signal level is decreased after two consecutive correct responses and increased after one incorrect response. The mean of the levels at the reversal points of the track provides an estimate of threshold at the 70.7% point on the psychometric function. If a three-down, one-up procedure is used (i.e., the signal level is decreased after three consecutive correct responses and increased after one incorrect response), then the estimate of threshold is at the 79.4% point on the psychometric function. The stopping rule used to terminate the track is set by the experimenter as a specified number of trials or number of track reversals. Typically between 50 and 80 trials are used to obtain a threshold estimate (Marshall, Hanna, & Wilson, 1996). The use of adaptive approaches has been shown to be effective in estimating speech thresholds for subjects with and without hearing loss. (Levitt, 1978, provides a good tutorial on adaptive techniques.)

Relations between Speech Thresholds and Pure-Tone Thresholds

There is a strong relationship between certain pure-tone thresholds and the speech-recognition threshold (SRT) - (Carhart, 1946a, 1946b; Fletcher, 1950; Hughson & Thompson, 1942; Jerger, Carhart, Tillman, & Peterson, 1959). The average pure-tone thresholds at 500, 1000, and 2000 Hz and the SRT should agree, ±6 dB, which is a normal relationship.

Fletcher (1929) advocated the use of the three-frequency pure-tone average (512, 1024, and 2048 Hz) in predicting the SRT. The first study to measure the SRT of patients with hearing loss was conducted by Hughson and Thompson (1942), who also demonstrated interdependence between the threshold for sentences and sensitivity for pure-tones in the mid-frequencies. Subsequent work by Carhart (1946a, 1946b) demonstrated a high correlation between the Fletcher three-frequency pure-tone average and the SRT in patients with flat or gradually sloping audiometric configurations, but lower correlations for patients with steeply sloping pure-tone threshold configurations. Fletcher (1950) suggested that the mean of the better two of the three thresholds correlated better with the SRT than did the three-frequency pure-tone average for patients with steeply sloping audiometric configurations. Carhart (1971) later recommended obtaining the average of the pure-tone thresholds at 500 and 1000 Hz minus 2 dB to predict the SRT. Wilson and colleagues (1973) examined the relationship between the various averaging methods (two- or three-frequency pure-tone average, and Carhart, 1971) and the SRT and found only small differences (0.3–3.1 dB) between methods. The use of multiple regression equations for predicting the SRT has also been evaluated and compared with averaging procedures (Carhart & Porter, 1971; Graham, 1960; Harris, Haines, & Myers, 1956). Results showed that regression procedures could be used to accurately predict the SRT. These statistically more complicated methods, however, were no better predictors of the SRT than the simpler pure-tone averaging procedures.

Discrepancies between the pure-tone average and SRT may occur for many reasons. In some cases the SRT is lower than would be predicted from the pure-tone average. This may be true in patients with atypical audiometric configurations such as normal hearing at frequencies above 8000 Hz (Berlin, Wexler, Jerger, Halperin, & Smith, 1978), or significant hearing loss with an island of normal hearing (Roeser, 1982). *Pseudohypacusis* (functional hearing loss) also can cause a disparity between pure-tone and speech thresholds, with typically lower SRTs than the pure-tone results would predict (Menzel, 1960; Ventry & Chaiklin, 1965). The basis for this discrepancy is the greater perceived loudness for speech than for pure-tones at the same hearing levels (Ventry, 1976). There are other cases in which the pure-tone average may be lower than the SRT. Intracranial tumors that exert pressure on the auditory nerve have been shown to cause marked deficits in word-recognition ability (Dirks, Kamm, Bower, & Bettsworth, 1977), resulting in an elevated SRT compared to the pure-tone average. Finally, discrepancies between the two metrics also may occur as a result of misunderstanding the instructions by the patient or may be due to cognitive and language disorders (Working Group on Speech Understanding and Aging, 1988). Regardless of the cause, the important point is that unexplained differences greater than ±6 dB between the two- or three-frequency, pure-tone average and the SRT warrant further investigation, reinstruction, and evaluation to resolve the discrepancy.

An important limitation of the relationship between pure-tone sensitivity and the SRT was noted by Wilson and Margolis (1983). They recognized that because of the relationship between the two measures, many investigators and clinicians refer to 500, 1000, and 2000 Hz as the "speech frequencies," leading to the misconception that the frequencies above 2000 Hz and below 500 Hz are unimportant for speech recognition. As early as 1929, Fletcher noted that frequencies above 3000 Hz are as important as frequencies below 1000 Hz for speech recognition. Research also indicates that the frequencies between 4000 and 6000 Hz are important for consonant recognition (Skinner, Pascoe, Miller, & Popelka, 1982). Consequently, the relationship between the speech-recognition threshold for spondaic words and the pure-tone average must be interpreted with consideration for the differences between the task of recognizing items from a small set of materials and the more complicated task of speech communication. Although the pure-tone average may predict the SRT (±6 dB), the pure-tone average does not adequately assess communicative ability or disability.

ASSESSMENT OF WORD-RECOGNITION ABILITIES

Word-recognition ability and word-recognition performance are used in this chapter to denote the assessment of how well a person understands speech both in quiet and in noise environments. Several types of word-recognition paradigms are used to assess the ability of a patient to understand speech, including nonsense syllables, monosyllabic words, and sentences. As was illustrated in Figure 2.9 from Miller and colleagues (1951), the most difficult materials for a patient to understand are nonsense syllables, and the easiest materials for a patient to understand are sentence materials with monosyllabic words between these two extremes.

Nonsense Syllables

Nonsense syllables were one of the earliest materials used in the assessment of speech recognition. The first nonsense syllable tests were developed by Fletcher and Steinberg (1929) for use in assessing communication systems, and they served as a model for future nonsense syllable tests designed for the evaluation of speech-recognition abilities of humans in the 1970s. Nonsense syllable tests were developed in an attempt to minimize contextual cues inherent in meaningful speech stimuli. As described in later sections, when using meaningful word and sentence tests to assess speech recognition, listeners do not have to perceive the entire stimulus to respond correctly because contextual cues aid in stimulus recognition. Clinicians often are hesitant to use nonsense syllable tests in clinical settings, however, because the material is not representative of everyday speech and also because of difficulties in eliciting appropriate responses from patients (Bess, 1983). This is especially true when evaluating elderly subjects.

The most commonly utilized nonsense syllable tests include the closed-set response *Nonsense Syllable Test (CUNY NST)* (Resnick, Dubno, Hoffnung, & Levitt, 1975; Levitt & Resnick, 1978) and the *Nonsense Syllable Test (NST)* developed by Edgerton and Danhauer (1979). The CUNY NST consists of 91 consonant-vowel (CV) or vowel-consonant (VC) syllables divided into 11 subtests, each containing 7, 8, or 9 syllables. The subtests are arranged so that each contains either voiced or voiceless consonants in the initial or final position, paired with one of three vowels /a, u, i/, (e.g., /af/, /ta/, /fa/ and /ap/). The syllables are presented within the carrier phrase "You will mark _____ please." The test, which was designed for use with adults with moderate-to-severe hearing loss, provides detailed information regarding syllable recognition and consonant error patterns. Dubno and Dirks (1982) and Dubno, Dirks, and Langhofer (1982) found with the CUNY NST materials that the responses of subjects with hearing impairment had good reliability.

The NST has two lists of 25 CVCV nonsense stimuli, with six randomizations of each list. The syllables are presented in an open-set format within the carrier phrase "Say _____." The NST was standardized on subjects with normal hearing and with impaired hearing. Psychometric functions for both populations have been obtained, and test-retest reliability has been examined. The NST, which has been used extensively in speech perception research, is useful in the evaluation of speech-recognition abilities of non-English-speaking listeners (Danhauer, Crawford, &

Edgerton, 1984) and in testing the speech-recognition ability of both children and adults in noisy and reverberant conditions (Johnson, Cosci, Brown, & Scroggins, 1995). [Track 5 (left channel) contains 10 examples of the NST. Courtesy of Auditec of St. Louis, Missouri.]

Monosyllabic Words in Quiet

The use of monosyllabic words in speech audiometry can be traced to the 20 lists of "phonetically balanced" (PB) words developed at the Harvard Psycho-Acoustic Laboratory (PAL) during World War II (Egan, 1948). The 50 monosyllabic words in each list supposedly were in common usage. An attempt was made to distribute the various speech sounds equally in each list. When the PAL PB-50 lists were recorded (Rush Hughes was the speaker) several words in each list were changed (e.g., on List 9 original words *cud, fluff,* and *pact* were replaced in the Rush Hughes recorded version with *skill, tax,* and *tub*). The PB-50 lists were used in hearing evaluations until the early 1950s when Hirsh and colleagues (1952) developed the CID W-22 lists that were modeled after the PB-50 with two improvements. First, the vocabulary was restricted to include only those words familiar to patients, which reduced the test items from 1200 words to 200 words. Of the 200 W-22 words, 120 words came from the PB-50 lists and 80 words came from other sources. Second, the materials were recorded on magnetic tape, which enabled the same word waveform to be used in each randomized version. The W-22 lists were recorded with Hirsh as the speaker and were available commercially on vinyl records (six randomizations). The carrier phrase "You will say" preceded each word. [Track 6 contains 10 items of the PB-50s recorded by Rush Hughes (left channel) and 10 items of the CID W-22s recorded by Hirsh (right channel). Courtesy of Technisonic Studios, Inc., St. Louis, Missouri.]

Several sets of monosyllabic materials are available on compact disc including the *CID W-22s* (Hirsh et al., 1952), the *Northwestern University Auditory Test No. 6 (NU No. 6)* (Tillman & Carhart, 1966), and the *Maryland CNCs* (Causey, Hermanson, Hood, & Bowling, 1983). In addition to the one syllable characteristic of these test words, the words used in these lists are all fairly common words. As was indicated earlier, the psychometric characteristics of the monosyllabic word lists are related to a particular recording of the word lists (Kruel et al., 1969). The functions in Figure 2.13 illustrate the influence that speaker has on the psychometric characteristics of a given set of materials, NU No. 6. The functions in the top panel of Figure 2.13 are from three studies that used the same recorded version of the NU No. 6 materials (Tillman as the speaker) (Tillman & Carhart, 1966; Wilson, Coley, Haenel, & Browning, 1976; Wilson, Zizz, Shanks, & Causey, 1990).

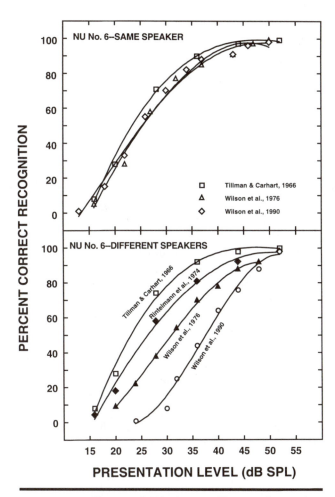

psychometric characteristics of the word lists. *When discussing any speech audiometry materials, the importance of identifying both the particular recording and the speaker of that recording cannot be overemphasized.* [Track 7 contains 12 items of NU No. 6 spoken by Tillman (left channel) and by the VA female speaker (right channel); Track 8 contains 11 items of NU No. 6 spoken by the male Auditec speaker (left channel) and items of the Maryland CNCs spoken by a male speaker (right channel). Courtesy of the Auditory Research Laboratory, Northwestern University, Evanston, Illinois; G. Donald Causey, VA Medical Center, Washington, D.C.; and Auditec of St. Louis, Missouri.]

The data in Figure 2.14 are normative functions for the CID W-22 materials spoken by Hirsh (Heckendorf et al., 1997; Hirsh et al., 1952), for the PB-50s spoken by Rush Hughes (Heckendorf et al., 1997), and for the Maryland CNCs spoken by a male speaker (Causey et al., 1983). There are three main points of interest in Figure 2.14. First, the two functions for the Hirsh recording of the W-22s (1952, filled squares; 1997, open squares) are displaced by about 10 dB. As Heckendorf and colleagues and others (e.g., Gengel & Kupperman, 1980) have noted, this difference probably is owing to differences in calibration. Hirsh and colleagues calibrated to the average level of the materials, whereas the current versions of the materials used by Heckendorf and colleagues are calibrated to the peaks of the carrier phrases. Second, the functions for the current

FIGURE 2.13 *Top panel:* Word-recognition psychometric functions for the NU No. 6 materials spoken by the same speaker (Tillman) from three studies (Tillman & Carhart, 1966; Wilson et al., 1976; Wilson, Preece, & Thornton, 1990; Wilson, Zizz, et al., 1990). *Bottom panel:* Word-recognition psychometric functions for the NU No. 6 materials spoken by four speakers—Tillman (Tillman & Carhart, 1966), Rintelmann (Rintelmann & Associates, 1974), Auditec of St. Louis male (Wilson et al., 1976), and VA female (Wilson, Preece, & Thornton, 1990; Wilson, Zizz, et al., 1990).

When the same recorded version was used in three studies, differences among the psychometric functions were on the order of 2 to 3 dB. The functions in the bottom panel of Figure 2.13 are from four studies that used different speakers for each of the four versions of NU No. 6. The speakers for the four versions were Tillman (Tillman & Carhart, 1966), Rintelmann (Rintelmann & Associates, 1974), Auditec of St. Louis male (Wilson et al., 1976), and VA female (Wilson, Zizz, et al., 1990). When different recorded versions were compared, differences among the psychometric functions were on the order of 2–3 to 18–20 dB. The point is that the speaker makes a substantial contribution to the

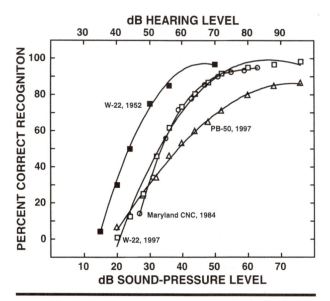

FIGURE 2.14 Psychometric functions for four lists of monosyllabic word-recognition materials spoken by three speakers—Hirsh (W-22s, Hirsh et al., 1952; Heckendorf et al., 1997), VA male (Maryland CNCs, Causey et al., 1983), and Rush Hughes (PB-50s, Heckendorf et al., 1997).

Hirsh version of the W-22s (Heckendorf et al., 1997) and the Maryland CNCs (Causey et al., 1983) are almost the same. This relation demonstrates that two speakers, speaking different word lists (both on compact disc) can produce psychometric functions that are nearly identical. Third, the function for the PB-50s (triangles) has a slope that is more gradual than the slopes of the other functions and is for the most part displaced to the higher presentation levels. The lower portion of the PB-50 function from 0% to 30% correct, however, overlays the functions for the W-22s and Maryland CNCs. The reason for the overlap is that some of the PB-50 words are just as easy to recognize as are some of the words from the other two sets of materials. The majority of the PB-50 words, however, are more difficult to recognize than are the words from the other materials, thus reduced performance is observed on the PB-50 function at the higher presentation levels. From the homogeneity perspective, the PB-50s are less homogenous with respect to word-recognition than are the W-22s (Hirsh) and the Maryland CNCs, hence the more gradual slope for the PB-50 function.

Boothroyd (1968) described isophonemic word lists comprised of 15 lists of CVC words that are phonemically balanced. Each list consists of 10 words, with the same 20 consonants and 10 vowels occurring once in each list. The phonemes chosen were those occurring most frequently in CVC words, but no attempt was made to relate the frequency of individual phonemes in the list to their frequency of occurrence in spoken English. Each phoneme is scored individually rather than scoring each of the 10 words as correct or incorrect. Boothroyd advocated that the advantage of scoring phonemes rather than words is that phoneme scores give a more valid estimate of the ability of a subject to recognize the acoustic features of speech sounds. Reported advantages of this test is that it allows for phonemic analysis and may be administered in a short period of time (Olsen & Matkin, 1979).

Monosyllablic Words in Noise

The discussion in the previous section of monosyllabic word-recognition was restricted to presentation of the stimulus words in quiet, which currently is the listening condition most often used to assess the word-recognition abilities of a patient. Most patients do not complain that they have trouble understanding speech in a quiet environment, but rather that they have trouble understanding speech in noisy environments. Unfortunately, this complaint of a patient unable to understand speech in a noisy background typically is not addressed in the course of most audiologic evaluations. The reasons for this probably are related to academic/historical factors (word-recognition testing has always been conducted in quiet) and to pragmatic factors (noisy conditions are not standardized). We contend that for diagnostic and rehabilitative purposes each patient with hearing loss should have their word-recognition abilities evaluated in some type of background noise. It is common knowledge that patients with hearing loss have more trouble understanding speech in noise than do listeners with normal hearing (Beattie, 1989; Carhart & Tillman, 1970; Dubno et al., 1984; Keith & Talis, 1970; Olsen, Noffsinger, & Kurdziel, 1975; Pekkarinen, Salmivalli, & Suonpää, 1990; Souza & Turner, 1994). Patients with identical pure-tone hearing losses can have vastly different word-recognition abilities in quiet listening conditions. Likewise, patients with identical word-recognition abilities in quiet can have vastly different word-recognition abilities in noisy listening conditions (Beattie, Barr, & Roup, 1997; Norwood-Chapman, Wilson, & Thelin, 1997; Wilson, Oyler, & Sumrall, 1996).

Noise as used in this section refers to any unwanted sound that interferes with the understanding of speech. Noise can take the form (1) of generated noises such as broadband (white) noise or speech-spectrum noise that are continuous or amplitude-modulated; (2) of various environmental noises such as traffic, restaurants, factories; and (3) of speech noises that range from a single speaker to a group of speakers. Clinically for a speech-in-noise test paradigm, there are advantages and disadvantages to each of these forms of noise. With regard to level and modulation characteristics, broadband and speech-spectrum noises can be controlled with precision. The effect of ipsilateral broadband or speech-spectrum noise on word-recognition is predictable and linear as the noise level increases (Hawkins & Stevens, 1950) and is stimulus dependent, that is, the effectiveness of the noise varies with the type of speech material and the speaker. With spondaic words, speech-spectrum noise, which is about 8 dB more effective than broadband noise, produces 50% correct thresholds for listeners with normal hearing at about −6 dB signal-to-noise ratio (Konkle & Berry, 1983). For monosyllabic words like NU No. 6, the 50% correct point in broadband noise is dependent upon the particular recording and speaker. The 50% points for the NU No. 6 in broadband noise are at signal-to-noise ratios of −3.1 dB, 0.3 dB, and 13.5 dB for the Tillman recording, the Auditec recording, and the VA female recording, respectively (Wilson et al., 1976; Wilson, Zizz, et al., 1990). The disadvantage of using broadband or speech-spectrum noise is they are not encountered in everyday life. While environmental noises are encountered more often, environmental noises are difficult to control and are very listener specific, that is, each listener has unique acoustic environments making widespread application of any particular environmental noise difficult at best.

Most people throughout the day encounter listening in noisy situations in which the noise is composed of speech from other speakers. When one speaker provides the noise, the noise is termed a *competing message*. The NU No. 20 (Olsen & Carhart, 1967) is an example of a word-recognition task in a competing message paradigm that was developed for use in hearing aid evaluations. With NU No. 20, the Bell Telephone Sentences were the competing messages with the NU No. 6 words serving as the primary message. NU No. 20 could be used either in a binaural mode (words in one ear and competing sentences in the other ear) or in a monaural mode (words and competing sentences in the same ear).

Another form of competing message noise occurs when several speakers are talking simultaneously and the listener selectively can attend to and understand any of the messages, which is the so-called *cocktail-party effect* (Broadbent, 1958; Cherry, 1966). When several speakers are talking simultaneously and none of the messages are understandable to the listener, the noise is termed *multi-talker babble*. In addition to being the most commonly encountered noise, multi-talker speech noise creates a difficult listening environment because it is (1) a speech-spectrum shape, (2) minimally amplitude-modulated, and (3) aperiodic. [Tracks 9 and 10 contain two versions of NU No. 20 with the left channels containing the target words (VA female speaker and Tillman, respectively), and the right channels containing the competing sentences (VA male speaker and Matkin, respectively). Courtesy of the Auditory Research Laboratories, Northwestern University, Evanston, Illinois, and Mountain Home, Tennessee.]

There are several approaches that can be used to evaluate word-recognition performance in a noisy background. The speech stimuli can be presented (1) at one or two signal-to-noise ratios (e.g., 0 and 10 dB) with the noise fixed at a predetermined (standard) level (e.g., 50 dB SPL or 70 dB SPL), or (2) at a multitude of signal-to-noise ratios from which the psychometric function, or a segment thereof, can be generated. An example of this latter scheme is provided on Track 11 (left channel) of the compact disc. Track 11 contains the NU No. 6 words (VA female speaker) mixed in multi-talker babble at 7 signal-to-noise ratios in 5 dB steps (the same words in quiet but at the various levels are on the right channel of Track 11). NU No. 6 data using this scheme are depicted in Figure 2.15 in which the percent correct word recognition obtained in quiet at 50 dB HL (ordinate) is plotted against the signal-to-babble ratio (dB) at which the 50% word recognition was obtained from the same speaker in multi-talker babble presented at 50 dB HL (Norwood-Chapman et al., 1997). Data for both listeners with normal with normal hearing (filled circles) and listeners with mild-to-moderate sensorineural hearing losses (squares) are shown. The data for the listeners with normal hearing are grouped in the upper left corner and indicate little intersubject variability. The data for the listeners with impaired hearing are not systematic in that there is no relation between word-recognition abilities in quiet and in multi-talker babble. The linear regression fit to the data (solid line) had a slope

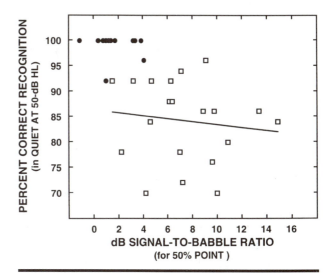

FIGURE 2.15   The correct word recognition in quiet as a function of the 50% correct point in dB signal-to-babble ratio for listeners with normal hearing (solid circles) and listeners with mild-to-moderate sensorineural hearing loss (squares). The solid line is the linear regression used to describe the data. (Adapted from Norwood-Chapman et al., 1997)

that approximated zero and a very poor fit ($r^2 = 0.0017$). The data in Figure 2.15 demonstrate the difficulty of predicting word-recognition abilities in a noisy background from word-recognition abilities in quiet.

Use of 25 versus 50 Word Lists.   Ideally, the audiologist would like to know how the patient understands speech at a variety of presentation levels and under a variety of listening conditions (e.g., quiet and noise). Such a scheme could involve many 50-word lists of materials that, at 4 to 5 minutes per list, could consume 30 to 60 minutes during an evaluation. Pragmatically, both economic and patient fatigue factors drive audiologists to shorten test procedures. With speech audiometry, many clinics use half-lists of 25 words to assess the word-recognition abilities of patients. The use of 25-word lists has been the topic of study for a number of years (Beattie, Svihovec, & Edgerton, 1978; Elpern, 1961; Grubb, 1963a, 1963b; Resnick, 1962; Rintelmann et al., 1974) and continues to lack consensus. According to the various sampling theorems and the binomial distribution, which is discussed below, more reliable and perhaps more valid word-recognition data are obtained with 50 words as opposed to 25 words. If the word-recognition ability of the patient is evaluated at one presentation level, then the full complement of 50 words should be used. If on the other hand, multiple listening conditions are used in the evaluation (i.e., different presentation levels in quiet and/or in noise), then consideration must be given to the use of

25 words per condition. Audiologists often forget how fatiguing an audiological assessment is, especially for older listeners. The demands of listening to pure-tone and speech signals around threshold followed by repeating multiple word lists can have a substantial impact on the validity of the data obtained, especially during the latter part of the test session when patient fatigue becomes a factor.

Binomial Characteristics of Speech Recognition.   An important characteristic for any speech-recognition test is that the instrument yield good test-retest reliability. The reliability of a speech-recognition score is influenced by two variables, the performance of the listener and the number of test items. Egan (1948) noted that the reliability of a given score is dependent, in part, on the location of the score of the listener on the scoring interval. He observed that variability is at a minimum near the extremes of the percentage scale (0% and 100%) and at a maximum in the middle of the range. Egan also recognized that variability was related inversely to the number of test items, that is, the larger the number of test items, the smaller the variability.

Thirty years later, Thornton and Raffin (1978) suggested that variability between test forms could be estimated using a probabilistic model. The model is appropriate for open-set word-recognition tests in which responses to test items are scored as correct or incorrect, the total score is reported as the number of correct responses, and the alternate forms of the test have an equal number of test items. Since the response to each speech stimulus is independent of those for the other stimuli, Thornton and Raffin contended that the test responses could be evaluated as a binomial distribution. The standard deviation of the binomial distribution is expressed as:

$$SD = \frac{(\% \text{ correct}) \times (\% \text{ incorrect})}{\sqrt{\# \text{ test items})}}$$

As can be seen in Figure 2.16, when this formula is applied to test scores obtained with traditional word-recognition tests of various lengths, the standard deviations vary as a function of the sample size and the probability of a binary event being <100% or >0%. As Egan (1948) initially observed, the largest standard deviations occur with small sample sizes and scores that approach the middle range of the percentage scale.

Once the standard deviation of the distribution is known, the critical differences at various levels of confidence can be estimated for tests with various numbers of items. Table 2.2 shows some of the 95% critical differences developed by Thornton and Raffin (1978) associated with each percentage score for 50-, 25-, and 10-item words lists. For example, if the score is 80% correct, then there is a 95% probability that the score on another form of the test would

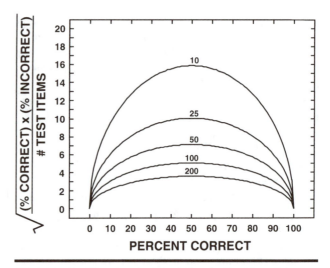

FIGURE 2.16   The standard deviation for the binomial distribution (ordinate) for the various percent correct scores for 10-, 25-, 50-, 100-, and 200-word lists.

fall between 64 and 92% on a 50-item test, between 56 and 96% on a 25-item test, or 40 and 100% on a 10-item test. If the actual score obtained on a second test is outside the predicted range, then the two scores may be considered significantly different. Clearly, the smaller the test list, the larger the test-retest difference score needed to exceed the confidence limits. Tables of critical differences are available for comparing scores from word lists of both equal and unequal length (Raffin & Thornton, 1980).

Word Recognition in Hearing Loss.   The psychometric functions for the various word-recognition materials from subjects with normal hearing indicate that when the materials are presented 30 dB or so above their speech-recognition threshold or three-frequency, pure-tone average a score of 90% correct or better can be expected. Hearing loss produces the gamut of performances on word-recognition tasks from 100% correct to 0% correct. That is, patients with hearing loss may have word-recognition abilities that range from understanding everything, just as individuals with normal hearing do, to not understanding

TABLE 2.2   Lower and upper limits of the 95% critical differences for percentage scores as a function of test sample size (Thornton & Raffin, 1978).

SCORE (%)	50 ITEMS (RANGE)	25 ITEMS (RANGE)	10 ITEMS (RANGE)
20	8–36	4–44	0–60
50	32–66	28–76	10–90
80	64–92	56–96	40–100
100	96–100	92–100	80–100

anything at any presentation level. Within limits, however, certain word-recognition performances can be expected with certain hearing losses. The psychometric functions in the three panels of Figure 2.17 illustrate this point. For

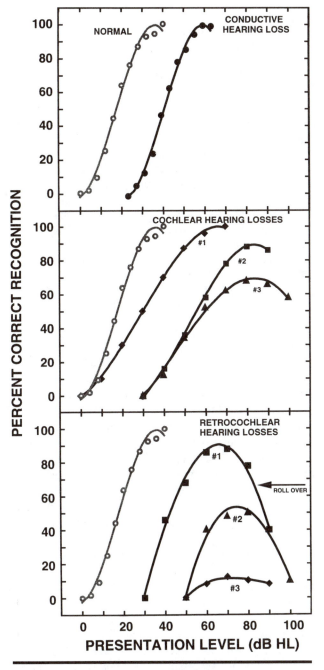

FIGURE 2.17 Example word-recognition psychometric functions for conductive (top), cochlear (middle), and retrocochlear (bottom) hearing losses. The shaded function in each panel represents performance of a listener with normal hearing. (Adapted from Department of Veterans Affairs, *The Audiology Primer for Students and Health Care Professionals,* 1997)

reference purposes in Figure 2.17, the psychometric function for an individual with normal hearing is shown. First, as depicted in the top panel of Figure 2.17, conductive hearing losses produce a psychometric function for word-recognition that is shifted to higher presentation levels by the amount of the conductive component. A patient with a 25 dB conductive hearing loss will have the same word-recognition function as a subject with normal hearing except it will be located 25 dB higher on the abscissa. Second, with pure cochlear hearing losses (i.e., cochlear hearing losses not compounded by such variables as aging), any range of word-recognition performances can be obtained at any range of presentation levels. As shown in the middle panel of Figure 2.17, typically word-recognition performances for patients with cochlear hearing losses are poorer than word-recognition performance for subjects with normal hearing, even when compensation is made for threshold differences. Within the dynamics of the cochlear hearing loss, word-recognition performance generally improves as the presentation level is increased. As the presentation level is increased to the higher levels (e.g., 90 dB HL) with some patients with cochlear hearing loss (case #3 for example), it is not uncommon for word-recognition performance to decrease or *roll over* (discussed in a subsequent section). The improvement in performance (or slope of the psychometric function) for patients with cochlear hearing loss is not as fast (steep) as that observed in subjects with normal hearing. In part, the disparity in word-recognition performance between the people with normal hearing and patients with cochlear hearing loss is due to the differential sensitivity across frequency that is characteristic of cochlear hearing loss. As the cochlear hearing loss involves progressively lower frequencies, performance on word-recognition tasks typically is reduced, especially as the frequency region around and below 2000 Hz becomes involved. The extreme in this progression of hearing loss is most often observed with the patient presenting with a sudden onset hearing loss caused by some type of cochlear episode. These patients have flat, pure-tone threshold configurations around 60 dB HL and 10 to 20% word-recognition scores. Third, patients with retrocochlear (CNVIII) hearing loss exhibit word-recognition abilities that range from 0% to 100% correct, depending upon the stage of the disease process (see Figure 2.17, bottom panel). Generally, as the patients become more symptomatic, word-recognition performance decreases disproportionate to the loss in pure-tone sensitivity. Often with these patients, word-recognition performance at the higher levels decreases substantially (roll over) instead of increasing.

Word lists designed for use in evaluation of high-frequency hearing losses have been devised (Gardner, 1971; Pascoe, 1975). Both tests are comprised of monosyllabic words that focus on sound elements that typically cause difficulty for patients with high-frequency hearing loss. The Gardner High Frequency Word Lists consist of two lists of 25 monosyllables each using only voiceless plosives [*p, t, k*], the fricatives [*s, f, th*], and the aspirate [*h*], paired with the vowel [*ɪ*]. Examples of test words include *kits*, *sick*, and *tip*. Stimuli for the Pascoe High Frequency Test include 50 monosyllables that contain three vowels [*ɪ, a ɪ, ou*] and 63% of the consonant sounds are voiceless fricatives and voiceless plosives. Examples of test items include *hits*, *chip*, and *road*. The high-frequency lists appear to have potential, however, there is limited information concerning the clinical applicability of these tests. Although no normative data has been published for the high-frequency word tests, data are available showing that these tests appear to be useful in the evaluation of word-recognition ability (Gravel, Ochs, Konkle, & Bess, 1981) and in hearing aid selection (Dennison & Kelly, 1978; Skinner & Miller, 1983) for individuals with high-frequency hearing loss.

Several authors have proposed that word-recognition ability can be predicted without actually conducting word-recognition testing (Humes, Dirks, Bell, Ahlstrom, & Kincaid, 1986; Pavlovic, Studebaker, & Sherbecoe, 1986), regardless of the degree of hearing loss. The *articulation index (AI)* (ANSI S3.5, 1969) is a calculation designed to predict what part of the total speech signal is available (audible) to the listener. The AI is expressed in values ranging from 0.0 to 1.0; the higher the value, the more speech information available to the listener. The AI is calculated as the sum of a number of contiguous frequency bands that are weighted according to their contribution to the overall intelligibility of the speech signal. The original version of the AI was presented by Fletcher (1953); however, several other methods have been proposed for calculating the AI, each using slightly different frequency bands and weighting (ANSI S3.5, 1969; French & Steinberg, 1947; Pavlovic, 1988, 1991). The most frequently used calculation is the ANSI S3.5, a simplified version of articulation theory based on the work of French and Steinberg (1947), which is a substantial reduction of Fletcher's original calculations. Rankovic (1997, in press) compared the ANSI S3.5 AI calculation with the original version of articulation theory presented by Fletcher and reported that the Fletcher calculation was superior to ANSI S3.5 for predicting nonsense syllable recognition scores of subjects with hearing impairment presented in both quiet and noise backgrounds. Figure 2.18 displays the nonsense syllable recognition data in noise. The crosses (+) represent consonant recognition as a function of ANSI S3.5, and the open circles represent the same scores plotted as a function of the Fletcher AIs. The solid lines represent mean consonant recognition scores obtained from subjects with normal hearing for the same nonsense syllable test. The comparison shows that the performance of subjects with hearing impair-

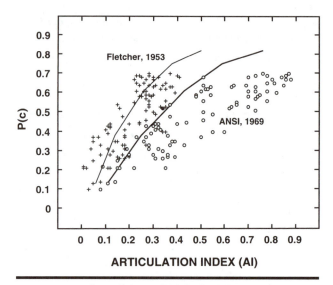

FIGURE 2.18   Comparison of ANSI S3.5 Fletcher AI calculations. The solid lines represent the averaged consonant recognition of five normal-hearing subjects for nonsense syllables presented in noise. (Reprinted with permission from C. M. Rankovic, "Factors governing speech reception benefits of adaptive linear filtering for listeners with sensorineural hearing loss." *Journal of the Acoustical Society of America*, *103*(2), February 1998.)

ment is predicted more accurately from the curves defined for normal-hearing subjects when the Fletcher calculation is used. This is indicated by how well the solid line describes the open circles. The ANSI S3.5 calculation overestimates the performance of the listeners with hearing impairment.

The reported advantage of the AI is that it can provide a reasonable estimate of communication ability using audiogram data. Given the unreliability of some listeners (e.g., children, aphasic patients) on word-recognition tasks, it is possible that for some individuals, the AI may be a better predictor of average speech understanding ability than the actual results of speech testing. Clinicians should be aware, however, that simple audibility of a speech signal does not guarantee understanding. For example, numerous studies have indicated that word-recognition ability in elderly listeners is poorer than would be expected based on pure-tone findings (Dubno et al., 1984; Gelfand, Piper, & Silman, 1985). Thus, in a group of listeners with similar audiometric configurations, word-recognition scores will vary considerably. Nonetheless, investigations have shown that the AI can be used as a successful predictor of word-recognition performance in listeners with hearing impairment (Humes et al., 1986; Kamm, Dirks, & Bell, 1985). The AI has also been used successfully in the selection and fitting of hearing aids (Fabry & Van Tasell, 1990; Mueller & Killion, 1990; Rankovic, 1991).

Word Recognition with Nonverbal Patients. Audiologists, especially in medical environments, encounter patients who are unable to respond verbally to word-recognition materials. These patients cover the gamut of medical conditions from laryngectomy to cerebral vascular accidents. For these patients, the response task for word-recognition needs to be modified to meet the abilities of the patient. These response modifications range from simple to complex. For example, a nonverbal patient who can write can simply write the responses to the word-recognition task. The written response maintains the recognition task but might require additional time between word presentations. More complicated techniques involve a word-pointing or picture-pointing response in which the target word or picture is grouped with a number of rhyming alternatives (see Figure 2.7). As was discussed earlier in the Response Mode Section, the word- or picture-pointing response is a closed-set response and changes the response from recognition to identification, which is the basis of tests such as the *Word Intelligibility from Picture Identification (WIPI)* (Ross & Lerman, 1970) developed for use with children (see Chapter 10) and the *Picture Identification Task (PIT)* (Wilson & Antablin, 1980) devised for use with adults. [Track 12 presents 10 examples of the WIPI (left channel) and 10 examples of the PIT (right channel). Courtesy of Richard Harris, Brigham Young University, Provo, Utah, and the Auditory Research Laboratory, Mountain Home, Tennessee.]

Word Recognition with Multilingual Patients. Many audiologists are encountering the effects of the growing ethnic diversity of the population in the United States. As many of the recent migrants speak little or no English, establishing the word-recognition abilities of these patients is next to impossible, unless the audiologist is fluent in the particular foreign language. To obviate this situation, a computerized, multimedia approach to word recognition has been proposed and evaluated (McCullough, Wilson, Birck, & Anderson, 1994). The concept, which is used with English-speaking patients who are unable to respond verbally, involves using an identification task in which the stimulus words are presented to the patient in their native language. The patient responds by pointing to a picture (or word) on a response foil. The response foil typically contains four response options, one of which is the target word. To score the responses, the audiologist performs a word-to-place transformation that requires no knowledge of the language in which the stimulus is presented. The technology (including touch-screen monitors) is now available to automate completely stimulus delivery and scoring in any foreign language. To our knowledge, materials in only Spanish and Russian have been developed (Aleksandrovsky, McCullough, & Wilson, in press). Information

on Spanish materials are available from several sources (Weislender & Hodgson, 1989). [Track 13 presents examples of Spanish lists (left channel) and of Russian lists (right channel). Courtesy of the Auditory Research Laboratory, Mountain Home, Tennessee, and June McCullough, San José State University, San José, California.]

Sentences

Traditionally, single syllables or single words have been used for tests of speech recognition. The use of sentence materials is an important, attractive consideration, however, since sentences provide a more realistic listening condition for everyday communication. The increased redundancy and contextual cues in sentence materials typically produces a psychometric function with a steep slope. Because of this, when using sentence materials to measure word-recognition (or identification), it is difficult to determine whether subject responses are a result of perceiving the entire sentence or just a few key words that convey the meaning of the sentence to allow the recognition (or identification) of the rest of the sentence. In addition, many sentence tests measure performance of a single target word or reflect the least intelligible word in the sentence if the sentence is scored as a unit. Another complication is that as sentence materials exceed 7 to 9 syllables, memory considerations become a problem with older adult listeners when the listening task is to shadow the sentence (i.e., repeat the sentence verbatim).

The use of sentence materials dates to the 1930s, when Fletcher and Steinberg devised sentence intelligibility lists following the format of simple interrogative or imperative sentences. The sentences never became widely used clinically because of problems related to familiarity and difficulty of the test materials (Hirsh, 1952). Some time later, during World War II, articulation testing methods were developed to evaluate military communications equipment. These efforts led to the development of the PAL Auditory Test No. 12 (Hudgins et al., 1947), which was designed as a threshold measure, but subsequently adapted for suprathreshold word-recognition tasks. PAL Auditory Test No. 12 uses interrogative sentences presented in an open-set format. Example test items include *What letter comes between A and C?* and *What day comes after Sunday?* Concurrently, the PAL Auditory Test No. 8 was developed (Hudgins et al., 1947) as an identification task. The Auditory Test No. 8 used interrogative sentences with four one-word multiple choice responses (e.g., *Butter is made from: Cheese Churns Dairies Milk*). Because there are no standardized data available for either of the PAL sentence tests, their clinical use is limited.

One of the first sentence tests to receive widespread clinical acceptance was the *Central Institute for the Deaf*

(CID) Everyday Sentences Test developed by Silverman and Hirsh (1955). The CID test uses a target-word format, meaning that although the subject must repeat the entire sentence during testing, scoring is based on correct recognition of key words (e.g., *It would be much easier if everyone would help*). Most sentence tests follow this format for scoring. [Track 5 (right channel) contains 10 examples of the CID Everyday Sentences. Courtesy Auditec of St. Louis, Missouri.]

The *Speech Perception in Noise (SPIN)* test (Bilger, Nuetzel, Rabinowitz, & Rzeczkowski, 1984; Kalikow, Stevens, & Elliot, 1977) makes use of the concept of redundancy by controlling the predictability of the target word, which is always the final word of the SPIN sentence. For half of the sentences, the final word has high predictability, meaning that recognition of the target word is aided by surrounding contextual cues in the sentence including syntactic, semantic, and prosodic information (e.g., *The watchdog gave a warning growl*). The other half of the sentences are rated as having low predictability, meaning that the listener receives only minimal contextual cues and, therefore, must rely on the acoustical properties of the target word for correct recognition (e.g., *I had not thought about the growl*). Sentences are presented monotically in the presence of multi-talker babble. Hutcherson, Dirks, and Morgan (1979) investigated the effects of signal-to-babble ratio and presentation level on a group of listeners with normal hearing. The functions at 10 dB signal-to-babble ratio for the listeners with normal hearing is shown in Figure 2.19. As expected, recognition performance on the high-predictability items was better than performance on the low-predictability items. Likewise, the

slope of the high-predictability function (9%/dB) was twice as steep as the slope of the low-predictability function (4%/dB). Both the better performance and steeper slope on the high-predictability items reflect the contributions made by contextual cues to recognition of the target word. [Track 14 presents examples of the SPIN test (left channel) and multi-talker babble (right channel). Sentences 2, 5, 6, 9, and 10 are examples of high-predictability sentences. Sentences 3, 4, 7, 8, and 11 are examples of low-predictability sentences. Courtesy of Robert Bilger, Department of Speech and Hearing Science, University of Illinois, Champaign, Illinois.]

The *Connected Speech Test (CST)* is a sentence test that is also based on correct recognition of target words (Cox, Alexander, & Gilmore, 1987). The CST consists of 48 passages of connected speech. Each passage contains 10 sentences, 7 to 10 words in length, pertaining to a familiar topic. For example, the following are 2 of the 10 sentences from the NAILS passage: (1) *Nails are used to fasten wood together*, and (2) *Pioneers used wooden pegs instead of nails*. The listener is informed of the topic of the passage, and sentences are presented one at a time at an individually determined signal-to-babble ratio. Typically, pairs of passages are presented (i.e., *lawn/cactus; dice/eagle*), with 50 key words available for scoring. The CST was developed primarily for use as a criterion measure in investigations of hearing aid benefit. Substantial standardization information has been collected for the CST including psychometric functions, testing in noise, and evaluation of listeners with and without hearing loss (Cox, Alexander, Gilmore, & Pusakulich, 1988, 1989). [Track 15 presents the 10 sentences from the *UMBRELLA* passage and 10 sentences from the *GIRAFFE* passage of the CST (left channel) presented in multi-talker babble (right channel). Courtesy of Robyn Cox, Hearing Aid Research Laboratory, Memphis, Tennessee.]

In an effort to overcome the problem of sentence recognition (or identification) through recognition (or identification) of key words, synthetic sentences were developed that provide minimal contextual cues and minimal redundancy compared to actual English sentences. The *Synthetic Sentence Identification (SSI)* test (Jerger, Speaks, & Trammell, 1968; Speaks & Jerger, 1965) consists of 10 third-order approximations of English sentences presented in a closed-set format. The task of the listener is to select (identify) the target sentence by pointing to 1 of the 10 sentences displayed on a response form. Examples of sentences include *Forward march said the boy had a* and *Small boat with a picture has become*. For testing purposes, sentences are presented against a competing story describing the life of Davy Crockett. Identification performance is measured at several message-to-competition ratios (MCR) for both contralateral competing message (CCM) and ipsilateral competing message (ICM) conditions. For

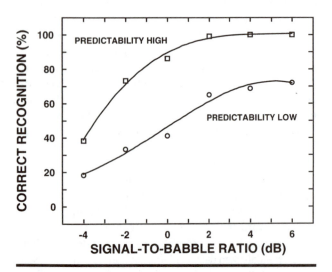

FIGURE 2.19 The percent correct recognition on the SPIN high predictability (squares) and low predictability (circles) items in competing babble by listeners with normal hearing. (Adapted from Hutcherson et al., 1979)

the CCM, the test is administered at MCRs of 0, –20, and –40 dB. For the ICM condition, the test is administered at MCRs of 10, 0, –10, and –20 dB. For SSI-CCM, normal performance is typically between 90 and 100% for all MCRs. Identification performance on the SSI-ICM is represented by the mean of the 0, –10, and –20 MCR conditions, with a mean normal performance of 77% (Jerger & Jerger, 1975). An example of a normal SSI function for CCM and ICM conditions is illustrated in Figure 2.20. [Track 16 presents the SSI in the CCM paradigm with 10 SSI sentences on the left channel and the competing message story on the right channel. Track 17 presents 10 SSI sentences in the ICM paradigm; different S/N ratios are presented on the two channels. Courtesy of James Jerger, The University of Texas at Dallas.]

Interest in the use of sentence materials has resurfaced in recent years (Bell, Wilson, Wright, & Stabinsky, 1993, Killion & Villchur, 1993; Lilly & Vernon, 1997), with a focus on maintaining the naturalness of conversational speech while minimizing the availability of contextual cues. These include the *Experimental Sentence Materials* (Lilly & Vernon, 1997), the *Speech in Noise (SIN)* test (Killion & Villchur, 1993), and the *VA Sentence Test (VAST)* (Bell et al., 1993).

The Experimental Sentence Materials use a version of the original *Sentence-Intelligibility (SI)* test (IEEE, 1969) that was developed at the Harvard Psycho-Acoustic Laboratory during World War II (Egan, 1944). The SI sentences were selected because they sound like conversational speech and it is difficult to identify the key words from the

context of the sentence (Killion & Villchur, 1993). Additionally, each test sentence is short, which reduces some problems for subjects with limited short-term memory. Sentences in the Experimental Sentence Materials each contain five key words, four monosyllables and one dissyllable (e.g., *A rod is used to catch pink salmon* and *The coffee stand is too high for the couch*). Sentences are presented in the sound field at S/N ratios ranging from –4 to 10 dB in 2 dB steps. Using an open-set format, the listener is instructed to repeat the entire sentence, and recognition performance is determined by scoring the number of key words in each sentence that are repeated correctly. The sentences are processed to provide three temporal paradigms: (1) at a natural speaking rate, (2) an expanded speaking rate created by doubling the silent intervals between utterances in the test sentences, and (3) at a compressed speaking rate created by halving the silent intervals between utterances. [Track 18 presents 10 examples of the Experimental Sentence Materials at the normal rate (left channel) and at the expanded rate (right channel). Track 19 presents 10 examples of the Experimental Sentence Materials at the normal rate (left channel) and at the compressed rate (right channel). Courtesy of David J. Lilly, Oregon Hearing Research Center, Portland, Oregon.] Preliminary findings using the Experimental Sentence Materials indicate that for test sentences spoken at a natural rate, elderly subjects require a better S/N ratio than younger subjects to repeat correctly the same number of key words. In addition, subjects generally are able to repeat a greater percentage of the key words in the expanded speech condition versus naturally spoken or compressed speech materials (Lilly & Vernon, 1997).

The Speech in Noise (SIN) test consists of a series of female-talker recordings of the IEEE sentences as the target speech, and four-talker babble (three women and one man) as the noise source (Killion & Villchur, 1993). Five sentences are recorded at four signal-to-noise ratios (15, 10, 5, and 0 dB), with reference to 0 vu, followed by a similar series recorded 30 dB lower. With the audiometer set to 70 dB HL, these levels approximate 83 dB SPL and 53 dB SPL in the sound field with the patient seated at a 45° azimuth. The SIN test is divided into blocks of 20 sentences at each of the two levels. Typically, two blocks are presented for each test condition, and the results averaged. Five key words in each sentence are scored, and half-word credit is given for nearly correct answers such as *tasks* instead of *task*. Examples of SIN sentences include *Oak is strong and also gives shade* and *The Navy attacked the big task force*. A spreadsheet for scoring the SIN is available or results may be recorded manually by plotting the word-recognition score obtained at each signal-to-noise ratio at the two presentation levels. The SIN has been demonstrated as useful in determining whether and how much a given hearing aid or pair of hearing aids

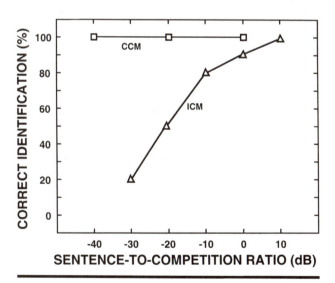

FIGURE 2.20 The percent correct identification of the SSI materials for listeners with normal hearing under the contralateral competing message (CCM) and ipsilateral competing message (ICM) conditions. (Adapted from Jerger & Jerger, 1974)

helps an individual understand speech in noise, compared to listening unaided or with other hearing aids (Killion & Villchur, 1993). [Track 20 presents examples of the SIN materials with the sentences and multi-talker babble on both channels. Four sentences are presented at each S/N ratio (15, 10, 5, and 0 dB, respectively). Courtesy of Mead Killion, Etymotic Research, Inc.]

The *VA Sentence Test (VAST)* (Bell et al., 1993) was constructed by embedding three key words in each sentence, which were similar in their lexical characteristics, word usage (frequency of usage in everyday language), and lexical-phonetic confusibility (Pisoni, 1985). The Kucera and Francis *Computational Analysis of Word Usage in Present Day English* (1969) was used to categorize stimuli as either *high usage* or *low usage* (re: a median value). Phonetic confusibility was defined as the number of other words in the language that were phonetically similar to a target word. A word was considered to be similar to the target word if it differed by only one phoneme. The terminology advanced by Luce (1986) in his *Neighborhood Activation Model* was used. *Sparse* words are phonetically unique words (words that sound like few other words), whereas *dense* words are those that are phonetically similar to many other words.

A corpus of 850 sentences was composed, each 9 to 11 syllables in length and containing three key words selected on the basis of phonetic content and frequency of usage in everyday language (e.g., *They put a loud pump near the drain* and *The yarn in the box was soft*). Preliminary findings shown in Figure 2.21 illustrate three points of interest. First, high-usage words are more intelligible than low-usage words under equivalent acoustical conditions.

Second, words with high lexical-phonetic confusibility have significantly higher thresholds under equivalent acoustical presentation conditions. Third, there is a tendency for the lexical density effect to dissipate at suprathreshold levels (above 50%). [Track 21 presents 10 examples of the VA Sentence Test materials. Sentences on the left channel are made up of high usage/sparse words. Sentences on the right channel contain low usage/dense words. Courtesy of the Human Auditory Research Laboratory at UCLA and the Auditory Research Laboratory, Mountain Home, Tennessee.]

Degraded Speech Tests

Monaural speech stimuli may be degraded by electroacoustically modifying the frequency, temporal, or level characteristics of the speech signal. These parameters may be manipulated singly or in any combination. As was mentioned earlier, degradation of the speech material reduces the extrinsic redundancies in the materials and increases the uncertainty about the stimulus materials that is imposed on the listener. Three monaural degraded auditory tasks are discussed in this section including *filtered speech*, *time compressed speech*, and *reverberated speech*. Degraded speech tests are used extensively in the assessment of central auditory problems (see Chapter 13).

Filtered Speech. Speech can be distorted by eliminating a portion of the frequency spectrum through electronic or digital filtering. Although speech can be processed through a low-pass, high-pass, or band-pass (both low-pass and high-pass) filter system, most applications of monaural filtered speech tasks use low-pass filtering. The effects of filtering on the word-recognition scores of young normal adult listeners has been studied rather extensively since first described by Bocca and colleagues in the mid-1950s (Bocca, Calearo, & Cassinari, 1954; Bocca, Calearo, Cassinari, & Migliavacca, 1955).

The degradation of the speech signal that is produced by filtering is affected by the cut-off frequency of the filter and by the rejection rate of the filter. Bornstein, Wilson, and Cambron (1994) summarized three generalizations that may be applied to filtered speech: (1) for low-pass filtered materials, the lower the cut-off frequency, the poorer the word-recognition performance; (2) for high-pass filtered materials, the higher the cut-off frequency, the poorer the word-recognition performance; and (3) for both low-pass and high-pass filtering techniques, the steeper the rejection rate of the filter, the poorer the word-recognition performance. The relationship between recognition performance and cut-off frequency for low-pass and high-pass filtered NU No. 6 materials is shown in Figure 2.22 (Bornstein et al., 1994). Results plotted in this figure illustrate that as the low-pass cut-off was increased from

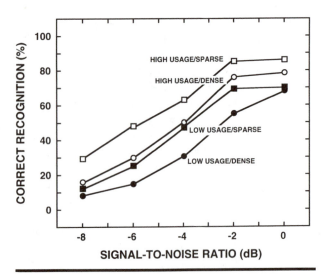

FIGURE 2.21 The lexical categories of words used to develop the VA Sentences. The numbers in parentheses indicate the usage value and the similarity value of each corresponding word. (Adapted from Bell et al., 1993)

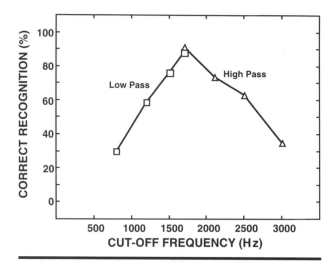

FIGURE 2.22 The percent correct recognition by listeners with normal hearing on the NU No. 6 materials low-pass filtered at 800, 1200, 1500, and 1700 Hz cut-offs and high-pass filtered at 1700, 2100, 2500, and 3000 Hz cut-offs (115 dB/octave rejection). (Adapted from Bornstein et al., 1994)

routine. The amount of compression is expressed as the percent of the original signal that is eliminated. For example, a 750 ms signal compressed by 40% would result in a 450 ms signal, whereas a 750 ms signal compressed by 70% would result in a 225 ms signal.

Various stimuli have been used in studies involving time-compressed speech, with monosyllabic words and sentences being the most frequent. For clinical purposes, time-compressed monosyllabic test materials are used (Beasley, Forman, & Rintelmann, 1972; Beasley, Schwimmer, & Rintelmann, 1972; Wilson, Preece, Salomon, Sperry, & Bornstein, 1994). As shown in Figure 2.23, word-recognition

800 Hz to 1700 Hz, there was a corresponding increase in performance. Similarly, as the high-pass cut-off was decreased from 3000 Hz to 1700 Hz, there was a corresponding increase in performance. Although individual findings have varied depending on the filter characteristics and the speech stimuli used, normal scores at high sensation levels (e.g., 35 to 50 dB) typically range from 60% to 90%. [Track 22 presents 12 examples of the NU No. 6 materials spoken by the VA female speaker, low-pass filtered (1500 Hz cut-off) (left channel) and of high-pass filtered (2100 Hz cut-off) (right channel). Courtesy of the Auditory Research Laboratory, Mountain Home, Tennessee.]

Time Compressed Speech. The rate of speech can be altered in several ways. First, the rate of speech may be increased (or decreased) by having the speaker talk faster (or slower). Second, the rate can be altered by changing the rate of the analog or digital playback with respect to the rate of the recording (Bocca, 1958; Calearo & Lazzaroni, 1957). Speech changed by acceleration or deceleration of the playback rate has a power spectrum and pitch that vary directly with the rate change. Third, portions of the speech waveform can be added or deleted, thereby altering the rate of the signal without altering the power spectrum of the speech sample. Originally this was accomplished with an electromechanical device whose algorithm was not disseminated (Fairbanks, Everitt, & Jaeger, 1954). Now, waveform editing software available with computers makes alterations in the time-course of a speech waveform somewhat

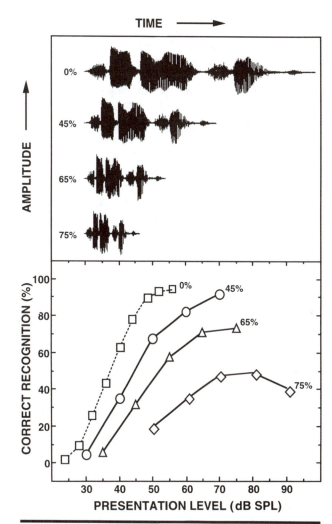

FIGURE 2.23 *Top panel:* An example of a digitized waveform, "Say the word chief." The top waveform is 0% compressed, contrasted to the lower three waveforms that have been compressed by 45%, 65%, and 75%. *Bottom panel:* Psychometric functions for the NU No. 6 materials 45%, 65%, and 75% compressed (0% is the uncompressed condition). The data are from 18 listeners with normal hearing. (Adapted from Wilson et al., 1994)

performance is inversely related to the percent of compression. The data in the figure are based on listeners with normal hearing responding to NU No. 6 materials compressed 45%, 65%, and 75% (0% is uncompressed). The top panel of the figure is an amplitude (Y) by time (X) display of the digitized waveform *Say the word chief*, for the uncompressed condition and for three compression ratios. The bottom panel shows percent correct recognition at the various presentation levels. As the amount of compression of the signal increases, recognition performance of the listeners decreases. [Track 23 presents 12 examples of NU No. 6 materials spoken by the VA female speaker 45% compressed (left channel) and 45% compressed with 0.3 s reverberation (right channel). Track 24 presents 12 examples of NU No. 6 materials spoken by the VA female speaker 65% compressed (left channel) and 65% compressed with 0.3 s reverberation (right channel). Courtesy of the Auditory Research Laboratory, Mountain Home, Tennessee.]

Reverberated Speech.   *Reverberation* refers to the persistence of an acoustic signal in an enclosure after the sound source has stopped and is quantified as the time required for the amplitude of a signal to decay 60 dB after signal offset. The effects of reverberation on word-recognition performance have been studied for a number of years (Knudsen, 1929). Because the persistent sound becomes a masker of later sounds, the general case is that as reverberation time increases, there is a corresponding decrease in word-recognition performance (Harris & Swenson, 1990; Moncur & Dirks, 1967; Nabelek & Robinson, 1982). Figure 2.24 depicts this relationship for young adult listeners with and without hearing loss for nonsense syllables at

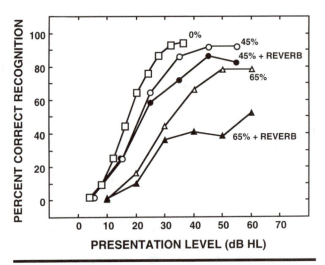

FIGURE 2.25   Psychometric functions for the NU No. 6 materials compressed 45% plus 0.3 ms of reverberation and compressed 65% plus 0.3 ms of reverberation. The 0% function is the normal function that is not compressed and not reverberated. Each datum point represents 20 listeners with normal hearing. (Adapted from Wilson et al., 1994)

four reverberation times. Specific effects of reverberation on the speech signal include the masking of adjacent phonemes, smearing of speech elements in the time domain, and smoothing of the temporal envelope of speech (Houtgast & Steeneken, 1973). Reverberation typically affects the recognition of consonants more than vowels. [Track 25 presents the NU No. 6 materials spoken by the VA female speaker normally (left channel) and reverberated 0.3 s (right channel). Courtesy of the Auditory Research Laboratory, Mountain Home, Tennessee.]

Many investigations have shown that combinations of speech degradation techniques (e.g., low-pass filtering, time compression, masking, and reverberation) produce word-recognition performance that is poorer than the simple additive affects of the degradation techniques (Harris, 1960; Licklider & Pollack, 1948). Figure 2.25 shows percent correct recognition obtained for four degraded conditions of NU No. 6 word lists including 45% compression, 45% compression plus 0.3 s reverberation, 65% compression, and 65% compression plus 0.3 s reverberation (Wilson et al., 1994). The normal psychometric function for the NU No. 6 materials is also depicted (Wilson, Zizz, et al., 1990). Results illustrate that as the signal is increasingly degraded, the psychometric functions are displaced to higher presentation levels and the slope of the function becomes more gradual.

Dichotic Tests

The term *dichotic* refers to a condition in which the sound stimulus presented at one ear differs from the sound

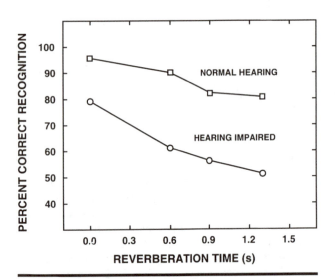

FIGURE 2.24   The mean percent correct recognition on the NST at four reverberation times for groups (n = 8) of young adults (<36 years) with normal hearing (squares) and with hearing impairment (circles). (Adapted from Helfer & Wilber, 1990)

stimulus presented simultaneously at the other ear. This is contrasted with *diotic* conditions in which the sound stimulus simultaneously presented at each ear is identical. Both dichotic and diotic conditions fall under the more general category of *binaural* hearing, defined as hearing by use of two ears (ANSI, 1995).

When different auditory stimuli are presented concurrently to the two ears, most listeners correctly perceive more of the messages presented to the right ear than to the left ear (Kimura, 1961). This right-ear superiority is often termed the *right-ear advantage (REA)*. A commonly accepted explanation for the REA derives from two principles. First, the left hemisphere is specialized for the processing of verbal materials. Second, the right ear is directly connected to the left hemisphere via the crossed afferent auditory pathway, whereas the left ear, connected directly to the right hemisphere, has access to the left hemisphere only via the interhemispheric connecting pathways mainly in the corpus callosum. The magnitude of the REA is dependent upon the difficulty of the listening task, ranging from less than 10% with dichotic digit materials to 15% with dichotic nonsense syllables. The REA is typically present for both right- and left-handed subjects, although is smaller for left-handed subjects (Bryden, 1988).

Dichotic listening procedures were developed initially by Broadbent (1954) to address attentional problems faced by air traffic controllers who often experienced difficulty when receiving flight information from more than one airplane at a time. Broadbent found differences in the order in which subjects recalled digit materials based on rate of presentation. When pairs of digits were presented at a fast rate, subjects most often recalled all digits heard in one ear before recalling digits presented to the other ear. When digits were presented at much slower rates, subjects were able to identify items in their temporal order of presentation. This led to the development of an early information-processing model to account for varying order of recall (Broadbent, 1958). Based on his findings, most early research focused on attentional and short-term memory aspects of dichotic listening, as well as the effects of changing the rate of presentation, type of material, and number of items in the test set (Bryden, 1962, 1964; Moray, 1960). Kimura (1961), following Broadbent's procedure, carried out several investigations of the deficits associated with temporal lobe lesions, and was the first to document the presence of the REA for verbal materials using dichotic digits as stimuli. This early work with dichotic digits stimulated the development of other dichotic materials including dichotic nonsense syllables, words, and sentence materials. For a comprehensive review of dichotic listening, the reader is directed to Hugdahl (1988).

Dichotic Digits. Stimuli for dichotic digit tasks typically include digits from *1* through *10* with the exception of bisyllabic *7*. There are a variety of ways the test can be administered. Perception can be made easy or difficult based on how many pairs of digits the listener is required to repeat. An easy dichotic task is one pair of digits (e.g., simultaneous presentation of *3* to the left ear and *4* to the right ear). A difficult task is the presentation of four pairs of digits (e.g., the sequential presentation of *2, 6, 8, 9* to the left ear simultaneous with the sequential presentation of *1, 5, 10, 3* to the right ear). Research has been done using one-pair digit materials that are currently available on compact disc. Normal young adults typically score close to 100% on these materials (Noffsinger, Martinez, & Wilson, 1994). Although two pairs of digits begin to increase the difficulty of the task, subjects are still able to respond with good accuracy. The criterion for abnormal results on the two-pair dichotic digits test, based on results from patients with normal hearing, is considered to be a score below 90% for either ear. If pure-tone hearing loss is present, then an 80% criterion is used (Musiek, Gollegly, Kibbe, & Verkest-Lenz, 1991).

Kimura (1961) showed that mean recognition performance for three-pair digits was 90% for the left ear and 93% for the right ear. Similar results for three-pair digit materials were reported by Wilson, Dirks, and Carterette (1968) (91% left-ear performance; 94% right-ear performance). Bryden (1963) found recognition performance using four-pair digits was 77% for the left ear and 82% for the right ear. He also evaluated the effect of order of report when subjects were told to report materials presented to one ear before reporting any materials presented to the other ear. Results showed a tendency for subjects to make more errors when instructed to recall materials presented to the left ear first. In a more recent investigation, Wilson and Jaffe (1996) studied recognition performance using a hierarchy of one-pair, two-pair, three-pair, and four-pair dichotic digits. The mean data for the four dichotic conditions for young adult subjects are shown in Figure 2.26. The results demonstrate that as the dichotic task progressed from the easiest to the most difficult conditions, recognition performance decreased. Data also demonstrated a right-ear advantage similar to that reported by earlier investigators. Collectively, findings on dichotic digit tasks show that (1) the REA is present in most subjects no matter what variations are introduced; (2) as the dichotic digit task progresses from easy (one-pair) to difficult (four-pair) conditions, recognition performance decreases. In most studies, young adults with normal hearing have little difficulty recalling one- to three-pair digits; and (3) items recalled early are more accurately reported than those reported later in the digit sequence, thus there is an effect of presentation position (Bartz, 1968; Bryden, 1967). [Track 26 presents on both left and right channels 5 stimulus pairs each of one-pair, two-pair, three-pair, and four-pair dichotic digits presented sequentially. Track 27 contains 10 items of one- to three-pair digits presented randomly. Courtesy of Charles Martinez, VA Medical Center, West

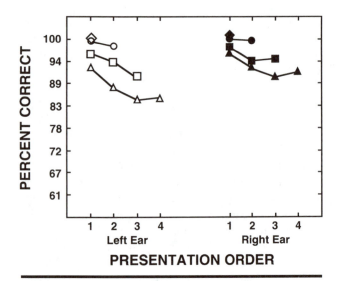

FIGURE 2.26 The percent correct recognition by 20 listeners with normal hearing for one-, two-, three-, and four-pair dichotic digits by ear and by presentation order. (Adapted from Wilson & Jaffe, 1996)

Los Angeles, California, and the Auditory Research Laboratory, Mountain Home, Tennessee.]

Dichotic Consonant Vowels (CVs). The *dichotic consonant-vowel (CV)* test is a more difficult task than dichotic digits. Dichotic CV materials are nonsense syllables presented to the two ears either simultaneously or with varied onsets. Much of the background research and current understanding of dichotic CV material was initiated by Shankweiler and Studdert-Kennedy (1967) and elaborated on by Berlin and his colleagues.

Stimuli for dichotic CVs consist of a set of six syllables formed by the combination of a stop plosive and the vowel /a/, including *ba, pa, da, ta, ga, ka*. Various presentation levels have been used such as 55 dB SL (Collard, Lesser, Luders, Dinner, Morris, Hahn, & Rothner, 1986), most comfortable listening level (Jacobson, Deppe, & Murray, 1983), 75 dB SPL (Lowe, Cullen, Berlin, Thompson, & Willett, 1970), and 80 dB SPL (Berlin, Cullen, Hughes, Berlin, Lowe-Bell, & Thompson, 1975). Subjects usually respond in an open report strategy, indicating the appropriate CV syllables either through verbal report, written report (recognition task), or selection from multiple choices (an identification task). For one test, 30 possible pairings of the six syllables are precisely aligned at the onset so that stimuli are presented to each ear simultaneously. For a second test condition, the onset time is aligned so that one ear receives the syllable a fixed number of milliseconds before the other. Onset lags of 15, 30, 60, and 90 ms have been used. The simultaneous and 90 ms lag condition are most widely used clinically.

Berlin and colleagues found that under simultaneous dichotic listening conditions, right-ear scores were better than left-ear scores. In normal subjects, the right-ear score was usually between 70% and 80% correct and the left-ear score between 58% and 70% correct (Berlin, Lowe-Bell, Cullen, Thompson, & Loovis, 1973). Results of time-staggered dichotic CV tests revealed that perception was better for the lagging than for the leading ear, that is, for the ear receiving the second syllable (Berlin et al., 1973; Porter, Shankweiler, & Liberman, 1969). This is termed the *lag effect*. Wilson and Leigh (1996) investigated identification performance by right- and left-handed listeners on dichotic CV materials in simultaneous 90 ms right-ear lag and 90 ms left-ear lag alignments. The top panel of Figure 2.27 shows an amplitude (Y) by time (X) display of digital CV waveforms in the three temporal listening conditions. Mean percent correct identification and standard deviations (dashed and solid lines) of CV syllables for both ears in the three conditions are displayed in the bottom panels of Figure 2.27. Mean percent correct scores for the simultaneous

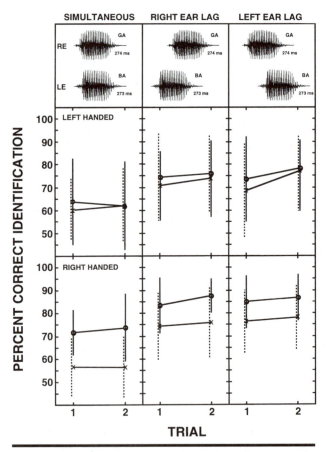

FIGURE 2.27 *Top panel:* Representative digital waveforms of dichotic CVs in three onset conditions (simultaneous, 90 ms right-ear lag, and 90 ms left-ear lag). *Bottom panels:* The percent correct identification and standard deviations (dashed and solid lines) by 24 left-handed and 24 right-handed listeners with normal hearing for dichotic CVs under the three onset conditions for two trials. (Adapted from Wilson & Leigh, 1996)

condition (72.8% for the right ear, 56.5% for the left ear), were similar to normative data reported by Berlin and colleagues and by Noffsinger (1985). For both lag conditions in the right-handed group, the mean performance on materials presented to the right ear (86% correct) was better than that of the left ear (76% correct). This relation is contrary to the lag effect reported by Berlin and colleagues; however, it is consistent with additional data reporting a right-ear advantage for right-handed subjects for both the right-ear lag and left-ear lag conditions (Gelfand, Hoffman, Waltzman, & Piper, 1980; Noffsinger, 1985). Left-handed subjects in the Wilson and Leigh study also showed a mean right-ear advantage; however, the effect was smaller than with the right-handed listeners. In addition, intersubject variability among left-handers was larger than that of right-handed subjects. [Track 28 presents 8 dichotic CVs with simultaneous onsets, followed by 8 dichotic CVs with the materials in the left channel lagging the materials in the right channel by 90 ms. Courtesy of Charles I. Berlin and staff, Kresge Hearing Research Laboratory of the South, New Orleans, Louisiana.]

Dichotic Words. Both monosyllabic words (Dirks, 1964) and spondaic words (Katz, 1962) have been evaluated in the dichotic paradigm. As described previously, the NU No. 20 (Olsen & Carhart, 1967) is an example of a word-recognition task that can be presented dichotically, with the NU No. 6 words (primary message) and the Bell Telephone Sentences (competing message) presented in the same ear. The *Staggered Spondaic Word (SSW)* test developed by Katz is a measure of dichotic listening that utilizes spondaic words presented to each ear in an overlapping fashion. As shown below, the first syllable of the first word is presented to one ear with no competing signal; the second syllable of the first word is presented simultaneous with the first syllable of the second word, which is presented to the opposite ear. Finally, the second syllable of the second word is presented to the opposite ear with no competition. The test stimuli are alternated between the two channels of the audiometer so that the ear receiving the first spondaic word is alternated. During the SSW test, the subject must simply repeat both words. The test contains 40 items. Scoring and interpreting SSW results is rather complicated, and the scoring procedures used are not uniform. The reader is directed to Chapter 13 as well as to Brunt (1978) for detailed information on the administration and scoring of the SSW.

	1	2	3
Right ear	up	stairs	
Left ear		down	town

Dichotic Sentences. Several dichotic procedures involve sentence stimuli. As discussed in a previous section, the SSI-CCM, described by Jerger and Jerger (1974, 1975) may be used as a dichotic test, with sentences presented to one ear and the Davy Crockett competing message presented to the contralateral ear (refer to Figure 2.20).

The SSI materials have also been adapted into a dichotic test called the *Dichotic Sentence Identification (DSI)* test. The DSI was developed in an attempt to devise a dichotic listening test that would be only minimally affected by peripheral hearing loss (Fifer, Jerger, Berlin, Tobey, & Campbell, 1983). The test is applicable for use in auditory assessment of persons with pure-tone averages up to 50 dB HL. The test consists of 30 sentence pairs and uses six of the ten synthetic sentences developed for the SSI as stimuli. Two different sentences are presented simultaneously to the two ears. Onsets and offsets of the two sentences are aligned with an accuracy of 100 ms. As with the SSI, the listener is given a list of response alternatives and reports the number of the sentence heard in each ear. Test items are presented at 50 dB SL relative to the pure-tone average for the respective ears.

Traditionally, the DSI has been administered in a free report format in which the subject identifies both sentences in any order. When administered in this format, normal performance is a score of 75% or better for each ear. There are also norms provided for individuals with hearing loss (Fifer et al., 1983). To interpret interaural scores, DSI results are considered abnormal if there is more than a 16% difference in scores between ears if the pure-tone average is less than 40 dB HL in both ears. If the pure-tone average in either ear exceeds 40 dB HL, then the criterion for abnormality is ear differences greater than 37%. Although the DSI is presumably insensitive to peripheral hearing loss, Cokely and Humes (1992) found that scores in a group of older adults were strongly related to degree of hearing loss and also noted large test-retest variability among their subjects.

More recently, investigators have utilized a directed report format with the DSI test, in which the listener is instructed to identify the sentence in one ear while ignoring the sentence heard in the opposite ear (Chmiel & Jerger, 1993; Jerger, Chmiel, Allen, & Wilson, 1994). The reasoning behind this test format is that a comparison of performance in the free recall and the directed report conditions may differentiate auditory from cognitive influences on the dichotic performance score. DSI results are interpreted as a problem in the cognitive domain when performance is poor in the free recall condition but improves substantially in the directed report condition. When performance is poor in both free recall and directed report conditions, then the problem is interpreted to be primarily in the auditory domain since the deficit is not eased by lessening of cognitive requirements. [Track 29 on both left and right channels contains 7 examples of the DSI. Courtesy of James Jerger, The University of Texas at Dallas.]

Masking-Level Difference for Spondaic Words. Spondaic words often are used to measure the *masking-level difference (MLD)* for speech, the clinical application for which is discussed in Chapter 13. The MLD is a binaural phenomenon originally described by Hirsh (1948) for pure-tones and by Licklider (1948) for speech. The MLD is the difference between thresholds established in homophasic and antiphasic listening conditions (see Figure 2.28). If the phase of either the signal or noise is in-phase (the same) in the ears (top panel of Figure 2.28), then the condition is homophasic and is denoted with the subscript o (S_o = homophasic signal; N_o = homophasic noise). If the phase of either the signal or noise is 180° out-of-phase in the ears (bottom panel of Figure 2.28), then the condition is antiphasic and is denoted with the subscript π (S_π = antiphasic signal; N_π = antiphasic noise). The two MLD conditions most commonly used in audiologic evaluations are S_oN_o (homophasic) and $S_\pi N_o$ (antiphasic) (Olsen, Noffsinger, & Carhart, 1976; Stubblefield & Goldstein, 1977; Sweetow & Reddell, 1978; Wilson, Shanks, & Koebsell, 1982). The psychometric functions in Figure 2.29 are representative of the detection performance (filled symbols) and recognition performance (open symbols) with spondaic words for $S_\pi N_o$ (triangles) and S_oN_o (circles) listening conditions. The data are based on the Hirsh recording of the CID W-1 spondaic words masked with 70 dB SPL speech-spectrum noise; 36 young adults with normal hearing participated in the study (Wilson, Hopkins, Mance, & Novak, 1982). Thresholds for each subject were calculated with the Spearman-Kärber formula and

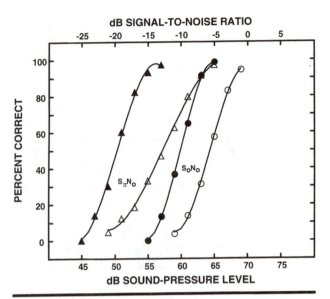

FIGURE 2.29 Psychometric functions for detection (filled symbols) and recognition (open symbols) response tasks under S_oN_o (circles) and $S_\pi N_o$ (triangles) listening conditions. The data (n = 36) are based on the Hirsh recording of the spondaic words. (Adapted from Wilson et al., 1982)

are listed in Table 2.3 along with the masking-level differences. From Figure 2.29, in comparison to the recognition functions, the detection functions are displaced 4 to 7 dB to the lower sound-pressure levels, which is a relation observed in other reports (Carhart, Tillman, & Johnson, 1967; Levitt & Rabiner, 1967). The slopes of the functions for the two response tasks are different from one another in two ways. First, the slopes of the detection functions are steeper than the slopes of the recognition functions. Second, the S_oN_o and $S_\pi N_o$ detection functions have almost identical slopes, whereas with recognition the slope for the $S_\pi N_o$ function is much more gradual than the slope for the S_oN_o function. This slope difference for the recognition functions produces an inverse relation between the magnitude of the MLD and the presentation level.

One final comment is in order regarding the psychometric functions for S_oN_o and $S_\pi N_o$ in Figure 2.29. Earlier

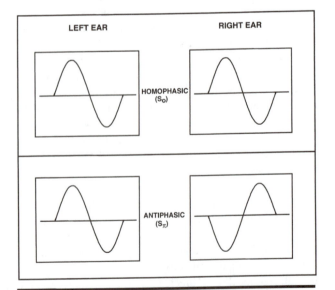

FIGURE 2.28 Sinusoids depicting the phase relations between homophasic signals presented to the left and right ears (top panel) and between antiphasic signals presented to the left and right ears (bottom panel).

TABLE 2.3 Mean detection and recognition thresholds (dB SPL) obtained from 36 listeners with normal hearing in speech-spectrum noise presented at 70 dB SPL. (From Wilson et al., 1982)

RESPONSE TASK	S_oN_o	$S_\pi N_o$	MLD
Detection	59.9	50.5	9.4
Recognition	64.3	57.1	7.2

in the discussion of psychometric functions the implied axiom was the easier the speech material, the steeper the slope of the function. The recognition functions in Figure 2.29 indicate that this axiom is not always true. The function for the easier $S_\pi N_o$ condition has a more gradual slope (7.8%/dB) than does the function for the more difficult, $S_o N_o$ condition (11.7%/dB). In this example the threshold (50% correct point) for the more gradual-sloping $S_\pi N_o$ function is 57.1 dB SPL, whereas the threshold for the steeper-sloping $S_o N_o$ function is 64.3 dB SPL. As expected, the interword threshold variability (standard deviation) was greater for the $S_\pi N_o$ condition (1.8 dB) than for the $S_o N_o$ condition (1.3 dB). These variability data support that the axiom that the more variable the data, the more gradual the slope of the psychometric function. Thus, there are instances in which the more gradual slope of a psychometric function can be related to an easier listening condition with a steeper slope related to a more difficult listening condition. [Track 30 presents 16 spondaic words in the $S_\pi N_o$ paradigm at S/N ratios of 0 to –30 dB, in 2 dB decrements. The level of the noise is constant, with each successive spondaic word decreased by 2 dB. The homophasic condition can be experienced by listening through one channel or by routing the same channel to both ear. The antiphasic condition can be appreciated when the two channels are presented to separate ears through earphones. Courtesy of the Auditory Research Laboratory, Mountain Home, Tennessee.]

Binaural Fusion. Tests of binaural fusion assess the ability of the central auditory nervous system to process different information cues presented to the two ears. Unlike dichotic tasks, the stimuli utilized in binaural fusion tasks are typically presented either in a nonsimultaneous, sequential condition, or the information presented to each ear is composed of a portion of an entire message, so that information must be integrated in order for the listener to perceive the whole message. Results of several investigations suggest that binaural fusion tasks are effective in detecting brainstem dysfunction (Calearo, 1957; Jerger, 1960; Lynn & Gilroy, 1972; Matzger, 1959), however, results have been somewhat inconsistent (see Chapter 13).

Both *binaural spectral fusion* and *binaural temporal fusion* paradigms have been used to assess the integrity of the central auditory system. Binaural spectral fusion paradigms involve filtering a speech signal into a low-pass band and a high-pass band. First described by Matzger (1959), the goal with these schemes is to present minimal information to each ear that, when combined (fused), produce recognition performance that is substantially better than the sum of the recognition performances on the two parts. One of the more popular binaural spectral fusion tests uses spondaic words that are filtered using 500 to 700 Hz and 1900 to 2100 Hz bandpass filters (Willeford, 1976, 1977). Results show that normal subjects are able to fuse the high

bandpass and low bandpass and correctly recognize the word. When only one of the bands is presented to an ear, normal subjects have difficulty correctly recognizing the word. A pilot project using normal-hearing young adults showed the intelligibility of the low bandpass segment to be 18% correct, and the high bandpass segment to be 29% correct (Ivey & Willeford, 1988). In the binaural condition, intelligibility was 94% correct. In most tests, normal binaural fusion scores usually surpass the highest monaural single band score by at least 50%.

Most of the research in binaural spectral fusion has involved the use of bisyllabic speech stimuli; however, Smith and Resnick (1972) believed that monosyllables would further reduce the redundancy of the speech signal and make the test more sensitive. They used CNC monosyllables filtered to obtain a low bandpass from 360-890 Hz and a high bandpass from 1750 to 2220 Hz. When either bandpass was presented alone, word-recognition performance for the listener with normal hearing was about 20% correct. When presented in the binaural paradigm with the low-pass signal to one ear and high-pass signal to the other ear, recognition performance improved to about 60% correct. [The binaural fusion of low-pass and high-pass materials can be experienced by listening to Track 22 binaurally under earphones.]

By design, the binaural spectral fusion paradigm simultaneously places predominately vowel information in one ear (low pass) and predominantly consonant information (high pass) in the other ear. Because substantial portions of the speech spectrum have to be eliminated in these binaural spectral fusion tasks, the materials are difficult to use with subjects with hearing loss.

Binaural temporal fusion paradigms differ from binaural spectral fusion paradigms in that they typically involve a speech signal that is alternated between ears with a 50% duty cycle up to 100 times/s. Examples of this paradigm include *rapidly alternating speech perception (RASP)* tests in which segments of sentences are presented to the subjects two ears in an alternating fashion (Bocca & Calearo, 1963; Cherry & Taylor, 1954; Jerger, 1960; Willeford, 1976). Segments delivered monaurally to either ear are unintelligible, but when the two parts are delivered simultaneously, the segments can be fused and the sentence can be understood. Lynn and Gilroy (1977) observed that normal adults have low monaural scores for each ear (0% to 10% correct) but 90 to 100% scores when the presentation was binaural. A disadvantage of this paradigm is that in addition to the degradation of the speech signal caused by the alterations, the distortion caused by the rapid switching introduces additional temporal and spectral degradation of the signal. [Track 31 on both the left and right channels contains 8 examples of the RASP recorded with a 600 ms period and a 50% duty cycle. Courtesy of Auditec of St. Louis, Missouri.]

The *segmented-alternated CVC* task is a binaural fusion test designed to maintain the spectral and temporal information of test stimuli, making the test materials relatively resistant to the confounding effects of hearing loss (Wilson, Arcos, & Jones, 1984). The test uses CVC words recorded with the Picture Identification Task materials (Wilson & Antablin, 1980) and involves presentation of the carrier phrase to both ears, the consonant segments of the target word to one ear and the vowel segment of the target word to the other ear. An example digital waveform of this paradigm is given in Figure 2.30 (top panel). The carrier phrase is *Show me,* and the target word is *yam.* The bottom panel of Figure 2.30 shows data obtained from 120 subjects with normal hearing on the segmented-alternated CVC task (Wilson, 1994). The percent correct recognition is displayed for the binaural condition in which the vowel segments were presented to one ear and the consonant segment to the other ear and for two monaural conditions, vowel segments and consonant segments. The normal, monaural psychometric function for the Picture Identification task materials is shown for reference (Wilson & Antablin, 1980). Several features are noteworthy from the data in the figure. First, the psychometric function for the segmented-alternated CVC task is essentially identical with that of the normative, monaural data for the materials. Second, results show that binaural-recognition performance was substantially better than monaural performance at all presentation levels. In this example, at 40 dB HL, binaural performance was about 100% correct, or 80% better than performance under either monaural condition. Humes, Coughlin, and Talley (1996) evaluated the segmented-alternated CVC task in elderly subjects with and without hearing loss. Their findings indicated good test-retest reliability and showed that the segmented-alternated CVC task is independent of degree of hearing loss. [Track 32 presents 13 examples of the segmented-alternated CVC task with the consonant segments on the left channel and the vowel segments on the right channel. Courtesy of the Auditory Research Laboratory, Mountain Home, Tennessee.]

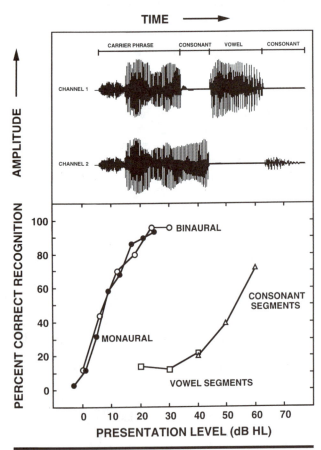

FIGURE 2.30 *Top panel:* An example of a digitized waveform developed for the segmented-alternated CVC task. The carrier phrase is *Show me,* and the target word is *yam. Bottom panel:* The percent correct recognition (n = 120) for normal monaural listening [filled circles, from Wilson and Antablin (1980) shown for reference], for binaural listening (open circles, the consonant segments to one ear and the vowel segments to the other ear), for the vowel segments presented to one ear (squares), and for the consonant segments presented to one ear (triangles). (Adapted from Wilson, 1994)

CONCLUSIONS

This chapter started with the thought that the language-based communications transmitted by speech are the most important sounds transduced by the ear. As such, an evaluation of the auditory system should include measures of how well the patient understands speech. Two of the most common complaints that individuals with hearing loss have are (1) *I can hear, but I can't understand,* and (2) *I can't understand when it is noisy.* Both of these complaints need to be evaluated with speech materials. The importance of using standardized recorded materials was emphasized. Basically, two types of speech measures have been described, threshold and supra-threshold. Since the beginnings of audiology, the speech-recognition threshold (SRT) has been one component of the audiologic evaluation. In the past ten to twenty years, as new test instruments have been developed (e.g., aural acoustic immittance, auditory evoked potentials, otoacoustic emissions), the SRT has become a secondary instrument in the typical audiologic evaluation but has retained its usefulness in certain types of difficult to test patients, for example, patients with pseudohypacusis.

Supra-threshold measures of word-recognition abilities are useful for both diagnostic and rehabilitative purposes. Unfortunately, the majority of these measures are made by most audiologists in a quiet environment, which is an acoustic environment in which most patients do not have trouble understanding speech, especially once the audibility factor is overcome. Just as pure-tone thresholds provide insight into the functioning of an auditory system, estimates of (spoken) word-recognition abilities in quiet, especially at multiple presentation levels, provide insight into the functioning of an auditory system. Patients with the same pure-tone thresholds can have word-recognition abilities in a quiet acoustic environment that are very similar or that are vastly different. Clinically, however, we need to go one step further with word-recognition testing. The ability of each patient to understand speech in a noisy background should be evaluated as part of the routine audiologic evaluation. Patients with the same pure-tone thresholds and with the same word-recognition abilities in quiet can have vastly different word-recognition abilities in a noisy acoustic environment. Quantifying how disruptive a background noise is on the ability of a patient to understand speech should be useful in hearing aid selection and in counseling the patient, particularly concerning expectations of hearing aid use.

One final note concerning standardization of materials for speech audiometry. As was emphasized earlier, each set of speech audiometric materials has its own unique psychometric characteristics. Not only are those characteristics unique to the specific materials but they are unique to a specific recording of the materials by a specific speaker. This means that materials presented via monitored-live voice can have different psychometric characteristics with each presentation. Thus, for reliability purposes recorded materials that have standardized data should be used. Finally, correct interpretation of the speech audiometric data, whether a typical word-recognition paradigm or one of the degraded speech paradigms, must be made with reference to a database that is applicable to the characteristics of the patient undergoing the evaluation.

APPENDIX 2A

TRACK	LEFT CHANNEL	RIGHT CHANNEL	TIME
1	Calibration tone (Not intended for precise calibration of various tracks)	Calibration tone	0:31
	[Courtesy of the Auditory Research Laboratory, Mountain Home, TN.]		
2	Broadband Noise	Speech Spectrum Noise	0:30
	[Courtesy of the Auditory Research Laboratory, Mountain Home, TN.]		
3	Spondaic words (12 items) VA female speaker	Spondaic words (12 items) Hirsh speaker	1:05
	[Courtesy of the Auditory Research Laboratory, Mountain Home, TN, G. Donald Causey, VA Medical Center, Washington, DC, and Technisonic Studios, Inc., St. Louis, MO.]		
4	Hearing in Noise Test (HINT) (10 items) (On the original HINT CD, items are recorded below the level of the calibration tone. This relationship was maintained in this sample) recording.)	Hearing in Noise Test (HINT) (10 items)	1:16
	[Developed by Michael Nilsson and Sigfrid Soli, copyright House Ear Institute, Los Angeles, CA.]		
5	Nonsense Syllable Test (10 items)	CID Everyday Sentences (10 items)	1:11
	[Courtesy of Auditec of St. Louis, MO]		

TRACK	LEFT CHANNEL	RIGHT CHANNEL	TIME
6	PB-50 words (10 items) Rush-Hughes	CID W-22 (10 items) VA male speaker	0:57
	[Courtesy of Technisonic Studios, Inc., St. Louis, MO.]		
7	NU No. 6 (12 items) Tillman	NU No. 6 (12 items) VA female speaker	1:00
	[Courtesy of Auditory Research Laboratory, Northwestern University, Evanston, Illinois; G. Donald Causey, VA Medical Center, Washington, DC, and Auditec of St. Louis, MO.]		
8	NU No. 6 (11 items) Auditec male speaker	Maryland CNC words (11 items) VA male speaker	0:51
	[Courtesy of Auditory Research Laboratory, Northwestern University, Evanston, Illinois; G. Donald Causey, VA Medical Center, Washington, DC, and Auditec of St. Louis, MO.]		
9	NU No. 6 (13 items) VA female speaker	Competing sentences (13 items) VA male speaker	1:05
	[Courtesy of the Auditory Research Laboratory, Mountain Home, TN.]		

(continued)

APPENDIX 2A   continued

TRACK	LEFT CHANNEL	RIGHT CHANNEL	TIME
10	NU No. 6 (12 items) Tillman	Competing sentences (12 items) Tillman	1:03
	[Courtesy of Auditory Research Laboratory, Northwestern University, Evanston, IL.]		
11	NU No. 6 in Babble, attenuated (21 items) (The words presented at the highest level of 20 dB S/N are reflected by the calibration tone.)	NU No. 6 in Quiet, attenuated (21 items)	2:09
	[Courtesy of the Auditory Research Laboratory, Mountain Home, TN.]		
12	WIPI (10 items)	Picture Identifica-tion Task (10 items)	0:52
	[Courtesy of Richard Harris, Brigham Young University, Provo, UT, and the Auditory Research Laboratory, Mountain Home, TN.]		
13	Spanish words (11 items) female speaker	Russian words (11 items) female speaker	1:02
	[Courtesy of the Auditory Research Laboratory, Mountain Home, TN, and June McCullough, San Jose State University, San Jose, CA.]		
14	SPIN sentences (Sentences 2, 5, 6, 9, and 10 = high predictability sentences. Sentences 3, 4, 7, 8, and 11 = low predictability sentences)	SPIN multi-talker babble	1:59
	[Courtesy of Robert Bilger, Department of Speech and Hearing Science, University of Illinois, Champaign, IL.]		
15	Connected Speech Test (10 sentences UMBRELLA, 10 sentences GIRAFFE)￼	CST multi-talker babble	1:08
	[Courtesy of Robyn Cox, Hearing Aid Research Laboratory, Memphis, TN.]		
16	SSI-CCM sentences (10 items)	Competing message story	1:47
	[Courtesy of James Jerger, The University of Texas at Dallas.]		
17	SSI-ICM (–20 dB S/N) (10 items)	SSI-ICM (0 dB S/N)	1:43
	[Courtesy of James Jerger, The University of Texas at Dallas.]		
18	Experimental Sentence Materials (10 items) Natural speech rate	Experimental Sentence Materials (10 items) Expanded speech rate	1:21
	[Courtesy of David J. Lilly, Oregon Hearing Research Center, Portland, OR.]		
19	Experimental Sentence Materials (10 items) Natural speech rate	Experimental Sentence Materials (10 items) Compressed speech rate	1:21
	[Courtesy of David J. Lilly, Oregon Hearing Research Center, Portland, OR.]		
20	Speech in Noise (SIN) test (16 items)	Speech in Noise (SIN) test (16 items)	2:13
	[Courtesy of Mead Killion, Etymotic Research, Inc.]		
21	VA Sentence Test (VAST) (10 items)	VA Sentence Test (VAST) (10 items)	1:37
	[Courtesy of the Auditory Research Laboratory, Mountain Home, TN, and the Human Auditory Research Laboratory at UCLA.]		
22	NU No. 6 Low-pass filtered (12 items) VA female speaker	NU No. 6 High-pass filtered (12 items) VA female speaker	1:00
	[Courtesy of the Auditory Research Laboratory, Mountain Home, TN.]		
23	NU No. 6 45% compressed (12 items) VA female speaker	NU No. 6 45% compressed + 3.5 s reverberated (12 items) VA female speaker	0:59
	[Courtesy of the Auditory Research Laboratory, Mountain Home, TN.]		
24	NU No. 6 65% compressed (12 items) VA female speaker	NU No. 6 65% compressed + 3.5 s reverberated (12 items) VA female speaker	0:58
	[Courtesy of the Auditory Research Laboratory, Mountain Home, TN.]		
25	NU No. 6 Normal (12 items) VA female speaker	NU No. 6 3.5 s reverberated (12 items) VA female speaker	0:57
	[Courtesy of the Auditory Research Laboratory, Mountain Home, TN.]		

TRACK	LEFT CHANNEL	RIGHT CHANNEL	TIME
26	Dichotic Digits 1-4 pair (20 pairs, 5 of each)	Dichotic Digits 1-4 pair (20 pairs, 5 of each)	2:46
	[Courtesy of the Auditory Research Laboratory, Mountain Home, TN, and Charles Martinez, VA Medical Center, West Los Angeles, CA.]		
27	Dichotic Digits, random 1-3 pair, random (10 items)	Dichotic Digits, random 1-3 pair, random (10 items)	1:15
	[Courtesy of the Auditory Research Laboratory, Mountain Home, TN, and Charles Martinez, VA Medical Center, West Los Angeles, CA.]		
28	Dichotic CVs (8 simultaneous followed by 8 with 90 ms lag)	Dichotic CVs	1:43
	[Courtesy of Charles I. Berlin and the staff of Kresge Hearing Research Laboratory at LSUMC in New Orleans, LA.]		
29	Dichotic Sentence Identification (7 items)	Dichotic Sentence Identification (7 items)	1:07
	[Courtesy of James Jerger, The University of Texas at Dallas.]		
30	Speech MLD (16 items)	Speech MLD (16 items)	1:21
	[Courtesy of the Auditory Research Laboratory, Mountain Home, TN.]		
31	RASP (8 items)	RASP (8 items)	1:03
	[Courtesy of Auditec of St. Louis, MO.]		
32	Segmented-Alternated CVCs Consonant segments (13 items)	Segmented-Alternated CVCs Vowel segments (13 items)	0:59
	[Courtesy of the Auditory Research Laboratory, Mountain Home, TN.]		
33	PSI words (6 items)	PSI competing sentences (6 items)	0:43
	[Courtesy of Susan Jerger, The University of Texas at Dallas.]		

TRACK	LEFT CHANNEL	RIGHT CHANNEL	TIME
34	PSI sentences (5 items)	PSI competing sentences (5 items)	0:46
	[Courtesy of Susan Jerger, The University of Texas at Dallas.]		
35	NU-CHIPS (12 items) Male speaker	NU-CHIPS (12 items) Female speaker	0:58
	[Courtesy of Auditec of St. Louis, MO.]		
36	PBK-50s (25 words)	Filtered speech (10 NU No. 6 words—500 Hz) (10 NU No. 6 words—1000 Hz)	1:50
	[Courtesy of Richard Harris, Brigham Young University, Provo, UT, and Auditec of St. Louis, MO.]		
37	Binaural fusion (15 spondaic words) Low-pass filtered	Binaural fusion (15 spondaic words) High-pass filtered	1:16
	[Courtesy of Auditec of St. Louis, MO.]		
38	Competing sentences (10 items)	Competing sentences (10 items)	1:18
	[Courtesy of Auditec of St. Louis, MO.]		
39	Pitch patterns (15 items)	Duration patterns (15 items)	1:25
	[Courtesy of the Auditory Research Laboratory, Mountain Home, TN.]		
40	Dichotic Chords (8 simultaneous followed by 8 with 90 ms lag)	Dichotic Chords	2:44
	[Courtesy of the Auditory Research Laboratory, Mountain Home, TN.]		
41	Carhart lecture, 1st half	Carhart lecture, 2nd half	19:52
	[Courtesy of Noel Matkin, Doug Noffsinger, and the Auditory Research Laboratory, Mountain Home, TN.]		
		TOTAL CD TIME	73:16

APPENDIX 2B

Resources

Auditec recordings
Auditec of St. Louis
2515 Big Ben Blvd.
St. Louis, MO 63143-2105
(800)-669-9065
WCARVER@AUDITEC.COM

Brigham Young University, Speech Audiometry
Materials
Richard W. Harris, Ph.D.
131 TLRB, Box 28653
Brigham Young University
Provo, UT 84602-8653
(801)-378-6460
RICHARD_HARRIS@BYU.EDU

Speech Recognition and Identification Materials,
Disc 1.1 Tonal and Speech Materials for Auditory
Perceptual Assessment
ETSU Foundation
Audiology (126)
VA Medical Center
Mountain Home, TN 38684
(423) 926-1171, ext. 7553
RICHARD.WILSON2@MED.VA.GOV

Q/MASS Speech Audiometry, Volume 2, Volume 3
(produced jointly by Qualitone and the
Massachusetts Eye and Ear Infirmary)
Qualitone, Inc.
4931 West 35th Street
Minneapolis, MN 55416
(800) 328-3897
TIM_SHEA@STARKEY.COM

Speech Intelligibility Tests
Robyn Cox, Ph.D.
Hearing Aid Research Laboratory
807 Jefferson Avenue
Memphis, TN 38105
(901) 678-5800
HARL@CC.MEMPHIS.EDU

Speech Perception In Noise (SPIN)
Robert Bilger, Ph.D.
Department of Speech and Hearing Science
901 South 6th Street
Champaign, IL 61820
(217) 244-4140
R-BILGER@UIUC.EDU

Hearing in Noise Test (HINT)
Starkey Laboratories, Inc.
6700 Washington Avenue
Eden Prairie, MN 55344
(800) 328-8602
SUE_PEHRINGER@STARKEY.COM

Speech Recognition Materials
National Acoustic Laboratories
126 Greville Street
Chatswood 2067
Australia

APPENDIX 2C

Equations expressing the line of best fit to a set of datum points such as orthogonal polynomials are useful because they enable any ordinate values *(y)* and slopes *(y′)* to be calculated for any abscissa value *(x)*. Likewise, any abscissa value can be calculated at any ordinal value. Orthogonal polynomials provide or define the following: (1) the *y*-intercept (i.e., where the function crosses the ordinal zero point), (2) the sum of the differences between the real data *(y)* and the idealized point on the best-fit line *(ÿ)* is zero, and (3) the r^2 statistic, which gives an indication of the goodness of fit of the function to the data.

Additionally, the first derivative of the polynomial equation provides the slope function. The left panels of Figure 2.31 illustrate three sets of data that were fit with a linear equation or first-degree polynomial (top panel), with a cubic equation or third-degree polynomial (middle panel), and with a quadratic equation or second-degree polynomial (bottom panel). The right panels depict the slope functions for the corresponding functions. *Top panels:* The linear equation or first-degree polynomial is expressed as $y = a + bx$, in which *a* is the *y*-intercept, and *b* is the coefficient and (in the linear case) the slope. The linear

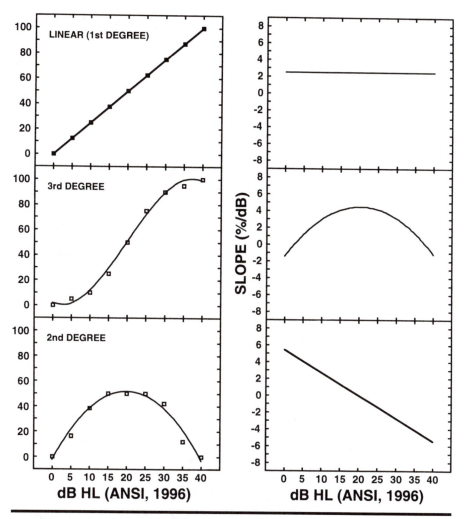

FIGURE 2.31 *Left panels:* Examples of first-degree (linear) (top panel), third-degree (middle panel), and second-degree (bottom panel) polynomials. *Right panels:* The slope functions for the corresponding polynomials calculated from the first derivatives of the polynomial equations.

regression fit to the data in the upper right panel is expressed as $y = 0 + 2.5x$. In this example, the y-intercept is at zero, the slope is 2.5%/dB, and r^2 is 1.0 (which is a perfect fit). The slope function for a linear regression is constant (upper right panel). Obviously, the linear function is the simplest function.

Middle panels: The cubic equation or third-degree polynomial ($y = a + bx + cx^2 + dx^3$) has a y-intercept and three coefficients (a, b, c) and is a two-bend curve or S-shaped. The equation for the function in Figure 2.31 is $y = 1.5152 - 1.4545x + 0.2909x^2 - 0.0048x^3$ with an r^2 of 0.9948. The first derivative of the third-degree polynomial ($y' = 3dx^2 + 2cx + b$) is used to compute the slope function shown in the middle right panel. The slope function is zero near the

extremes of the function and for the most part is between 0%/dB and 4%/dB with slightly negative slopes at the two extremes. The majority of mean word-recognition functions conform to this S-shaped function. *Bottom panels:* The quadratic equation or second-degree polynomial ($y = a + bx + cx^2$) has a y-intercept and two coefficients (a, b) and is a one-bend curve or U-shaped. The equation for the function shown in Figure 2.31 is $y = -2.8242 + 5.4308x - 0.1361x^2$ with an r^2 of 0.9607. The first derivative of the second-degree polynomial ($y' = 2cx + b$) was used to compute the slope function shown in the lower right panel. The slope function for the second-degree function is positive-going from 0 to 20 dB HL and negative going from 20 to 40 dB HL; at 20 dB HL the slope is zero.

REFERENCES

Aleksandrovsky, I. V., McCullough, J. K., & Wilson, R. H. (in press). Development of the Russian picture-identification test. *Journal of the American Academy of Audiology.*

American National Standards Institute. (1954). *Volume Measurements of Electrical Speech and Program Waves* (ANSI C16.5-1954). New York: Author.

American National Standards Institute. (1969). *American National Standards for Calculation of the Articulation Index* (ANSI S3.5-1969). New York: Author.

American National Standards Institute. (1995). *Bioacoustical Terminology* (ANSI S3.2-1995). New York: Author.

American National Standards Institute. (1996). *Specification for Audiometers* (ANSI S3.6-1996). New York: Author.

American Speech and Hearing Association. (1979). Guidelines for determining the threshold level for speech. *Asha, 21,* 353–356.

American Speech-Language-Hearing Association. (1988). Guidelines for determining threshold level for speech. *Asha, 30,* 85–88.

Bartz, W. H. (1968). Serial position effects in dichotic listening. *Perceptual and Motor Skills, 27,* 1014.

Beasley, D. S., Forman, B., & Rintelmann, W. F. (1972). Perception of time-compressed CNC monosyllables by normal listeners. *Journal of Auditory Research, 12,* 71–75.

Beasley, D. S., Schwimmer, S., & Rintelmann, W. F. (1972). Intelligibility of time-compressed CNC monosyllables. *Journal of Speech and Hearing Research, 15,* 340–350.

Beattie, R. C. (1989). Word recognition functions for the CID W-22 test in multitalker noise for normally hearing and hearing-impaired subjects. *Journal of Speech and Hearing Disorders, 54,* 20–32.

Beattie, R. C., Barr, T., & Roup, C. (1997). Normal and hearing-impaired word recognition scores for monosyllabic words in quiet and noise. *British Journal of Audiology, 31,* 153–164.

Beattie, R. C., Edgerton, B. J. & Svihovec, D. V. (1975). An investigation of Auditec of St. Louis Recordings of Central Institute for the Deaf Spondees. *Journal of the American Audiology Society, 1,* 97–101.

Beattie, R. C., Svihovec, S. A., & Edgerton, B. J. (1978). Comparison of speech detection and spondee thresholds for half- versus full-list intelligibility scores with MLV and taped presentations of NU-6. *Journal of the American Audiology Society, 3,* 267–272.

Bell, T. S., Wilson, R. H., Wright, R. A., & Stabinsky, T. (1993). *A New Word Recognition Test Using Sentence Materials.* Convention of the American Academy of Audiology, Phoenix, AZ.

Berlin, C. I., Cullen, J. K., Jr., Hughes, L. F., Berlin, H. L., Lowe-Bell, S. S., & Thompson, C. L. (1975). Acoustic variables in dichotic listening. In M. D. Sullivan (Ed.), *Proceedings of a Symposium on Central Auditory Processing Disorders* (pp. 36–46). Omaha: University of Nebraska Medical Center.

Berlin, C. I., Lowe-Bell, S. S., Cullen, J. K., Jr., Thompson, C. L., & Loovis, C. F. (1973). Dichotic speech perception: An interpretation of right-ear advantage and temporal offset effects. *Journal of the Acoustical Society of America, 53,* 699–709.

Berlin, C. I., Wexler, K. F., Jerger, J. F., Halperin, H. R., & Smith, S. (1978). Superior ultra-audiometric hearing: A new type of hearing loss which correlates highly with unusually good speech in the "profoundly deaf." *Archives of Otolaryngology, 86,* 111–116.

Bess, F. H. (1983). Clinical assessment of speech recognition. In D. F. Konkle & W. F. Rintelmann (Eds.), *Principals of Speech Audiometry* (pp. 127–201). Baltimore: University Park Press.

Bilger, R. C., Matthies, M. L., Meyer, T. A., & Griffiths, S. K. (in press). Psychometric equivalence of recorded spondaic words as test items. *Journal of Speech, Language, and Hearing Research.*

Bilger, R. C., Nuetzel, J. M., Rabinowitz, W. M., & Rzeczkowski, C. (1984). Standardization of a test of speech perception in noise. *Journal of Speech and Hearing Research, 27,* 32–48.

Bocca, E. (1958). Clinical aspects of cortical deafness. *The Laryngoscope, 68,* 301–309.

Bocca, E., & Calearo, C. (1963). Central hearing processes. In J. Jerger (Ed.), *Modern Developments in Audiology* (pp. 337–370). New York: Academic Press.

Bocca, E., Calearo, C., & Cassinari, V. (1954). A new method for testing hearing in temporal lobe tumors. *Acta-Otolaryngologica, 44,* 219–221.

Bocca, E., Calearo, C., Cassinari, V., & Migliavacca, F. (1955). Testing "cortical" hearing in temporal lobe tumors. *Acta-Otolaryngologica, 45,* 289–304.

Boothroyd, A. (1968). Developments in speech audiometry. *Sound, 2,* 2–10.

Bornstein, S. P., Wilson, R. H., & Cambron, N. B. (1994). Low-pass and high-pass frequency responses: Northwestern University Auditory Test No. 6 for monaural and binaural evaluation. *Journal of the American Academy of Audiology, 5,* 259–264.

Bowling, L. S., & Elpern, B. S. (1961). Relative intelligibility of items of CID Auditory Test W-1. *Journal of Auditory Research, 1,* 152–157.

Brandy, W. T. (1966). Reliability of voice tests of speech discrimination. *Journal of Speech and Hearing Research, 9,* 461–465.

Breakey, M. R. & Davis, H. (1949). Comparisons of thresholds for speech: Words and sentence tests; receiver vs. field and monaural vs. binaural listening. *The Laryngoscope, 59,* 236–250.

Broadbent, D. E. (1954). The role of auditory localization in attention and memory span. *Journal of Experimental Psychology, 47,* 191–196.

Broadbent, D. E. (1958). *Perception and Communication.* London: Pergamon Press.

Brunt, M. A. (1978). The staggered spondaic word test. In J. Katz (Ed.), *Handbook of Clinical Audiology* (2nd ed., pp. 262–275). Baltimore: Williams & Wilkins.

Bryden, M. P. (1962). Order of report in dichotic listening. *Canadian Journal of Psychology, 16,* 291–299.

Bryden, M. P. (1963). Ear preference in auditory perception. *Journal of Experimental Psychology, 65,* 103–105.

Bryden, M. P. (1964). The manipulation of strategies of report in dichotic listening. *Canadian Journal of Psychology, 18,* 126–138.

Bryden, M. P. (1967). An evaluation of some models of laterality effects in dichotic listening. *Acta Otolaryngologica, 63,* 595–604.

Bryden, M. P. (1988). An overview of the dichotic listening procedure and its relation to cerebral organization. In K. Hugdahl (Ed.), *Handbook of Dichotic Listening: Theory, Methods, and Research* (pp. 1–43). New York: John Wiley & Sons.

Calearo, C. (1957). Binaural summation in lesions of the temporal lobe. *Acta Otolaryngologica, 47,* 392–395.

Calearo, C., & Lazzaroni, A. (1957). Speech intelligibility in relation to the speed of the message. *The Laryngoscope, 67,* 410–419.

Cambron, N. K., Wilson, R. H., & Shanks, J. E. (1991). Spondaic word detection and recognition functions for female and male speakers. *Ear and Hearing, 12,* 64–70.

Carhart, R. (1946a). Monitored live voice as a test of auditory acuity. *Journal of the Acoustical Society of America, 17,* 339–349.

Carhart, R. (1946b). Speech reception in relation to pattern of pure tone loss. *Journal of Speech and Hearing Disorders, 11,* 97–108.

Carhart, R. (1971). Observations on the relations between thresholds for pure tones and for speech. *Journal of Speech and Hearing Disorders, 36,* 476–483.

Carhart, R., & Jerger, J. (1959). Preferred method for clinical determination of pure-tone thresholds. *Journal of Speech and Hearing Disorders, 24,* 330–345.

Carhart, R., & Porter, L. S. (1971). Audiometric configurations and prediction of thresholds for spondees. *Journal of Speech and Hearing Research, 14,* 486–495.

Carhart, R., & Tillman, T. W. (1970). Interaction of competing speech signals with hearing loss. *Archives of Otolaryngology, 91,* 273–279.

Carhart, R., Tillman, T., & Johnson, K. (1967). Binaural masking of speech by periodically modulated noise. *Journal of the Acoustical Society of America, 39,* 1037–1050.

Causey, G. D., Hermanson, C. L., Hood, L. J., & Bowling, L. S. (1983). A comparative evaluation of the Maryland NU-6 auditory test. *Journal of Speech and Hearing Disorders, 48,* 62–69.

Cherry, C. (1966). *On Human Communication* (2nd ed.). Cambridge, MA: MIT Press.

Cherry, E. C., & Taylor, W. K. (1954). Some further experiments upon the recognition of speech, with one and with two ears. *Journal of the Acoustical Society of America, 26,* 554–559.

Chmiel, R., & Jerger, J. (1993). Some factors affecting assessment of hearing handicap in the elderly. *Journal of the American Academy of Audiology, 4,* 249–257.

Cokely, C. G., & Humes, L. E. (1992). Reliability of two measures of speech recognition in the elderly. *Journal of Speech and Hearing Research, 35* (3), 654–660.

Collard, M. E., Lesser, R. P., Luders, H., Dinner, D. S., Morris, H. M., Hahn, J. F., & Rothner, A. D. (1986). Four dichotic speech tests before and after temporal lobectomy. *Ear and Hearing, 7,* 363–369.

Conn, M. J., Dancer, J., & Ventry, I. M. (1975). A spondee list for determining speech reception threshold without prior familiarization. *Journal of Speech and Hearing Disorders, 40,* 388–396.

Cox, R. M., Alexander, G. C., & Gilmore, C. (1987). Development of the connected speech test (CST). *Ear and Hearing, 8,* 119S–126S.

Cox, R. M., Alexander, G. C., Gilmore, C., & Pusakulich, K. M. (1988). Use of the connected speech test (CST) with hearing-impaired listeners. *Ear and Hearing, 9,* 198–207.

Cox, R. M., Alexander, G. C., Gilmore, C., & Pusakulich, K. M. (1989). The connected speech test version 3: Audiovisual administration. *Ear and Hearing, 10,* 29–32.

Creelman, C. D. (1957). Case of the unknown talker. *Journal of the Acoustical Society of America, 29,* 655.

Curry, E. T., & Cox, B. P. (1966). The relative intelligibility of spondees. *Journal of Auditory Research, 6,* 419–424.

Danhauer, J. L., Crawford, S., & Edgerton, B. J. (1984). English, Spanish, and bilingual speakers' performance on a nonsense syllable test (NST) of speech sound discrimination. *Journal of Speech and Hearing Disorders, 49,* 143–148.

Dennison, L. B., & Kelly, B. R. (1978). High frequency consonant word discrimination lists in hearing aid evaluation. *Journal of the American Auditory Society, 4,* 91–97.

Department of Veterans Affairs (1997). *The Audiology Primer for Students and Health Care Professionals.* Mountain Home, Tennessee: VA Medical Center.

Dirks, D. D. (1964). Perception of dichotic and monaural verbal material and cerebral dominance for speech. *Acta Otolaryngologica, 58,* 73–80.

Dirks, D. D., Kamm, C., Bower, D., & Bettsworth, A. (1977). Use of performance-intensity functions for diagnosis. *Journal of Speech and Hearing Disorders, 42,* 408–415.

Dirks, D. D., Stream, R. W., & Wilson, R. H. (1972). Speech audiometry: Earphone and sound field. *Journal of Speech and Hearing Disorders, 37,* 167–173.

Dubno, J. R., & Dirks, D. D. (1982). Evaluation of hearing-impaired listeners using a nonsense syllable test, I. Test reliability. *Journal of Speech and Hearing Research, 25,* 135–141.

Dubno, J. R., Dirks, D. D., & Langhofer, L. R. (1982). Evaluation of hearing-impaired listeners using a nonsense syllable test, II. Syllable recognition and consonant confusion patterns. *Journal of Speech and Hearing Research, 25,* 141–148.

Dubno, J. R., & Dirks, D. D., & Morgan, D. E. (1984). Effects of age and mild hearing loss on speech recognition in noise. *Journal of the Acoustical Society of America, 76,* 87–96.

Edgerton, B. J., & Danhauer, J. L. (1979). *Clinical Implications of Speech Discrimination Testing Using Nonsense Stimuli.* Baltimore: University Park Press.

Egan, J. (1944). *Articulation Testing Methods II.* OSRD Report No. 3802, Psychoacoustic Laboratory, Harvard University, Cambridge, MA.

Egan, J. (1948). Articulation testing methods. *The Laryngoscope, 58,* 955–991.

Egan, J., Greenberg, G. Z., & Schulman, A. I. (1961). Interval of time uncertainty in auditory detection. *Journal of the Acoustical Society of America, 33,* 771–778.

Elpern, B. (1961). The relative stability of half list and full list discrimination tests. *The Laryngoscope, 71,* 30–36.

Fabry, D. A., & Van Tasell, D. J. (1990). Evaluation of an articulation-index based model for predicting the effects of adaptive frequency response hearing aids. *Journal of Speech and Hearing Research, 33,* 676–689.

Fairbanks, G., Everitt, W. L., & Jaeger, R. P. (1954). Method for time or frequency compression expansion of speech. *Transactions of the Institute of Radio Engineers, 2,* 7–12.

Feldmann, H. (1960). A history of audiology: A comprehensive report and bibliography from the earliest beginnings to the present. *Translations for the Beltone Institute for Hearing Research, 22,* 1–111. [Translated by J. Tonndorf from Die Geschichtliche Entwicklung der Horprufungsmethoden, kuze Darstellung and Bibliographie von der Anfongen bis zur Gegenwart. In H. Leicher, R. Mittermaiser, & G. Theissing (Eds.), *Zwanglose Abhandungen aus dem Gebeit der Hals-Nasen-Ohren-Heilkunde.* Stuttgart: Georg Thieme Verlag, 1960.]

Fifer, R. C., Jerger, J. F., Berlin, C. I., Tobey, E. A., & Campbell, J. C. (1983). Development of a dichotic sentence identification test for hearing-impaired adults. *Ear and Hearing, 4,* 300–305.

Finney, D. J. (1952). *Statistical Method in Biological Assay.* London: C. Griffen.

Fletcher, H. (1929). *Speech and Hearing.* Princeton: Van Nostrand Reinhold.

Fletcher, H. (1950). A method of calculating hearing loss for speech from an audiogram. *Acta Otolaryngologica, Supplement 90,* 26–37.

Fletcher, H. (1953). *Speech and Hearing in Communication.* New York: Krieger.

Fletcher, H., & Steinberg, J. C. (1929). Articulation testing methods. *Bell System Journal, 8,* 806–854.

Frauenfelder, U. H., & Tyler, L. K. (Eds.) (1987). *Spoken Word Recognition.* Cambridge: The MIT Press.

French, N. R., & Steinberg, J. C. (1947). Factors governing the intelligibility of speech sounds. *Journal of the Acoustical Society of America, 19,* 90–119.

Gardner, H. J. (1971). Application of a high frequency consonant discrimination word list in hearing aid evaluation. *Journal of Speech and Hearing Disorders, 36,* 354–355.

Gelfand, S. A., Piper, N., & Silman, S. (1985). Consonant recognition in quiet as a function of aging among normal hearing subjects. *Journal of the Acoustical Society of America, 80,* 1589–1598.

Gelfand, S., Hoffman, S., Waltzman, S., & Piper, N. (1980). Dichotic CV recognition at various interaural temporal onset asynchronies: Effect of age. *Journal of the Acoustical Society of America, 68,* 1258–1261.

Gengel, R. W., & Kupperman, G. L. (1980). On the calibration of two commercially recorded versions of CID auditory test W-22. *Ear and Hearing, 1,* 229–231.

Graham, J. T. (1960). Evaluation of methods for predicting speech reception threshold. *Archives of Otolaryngology, 72,* 347–350.

Gravel, J. S., Ochs, M. G., Konkle, D. F., & Bess, F. H. (1981). *The Pascoe High Frequency Word List: Performance of Normal and Hearing-Impaired Listeners.* Convention of the American Speech-Language-Hearing Association, Los Angeles, CA.

Green, D. M. (1961). Detection of auditory sinusoids of uncertain frequency. *Journal of the Acoustical Society of America, 33,* 897–903.

Green, D. M. (1980). Detection of temporally uncertain signals. *Journal of the Acoustical Society of America, 67,* 1304–1311.

Green, D. M., & Weber, D. L. (1980). Detection of temporally uncertain signals. *Journal of the Acoustical Society of America, 67,* 1304–1311.

Grubb, P. A. (1963a). Phoneme analysis of half-list discrimination tests. *Journal of Speech and Hearing Research, 6,* 271–276.

Grubb, P. A. (1963b). Considerations in the use of half-list speech discrimination tests. *Journal of Speech and Hearing Research, 6,* 294–297.

Gruber, J. (1891). *A Text-book of the Diseases of the Ear.* (Translated by E. Law and C. Jewell from the second German edition). New York: D. Appleton and Company.

Hagerman, B. (1982). Sentences for testing speech intelligibility in noise. *Scandinavian Audiology, 11,* 79–87.

Harris, J. D. (1960). Combinations of distorted speech. *Archives of Otolaryngology, 72,* 227–232.

Harris, J. D., Haines, H. L., & Myers, C. K. (1956). A new formula for using the audiogram to predict speech hearing loss. *Archives of Otolaryngology, 63,* 158–176.

Harris, R. W., & Swenson, D. W. (1990). Effects of reverberation and noise on speech recognition by adults with various amounts of sensorineural hearing loss. *Audiology, 29,* 314–321.

Hawkins, J. E., & Stevens, S. S. (1950). Masking of pure tones and of speech by white noise. *Journal of the Acoustical Society of America, 22,* 6–13.

Heckendorf, A. L., Wiley, T. L., & Wilson, R. H. (1997). Performance norms for the VA compact disc versions of CID W-22 (Hirsh) and PB-50 (Rush Hughes) word lists. *Journal of the American Academy of Audiology, 8,* 163–172.

Helfer, K. A., & Wilber, L. A. (1990). Hearing loss, aging, and speech perception in reverberation and noise. *Journal of Speech and Hearing Research, 33,* 149–155.

Hirsh, I. (1947). The influence of interaural phase on summation and inhibition. *Journal of the Acoustical Society of America, 20,* 536–544.

Hirsh, I. J. (1952). Clinical application of two Harvard auditory tests. *Journal of Speech Disorders, 12,* 151–158.

Hirsh, I. J., Davis, H., Silverman, S. R., Reynolds, E. G., Eldert, E., & Benson, R. W. (1952). Development of materials for speech audiometry. *Journal of Speech and Hearing Disorders, 17,* 321–337.

Houtgast, T., & Steeneken, H. J. M. (1973). The modulation transfer function in room acoustics as a predictor of speech intelligibility, *Acustica, 28,* 66–73.

Hudgins, C. V., Hawkins, J. E., Jr., Karlin, J. E., & Stevens, S. S. (1947). The development of recorded auditory tests for measuring hearing loss for speech. *The Laryngoscope, 57,* 57–89.

Hugdahl, K. (1988). *Handbook of Dichotic Listening: Theory, Methods and Research.* New York: John Wiley & Sons.

Hughson, W., & Thompson, E. A. (1942). Correlation of hearing acuity for speech with discrete frequency audiograms. *Archives of Otolaryngology, 36,* 526–540.

Humes, L. E., Coughlin, M., & Talley, L. (1996). Evaluation of the use of a new compact disc for auditory perceptual assessment in the elderly. *Journal of the American Academy of Audiology, 7*, 419–427.

Humes, L. E., Dirks, D. D., Bell, T. S., Ahlstrom, C., & Kincaid, G. E. (1986). Application of the articulation index and the speech transmission index to the recognition of speech by normal-hearing and hearing-impaired listeners. *Journal of Speech and Hearing Research, 29*, 447–462.

Hutcherson, R. W., Dirks, D. D., & Morgan, D. E. (1979). Evaluation of the Speech Perception in Noise (SPIN) test. *Otolaryngology Head Neck Surgery, 87*, 239–245.

Institute of Electrical and Electronics Engineers. (1969). *IEEE Recommended Practice for Speech Quality Measurements.* New York: Author.

Institute of Electrical and Electronics Engineers. (1993). *The New IEEE Standard Dictionary of Electrical and Electronics Terms* (IEEE Std. 100-1992). New York: Author.

Ivey, R. G., & Willeford, J. A. (1988). Three tests of CNS auditory function. *Human Communication, 12,* 35–43.

Jacobson, J. T., Deppe, U., & Murray, T. J. (1983). Dichotic paradigms in multiple sclerosis. *Ear and Hearing, 4,* 311–318.

Jerger, J. (1960). Observations on auditory behavior in lesions of the central auditory pathways. *Archives of Otolaryngology, 71,* 797–806.

Jerger, J. F., Carhart, R., Tillman, T. W., & Peterson, J. L. (1959). Some relations between normal hearing for pure tones and for speech. *Journal of Speech and Hearing Research, 2,* 126–140.

Jerger, J., Chmiel, R., Allen, J., & Wilson, A. (1994). Effects of age and gender on dichotic sentence identification. *Ear and Hearing, 15,* 274–286.

Jerger, J., & Jerger, S. (1974). Auditory findings in brainstem disorders. *Archives of Otolaryngology, 99,* 342–349.

Jerger, J., & Jerger, S. (1975). Clinical validity of central auditory tests. *Scandinavian Audiology, 4,* 147–163.

Jerger, J., Speaks, C., & Trammell, J. L. (1968). A new approach to speech audiometry. *Journal of Speech and Hearing Disorders, 33,* 318–329.

Johnson, C. E., Cosci, S. M., Brown, J. W., & Scroggins, A. P. (1995). *Reverberation and Noise Effects on Word-Recognition: Preschool through First Grade Children.* Convention of the American Speech-Language-Hearing Association, Orlando, FL.

Kalikow, D. N., Stevens, K. N., & Elliot, L. L. (1977). Development of a test of speech intelligibility in noise using sentence materials with controlled word predictability. *Journal of the Acoustical Society of America, 61,* 1337–1351.

Kamm, C. A., Dirks, D. D., & Bell, T. S. (1985). Speech recognition and the articulation index for normal and hearing-impaired listeners. *Journal of the Acoustical Society of America, 77,* 281–288.

Kärber, G. (1931). Beitrag zue kollektiven behandlung pharmakologischer reihenversuche. *Archiv fur Experimentelle Pathologie und Pharmakologie, 4,* 480–483.

Katz, J. (1962). The use of staggered spondaic words in assessing the integrity of the central auditory system. *Journal of Auditory Research, 2,* 327–337.

Keith, R. W., & Talis, H. P. (1970). The use of speech in noise in diagnostic audiometry. *Journal of Auditory Research, 10,* 201–204.

Killion, M. C., & Villchur, E. (1993). Kessler was right—partly: But SIN test shows some aids improve hearing in noise. *Hearing Journal, 46,* 31–35.

Kimura, D. (1961). Cerebral dominance and the perception of verbal stimuli. *Canadian Journal of Psychology, 15,* 166–171.

Kirk, K. I., Pisoni, D. B., & Miyamoto, R. C. (1997). Effects of stimulus variability on speech perception in listeners with hearing impairment. *Journal of Speech, Language, and Hearing Research, 40,* 1395–1405.

Knudsen, V. O. (1929). The hearing of speech in auditoriums. *Journal of the Acoustical Society of America, 1,* 56–82.

Konkle, D. F., & Berry, G. A. (1983). Masking in speech audiometry. In D. F. Konkle & W. F. Rintelmann (Eds.), *Principles of Speech Audiometry* (pp. 285–319). Baltimore: University Park Press.

Konkle, D. F., & Rintelmann, W. F. (Eds.) (1983). *Principles of Speech Audiometry.* Baltimore: University Park Press.

Kruel, E. J., Bell, D. W., & Nixon, J. C. (1969). Factors affecting speech discrimination test difficulty. *Journal of Speech and Hearing Research, 12,* 281–287.

Kucera, F., & Francis, W. (1969). *Computational Analysis of Present Day English.* Providence: Brown University Press.

Levitt, H. (1971). Transformed up-down methods in psychoacoustics. *Journal of the Acoustical Society of America, 49,* 467–477.

Levitt, H. (1978). Adaptive testing in audiology. *Scandinavian Audiology, (Supplement 6),* 241–291.

Levitt, H., & Resnick, S. B. (1978). Speech reception by the hearing impaired: Methods of testing and the development of new tests. *Scandinavian Audiology, 6,* 199–239.

Levitt, H., & Rabiner, L. (1967). Binaural release from masking for speech and gain in intelligibility. *Journal of the Acoustical Society of America, 20,* 150–159.

Licklider, J. (1948). The influence of interaural phase relations upon the masking of speech by white noise. *Journal of the Acoustical Society of America, 20,* 150–159.

Licklider, J. C., & Pollack, I. (1948). Effects of differentiation, integration, and infinite peak clipping upon the intelligibility of speech. *Journal of the Acoustical Society of America, 20,* 42–51.

Lilly, D. J., & Vernon, J. A. (1997). Personal communication.

Lowe, S., Cullen, J., Berlin, C., Thompson, C., & Willett, M. (1970). Perception of simultaneous dichotic and monotic monosyllables. *Journal of Speech and Hearing Research, 13,* 812–822.

Luce, P. A. (1986). A computational analysis of uniqueness points in auditory word recognition. *Perception & Psychophysics, 39,* 155–159.

Lynn, G. W., & Gilroy, J. (1977). Evaluation of central auditory dysfunction in patients with neurological disorders. In R. W. Keith (Ed.). *Central Auditory Dysfunction* (pp. 177–221). New York: Grune & Stratton.

Marshall, L., Hanna, T. E., & Wilson, R. H. (1996). Effect of step size on clinical and adaptive 2IFC procedures in quiet and in a noise background. *Journal of Speech and Hearing Research, 39,* 687–696.

Martin, F., Woodrick-Armstrong, T., & Champlin, C. (1994). A survey of audiological practices in the United States. *American Journal of Audiology*, *3*, 20–26.

Martin, M. (Ed.). (1997). *Speech Audiometry* (2nd ed.). London: Whurr.

Matzger, J. (1959). Two methods for the assessment of central auditory functions in cases of brain disease. *Annals of Otology, Rhinology, and Laryngology*, *68*, 1185–1197.

McCullough, J. A., Wilson, R. H., Birck, J. D., & Anderson, L. G. (1994). A multimedia approach for estimating speech recognition of multilingual clients. *American Journal of Audiology*, *3*, 19–22.

Mendel, L. L., & Danhauer, J. L. (Eds.). (1997). *Audiologic Evaluation and Management and Speech Perception Assessment.* San Diego: Singular.

Menzel, O. J. (1960). Clinical efficiency in compensation audiometry. *Journal of Speech and Hearing Disorders*, *25*, 49–54.

Miller, G. A. (1951). *Language and Communication.* New York: McGraw-Hill.

Miller, G. A., Heise, G. A., & Lichten, W. (1951). The intelligibility of speech as a function of the context of the test materials. *Journal of Experimental Psychology*, *41*, 329–335.

Moncur, J. P., & Dirks, D. D. (1967). Binaural and monaural speech intelligibility in reverberation. *Journal of Speech and Hearing Research*, *10*, 186–195.

Moray, N. (1960). Broadbent's filter theory: Postulate H and the problem of switching time. *Quarterly Journal of Experimental Psychology*, *12*, 214–220.

Mueller, H. G., & Killion, M. C. (1990). An easy method for calculating the articulation index. *The Hearing Journal*, *43*, 14–17.

Mullennix, J. W., Pisoni, D. B., & Martin, C. S. (1989). Some effects of talker variability on spoken word recognition. *Journal of the Acoustical Society of America*, *85*, 365–378.

Musiek, F. E., Gollegly, K., Kibbe, K., & Verkest-Lenz, S. (1991). Proposed screening test for central auditory disorders: Follow-up on the dichotic digits test. *American Journal of Otolaryngology*, *12*, 109–113.

Nabelek, A., & Robinson, P. (1982). Monaural and binaural speech perception in reverberation for listeners of various ages. *Journal of the Acoustical Society of America*, *71*, 1242–1248.

Nelson, D. A., & Chaiklin, J. B. (1970). Writedown versus talk-back scoring and scoring bias in speech discrimination testing. *Journal of Speech and Hearing Research*, *13*, 645–654.

Nilsson, M., Soli, S. D., & Sullivan, J. A. (1994). Development of the Hearing in Noise Test for the measurement of speech reception thresholds in quiet and in noise. *Journal of the Acoustical Society of America*, *95*, 1085–1099.

Nilsson, M., Soli, S. D., & Sumida, A. (1995). Development of norms and percent intelligibility functions for the HINT. *House Ear Institute* (pp. 1–9). Los Angeles: House Ear Institute.

Noffsinger, D. (1985). Dichotic listening techniques in the study of hemispheric asymmetries. In D. F. Benson & E. Zaidel (Eds.), *The Dual Brain* (pp. 127–141). New York: Gilford.

Noffsinger, D., Martinez, C. D., & Wilson, R. H. (1994). Dichotic listening to speech: Background and normative data for digits, sentences, and nonsense syllables (CVs). *Journal of the American Academy of Audiology*, *5*, 248–254.

Norwood-Chapman, L., Wilson, R. H., & Thelin, J. W. (1997). *Clinical Evaluation of Word Recognition in Multi-talker Babble under Four Listening Conditions.* American Academy of Audiology Convention, Fort Lauderdale.

Olsen, W. O., & Carhart, R. (1967). Development of test procedures for evaluation of binaural hearing aids. *Bulletin of Prosthetics Research: Prosthetic and Sensory Aids Service* (pp. 22–49). Washington, DC: Department of Medicine and Surgery, Veterans Administration.

Olsen, W. O., & Matkin, N. D. (1979). Speech audiometry. In W. F. Rintelmann (Ed.), *Hearing Assessment*. Baltimore: University Park Press.

Olsen, W. O., & Matkin, N. D. (1991). Speech audiometry. In W. F. Rintelmann (Ed.), *Hearing Assessment* (2nd ed.). Austin: PRO-ED.

Olsen, W., Noffsinger, D., & Carhart, R. (1976). Masking level differences encountered in clinical populations. *Audiology*, *15*, 287–301.

Olsen, W. O., Noffsinger, D., & Kurdziel, S. (1975). Speech discrimination in quiet and in white noise by patients with peripheral and central lesions. *Acta Otolaryngologica*, *80*, 375–382.

Pascoe, D. P. (1975). Frequency responses of hearing aids and their effects on the speech perception of hearing-impaired subjects. *Annals of Otology, Rhinology and Laryngology (Supplement 23)*, *84*, 1–40.

Pavlovic, C. V. (1988). Articulation index predictions of speech intelligibility in hearing aid selection. *Asha*, *7/8*, 63–65.

Pavlovic, C. V. (1991). Speech recognition and five articulation indexes. *Hearing Instruments*, *42*, 20–23.

Pavlovic, C. V., Studebaker, G. A., & Sherbecoe, R. L. (1986). An articulation index based procedure for predicting the speech recognition performance of hearing-impaired individuals. *Journal of the Acoustical Society of America*, *80*, 50–57.

Pekkarinen, E., Salmivalli, A., & Suonpää, J. (1990). Effect of noise on word discrimination by subjects with impaired hearing, compared with those with normal hearing. *Scandinavian Audiology*, *19*, 31–36.

Pisoni, D. (1985). Speech perception: Some new directions in research and theory. *Journal of the Acoustical Society of America*, *78*, 381–388.

Plomp, R. (1986). A signal-to-noise ratio model for the speech-reception threshold of the hearing impaired. *Journal of Speech and Hearing Research*, *29*, 146–154.

Plomp, R., & Mimpen, A. M. (1979). Speech-reception threshold for sentences as a function of age and noise level. *Journal of the Acoustical Society of America*, *66*, 1333–1342.

Pollack, I. (1959). Message uncertainty and message reception. *Journal of the Acoustical Society of America*, *31*, 1500–1508.

Porter, R., Shankweiler, D., & Liberman, A. (1969). Differential effects of binaural time differences on perception of stop consonants and vowels. *Proceedings of the 77th Meeting of American Psychology Association* (pp. 15–16).

Raffin, M. J. M., & Thornton, A. R. (1980). Confidence levels for differences between speech discrimination scores. *Journal of Speech and Hearing Research, 23,* 5–18.

Rankovic, C. M. (1991). An application of the articulation index to hearing and fitting. *Journal of Speech and Hearing Research, 34,* 391–402.

Rankovic, C. M. (1997). Prediction of speech reception for listeners with sensorineural hearing loss. In W. Jesteadt (Ed.), *Modeling Sensorineural Hearing Loss.* New Jersey: Lawrence Erlbaum Associates.

Rankovic, C. M. (in press). Factors governing speech reception benefits of adaptive linear filtering for listeners with sensorineural hearing loss. *Journal of the Acoustical Society of America, 103* (2).

Resnick, D. M. (1962). Reliability of the twenty-five word phonetically balanced lists. *Journal of Auditory Research, 2,* 5–12.

Resnick, S. B., Dubno, J. R., Hoffnung, S., & Levitt, H. (1975). Phoneme errors on a nonsense syllable test. *Journal of the Acoustical Society of America, 58 (Supplement 1),* 114.

Rintelmann, W. F., & Associates. (1974). Six experiments on speech discrimination utilizing CNC monosyllables. *Journal of Auditory Research, 2,* 1–30.

Roeser, R. (1982). Moderate-to-severe hearing loss with an island of normal hearing. *Ear and Hearing, 3,* 284–286.

Rosenzweig, M. R., & Postman, L. (1957). Intelligibility as a function of frequency of usage. *Journal of Experimental Psychology, 54,* 412–422.

Ross, M., & Lerman, J. (1970). Picture identification test for hearing-impaired children. *Journal of Speech and Hearing Research, 13,* 44–53.

Shankweiler, D., & Studdert-Kennedy, M. (1967). Identification of consonants and vowels presented to left and right ears. *Quarterly Journal of Experimental Psychology, 19,* 59–63.

Silverman, S. R., & Hirsh, I. J. (1955). Problems related to the use of speech in clinical audiometry. *Annals of Otology, Rhinology and Laryngology, 64* (4), 1234–1244.

Skinner, M., & Miller, J. (1983). Amplification bandwidth and intelligibility of speech in quiet and noise for listeners with sensorineural hearing loss. *Audiology, 22,* 253–279.

Skinner, M., Pascoe, D., Miller, J., & Popelka, G. (1982). Measurements to determine the optimal placement of speech energy within the listener's auditory area: A basis for selecting amplification characteristics. In G. Studebaker & F. Bess (Eds.), *The Vanderbilt Hearing Aid Report State of the Art—Research Needs* (pp. 161–169). Upper Darby, PA: Monographs in Contemporary Audiology.

Smith, B. B., & Resnick, D. M. (1972). An auditory test for assessing brainstem integrity: Preliminary report. *The Laryngoscope, 82,* 414–424.

Souza, P. E., & Turner, C. W. (1994). Masking of speech in young and elderly listeners with hearing loss. *Journal of Speech and Hearing Research, 37,* 655–661.

Speaks, C., & Jerger, J. (1965). Performance-intensity characteristics of synthetic sentences. *Journal of Speech and Hearing Research, 9,* 305–312.

Spearman, C. (1908). The method of "right and wrong cases" ("constant stimuli") without Guass's formulae. *British Journal of Psychology, 2,* 227–242.

Stubblefield, J., & Goldstein, D. (1977). A test-retest reliability study on clinical measurement of masking level differences. *Audiology, 16,* 419–431.

Sweetow, R., & Reddell, R. (1978). The use of masking level differences in the identification of children with perceptual problems. *Journal of the American Auditory Society, 4,* 52–56.

Thornton, A., & Raffin, M. J. M. (1978). Speech discrimination scores modeled as a binomial variable. *Journal of Speech and Hearing Research, 21,* 507–518.

Tillman, T. W., & Carhart, R., (1966). *An Expanded Test for Speech Discrimination Utilizing CNC Monosyllabic words.* Northwestern University Auditory Test No. 6. Brooks Air Force Base, TX, USAF School of Aerospace Medicine Technical Report.

Tillman, T. W., & Jerger, J. F. (1959). Some factors affecting the spondee threshold in normal-hearing subjects. *Journal of Speech and Hearing Research, 2,* 141–146.

Tillman, T. W., Johnson, R. M., & Olsen, W. O. (1966). Earphone versus soundfield threshold sound pressure level for spondee words. *Journal of the Acoustical Society of America, 39,* 125–133.

Tillman, T. W., & Olsen, W. O. (1973). Speech audiometry. In J. Jerger (Ed.), *Modern Developments in Audiology* (2nd ed., pp. 37–74). New York: Academic Press.

Ullrich, K., & Grimm, D. (1976). Most comfortable listening level presentation versus maximum discrimination for word discrimination material. *Audiology, 15,* 338–347.

Ventry, I. M. (1976). Pure tone-spondee threshold relationship in functional hearing loss. *Journal of Speech and Hearing Disorders, 30,* 377–386.

Ventry, I. M., & Chaiklin, J. B. (1965). Multidiscipline study of functional hearing loss. *Journal of Auditory Research, 3,* 175–272

Ward, W. D. (1964). "Sensitivity" versus "acuity." *Journal of Speech and Hearing Research, 7,* 294–295.

Weislender, P., & Hodgson, W. R. (1989). Evaluation of four Spanish word-recognition-ability lists. *Ear and Hearing, 10,* 387–392.

Willeford, J. A. (1976). Differential diagnosis of central auditory dysfunction. In I. Bradford (Ed.), *Audiology: An Audio Journal for Continuing Education* (Vol. 2). New York: Grune & Stratton.

Willeford, J. A. (1977). Assessing auditory behavior in children: A test battery approach. In R. W. Keith (Ed.), *Central Auditory Dysfunction* (pp. 43–72). New York: Grune & Stratton.

Wilson, R. H. (1994). Word recognition with segmented-alternated CVC words: Compact disc trials. *Journal of the American Academy of Audiology, 5,* 255–258.

Wilson, R. H. & Antablin, J. K. (1980). A picture identification task as an estimate of word-recognition performance of nonverbal adults. *Journal of Speech and Hearing Disorders, 45,* 223–238.

Wilson, R. H., & Antablin, J. K. (1982). The Picture Identification Task—A reply to Dillon. *Journal of Speech and Hearing Disorders, 47,* 111–112.

Wilson, R. H., Arcos, J. T., & Jones, H. C. (1984). Word-recognition with segmented-alternated CVC words: A preliminary report on listeners with normal nearing. *Journal of Speech and Hearing Research, 27,* 378–386.

Wilson, R. H., Coley, K. E., Haenel, J. L., & Browning, K. M. (1976). Northwestern University Auditory Test No. 6: Normative and comparative intelligibility functions. *Journal of the American Audiology Society, 1,* 221–228.

Wilson, R. H., Dirks, D. D., & Carterette, E. (1968). Effects of ear preference and order bias on the reception of verbal materials. *Journal of Speech and Hearing Research, 11,* 509–522.

Wilson, R. H., Hopkins, J., Mance, C., & Novak, R. (1982). Detection and recognition masking-level difference for individual CID W-1 spondaic words. *Journal of Speech and Hearing Research, 25,* 235–242.

Wilson, R. H., & Jaffe, M. S. (1996). Interactions of age, ear, and stimulus complexity on dichotic digit recognition. *Journal of the American Academy of Audiology, 7,* 358–364.

Wilson, R. H., & Leigh, E. D. (1996). Identification performance by right- and left-handed listeners on the dichotic consonant-vowel (CVs) materials recorded on the VA-CD. *Journal of the American Academy of Audiology, 7,* 1–6.

Wilson, R. H., & Margolis, R. H. (1983). Measurements of auditory thresholds for speech stimuli. In D. F. Konkle & W. F. Rintelmann (Eds.), *Principles of Speech Audiometry* (pp. 79–126). Baltimore: University Park Press.

Wilson, R. H., Morgan, D. E., & Dirks, D. D. (1973). A proposed SRT procedure and its statistical precedent. *Journal of Speech and Hearing Disorders, 38,* 184–191.

Wilson, R. H., Oyler, A. L., & Sumrall, R. (1996). *Psychometric Functions for Northwestern University Auditory Test No. 6 in Quiet and Multi-talker Babble.* American Academy of Audiology Convention, Salt Lake City, UT.

Wilson, R. H., Preece, J. P., Salomon, D. L., Sperry, J. L., & Bornstein, S. P. (1994). Effects of time compression and time compression plus reverberation on the intelligibility of Northwestern University Auditory Test No. 6. *Journal of the American Academy of Audiology, 5,* 269–277.

Wilson, R. H., Preece, J. P., & Thornton, A. R. (1990). Clinical use of the compact disc in speech audiometry. *Asha, 32,* 3247–3251.

Wilson, R. H., Shanks, J. E., & Koebsell, K. A. (1982). Recognition masking-level differences for 10 CID W-1 spondaic words. *Journal of Speech and Hearing Research, 25,* 624–628.

Wilson, R. H., & Strouse, A. (in review). Factors that contribute to the slope of a psychometric function for word-recognition. *Journal of Speech and Hearing Research.*

Wilson, R. H., Zizz, C. A., Shanks, J. E., & Causey, G. D. (1990). Normative data in quiet, broadband noise, and competing message for Northwestern University Auditory Test No. 6 by a female speaker. *Journal of Speech and Hearing Disorders, 55,* 771–778.

Working Group on Speech Understanding and Aging, Committee on Hearing, Bioacoustics, and Biomechanics, Commission on Behavioral and Social Sciences and Education, National Research Council. (1988). Speech understanding and aging. *Journal of the Acoustical Society of America, 83,* 859–895.

Young, L. L., Dudley, B., & Gunter, M. B. (1982). Thresholds and psychometric functions of the individual spondaic words. *Journal of Speech and Hearing Research, 25,* 586–593.

CHAPTER 3

CLINICAL MASKING

JAY W. SANDERS
JAMES W. HALL III

Although auditory masking has been defined in various ways (Studebaker, 1973), it can be regarded, for clinical purposes, as the elevation in threshold of sensitivity for one signal (the test stimulus) by a second signal (the masking noise). The importance of appropriate and accurate masking in audiometry cannot be overemphasized. Without proper masking, test results can indicate a moderate conductive impairment in an ear with a profound sensorineural loss, reasonably good word recognition in an ear with severely impaired speech discrimination, or moderate tone decay in an ear with excessive auditory adaptation.

THE PROBLEM

The problem requiring the use of masking is posed by the patient with a unilateral hearing loss or an asymmetrical bilateral loss. In an attempt to reach threshold of sensitivity in the poorer ear of such a patient, the intensity of the test signal may be raised to such a level that it is transmitted across the skull and heard in the better ear before it reaches threshold level in the test ear. A number of investigators (Liden, 1954; Liden, Nilsson, & Anderson, 1959a; Zwislocki, 1953) have shown that a pure-tone stimulus presented by air conduction to an ear with a profound hearing loss may be heard in the nontest ear when the signal intensity is 50 to 60 dB above the sensorineural sensitivity of the nontest ear. Transmission of the test stimulus across the skull to the nontest ear is referred to as *cross-over*. The intensity reduction of 50 to 60 dB in an air-conduction signal from the test ear across the skull to the nontest ear is called *interaural attenuation*. For a signal presented by bone conduction, the interaural attenuation is essentially zero. Indeed, it is possible to obtain a cross-over bone conduction threshold response at a *better* hearing threshold level (HTL) than the actual bone-conduction sensitivity in the nontest ear (Sanders & Rintelmann, 1964; Studebaker, 1964). Thus, if hearing is normal in the nontest ear, cross-over response can be obtained at the 0 dB HTL to a bone-conduction signal presented to an ear with a profound sensorineural hearing loss. Furthermore, false air-conduction thresholds at 50 to 60 dB HTL can be obtained for an ear with profound sensorineural impairment

even when the nontest ear has a conductive loss of equal severity. In this case the test tone presented by air conduction has reached sufficient intensity to stimulate the nontest ear by bone-conduction.

Thus, without appropriate masking, the pure-tone audiogram may suggest a pure conductive hearing loss in an ear with a profound sensorineural impairment. In addition, false results may be obtained in other areas of auditory assessment, such as speech audiometry and diagnostic tests.

THE SOLUTION

The solution to the problem of cross-over of the auditory stimulus is to ensure that the response is from the ear being tested by eliminating the possibility of response from the nontest ear. This is accomplished by presenting a masking noise to the nontest ear at sufficient intensity to shift its sensitivity to a higher HTL, thus permitting presentation of the test signal to the test ear at higher intensities without a cross-over response from the nontest ear. The magnitude of the threshold shift in the masked ear is determined by the nature and intensity of the masking noise.

The use of a masking noise, however, introduces the possibility of a new problem. Just as the test signal may cross over to the nontest ear, so may the masking noise, presented to the nontest ear, cross over and elevate threshold in the test ear. This result is known as *overmasking*. Both clinical errors, undermasking and overmasking, may result in erroneous decisions in the audiometric assessment of a hearing disorder.

The effective application of clinical masking requires a good understanding of the answers to the following three questions:

1. When should masking be used?
2. What kind of masking noise should be used?
3. How much masking should be used?

The following sections of this chapter answer these questions through a discussion of the principles of masking based on experimental evidence.

WHEN SHOULD MASKING BE USED?

The answer to the question of when to mask is quite simple: Masking must be used whenever there is a possibility of the test signal being heard in the nontest ear. The possibility exists any time the test tone is presented with sufficient intensity to cross the skull and stimulate the nontest ear. Important factors in determining when to mask are:

1. The intensity of the test signal
2. Auditory sensitivity in the nontest ear
3. Interaural attenuation

Differences in interaural attenuation for the air- and bone-conduction stimuli require a different answer to the question of when to mask in air- and bone-conduction audiometry.

Air Conduction

In air-conduction audiometry, masking must be used whenever the intensity of the test tone exceeds auditory sensitivity in the nontest ear by an amount greater than the expected interaural attenuation. A critical factor is that a decision of when to mask must be based on *sensorineural sensitivity* in the nontest ear and not on the air-conduction thresholds of that ear. Even when the stimulus is presented by air conduction, *cross-over occurs by bone conduction* through the skull and not by air conduction around the skull. A cross-over response will be obtained from the nontest ear whenever the air-conduction stimulus in the test ear exceeds bone conduction thresholds in the nontest ear by about 50 dB, regardless of the air-conduction thresholds in that ear. With no masking in the nontest ear, false responses to an air-conduction signal will be obtained at 50 to 60 dB HTL in an ear with a more severe hearing loss, even with air-conduction thresholds in the nontest ear at 50 to 60 dB, if bone-conduction sensitivity in that ear is normal. Thus, in air-conduction testing, *interaural difference* refers to the difference between the intensity level of the test tone and bone-conduction sensitivity in the nontest ear.

Research has shown that for an air-conducted pure tone signal presented through a standard audiometer earphone, interaural attenuation ranges from 40 to about 80 dB, varying with the test frequency and subject (Liden et al., 1959a; Zwislocki, 1953). The use of a larger earphone cushion, such as the circumaural type having a larger contact area between the cushion and skull, will actually result in a decreased attenuation (Zwislocki, 1953). Because in some subjects interaural attenuation with a standard earphone may be as little as 40 dB, it seems wise to accept Studebaker's (1967) principle that whenever variability is a result of intersubject differences, the safest course is to adopt the extreme value, in this case the smallest reported interaural attenua-tion. Thus, the rule for when to mask in air-conduction pure-tone audiometry is:

> In air conduction audiometry, the nontest ear should be masked whenever the intensity of the signal presented to the test ear exceeds bone-conduction sensitivity in the nontest ear by more than 40 dB.

Although this approach may occasionally lead to unnecessary masking, it will ensure the use of masking whenever needed.

Bone Conduction

Research evidence has shown that the interaural attenuation for a pure-tone stimulus presented by bone conduction is essentially zero (Feldman, 1961; Liden et al., 1959a; Sanders & Rintelmann, 1964; Studebaker, 1964). Although some subjects show an attenuation of about 10 dB, the value varies from one subject to another and cannot be regarded as dependable. With an expectation of no interaural attenuation, some researchers have proposed that masking should always be used in bone-conduction audiometry (Glorig, 1965; O'Neill & Oyer, 1966). This approach, however, will lead to unnecessary masking in some patients. As pointed out by Studebaker (1964), whenever air- and bone-conduction thresholds are at the same HTL in the test ear without masking, the use of masking noise in the nontest ear should not affect the results.

A further factor affecting decisions regarding masking in bone-conduction audiometry is the effect of *central masking*. Central masking, probably mediated by the efferent pathways (Liden et al., 1959b), is an elevation in the test ear threshold as a result of a masking noise in the nontest ear, even though the intensity of the masking noise is not sufficient to cross over to the test ear. Zwislocki (1953) suggested that the central masking threshold shift is on the order of approximately 5 dB. Liden (1954), and Dirks and Malmquist (1964), found that central masking increases with increased intensity of the masking noise and may be as great as 10 to 12 dB. These findings suggest that with no masking in the nontest ear, bone-conduction thresholds may be 5 to 15 dB better than those obtained with masking, even when masking is not required to prevent cross-over of the test signal. Thus, because the bone-conduction system on the audiometer is usually calibrated with normal ear data obtained with masking in the opposite ear (ANSI, S3.13-1972; ANSI, S3.26-1981), unmasked bone-conduction thresholds may underestimate sensorineural loss even without false responses from test signal cross-over. That is, as a result of the central masking effect on the normative data used to determine calibration values for bone conduction, the test ear should always show an air-bone gap if bone-conduction thresholds are obtained without masking the nontest ear. With this in mind, we can accept Studebaker's (1964) rule for when to mask in bone-conduction audiometry:

> In bone-conduction audiometry, the nontest ear should be masked whenever the test ear exhibits an air-bone gap.

Masking and Insert Earphones

Guidelines for when to mask have traditionally been offered for audiometric procedures assuming presentation of a signal or masker via a supra-aural earphone. However, insert earphones, specifically the ER-3A earphone (Etymotics Research), are now employed regularly instead of supra-aural earphones by many clinical audiologists. The transducer (housed in a small box) is coupled to the ear by an acoustic tube and a foam cushion (E.A.R. plug). At least six general clinical advantages are recognized for properly placed insert versus conventional supra-aural earphones (Mueller & Hall, 1998), including:

1. *Patient comfort:* If the tension on the headband of your supra-aural earphones is correct, the earphones can become very uncomfortable during a test session. Insert earphones are as comfortable to wear as foam earplugs.
2. *Reduced occurrence of collapsing ear canals:* With supra-aural earphones, collapsing ear canals occur fairly often. When the insert earphone is placed correctly in the ear, it occupies the space where the ear canal is most likely to collapse.
3. *Attenuation of ambient noise:* The insert earphone, when placed deeply in the ear canal, acts like an earplug. This helps prevent ambient noise from influencing threshold measurements.
4. *Patient aural hygiene:* There's really no effective way to sanitize or sterilize the conventional supra-aural cushions. After they're used with a single patient, insert earphone plugs are discarded.
5. *Test-retest reliability:* The placement of the insert earphone in the ear canal increases precision of audiometric measures and eliminates much of the variability that is associated with placing a supra-aural earphone over the ear.
6. *Increased interaural attenuation:* Insert earphones provide significantly more interaural attenuation than their supra-aural counterparts, about 10 dB to 15 dB in the highs, and 25 dB to 30 dB in the lows. This reduces the need for masking during air-conduction testing.

This final advantage is of particular relevance to the discussion of masking. Consequently, the rule offered above for when to mask during pure-tone audiometry can be amended to read:

> In air-conduction audiometry, the nontest ear should be masked whenever the intensity of the signal presented to the test ear exceeds bone-conduction sensitivity in the nontest ear by more than 60 dB.

Clearly, the upper limit on how much masking can be used before interaural attenuation is exceeded and the masker crosses over to the test ear is similarly increased with insert earphones. In short, deeply placed insert earphones offer the clinician a distinct advantage and an additional measure of confidence in clinical masking decisions.

WHAT KIND OF MASKING NOISE SHOULD BE USED?

An important decision in masking is that of what type of masking noise to use. The masking effectiveness of a noise depends not only on the intensity of the noise but also on its nature. Although the results of Wegel and Lane (1924) showed that masking can be accomplished with a pure tone, their findings indicated that a sound composed of a range of frequencies is a more effective masker. Consequently, the masking signal available on audiometers is usually some form of acoustic energy in a band of frequencies. The clinical audiometer may provide two or more different masking noises, which requires the clinician to make a choice.

Available Masking Noises

Over the years, three basic types of masking noise have been available for masking in pure tone audiometry: complex noise, white noise, and narrowband noise. Because the clinician may have a choice among two or more masking noises or may be limited by equipment to one of the available maskers, it is important to understand the nature of the available noises.

Complex Noise.   Complex noise, sometimes referred to as sawtooth noise, is a broadband signal composed of a low-frequency fundamental plus the multiples of that fundamental. The acoustic spectrum of a typical complex noise is shown in Figure 3.1. For this particular noise, the fundamental frequency is 78 Hz, and the additional frequencies are multiples of that fundamental (156 Hz, 234 Hz, etc.) The line spectrum of Figure 3.1 demonstrates two basic problems in complex noise as a masker of pure tones. First, acoustic energy is present only at the frequencies designated by the lines and is not spread continuously across the frequency range of the noise. With energy only at discrete frequencies, it is possible for the frequency of a test pure tone to fall within three or four cycles of a frequency component of the noise, producing a "beat" or pulsing phenomenon in the ear of the listener. Liden and colleagues (1959a) pointed out that the fifth harmonic of a 50 Hz fundamental will beat with a test tone of 254 Hz. A 254 Hz tone is well within the permissible variability of an audiometer test tone (ANSI, S3.6-1996).

A second problem with complex noise as a masker in pure-tone audiometry is the significant decrease in acoustic

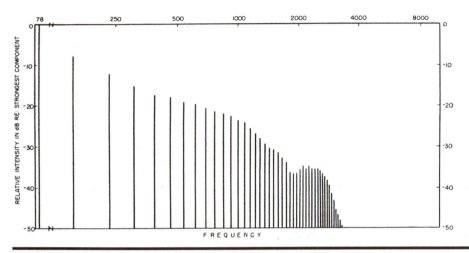

FIGURE 3.1   Acoustic spectrum of a sawtooth noise through a PDR-8 earphone. (From J. W. Sanders & W. F. Rintelmann, "Masking in audiometry: A clinical evaluation of three methods." *Archives of Otolaryngology, 8*, 541–556. Copyright 1964, American Medical Association.)

energy in the higher frequencies. For the noise shown in Figure 3.1, the energy present near 1000 Hz is down about 23 dB from the intensity level at 78 Hz. At 4000 Hz, the decrease in energy is greater than 50 dB. This characteristic suggests that complex noise may not be a very effective masker at least for test tones in the middle or higher frequencies. Although the spectrum may differ somewhat from one noise generator to another, the basic limitations of the complex noise as a masker are generally characteristic of the noise. Because of these limitations, complex noise is usually no longer provided on clinical audiometers. The noise is included here because some older units

still in use, particularly portable audiometers, may include it. Masking data on complex noise also helps to illustrate the critical band concept, to be discussed later.

White Noise.   White noise is a broadband signal containing acoustic energy at all frequencies in the audible spectrum at approximately equal intensities. As shown in Figure 3.2, however, the acoustic spectrum of the noise is determined by the frequency response of the transducer. Through a TDH-39 earphone, the spectrum is essentially flat to 6000 Hz but drops off rapidly beyond that point. The acoustic spectrum of white noise is constant from one

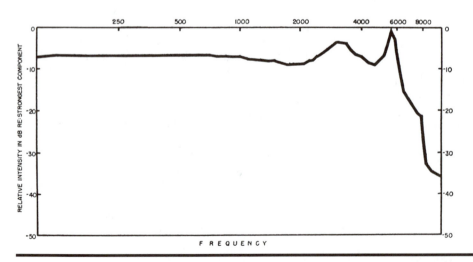

FIGURE 3.2   Acoustic spectrum of a broadband white noise through a TDH-39 earphone. (From J. W. Sanders & W. F. Rintelmann, "Masking in audiometry: A clinical evaluation of three methods." *Archives of Otolaryngology, 8*, 541–556. Copyright 1964, American Medical Association.)

audiometer to another, provided that the same earphone is used. In contrast to complex noise, white noise is essentially equal in intensity across the frequency range to about 6000 Hz. With the newer TDH-49, 49P, 50, and 50P earphones, the spectrum is more nearly flat at 3000 and 4000 Hz by 1 or 2 dB, but the bandwidth continues to be essentially 6000 Hz.

Narrowband Noise.   Narrowband noise is actually not a third type of noise but is rather white noise in limited bands of frequencies. It differs from white noise only in bandwidth. Within the frequency band, acoustic energy is continuous and essentially equal across the band. Narrowband noise has been produced and used in the laboratory for some time (Denes & Naunton, 1952; Dirks, 1963; Egan & Hake, 1950; Jerger, Tillman, & Peterson, 1960; Koenig, 1962b; Liden et al., 1959a; Sanders & Rintelmann, 1964; Studebaker, 1962).

For the purposes of pure-tone audiometry, the narrowband noise generator produces a separate noise band for each test frequency. For example, a 1000 Hz narrowband masker would be white noise in a limited band of frequencies with 1000 Hz at the center of the band. The acoustic spectra of narrowband noises at three test frequencies are shown in Figure 3.3. A given noise band is described in terms of its center frequency, its bandwidth (the span of frequencies whose intensities are no more than 3 dB below the peak component of the band), and its rejection rate (the decrease in intensity over a range of one octave on each side of the band). Because the latter two characteristics, bandwidth and rejection rates, are products of the generator and the transducer used, the acoustic spectra of the noise bands may vary from one audiometer to another.

Relative Masking Efficiency

A critical factor in the choice of a masking noise is that of *masking efficiency*. Masking efficiency is defined as the ratio of the obtained masking to the intensity of the noise (Denes & Naunton, 1952). That is, the most efficient masking noise is the one that produces the greatest threshold shift with the least overall intensity. Thus, if the three different masking noises—complex, white, and narrowband—are presented to an ear at equal overall intensity, the noise producing the greatest threshold shift could be regarded as the most efficient. Before actually measuring the threshold shift produced by each masker, let us consider the way in which masking noise affects auditory sensitivity and a method for predicting threshold shift.

The Critical Band Concept

The *critical band concept* is a statement of masking effect relative to a band of frequencies of critical width. A thorough understanding of the concept is extremely helpful in understanding how masking noise affects auditory sensitivity. The concept developed from the early work of Fletcher and Munson (1937) and Fletcher (1940) and was elaborated in the later investigations of Hawkins and Stevens (1950) and Egan and Hake (1950). The concept is stated in two parts:

1. In masking a pure tone with a broadband noise, the only components of the noise having a masking effect on the tone are those frequencies included in a restricted band with the test tone at its center.
2. When the pure tone is just audible in the presence of the noise, the acoustic energy in the restricted band of frequencies is equal to the acoustic energy of the pure tone.

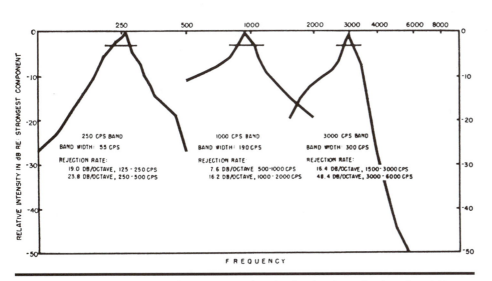

FIGURE 3.3   Acoustic spectra of three narrow bands of noise through a hearing aid type receiver. (From J. W. Sanders & W. F. Rintelmann, "Masking in audiometry: A clinical evaluation of three methods." *Archives of Otolaryngology, 8,* 541–556. Copyright 1964, American Medical Association.)

The width of the frequency band responsible for masking the pure tone is critical. If a band is narrowed to less than critical width without increasing intensity, the *masking effect* is decreased. If the band is widened to more than critical width, the *masking efficiency* is decreased, because the added frequencies in the band increase the overall intensity without producing a further shift in threshold. According to the first part of the critical band concept, in the masking of a 1000 Hz pure tone with white noise, the only components of the noise having a masking effect are the frequencies included in a band from 968 Hz to 1032 Hz, inclusive: that is, 32 cycles (Hz) on either side (above and below) of the 1000 Hz center frequency (see Table 3.1). The acoustic energy in the frequencies above and below that band could be removed without affecting the masking produced by the noise.

According to the second part of the critical band concept, it is the acoustic energy within the critical band of frequencies and not the overall intensity of the noise that determines the masking produced, because the overall level includes the energy in the frequencies above and below the critical band—energy that has no masking effect. In a comparison of masking efficiency for several masking noises, our concern is for the spectrum level within the critical band, often referred to as the *level per cycle*—the intensity of each individual cycle of the noise. The critical band concept can be very helpful in a comparative evaluation of noises for masking in pure tone audiometry.

Predicting Masking Efficiency

With the information supplied by the critical band concept, it is possible to make predictions regarding the efficiency of a masking noise. Although the concept will not hold entirely true for complex noise, given that the concept is specific to a noise of continuous and flat spectrum and complex noise is neither, we can make a general application,

because the components of the noise will in effect combine their acoustic energies in masking.

According to part 1 of the critical band concept, we can expect both complex and white noise to be inefficient to some extent, because for a given pure tone, both noises include considerable energy outside the critical band. Of the two noises, however, we should expect greater masking efficiency for white noise, because its spectrum is essentially flat; whereas in the complex noise, energy is concentrated in the lower frequencies with a rapid dropoff of energy in the higher frequencies. In the masking of a pure tone in the higher frequencies with complex noise, the high intensity in the lower frequencies of the noise contributes significantly to the overall intensity of the noise but not at all to the masking of the tone.

If, as stated in the critical band concept, the important factor in masking is the level per cycle within the critical band rather than the overall intensity of the noise, then narrowband noise should show the greatest masking efficiency. If, for example, we produce each noise at a sound pressure level (SPL) of 80 dB, the level per cycle should be highest in the narrowband noise, because 80 dB are concentrated in a more restricted range of frequencies. This expectation can be demonstrated mathematically for white noise and narrowband noise, because the level per cycle can be computed for a noise of continuous, flat spectrum. The level per cycle (energy in each individual cycle) is the overall intensity of the noise divided by the number of cycles in the noise band. For the white noise in our example, this would be 80 dB divided by 6000 Hz (the bandwidth of white noise through a standard audiometer earphone). In order to carry out the computation, given that intensity in dB is a logarithm, frequency must be converted to its logarithm, and the function becomes one of subtraction.

Level per cycle = overall intensity (OA SPL) minus 10 times the logarithm of the bandwidth (BW).

Since the logarithm of 6000 is 3.78, the formula for determining the level per cycle (LPC) of a white noise of 80 dB would be

$$LPC = OA\ SPL - 10 \log BW$$
$$LPC = 80 - 37.8$$
$$LPC = 42.2\ dB\ SPL$$

Applying the same formula to a narrowband noise having a band width of, let us say, 200 Hz (log of 200 is 2.3) and an overall intensity of 80 dB, the result would be

$$LPC = OA\ SPL - 10 \log BW$$
$$LPC = 80 - 23$$
$$LPC = 57\ dB\ SPL$$

Thus, for white and narrowband noises at an overall intensity of 80 dB, the spectrum level would be 14.8 dB greater in

TABLE 3.1 Critical band widths* for 11 test frequencies.

CENTER FREQUENCY IN Hz	CRITICAL BAND WIDTH	
	In Hz	*10 log CBW*
125	70.8	18.3
250	50	17
500	50	17
750	56.2	17.5
1000	64	18
1500	79.4	19
2000	100	20
3000	158	22
4000	200	23
6000	376	25.75
8000	501	27

*Critical band widths from Hawkins and Stevens (1950)

the narrowband noise. According to the second part of the critical band concept, we would expect the threshold shift to be 14.8 dB greater with the narrowband noise.

Computation of the level per cycle for a narrowband noise indicates that the narrower the band the greater the masking efficiency, as long as the band is no less than the critical width. Because the bandwidth is determined by the characteristics of the noise generator, the efficiency of narrowband masking may vary from one audiometer to another.

Experimental Verification.   The prediction of masking efficiency with the critical band concept can be verified through the direct measurement of masked thresholds. The masking noise and the test tone are mixed in the same earphone, and hearing threshold level is determined in the presence of the masking noise. A number of investigations (Denes & Naunton, 1952; Liden et al., 1959a; Sanders & Rintelmann, 1964; Studebaker, 1962) have carried out this kind of measurement with essentially the same results. Typical data from such a measurement are shown in Figure 3.4. The masked thresholds shown are the mean hearing threshold levels (according to ASA, 1951, specifications) for 10 normal-hearing subjects in the presence of the three masking noises at three different overall sound pressure levels. The acoustic spectra of the noises used for these measurements are those shown in Figures 3.1, 3.2, and 3.3.

The results shown in Figure 3.4 clearly support our predictions of relative masking efficiency. For a given overall intensity level, narrowband noise showed the greatest masking efficiency. Of the two broadband noises, white noise had considerably greater masking efficiency than did the complex noise, at least in the middle and higher frequencies.

Figure 3.4 also demonstrates two additional factors of importance in clinical masking. First, for both white and narrowband noise, masking is least effective in the lower frequencies. This is because auditory sensitivity is poorest in this frequency range, and greater intensity is required to reach hearing threshold level. Second, for both white and narrowband noise, masking is *linear*. That is, beyond a certain minimal level, for each additional dB of noise there is an additional dB of threshold shift. This linearity is not obtained with complex noise.

Choice of Masking Noise.   With a verified prediction of relative masking efficiency, the question of what kind of masking noise to use has been answered. Whenever the clinician has a choice of masking noise for pure-tone audiometry, narrowband noise should be selected for its superior masking efficiency. The second choice is white noise. Although not as efficient as narrowband noise, white noise is clearly superior to complex noise and will provide adequate and predictable masking in most cases if the output of the noise generator is sufficiently high.

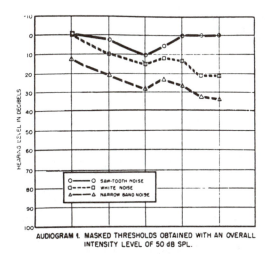

AUDIOGRAM 1. MASKED THRESHOLDS OBTAINED WITH AN OVERALL INTENSITY LEVEL OF 50 dB SPL.

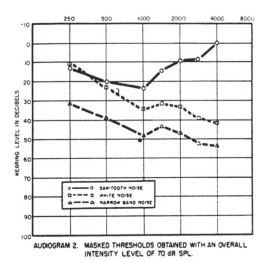

AUDIOGRAM 2. MASKED THRESHOLDS OBTAINED WITH AN OVERALL INTENSITY LEVEL OF 70 dB SPL.

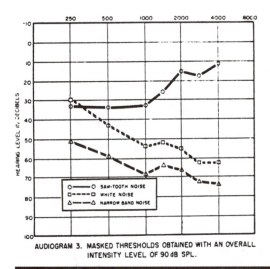

AUDIOGRAM 3. MASKED THRESHOLDS OBTAINED WITH AN OVERALL INTENSITY LEVEL OF 90 dB SPL.

FIGURE 3.4   Masking audiograms obtained with three types of masking noise at three intensity levels. (From J. W. Sanders & W. F. Rintelmann, "Masking in audiometry: A clinical evaluation of three methods." *Archives of Otolaryngology, 8,* 541–556. Copyright 1964, American Medical Association.)

HOW MUCH MASKING SHOULD BE USED?

With the answers to our first two questions of when to mask and what kind of masking noise to use, we can turn to the important third question of how much masking to use. Basically, the masking noise must be sufficient to prevent a response from the nontest ear without affecting sensitivity in the test ear. The least intensity required to effect the needed threshold shift in the nontest ear has been called the *minimum effective masking level* (Liden et al., 1959b) or the *minimum masking level* (Studebaker, 1962) and is defined as the masking level just sufficient to mask the test signal in the masked ear. The *maximum effective masking level* or *maximum masking level* is defined as the masking noise intensity just insufficient to mask the signal in the test ear (Studebaker, 1967). The intensity of the masking noise, then, must be at or beyond the minimum effective level without exceeding the maximum effective level. Several investigators have proposed mathematical formulas for determination of the minimum and maximum effective levels.

The Formula Approach

As an example of the formula approach to determining minimum and maximum effective masking levels, Liden and colleagues (1959a) suggested the following for air conduction testing:

$$Mmin = At - 40 + (Am - Bm)$$

$$Mmax = Bt + 40, \text{ provided Mmax is less than D}$$

That is, the minimum masking level is equal to the air-conduction threshold in the test ear (At) minus the attenuation factor of 40 dB, plus the difference between the air- and bone-conduction thresholds in the masked ear (Am and Bm). The maximum masking level is the bone-conduction threshold in the test ear (Bt) plus the attenuation factor, providing the result does not exceed the patient's discomfort level (D).

For masking in bone-conduction audiometry, the following formulas were proposed:

$$Mmin = Bt + (Am - Bm)$$

$$Mmax = Bt + 40, \text{ provided Mmax is less than D}$$

Minimum masking level is the bone-conduction threshold in the test ear plus the difference between the air- and bone-conduction thresholds in the masked ear. The maximum level, like that for air-conduction audiometry, is the bone-conduction threshold in the test ear plus the attenuation factor of 40 dB for the masking noise, providing the maximum level does not exceed the patient's discomfort level.

Although these formulas will provide the clinician with minimum and maximum effective masking levels, the approach would be extremely cumbersome and time-consuming in clinical audiometry. The clinician would be required to carry out the arithmetic of four formulas in order to obtain air- and bone-conduction thresholds at one test frequency. Although Studebaker (1964) simplified the process somewhat by combining air- and bone-conduction testing into a single formula, he recognized the problems in the formula approach and suggested that this method, although perhaps desirable in laboratory research, is not suited to clinical audiometry.

The Effective Masking Level Approach

A direct approach to the question of how much masking to use is through the determination and use of the *effective masking level*. The effective masking level is defined as the number of dB by which the total energy in the critical band exceeds the threshold energy for a pure tone whose frequency is at the center of the band. Effective level can also be regarded as the threshold shift in dB produced in the masked ear by a given noise intensity. That is, if a masking noise shifts threshold in the masked ear from 0 dB to 30 dB hearing threshold level, the noise has produced 30 dB of effective masking, and threshold in the masked ear has been shifted to a hearing threshold level of 30 dB. Thus, the effective masking level for an ear with normal sensitivity expressed in dB on the hearing threshold level scale can be regarded as the hearing level to which an ear will be shifted by a given amount of masking noise. Applying the concept of the effective masking level in this manner can greatly simplify masking procedures in audiometry.

If the numbers on the audiometer masking-noise intensity dial can be translated into effective masking levels re normal thresholds, we can predict the masked thresholds that will be produced by each setting of the dial. With this information, we can answer the question of how much masking noise to use through a direct inspection of the audiogram. If, for example, we wish to produce a minimum masking level of 10 dB in an ear with air- and bone-conduction thresholds of 0 dB HTL, we can simply turn the masking-noise intensity dial to a setting that will produce an effective masking level of 10 dB. At this masking-noise intensity, the masked air and bone threshold in the nontest ear will be at the 10 dB HTL.

The Masking-Noise Intensity Dial

In past years there has been little or no relationship between the masking effect and the numbers on the audiometer dial controlling the intensity of the masking noise. In an informal survey of eight older audiometers (portable, clinical, and research), we found that with the dial set to "60," the intensity of the masking noise (complex or white) ranged from 60 to 120 dB SPL. Obviously, on these instruments no assumptions could be made regarding the masking effect at a given setting on the dial. On the more recent audiometers, those providing narrowband masking noise, the dial controlling the intensity of the narrowband noise is calibrated in effective masking level re 0 dB HTL. This is possible because narrowband masking requires a different noise band for each test frequency. Unfortunately, the dial cannot be calibrated in effective level for white noise masking, even though some audiometers providing white noise label the intensity dial "effective masking." The dial numbers may be in effective masking for one or two frequencies, but this cannot apply at all test frequencies because the sound pressure level for effective masking with white noise varies with the frequency of the test tone. A possible exception to this problem would be an audiometer in which a change on the frequency dial also effects a change in the output of the masking circuit. Even without this special equipment feature, however, it is possible for the clinician to determine the relationship between dial numbers and their masking effect with white noise.

Determining Effective Masking Level

There are two methods available to the clinician for determining effective masking levels for either white noise or narrowband noise and relating those levels to the numbers on the masking-noise intensity dial. The first method is through computation with the critical band data.

Effective Level through Computation.   Part 2 of the critical band concept, presented earlier, states:

> When the pure tone is just audible in the presence of the masking noise, the acoustic energy in the restricted band of frequencies (the critical band) is equal to the acoustic energy in the test tone.

From this part of the critical band concept, we can see that if the acoustic energy in a given critical band of white noise can be determined, that information can be used to predict the masking effect of the noise. As we have already seen, the spectrum level, or level per cycle, within a given band of white noise can be computed from the overall intensity of the noise and the width of the band. If we also know the width of the critical band, we can determine the acoustic energy in the critical band for a given overall intensity. The critical bandwidths from the data of Hawkins and Stevens (1950) are shown in Table 3.1. Each bandwidth is reported in frequency and in 10 times the logarithm of the frequency. The total energy in a critical band is the level per cycle (energy in each individual cycle) multiplied by the number of cycles in the critical band. In the critical band having 1000 Hz as a center frequency, for example, if the level per cycle is 42.2 dB (from the

example given earlier for the computation of level per cycle), and the critical band is 64 cycles in width, the total energy in the critical band would be 42.2 dB multiplied by 64 cycles. Here again, we must convert the bandwidth to its logarithm, and the function becomes one of addition:

> Energy in the critical band (CB) is equal to the level per cycle (LPC) plus 10 times the logarithm of the critical band (CBW).

As shown earlier, the level per cycle for a given white noise, broad- or narrowband, is the overall sound pressure of the noise minus 10 times the logarithm of the bandwidth of the noise. In an earlier computation, we found that for white noise through a standard earphone at a sound pressure level of 80 dB, the level per cycle was as follows:

$$LPC = OA\ SPL - 10 \log BW$$
$$LPC = 80 - 37.8$$
$$LPC = 42.2\ dB\ SPL$$

Thus, for white noise at an overall intensity of 80 dB and the critical band at 1000 Hz (see Table 3.1), the computation of the energy (E) in the critical band is as follows:

$$E\ in\ CB = LPC + 10 \log CBW$$
$$E\ in\ CB = 42.2 + 18$$
$$E\ in\ CB = 60.2\ dB\ SPL$$

In this example, the total energy in the 1000 Hz critical band is 60.2 dB SPL. The magnitude of the difference between the energy in that critical band and the intensity necessary to reach threshold at 1000 Hz in a given ear is the effective level of the noise at that frequency in that ear. Thus, effective level, often designated as Z, can be determined as follows:

$$Z = LPC + 10 \log CBW - threshold\ in\ quiet$$

In this computation, threshold in quiet must be expressed in dB sound pressure level. According to ANSI S 3.6-1996, 0 dB HTL for the TDH-39 earphone at 1000 Hz = 7 dB SPL. Thus, the effective level for white noise at a sound pressure level of 80 dB in a TDH-39 earphone in a normal ear would be:

$$Z = 42.2 + 18 - 7$$
$$Z = 53.2\ dB$$

That is, the energy in the critical band (42.2 + 18) exceeds the energy required to reach threshold in quiet (7 dB) by 53.2 dB. With an effective level of 53.2 dB, we would expect 53.2 dB of masking in a normal ear for a 1000 Hz tone. Furthermore, this masking would shift threshold to a hearing level of 53.2 dB.

Because our prediction is based entirely on computation with the critical band data, we might well ask at this point for verification. Does 80 dB of white noise actually produce a threshold shift of 53.2 dB for a 1000 Hz tone in the normal ear? The relationship between effective masking levels predicted through computation and the masking actually obtained with white noise at three different sound pressure levels in 10 normal ears is shown in Figure 3.5. Figure 3.6 reports the same data (predicted and obtained masking) for narrowband noise. In each figure, for a given overall intensity of the masking noise, one set of data points shows the masked thresholds predicted with the critical band data computations, and the second set of data reports the mean hearing threshold levels (re ASA, 1951) to which the 10 normal hearers were actually shifted. Converting the measured and predicted masked thresholds to hearing threshold levels re the ANSI S3.6-1996 standard would not, of course, alter the relationship shown.

The data shown in Figure 3.5 and 3.6 verify the prediction of effective masking level through computation. The figures show further that if the overall intensity of the noise (white or narrowband) is known, the hearing threshold levels to which an ear will be shifted by a given noise can

be determined. This information will permit the clinician to establish the effective masking level at each test frequency for each setting of the masking-noise intensity dial.

The Effective Masking Table. For the audiometer having a masking-noise intensity dial that is not calibrated in effective masking level, the relationship between dial setting and effective masking can be established through the construction of an *effective masking table*, which should be posted at the audiometer. The first step is to measure the acoustic output of the masking noise in sound pressure level at the maximum dial setting with a sound level meter. If the clinician does not have such equipment, the measurement can be made by the people who service and calibrate the audiometer. For the maximum noise output, the level per cycle and the energy in the critical bands can be determined with the formulas given, using the critical band data from Table 3.1. Finally, the effective masking levels re audiometric zero can be determined for each test frequency by subtracting the appropriate sound pressure levels at audiometric zero (ANSI, 1996) for the earphones in use from

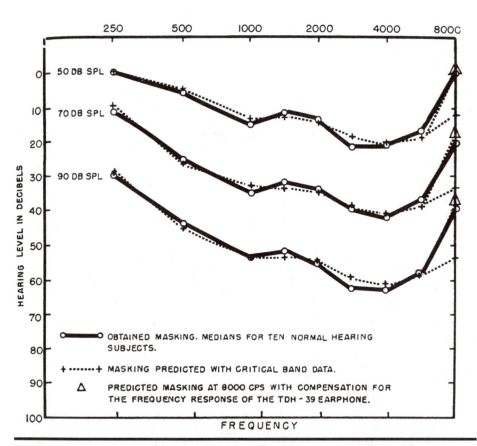

FIGURE 3.5 Comparison of the masking obtained with white noise at three different intensity levels for 10 normal hearing subjects and the masking predicted with the critical band data of Fletcher (1940). (From J. W. Sanders & W. F. Rintelmann, "Masking in audiometry: A clinical evaluation of three methods." *Archives of Otolaryngology, 8,* 541–556. Copyright 1964, American Medical Association.)

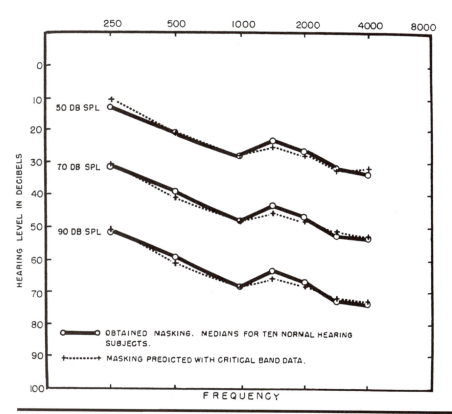

FIGURE 3.6   Comparison of the masking obtained with narrowband noise at three different intensity levels for 10 normal hearing subjects and the masking predicted with the critical band data of Fletcher (1940). (From J. W. Sanders & W. F. Rintelmann, "Masking in audiometry: A clinical evaluation of three methods." *Archives of Otolaryngology, 8*, 541–556. Copyright 1964, American Medical Association.)

the energy in the critical bands. The resulting values are the effective levels re normal hearing at each test frequency for the maximum output of the masking noise.

The next step is to check the linearity of the masking-noise intensity dial. That is, does each 10 dB change on the dial bring about a 10 dB change in the intensity of the noise? On most clinical audiometers, masking-noise intensity is controlled by an attenuator that should provide satisfactory linearity. Some older instruments and most portable audiometers, however, are equipped with potentiometers that do not provide linear control. The linearity check can be made with a sound level meter, but it is done more satisfactorily with a voltmeter. If the dial departs significantly from linearity (1 or 2 dB per 10 dB step and/or a cumulative error greater than 4 or 5 dB), use the voltmeter to establish 10 dB steps and mark those on the dial. If a voltmeter is not available, this measurement can be made by the people who service the audiometer. Actually, measurement of the masking-noise intensity and a determination of masking-noise dial linearity should be part of the routine calibration

of the audiometer. With linearity of the dial assured, the effective level for each dial setting can be established simply by subtracting 10 dB for each 10 dB reduction on the dial.

For example, suppose that on an audiometer equipped with white noise through a TDH-50P earphone, the maximum setting on the masking-noise intensity dial is 100 and the noise intensity at that setting is 110 dB SPL. The level per cycle of the noise would be 110 dB minus 37.8 (10 times the logarithm of 6000 Hz) or 72.2 dB. With this level per cycle and the data from Table 3.1, effective masking levels would be computed as shown for three test frequencies in Table 3.2. These are the effective levels for normal hearers and thus are the hearing levels to which an ear will be shifted with the noise-intensity dial setting of 100. These levels, *rounded off to the next lower 5 dB level,* are entered into a table of effective masking opposite the dial setting of 100. Next, for each linear setting of the masking dial, effective levels can be entered for each dial setting by subtracting 10 dB from the maximum effective levels for

TABLE 3.2 An illustration of the computation of effective masking levels at three test frequencies.

FREQUENCY IN Hz	COMPUTATION	EFFECTIVE LEVEL
250	Z = 72.2 + 17 − 26.5* =	62.7
1000	Z = 72.2 + 18 − 7.5* =	82.7
4000	Z = 72.2 + 23 − 10.5* =	84.7

*Audiometric zero for the TDH-50P earphone according to the ANSI standards

each 10 dB reduction on the dial. Table 3.3 illustrates the effective masking table, using the data for the three frequencies computed in Table 3.2. A table for clinical use would, of course, include effective masking levels for all test frequencies. The completed table provides for each test frequency the hearing threshold level to which a masked ear will be shifted by the masking noise at each setting of the intensity dial on a given audiometer.

Effective Level by Measurement.   A second method for determining effective masking levels is through direct measurement with normal hearers. Although this approach is time-consuming, it will provide accurate masking data and may be necessary if any of the information for computation of effective masking levels cannot be obtained. In this method, the masking noise and the test tone are mixed in the same earphone. At several settings of the masking-noise intensity dial, thresholds are determined at each test frequency in the presence of the noise for 8 or 10 normal hearers. For each dial setting, the mean masked threshold at each frequency is the effective masking level for normal hearers and represents the hearing threshold level to which an ear will be shifted by noise at that dial setting. If the masking dial is linear, the effective masking levels for those dial settings not used for measurement can be interpolated from the obtained results, and a complete masking table can be constructed, which provides effective masking level

TABLE 3.3 Illustration of an effective masking table.

DIAL SETTING	EFFECTIVE LEVELS IN dB		
	250 Hz	*1000 Hz*	*4000 Hz*
30		10	10
40		20	20
50	10	30	30
60	20	40	40
70	30	50	50
80	40	60	60
90	50	70	70
100	60	80	80

for each frequency at each setting of the masking noise dial. If the dial is not linear, the alternative is to mark linear points on the dial as described earlier to measure masking in the normal ears at each dial setting.

This approach to the determination of effective masking levels assumes that the noise and the test tone can be presented in the same earphone. This is not true on most one-channel audiometers. The same thing can be accomplished, however, through a simple mixing network described by Studebaker (1967) and shown in Figure 3.7. If the clinician cannot construct the network, it can be made from the diagram in a radio-television repair shop.

Effective Masking and Complex Noise.   As indicated earlier, complex noise is no longer included on clinical audiometers and has been replaced by white noise on most portable instruments. If, for whatever reason, the clinician is limited to complex noise, he or she should be fully aware of its limitations. First, masking with complex noise is not linear. That is, each additional dB of noise does not necessarily produce an additional dB of masking (see Figure 3.4). Furthermore, the critical band data cannot be applied to complex noise because its spectrum is neither continuous nor flat. The only approach to a determination of effective masking levels is through actual measurement with normal hearers, and that measurement must be made at each setting of the masking dial. Even with an effective masking chart, the clinician must remain aware of the possibility of a beat phenomenon between the test tone and a component of the noise.

Using Effective Masking Levels

With a masking-noise intensity dial calibrated in effective masking level, directly or through the use of a table relating effective masking to dial setting, the clinician has an immediate indication of the hearing threshold level to which the masked ear will be shifted by each setting of the masking noise dial. To use that information appropriately, however, the clinician must be aware of several additional factors.

Effective Level Refers to Any Ear.   The effective masking level has been defined as the number of dB by which the energy in the critical band exceeds the threshold energy of a pure tone whose frequency is at the center of the band. Because effective levels on the calibrated dial or in the masking table are re normal hearing (audiometric zero), they can be regarded as the hearing threshold level to which the masked ear will be shifted. This will be true for the impaired ear as well as the normal ear, provided threshold in the impaired ear is at a lower HTL than the effective level. For example, in the illustration used earlier, white noise at an overall intensity of 80 dB through a TDH-39 earphone was found to produce an effective level in the

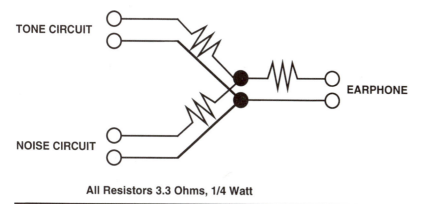

All Resistors 3.3 Ohms, 1/4 Watt

FIGURE 3.7   Combining network for mixing the pure tone and the masking noise into the same earphone. (From G. A. Studebaker, "Clinical masking of the nontest ear." *Journal of Speech and Hearing Disorders, 32*, 360–371, 1967. Reprinted by permission of the American Speech-Language-Hearing Association.)

normal ear of 53.2 dB at 1000 Hz. A threshold shift of 53.2 dB in the normal ear would produce, of course, a masked hearing threshold level of 53.2 dB. If we apply that 80 dB SPL white noise to an impaired ear with HTL at, let us say, 40 dB, the threshold shift would be smaller, but the masked threshold would still be 53.2 dB HTL. Recall that the computation of effective level for a given ear requires us to subtract that ear's threshold in quiet, expressed in sound pressure level, from the total energy in the critical band. Computation of the effective masking level with white noise at an overall SPL of 80 dB for a 1000 Hz pure tone in an ear with a 40 dB hearing loss would be:

$$Z = LPC + 10 \log CBW - \text{threshold in quiet}$$
$$Z = 42.2 + 18 - 47$$
$$Z = 13.2 \text{ dB}$$

The value of 47 in the computation is the 40 dB hearing loss at 1000 Hz expressed in sound pressure level with a TDH-39 earphone (7 dB at audiometric zero plus the 40 dB HTL). The effective level, and thus the threshold shift, in this ear would be 13.2 dB. A threshold shift of 13.2 dB from a hearing threshold level of 40 dB would result in a masked hearing threshold level of 53.2 dB, the same HTL to which the normal ear is shifted at 1000 Hz by 80 dB of white noise. Thus, we can interpret effective masking levels re normal ears as the HTL to which any ear will be shifted, regardless of hearing loss in the ear, as long as the hearing loss does not exceed the effective level.

The foregoing assumes that the impaired ear will give the same linear response to white noise as will the normal ear. Although clinical experience suggests that undermasking is not a problem with the effective masking approach, there may be instances where masking an ear with sensorineural impairment produces questionable results. In such cases, the clinician should combine the effective masking level approach with the Hood technique to be described later.

Effective Level Is by Air Conduction.   In using the concept of effective masking level in clinical audiometry, it is important to recognize that the masked threshold produced by the noise is by air conduction, not bone conduction. For example, if we present masking noise at an effective level of 50 dB to an ear with air-conduction threshold at 40 dB and bone-conduction threshold at 0 dB HTL, the air-conduction threshold on that ear will be shifted to 50 dB, but the bone-conduction threshold in that ear will be shifted to only 10 dB HTL. Increasing the effective masking level to 60 dB will shift the air threshold to 60 dB but the bone threshold to only 20 dB. The introduction of masking noise does not change the air-bone relationship in the masked ear. In an attempt to shift bone-conduction threshold in an ear with a conductive impairment, effective masking is reduced by the amount of the air-bone gap. This is why in the formula approach to masking described earlier, Liden and colleagues (1959a) included subtraction of the air-bone gap in the masked ear. Given that bone-conduction sensitivity is the most important concern in masking, the clinician must remain aware of the loss of effective masking due to an air-bone gap.

The Occlusion Effect.   The *occlusion effect*, described by Liden and colleagues (1959b), Feldman (1961), Studebaker (1962), Dirks and Swindeman (1967), and others, is an improvement in bone-conduction responses in an ear covered (occluded) by an earphone. The improved responses are a result of sound pressure generated in the enclosed external auditory canal and transmitted through the conductive mechanism; the effect does not occur in the ear with conductive impairment. The effect might be as great as 25 dB (Dirks & Swindeman, 1967) but is limited to the lower frequencies, primarily 250 and 500 Hz. To overcome the occlusion effect, the minimum effective level must be increased by 30 dB when testing at these frequencies, unless the masked ear is known to have a conductive impairment.

Some Illustrative Cases.   The following cases are presented to illustrate the use of effective masking levels re the normal ear. Audiometric data for the cases are shown in Figure 3.8.

Case A.   An air-conduction response for a 1000 Hz tone is obtained in the right ear at 60 dB after air- and bone-conduction thresholds have been established at that frequency in the left ear at 0 dB. As we have already seen in our discussion of when to mask, the right ear response could be a result of cross-over of the test tone to the left ear, because the intensity of the tone at 60 dB exceeds bone-conduction sensitivity in the nontest ear by more than the interaural attenuation value of 40 dB. The minimum

effective masking level is 10 dB. The maximum effective level is 40 dB, assuming the possibility of bone-conduction threshold in the right ear at 0 dB. If the right ear response is a result of cross-over, shifting the left ear sensitivity by 10 dB should cause the right ear response to disappear. In this case, however, we can use an effective level greater than the minimum. An effective level of 40 dB would bring about a considerable shift in the left ear without danger of masking cross-over to the right ear, even if bone-conduction sensitivity in the right ear is at 0 dB. With 40 dB of effective masking in the left ear, threshold in the right ear is redetermined. If the response continues at 60 dB, we can accept it as a true threshold, because the difference between the test signal and bone-conduction sensitivity in the masked left ear is now only 20 dB, considerably less than the interaural attenuation of 40 dB. A disappearance of the right ear response with the masking at a 40 dB effective level in the left ear, however, does not guarantee that the response was a result of cross-over, because it could disappear due to central masking. If, in the presence of the masking noise, the response reappears at 70 dB, this can be accepted as correct, given that the interaural difference is now only 30 dB and still not in excess of interaural attenuation. If, however, the redetermined response is at 85 dB HTL or higher (interaural difference of 45 dB or more), masking must be increased and threshold search continued until a stable response is obtained with effective level in the left ear no more than 40 dB below presentation level in the right ear. In some instances, of course, a stable response might never occur. If the actual threshold in the right ear is so poor as to be beyond the limits of the audiometer output, we would eliminate response entirely with increasing levels of masking and thus demonstrate the profound nature of the hearing loss. If, however, our masking noise output is limited to an effective level no greater than 60 dB, we might continue to obtain a right ear response at 105 or 110 dB HTL that does not meet our criterion of acceptability. Under these circumstances, we would have to conclude that threshold in the right ear is at least as poor and probably poorer than the last obtained response.

Case B.   In this case, with left ear thresholds established at 30 dB by air conduction and 0 dB by bone conduction, an air-conduction response is obtained in the right ear at 60 dB HTL for a 4000 Hz tone. Here again, this right ear response must be checked with masking in the left ear, because the difference between the presentation level in the test ear and bone-conduction sensitivity in the nontest ear is 60 dB, considerably greater than the interaural attenuation of 40 dB. As in Case A, the minimum threshold shift required in the nontest ear is 10 dB. In this case, however, we cannot use an effective masking level of 10 dB, because of the air-bone gap in the nontest ear. In order to shift bone-conduction sensitivity in the left ear to 10 dB HTL, we must use an effective level of 40 dB, shifting air-conduction

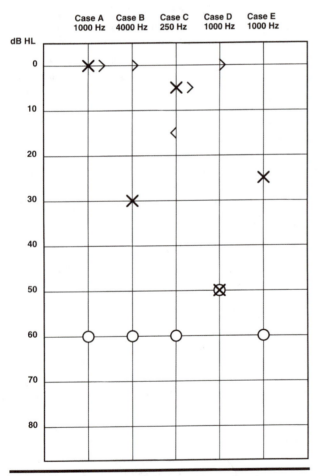

FIGURE 3.8   Five hypothetical cases illustrating the application of effective masking.

threshold to 40 dB and thus shifting bone-conduction threshold to 10 dB. With 40 dB of interaural attenuation for the masking noise, an effective level of 40 dB would not result in overmasking, even if bone-conduction threshold in the right ear is at 0 dB. If the right ear response continues at 60 dB with masking at an effective level of 40 dB in the left ear, it can be accepted as threshold. If it disappears, the procedure outlined for Case A must be followed until a response that meets our criterion is obtained. In this case the chances of failure to obtain an acceptable response because of insufficient masking noise output are increased by the presence of the air-bone gap in the nontest ear. It should be remembered that masking effect is decreased by an amount equal to the difference between air- and bone-conduction thresholds in the masked ear.

Case C. This case illustrates masking in bone-conduction testing with the added complication of the occlusion effect. The response in question is the unmasked bone-conduction response at 250 Hz in the right ear, with air-conduction threshold in that ear already established at 60 dB and air- and bone-conduction thresholds in the left ear at 5 dB with no air-bone gap. With no interaural attenuation expected in bone-conduction testing and with an air-bone gap in the test ear, the right ear bone-conduction response must be checked with masking in the left ear. In this case, a 10 dB threshold shift in the nontest ear is not acceptable as a minimum. With the test signal at a low frequency and no conductive component in the masked ear, we must add 30 dB of effective masking to compensate for the occlusion effect in that ear, which brings the minimum effective level to 45 dB. In this case, however, we can exceed the minimum level by 10 dB without danger of overmasking, because an effective level of 55 dB is only 40 dB above the bone-conduction response level in the test ear.

Case D. In this case, an air-conduction response is obtained at 50 dB in the right ear for a 1000 Hz tone with unmasked responses in the left ear, which indicate air-conduction threshold at 50 dB and bone-conduction threshold at 0 dB. The need for checking the right ear response with masking in the left ear is apparent. In order to overcome the air-bone gap in the left ear and bring about a shift of 10 dB in bone-conduction response, we must use an effective masking level of 60 dB. If, however, the undetermined bone-conduction sensitivity in the right ear is actually at 0 or even 5 dB, an effective level of 60 dB would be overmasking, since that noise level in the nontest ear would exceed that hypothetical bone-conduction sensitivity by more than 40 dB. If we attempt to solve the problem by establishing a bone-conduction threshold in the right ear, we face the same problem. Sufficient masking in the left ear to produce a minimum shift of 10 dB of bone-conduction response in that ear would also eliminate a true bone-conduction threshold response in the right ear, if

bone-conduction threshold in that ear is actually at 0 to 10 dB. Furthermore, if we obtain an unmasked bone-conduction threshold in the right ear at 0 dB, we have no way of knowing whether 0 dB bone-conduction thresholds are correct in both ears or correct in one with cross-over response in the other. If one is due to cross-over, we have no way of telling which. Finally, the same problem exists for the air-conduction responses. The obtained response in one ear might be a result of cross-over, and as with the bone-conduction responses, we cannot tell which. This problem, described by Carhart (1960) and by Feldman (1961), and aptly labeled a "masking dilemma" by Naunton (1960), cannot be solved with standard masking procedures. The only masking solution to the problem is to increase the interaural attenuation for the masking noise by transducing the noise in an insert receiver (Koenig, 1962a; Zwislocki, 1953). Because the insert receiver results in a much smaller contact area between transducer and skull, the interaural attenuation may be increased to as much as 70 to 90 dB.

In cases like this in which masking limitations preclude an accurate assessment, an excellent procedure for determining the true nature of the hearing loss is acoustic immittance measurement. This procedure is discussed in Chapter 4.

Case E. In Cases A, B, and C, we considered the amount of masking to be used when air- and bone-conduction thresholds are known for the nontest ear. This is usually not the case, however, because most clinicians complete air-conduction testing for both ears before turning to bone-conduction audiometry. In Case E, then, air-conduction responses are obtained at 60 dB in the right ear with air-conduction threshold previously established for the left ear at 25 dB. Although bone-conduction sensitivity in the left ear is unknown, it could be as low as 0 dB, and the right ear response could be a result of cross-over. In this situation the clinician has two choices. First, the right ear air response at 60 dB can be accepted temporarily and a final decision as to the need for masking made after bone-conduction testing. The second choice is to assume a bone-conduction threshold of 0 dB in the left ear and mask accordingly.

These illustrative cases certainly do not cover every problem encountered in masking in clinical audiometry. They should, however, present the principles of effective masking in a manner that will permit the clinician to reason from them to situations not included here.

The Hood Technique. As shown in several of the illustrative cases, whenever a suspect response disappears in the presence of appropriate masking, the clinician must search for the true threshold at higher hearing levels. This search may also involve increasing the effective masking level to ensure a continued nonparticipation by the nontest ear. As the intensity of the masking noise is increased, so are the chances for overmasking. An excellent procedure for ensuring sufficient masking without overmasking in the threshold search is a technique described by Hood (1960) and referred to by various terms, such as the *plateau method*, the *threshold shift method*, or the *shadowing method*. In this procedure, a questionable unmasked threshold is checked with masking in the nontest ear at the minimum effective masking level. If the response disappears, the effective masking level is increased in 10 dB steps with a redetermination of threshold at each step until a plateau of threshold response is reached—a level at which threshold response shows no further increase with increase in masking over a range of at least 20 to 30 dB of masking noise. One or more of the responses on the plateau will meet the criterion for a true threshold response. That is, the interaural difference will be 40 dB or less. The Hood technique is demonstrated with the two illustrative cases outlined in Table 3.4 and Figure 3.9.

Case 1. In this case, as shown in the figure, left ear air- and bone-conduction thresholds have been established at 0 dB. An air-conduction threshold response has been obtained in the right ear at 50 dB, although, unknown to the clinician, the actual threshold is at 80 dB. Because the unmasked response at 50 dB is a result of cross-over of the test tone to the nontest ear, masking at an effective level of 10 dB will shift bone-conduction sensitivity in the left ear to 10 dB HTL, and the cross-over response in the right ear will shift to 60 dB, as shown in Table 3.4. This response is also unacceptable, of course, because the difference between the test tone presentation level of 60 dB exceeds the masked bone-conduction threshold in the left ear by more than 40 dB. The next step is to increase the effective masking level to 20 dB. At this masking level, response in the right ear will shift to 70 dB, which is also unacceptable, because the interaural difference still exceeds 40 dB. Continuing the procedure of increasing the

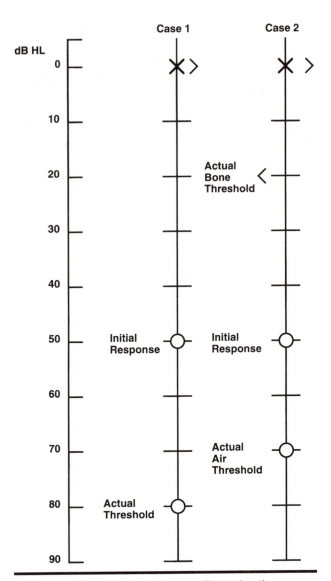

FIGURE 3.9 Two hypothetical cases illustrating the application of the Hood technique in masking.

effective masking level in 10 dB steps with redetermination of threshold at each step will bring us to a threshold response at 80 dB. At this point, we will observe no further shifts in hearing threshold response with increase in masking level, because the response is no longer due to cross-over but rather is the true right ear threshold. Further shifts in left ear threshold with masking will not affect the response.

Case 2. This case presents a somewhat different situation. Left ear thresholds have been established at 0 dB. In the right ear, air-conduction threshold response is obtained at 50 dB. This response is due to cross-over, because, again unknown to the clinician, actual threshold in the right ear is at 70 dB. Also unknown to the clinician, bone-conduction

TABLE 3.4 Two illustrative cases of the Hood technique for bone conduction threshold measurement.

CASE 1		CASE 2	
Threshold Response	Effective Level	Threshold Response	Effective Level
50	0	50	0
60	10	60	10
70	20	70	20
80	30	70	30
80	40	70	40
80	50	70	50
80	60	70	60
		80	70
		90	80

threshold in that ear is at 20 dB. With the Hood technique, we will find a response plateau in this case at 70 dB HTL in the test ear. As shown in the table, this response will remain stable over a range of effective masking levels from 20 to 60 dB. If we continue to increase the masking noise level in this case, however, we will eventually observe a further shift in threshold response. As shown in the table, at an effective level of 70 dB, threshold response will shift to 80 dB, because at this point the masking noise is more than 40 dB greater than bone-conduction sensitivity in the test ear, and overmasking has occurred. This further shift of threshold response at higher levels of masking noise should not constitute a problem, however, so long as the clinician recognizes the response plateau when it occurs. As in Case 1, responses on the plateau occurred at several effective masking levels sufficient to preclude a response from the nontest ear.

MASKING IN SPEECH AUDIOMETRY

With a few notable exceptions, the attention given to masking in the literature has been directed primarily toward masking in pure tone audiometry, with considerably less said about the equally important subject of masking in speech audiometry. Although both the signal and the task are different in speech audiometry, given that we are seeking recognition of spoken language rather than detection of a pure tone, the problem is the same—that is, the possibility of a false and inaccurate response as a result of crossover of the test signal to the nontest ear. Indeed, as pointed out by Studebaker (1967), the danger is increased in word recognition testing, because the signal to the test ear is presented at suprathreshold level, increasing even further the interaural difference.

When to Mask

The answer to the question of when to mask in speech audiometry is the same as that for pure-tone audiometry. Masking must be used whenever the intensity of the test signal exceeds bone-conduction sensitivity for that signal by more than the expected interaural attenuation. Liden (1954) and Liden and colleagues (1959b) indicated that the interaural attenuation for speech by air conduction is 50 dB. Konkle and Berry (1983), however, present a convincing argument for an interaural attenuation of only 45 dB for threshold assessment with spondee words. They also point out that, because of differences in the nature of the tasks, interaural attenuation for word recognition tests should be regarded as 35 dB. In deciding when to mask, it must be remembered that the interaural difference must be determined as the difference between presentation level to the test ear and bone-conduction sensitivity in the nontest ear. If an air-bone gap is present in the nontest ear, bone-conduction sensitivity for speech can be taken as the pure tone average (500, 1000, and 2000 Hz) by bone conduction. If the nontest ear does not have a conductive loss, interaural difference can be based on the air-conduction pure-tone average if the speech recognition threshold (SRT) has not been obtained. If the interaural difference is based on the pure tone average in the nontest ear, a higher effective masking level might be needed if the audiogram is irregular in configuration. In such cases, the clinician might use either the 500 and 1000 Hz average or simply the pure-tone threshold at either 500 or 1000 Hz, whichever is better. Carhart (1971) reported correlation coefficients for SRT and pure-tone thresholds of 0.90 for 500 Hz and 0.92 for 1000 Hz. The correlation coefficient between SRT and pure-tone threshold at 2000 Hz was 0.78.

What Kind of Noise?

The question of what kind of noise to use for masking in speech audiometry is usually not a problem. Narrow bands of noise, like those used with significant advantage in pure-tone audiometry, are too limited in frequency response for the relatively broad spectrum speech signal (Hirsh & Bowman, 1953; Miller, 1947; Setliff, 1971). Complex noise suffers the same deficiency it exhibits as a pure-tone masker (energy concentration in the lower frequencies). On audiometers permitting speech audiometry, the clinician usually has a choice between white noise as described earlier in this chapter and *speech spectrum noise.* Speech spectrum noise is white noise filtered to a low- and middle-frequency band, simulating the long-term average spectrum of conversational speech. Because of its more limited band, speech spectrum noise is somewhat more efficient than white noise, with a masking advantage of about 8 dB (Konkle & Berry, 1983). Hawkins and Stevens (1950), Liden (1954), and Liden and colleagues (1959b) have shown that the relationship between white noise intensity level and threshold for speech is a linear function. That is, beyond a certain minimum level, each additional dB of noise produces an additional dB of shift in threshold for speech. This same linearity is found for speech spectrum noise (Konkle & Berry, 1983).

How Much Masking?

In deciding how much masking noise to use, the well-established one-to-one relationship between pure-tone average and SRT can be used to advantage. In demonstrating the linearity of white noise masking in speech audiometry by obtaining speech thresholds in normal hearers at three different noise intensity levels, Hawkins and Stevens (1950) also found good agreement between masked thresholds for speech and masked pure-tone averages. Their results are compared in Table 3.5 with masked SRTs and

TABLE 3.5 Masked speech and pure tone thresholds in normal hearers obtained with white noise at three intensity levels expressed in level per cycle.

MEASURES	LEVEL PER CYCLE		
	40	*50*	*60*
Average TD and TI[1]	50.9	60.4	69.8
Speech reception threshold[2]	49.8	59.8	69.8
Speech reception threshold[3]	48.4	58.4	68.3
Pure-tone average[4]	51.0	60.8	69.7
Pure-tone average[5]	49.2	59.0	69.0

[1]Average of threshold of detectability (TD) and threshold of intelligibility (TI) for connected discourse re threshold in quiet for the subjects tested (Hawkins & Stevens, 1950)

[2]Speech reception thresholds in dB re: 22 dB SPL (Lizar, Peck, Schwartz, & Stockdell, 1969)

[3]Speech reception thresholds in dB: 20 dB SPL (Setliff, 1971)

[4]Average masked thresholds for pure tones re: thresholds in quiet for the subjects tested (Hawkins & Stevens, 1950)

[5]Average masked thresholds for pure tones re: the ANSI-1969 standard (Sanders & Rintelmann, 1964)

TABLE 3.6 Masked thresholds for speech predicted with the critical band data and masked speech reception thresholds at three intensity levels expressed in level per cycle.

MEASURES	LEVEL PER CYCLE		
	40	*50*	*60*
Pure-tone average[1]	49.1	59.1	69.1
Speech reception threshold[2]	49.8	59.8	69.8
Speech reception threshold[3]	48.4	58.4	68.3

Note: 68.3 agrees with Table 5
See speech reception thresholds[3], Level per Cycle at 60

[1]Average masked threshold at 500, 1000, and 2000 Hz predicted with the critical band data.

[2]Speech reception thresholds in dB re 22 dB SPL (Lizar et al., 1969)

[3]Speech reception thresholds in dB re 20 dB SPL (Setliff, 1971)

pure-tone averages from several other reports. Regarding the masked pure-tone averages in the table derived from the results reported by Sanders and Rintelmann (1964), it should be pointed out that the masked thresholds obtained in their study were in hearing level according to the 1951 ASA standard; whereas the pure-tone thresholds of Hawkins and Stevens (1950) were sensation levels re their subjects' thresholds in quiet. Because the thresholds in quiet were within 1 or 2 dB of the 1969 ANSI standard, the data of Sanders and Rintelmann were converted to that standard for comparison purposes here. The data in Table 3.5 show excellent agreement among the studies and demonstrate the linear nature of speech masking with white noise as well as the close agreement between masked hearing for speech and for the pure-tone average. This agreement permits us to determine effective masking levels for speech from those computed for pure tones.

On at least some of the newer speech audiometers, the masking-noise intensity dial is calibrated in effective masking level for speech. For those that are not, effective levels can be related to the numbers on the dial in either of two ways.

First, effective masking levels for speech can be derived from a table of effective masking for pure tones with white noise by averaging the effective levels for 500, 1000, and 2000 Hz for each dial setting. The construction of an effective masking level table for pure tones was described earlier in this chapter. Table 3.6 is a comparison of the effective masking levels for speech based on the mean effective levels computed for pure tones at 500, 1000, and 2000 Hz and the masked SRTs measured for normal hearers at three white noise intensities. The table shows an excellent agreement between the effective masking levels for speech predicted with the critical band data for pure tones and the effective levels obtained through direct measurement.

Second, effective levels can be obtained through actual measurement with a group of normal hearers. The speech signal and the masking noise are mixed into the same earphone, and SRTs are determined at three different settings of the masking dial. If the dial is linear, the average thresholds will show a linear relationship, and effective levels at other dial settings can be interpolated to complete the table. Just as with the effective masking table for pure tones, the values in the table indicate the hearing threshold levels to which the ear will be shifted with masking noise at the corresponding dial setting.

THE SENSORINEURAL ACUITY LEVEL (SAL) PROCEDURE

The SAL procedure is among the least used and appreciated of clinical audiometric procedures. In the early 1960s, Jerger and colleagues (Jerger & Jerger, 1965; Jerger & Tillman, 1960) described a modified, and clinically feasible, version of a technique originally introduced by Rainville several years earlier (Rainville, 1955). This technique was not based on the principles of conventional bone-conduction audiometry. Rather, air-conduction pure-tone thresholds are first measured for each ear without any masking. Then, a masking noise is presented via a bone vibrator placed on the forehead at an intensity level approximating 2 volts RMS. Clinically, this level is produced by presenting masking noise by bone conduction near the output limit of the audiometer, typically about 55 dB HL for 500 Hz, and 60 or 65 dB HL for 1000, 2000, and 4000 Hz test frequencies. To perform the SAL test, therefore, one must have access to an audiometer that permits the presentation of masking noise via bone conduction. Before the SAL test is applied in a clinical facility, the average shift in air-conduction thresholds produced by this amount of masking noise at each test frequency is determined for a group of normal-hearing subjects.

In analysis of SAL test data, the clinician compares the air-conduction hearing threshold shift in the bone-conduction masking condition to the air-conduction hearing level without masking (Figure 3.10). If a patient's hearing loss is entirely conductive (normal bone-conduction thresholds), this shift will equal the normal shift value. That is, the bone-conduction masking will have the full effect on the normal cochlea of the patient with a purely conductive hearing loss. Normal bone conduction is presumed. If, on the other hand, the hearing loss is partially or completely sensory, masking noise will have no effect on air-conduction hearing thresholds until the intensity level of the masking signal exceeds bone-conduction hearing thresholds. There will be no masking-induced shift in hearing thresholds if

Patient Name: Age: Gender:

Date of Test: Tester:

Ear	Condition	500	1000	2000	4000	SRT
		Test Frequency in Hz				
Right	Quiet (dB HL)					
Right	Noise (dB HL)					
	SAL Shift Normal Value	45	45	50	55	
	Noise - SAL (Air-bone gap)					
Left	Quiet (dB HL)					
Left	Noise (dB HL)					
	SAL Shift Normal Value	45	45	50	55	
	Noise - SAL (Air-bone gap)					

Masking noise by bone-conduction (at forehead)

500 Hz   45 dB HL
1000 Hz   55 dB HL
2000 Hz   70 dB HL
4000 Hz   70 dB HL

FIGURE 3.10   Response record form used with the sensorineural acuity level (SAL) procedure for assessing bone-conduction hearing in patients posing masking problems. SAL shift normative values were obtained from a group of young, normal-hearing adults using a GSI 16 audiometer with TDH-39 earphones.

bone-conduction thresholds exceed 50 to 60 dB HL. The SAL procedure is most helpful clinically with patients demonstrating apparently large air-bone gaps in pure-tone audiometry and for whom the adequacy of masking in conventional air- or bone-conduction audiometry is questioned. Although infrequently used, SAL is an excellent test for pseudohypacusis (see Chapter 14).

DIAGNOSTIC AUDIOMETRY AND AUDITORY BRAINSTEM RESPONSE (ABR)

Although diagnostic audiometric tests, directed toward qualitative rather than quantitative results, are perhaps used less frequently than in the past, the clinician using these procedures must recognize that they often present the situation in which masking is required to ensure response from the ear being tested. And, although questions have been raised regarding the possibility of unusual effects when masking is used in diagnostic audiometry (Goldstein & Newman, 1985), there is no question that the failure to use masking will lead to erroneous results in at least some diagnostic tests. Particularly vulnerable to participation from the nontest ear are procedures such as the *Carhart Tone Decay Test* (Carhart, 1957; Jerger, Carhart, & Lassman, 1958) and the *Performance-Intensity Tests* (Jerger & Hayes, 1977; Jerger & Jerger, 1971). Tests such as these that involve presentation of the test signal at high intensity, often to an ear with unilateral sensorineural hearing loss, almost ensure a very large interaural difference with certain cross-over to the nontest ear. If tests such as these are to be used, the clinician must ensure against nontest ear response through the use of appropriate masking.

The principles of masking described in this chapter are not applied in ABR measurement. In fact, masking is required far less often in ABR measurement than in routine clinical audiometry. A complete discussion of masking in ABR measurement is beyond the scope of this chapter. The reader is referred to Hall (1992) for a detailed review of the indications for masking, and strategies for verifying ear-specific findings with air- and bone-conduction stimulation during ABR assessment. It is important to point out, however, that with appropriate ABR recording technique, and skillful analysis of ABR waveforms, one may obtain ear-specific findings with air- or bone-conduction stimulation even in patients with severe bilateral conductive hearing loss who present the traditional masking dilemma. ABR is particularly valuable for ear-specific assessment of sensorineural hearing status in infants and young children (refer to Chapters 7 and 11).

COMMENT

In 1972 the following statement was made to introduce a chapter on clinical masking:

> Of all the clinical procedures used in auditory assessment, masking is probably the most often misused and the least understood. For many clinicians the approach to masking is a haphazard, hit-or-miss bit of guess work with no basis in any set of principles. (Sanders, 1972, p. 111)

The problem leading to the masking difficulties at that time was twofold. First, although the basic principles of accurate and effective masking were well established through experimental research, the studies reporting those principles were published in a wide range of literature, much of which was generally unavailable to the clinician and even to many professionals and students in educational programs. Second, the masking equipment available was either inadequate or required special procedures for appropriate application. Both of those difficulties have now been overcome. Research findings have been brought together in a number of single sources that are readily available, and clinical audiometers now provide efficient masking noises calibrated in effective masking levels. Although clinical masking continues to pose challenging difficulties, the clinician now has ready access to the knowledge and equipment to solve whatever problems may arise in clinical masking.

REFERENCES

American National Standards Institute. (1972). *Artificial Headbone for the Calibration of Audiometer Bone Vibrators* (ANSI S3.13-1972). New York: Author.

American National Standards Institute. (1981). *Reference Equivalent Threshold Force Levels for Audiometric Bone Vibrators* (ANSI S3.26-1981). New York: Author.

American National Standards Institute. (1996). *Specifications for Audiometers* (ANSI S3.6-1996). New York: Author.

American Standards Association. (1951). *American Standard Specifications for Audiometers for General Diagnostic Purposes* (ASA Z24.5-1951). New York.

Carhart, R. (1957). Clinical determination of abnormal auditory adaptation. *Archives of Otolaryngology, 65,* 32–39.

Carhart, R. (1960). Assessment of sensorineural response in otosclerosis. *Archives of Otolaryngology, 71,* 141–149.

Carhart, R. (1971). Observations on relations between thresholds for pure tones and for speech. *Journal of Speech and Hearing Disorders, 36,* 476–483.

Denes, P., & Naunton, R. F. (1952). Masking in pure tone audiometry. *Proceedings of the Royal Society of Medicine, 45,* 790–794.

Dirks, D. (1963). *Factors Related to Reliability of Bone Conduction.* Unpublished doctoral dissertation, Northwestern University.

Dirks, D. (1964). Bone-conduction measurements. *Archives of Otolaryngology, 79,* 594–595.

Dirks, D., & Malmquist, C. (1964). Changes in bone-conduction thresholds produced by masking in the nontest ear. *Journal of Speech and Hearing Research, 7,* 271–278.

Dirks, D., & Swindeman, J. G. (1967). The variability of occluded and unoccluded bone-conduction thresholds. *Journal of Speech and Hearing Research, 10,* 232–249.

Egan, J. P., & Hake, H. W. (1950). On the masking pattern of a simple auditory stimulus. *Journal of the Acoustical Society of America, 22,* 622–630.

Feldman, A. S. (1961). Problems in the measurement of bone conduction. *Journal of Speech and Hearing Disorders, 26,* 39–44.

Fletcher, H. (1940). Auditory patterns. *Review of Modern Physics, 12,* 47–65.

Fletcher, H., & Munson, W. A. (1937). Relation between loudness and masking. *Journal of the Acoustical Society of America, 9,* 1–10.

Glorig, A. (1965). *Audiometry: Principles and Practices.* Baltimore: Williams & Wilkins.

Goldstein, B. A., & Newman, C. W. (1985). Clinical masking. In J. Katz (Ed.), *Handbook of Clinical Audiology* (3rd. ed., pp. 170–201). Baltimore: Williams & Wilkins.

Hall, J. W. III. (1992). *Handbook of Auditory Evoked Responses* (pp. 156–160, 169–176). Boston: Allyn & Bacon.

Hawkins, J. E., & Stevens, S. S. (1950). Masking of pure tones and of speech by white noise. *Journal of the Acoustical Society of America, 22,* 6–13.

Hirsh, I. J., & Bowman, W. D. (1953). Masking of speech by bands of noise. *Journal of the Acoustical Society of America, 25,* 1175–1180.

Hood, J. D. (1960). Principles and practices of bone conduction audiometry. *The Laryngoscope, 70,* 1211–1228.

Jerger, J., Carhart, R., & Lassman, J. (1958). Clinical observations on excessive threshold adaptation. *Archives of Otolaryngology, 99,* 409–413.

Jerger, J., & Hayes, D. (1977). Diagnostic speech audiometry. *Archives of Otolaryngology, 103,* 216–222.

Jerger J., & Jerger S. (1965). Critical evaluation of SAL audiometry. *Journal of Speech and Hearing Research, 8,* 103–128.

Jerger, J., & Jerger, S. (1971). Diagnostic significance of PB word functions. *Archives of Otolaryngology, 93,* 573–580.

Jerger, J., & Tillman, T. (1960). A new method for the clinical determination of sensorineural ears. *Archives of Otolaryngology, 71,* 948–955.

Jerger, J. F., Tillman, T. W., & Peterson, J. L. (1960). Masking by octave bands of noise in normal and impaired ears. *Journal of the Acoustical Society of America, 32,* 385–390.

Koenig, E. (1962a). On the use of hearing-aid type phones in clinical audiometry. *Acta Otolaryngologica, 55,* 131–143.

Koenig, E. (1962b). The use of masking noise and its limitations in clinical audiometry. *Acta Otolaryngologica, (Supplement 180),* 1.

Konkle, D. F., & Berry, G. A. (1983). Masking in speech audiometry. In D. F. Konkle & W. F. Rintelmann (Eds.), *Principles of Speech Audiometry* (pp. 285–319). Baltimore: University Park Press.

Liden, G. (1954). Speech audiometry. *Acta Otolaryngologica (Supplement 114),* 72–76.

Liden, G., Nilsson, G., & Anderson, H. (1959a). Narrow-band masking with white noise. *Acta Otolaryngologica, 50,* 116–124.

Liden, G., Nilsson, G., & Anderson, H. (1959b). Masking in clinical audiometry. *Acta Otolaryngologica, 50,* 125–136.

Lizar, D., Peck, J., Schwartz, A., & Stockdell, K. (1969). *Masking in Speech Audiometry.* Unpublished report, Vanderbilt University.

Miller, G. A. (1947). The masking of speech. *Psychology Bulletin, 44,* 105–129.

Mueller, H. G. III, & Hall, J. W. III. (1998). *Audiologists' Desk Reference Volume II.* San Diego: Singular.

Naunton, R. F. (1960). A masking dilemma in bilateral conduction deafness. *Archives of Otolaryngology, 72,* 752–757.

O'Neill, J. J., & Oyer, H. J. (1966). *Applied Audiometry.* New York: Dodd, Mead.

Rainville, M. J. (1955). Nouvelle méthode d'assourdissement pour le releve des courbes de conduction osseuse. *Journal de Francais Oto-laryngologie, 4,* 851–858.

Sanders, J. W. (1972). Masking. In J. Katz (Ed.), *Handbook of Clinical Audiology* (pp. 111–142). Baltimore: Williams & Wilkins.

Sanders, J. W., & Rintelmann, W. F. (1964). Masking in audiometry: A clinical evaluation of three methods. *Archives of Oto-Laryngology, 80,* 541–556.

Setliff, W. M. (1971). *A Comparison of Four Noises for Masking Speech.* Unpublished master's thesis, Vanderbilt University.

Studebaker, G. A. (1962). On masking in bone-conduction testing. *Journal of Speech and Hearing Research, 5,* 215–227.

Studebaker, G. A. (1964). Clinical masking of air- and bone-conduction stimuli. *Journal of Speech and Hearing Disorders, 29,* 23–35.

Studebaker, G. A. (1967). Clinical masking of the nontest ear. *Journal of Speech and Hearing Disorders, 32,* 360–371.

Studebaker, G. A. (1973). Auditory masking. In J. Jerger (Ed.), *Modern Developments in Audiology* (2nd ed., pp. 117–154). New York: Academic Press.

Wegel, R. L., & Lane, C. E. (1924). Auditory masking of one pure tone by another and its probable relation to dynamics of inner ear. *Physics Review, 23,* 266–285.

Zwislocki, J. (1953). Acoustic attenuation between ears. *Journal of the Acoustical Society of America, 25,* 752–759.

Zwislocki, J. (1966). Eine verbesserte vertaubungsmethode fur die audiometrie. *Translations of the Beltone Institute for Hearing Research. Acta Otolaryngologica, 39,* 338–356.

CHAPTER 4

TYMPANOMETRY: BASIC PRINCIPLES AND CLINICAL APPLICATIONS

ROBERT H. MARGOLIS
LISA L. HUNTER

INTRODUCTION AND A LITTLE HISTORY

Tympanometry is unique among audiologic procedures. While most of our tests are rather logical applications of methods that were developed for behavioral or physiologic assessment—audiometry from auditory psychophysics, ABR from electrophysiology—the roots of tympanometry are as diverse as the principles governing transoceanic transmission lines, research on early telephone transducers, and observations of the effects of air pressure on hearing. An understanding of the clinical application of tympanometry does not come naturally from knowledge of the anatomy, physiology, and pathology of the middle ear. A different set of underlying principles is required—one that is usually better understood by physicists and acoustical engineers than by clinicians concerned with ear disease. In this chapter we review the physical principles of aural acoustic immittance measurement that form the basis for the clinical test we call tympanometry.

The history of the development of tympanometry, reviewed elsewhere (Shallop, 1976; Van Camp, Margolis, Wilson, Creten, & Shanks, 1986), might begin with informal observations of the effects of air pressure on hearing, published early in the nineteenth century in England by William Hyde Wollaston and Sir Charles Wheatstone. Although these papers described some perceptive observations and predate any real research in the area, they are not the tightly controlled research papers found in our contemporary journals. In fact, it is hard to imagine that anything like them would be published by any present-day scientific journal. But the observation that air pressure on either side of the tympanic membrane alters the function of the ear would be applied to clinical problems as early as the latter half of the nineteenth century by the pioneers of otology, Toynbee and Politzer.

At about the same time, Wheatstone's uncle, Oliver Heaviside (1850–1925), who was unemployed from the time he was 24 until his death at age 75, wrote prolifically on a variety of physical and mathematical topics, including the age of the earth, operational calculus, and electrical circuit theory. He was probably best known for his theoretical work on long electrical transmission lines, an important topic at that time because of the need for transoceanic telephone cables. In the process of defining the characteristics of long transmission lines, Heaviside coined the term *impedance*, wrote its defining equations for electrical circuits, and demonstrated the usefulness of vector mathematics for circuit analysis. Precisely the same principles would be applied to acoustic systems by the early telephone engineers in this century (West, 1928), and a powerful tool, acoustic impedance measurement, was born. That tool would be used to design loudspeakers for acoustic systems as large as a sports stadium and as small as the space in front of a CIC hearing aid. And it would form the basis for the clinical test we call tympanometry. (By the way, Heaviside was hearing impaired, perhaps the reason for his reclusive lifestyle [Nahin, 1988].)

The clinical application of acoustic impedance measurement was born in the Rigshospitalet (State Hospital) in Copenhagen, Denmark in the 1940s. There Otto Metz produced his landmark work on the acoustic impedance of normal and pathological ears (Metz, 1946). Using an ingenious, pre-electric device (Figure 4.1), Metz developed the theory of acoustic impedance of the ear and tested a large number of normal subjects and patients with ear disease. He was also the first to study the acoustic stapedius reflex in patients with ear disease.

The method that Metz developed would be further refined by several of his colleagues at the same hospital. Acoustic impedance measurement would not be useful for routine clinical evaluation until an additional dimension, ear canal air pressure, was added to the measurement. By measuring impedance as a function of ear canal pressure, it was possible to estimate the impedance of the middle ear without the contaminating influence of the ear canal. In addition, the tympanometric patterns that were observed in normal and abnormal ears were quickly found to have

Acknowledgment: This work was supported by grant no. P50 DC03093 from the NIH National Institute of Deafness and Other Communication Disorders.

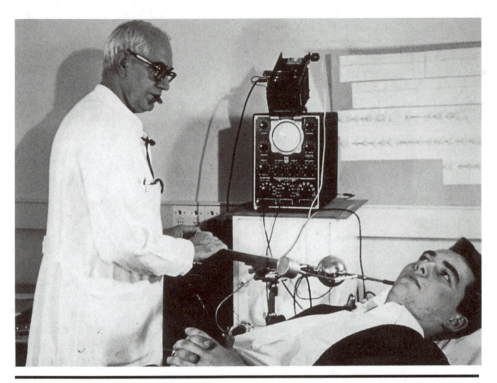

FIGURE 4.1 Otto Metz testing a patient with the Metz bridge (c. 1955).

diagnostic significance. Although several investigators contributed to this refinement, it was Terkildsen (Terkildsen & Nielsen, 1960; Terkildsen & Thomsen, 1959) who developed the method that would be incorporated in the first commercially produced clinical instrument (see Figure 5.1 in Chapter 5).

The advent of clinical instruments in the 1960s and 1970s led to many observations of the effects of specific ear pathologies on tympanograms. A variety of tympanometric patterns were described for patients of different ages, for different probe frequencies, and for different ear diseases. The wide variety of patterns was not well understood until a group of physicists at the University of Antwerp took an interest in understanding the relations between tympanometric patterns and the physics of the middle ear. The result was the *Vanhuyse model* (pronounced VAN-EYES-UH), perhaps the most important single contribution to understanding tympanograms (Vanhuyse, Creten, & Van Camp, 1975). The model provides a basis for understanding the effects of frequency, pathology, and middle ear development on tympanometric patterns. It is the basis for clinical interpretation of tympanograms and a tool for experimental studies of pathology on middle ear function.

There are other significant characters in the story—Bekesy, Zwislocki, Jerger, Colletti, and Van Camp, to name a few of the most significant contributors. Although much has been learned about the acoustic immittance characteristics of normal and pathological ears, the usual clinical approach to tympanometry is not substantially different than that used by the first clinicians to use this tool in the late 1960s and early 1970s. Although that approach is adequate for most patients, a more systematic and quantitative approach, based on an understanding of the underlying physical principles, can enhance the usefulness of the technique and make us better clinicians.

PHYSICAL PRINCIPLES OF AURAL ACOUSTIC IMMITTANCE[1]

The middle ear is a transducer that converts acoustic energy into mechanical energy. It is so efficient that eardrum vibrations for sounds that are near threshold cannot be detected by the most sensitive instruments. Yet it responds with almost unmeasurable distortion to sound pressures that are a million times greater than the sound pressure at threshold. This remarkable system achieves its sensitivity and dynamic range by a delicate mechanical balance of anatomic structures that exist in an equally delicate physiologic environment. It is not surprising that pathologic disturbances of the middle ear produce changes in its mechanical properties. With ingenious electroacoustic devices, and an

---

[1]See also Margolis (1981), Van Camp et al. (1986), and Wiley and Fowler (1997).

understanding of some basic physical principles, pathologic changes in middle ear function can be measured, and these measurements can be used to diagnose ear disease and understand the effect of disease on middle ear function.

The direct approach to the evaluation of a mechanical system is to observe the effect that a known force has on the system. With a procedure as simple and direct as deforming the basilar membrane with a hair, Bekesy determined some of the mechanical characteristics of the cochlear partition. If we could use a similar direct approach to examine the response of the middle ear, we could probably improve our ability to evaluate middle ear function. Because it is not feasible to directly probe the eardrum or ossicles, an indirect method has been developed based on measurements of the *acoustic immittance* in the ear canal. The acoustic immittance measured in the ear canal is a result of the combined effects of the air volume in the canal and the characteristics of the middle ear. If we know the effect of the ear canal, we can evaluate the middle ear. Studies of the acoustic immittance of normal ears form a basis for determining abnormal middle ear conditions.

Acoustic immittance is a generic term that refers to *acoustic impedance* and *acoustic admittance* and all of their components. Acoustic immittance measurement is a method for analyzing the responses of acoustic systems to sound. Other kinds of systems (e.g., mechanical and electrical systems) can be analyzed using similar techniques. Because mechanical systems are simpler and more familiar, the concept of *mechanical immittance* will be developed in this chapter, and then the same principles will be applied to acoustic systems, specifically, the ear. The immittance of a mechanical system is determined by exerting a force on the system and observing its response. We will begin with the concept of *force*.

Force

An action that is capable of moving a body or changing the motion of a body is a force. In the international unit system (*Système Internationale*, SI)[2] the unit of force is the Newton (N). One N is the force required to change the velocity of a mass of 1 kilogram (kg) by 1 meter/second (m/s) in one second. For example, if a 1 kg mass at rest is set into motion accelerating to a velocity of 1 m/s in one second, the force was 1 N.

Force can be static (constant) or dynamic (changing with time). Of course, there are an infinite number of ways that a force could change in time. The simplest time-varying pattern is one that changes sinusoidally, illustrated in Figure 4.2. A sinusoidally changing force can be described mathematically by

$$F(t) = A \sin (2\pi ft) \qquad (4.1)$$

where F(t) is the force at any instant in time, A is the peak amplitude, f is the frequency of the sinusoidal change, and t is the time at which the measurement is made. The period of a sinusoidal waveform, denoted T, is the time elapsed during one cycle. It is convenient to express a sinusoidally changing force with one number that expresses its magnitude. This is typically done by calculating the root mean square (rms) value of the sinusoidally changing force. That is, each instantaneous force is squared, the squared values are averaged, and the square root of the average is the rms force. We commonly employ this rms method to express the sound pressure of an acoustic signal.

Mechanical Immittance

When a force is applied to an object, the object moves with a velocity that is proportional to the applied force. The relationship between the velocity and the applied force provides the basis for quantitative analysis of the mechanical characteristics of the system. There are a number of ways that this relationship can be expressed. Recall that *immittance* is a generic term that includes a number of quantities with different units of measurement. The two approaches to immittance measurement are *impedance* and *admittance*.

Mechanical Impedance

Mechanical impedance is the opposition offered by an object to the flow of energy. In simple terms, the mechanical impedance of an object is an expression of how difficult it is to move. If the same force moves one object faster than another, the first object has a lower mechanical

---

[2]See Van Camp et al. (1986) for a discussion of units and unit systems.

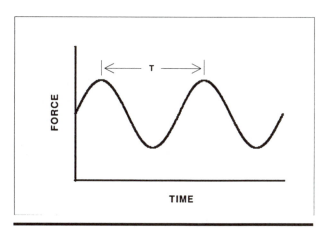

FIGURE 4.2   Sinusoidally varying force with period T.

impedance than the second. Stated more formally, mechanical impedance Z_m is the ratio of the applied force F to the resulting velocity V:

$$Z_m = F/V\angle\emptyset_z \qquad (4.2)$$

Since the unit of force is the Newton (N) and the unit of velocity is meters/second (m/s), mechanical impedance has units N/m/s, or more simply, N•s/m. One N•s/m is a mechanical ohm.

The force may be static or dynamic. A dynamic force is usually expressed as an rms value. In a linear system, a sinusoidal force results in a sinusoidally changing velocity, also expressed as an rms value. The frequency of the sinusoidally changing velocity is identical to that of the force. $\angle\emptyset_z$ is the impedance phase angle and represents the time relationship between F and V. The phase angle gives important information about the characteristics of *mass, compliance,* and *friction* that contribute to the impedance of the system.

The mass, compliance, and friction of a mechanical system determine its impedance. *Ideal* mass, compliance, and friction elements are those that possess only one of these characteristics. Ideal elements do not exist in the real world but they are useful concepts. The three types of ideal elements respond in a unique manner when acted upon by a force.

When a force is applied to an ideal mass, it moves in the direction of the applied force until another force stops it. In the real world, it does not move indefinitely because it encounters friction, which eventually stops the motion. The impedance offered by a mass is its *mass reactance* X_m.

A compliant element is a spring. Compliance is the ability of the spring to be compressed, the inverse of stiffness. When a force is applied to an ideal spring, it is compressed and returns to its original position when the applied force is removed. The impedance offered by a spring is its *compliant reactance* X_c.

The *total reactance* of a system is the combination of all the component mass and spring elements. That is,

$$X_{total} = X_m + X_c \qquad (4.3)$$

A system that has both mass and spring elements can be characterized as a mass *or* a spring, depending on which type of reactance is greater. Because values of X_c are negative, a negative total reactance indicates that the system is dominated by spring elements, and a positive total reactance indicates that the system is dominated by mass elements.

The impedance that results from friction is called *resistance* R. Friction causes energy loss through dissipation as heat. Thus, mass and spring elements (*reactive* elements) store energy and friction dissipates energy.

The total impedance of a mechanical system composed of mass, spring, and friction elements is

$$Z_m = R + jX_{total} \qquad (4.4)$$

The j mathematically represents $\sqrt{-1}$ in complex number notation and indicates that resistance and reactance cannot be combined by simple arithmetic.[3]

Eqs. 4.2 and 4.4 represent two ways to define the mechanical impedance of a system. Eq. 4.2 defines impedance as a force/velocity ratio with a specific time relationship between the force and velocity. Eq. 4.4 expresses impedance as the combined contributions of mass and spring elements (X_{total}) and friction (R). Because Eq. 4.2 can be represented by a vector with a specific length and angle, it is referred to as *polar notation*. Eq. 4.4 represents the vector in terms of its rectangular components (R and X_{total}) and is referred to as *rectangular notation*.

Vector Analysis

The relations expressed in Eqs. 4.2 and 4.4 indicate that impedance is a *vector*, a two-dimensional quantity that can be analyzed into polar or rectangular components.

Vector analysis is a useful way to understand the concept of *complex impedance*. A complete description of the impedance of a system requires two numbers—either magnitude and phase (Eq. 4.2) or resistance and reactance (Eq. 4.4). A graphic representation of a vector plot shows how these representations are related. Consider the complex mechanical system schematized in Figure 4.3. In order to move the system, a mass has to be set into motion, a spring has to be compressed, and friction is encountered when the components move. Similar processes need to occur to set the middle ear into vibration. This system,

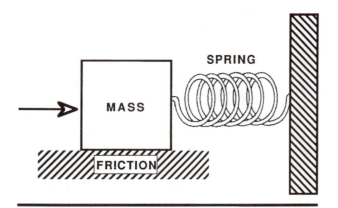

FIGURE 4.3 A complex mechanical system composed of a mass and spring. Friction is encountered when the mass and spring move. The impedance of the system is the vector sum of the effects of the mass, spring, and friction.

---

[3]See Nahin (1988) Tech Note 1, p. 204, for the mathematical basis for $\sqrt{-1}$ in vector analysis.

then, has compliant reactance associated with the spring, mass reactance associated with the mass, and resistance resulting from friction. In the vector system illustrated in Figure 4.4A, compliant reactance X_c is shown as a negative value on the y-axis, mass reactance X_m is shown as a positive value on the y-axis, and resistance R is shown as a positive value on the x-axis. Total reactance X_{total} is the sum of X_c and X_m. X_{total} and R can be thought of as vectors that produce a resultant vector, impedance Z with a phase angle $\emptyset_z$. From Eq. 4.2 it is evident that $|Z| = F/V$. (When the impedance magnitude is given without the phase angle it is placed in absolute value signs.)

Mechanical Admittance

For reasons that will be discussed below, it is convenient to characterize the immittance of the ear as an admittance rather than impedance. The mechanical admittance Y of a system is the reciprocal of impedance:

$$Y = V/F \;\angle\emptyset_Y \qquad (4.5)$$

Just as impedance has components representing mass, compliance, and friction, admittance can be analyzed into similar components. The admittance associated with a mass is *mass susceptance* B_m. The admittance associated with

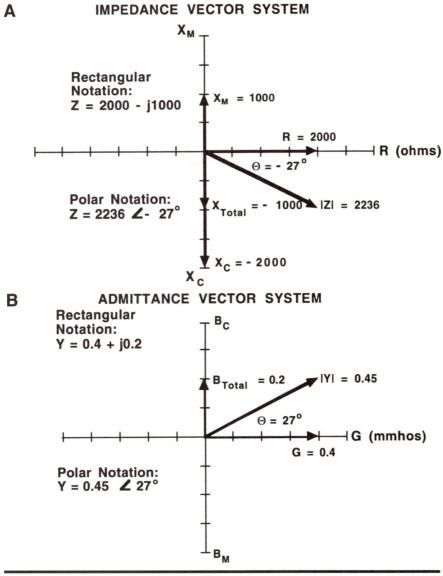

FIGURE 4.4 Impedance and admittance vector systems. (A) The impedance vector system is composed of mass reactance X_m and compliant reactance X_c, which sum to total reactance X_t and resistance R. X_t and R combine to form Z, the impedance magnitude that has a phase angle Θ. (B) The admittance vector system is calculated from the impedance vector values by the conversion equations given in Table 4.2.

spring elements is *compliant susceptance* B_c. The admittance resulting from friction is *conductance* G. The total susceptance B_{total} is the sum of the mass and compliant susceptances:

$$B_{total} = B_m + B_c \qquad (4.6)$$

Admittance can be stated in terms of susceptance and conductance:

$$Y = G + jB_{total} \qquad (4.7)$$

Eqs. 4.5 and 4.7 represent the polar and rectangular forms of admittance. Just as impedance can be graphically represented as a vector system, admittance can also be represented as a pair of vectors representing conductance on the *x*-axis and susceptance on the *y*-axis. Figure 4.4B illustrates the vector representation of admittance.

Table 4.1 presents a summary of immittance quantities, their definitions, and their units. Table 4.2 presents the formulae defining the relationships among immittance quantities. For further discussion of immittance quantities, their

TABLE 4.1   Immittance quantities.

QUANTITY	SYMBOL	UNIT	DEFINITION
Force	F	Newton (N)	An action that is capable of moving a body or changing the motion of a body.
Pressure	P	Pascal (Pa)	Force per unit area. 1 Pa = 1 N/m^2.
Volume Velocity	U	m^3/s	Volume of a medium (e.g., air) that moves past an imaginary plane per unit time.
Acoustic Mass	M_a	Pa•s^2/m^3	Ratio of sound pressure to the resulting change in volume velocity. An acoustic mass element is a volume of air that moves as a unit in response to sound, such as the air in an open tube.
Acoustic Stiffness	K_a	Pa/m^3	Ratio of change in sound pressure to the resulting change in volume displacement. An acoustic stiffness element is a volume of air that is alternately compressed and expanded by sound, such as the air in rigid enclosure.
Acoustic Compliance	C_a	m^3/Pa	The inverse of acoustic stiffness.
Acoustic Immittance	None	None	A generic term referring to acoustic impedance, acoustic admittance, and all of their rectangular and polar components.
Acoustic Impedance	Z_a	Acoustic ohm	Opposition offered by a system to the flow of acoustic energy; the reciprocal of acoustic admittance.
Acoustic Reactance	X_a	Acoustic ohm	The impedance offered by acoustic mass and acoustic compliance elements.
Compliant (Stiffness) Reactance	X_c	Acoustic ohm	The impedance offered by acoustic compliance elements.
Mass Reactance	X_m	Acoustic ohm	The impedance offered by mass elements.
Acoustic Resistance	R_a	Acoustic ohm	The impedance resulting from friction.
Acoustic Admittance	Y_a	Acoustic millimho (mmho)	The ease with which energy flows through an acoustic system; the reciprocal of acoustic impedance.
Acoustic Susceptance	B_a	Acoustic millimho (mmho)	The admittance offered by acoustic compliance and acoustic mass elements.
Compliant Susceptance	B_c	Acoustic millimho (mmho)	The admittance offered by acoustic compliance elements.
Mass Susceptance	B_m	Acoustic millimho (mmho)	The admittance offered by acoustic mass elements.
Acoustic Conductance	G_a	Acoustic millimho (mmho)	The admittance associated with friction in an acoustic system.

TABLE 4.2 Relations among acoustic immittance quantities.

DEFINING EQUATIONS

$$Z_a = P/U \angle \emptyset_z \qquad Y_a = U/P \angle \emptyset_Y$$

$$Z_a = R_a + jX_a \qquad Y_a = G_a + jB_a$$

COMPUTATIONAL EQUATIONS

$$|Z_a| = \sqrt{R_a^2 + X_a^2} \qquad |Y_a| = \sqrt{G_a^2 + B_a^2}$$

$$\emptyset_Z = \arctan(X_a/R_a) \qquad \emptyset_Y = \arctan(B_a/G_a)$$

CONVERSION EQUATIONS

$$R_a = \frac{G_a}{G_a^2 + B_a^2} \qquad G_a = \frac{R_a}{R_a^2 + X_a^2}$$

$$X_a = \frac{-B_a}{G_a^2 + B_a^2} \qquad B_a = \frac{-X_a}{R_a^2 + X_a^2}$$

$$\emptyset_Z = -\emptyset_Y \qquad \emptyset_Y = -\emptyset_Z$$

relationships, and their units see American National Standards Institute (1987) and Van Camp and colleagues (1986).

Acoustic Immittance

The principles governing mechanical systems can be applied to acoustic systems. Like mechanical systems, the acoustic immittance of a system is determined by its mass, compliance, and friction. An acoustic mass is a volume of air that moves as a unit without compression, such as the air in an open tube. An acoustic spring (compliance) is a volume of air that is alternately compressed and expanded, such as a rigidly enclosed volume of air. Friction occurs as a result of collisions of molecules in the medium (such as air) and between the medium and surrounding structures.

We can define acoustic impedance Z_a by modifying Eq. 4.2. *Sound pressure* P is substituted for force and *volume velocity* U is substituted for velocity:

$$Z_a = P/U \angle \emptyset_z \qquad (4.8)$$

Eq. 4.8 is the polar form of acoustic impedance. In rectangular form,

$$Z_a = R_a + jX_a \qquad (4.9a)$$

X_a (or X_{total}) is the sum of the compliant reactance and mass reactance. When X_a has a positive value, the reactance associated with mass elements is greater than the reactance associated with spring elements and the system is said to be mass controlled. When X_a is negative, the system is stiffness controlled or compliance controlled.

Acoustic admittance is the reciprocal of acoustic impedance. From Eq. 4.8,

$$Y_a = U/P \angle \emptyset_Y \qquad (4.9b)$$

or in rectangular form

$$Y_a = G_a + jB_a \qquad (4.10)$$

When B_a is positive, the system is compliance controlled or stiffness controlled. A negative B_a indicates a mass-controlled system.

Measurements of acoustic immittance in the ear canal are influenced by both mechanical and acoustic elements. Because the middle ear is a transducer, converting acoustic energy to mechanical energy, both acoustic and mechanical structures comprise the system. The enclosed volumes of air on both sides of the tympanic membrane act as acoustic compliance elements (acoustic springs). At high frequencies there are significant acoustic-mass effects associated with these air volumes. The eardrum, ligaments, tendons, and muscles of the middle ear act as mechanical springs that return to their original position when stretched and released. The ossicles are mechanical masses. Although tympanometry is based on the measurement of acoustic impedance in the ear canal, it is really the *mechanoacoustic* middle ear system that we are evaluating.

Acoustic Immittance Units

From Eq. 4.8 we can determine the units for acoustic impedance. Sound pressure P is force per unit area and has units N/m^2. One N/m^2 is a Pascal (Pa). Volume velocity is the rate at which a volume of air moves past an imaginary plane and has units m^3/s. Acoustic impedance, then, has units $N/m^2/m^3/s$, or $Pa/m^3/s$, or more simply, $Pa \cdot s/m^3$. One $Pa \cdot s/m^3$ is one acoustic ohm in the mks unit system. It has become conventional in tympanometry to use the cgs unit system. One cgs ohm is equal to 10,000 mks ohms. One cgs ohm, then, is $10^5 \, Pa \cdot s/m^3$.

The unit of admittance is the mho, the inverse of the ohm. One mks mho is one $m^3/Pa \cdot s$ and one cgs mho is one $m^3/10^5 Pa \cdot s$ or $10^{-5} m^3/Pa \cdot s$. Because the admittance of the ear is a fraction of a mho, it is convenient to use the millimho (mmho) which is one-thousandth of a mho. One cgs millimho is $10^{-8} m^3/Pa \cdot s$.

Frequency Dependence of Acoustic Immittance

We know that virtually every measure of auditory function depends on the frequency of the stimulus. Audiometric thresholds are typically measured over a 5-octave range because hearing sensitivity in normal and impaired ears is frequency dependent. One of the sources of the frequency dependence of auditory sensitivity is the frequency dependence of the transmission of sound through the middle ear.

Of the three types of mechanical and acoustic elements, one—acoustic resistance—is independent of frequency. The immittance associated with springs and masses, however, is strongly dependent on frequency. This is evident in the next two equations.

$$X_m = 2\pi fM \qquad (4.11)$$

$$X_c = \frac{-\rho c^2}{2\pi fV} \qquad (4.12)$$

where M is mass, ρ is the density of the medium (usually air), c is the velocity of sound, and V is the volume of an enclosed quantity of air (an acoustic spring). Eq. 4.11 expresses the relationship between mass reactance X_m, mass M, and frequency f. The reactance of a mass increases in direct proportion to frequency. Mass elements, then, have a low reactance at low frequencies and a high reactance at high frequencies. In contrast, Eq. 4.12 shows that the reactance of a spring is inversely proportional to frequency so that spring elements have a high reactance at low frequencies and a low reactance at high frequencies.

Because mass reactance increases with frequency, adding mass to a system will have a greater effect at high frequencies than at low frequencies. A mass on the tympanic membrane causes a downward sloping hearing loss (mass tilt). Because stiffness reactance decreases with frequency, adding stiffness to a system has a greater effect at low frequencies. Conditions that stiffen the middle ear,

such as ossicular adhesion or negative middle ear pressure, cause an upward sloping hearing loss (stiffness tilt).

If the reactance of spring elements decreases with frequency and the reactance of mass elements increases with frequency, then a system composed of a combination of mass and spring elements will be maximally efficient at one frequency at which the compliant and mass suspectance are in balance. This is called the *resonant frequency*. At the resonant frequency $X_{total} = 0$ and $Z = R$. That is, the reactances associated with the masses and springs cancel and the impedance of the system consists solely of the resistive component.

Acoustic Immittance of Complex Systems

Complex systems are those comprised of a combination of mass, compliance, and resistive elements. The middle ear system has been modeled as a complex network of elements representing the various anatomical structures of the ear (Goode, Killion, Nakimura, & Nashihara, 1994; Kringlbotn, 1988; Zwislocki, 1962). These models predict the input and output characteristics of the middle ear and can be used to predict the effects of pathology on middle ear function. The Zwislocki model is shown in Figure 4.5.

The Zwislocki model represents the transmission pathway from the ear canal to the cochlea and is composed of series elements (components 1, 3, 5, and 7) and parallel, or shunt, elements (components 2, 4, and 6). In order for sound to reach the cochlea it must travel through the series elements. Sound that passes through the shunt elements does not reach the cochlea and represents energy that does not contribute to hearing. Note that the middle ear cavities are shown as the first element (component 1), preceding the eardrum (components 2 and 3). This seems counterintuitive since we know that anatomically the eardrum precedes the

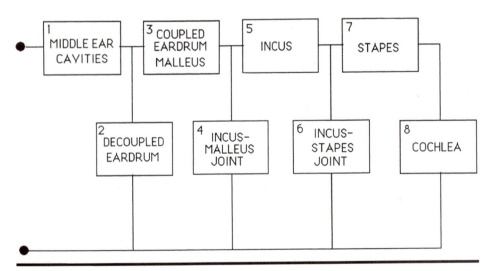

FIGURE 4.5 *Zwislocki middle ear model.*

middle ear cavities. However, in order for the eardrum to move, the air in the middle ear must expand or contract. Functionally, then, the middle ear cavities represent a series element at the input to the system.

The eardrum appears in two locations, as a shunt element (component 2) and as a series element (component 3). This indicates that some of the vibration of the eardrum is coupled to the ossicular chain and some of its vibration is energy that is not transmitted through the middle ear.

The incus-malleus joint (component 4) and the incus-stapes joint (component 6) are shown as shunt elements because there is some energy loss at the joints.

The model helps us understand why the relationship between tympanometry and hearing is complex. Because tympanometry is a measure of the *input immittance* of the system, it is influenced by both shunt and series elements. Sound that is heard is transmitted through only the series elements. The components that most influence the input immittance are those series and shunt elements that are closest to the input. Thus, the tympanogram is dominated by the middle ear cavities, the eardrum, and the malleus. A substantial change at the output of a complex system can have a small or negligible effect on the input immittance. An example of this is otosclerosis in which the impedance of the stapes becomes virtually infinite but it has little effect on the tympanogram (Shahnaz & Polka, in press).

The goal of tympanometry is to determine the input characteristics of the middle ear, independent of the ear canal. The ear canal and middle ear can be modeled as a system with two impedances which may be either in series or in parallel. Network representations of series and parallel systems are shown in Figure 4.6.

The input impedance of the series system shown in Figure 4.6 is

$$Z_i = Z_1 + Z_2 \qquad (4.13)$$

The input impedance of the parallel system shown in Figure 4.6 is given by

$$\frac{1}{Z_i} = \frac{1}{Z_1} + \frac{1}{Z_2} \qquad (4.14)$$

Solving for Z_i

$$Z_i = \frac{Z_1 Z_2}{Z_1 + Z_2} \qquad (4.15)$$

Because admittance is the reciprocal of impedance Eq. 4.14 can be rewritten as follows:

$$Y_i = Y_1 + Y_2 \qquad (4.16)$$

Eqs. 4.13 and 4.16 reveal two simple rules governing the immittance of series and parallel systems. The input impedance of a series system is the sum of the impedances

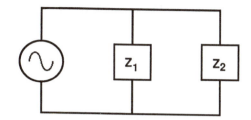

PARALLEL SYSTEM

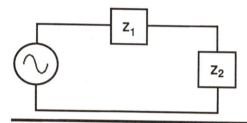

SERIES SYSTEM

FIGURE 4.6 Parallel and series systems. *Top panel:* A parallel circuit composed of a sinusoidal source of energy and two impedances (Z_1 and Z_2) configured in parallel. *Bottom panel:* A series circuit composed of a sinusoidal source of energy and two impedances (Z_1 and Z_2) configured in series.

of its components. The input admittance of a parallel system is the sum of the admittances of its components.

If we view the ear as a system consisting of two components, we can use these rules to determine the interaction between the ear canal and the middle ear. Anatomically, the ear canal and middle ear appear to be in series. However, acoustically, they behave as parallel elements.

From Eq. 4.13 we see that the input impedance Z_i of a series system is greater than the impedance of either component. Not so obviously, Eq. 4.14 and 4.15 indicate that the input impedance of a parallel system is less than either component. Acoustic impedance measurements have shown that the input impedance at the entrance to the ear canal is less than the impedance of either the ear canal volume or the middle ear measured separately. This suggests that the ear canal and middle ear are configured as a parallel acoustic system. Another characteristic of a parallel acoustic system is that the sound pressure delivered to each element is the same. At the low frequencies typically used for aural acoustic impedance measurements, the sound pressure at the entrance to the eardrum and the sound pressure at the tympanic membrane are virtually identical. This again suggests that the ear canal and middle ear can be represented as a parallel acoustic system.

If we let Z_1 represent the ear canal and Z_2 represent the middle ear, we can solve Eq. 4.15 for the middle ear impedance. Denoting the ear canal impedance as Z_{ec}, the middle ear impedance as Z_{me}, and the measured impedance at the lateral end of the ear canal as Z, we can rewrite Eq. 4.15 as follows:

$$Z = \frac{Z_{ec}Z_{me}}{Z_{ec} + Z_{me}} \qquad (4.17)$$

Solving for Z_{me}

$$Z_{me} = \frac{Z_{ec}Z}{Z_{ec} - Z} \qquad (4.18)$$

Alternatively, we can determine the input admittance from Eq. 4.16. First, let us rewrite Eq. 4.16 in terms of the admittance of the ear canal Y_{ec}, the admittance of the middle ear Y_{me}, and the admittance at the lateral end of the ear canal Y.

$$Y = Y_{ec} + Y_{me} \qquad (4.19)$$

Solving for Y_{me}

$$Y_{me} = Y - Y_{ec} \qquad (4.20)$$

The point of this exercise is to demonstrate that the admittance measured at the lateral end of the ear canal is more easily corrected for ear canal volume than the impedance. Eq. 4.18 is a complex relationship where Eq. 4.20 is a simple one. Eq. 4.20 tells us that a simple subtraction of the admittance associated with ear canal volume from the measured admittance will yield the admittance of the middle ear. *The simpler relationship expressed in Eq. 4.20 compared to Eq. 4.18 is the reason that tympanometric measurements are made in admittance rather than impedance.*

Determining the Admittance of the Ear Canal

Eq. 4.20 provides a method for determining the admittance of the middle ear from the measured admittance Y and the admittance of the ear canal Y_{ec}. How can we estimate Y_{ec}? If we know the ear canal volume V, we can calculate Y_{ec}. Since the susceptance of a volume of air is the reciprocal of its reactance, we can rewrite Eq. 4.12 in terms of compliant susceptance B_c and volume V:

$$B_c = \frac{2\pi fV}{\rho c^2} \qquad (4.21)$$

where the unit of B_c is the mho (the inverse of an ohm) and volume V is in in cm^3. At 226 Hz, $2\pi f/\rho c^2 = 0.001$, so we can write Eq. 4.21 as follows:

$$B_c = 0.001 \, V \qquad (4.22)$$

Converting to mmhos,

$$B_c \text{ (in mmhos)} = V \qquad (4.23)$$

That is, at 226 Hz, the susceptance (in mmho) of an enclosed volume of air that conforms to certain constraints on its geometry is numerically equal to its volume (in cm^3). So the susceptance of a volume of air of 1 cm^3 is 1 mmho. This is a convenient relationship that simplifies the calibration of instruments that use a 226 Hz probe frequency. In fact, that is precisely why the 226 Hz probe frequency was selected.

Now we can calculate the susceptance of the ear canal if we know its volume. Because an enclosed volume of air has no resistive (or conductance) component, we also know its admittance. The G term in Eq. 4.10 is zero, so at 226 Hz, $Y_{ec} = B = V$.

How do we determine the volume of the ear canal? The first commercially available instrument for measurement of aural acoustic immittance, the Zwislocki acoustic impedance bridge, manufactured by Grason-Stadler, Inc., obtained an estimate of the ear canal volume by pouring alcohol into the ear canal from a calibrated syringe (Zwislocki, 1963). This approach produces a good measurement of ear canal volume but is not practical in the clinic. An alternative approach was suggested by Terkildsen and Thomsen (1959) in the very first article on tympanometry. By pressurizing the ear canal, the middle ear could be stiffened to the point that the middle ear admittance becomes nearly zero. From Eq. 4.20 it is evident that the measured admittance in that condition becomes the admittance of the ear canal. This acoustic method provides a reasonably accurate measure of the ear canal volume (Shanks & Lilly, 1981) and provides the basis for measurement of the middle ear impedance from tympanometry. This method has been shown to produce estimates of middle ear impedance that are comparable to those obtained by laboratory methods (Margolis, Van Camp, Wilson, & Creten, 1985).

Calculating the Admittance of the Middle Ear

Using Eq. 4.20 we can calculate the admittance of the middle ear by subtracting the admittance of the ear canal from the measured admittance. The measured admittance that we are most interested in is the one corresponding to the peak of the tympanogram. The admittance of the ear canal is taken from the positive or negative tail of the tympanogram. The negative tail provides the more accurate estimate of ear canal volume (Shanks & Lilly, 1981). Many instruments, however, use the positive tail value. From the tympanogram in Figure 4.7, the admittance of the middle ear is 0.52 mmho using the negative tail and 0.45 using the positive tail. Because of the asymmetry of tympanograms, the middle ear admittance using the negative tail value is almost always greater than that obtained using the positive tail (Margolis & Smith, 1977). It is necessary, therefore, to use different norms for admittance calculated using the positive tail and that obtained using the negative tail.

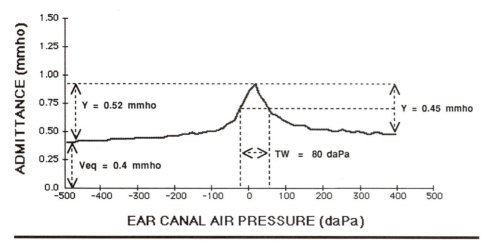

FIGURE 4.7 Single-component, single-frequency (226 Hz) tympanogram. This tympanogram, from a normal adult ear, has a compensated static admittance (Y) of 0.45 mmho compensated from the positive tail, 0.52 mmho compensated from the negative tail, tympanometric width (TW) of 80 daPa calculated from the positive tail, and an equivalent volume V_{eq} of 0.4 mmho calculated from the negative tail.

The admittance calculated in this manner is referred to as the *peak compensated static acoustic admittance* (American National Standards Institute, 1987) or more concisely, the *static admittance*.

The static admittance can be accurately determined from the admittance tympanogram only if there are no significant phase shifts that occur when the ear is pressurized. In fact, the admittance phase changes during pressurization, becoming larger at the tails of the tympanogram than at the peak. At 226 Hz, these phase shifts are usually small enough that the error is negligible. At higher frequencies it is necessary to calculate compensated conductance and susceptance separately. From the compensated conductance and susceptance, the compensated admittance can be determined. The compensated conductance G_{tm} and susceptance B_{tm} are

$$G_{tm} = G_{peak} - G_{tail} \quad (4.24)$$

$$B_{tm} = B_{peak} - B_{tail} \quad (4.25)$$

Compensated admittance is calculated from compensated conductance and susceptance with the computational equation in Table 4.2:

$$Y_{tm} = \sqrt{G_{tm^2} + B_{tm^2}} \quad (4.26)$$

INSTRUMENTATION

Design Principles of Clinical Acoustic Immittance Instruments

The earliest devices for evaluation of middle ear function were acoustic instruments that presented a sound to the ear

and evaluated the sound energy that was developed in the ear canal. From Eq. 4.8 we see that if we present a sound (probe tone) with a certain volume velocity, the impedance is proportional to the sound pressure. A probe tone presented to a system with high impedance has a high sound pressure; if the impedance is low, the probe tone sound pressure will be low. This is a convenient method for measuring the impedance of a system. A constant volume velocity probe tone is presented to the ear and the sound pressure is measured in the ear canal. A calibration procedure provides a conversion from sound pressure to impedance.

Alternatively, the probe tone sound pressure could be held constant and the volume velocity could be measured. This approach has been adopted by most commercially produced acoustic immittance systems.

Figure 4.8 illustrates the design of a typical probe for acoustic immittance measurement. A tube is used to couple an air pump and manometer to the probe to pressurize the ear canal. A miniature loudspeaker delivers the probe tone to the ear. A microphone picks up the acoustic signal in the

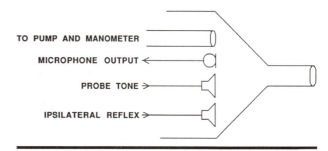

FIGURE 4.8 Components of a tympanometric probe.

ear canal and converts it to an electrical signal that is used to measure the acoustic immittance. Some systems have a second transducer used for delivering a stimulus for ipsilateral acoustic reflex measurement.

Figure 4.9 shows a block diagram of an admittance meter. A sinusoidal electrical signal is generated, amplified, and delivered to the miniature loudspeaker housed in the probe. The microphone picks up the probe tone in the ear canal and converts it to an electrical signal. An automatic gain control (AGC) keeps the probe tone at a constant sound pressure by controlling the gain of the probe tone amplifier. The voltage that is required to keep the probe tone at a fixed level is proportional to the admittance of the ear. The electrical signal that drives the probe tone transducer is also delivered to a comparator along with the amplified output of the microphone. The comparator provides a measurement of the magnitude of the probe tone signal and the phase of the microphone signal. Once the system is calibrated, the magnitude and phase are identical to $|Y|$ and $\varnothing_Y$, the polar components of acoustic admittance.

The first electroacoustic admittance meters were analog electrical systems similar to that depicted in Figure 4.9. Current instruments employ microprocessors that perform the same functions by digital signal processing. Many of the functions of the components in Figure 4.9 are accomplished in software. The block diagram in Figure 4.9, however, is a good representation of the functions designed into these digital acoustic immittance systems.

ANSI Standard for Acoustic Immittance Instruments

The American National Standards Institute (ANSI) published a standard in 1987 describing the desirable characteristics of clinical acoustic immittance systems (American National Standards Institute, 1987). Manufacturers of these systems generally design their instruments to comply with the standard. The goal of the standard is to ensure that aural acoustic immittance measurements, using a 226 Hz probe tone, are equivalent when measured with any instrument that meets the specifications of the standard. In addition, the standard helps to promote uniform terminology and plotting formats. However, compliance with a standard is entirely voluntary, unless there is a stipulation in statute that requires conformity to a standard.

Measurement Units and Terminology. The ANSI standard recommends the use of the international units system (*Système Internationale*, SI). The SI unit of pressure is the dekapascal (daPa). Another pressure unit that has been commonly used for tympanometry is the mm H_2O. These units are related in the following manner.

$$1 \text{ mm } H_2O = 0.98 \text{ daPa}$$
$$1 \text{ daPa} = 1.02 \text{ mm } H_2O$$

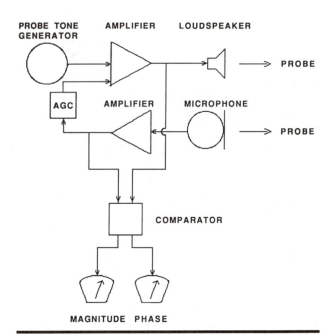

TWO-COMPONENT ADMITTANCE METER

FIGURE 4.9 Block diagram of an acoustic immittance measurement system. The probe tone is produced by the signal generator, amplified, and delivered to the miniature loudspeaker in the probe (Figure 4.8). The acoustic signal in the ear canal is picked up by the microphone, converted to an electrical signal, and amplified. The automatic gain control (AGC) dynamically adjusts the gain of the probe tone amplifier to keep the sound pressure in the ear canal constant. The comparator compares the amplified microphone signal and the probe signal to determine the relative amplitude and phase in the ear canal. The calibration process allows the amplitude and phase to be converted to admittance units.

For practical purposes, the two units can be considered to be equivalent.

Because clinical acoustic immittance measurement was widely employed before the existence of the standard, inconsistent and sometimes confusing terminology has been used. The standard provides the following definitions of terms, many of which are frequently misused by manufacturers and in published reports.

Acoustic immittance refers collectively to acoustic impedance, acoustic admittance, and all of their components.

Acoustic compliance, the reciprocal of acoustic stiffness, is the ratio of a change in volume displacement to a change in sound pressure. Compliance is a characteristic of a spring. This term has been improperly used for measurements that are actually admittance magnitude values. A variety of units have been used in conjunction with incorrectly reported "compliance" values, including "arbitrary units" and cubic centimeters. Since most instruments are actually admittance meters, the correct unit is the millimho (mmho).

Compensated static acoustic immittance is the immittance that has been compensated (or corrected) for the acoustic immittance of the ear canal. This value represents the acoustic immittance of the middle ear at the tympanic membrane.

Peak compensated static acoustic immittance is the static immittance obtained with the ear canal air pressure adjusted to produce a peak in the measured immittance. This is frequently referred to as the static admittance or the peak admittance.

Measurement-plane tympanometry is a measurement of acoustic immittance at the probe tip and represents the combined acoustic immittance of the ear canal and middle ear.

Compensated tympanometry is a measurement of acoustic immittance that has been compensated (or corrected) for the acoustic immittance of the ear canal.

Plotting Format. The appearance of a tympanogram is affected by the scale proportions (aspect ratio) of the plot. Just as the audiometer standard (American National Standards Institute, 1996) describes the specifications for an audiogram, the acoustic immittance standard provides a standard format for plotting 226 Hz tympanograms. The standard recommends an aspect ratio of 300 daPa to 1 mmho. Note in Figure 4.7 that a distance corresponding to 300 daPa on the *x*-axis is equivalent to the distance corresponding to 1 mmho on the *y*-axis.

The standard also recommends the following axis labels. The *y*-axis should be labeled with one of the following:

Acoustic Admittance (10^{-8} m^3/Pa•s [Acoustic mmho])
Acoustic Admittance of an Equivalent Volume of Air (cm^3)
Acoustic Impedance (10^8 Pa•s/m^3 [Acoustic kohm])

The *x*-axis should be labeled as follows:

Air Pressure (daPa) (1 daPa = 1.02 mm H$_2$O)

These rather cumbersome labels were recommended because of the confusion that existed resulting from inconsistent use of terminology and units. The ANSI working group wanted to be as specific as possible so that there would be no ambiguity in the quantities that are represented on tympanograms. Perhaps because the recommended labels are quite cumbersome, they have not been used consistently. We recommend the following axis labels for tympanograms. These are adequately specific but not as unwieldy as those recommended by ANSI.

y-axis: Acoustic Admittance (mmho)
x-axis: Ear Canal Air Pressure (daPa)

Calibration. There are many features of an acoustic immittance instrument that must be calibrated. These include the probe tone, the admittance measurement system, the air pressure measurement system, and the ipsilateral and contralateral reflex stimuli. All of these features should be calibrated on a regular basis.

Probe Tone. The standard is applicable to instruments that employ a 226 Hz probe tone. Although that frequency is not necessarily the one that is best for clinical diagnosis, it has been widely used, and more is known about tympanograms obtained at that frequency than other frequencies. It is a convenient frequency because of the simple relationship between acoustic admittance and the volume of air-filled calibration cavities.

The standard specifies that the actual frequency of the probe tone should be within 3% of the nominal frequency. That is, the actual frequency of the 226 Hz probe tone must be between 219 and 233 Hz. The sound pressure level must be ≤90 dB measured in a 2 cm^3 (HA-1) coupler.

Admittance Measurement System. The admittance measurement section of the acoustic immittance instruments are calibrated by placing the probe into a known acoustic admittance. An enclosed volume of air can be used as the known admittance because its admittance can be calculated from the volume of the enclosure. At 226 Hz, the admittance of an air-filled enclosure is equal to its volume. That is, the admittance of a 1 cm^3 volume is 1 mmho. This simple relationship holds if the cavity dimensions are within certain limits (the length can't be much greater than the diameter) and the atmospheric conditions (temperature and pressure) are not extreme.

Because the admittance of a volume of air is dependent on atmospheric conditions, it may be necessary to adjust the calibration in cities where the altitude is significantly different from sea level. At an elevation of 1 mile (e.g., Denver), the admittance of a volume of air is 22% higher than at sea level. This requires a correction in the calibration that is usually incorporated into the software calibration routine that is built into the instrument.

The standard specifies that the acoustic immittance measurement system should be calibrated in three calibration cavities with volume of 0.5, 2.0, and 5.0 cm^3. The admittance magnitude and phase indicators (Figure 4.9) are adjusted to read 0.5, 2.0, and 5.0 mmho with phase angles of 90° for all three cavities. The 90° phase angle results from the fact that an enclosed cavity is nearly an ideal compliant element. That is, the admittance is composed of a positive (compliant) susceptance value that is equal to the volume and a conductance of 0 mmho.

For instruments that measure admittance at other frequencies the calibration method is similar. Instead of the admittance being equal to the volume, the admittance is determined from the following formula:

$$Y = V \frac{f_p}{226} \angle 90° \qquad (4.27)$$

where V is the volume of the calibration cavity and f_p is the probe frequency. Eq. 4.27 tells us that the admittance of an enclosed volume increases in proportion to the frequency and the phase angle remains $90°$.

CLINICAL APPLICATIONS OF TYMPANOMETRY

The Vanhuyse Model

As clinical experience with tympanometry accumulated in the 1970s, a variety of tympanometric patterns were observed. A few investigators, experimenting with higher frequency probe tones, observed that tympanometric patterns are more complex at higher frequencies (Alberti & Jerger, 1974; Colletti, 1976; Liden, Bjorkman, Nyman, & Kunov, 1977; Liden, Harford, & Hallen, 1974a, 1974b; Margolis & Popelka, 1977; Van Camp, Raman, & Creten, 1976). The first studies of tympanometry in neonates revealed that newborns have complex tympanometric shapes even at low frequencies (Bennett, 1975; Keith, 1973, 1975). Although certain patterns appeared to be associated with certain ear conditions, it was the model developed at the University of Antwerp that would provide a framework for understanding the variety of tympanometric shapes (Vanhuyse et al., 1975).

The Vanhuyse model is based on assumptions of the shapes of resistance and reactance tympanograms. Because admittance, conductance, and susceptance tympanograms are simply mathematical transformations of impedance components (resistance and reactance) (see Table 4.2), impedance can be manipulated and the effects on admittance, conductance, and susceptance can be observed. The reason that this approach is informative is that simple changes in impedance quantities produce complex changes in admittance quantities.

The Vanhuyse model is represented graphically in Figure 4.10. Based on acoustic impedance measurements that had been made in the cat (Moller, 1965a), the resistance tympanogram was assumed to be a monotonically decreasing function of air pressure, with a higher resistance for negative pressure than for positive pressure and reactance is a single-peaked function that is symmetric around ambient ear canal pressure (upper left panel of Figure 4.10A). The reactance values are negative because at low frequencies the ear is stiffness controlled. The absolute values of reactance are greater than resistance at all pressures. (Compare the reactance X tympanogram with the dashed line in Figure 4.10A.)

As the reactance tympanogram shifts from negative to positive values, four tympanometric patterns occur. These were named by Vanhuyse and colleagues according to the number of positive and negative peaks (extrema) in the susceptance and conductance patterns.

1B1G. In the 1B1G pattern both susceptance B and conductance G are single peaked. The admittance Y tympanogram is also single peaked. This pattern occurs when acoustic reactance is negative at all ear canal pressures and greater in absolute value than resistance (Figure 4.10A). That is, $X < 0$ and $|X| > R$.

3B1G. In the 3B1G tympanogram, conductance G is single peaked and there is a central notch in susceptance B, resulting in three extrema. This occurs when the reactance tympanogram is shifted toward zero so that at low pressures the absolute value of reactance is less than resistance ($X < 0$ and $|X| < R$) and at high pressures the absolute value of reactance is greater than resistance ($X < 0$ and $|X| > R$). The model predicts that the admittance Y tympanogram is single peaked. In some cases, however, admittance can be notched in the 3B1G pattern (Margolis et al., 1985).

3B3G. In the 3B3G pattern conductance G and susceptance B are both notched. This occurs when reactance at low pressure becomes positive but remains less than resistance ($0 < X < R$). That is, the ear becomes mass controlled. When the ear is pressurized, the system is stiffened and reactance is negative. The susceptance B notch dips below the tail values resulting in a negative compensated susceptance indicating a mass controlled ear. The admittance Y tympanogram is also notched.

5B3G. In the 5B3G pattern, the conductance G tympanogram is notched and the susceptance B tympanogram has five extrema. This occurs when the reactance X tympanogram shifts further into positive values so that at low pressures reactance is positive and greater than reactance ($X > R$). Pressurizing the ear has a stiffening effect and at high pressures the reactance is negative (stiffness controlled).

Resonant Frequency. The resonant frequency is the frequency at which the total reactance is 0. At that frequency, the stiffness reactance and mass reactance are equal but of opposite sign so the total is zero. According to the Vanhuyse model, the resonant frequency of the middle ear is the transition frequency from 3B1G to 3B3G. Another way to identify the resonant frequency is to locate the frequency at which the compensated susceptance is zero. A number of methods for estimating resonant frequencies have been compared (Margolis & Goycoolea, 1993; Hanks & Rose, 1993). The method that appears to be optimal is the frequency at which the minimum susceptance (in the notch) is equal to the positive tail value.

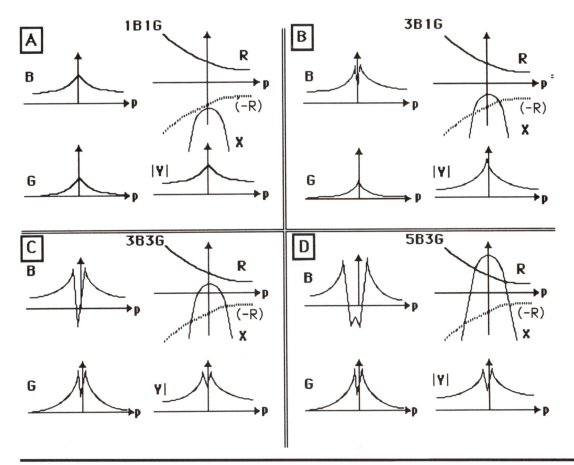

FIGURE 4.10 Graphic representation of the Vanhuyse model (Vanhuyse et al., 1975). The model determines the shapes of susceptance [B] and conductance [G] tympanograms from assumptions of the shapes and locations of reactance [X] and resistance [R] tympanograms using the conversion equations shown in Table 4.2. The upper right corner of each panel shows the reactance and resistance tympanograms. The resistance tympanogram is also shown as negative values [–R] to compare its magnitude with the reactance tympanogram. The corresponding susceptance [B], conductance [G], and admittance [Y] tympanograms are also shown in each panel. (A) The 1B1G pattern occurs when reactance is negative (stiffness controlled) and its absolute value is greater than resistance at all pressures. (B) The 3B1G pattern occurs when the reactance is negative and its absolute value is less than resistance at low pressures but greater than resistance at high pressures. (C) The 3B3G pattern occurs when reactance is positive (mass controlled) and less than resistance at low pressures and negative at high pressures. (D) The 5B3G pattern occurs when reactance is positive and greater than resistance at low pressures and negative at high pressures.

The model provides an understanding of the greater complexity of tympanometric patterns as frequency increases. We know that the reactance of the ear shifts from large negative values toward zero with increasing frequency. The effect of probe frequency on tympanometric shapes can be predicted by shifting the reactance tympanogram accordingly. Shifting the reactance tympanogram from large negative values to positive values results in a sequence beginning with 1B1G and progressing through 5B3G. This is the sequence that occurs in a typical normal adult ear (Margolis & Goycoolea, 1993; Margolis et al., 1985).

The effects of some pathologies can also be predicted. A stiffening of the middle ear is expected to shift the reactance tympanogram toward larger negative values while an ossicular discontinuity would have the opposite effect. This approach has been found to account for the effects of frequency and many pathologies on tympanometric shapes.

The Vanhuyse model is useful for interpreting tympanometric shapes at any frequency. However, since more complex shapes occur at higher frequencies, the model is most useful for interpreting multifrequency tympanograms.

Single-Frequency (226 Hz) Tympanometry

Tympanometric Features. A number of features of the 226 Hz tympanogram have been used for qualitative and quantitative analysis in the evaluation of middle ear function. These include tympanometric shape, static acoustic admittance, tympanometric width (gradient), tympanometric peak pressure, and equivalent ear canal volume.

Tympanometric Shapes.   Two approaches have been taken to the interpretation of 226 Hz tympanograms—qualitative and quantitative. Many of the early instruments that were used for tympanometry were uncalibrated and presented tympanometric results as "arbitrary compliance units." Because it was not appropriate to quantitatively measure tympanometric characteristics from such data, qualitative methods were employed based on judgments of the shapes of tympanograms. The most popular of these methods was the classification scheme originally described by Liden (Liden, 1969; Liden et al., 1974b) and Jerger (1970). Tympanograms are classified according to the height and location of the tympanometric peak. A Type A tympanogram has a normal peak height and location on the pressure axis. A Type B tympanogram is flat. A Type C tympanogram has a peak that is displaced toward negative pressure. Liden also described a Type D pattern characterized by a double peak. Later, subtypes A_d and A_s were added (Feldman, 1976), indicating a high-peaked and a low-peaked Type A pattern, respectively. Although this approach is useful for identifying abnormal tympanometric features, its lack of precision leads to occasional errors and misinterpretations. For example, without quantitative criteria, there is no rule for distinguishing Types A, A_s, and A_d. Even the Type B and Type A designations are not always agreed upon when small peaks occur.

After the publication of the ANSI standard, manufacturers began to conform with the requirement that the immittance indicator must be calibrated in physical units. Virtually all clinical instruments produced since then have been admittance meters. Although some have labeled the y-axis cm^3, the units are equivalent to the millimho. With the current calibrated instruments it is possible to present results quantitatively and determine pass-fail criteria for tympanometric features. There are four features that are useful to consider in the clinical interpretation of 226 Hz tympanograms.

Static Admittance.   The peak compensated static acoustic admittance, or static admittance, is perhaps the most important feature of the 226 Hz tympanogram. Static admittance is sensitive to many middle ear conditions, including otitis media with effusion, some chronic otitis media sequelae such as cholesteatoma and ossicular adhesions, space-occupying lesions of the middle ear that are in contact with the eardrum or ossicular chain such as glomus tumor, ossicular discontinuity, eardrum perforation, and ear canal occlusion. Table 4.3 includes normative values for children and adults.

Tympanometric Width.   A number of studies demonstrated that the sharpness of the tympanometric peak is an indicator of middle ear pathology (Fiellau-Nikolajsen, 1983; Haughton, 1977; Nozza, Bluestone, & Kardatze, 1992a; Nozza, Bluestone, Kardatze, & Bachman, 1994; Paradise, Smith, & Bluestone, 1976). Brooks (1968) introduced the term *gradient* for this tympanometric characteristic.

TABLE 4.3   Norms for static admittance (Y), tympanometric width (TW), equivalent ear canal volume (V_{ea}), and resonant frequency (Res F) determined from sweep frequency (SF) and sweep pressure (SP) methods.

AGE GROUP		Y (mmho)	TW (daPa)	V_{ea} (cm³)	Res F SF (Hz)	Res F SP (Hz)
Children (3–10 years)	Mean	0.52[*1]	114[1]	0.58[4]	1153[1]	1041[1]
	90% Range	(0.25–1.05)[*1]	(80–159)[1]	(0.3–0.9)[4]	(850–1525)[1]	(755–1425)[1]
	Fail	≤0.2*	≥160	≥1.0	<850 Hz	<755 Hz
	Criteria	≤0.3**			>1525 Hz	>1425 Hz
Adults (≥ 18 years)	Mean	0.79[*2]	77[3]	1.36[5]	1135[2]	990[2]
	90% Range	(0.30–1.70)[*2]	(51–114)[3]	(0.9–2.0)[5]	(800–2000)[2]	(630–1400)[2]
	Fail	≤0.3*	≥115	≥2.0	<800 Hz	<630 Hz
	Criteria	≤0.4**			>2000 Hz	>1400 Hz

[1] Hunter (1993)

[2] Margolis & Goycoolea (1993)

[3] Margolis & Heller (1987)

[4] Shanks, Stelmachowicz, Beauchaine, & Schulte (1992)

[5] Wiley, Cruikshanks, Nondahl, Tweed, Klein, & Klein (1996)

*+200 daPa compensation

**negative tail compensation

Methods for quantifying the gradient were proposed by Brooks (1968), Paradise and colleagues (1976), and Liden, Peterson, and Bjorkman (1970). Two studies have compared gradient measures obtained with the various techniques in normal children and adults (DeJonge, 1986; Koebsell & Margolis, 1986). These studies concluded that the preferred method is the tympanometric width. Figure 4.7 illustrates the calculation of this measure. The distance from the peak to the positive tail of the tympanogram is bisected. The width of the tympanogram at that point is determined in daPa. Although it has been suggested that abnormally narrow width may indicate stapes fixation (Ivey, 1975), this has not been confirmed. Only abnormally wide tympanometric width should be considered an indication of middle ear dysfunction. Normative data for tympanometric width are presented in Table 4.3. Figure 4.11 shows a tympanogram from a patient with otitis media in which static admittance is normal but tympanometric width is abnormal.

Tympanometric Peak Pressure.   The ear canal air pressure at which the peak of the tympanogram occurs is the *tympanometric peak pressure* (TPP). TPP is an indicator of the pressure in the middle ear space. Although TPP overestimates the actual middle ear pressure, sometimes by as

much as 100% (Elner, Ingelstedt, & Ivarsson, 1971; Renvall & Holmquist, 1976), it is an indicator of the status of the middle ear pressure. A TPP of –300 daPa, for example, indicates a significant negative middle ear pressure, but the actual middle ear pressure may be quite different in two ears having the same TPP.

TPP has been widely used to evaluate middle ear pressure. In fact, the first tympanometry paper was subtitled "A method for objective determination of the middle-ear pressure" (Terkildsen & Thomsen, 1959). Since then, it has been used in the classification of tympanometric shapes (Jerger, 1970; Liden, 1969; Paradise et al., 1976), as a pass-fail criterion for screening for middle ear disease (American Speech-Language-Hearing Association, 1979), and as a diagnostic indicator for otitis media (Renvall, Liden, Jungert, & Nilsson, 1975).

The clinical use of TPP has been based on the *ex vacuo* theory of middle ear function. (See Magnuson, 1983, for a review.) The theory holds that the absorption of gases by the middle ear mucosa results in negative middle ear pressure that accumulates until the eustachian tube opens, restoring the middle ear pressure to ambient. If the eustachian tube fails to open, the negative pressure continues to build, resulting in the large negative pressures that are frequently observed in children.

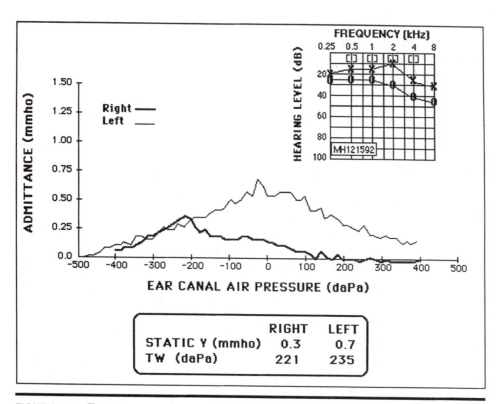

FIGURE 4.11   Tympanograms from a child with bilateral otitis media. The static admittance is normal but tympanometric widths are abnormal in both ears.

Recent observations indicate that the gas exchange mechanism for the middle ear is more complex than previously thought (Ostfeld & Silberberg, 1992). The diffusion of gases depends on many factors related to gas concentrations in the middle ear, mucosa, and blood. Diffusion is bidirectional and, under certain circumstances, can produce positive middle ear pressures (Hergils & Magnuson, 1985, 1987). Experimental evidence has failed to verify that chronic closure of the eustachian tube leads to large negative middle ear pressures (Cantekin, Doyle, Phillips, & Bluestone, 1980; Proud, Odoi, & Toledo, 1971).

Other mechanisms may be responsible for the large negative pressures observed in patients. The ciliary action of the eustachian tube may lower the middle ear pressure as it moves fluid through the closed tube (Hilding, 1944; Murphy, 1979). Alteration of middle ear gas composition may also contribute to negative middle ear pressure (Cantekin, Doyle, et al., 1980; Yee & Cantekin, 1986). In some patients, particularly in children, sniffing may produce large negative middle ear pressures (Falk, 1981, 1983; Magnuson, 1981). The negative pressure that occurs in the nasopharynx during sniffing can cause evacuation of air through the eustachian tube. Rather than indicating chronic closure of the eustachian tube, negative pressure due to sniffing may result from an abnormally compliant tube that is too easily opened by the rush of air in the nasopharynx.

Perhaps because of the multiple mechanisms that produce middle ear pressure, TPP is not a reliable indicator of medically significant middle ear disease. Several studies have revealed that TPP is not a good predictor of middle ear effusion (Fiellau-Nikolajsen, 1983; Haughton, 1977; Nozza, Bluestone, Kardatze, & Bachman, 1994; Paradise et al., 1976). In the absence of other tympanometric, audiometric, or otoscopic abnormality, negative middle ear pressure probably does not indicate a significant middle ear disorder.

Positive middle ear pressure has been reported in patients with acute otitis media (Margolis & Nelson, 1992; Ostergard & Carter, 1981). Although only a few cases have been reported in the literature, positive TPP (>50 daPa) should raise a suspicion of AOM, and should be followed with a careful history, otoscopic examination, audiometric evaluation, and, if appropriate, medical referral.

Equivalent Ear Canal Volume.   In the presence of a flat tympanogram, an estimate of the volume of air in front of the probe can be useful for detecting eardrum perforations and evaluating the patency of tympanostomy tubes. Although a normal equivalent volume (V_{ea}) does not rule out a perforation, a flat tympanogram with a large volume is evidence of an opening in the tympanic membrane.

Acoustic immittance measurements using a 226 Hz probe tone are useful for estimating the volume of air in front of the probe (Lindeman & Holmquist, 1982; Shanks, Stelmachowicz, Beauchaine, & Schulte, 1992). In normal ears, the admittance at high positive or negative pressure is primarily determined by the ear canal volume. However, because the eardrum and ear canal walls are not perfectly rigid when the ear is pressurized, the admittance at 226 Hz, expressed as an equivalent volume, overestimates the actual ear canal volume by about 25% in adults (Shanks & Lilly, 1981). The average tympanometrically measured equivalent ear canal volume is about 0.3 cm^3 in 4-month infants (Holte, Margolis, & Cavanaugh, 1991), 0.75 cm^3 in preschool-aged children (Margolis & Heller, 1987), and 1.0 to 1.4 cm^3 in adults (Margolis & Heller, 1987; Wiley, Cruikshanks, Nondahl, Tweed, Klein, & Klein, 1996). An opening in the tympanic membrane adds the volume of the middle ear space and contiguous mastoid air cells to the volume of the ear canal. Estimates of the size of the middle ear and mastoid vary considerably among studies. Estimates of 2.0 and 4.7 cm^3 have been reported for 1-year-old infants (Palva & Palva, 1966; Rubensohn, 1965); 6.5, 8.6, and 12.0 cm^3 for adults (Diamant, Rubensohn, & Walander, 1958; Moller, 1965b; Zwislocki, 1962). Within studies, a wide range of volumes have been reported, with a range of 2 to 22 cm^3 in one study of adults (Molvaer, Vallersnes, & Kringlbotn, 1978).

Based on these measurements, it should be possible to distinguish between ears with intact eardrums and those with perforations without difficulty. However, ears with past or present middle ear disease have smaller middle ear/mastoid volumes than normal ears for several reasons. First, an ear with active disease may contain fluid, inflammation, granulation, fibrosis, and cholesteatoma, which displace air volume, reducing the middle ear/mastoid volume. Second, ears with active disease may have obstructions of the mastoid air cell system, reducing the total mastoid volume. Third, when chronic disease occurs in infancy, there is an interruption of the pneumatization process, resulting in a smaller air-filled space (Palva & Palva, 1966). Fourth, chronic disease is more prevalent in ears with poorly pneumatized mastoids (Diamant et al., 1958).

Shanks (1985) demonstrated that ears with perforations have abnormally large volumes when they are free of active disease. However, when perforations occurred in the presence of active disease, V_{ea} was often normal. The data from that study are shown in Figure 4.12. The subjects were older male adults so the volumes are larger than would be obtained from the general population. A criterion of 6 cm^3 results in a specificity of 95%. That is, 95% of the normal subjects had equivalent volume ≤6 cm^3. For subjects with eardrum perforations who were free of active middle ear disease, equivalent volume exceeded 6 cm^3 in 92% of the cases. That is, the sensitivity was 92%. For

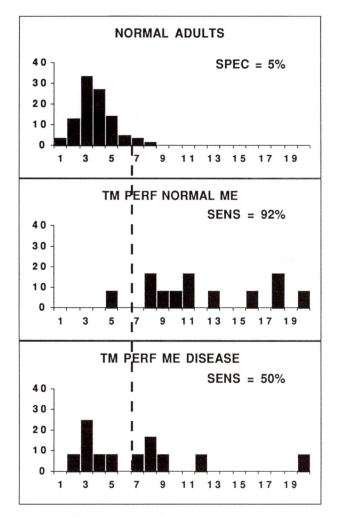

FIGURE 4.12 Equivalent volume measures for three groups of adult male patients. *Top panel:* Normal middle ear, intact tympanic membrane. *Middle panel:* Tympanic membrane perforation with otherwise normal middle ear. *Bottom panel:* Tympanic membrane perforation with middle ear inflammation. (Data from Shanks, 1985)

subjects with perforations and active middle ear disease, the sensitivity dropped to 50%. Thus, a normal volume in the presence of a flat tympanogram may indicate an intact eardrum or a perforation with active middle ear disease. An abnormally large volume suggests a perforation and a normal middle ear/mastoid air space. This study demonstrates a very important point—a normal volume does not rule out an eardrum perforation.

Shanks and colleagues (1992) recommended an abnormal criterion of 1.0 cm³ for children. For adults, a value of 2.0 cm³ appears to effectively separate ears with intact

eardrums from those with perforations but without active disease (Margolis & Heller, 1987; Wiley et al., 1996).

Another useful clinical application for equivalent volume is to monitor the course of middle ear disease after the insertion of tympanostomy tubes. It has been shown that equivalent volume correlates highly with indices of disease severity (Hunter, Margolis, Daly, & Giebink, 1992) and with recurrence of otitis media (Takasaka, Hozawa, Shoji, Takahashi, Jingu, Adachi, & Kobayashi, 1996). A progressively larger equivalent volume following tube insertion is an indication of recovery from otitis media. When the equivalent volume remains small, it is an indication of persistent disease. In a study of 157 children aged 6 months to 8 years, treated with tympanostomy tubes for chronic OME, Hunter and colleagues (1992) found that ears with post-operative equivalent volumes of less than 1.5 cc had recurrences of otitis media on average 9.5 months following surgery, while ears with equivalent volumes of 3.0 cc or more were otitis free twice as long after surgery (17.5 months on average). This difference was highly significant. Therefore, it appears that equivalent volume can be a useful predictor of post-operative recovery, and that ears with equivalent volumes of 1.5 cc or less should be followed more closely for recurrence of otitis media.

Sensitivity and Specificity of Tympanometry and Otoscopy. In order to gauge the clinical usefulness of any diagnostic test, a complete understanding must be developed of the test's performance in various populations at high and low risk for the disease of interest. Tympanometry is no different in this regard. Tympanometry is one of the most highly utilized diagnostic tests for diagnosing a specific disease in audiologic practice. However, we have had adequate information about sensitivity and specificity of tympanometry obtained with calibrated instruments for well described populations only within the past few years.

Pneumatic otoscopy requires skill, experience, and the proper equipment. With the proper equipment and a highly trained, experienced otoscopist, pneumatic otoscopy is about 94% sensitive and 78% specific, using myringotomy as the gold standard (Gates, Avery, Cooper, Hearne, & Holt, 1986). Tympanometry is generally less sensitive, but more specific than otoscopy. This fact makes tympanometry a good adjunct to pneumatic otoscopy. It is important for the audiologist and physician to understand that the two procedures will not always agree, and that the combination in this case is stronger than either procedure alone.

In most studies prior to 1990, tympanometry was measured with arbitrary units and, therefore, qualitative types were compared with otoscopic examination or surgery. For example, Bluestone, Beery, and Paradise (1973) correlated tympanogram types with the presence of OME at surgery in ears at high risk for OME (all had surgery due to suspected fluid). Flattened or extremely rounded tympanograms were associated with OME in 82% of ears, while normal, sharply peaked tympanograms were associated with absence of fluid in 100% of ears. Paradise and colleagues (1976) expanded the familiar Liden-Jerger classification of tympanogram types into fourteen types based on arbitrary "compliance" units and gradient. They studied 280 subjects aged 10 days to 5 years, 11 months. These infants and children were from two groups: 107 were scheduled to receive myringotomy and tubes, and 173 were selected from various outpatient clinics. Tympanometry and otoscopy were completed within one hour, and within two hours of myringotomy for the surgical group. Overall, agreement between otoscopy and surgery was 86%. Sensitivity of otoscopy for presence of OME was 91%, and specificity was 75%. Percentage of ears with OME varied by type of tympanogram, with the highest prevalence of fluid (89%) found in the flat or rounded tympanogram. Normal tympanograms were associated with no OME in 95% of ears. In tympanograms with pressure peaks at or less than −100 daPa, presence of OME depended highly on the gradient, or width of the tympanogram. If gradient alone was considered, then sensitivity was 95% and specificity was 76% for presence of OME, similar to the test performance of otoscopy. Cantekin and colleagues (1980) combined otoscopy and tympanometry into an algorithm and found that tympanometry in combination with otoscopy resulted in better test performance than either test alone. The combined sensitivity of otoscopy and tympanometry was 97%, and specificity was 90%. Gates and colleagues (1986) used the fourteen tympanogram types suggested by Paradise and colleagues (1976). Five of these types were found to be associated with a low prevalence of OME (8% of ears with these tympanogram types had OME at surgery). Three types were highly associated with OME with a prevalence of 88%. The other six types were intermediate, with prevalences varying from 20 to 54%.

Because otitis media is a continuum of middle ear conditions with tympanometric results also varying along a continuum, it is highly unlikely that any criterion, no matter how carefully selected, will identify all affected ears. This fact was demonstrated by Le and colleagues in two studies of tympanometry in ears prior to and after intubation (Le, Daly, Margolis, Lindgren, & Giebink, 1992; Le, Hunter, Margolis, Daly, Lindgren, & Giebink, 1994).

As in the Le studies, more recent investigators have utilized calibrated equipment that allows static admittance and tympanometric width to be quantified and compared among groups of individuals. Silman, Silverman, and Arick (1992) investigated several protocols for sensitivity and specificity of detection of middle ear OME in children. Children were identified with OME based on pneumatic otoscopy by an experienced otolaryngologist. Sensitivity

and specificity of four combinations of immittance variables were estimated. Variables included static admittance, tympanometric width, tympanometric peak pressure, and ipsilateral acoustic reflex. The sensitivity of the various combinations ranged from 76% to 95%.

Performance of two screening procedures was also assessed by Roush, Drake, and Sexton (1992) in 374 ears of 3- to 4-year-old children in a preschool program. A "traditional" procedure, based on TPP < −200 daPa or absent ipsilateral acoustic reflex was compared with the interim norms published in the 1990 ASHA Guidelines (American Speech-Language Hearing Association, 1990). The gold standard was pneumatic otoscopy performed by an experienced, validated otoscopist. The "traditional" procedure had high sensitivity (95%), but low specificity (65%). While the negative predictive value was high (99%), the positive predictive value was low (27%). The ASHA interim norms had high sensitivity (84%) and specificity (95%), with a positive predictive value of 69% and a negative predictive value of 98%. The guidelines will perform differently in different populations, and other variables such as the time interval between screening and medical examination, personnel used for screening, and use of case history and visual inspection will all affect the performance of the screening protocol.

Nozza and colleagues (1992b) have made some very important contributions in their studies of acoustic immittance in various populations of children (Nozza et al., 1992b; Nozza et al., 1994). In the first study, two groups of children were studied. One group (n = 61, aged 1 to 8 years) received myringotomy and intubation and thus was at high risk for OME. Tympanometry was performed no more than 30 minutes prior to surgery. The surgeon was unaware of the results of tympanometry. Six different protocols were evaluated; three of these included ipsilateral acoustic reflexes. Sensitivity, specificity, positive and negative predictive values were all measured. Positive and negative predictive values are influenced by the prevalence of the disease in the population, which was very high in this sample (73%). Sensitivity (90%) and specificity (86%) were highest for gradient combined with acoustic reflexes. Gradient combined with static admittance also produced relatively high sensitivity (83%) and specificity (87%). A second group of children (n = 77, aged 3 to 16 years) who attended an allergy clinic and were unselected with regard to otitis media history were also studied and reported in the same paper (Nozza et al., 1992b). The same six immittance protocols were compared against a validated otoscopist. In this sample, sensitivity was 78% for all protocols except ipsilateral reflex alone (sensitivity = 88%) and gradient or static admittance < 0.1 mmho (sensitivity = 67%). Gradient + ipsilateral reflex and gradient + static admittance performed equally well for specificity (99%). Positive predictive value was higher for gradient + static admittance

(88%) than it was for gradient + ipsilateral reflex (78%). In a subsequent study (Nozza et al., 1994), a group of children (n = 171, aged 1 to 12 years) with recurrent or chronic OME, who were scheduled for myringotomy and tubes, received otoscopy by a validated otoscopist and tympanometry by a certified audiologist. The prevalence of OME in this group was 55%. Eleven criteria, with various cut-points for each criterion were evaluated. As expected, there was a tradeoff so that as sensitivity increased with changes in cut-point, specificity decreased. Sensitivity and specificity for various criteria are depicted on a receiver-operator curve (ROC) in Figure 4.13. Sensitivity is depicted on the *y*-axis and the false positive rate (1 – specificity) is depicted on the *x*-axis. Points that fall closest to the upper left corner show best test performance (high sensitivity and low false positive rate). It can be seen that tympanometric width >275 daPa performs best as a single criterion, but width combined with otoscopy performs slightly better. The study also evaluated tympanometric criteria against otoscopy findings based on the child, rather than the ear. TW of >250 daPa performed better than cutoffs of 150 or 200 when judged against otoscopy.

These studies demonstrate that the choice of cut-off criteria affect test performance greatly. It appears that combinations of criteria, such as otoscopy and TW, perform better than single criteria. Static admittance alone has low sensitivity but good specificity. Use of either ipsilateral reflex or tympanometric width combined with static admittance provides good test performance, as does otoscopy combined with width. However, all studies have used highly experienced, validated otoscopists, and results may be very different with less experienced or knowledgeable personnel. Prevalence of the disease in the population will affect negative and positive predictive values. With lower prevalence, the positive predictive value goes down; that is, fewer referrals will turn out to have real problems. As the positive predictive value decreases, the number of unnecessary referrals increases. Cut-off criteria may need to be more stringent when prevalence is lower, and more lax when prevalence or risk of the disease is greater. Therefore, it is very helpful to estimate the prevalence of the disease in the population of interest when choosing pass/fail criteria.

The results of these studies indicate that both tympanometry and pneumatic otoscopy are good tests for identifying otitis media with effusion. It is important to remember that highly skilled otoscopists were used in the evaluation of otoscopy and that most clinicians who examine ears are probably not as skilled as those used in the studies. Most patients with middle ear disease are initially evaluated by primary care physicians who are less experienced in ear examination and in cleaning the ear canal in order to perform an adequate evaluation of the ear. In view of the fact that otoscopy and tympanometry are both effective screening tests, tympanometry would appear to be a very useful adjunct to otoscopy for evaluation of the ear by primary care physicians and by audiologists.

Screening Tympanometry. Tympanometry has been widely used in screening programs, primarily for identifying middle ear disease in pediatric populations. (See Holte & Margolis, 1987, and Roush, 1990, for discussions.) The value of mass screening programs for identifying middle ear disease has been controversial (American Academy of Audiology, 1997b; Bluestone, Fria, Arjona, Casselbrant, Schwartz, Ruben, et al., 1986). Although various conferences, organizations, and agencies have been hesitant to recommend large-scale screening programs, many programs for preschool and school-age children have incorporated tympanometric screening into the protocol. Most programs combine audiometric screening with tympanometric screening to detect both sensorineural hearing loss and middle ear disorders (American Speech-Language-Hearing Association, 1990; American Academy of Audiology, 1997a).

Margolis and Heller (1987) developed a screening protocol that was later incorporated into the 1990 ASHA Guideline. That protocol, shown in a flowchart format in Figure 4.14, utilizes case history information, visual inspection of

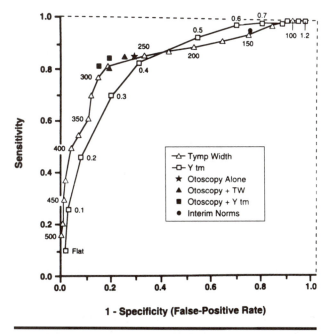

FIGURE 4.13 Receiver operating characteristics for tympanometric measures alone and in combination with otoscopy. (From Nozza, Bluestone, Kardatze, & Bachman, "Identification of middle ear effusion by aural acoustic admittance and otoscopy." *Ear and Hearing, 15*, 310–323, Figure 1, 1994. Reprinted with permission.)

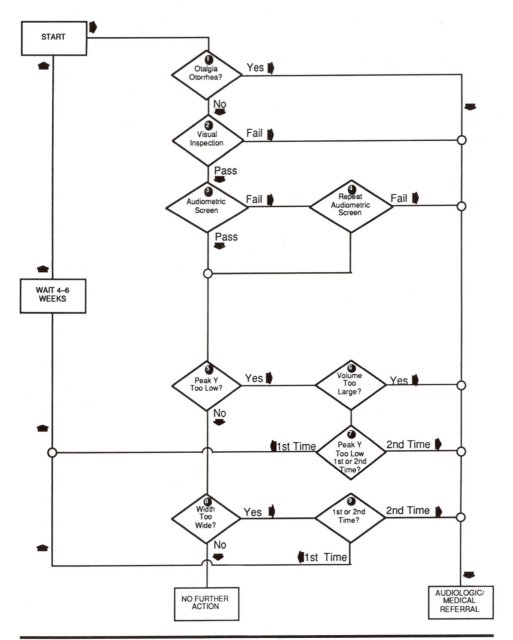

FIGURE 4.14 Flow chart for screening for hearing loss and middle ear disease. (Adapted from Margolis & Heller, 1987)

the ear, audiometric screening, and tympanometry to identify significant hearing loss and middle ear disorders requiring medical referral.

Case History. In a screening program, there is not sufficient time to take a complete history. However, certain information warrants a medical referral without the need to perform any tests. This includes a recent history of otalgia (ear pain) or otorrhea (ear discharge).

Visual Inspection. Personnel who administer screening tests vary widely in their skills for examining the ear. Some may be quite experienced otoscopists while others may not be able to visualize the tympanic membrane and reliably evaluate its appearance. However, every screening program should include an inspection of the ear to identify obvious signs of active disease. The visual inspection should include examination of the head and neck and otoscopic inspection of the ear canal and tympanic membrane.

Conditions that warrant additional testing or medical referral include developmental defects, ear canal occlusion or inflammation, and tympanic membrane abnormalities associated with ear disease including inflammation, perforation, and abnormal landmarks or color.

Audiometric Screening. Guidelines for audiometric screening have been recommended by various professional associations (American Speech-Language-Hearing Association, 1990; American Academy of Audiology, 1997a). Typically these involve a three-frequency screen at a fixed hearing level, such as 20 dB HL at 1, 2, and 4 kHz. Failure to respond to one or more frequencies in either ear constitutes a fail and results in further testing, audiologic evaluation, or medical referral.

Tympanometry. Variables that have been used in screening programs include qualitative assessment of tympanometric shapes, static admittance, tympanometric width, tympanometric peak pressure, and equivalent volume. Because tympanometric peak pressure has been shown to be weakly related to significant middle ear disease, it has been largely abandoned as a screening indicator. Early studies indicated that tympanometric screening resulted in an unacceptably high rate of referrals (Roush & Tait, 1985). More recent protocols have incorporated a rescreening requirement to reduce the number of false positive failures (Margolis & Heller, 1987). Adequate normative data are available to set reasonable fail criteria for static admittance, tympanometric width, and equivalent ear canal volume. Table 4.3 includes fail criteria for these variables for children and adults.

The flow chart in Figure 4.14 illustrates the logic used to determine the need for an audiologic or medical referral, not necessarily the order in which the tests are performed. A positive history or visual inspection results in an immediate referral, most likely to a physician. The audiometric screen requires a second test before a referral is made. The second test can be performed on the same day as the screen or at a later date. Failure of both audiometric screening tests is required to result in a referral. The tympanometric portion of the protocol utilizes equivalent ear canal volume, static admittance, and tympanometric width. A flat tympanogram with a large volume is an indication of a perforation and warrants an immediate referral if the patient is not already under the care of a physician. Patent tympanostomy tubes, for example, do not require a referral because the patient is obviously in medical treatment. Failure on static admittance or tympanometric width requires a second screening 4 to 6 weeks after the first screen. Failure on both occasions is required for a referral.

The nature of the referral will depend on the circumstances of the screening program. In some cases, patients may be referred to an audiologist for complete audiologic evaluation, the outcome of which will determine the need for medical referral. Those referred for medical evaluation may be referred to a primary care physician or to an otolaryngologist. This is determined by the available resources, the requirements of the health care provider, and the relationships between the screening program and other clinical facilities.

Multifrequency Tympanometry

High Impedance Pathologies. High impedance pathologies are conditions that increase the impedance of the middle ear, ranging from simple middle ear effusion to invasive neoplasms. Otitis media with effusion (OME) increases the impedance of the middle ear space, in direct proportion to the quantity of fluid occupying the normally air-filled space. With large quantities of fluid, varying the ear canal air pressure does not change the impedance at the eardrum, so the tympanogram is flat. A typical 226 Hz admittance tympanogram in an ear with OME is shown in Figure 4.15A. Because the tympanogram is flat, tympanometric width and tympanometric peak pressure are not measurable. Equivalent volume is within the normal range, indicating that the probe tip is not obstructed by the ear canal wall. A flat tympanogram at low frequencies is strong evidence for OME, but some high impedance pathologies may be evident only at higher frequencies. In various stages of OME, impedance may be altered by increased mass due to thick effusion in contact with the ossicles, or decreased compliance due to reduction of the air volume of the mastoid and middle ear space. In these stages, the 226 Hz tympanogram may not be flat, but it likely will be more rounded and broader than normal. Tympanometric width is more sensitive than static admittance for some of these conditions. However, even width can be normal in some cases of OME. Examination of the higher frequencies may be necessary to reveal impedance changes in some stages of OME. A 226 Hz tympanogram from a patient with chronic OME is shown in Figure 4.15B. The tympanic membrane was retracted and thickened with reduced mobility on pneumatic otoscopy. She had been treated for acute otitis media three month earlier. Static admittance is within normal limits but the tympanogram is abnormally wide. Multifrequency tympanograms for the same patient are shown in Figure 4.16. At all frequencies above 226 Hz, tympanograms are nearly flat and do not progress through the normal Vanhuyse sequence.

As with other sequelae of otitis media, tympanic membrane retraction occurs on a continuum (Maw & Bawden, 1994; Sade & Berco, 1976), ranging from slight retraction of pars tensa without atrophy to collapse of the eardrum onto the ossicles and promontory of the middle ear. Figure 4.15C shows a 226 Hz tympanogram from an ear with

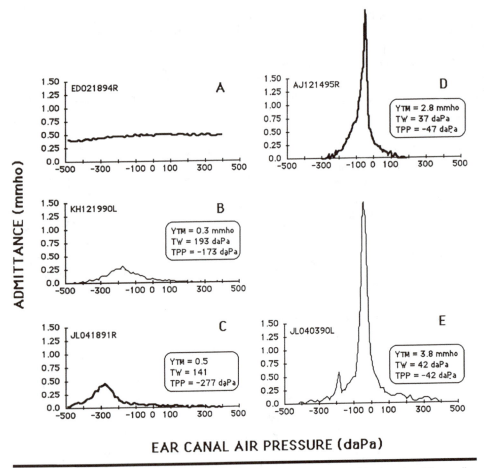

FIGURE 4.15 226 Hz admittance tympanogram from two patients with chronic otitis media with effusion (A and B), a patient with tympanic membrane retraction (C), a patient with tympanic membrane atrophy (D), and a patient with an ossicular discontinuity (E).

retraction due to negative middle ear pressure. Multifrequency tympanograms for the same patient are shown in Figure 4.17. The patterns are normal Vanhuyse patterns with a tympanometric peak pressure of –277 daPa and a resonant frequency of 1250 Hz. Retraction by itself results only in a shift of the tympanogram on the pressure axis. When retraction occurs with atrophy, tympanosclerosis, or other middle ear sequelae, other tympanometric abnormalities may be present.

Another high-impedance pathology, cholesteatoma (keratoma) is a collection of epithelial debris that usually originates in the lateral epithelial layer of the eardrum and migrates into the middle ear. In severe cases, cholesteatoma can result in destruction of ossicles and invasion of the mastoid air cell system (Proctor, 1991). In a study of acquired cholesteatoma in 1024 children and adults, Sheehy, Brachmann, and Graham (1977) found that the majority occurred in the attic or the posterosuperior quadrant (73%), while 18% had a complete marginal perforation, 6% had a partial, central perforation, and only 3% had an intact TM. Cholesteatomas are rare, even among people with histories of chronic OME. In children treated with tympanostomy tubes, prevalence of cholesteatoma six to twenty years later is approximately 1% (Daly, Hunter, Levine, Lindgren, & Giebink, 1997). A case study of a patient with cholesteatoma is presented in the last section of this chapter.

Otosclerosis is a high-impedance pathology that has defied attempts to develop a definitive diagnostic test. Although 226 Hz tympanograms tend to show low static admittance in otosclerotic ears, the overlap between normals and otosclerotics has prevented this measure from being an effective diagnostic test (Alberti & Jerger, 1974; Jerger, 1970; Jerger, Jerger, Maudlin, & Segal, 1974). In a study of experimentally produced stapes fixation in cats (Margolis, Osguthorpe, & Popelka, 1978), there was a clear separation of static impedance at 220 and 660 Hz between cats with stapes fixation and normals. This clear separation is not apparent between otosclerotic patients and normal subjects. Because the site of lesion is at the stapes footplate, where the input impedance to the cochlea

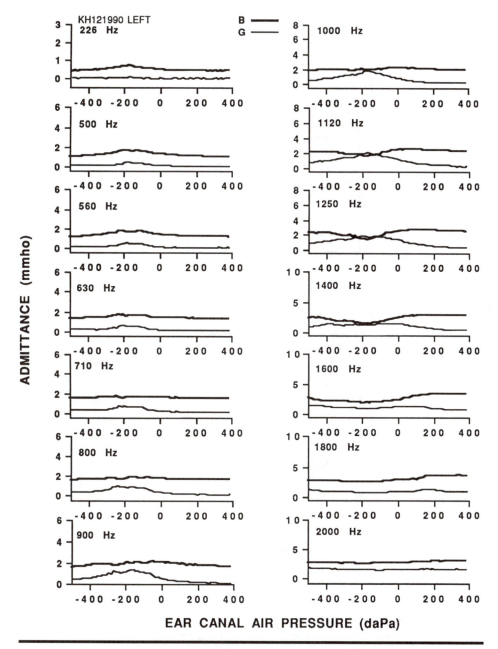

FIGURE 4.16   Multifrequency tympanograms from a patient with chronic otitis media with effusion. The 226 Hz admittance tympanogram is shown in Figure 4.15B.

is very high, increasing the impedance at that point has little effect on the impedance at the tympanic membrane. In addition, the wide normal variability among human individuals makes it more difficult to detect small impedance changes in clinical populations than in a controlled experiment.

Multifrequency tympanometry does not appear to increase the sensitivity of tympanometry for otosclerosis (Colletti, 1976; Shahnaz & Polka, in press). Shahnaz and Polka (in press) compared static admittance, tympanometric

width, resonant frequency, and the frequency corresponding to an admittance phase angle of 45° in 36 normal-hearing adults and 14 patients diagnosed with otosclerosis. Results showed no statistically significant difference in static admittance or width between normal and otosclerotic ears. There was a significant difference between normal and otosclerotic ears for resonant frequency, and for the frequency corresponding to an admittance phase angle of 45°. However, the sensitivity was only 79% and the specificity was 71%. Thus, multifrequency tympanometry does not perform particularly

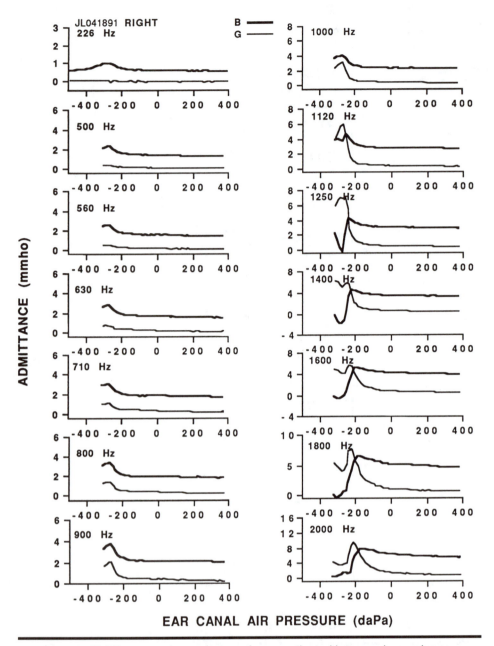

FIGURE 4.17 Multifrequency tympanograms from a patient with tympanic membrane retraction due to negative middle ear pressure. The 226 Hz admittance tympanogram is shown in Figure 4.15C.

well as a diagnostic test for otosclerosis. The combination of absent acoustic reflexes, conductive hearing loss, relatively normal 226 Hz tympanogram, and normal eardrum appearance in an adult with an otherwise unremarkable history for ear disease remains the best indication of otosclerosis.

Low Impedance Pathologies. Low impedance pathologies are those that decrease the impedance at the eardrum. Tympanometry is very effective for identifying these pathologies, because they cause a large impedance change

at the tympanic membrane. However, clinically significant low impedance pathologies are more rare than high impedance pathologies. The most common low impedance pathology is tympanic membrane atrophy, often called a monomeric or dimeric membrane. Thinning or destruction of the middle fibrous layer (lamina propria) of the tympanic membrane secondary to otitis media, traumatic perforation, or surgical placement of tympanostomy tubes results in decreased stiffness and hypermobility. Atrophy can occur in small, focal areas, often at a previous myringotomy site, or may be more generalized across the eardrum. Atrophy may lead to atelectasis (collapse of the eardrum into the ossicles and middle ear promontory) when combined with Eustachian tube dysfunction and otitis media, resulting in clinically significant pathology. Tympanic membrane atrophy is associated with increased static admittance, narrow tympanometric width, and decreased resonant frequency. Atrophy does not, however, appear to be associated with conductive hearing loss unless it is also accompanied by retraction of the tympanic membrane or ossicular erosion. Figure 4.15D

shows a 226 Hz tympanogram from a patient with a history of otitis media and generalized tympanic membrane atrophy. Note the high static admittance (2.8 mmho) and narrow width (37 daPa). Figure 4.18 shows multifrequency tympanograms for the same patient. The resonant frequency is abnormally low (<500 Hz). Tympanometric patterns are normal Vanhuyse patterns through 1400 Hz. The transitions from one Vanhuyse pattern to the next are all shifted toward lower frequencies. The 3B1G pattern at 500 Hz, 3B3G pattern at 710 Hz, and 5B3G pattern at 900 Hz are

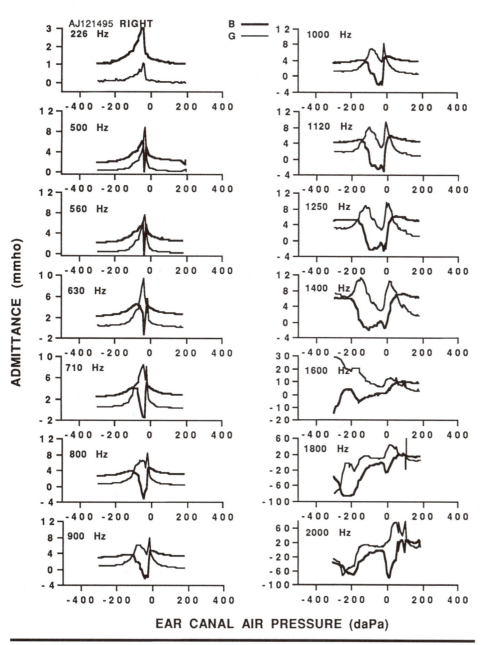

FIGURE 4.18 Multifrequency tympanograms from a patient with an atrophic tympanic membrane. The 226 Hz admittance tympanogram is shown in Figure 4.15D.

not observed in normal ears at those low frequencies. This indicates a decreased stiffness resulting in a decreased resonant frequency. At the highest frequencies (>1400 Hz) the patterns become very high amplitude and irregular, probably indicating that the measurement system is not capable of measuring such high admittance values. Because hearing is normal, it can be surmised that the changes are due to tympanic membrane atrophy, and not to ossicular disarticulation, which would result in conductive hearing loss.

The effect of ossicular erosion and disarticulation is similar to atrophy, though the effects can be more marked. Typically, complete disarticulation results in extremely high static admittance at 226 Hz and extremely low resonant frequency. Figure 4.15E shows the 226 Hz tympanogram from a patient with surgically confirmed traumatic disarticulation. Like the patient with tympanometric atrophy, the static admittance is high (3.8 mmho) and the tympanometric width is narrow (42 daPa). Figure 4.19 shows multifrequency tympanograms for the same patient. At 355 Hz the pattern is 3B1G and the depth of the susceptance notch indicates that the ear is beyond the resonant frequency. This is an extremely low resonant frequency and an unusually low frequency for a 3B1G pattern. 3B3G and 5B3G patterns occur at 450 and 1000 Hz, respectively, again, very low frequencies for these complex patterns.

A careful otologic examination is required to discover the cause of the hearing loss, when present, and the tympanometric abnormalities. Multiple pathologic conditions can coexist, obscuring the true etiology of hearing loss. For example, when otosclerosis coexists with atrophy of the tympanic membrane, the more lateral and less significant pathology dominates the tympanogram. Thus, an ear with both otosclerosis and atrophy may be confused with ossicular discontinuity.

Tympanometry in Infants

Tympanograms recorded from normal ears of newborn infants are very different from those obtained from older infants, children, and adults. In neonate ears with confirmed middle ear disease, 226 Hz tympanograms are not reliably different from those obtained from normal ears. For these reasons, the 226 Hz tympanometry is not an effective test for middle ear disease in newborns.

The earliest tympanometric recordings from neonate ears were made with single-component instruments that used a 220 Hz probe tone and expressed the results as "arbitrary compliance units" (Bennett, 1975; Keith, 1973, 1975; Poulsen & Tos, 1978). These studies reported a frequent occurrence of double-peaked tympanograms, indicating that the newborn ear is very different from the adult ear. Recall from the Vanhuyse model that double-peaked admittance tympanograms occur in 3B1G, 3B3G, or 5B3G

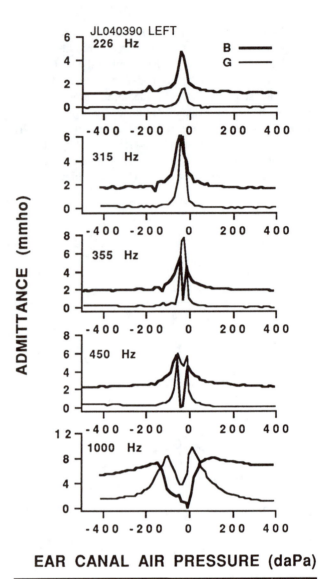

FIGURE 4.19 Multifrequency tympanograms from a patient with a complete disarticulation of the ossicular chain. The 226 Hz admittance tympanogram is shown in Figure 4.15E.

patterns, that is, when the absolute value of reactance is less than resistance or when reactance becomes positive (mass controlled). This condition never exists in the normal adult ear at 220 or 226 Hz because at low frequencies reactance is a large negative value indicating a stiffness-controlled system.

Later studies recorded two-component tympanograms at two probe frequencies, 220 and 660 Hz (Himelfarb, Popelka, & Shanon, 1979; Sprague, Wiley, & Goldstein, 1985). These two-component recordings permit an analysis of the components of immittance. These studies indicated that at low frequencies, the newborn ear is characterized by a large resistive component and a very low reactance. The low reactance suggests a significant mass effect that offsets the stiffness of the middle ear system. The patterns, particularly at 660 Hz, were generally not consistent with the Vanhuyse model.

Holte, Margolis, and Cavanaugh (1991) recorded multifrequency tympanograms (226 to 900 Hz) from newborns and, from the same babies, at several ages up to four months. Tympanometric patterns were classified by shape using the four categories of the Vanhuyse model and "other" for patterns that do not conform to any of the Vanhuyse categories. For newborns (1 to 7 days) at 226 Hz, all tympanograms conformed to the Vanhuyse categories, approximately equally distributed among the four patterns. Recall that adult ears are all 1B1G at that frequency. As frequency increases from 226 Hz to 900 Hz, the proportion of "other" patterns increases, reaching 100% at 900 Hz. With increasing age, the proportion of "other" patterns decreases and the tympanograms conform more consistently to the Vanhuyse model. By 3 to 4 months, the majority of patterns conformed to the Vanhuyse model with 100% 1B1G patterns at 226 Hz and 82% either 1B1G or 3B1G at 900 Hz. The results of that study indicated that tympanograms of newborns do not progress in an orderly sequence with changes in probe frequency and are apparently influenced by mass and resistive elements that are not present in older subjects. By 4 months of age tympanometric patterns behave in a manner that is consistent with the Vanhuyse model, although developmental changes are not yet complete.

Figure 4.20 shows multifrequency tympanograms from a two-day-old infant (left panel) and from the same infant at age 4 months (right panel). At two days, the 226 Hz tympanogram is a 1B1G pattern, but the peak susceptance is lower than conductance, a reversal of the relationship seen in older infants and adults. At higher frequencies, the patterns are irregular and do not conform to the Vanhuyse model. At 4 months, the patterns are regular 1B1G patterns up to 900 Hz where a 3B1G pattern is observed. These patterns are very similar to those seen in older children and indicates a rapid maturation of the external and/or middle ear.

The reasons for the disorganized behavior of tympanograms in newborns are not clear. Because the osseous portion of the ear canal wall of the newborn is not rigid as it is in adults, it has been suggested that movement of the canal wall influences tympanometric recordings (Keefe, Bulen, Arehart, & Burns, 1993; Paradise et al., 1976). There is evidence for and against this hypothesis. Holte, Cavanagh, and Margolis (1990) found no relationship between canal wall movement of neonates measured with video otomicroscopy and tympanometric patterns. Hsu, Margolis, Schachern, Sutherland, and Javel (1996) found similarly chaotic tympanometric patterns in newborn chinchillas despite the fact that the canal wall appeared to be

fully ossified on histologic analysis. On the other hand, Keefe and colleagues (1993) measured complex impedance in infants at various ages and found a mass effect that appeared to be similar to the acoustic properties of soft tissue elsewhere in the body. Because this effect dominates at low frequencies, they argued that probe tones below 1000 Hz would probably not be effective for evaluating middle ear function in newborns. While a mass component of ear canal wall vibration in newborns is certainly a possibility, it does not account for the irregular (non-Vanhuyse) patterns that are prevalent in that age group.

Another possible source of the differences between infants and older subjects is the presence of material in the middle ear. Mesenchyme (unresorbed fetal tissue), amniotic fluid, and other cellular debris have been observed in the middle ears of infant temporal bones (Eavey, 1993; Paparella, Shea, Meyerhoff, et al., 1980). Abnormal tissue that is in contact with the ossicles and eardrum have been shown to produce irregular tympanometric patterns in chinchillas (Margolis, Schachern, & Fulton, 1998). On the other hand, the middle ears of newborn chinchillas with irregular tympanometric patterns were free of debris and appeared mature in structure (Hsu et al., 1996).

Although the reasons for the chaotic nature of tympanometric patterns in newborns are not clear, it is evident that low-frequency tympanometry is not effective for detecting middle ear pathology in the neonate. Balkany, Berman, Simmons, and Jafek (1978) reported that 30% of 125 consecutively examined NICU infants had MEE, based on otoscopy and/or tympanocentesis. All were judged to have normal 226 Hz tympanograms. Others also have reported normal 226 Hz tympanograms in the presence of confirmed MEE in neonates (Hunter & Margolis, 1992; Paradise et al., 1976). Figure 4.21 shows tympanograms from a newborn intensive care nursery patient with confirmed acute otitis media with effusion. The 226 Hz tympanogram appeared to be normal and similar to that of the unaffected ear. Using a higher probe tone frequency, however, the tympanogram was clearly abnormal. Evidence is mounting that tympanograms obtained with probe tone frequencies that are higher than the conventional 226 Hz are more sensitive to middle ear disease in newborns than conventional tympanometry (Marchant, McMillan, Shurin, Johnson, Turczyk, Feinstein, & Panek, 1986; Rhodes, 1996).

Wideband Reflectance

A new technique has been used recently to evaluate middle ear function. *Energy reflectance* is the ratio of energy reflected from a surface to the energy that strikes the surface (incident energy). This is a useful concept for evaluating middle ear function because it tells us how much energy is reflected from the eardrum and how much is absorbed by the middle ear. Recall that because of the complexity of the

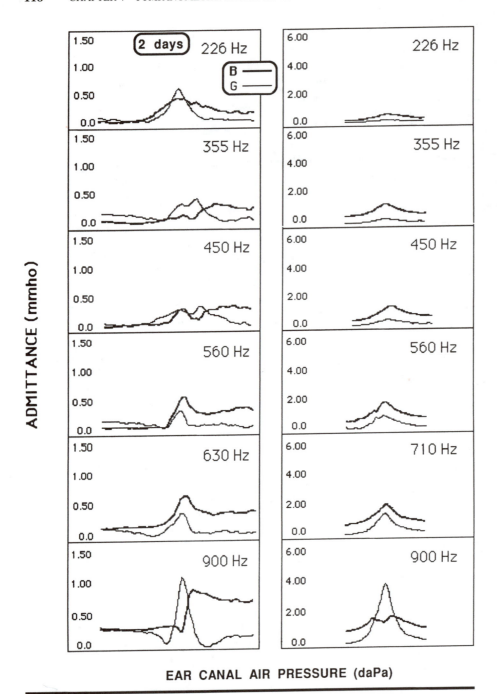

FIGURE 4.20 Tympanogram from a full-term 2-day-old infant (left panel) and from the same infant at age 133 days (right panel).

middle ear system, the amount of energy absorbed by the middle ear is not the same as the energy delivered to the cochlea. Consequently, although energy reflectance indicates how much energy is transmitted into the middle ear, it may not always correlate with hearing sensitivity.

Measurement systems used to measure energy reflectance are calibrated differently than those used for multifrequency tympanometry. Whereas multifrequency tympanometry is restricted to frequencies below 2 kHz, energy reflectance systems can measure over a much wider frequency range. Because energy reflectance is mathematically related to impedance and admittance, it is possible to derive any immittance quantity from measures of reflectance.

Keefe and colleagues (1993) measured energy reflectance from normal subjects aged 1 month to adult. The

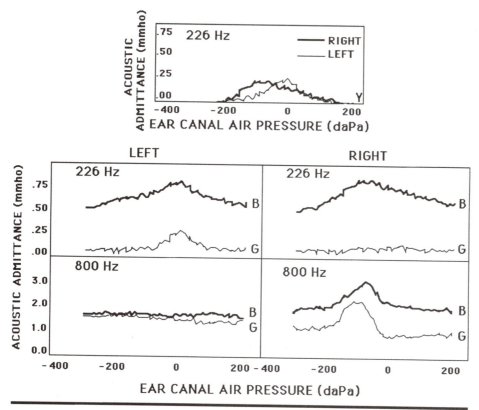

FIGURE 4.21 Tympanograms from a 2-week-old infant with acute otitis media in the left ear. The 226 Hz tympanograms appear to be normal and bilaterally similar. The 800 Hz tympanogram is flat in the involved ear and normal in the uninvolved ear.

results are shown in Figure 4.22. In normal adult ears, more than 90% of low-frequency energy is reflected, accounting for our relatively poor auditory sensitivity below 500 Hz. As frequency increases above 500 Hz, reflectance decreases forming a broad minimum near 3000 Hz. It is in this range that energy is most efficiently transmitted into the middle ear. Infants show roughly the same pattern. The youngest infants in the study (1 month) show an additional dip near 400 Hz, possibly an effect of the incomplete development of the ear canal wall. A compliant ear canal wall would absorb energy, decreasing the reflectance of the ear. The authors suggested that the 400 Hz frequency is the expected location of a reflectance dip due to the vibration of soft tissue in the ear canal.

Keefe and Levi (1996) introduced the concept of the reflectance tympanogram. Using a multifrequency tympanometry instrument they calculated reflectance from admittance and plotted it against ear canal air pressure. Margolis, Saly, and Keefe (in press) recorded reflectance tympanograms from normal adult subjects. Figure 4.23 shows the average reflectance for three ear canal pressures (0, +300, –300 daPa). Pressurizing the ear canal changes the reflectance pattern in several ways. At low frequencies reflectance is increased. The broad minimum that occurs

around 3 kHz becomes narrower, deepens, and shifts up in frequency, forming a narrow minimum around 5000 Hz. At this frequency, pressurizing the ear *increases* the sound absorption by the middle ear. This would be expected to *improve* hearing in a narrow, high-frequency region. This is consistent with observations made as early as 1820 by Wollaston that middle ear pressure significantly decreases the loudness of low-frequency sounds with little effect on higher frequencies.

Figure 4.24 shows mean reflectance tympanograms from 20 normal adult subjects for frequencies ranging from 100 to 11,000 Hz. As frequency increases, reflectance tympanograms progress through a sequence of three patterns. At low frequencies where reflectance is increased by positive and negative pressure, the reflectance tympanogram shows a single minimum near ambient pressure. At higher frequencies, where reflectance decreases with pressure, the pattern is inverted with a single maximum. At the highest frequencies the pattern is nearly flat, indicating that pressure has little effect on reflectance. This sequence of patterns may form the basis for evaluating ears with middle ear pathology, much the same as the Vanhuyse model is used for multifrequency tympanometry.

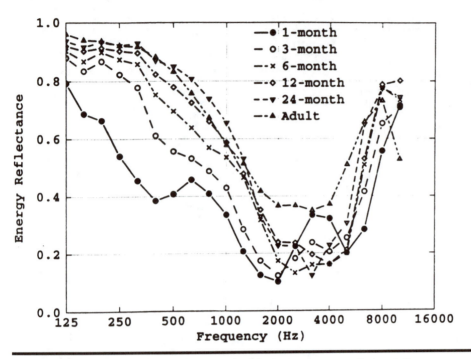

FIGURE 4.22   Energy reflectance for normal subjects aged one month to adult. (From Keefe, Bulen, Arehart, & Burns, "Ear-canal impedance and reflection coefficient in human infants and adults." *Journal of the Acoustical Society of America, 94*(5), 2617–2638, Figure 4, 1993. © Acoustical Society of America.)

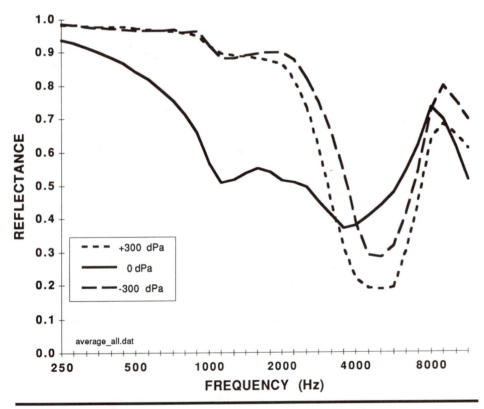

FIGURE 4.23   Average energy reflectance for 20 normal subjects at three ear canal air pressures (0, 300, −300 daPa).

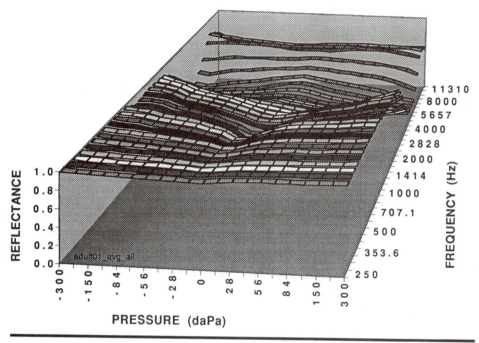

FIGURE 4.24 Average reflectance tympanograms for 20 normal adult subjects. As the test frequency progresses from low to high, tympanometric patterns progress from V-shaped, to inverted V, to flat.

CASE STUDIES

The following cases are patients in a long-term prospective study of otitis media. Children were recruited into the study at the time they were scheduled for surgery (myringotomy with tympanostomy tubes). Patients were tested preoperatively, postoperatively (2 weeks), and then quarterly for three years, semiannually for the next three years, and annually thereafter. See Giebink, Daly, Lindgren, Hunter, Westover, Grant, & Le, 1996, for additional information.

Recurrent Otitis Media

SR is a 10-year-old boy who has been followed since early childhood. He had frequent episodes of otitis media in his first two years and had bilateral myringotomy with tympanostomy tubes at age 2 and again at age 3. After the second surgery he responded well and his hearing was normal. At ages 6 and 7 he had several episodes of acute otitis media that were treated with antibiotics. Although his 226 Hz tympanograms returned to normal, the hearing in the left ear continued to show a mid-frequency conductive hearing loss, which has persisted to age 10. At his ten-year study visit the audiogram (Figure 4.25) showed a 35 dB conductive loss on the left in the mid frequencies (0.5 to 2.0 kHz). The eardrum on the left was retracted and showed areas of atrophy and fibrosis but there was no evidence of inflammation or effusion.

The 226 Hz tympanograms, shown in Figure 4.25, showed negative tympanometric peak pressure (–170 daPa), indicating negative middle ear pressure, and high static admittance, probably due to the atrophic areas on the eardrum. Multifrequency tympanograms (Figure 4.26) were

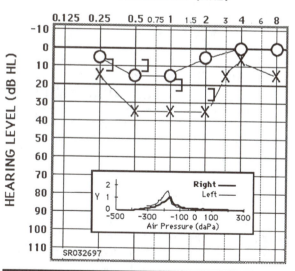

FIGURE 4.25 Audiogram and 226 Hz tympanograms from a 10-year-old boy with recurrent otitis media.

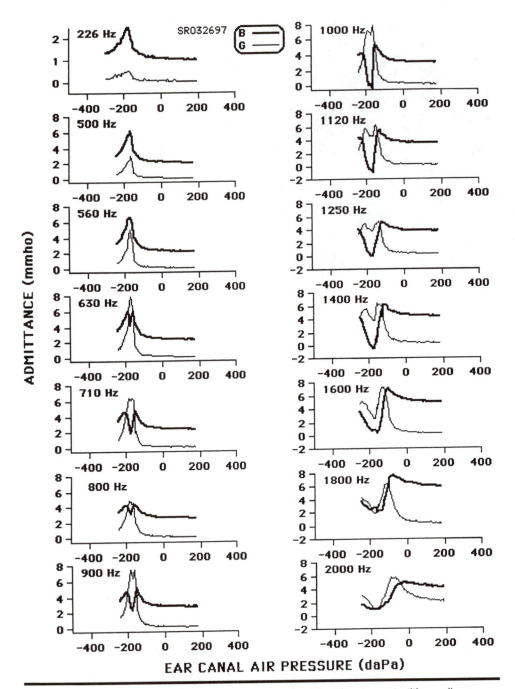

FIGURE 4.26 Multifrequency tympanograms for patient SR with recurrent otitis media. The patterns are 1B1G for frequencies ≤ 560 Hz, 3B1G at 630 Hz, and 3B3G at frequencies above 630 Hz.

characterized by regular Vanhuyse patterns, shifted toward negative pressure. The resonant frequency was low normal (710 Hz), with 3B3G and 5B3G patterns occurring at unusually low frequencies (900 and 1000 Hz, respectively). Above 1000 Hz, the patterns were 3B3G.

Wideband reflectance is shown in Figure 4.27. The measurements were made with the ear canal air pressure set to compensate for the middle ear pressure, that is, at tympanometric peak pressure. Also shown are the mean, 5th percentile, and 95th percentile from normal adult

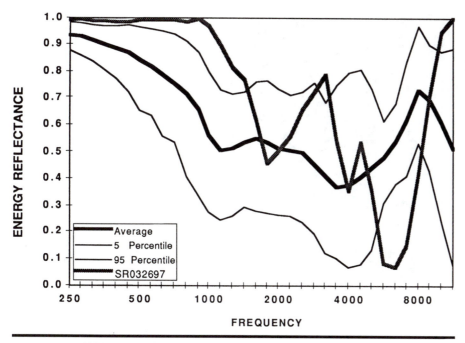

FIGURE 4.27 Wideband reflectance for patient SR with recurrent otitis media and conductive hearing loss. The mean, 5th, and 95th percentiles are shown for 20 normal adult subjects. The patient has a region of abnormal reflectance from 250 to 1500 Hz and a region of abnormally low reflectance from about 5 to 7 kHz.

subjects. There are two frequency regions in which reflectance is abnormal. Below 1500 Hz, reflectance is abnormally high. Below 1200 Hz reflectance is nearly 1.0 indicating that almost all the energy is reflected. This region of abnormality corresponds roughly to the region of hearing loss. Between 5 and 8 kHz, reflectance is abnormally low, indicating more than the normal sound absorption, perhaps due to the atrophic eardrum.

Reflectance tympanograms are shown in Figure 4.28. The patterns appear to be quite disorganized compared to normal subject data in Figure 4.24. In this case, reflectance tympanograms seem to more clearly identify the middle ear pathology than either the 226 Hz tympanograms or multifrequency tympanograms. The data shown in tympanogram format (Figure 4.28) appear more clearly abnormal than the same data displayed as reflectance plotted against frequency (Figure 4.27).

This case illustrates the complex relationship between acoustic admittance as measured by multifrequency tympanometry and energy reflectance. Multifrequency tympanograms indicate a high admittance system that has reduced stiffness, resulting in a low resonant frequency and the occurrence of 3B3G and 5B3G patterns at relatively low frequencies. The reflectance results, however, indicate an abnormally high reflectance at frequencies roughly corresponding to the frequency range of the hearing loss (Figure 4.25) and a rather disorganized response to ear canal air pressure (Figure 4.28).

The hearing loss is probably not accounted for by the abnormal otoscopic features. It is likely that middle ear adhesions have been formed as a result of recurrent otitis media. (See Margolis et al., 1998, for an example.) The multifrequency tympanograms show the expected effects of the atrophic eardrum. The correspondence of the frequency region of high reflectance and the hearing loss suggests that reflectance may be a useful diagnostic indicator for this type of pathology. More cases like this are required to determine the relative value of multifrequency tympanometry and wideband reflectance for detecting middle ear pathology.

Cholesteatoma

SP had bilateral myringotomy and tubes when he was 18 months old. On the preoperative examination, the right ear was thick and immobile and the left ear had a retraction pocket. There was no fluid at the time of surgery. At the seven-year study visit video otomicroscopy indicated two areas of crusted debris on the right eardrum. The otologist attempted to remove them by suction without success. Two weeks later the patient underwent exploratory surgery of

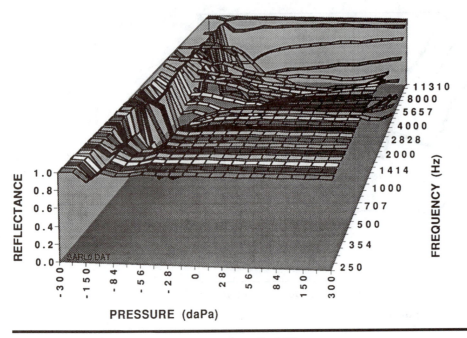

FIGURE 4.28 Reflectance tympanograms for patient SR.

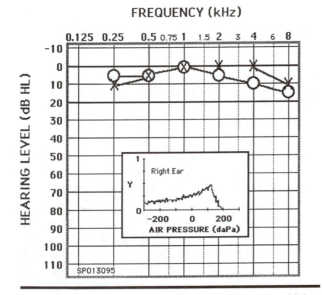

FIGURE 4.29 Audiogram and 226 Hz tympanogram (right ear) for patient SP with a cholesteatoma originating from the tympanic membrane and invading the middle ear.

the right ear and a cholesteatoma, adherent to one of the areas of debris on the eardrum, was removed from the middle ear.

The audiogram indicated normal hearing (Figure 4.29). The 226 Hz tympanogram (Figure 4.29 inset) had a distinct peak with static admittance in the normal range,

although the morphology was unusual. Multifrequency tympanograms were clearly abnormal at every frequency (Figure 4.30).

The case illustrates the superiority of multifrequency tympanometry over 226 Hz tympanometry for detecting some middle ear pathologies. Although the 226 Hz tympanogram was a bit odd, the static admittance was normal and it probably would be categorized as a Type A with positive pressure. Multifrequency tympanograms are unambiguous in suggesting abnormal middle ear function.

Chronic Otitis Media

JT was 10 months old when he had his first surgery and a second set of tubes was inserted at age 27 months. After each surgery he responded well but then developed recurrent episodes of otitis media. After the second surgery, the tube in the right ear extruded within the first postoperative month. He developed otitis media in that ear by the fifth postoperative month and had frequent episodes over the next twenty-two months. On subsequent examinations, the right eardrum appeared progressively retracted without

active disease. At his seven-year study visit he had normal hearing and there was no indication of recent symptoms. His audiogram and 226 Hz tympanograms were normal (Figure 4.31).

The otomicroscopic examination showed a complete absence of identifiable landmarks on the right eardrum. There was a deep retraction pocket anteriorly and a tympanosclerotic region in the anterior-superior region. Most of the drum was retracted against the promontory of the middle ear and was immobile on pneumatic stimulation. Only a small portion of the drum was mobile.

Multifrequency tympanograms (Figure 4.32) show an abnormally low resonant frequency (500 Hz) and broad, flat patterns at high frequencies. 3B3G patterns occur at abnormally low frequencies (≥ 560 Hz).

Considering the severity of the pathology, it is surprising that there are not more abnormal test results. The normal hearing and 226 Hz tympanogram are particularly unexpected. Only the multifrequency tympanograms indicated the presence of middle ear pathology. This type of middle ear pathology frequently leads to chronic sequelae like atelectasis, cholesteatoma, ossicular erosion, and conductive hearing loss. It is important to identify this condition and make the appropriate referral for otologic management. In this case, audiometry and single-frequency tympanometry did not reveal the middle ear pathology.

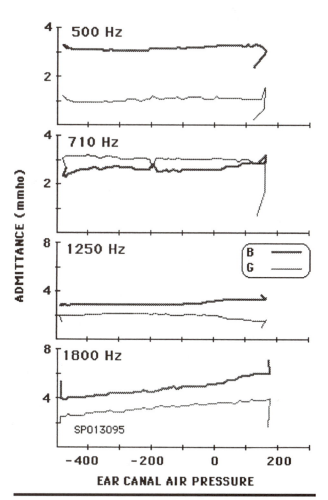

FIGURE 4.30 Multifrequency tympanograms from patient SP with a cholesteatoma. At approximately 200 daPa the values went out of range of the measurement instrument.

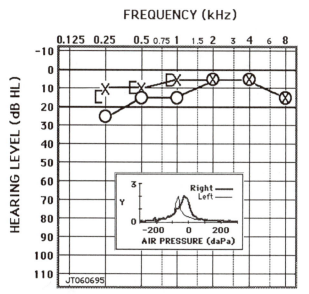

FIGURE 4.31 Audiogram and 226 Hz tympanograms from patient JT with chronic otitis media.

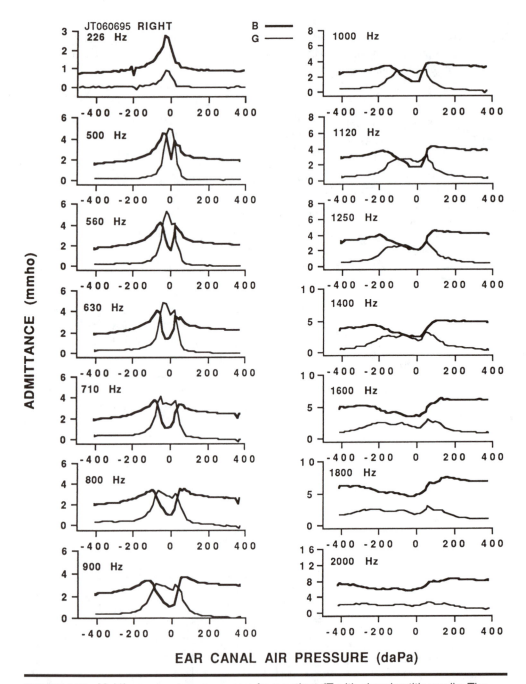

FIGURE 4.32   Multifrequency tympanograms from patient JT with chronic otitis media. The 226 Hz tympanograms are normal. At 500 Hz the pattern is 1B1G and the susceptance notch reaches the positive tail indicating resonance at that frequency. The 3B3G pattern occurs at an abnormally low frequency (560 Hz) and the high-frequency patterns are abnormally flattened.

REFERENCES

Alberti, P. W., & Jerger, J. F. (1974). Probe-tone frequency and the diagnostic value of tympanometry. *Archives of Otolaryngology, 99*, 206–10.

American National Standards Institute (1987). *American National Standard Specifications for Instruments to Measure Aural Acoustic Impedance and Admittance* (ANSI S3.39-1987). New York: Author.

American National Standards Institute (1996). *American National Standard Specification for Audiometers* (ANSI S3.6-1989). New York: Author.

American Speech-Language-Hearing Association (1979). Guidelines for acoustic immittance screening for middle-ear function. *Asha, 21*, 283–288.

American Speech-Language-Hearing Association (1990). Guidelines for screening for hearing impairment and middle-ear disorders. *Asha, 32* (Suppl 2), 17–24.

American Academy of Audiology (1997a). Identification of hearing loss and middle ear dysfunction in children. *Audiology Today, 9*, 18–20.

American Academy of Audiology (1997b). Identification of hearing loss and middle-ear dysfunction in preschool and school-age children. *Audiology Today, 9*, 21–23.

Balkany, T. J., Berman, S. A., Simmons, M. A., & Jafek, B. W. (1978). Middle ear effusion in neonates. *Laryngoscope, 88*, 398–405.

Bennett, M. (1975). Acoustic impedance bridge measurements with the neonate. *British Journal of Audiology, 9*, 117–124.

Bluestone, C. D., Beery, Q. C., & Paradise, J. L. (1973). Audiometry and tympanometry in relation to middle-ear effusions in children. *Laryngoscope, 83*, 594–604.

Bluestone, C. D., Fria, T. J., Arjona, S. K., Casselbrant, M. L., Schwartz, D. M., Ruben, R. J., Gates, G. A., Downs, M. P., Northern, J. L., Jerger, J. F., et al. (1986). Controversies in screening for middle ear disease and hearing loss in children. *Pediatrics, 77*, 57–70.

Brooks, D. N. (1968). An objective method of determining fluid in the middle ear. *International Journal of Audiology, 7*, 280–286.

Cantekin, E. I., Bluestone, C. D., Fria, T. J., Stool, S. E., Beery, Q. C., & Sabo, D. L. (1980). Identification of otitis media with effusion in children. *Annals of Otology, Rhinology and Laryngology, 89* (Supplement 68), 190–195.

Cantekin, E. I., Doyle, W. J., Phillips, D. C., & Bluestone, C. D. (1980). Gas absorption in the middle ear. *Annals of Otology, Rhinology and Laryngology, 89* (Supplement 68), 71–75.

Colletti, V. (1976). Tympanometry from 200 to 2000 Hz probe tone. *Audiology, 15*, 106–119.

Daly, K., Hunter, L. L., Levine, S., Lindgren, B., & Giebink, G. (1997). Sequelae of otitis media from childhood through young adulthood. In *Midwinter Meeting of the Association for Research in Otolaryngology,* 20 (pp. 698). St. Petersburg Beach, FL.

DeJonge, R. R. (1986). Normal tympanometric gradient: A comparison of three methods. *Audiology, 25*, 299–308.

Diamant, M., Rubensohn, G., & Walander, A. (1958). Otosalpingitis and mastoid pneumatization. *Acta Otolaryngologica, 49*, 381–388.

Eavey, R. D. (1993). Abnormalities of the neonatal ear: Otoscopic observations, histologic observations, and a model for contamination of the middle ear by cellular contents of amniotic fluid. *Laryngoscope, 103* (Supplement 58), 1–31.

Elner, A., Ingelstedt, S., & Ivarsson, A. (1971). The elastic properties of the tympanic membrane. *Acta Otolaryngologica, 72*, 397–403.

Falk, B. (1981). Negative pressure induced by sniffing, a tympanometric study in healthy ears. *Journal of Otolaryngology, 10*, 299–305.

Falk, B. (1983). Variability in the tympanogram due to eustachian tube closing failure. *Scandinavian Audiology, Supplement 17*, 11–17.

Feldman, A. S. (1976). Tympanometry—procedures, interpretations, and variables. In A. S. Feldman & L. A. Wilber (Eds.), *Acoustic Impedance and Admittance—The Measurement of Middle Ear Function* (pp. 103–155). Baltimore: Williams & Wilkins.

Fiellau-Nikolajsen, M. (1983). Tympanometry and secretory otitis media. Observations on diagnosis, epidemiology, treatment, and prevention in prospective cohort studies of three-year-old children. *Acta Otolaryngologica* (Supplement 394), 1–73.

Gates, G. A., Avery, C., Cooper, J. C., Hearne, E. M., & Holt, G. R. (1986). Predictive value of tympanometry in middle ear effusion. *Annals of Otology, Rhinology and Laryngology, 95*, 46–50.

Giebink, G., Daly, K., Lindgren, B., Hunter, L., Westover, D., Grant, S., & Le, C. (1996). Seven-year prospective study of tympanic membrane pathology after tympanostomy tube treatment of chronic otitis media with effusion. In D. J. Lim (Ed.), *Recent Advances in Otitis Media: Proceedings of the 6th International Symposium* (pp. 380–383). Hamilton, Ontario: Decker Periodicals.

Goode, R. L., & Killion, M. C. (1994). New knowledge about the function of the human middle ear: Development of an improved analog model. *American Journal of Otology, 15*, 145–154.

Hanks, W. D., & Rose, K. J. (1993). Middle ear resonance and acoustic immittance measures in children. *Journal of Speech and Hearing Research, 36* (1), 218–221.

Haughton, P. M. (1977). Validity of tympanometry for middle ear effusions. *Archives of Otorhinolaryngology, 103*, 505–513.

Hergils, L., & Magnuson, B. (1985). Morning pressure in the middle ear. *Archive of Otolaryngology, 111*, 86–89.

Hergils, L., & Magnuson, B. (1987). Middle-ear pressure under basal conditions. *Archives of Otolaryngology—Head and Neck Surgery, 113*, 829–832.

Hilding, A. C. (1944). Role of ciliary action in production of pulmonary atelectasis, vacuum in paranasal sinuses, and in otitis media. *Transactions of the American Academy of Ophthalmology and Otolaryngology,* 367–378.

Himelfarb, M. Z., Popelka, G. R., & Shanon, E. (1979). Tympanometry in normal neonates. *Journal of Speech and Hearing Research, 22*, 179–191.

Holte, L. A., Cavanaugh, R. M., & Margolis, R. H. (1990). Ear canal wall mobility and tympanometric shape in young infants. *Journal of Pediatrics, 117*, 77–80.

Holte, L. A., & Margolis, R. H. (1987). Screening tympanometry. *Seminars in Hearing, 8,* 329–338.

Holte, L. A., Margolis, R. H., & Cavanaugh, R. M. (1991). Developmental changes in multifrequency tympanograms. *Audiology, 30,* 1–24.

Hsu, G. S., Margolis, R. H., Schachern, P. L., Sutherland, C., & Javel, E. (1996). The development of hearing and middle ear function in neonatal chinchillas. In *Association for Research in Otolaryngology,* St. Petersburg Beach, FL.

Hunter, L. L., & Margolis, R. H. (1992). Multifrequency tympanometry: Current clinical application. *American Journal of Audiology, 1,* 33–43.

Hunter, L. L., Margolis, R. H., Daly, K. A., & Giebink, G. S. (1992). Relationship of tympanometric estimates of middle ear volume to middle ear status at surgery. In *15th Midwinter Research Meeting of the Association for Research in Otolaryngology,* St. Petersburg Beach, FL.

Ivey, R. (1975). Tympanometric curves and otosclerosis. *Journal of Speech and Hearing Research, 18,* 554–558.

Jerger, J. (1970). Clinical experience with impedance audiometry. *Archives of Otolaryngology, 92,* 311–324.

Jerger, J., Jerger, S., Mauldin, L., & Segal, P. (1974). Studies in impedance audiometry: II. Children less than six years old. *Archives of Otolaryngology, 99,* 1–9.

Keefe, D. H., Bulen, J. C., Arehart, K. H., & Burns, E. M. (1993). Ear-canal impedance and reflection coefficient in human infants and adults. *Journal of the Acoustical Society of America, 94*(5), 2617–2638.

Keefe, D. H., & Levi, E. (1996). Maturation of the middle and external ears: Acoustic power-based responses and reflectance tympanometry. *Ear and Hearing, 17,* 361–373.

Keith, R. W. (1973). Impedance audiometry with neonates. *Archives of Otolaryngology, 97,* 465–476.

Keith, R. W. (1975). Middle ear function in neonates. *Archives of Otolaryngology, 101,* 376–379.

Koebsell, K. A., & Margolis, R. H. (1986). Tympanometric gradient measured from normal preschool children. *Audiology, 25,* 149–157.

Kringlbotn, M. (1988). Network model for the human middle ear. *Scandinavian Audiology, 17,* 75–85.

Le, C. T., Daly, K. A., Margolis, R. H., Lindgren, B. R., & Giebink, G. S. (1992). A clinical profile of otitis media. *Archives of Otolaryngology—Head and Neck Surgery, 118,* 1225–1228.

Le, C. T., Hunter, L. L., Margolis, R. H., Daly, K. A., Lindgren, B. R., & Giebink, G. S. (1994). A clinical profile of otitis media without an intact tympanic membrane. *Archives of Otolaryngology—Head and Neck Surgery, 120,* 513–516.

Liden, G. (1969). The scope and application of current audiometric tests. *Journal of Laryngology and Otology, 83,* 507–520.

Liden, G., Bjorkman, G., Nyman, H., & Kunov, H. (1977). Tympanometry and acoustic impedance. *Acta Otolaryngologica, 83,* 140–145.

Liden, G., Harford, E., & Hallen, O. (1974a). Automatic tympanometry in clinical practice. *Audiology, 13,* 126–139.

Liden, G., Harford, E., & Hallen, O. (1974b). Tympanometry for the diagnosis of ossicular disruption. *Archives of Otolaryngology, 99,* 23–29.

Liden, G., Peterson, J., & Bjorkman, G. (1970). Tympanometry. *Archives of Otolaryngology, 92,* 248–257.

Lindeman, P., & Holmquist, J. (1982). Volume measurement of middle ear and mastoid air cell system with impedance audiometry on patients with ear-drum perforations. *Acta Otolaryngologica, Supplement 386,* 70–73.

Magnuson, B. (1981). On the origin of the high negative pressure in the middle ear space. *American Journal of Otolaryngology, 2,* 1–12.

Magnuson, B. (1983). Eustachian tube pathophysiology. *American Journal of Otolaryngology, 4,* 123–130.

Marchant, C. D., McMillan, P. M., Shurin, P. A., Johnson, C. E., Turczyk, V. A., Feinstein, J. C., & Panek, D. M. (1986). Objective diagnosis of otitis media in early infancy by tympanometry and ipsilateral acoustic reflex thresholds. *Journal of Pediatrics, 109*(4), 590–595.

Margolis, R. H. (1981). Fundamentals of acoustic immittance. In G. R. Popelka (Ed.), *Hearing Assessment with the Acoustic Reflex* (pp. 117–144). New York: Grune & Stratton.

Margolis, R. H., & Goycoolea, H. G. (1993). Multifrequency tympanometry in normal adults. *Ear and Hearing, 14,* 408–413.

Margolis, R. H., & Heller, J. W. (1987). Screening tympanometry: Criteria for medical referral. *Audiology, 26,* 197–208.

Margolis, R. H., & Nelson, D. A. (1992). Acute otitis media with transient sensorineural hearing loss: A case study. *Archives of Otolaryngology—Head and Neck Surgery, 119,* 682–686.

Margolis, R. H., Osguthorpe, J. D., & Popelka, G. R. (1978). The effects of experimentally produced middle ear lesions on tympanometry in cats. *Acta Otolaryngologica, 86,* 428–436.

Margolis, R. H., & Popelka, G. R. (1977). Interactions among tympanometric variables. *Journal of Speech and Hearing Research, 20,* 447–62.

Margolis, R. H., Saly, G. L., & Keefe, D. H. (in press). Wideband reflectance tympanometry in normal adults. *Journal of the Acoustical Society of America.*

Margolis, R. H., Schachern, P. L., & Fulton, S. (1998). Multifrequency tympanometry and histopathology in chinchillas with experimentally produced middle-ear pathologies. *Acta Otolaryngologica, 118,* 216–225.

Margolis, R. H., & Smith, P. (1977). Tympanometric asymmetry. *Journal of Speech and Hearing Research, 20,* 446.

Margolis, R. H., Van Camp, K. J., Wilson, R. H., & Creten, W. L. (1985). Multifrequency tympanometry in normal ears. *Audiology, 24,* 44–53.

Maw, A. R., & Bawden, R. (1994). Tympanic membrane atrophy, scarring, atelectasis and attic retraction in persistent untreated otitis media with effusion and ventilation tube insertion. *International Journal of Pediatric Otorhinolaryngology, 30,* 189–204.

Metz, O. (1946). The acoustical impedance measured on normal and pathological ears. *Acta Otolaryngologica (Stockholm), Supplement 63,* 3–254.

Moller, A. (1965a). An experimental study of the acoustic impedance of the middle ear and its transmission properties. *Acta Otolaryngologica (Stockholm), 60,* 129–149.

Moller, A. R. (1965b). Network model of the middle ear. *Journal of the Acoustical Society of America, 33,* 168–176.

Molvaer, O., Vallersnes, F., & Kringlbotn, M. (1978). The size of the middle ear and the mastoid air cell. *Acta Otolaryngologica*, *85*, 24–32.

Murphy, D. (1979). Negative pressure in the middle ear by ciliary propulsion of mucus through the Eustachian tube. *Laryngoscope*, *89*, 954–961.

Nahin, P. J. (1988). *Oliver Heaviside: Sage in Solitude*. New York: IEEE Press.

Nozza, R. J., Bluestone, C. D., & Kardatze, D. (1992a). Sensitivity, specificity, and predictive value of immittance measures in the identification of middle-ear effusion. In F. H. Bess & J. W. Hall (Eds.), *Screening Children for Auditory Function* (pp. 315–329). Nashville: Bill Wilkerson Center Press.

Nozza, R. J., Bluestone, C. D., Kardatze, D., & Bachman, R. (1992b). Towards the validation of aural acoustic immittance measures for diagnosis of middle ear effusion in children. *Ear and Hearing*, *13*, 442–453.

Nozza, R. J., Bluestone, C. D., Kardatze, D., & Bachman, R. (1994). Identification of middle ear effusion by aural acoustic admittance and otoscopy. *Ear and Hearing*, *15*, 310–323.

Ostergard, C. A., & Carter, D. R. (1981). Positive middle ear pressure shown by tympanometry. *Archives of Otolaryngology*, *107*, 353–356.

Ostfeld, E. J., & Silberberg, A. (1992). Theoretic analysis of middle ear gas composition under conditions of nonphysiologic ventilation. *Annals of Otology, Rhinology and Laryngology*, *101*, 445–451.

Palva, T., & Palva, A. (1966). Size of the human mastoid air cell system. *Acta Otolaryngologica*, *62*, 237–251.

Paparella, M. M., Shea, D., Meyerhoff, W. L., et al. (1980). Silent otitis media. *Laryngoscope*, *90*, 1089–1098.

Paradise, J. L., Smith, G. C., & Bluestone, C. D. (1976). Tympanometric detection of middle ear effusion in infants and children. *Pediatrics*, *58*, 198–210.

Poulsen, G., & Tos, M. (1978). Screening tympanometry in newborn infants and during the first six months of life. *Scandinavian Audiology*, *7*, 159–166.

Proctor, B. (1991). Chronic otitis media and mastoiditis. In M. M. Paparella, D. A. Shumrick, J. L. Gluckman, & W. I. Meyerhoff (Eds.), *Otolaryngology* (pp. 1349–1376). Philadelphia: W. B. Saunders.

Proud, G. O., Odoi, H., & Toledo, P. S. (1971). Bullar pressure changes in eustachian tube dysfunction. *Annals of Otology, Rhinology and Laryngology*, *80*, 835–837.

Renvall, U., & Holmquist, J. (1976). Tympanometry revealing middle ear pathology. *Annals of Otology, Rhinology and Laryngology*, *85 (Supplement 25)*, 209–215.

Renvall, U., Liden, G., Jungert, S., & Nilsson, E. (1975). Impedance audiometry in the detection of secretory otitis media. *Scandinavian Audiology*, *4*, 119–124.

Rhodes, M. C. (1996). *Multifrequency Tympanometry, Acoustic Stapedius Reflexes, and Evoked Otoacoustic Emissions in Infant Hearing Screening*. M.S. Thesis, University of Minnesota.

Roush, J. (1990). Identification of hearing loss and middle ear disease in preschool and school-age children. *Seminars in Hearing*, *11*, 357–371.

Roush, J., Drake, A., & Sexton, J. E. (1992). Identification of middle ear dysfunction in young children: A comparison of tympanometric screening procedures. *Ear and Hearing*, *13*(2), 63–69.

Roush, J., & Tait, C. A. (1985). Pure-tone and acoustic immittance screening of preschool-aged children: An examination of referral criteria. *Ear and Hearing*, *6*, 245–249.

Rubensohn, G. (1965). Mastoid pneumatization in children at various ages. *Acta Otolaryngologica*, *60*, 11–14.

Sade, J., & Berco, E. (1976). Atelectasis and secretory otitis media. *Annals of Otology, Rhinology and Laryngology*, *85 (Supplement 25)*, 66–72.

Shahnaz, N., & Polka, L. (in press). Standard and multifrequency tympanometry in normal and otosclerotic ears. *Ear and Hearing*.

Shallop, J. K. (1976). The historical development of the study of middle ear function. In A. S. Feldman & L. A. Wilber (Eds.), *Acoustic Impedance and Admittance—The Measurement of Middle Ear Function* (pp. 8–48). Baltimore: Williams & Wilkins.

Shanks, J. E. (1985). Tympanometric volume estimates in patients with intact and perforated eardrums. *Asha*, *27*, 78.

Shanks, J. E., & Lilly, D. J. (1981). An evaluation of tympanometric estimates of ear canal volume. *Journal of Speech and Hearing Research*, *24*, 557–566.

Shanks, J. E., Stelmachowicz, P. G., Beauchaine, K. L., & Schulte, L. (1992). Equivalent ear canal volumes in children pre- and post-tympanostomy tube insertion. *Journal of Speech and Hearing Research*, *35*, 936–941.

Sheehy, J., Brachmann, D., & Graham, M. (1977). Complications of cholesteatoma: A report on 1024 cases. In B. McCabe, J. Sade, & M. Abramson (Eds.), *Cholesteatoma: First International Conference* (pp. 420–429). Birmingham, AL: Aesculapius.

Silman, S., Silverman, C. A., & Arick, D. S. (1992). Acoustic-immittance screening for detection of middle-ear effusion in children. *Journal of the American Academy of Audiology*, *3*, 262–268.

Sprague, B. H., Wiley, T. L., & Goldstein, R. (1985). Tympanometric and acoustic reflex studies in neonates. *Journal of Speech and Hearing Research*, *28*, 265–272.

Takasaka, T., Hozawa, K., Shoji, F., Takahashi, Y., Jingu, K., Adachi, M., & Kobayashi, T. (1996). Tympanostomy tube treatment in recurrent otitis media with effusion. In D. J. Lim, C. D. Bluestone, M. Casselbrant, J. O. Klein, & P. L. Ogra (Eds.), *Recent Advances in Otitis Media* (pp. 197–199). Hamilton, Ontario: B.C. Decker.

Terkildsen, K., & Nielsen, S. (1960). An electroacoustic impedance measuring bridge for clinical use. *Archives of Otolaryngology*, *72*, 339–346.

Terkildsen, K., & Thomsen, K. A. (1959). The influence of pressure variations on the impedance of the human ear drum. *Journal of Laryngology and Otology*, *73*, 409–418.

Van Camp, K. J., Margolis, R. H., Wilson, R. H., Creten, W. L., & Shanks, J. E. (1986). Principles of tympanometry. *ASHA Monographs* (24), 1–88.

Van Camp, K. J., Raman, E. R., & Creten, W. L. (1976). Two-component versus admittance tympanometry. *Audiology*, *15*, 120–127.

Vanhuyse, V. J., Creten, W. L., & Van Camp, K. J. (1975). On the W-notching of tympanograms. *Scandinavian Audiology, 4,* 45–50.

West, W. (1928). Measurements of the acoustical impedances of human ears. *Post Office Elect Engineering, 21,* 293.

Wiley, T. L., Cruikshanks, K. J., Nondahl, D. M., Tweed, T. S., Klein, R., & Klein, B. E. K. (1996). Tympanometric measures in older adults. *Journal of the American Academy of Audiology, 7,* 260–268.

Wiley, T. L., & Fowler, C. G. (1997). *Acoustic Immittance Measures in Clinical Audiology.* San Diego: Singular Publishing.

Wollaston, W. H. (1820). On sounds inaudible to certain ears. *Philosophical Transactions of the Royal Society of London, 110,* 306–314.

Yee, A. L., & Cantekin, E. I. (1986). Effect of changes in systemic oxygen tension on middle ear gas exchange. *Annals of Otology, Rhinology and Laryngology, 95,* 369–372.

Zwislocki, J. (1962). Analysis of the middle-ear function. I. Input impedance. *Journal of the Acoustical Society of America, 34,* 1514–1523.

Zwislocki, J. J. (1963). An acoustic method for clinical examination of the ear. *Journal of Speech and Hearing Research, 6,* 303–314.

CHAPTER 5

ACOUSTIC-REFLEX MEASUREMENTS

RICHARD H. WILSON
ROBERT H. MARGOLIS

The acoustically evoked contraction of the stapedius muscle, which is called the *acoustic reflex*, has been the topic of considerable experimental and clinical research, beginning with the observation by Hensen (1878) that the stapedius and tensor tympani muscles in dogs contract in response to acoustic stimulation. Although debated since the work of Hensen, the function of the middle-ear muscles will not be discussed in this chapter. (Borg, Counter, and Rösler [1984] provide an excellent review of the theories of middle-ear muscle function.) In this chapter, the basis and methods for the clinical application of acoustic-reflex measurements will be reviewed.[1]

Lüscher made the first direct observations of the acoustic reflex in humans in 1929 (Potter, 1936). He viewed the movement of the stapedius tendon through a perforation in the tympanic membrane of a patient who had an otherwise normal middle ear. Lüscher observed the following: (1) the bilateral (consensual) nature of the acoustic reflex to monaural stimulation, (2) the frequency range of effective reflex eliciting stimuli, (3) the greater sensitivity of the reflex to complex signals in comparison to tonal signals, (4) the graded nature of the reflex, (5) the "anticipatory" characteristic of the reflex, (6) the responsiveness to certain nonacoustic stimuli, and (7) the relative independence of the muscle response to movement of the tympanic membrane.

Subsequently, several other investigators observed the acoustic reflex in patients with tympanic membrane perforations (Kobrak, 1948; Lindsay, Kobrak, & Perlman, 1936; Potter, 1936). In an attempt to develop a more widely applicable method of observation, Kobrak tried, with limited success, to induce transparency of the anesthetized tympanic membrane by coating the intact membrane with a mixture of glycerin, water, and potassium iodide. Visual observation of the acoustic reflex through the coated membrane proved to be impractical for general clinical application. Thus, several early reports expressed the view that,

> The importance of the acoustic stapedius reflex for practical clinical purposes is, at present at least, very limited. Observation of the reflex can be used, however, to determine the presence of hearing in persons suspected of malingering or in children. (Lindsay et al., 1936, p. 677)

In 1946, Metz reported the development of a mechano-acoustic bridge for middle-ear measurement that would eventually permit inexpensive, noninvasive recordings of the effect of the acoustic reflex on the input immittance of the middle ear. In the same report that provided the basic foundation for tympanometry, Metz (1946) also presented the first acoustic-reflex measurements that were obtained by monitoring changes in the acoustic immittance of the ear coincident with acoustic stimulation. By testing patients with a variety of otologic disorders, Metz determined the relations between acoustic-reflex thresholds and ear disease that have been only modestly refined since his pioneering efforts. The work by Metz is truly the origin of the clinical application of acoustic-reflex measurements.

The role of the tensor tympani muscle in humans was not clear to the early investigators. Hensen (1878) observed that both the stapedius and tensor tympani muscles in dogs contracted in response to acoustic stimulation, which led to the supposition that both muscles in humans must contract in response to acoustic stimulation. Kato (1913) reported, however, that only the stapedius muscle in monkeys was activated by acoustic stimulation. Metz (1946, 1952) was noncommittal as to which muscles were involved in the acoustic reflex, referring to the reflex as the intra-aural muscle reflex. Jepsen (1955), with the same Metz acoustic bridge, observed that patients with unilateral facial paralysis had no measurable acoustic reflex on the affected side. This evidence convinced Jepsen that only the stapedius muscle in humans was activated acoustically, and he referred to the response as the acoustic stapedius reflex. His colleague, Terkildsen, however, was unconvinced. Terkildsen (1957) reported acoustic-reflex

Acknowledgments: Appreciation is extended to Cynthia G. Fowler and Janet E. Shanks for their comments on the various drafts of this manuscript. Carol Zizz contributed to the project in several ways. Portions of this project were funded by the Rehabilitation Research and Development Service and by the Medical Research Service of the Department of Veterans Affairs.

[1] See Djupesland (1976) and Wiley and Block (1984) for a review of non-acoustic-reflex measurements.

measurements obtained manometrically, that is, by measuring air pressure changes in the ear canal. Terkildsen thought that the inward motion of the tympanic membrane and the resulting pressure decrease in the ear canal, was *prima facie* evidence of tensor tympani contraction. Terkildsen concluded that "the existence of an acoustic reflex of the musculus tensor tympani in the human being is established . . ." (p. 487). More recently, Brask (1978) demonstrated that the acoustic reflex produces outward, inward, or diphasic motion of the tympanic membrane. In some people there appears to be a tensor tympani reflex that is characterized by a response morphology that is different from the response morphology of a stapedius reflex. In comparison to the stapedius reflex, the tensor tympani reflex (1) is elicited at higher levels of the reflex-activator signal, (2) has a longer latency, (3) is monitored as an acoustic immittance change in the opposite direction, and (4) is associated with general body movements and the startle response (Brask, 1978; Davis, 1948; Djupesland, 1965; Salomon & Starr, 1963; Stach, Jerger, & Jenkins, 1984).

The initial clinical application of acoustic-reflex measurements was in the detection of hearing loss in difficult to test populations, an application that was abandoned and taken up again 35 years later (see Lindsay et al.,

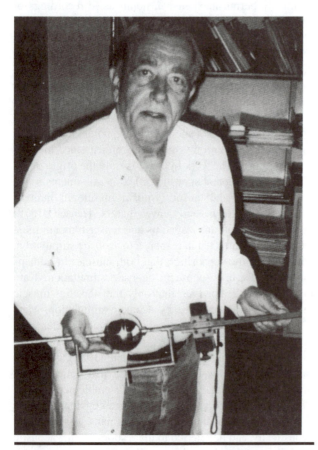

FIGURE 5.1 Knut Terkildsen (1918–1984) with the Metz mechano-acoustic bridge (ca. 1980).

1936, quotation above). Metz (1946), however, had greater ambitions for the use of acoustic-reflex data. His studies of a wide variety of patients with conductive, sensorineural, and facial nerve lesions provided the basis for the use of the acoustic reflex in the differential diagnosis of auditory and neurologic disorders. His work was extended by his colleagues (Kristensen & Jepsen, 1952; Jepsen, 1953, 1955, 1963), but the routine use of acoustic-reflex measurements was not possible until a more clinically feasible measurement method was available. Metz recognized the limitations of his mechano-acoustic bridge and anticipated the electroacoustic devices that soon would be developed. He stated, "it would be a great advantage if it would be sufficient to connect a small apparatus (telephone) with the ear, and make the measurements on a possibly bigger apparatus placed on a table alongside the patient" (Metz, 1946, p. 233). The instrument that Metz described was developed in the same State Hospital (Rigshospitalet) in Copenhagen by Terkildsen and Scott-Nielsen (1960). Their electroacoustic instrument was the prototype of the first commercially available electroacoustic immittance instrument, the Madsen ZO-61, that made possible routine measurements of the acoustic reflex. There is no question that the clinical applications of the acoustic reflex originated at Rigshospitalet in Copenhagen (Figure 5.1).

ANATOMY AND PHYSIOLOGY OF THE ACOUSTIC REFLEX

Understanding the anatomy and physiology of the human acoustic reflex is severely limited by the inaccessibility of the stapedius muscle and the reflex pathways. Even in animals, the available information on the reflex pathways is incomplete. The situation is complicated further by the likelihood that substantial interspecies differences occur in the anatomy and function of the acoustic reflex. The interspecies differences that are known to exist in the acoustic tensor tympani reflex warn against assuming that the animal data accurately reflect the characteristics of the human acoustic reflex.

The Borg (1973) study of the neural pathways involved in the acoustic reflex of rabbits provides much of the available information on the acoustic-reflex arc. Borg produced brainstem lesions and measured the resultant changes in the ipsilateral and contralateral acoustic reflexes.[2] Figure 5.2 is a schematic of the neural pathways of the acoustic-reflex arc proposed by Borg. The afferent portion of the

---

[2] For the ipsilateral (or uncrossed) acoustic reflex, the reflex-activator signal and the probe signal are in the same ear. For the contralateral (or crossed) acoustic reflex, the reflex-activator signal and the probe signal are in opposite ears. The ear in which the probe signal is located is referred to as the "probe ear."

ACOUSTIC-REFLEX ARC

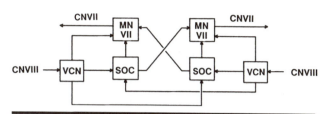

FIGURE 5.2   A schematic of the acoustic-reflex arc based on the rabbit (Borg, 1973). The arc involves input through CNVIII to the ventral cochlear nucleus (VCN) from which there are neural pathways through the two superior olivary complexes (SOC) to the motor nuclei of CNVII (MN VII) and the CNVII that innervates the stapedius muscle.

acoustic-reflex arc consists of a first order neuron in the cochlear branch of the eighth cranial nerve (CNVIII). At this stage the reflex pathways probably are undifferentiated, that is, there are no special neurons in the afferent branch of CNVIII that are devoted to the acoustic reflex. The central portion of the reflex arc consists of neurons located in the ventral cochlear nucleus (VCN) and axonal projections that are (1) primarily through the trapezoid body to the contralateral superior olivary complex (SOC) and (2) direct ipsilateral pathways to the region of the motor nucleus

(MN) of the seventh cranial nerve (CNVII). From the cell bodies in the superior olivary complex, axons project to the ipsilateral and contralateral motor nuclei of CNVII to synapse with stapedius motoneurons. The axons of the stapedius motoneurons join the trunk of CNVII, project through the internal auditory meatus, and collect into the stapedial branch of CNVII. The stapedial nerve separates from CNVII just inferior to the posterior genu (Figure 5.3) and courses anteriorly to the stapedius muscle, which is contained within a bony canal that runs roughly parallel to the facial nerve canal just inferior to the posterior genu. In addition to the "direct" pathways of the acoustic-reflex arc depicted in Figure 5.2, there may be indirect, multisynaptic pathways involving other sites in the central nervous system. For example, Borg (1973) presented evidence for a pathway involving the reticular formation. Borg and Møller (1975) suggested that the effect of central nervous system depressants on the acoustic reflex may implicate a central, multi-synaptic pathway. The function of these indirect reflex pathways is unknown, but they may be involved in complex acoustic-reflex characteristics such as the "anticipatory" response, that is, the enhanced acoustic-reflex response that occurs when the reflex-activator signal is preceded by a warning signal.

The locations of the cell bodies of the efferent neurons of the acoustic-reflex arc have been studied by a number of investigators (Joseph, Guinan, Fullerton, Norris, &

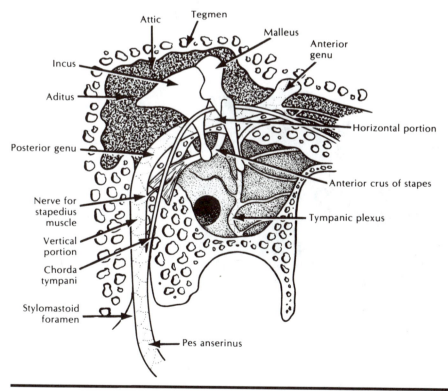

FIGURE 5.3   The course of CNVII (facial nerve) through the middle ear. (From Goodhill, 1981, with permission)

Kiang, 1985; Lyon, 1978, 1979; Shaw & Baker, 1983). These studies demonstrated that motoneurons of the reflex arc are located in several regions near, but not in, the motor nucleus of CNVII. Kobler, Vacher, and Guinan (1985, 1987) provide evidence from cats that motoneurons of the reflex arc are organized into regions with unique response properties. The following four types of neurons were identified: (1) contralateral units that respond only to contralateral stimuli, (2) ipsilateral units that respond only to ipsilateral stimuli, (3) "binaural and" units that respond only to binaural stimuli, and (4) "binaural or" units that respond to either ipsilateral or contralateral stimuli. These classes of motoneurons have distinctly different thresholds to acoustic stimulation (Kobler et al., 1987). In addition, there may be stapedius motoneurons that do not respond to sound (McCue & Guinan, 1983, 1988). McCue and Guinan (1988) presented evidence that these functionally distinct motoneuron groups are organized into anatomically distinct brainstem pathways. McCue and Guinan produced brainstem lesions in cats and observed the effects of the lesions on ipsilateral and contralateral acoustic reflexes. The findings suggested that the axons of the stapedial motoneurons are arranged in three distinct pathways originating from different sites in the brainstem. The three pathways are differentiated on the basis of responsiveness to stimulation of the two ears, with one pathway responsive to ipsilateral stimulation, one to contralateral stimulation, and one to stimulation of either ear. A fourth pathway may exist that is not acoustically excitable. The peripheral, efferent portion of the acoustic-reflex arc at the level of the middle ear apparently is not topographically organized in the same manner (Kobler et al., 1985). The peripheral processes of the various motoneuron groups appear to be distributed randomly within the stapedial branch of CNVII.

Because the clinical measurement of the acoustic reflex almost always is performed by measuring changes in middle-ear immittance, it is important to understand the relationship between the immittance changes of the middle ear and the more direct measurement of acoustic-reflex activity. Perhaps the most direct method for measuring the acoustic reflex is the electromyographic (EMG) response that is measured directly from the stapedius muscle or tendon. Zakrisson, Borg, and Blom (1974) compared EMG responses and immittance changes produced by the acoustic reflex in patients with unilateral perforations of the tympanic membrane that allowed insertion of an electrode into the stapedial tendon. Figure 5.4 presents a sample recording. The top tracings are the integrated EMG activity, in a sense, the sum of all of the individual motor unit discharges and an indication of the total muscle response. The middle tracings are EMG action potentials, in which each spike represents the discharge of a single motor unit. The lower panels show impedance changes in the opposite ear. Figure 5.5 shows magnitude-intensity level functions for contralateral EMG responses and for ipsilateral and contralateral impedance changes. The data, which are expressed in relative units, indicate that EMG responses and impedance changes are similarly dependent on the level of the reflex-activator signal (i.e., the stimulus used to elicit the acoustic reflex).

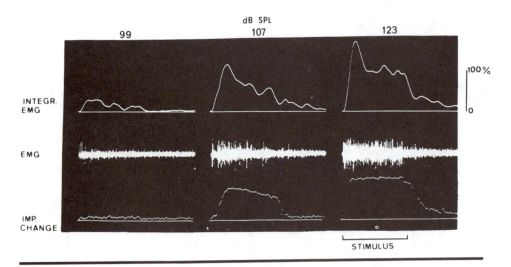

FIGURE 5.4 Simultaneously recorded responses of the human stapedius muscle to a 1 s, 2000 Hz tonal stimulus. The top panel depicts the integrated EMG response, a method of averaging the muscle activity. The middle panel shows the raw electromyographic (EMG) response recorded from the stapedial tendon showing individual muscle action potentials. The bottom panel illustrates the acoustic impedance change in the opposite ear. (From Zakrisson, Borg, & Blom, 1974, with permission)

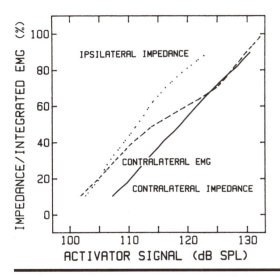

FIGURE 5.5 Acoustic reflex growth functions. The dashed line shows the reflex growth function obtained from the integrated EMG response to contralateral stimulation. The dotted and solid lines show reflex growth functions for ipsilateral and contralateral impedance changes, respectively. (From Zakrisson, Borg, & Blom, 1974, with permission)

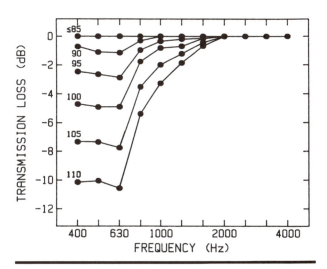

FIGURE 5.6 The frequency dependent attenuation characteristics (transmission loss in dB) of the acoustic reflex from four subjects in response to 85 to 110 dB SPL reflex-activator signals. (From Rabinowitz, 1977, with permission)

Recent data suggest that the differences between the ipsilateral and contralateral acoustic reflexes are greater when measured with EMG techniques than when measured with acoustic immittance procedures. In cats, Guinan and McCue (1987) observed that the EMG activity of the ipsilateral stapedius muscle was two to three times greater than the EMG activity of the contralateral stapedius muscle. In humans, the ipsilateral immittance change is only about one and one-half times greater than the contralateral immittance change (Hall, 1982).

When the stapedius muscle contracts, the stapes footplate is moved or rocked laterally from the oval window, the ossicular chain is stiffened, and the tympanic membrane is moved slightly in a direction that is dependent upon the movement of the stapes. These mechanical changes in the middle ear produce frequency-dependent changes in the sound transmission characteristics of the middle ear. As illustrated in Figure 5.6, the acoustic reflex acts as a high-pass filter on the transmission of sound through the middle ear. Stapedius contraction attenuates low-frequency signals with the maximum effect at about 600 Hz. Above 1000 Hz, there is little, if any, effect of the acoustic reflex on the sound level that reaches the inner ear (Rabinowitz, 1977). The ipsilateral acoustic reflex probably exhibits the same high-pass filter characteristic as does the contralateral reflex, but the attenuation produced by the ipsilateral reflex may be twice as large (in dB) as the attenuation produced by the contralateral reflex.

MEASUREMENT OF THE ACOUSTIC REFLEX

Measurement Methods

Several methods have been used to quantify the effect of stapedial muscle contraction. The early investigators of stapedius muscle activity in response to acoustic stimulation (1) recorded the change in either EMG activity (Perlman & Case, 1939) or tension (Lorente de Nó, 1935; Wersäll, 1958) from the stapedial muscle or tendon, (2) observed the movement of the stapedial tendon through perforations in the tympanic membrane (Lindsay et al., 1936), and (3) recorded air pressure changes in the ear canal caused by displacement of the tympanic membrane that coincided with stapedial contraction (Holst, Ingelstedt, & Örtegren, 1963; Terkildsen, 1957). When Otto Metz developed his impedance bridge and recorded acoustic-reflex responses as acoustic-immittance changes, he demonstrated that the acoustic reflex could be recorded in a clinically feasible, noninvasive manner. The method that Metz developed required the measurement of acoustic immittance during the presentation of a reflex-activator signal. In either the contralateral or ipsilateral condition, the activator signal may interact with the probe signal to produce measurement artifacts. Because the head provides isolation of the reflex-activator and probe signals in the contralateral condition, the interaction of the activator signal and the probe signal is less in the contralateral condition than when both signals are presented to the same ear

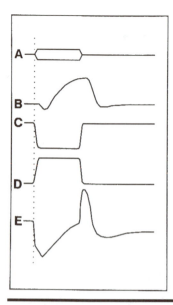

FIGURE 5.7 Schematic representation of (A) a reflex-activator signal, (B) an acoustic reflex measured as an impedance change, (C) an eardrum artifact, (D) an additive artifact, and (E) a simultaneously occurring eardrum artifact and acoustic reflex. (From Green & Margolis, 1984, with permission)

(ipsilateral). For this reason, the early clinical instruments measured only the contralateral acoustic reflex.

Two kinds of artifacts can result from interaction of the reflex-activator signal and the probe signal. Both artifacts can occur during ipsilateral or contralateral recording, but both artifacts are much more difficult to avoid in ipsilateral measurement. The *additive artifact* results from the addition of the energy in the reflex-activator signal to the energy of the probe signal. Because immittance instruments bandpass filter the probe tone, only the activator signal energy that is passed by the filter is problematic. The closer in frequency the reflex-activator signal is to the probe tone signal, the greater the likelihood is that the two signals will interact, causing an additive artifact. The additive artifact takes the form of an increase in impedance (a decrease in admittance), which can be misinterpreted as a true reflex (Margolis & Gilman, 1977; Popelka & Dubno, 1978). Because the additive artifact has no latency except for delays in the recording apparatus, it usually can be distinguished from a real acoustic reflex on the basis of latency. The *eardrum artifact* occurs primarily during ipsilateral recording with a low-frequency (226 Hz) probe tone (Kunov, 1977; Lutman & Leis, 1980; Møller, 1978). The eardrum artifact results from a nonlinear interaction between the reflex-activator signal and the probe signal and is not related to the frequency separation between the two signals. The artifact takes the form of a decrease in impedance (increase in admittance), the opposite immittance

change of a real reflex. Green and Margolis (1984) suggested that the eardrum artifact may be related to nonlinear properties of the tympanic membrane. Figure 5.7 presents a schematic representation of the additive and eardrum artifacts, a real acoustic reflex, and the simultaneous occurrence of an eardrum artifact and an acoustic reflex.

Quantification of the Amplitude of the Acoustic Reflex

Several parameters of the acoustic reflex can be quantified with the acoustic immittance method, including threshold, temporal, and amplitude characteristics. The following discussion focuses on the measurement parameters and computations that must be considered when quantifying the amplitude of the acoustic reflex. Recall from Chapter 4 that the acoustic admittance at the probe tip (Y_a) is the complex sum of the real component of admittance, acoustic conductance (G_a), and the imaginary component of admittance, acoustic susceptance (B_a), which is expressed as

$$Y_a = G_a + jB_a \qquad (5.1)$$

Further, the acoustic admittance at the probe tip (Y_a) is the sum of the admittance of the ear canal between the probe tip and the tympanic membrane (Y_{ec}) and the admittance at the tympanic membrane (Y_{tm}) that is expressed as

$$Y_a = Y_{ec} + Y_{tm} \qquad (5.2)$$

Although Eq. 5.2 and the equations that follow involve the addition of vectors without regard to the phase angle, the errors encountered with a low-frequency probe tone (e.g., 226 Hz) are slight. The effect of the acoustic reflex is to produce a change in the admittance (ΔY) at the tympanic membrane. The admittance at the probe tip when the stapedius muscle is contracted (Y_r) is the sum of the admittance of the ear canal (Y_{ec}), the admittance at the tympanic membrane (Y_{tm}), and the admittance change produced by the acoustic reflex (ΔY), which is expressed as

$$Y_r = Y_{ec} + Y_{tm} + \Delta Y \qquad (5.3)$$

Solving Eq. 5.3 for ΔY gives

$$\Delta Y = Y_r - (Y_{ec} + Y_{tm}) \qquad (5.4)$$

Substituting from Eq. 5.2, Eq. 5.4 reduces to

$$\Delta Y = Y_r - Y_a \qquad (5.5)$$

Because the admittance of the ear canal is a simple additive component of both Y_a (Eq. 5.2) and Y_r (Eq. 5.3), ΔY is not affected by ear-canal volume.

The relation between impedance change (ΔZ) and ear-canal volume is more complex than the relation between admittance change and ear-canal volume. Substituting from Eq. 4.15 in Chapter 4, Eq. 5.3 can be rewritten in impedance as follows:

$$Z_r = \frac{Z_{ec}(Z_{tm} + \Delta Z)}{Z_{ec} + (Z_{tm} + \Delta Z)} \qquad (5.6)$$

ΔZ is expressed as follows:

$$\Delta Z = \frac{Z_{ec}Z_{tm} - Z_r Z_{ec} - Z_r Z_{tm}}{Z_r - Z_{ec}} \qquad (5.7)$$

The point of this exercise is that Eqs. 5.3 and 5.5 express a simple relation between the admittance of the ear canal and the amplitude of the acoustic reflex (i.e., $\Delta Y_a = \Delta Y_{tm}$), whereas Eqs. 5.6 and 5.7 express a complex relation between the impedance of the ear canal and the amplitude of the acoustic reflex (i.e., $\Delta Z_a \neq \Delta Z_{tm}$). Although Z_{ec} must be known precisely to determine ΔZ_{tm}, Y_{ec} need not be determined to measure ΔY_{tm}.

Eqs. 5.4 and 5.7 produce reasonable estimates of the amplitude of the acoustic reflex only if, as was previously indicated, the admittance (or impedance) phase angle is not substantially altered by the reflex. In normal subjects >4 months of age and at a low-probe frequency (e.g., 226 Hz), only a small change in phase angle occurs when the stapedius muscle contracts. A typical acoustic reflex expressed as an admittance vector at a probe frequency of 226 Hz is depicted in the left panel of Figure 5.8. The length of the line segment from the origin to Y_{tm} is the static admittance at the tympanic membrane. The length of the line segment from the origin to Y_r is the admittance at the tympanic membrane with the stapedius muscle contracted. The difference between the lengths of the two line segments is ΔY defined in Eq. 5.5. The actual effect of the reflex, however, is the distance from point Y_{tm} to point Y_r,

which is almost exactly equivalent to ΔY because there is very little phase shift.

A typical acoustic reflex for a 678 Hz probe frequency is presented as an admittance vector in the right panel of Figure 5.8. Note that a substantial phase shift occurs when the stapedius muscle contracts. In this example, Eq. 5.5 underestimates the admittance change produced by the reflex by 24%. To avoid underestimating the admittance change at 678 Hz, ΔY must be determined from the admittance components expressed as

$$\Delta G = G_r - G_a \qquad (5.8)$$

and

$$\Delta B = B_r - B_a \qquad (5.9)$$

where ΔG and ΔB are the changes in conductance and susceptance produced by the acoustic reflex, G_r and B_r are the conductance and susceptance when the stapedius is contracted, and G_a and B_a are the conductance and susceptance in the uncontracted (relaxed) state. The admittance change then is expressed as

$$\Delta Y = \sqrt{\Delta G^2 + \Delta B^2} \qquad (5.10)$$

Eq. 5.10 produces a better estimate of reflex magnitude than does Eq. 5.5. To determine ΔG and ΔB, a two-component admittance meter is required. When a one-component admittance meter is used, the reflex magnitude must be determined from Eq. 5.5. Accurate estimates of ΔY can be obtained only at low probe frequencies (e.g., 226 Hz) in normal subjects who do not exhibit a significant phase shift

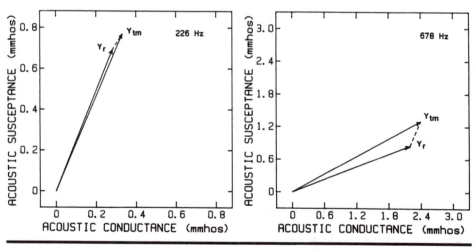

FIGURE 5.8 Acoustic reflex responses to a 100 dB SPL, 1000 Hz reflex-activator signal measured with two probe frequencies (226 and 678 Hz) expressed as admittance vector. Y_{tm} represents the baseline (static) admittance. Y_r is the admittance during stimulation. The reflex magnitude is represented by the dashed line between the two admittance vectors.

when the stapedius muscle contracts. That is, vectors can be added only if the vectors are identical in phase.

Several methods for quantifying the amplitude of the acoustic reflex are illustrated in Figure 5.9. The data for two subjects (S4 and S8) are based on compensated (i.e., corrected for ear-canal volume) admittance measures for a 226 Hz probe. The admittance data in acoustic mmhos (Figure 5.9A) show that the two subjects have different static admittance, evident from the different baseline values (filled symbols), but a similar change in admittance amplitude with increases in activator signal level (open symbols). In Figure 5.9B, the reflex data are plotted in

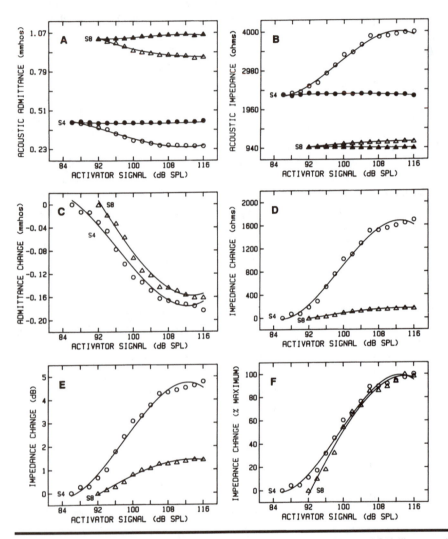

FIGURE 5.9. Acoustic-reflex growth functions for two subjects (S4 and S8) illustrated in various quantification units. The filled symbols represent a control baseline condition in which no reflex-activator signal was presented and the open symbols represent the admittance magnitude during stimulation at various sound-pressure levels. *Panel A:* Reflex growth functions expressed as absolute acoustic admittance magnitude. *Panel B:* Reflex growth functions expressed as absolute impedance magnitude. *Panel C:* Reflex growth functions expressed as the change in admittance between the baseline admittance and the admittance during muscle contraction shown in Panel A. *Panel D:* Reflex growth functions expressed as the change in impedance between the baseline impedance and the impedance during muscle contraction shown in Panel B. *Panel E:* Reflex growth functions expressed as an impedance change in decibels, which is equivalent to the change in sound-pressure level of the probe tone. *Panel F:* Reflex growth functions expressed as a percentage of the maximum impedance change for each subject. (Based on Figure 9, Wilson, 1981)

impedance (acoustic ohms). In impedance units, the static values for the two subjects (filled symbols) are different, and the reflex-growth functions (open symbols) are substantially different in slope. In the middle panels of Figure 5.9, the reflex data from the two subjects are plotted as the change in immittance between the pre-stimulus or baseline admittance, which is a "static" measure, and the peak values of each reflex response in admittance (Figure 5.9C) and in impedance (Figure 5.9D). Again, the reflex-growth functions for the two subjects expressed as an admittance change are similar, whereas the growth functions expressed as an impedance change are very different. In Figure 5.9E, the reflex data are expressed as the impedance change in dB (ΔdB)

$$\Delta dB = 20 \log_{10} (Z_r/Z_{tm}) \qquad (5.11)$$

where Z_r is the impedance at the tympanic membrane during stapedial contraction and Z_{tm} is the static or baseline impedance. Note again that the reflex-growth functions are very different for the two subjects. The reflex-growth functions expressed in decibels are very similar in form to the functions expressed as an impedance change in ohms (Figure 5.9D). Because the range of the data plotted in decibels is small ($\leq$5 dB), the log transformation has very little effect on the shape of the reflex-growth function. In Figure 5.9F, the reflex data are plotted as percent of the maximum impedance change. Because the largest change recorded is 100%, the two growth functions converge at the highest activator level used. When reflex magnitude is expressed in percent of maximum, the growth functions for the two subjects are very similar.

Another quantity that has been used to express the reflex magnitude is the change in the sound-pressure level of the probe tone, ΔdB, that is related to the impedance of the middle ear in the following manner:

$$\Delta dB = 20 \log_{10} (Z_r/Z_a) \qquad (5.12)$$

where Z_r is the impedance at the probe tip during stapedial contraction and Z_a is the impedance at the probe tip in the uncontracted state. Eqs. 5.11 and 5.12 are equivalent only in the hypothetical condition of an ear-canal volume of zero. As illustrated in Figure 5.10, however, ear-canal volume has a substantial effect on the reflex amplitudes expressed as a change in the sound-pressure level of the probe tone (Eq. 5.12). The growth function for subject S4 (from Figure 5.9E) is replotted with four ear-canal volumes [0.5, 1.0, 1.5 cm³ and corrected to the tympanic membrane (TM), i.e., a 0 cm³ volume]. The substantial effect of ear-canal volume on the amplitude of acoustic reflex plotted in acoustic impedance is obvious. The data demonstrate that comparisons between ears or between measures obtained at different times from the same ear, cannot be compared in absolute terms when reflex magnitudes are expressed as changes in the sound-pressure level

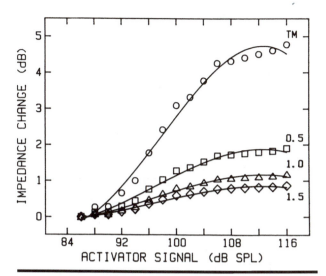

FIGURE 5.10   Acoustic reflex growth functions expressed as an impedance change (in dB) showing the effect of ear-canal volume on the amplitude of the acoustic reflex. The growth function is shown corrected to the plane of the tympanic membrane (TM), that is, an ear-canal volume of zero. The data also are presented with assumed ear-canal volumes of 0.5, 1.0, and 1.5 cm³.

of the probe tone because of the effects of variations in ear-canal volume.

ACOUSTIC-REFLEX THRESHOLD

The amplitude of the acoustic reflex is dependent both upon the level of the reflex-activator signal and upon the characteristics of the middle-ear transmission system(s). As a relative measure, the amplitude of the change in the acoustic immittance of the middle ear during contraction of the stapedius muscle is related directly to the level of the reflex-activator signal. As an absolute measure, the amplitude of the acoustic immittance of the middle ear during contraction of the stapedius muscle is related either directly to the level of the activator signal when measured in acoustic impedance (i.e., the higher the activator level, the higher the acoustic impedance) or inversely to the activator level when measured in acoustic admittance (i.e., the higher the activator level, the lower the acoustic admittance).

Nomenclature

The relation between the level of the reflex-activator signal and the magnitude of the acoustic reflex, measured as the change in acoustic admittance, is illustrated in Figure 5.11. The top panel depicts the 1 s activator signals that increment from 80 to 110 dB HL and the acoustic reflexes elicited by the activator signals. The bottom panel of Figure 5.11 depicts the admittance change (acoustic mmhos)

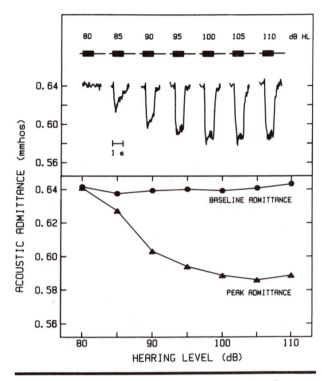

FIGURE 5.11 The top panel shows the acoustic-reflex responses in acoustic mmhos monitored with a 226 Hz probe and corrected for ear-canal volume. The 1 s, 1000 Hz activator signals were presented from 80 to 110 dB HL. The bottom panel depicts an acoustic-reflex growth function with baseline admittance (circles) representing the acoustic admittance of the middle ear 100 ms prior to presentation of the activator signal (Y_{tm}) and peak admittance (triangles) representing the acoustic admittance during the last 500 ms of the activator signal (Y_r). (Modified from Wilson & McBride, 1978)

during contraction of the stapedius muscle. In this plot, which is an *acoustic-reflex growth function*, the *baseline admittance* data represent the acoustic admittance of the middle ear during the 100 ms prior to presentation of each reflex-activator signal (Y_{tm}) and the *peak admittance* data represent the acoustic admittance of the middle ear during the last 500 ms of each activator signal (Y_r). The acoustic admittance data [baseline (Y_{tm}) and peak (Y_r)] and corresponding acoustic impedance data for the seven activator signals also are listed in Table 5.1 along with the acoustic admittance (and impedance) changes that occurred between the respective baseline and peak values.[3] Both

---

[3] The acoustic-admittance data in Table 5.1 are the average of 11 samples of the acoustic admittance of the middle ear during a 100 ms interval before the activator signal (Y_{tm}) and during a 500 ms interval during presentation of the activator signal (Y_r). In this manner the data were generated to three decimal points, which is beyond the measurement accuracy of instruments. To maintain simplicity, the phase angle data are omitted.

the reflex tracings and the reflex magnitude data demonstrate that with a 226 Hz probe, the acoustic admittance of the middle ear in the reflexive state decreases as the level of the reflex-activator signal increases from 80 to 100 dB SPL. Increases in the level of the activator signal above 100 dB SPL do not produce continued increases in the amplitude of the reflex. Above 100 dB SPL, the reflex growth function is saturated. Table 5.1 also contains the baseline (Z_{tm}), peak (Z_r), and change (ΔZ) data converted to acoustic impedance units (ohms). As the level of the activator signal increases from 80 to 100 dB HL, the Z_{tm} values fluctuate slightly around 1560 acoustic ohms, whereas the Z_r values grow consistently from 1560 acoustic ohms (no reflex at 80 dB HL) to 1698 acoustic ohms at 100 dB HL. The data expressed in acoustic ohms demonstrate that with a 226 Hz probe, the acoustic impedance of the middle ear in the reflexive state increases as the level of the reflex-activator signal increases.

With the exception of recent developments that are described in a subsequent section (Other Supra-Threshold Measures of the Acoustic Reflex), the acoustic-reflex growth function is not used widely as a clinical diagnostic procedure. One point on the acoustic-reflex growth function, however, the *acoustic-reflex threshold*, is used extensively in the evaluation of the auditory system. The acoustic-reflex threshold is the lowest sound-pressure level or hearing level of a reflex-activator signal that elicits a measurable immittance change that is coincident with presentation of the activator signal. In the example given in Figure 5.11, 85 dB HL is the lowest level at which an acoustic reflex was measured.

The level of the activator signal at which an acoustic-reflex threshold is measured is dependent upon the *sensitivity* of the measurement system. Reflex thresholds measured with a 678 Hz probe typically are 2 to 6 dB lower than reflex thresholds established with a 226 Hz probe (Beattie &

TABLE 5.1 The acoustic admittance and impedance values[3] for the acoustic reflexes elicited by 1000 Hz, 80 to 110 dB HL activator signals. These are the numeric data (226 Hz) for the acoustic reflexes depicted in Figure 5.11.

dB HL	ACOUSTIC ADMITTANCE (mmhos)			ACOUSTIC IMPEDANCE (ohms)		
	Y_{tm}	Y_r	ΔY	Z_{tm}	Z_r	ΔZ
80	0.642	0.641	−0.001	1558	1560	2
85	0.638	0.627	−0.011	1567	1595	28
90	0.639	0.603	−0.036	1565	1658	93
95	0.640	0.594	−0.046	1563	1684	121
100	0.639	0.589	−0.050	1565	1698	133
105	0.641	0.586	−0.055	1560	1707	147
110	0.643	0.589	−0.054	1555	1698	143

Leamy, 1975; Burke & Herer, 1973; Porter, 1972; Wilson & McBride, 1978). In all probability, the difference in reflex threshold levels obtained with the two probe frequencies is because the 678 Hz probe frequency is closer to the lowest resonance frequency of the middle ear than is the 226 Hz probe frequency. Reflex thresholds that are measured on a strip chart recorder, an oscilloscope, or a computer tend to be 3 to 7 dB lower than reflex thresholds visualized on a meter (Wilson & McBride, 1978; Wilson, Morgan, & Dirks, 1972). Many of the currently marketed immittance instruments feature CRT or stripchart displays that provide superior sensitivity compared to the visual observation of a needle on a meter.

Normal Reflex Thresholds

There are no standards that describe procedures for the measurement of the various parameters of the acoustic reflex, including reflex threshold, or that define the normal range of levels for acoustic-reflex thresholds. Anderson and Wedenberg (1968, Figure 3) considered reflex thresholds to be abnormal if the thresholds were at levels >90 dB HL. More recently, Jerger, Oliver, and Jenkins (1987) considered reflex thresholds to be abnormal if the reflex thresholds were >100 dB HL. The threshold data in Table 5.2 are representative of the normative values for contralateral acoustic-reflex thresholds for adults with normal hearing. The data for the pure-tone activator signals are in decibels hearing level (ANSI, 1969 or ISO, 1964), whereas the threshold data for the broadband noise activator signals are in decibels sound-pressure level (re: 20 μPa). Several relations emerge from the data in the table. First, although there are slight variations among studies, the mean/median reflex thresholds for 250, 500, 1000, 2000, and 4000 Hz activator signals range from 80 to 90 dB HL. The Handler and Margolis (1977) and Wilson (1981) investigations reported standard deviations that can be used to define the normal range. With two standard deviations used to define the normal limits and rounding up to a 5 dB interval (the most commonly used attenuator step size), the upper limit of the normal reflex thresholds is 95 dB HL for pure tones from 250 to 2000 Hz. At 4000 Hz, the upper limit of the normal range is between 100 dB HL (Wilson, 1981) and 105 dB HL (Handler & Margolis, 1977). Second, the mean reflex threshold for the broadband noise reflex activator ranges from 70 to 75 dB SPL. Again using two standard deviations from the Wilson and Handler and Margolis studies, 90 to 95 dB SPL is the upper limit of the normal reflex threshold for broadband noise. Third, in terms of sound-pressure level, the reflex threshold for the broadband

TABLE 5.2 The mean (or median) contralateral, 226 Hz acoustic-reflex thresholds (dB HL re: ANSI, 1969 or ISO, 1964 for the pure-tone activators and dB SPL re: 20 μPa for the broadband noise activators) from seven studies.

STUDY NUMBER, STATISTIC	REFLEX-ACTIVATOR SIGNAL (Hz)					
	250	500	1000	2000	4000	Noise
Anderson & Wedenberg, 1968						
N = 200, median	84.2	87.4	85.6	85.5	90.7	
Chiveralls, 1977						
N = 100, median	89.8					
N = 222, median		83.6	82.8	81.5	82.8	
Gelfand & Piper, 1981						
N = 12, mean		81.5	82.4	83.1		76.2
SD		(4.2)	(5.2)	(4.9)		(6.5)
Handler & Margolis, 1977						
N = 17, mean		82.5	83.0	83.0	86.5	75.0
SD		(6.1)	(5.1)	(5.2)	(9.0)	(8.4)
Osterhammel & Osterhammel, 1979						
N = 65, mean		90.1	90.2	89.8	93.8	
Peterson & Lidén, 1972[a]						
N = 88, mean	84.6	85.2	85.4	84.0	84.4	
SD	(7.1)	(7.0)	(6.7)	(5.5)	(7.2)	
Wilson, 1981						
N = 18, mean	78.8	79.4	82.8	82.1	83.3	71.7
SD	(6.3)	(4.7)	(4.5)	(4.6)	(5.9)	(8.6)

[a] 800 Hz probe, ascending, amplitude measurement

noise activator is 10 to 20 dB lower than the reflex thresholds in sound-pressure level[4] for 500, 1000, and 2000 Hz activators.

The interaural reflex threshold differences also may be useful diagnostically (Chiveralls, 1977). Contralateral reflex threshold data for the left ear and right ear of 48 young adults with normal hearing are listed in Table 5.3 (top panel) along with the absolute difference between thresholds (Wilson, Shanks, & Velde, 1981). The data, which were based on measurements made in 2 dB steps, indicate no significant difference between the reflex thresholds for the left and right ears, with an absolute difference between ears that ranged from 3.4 to 5.1 dB. The lower panel of Table 5.3 shows the cumulative percent for the absolute threshold differences between the 48 subjects for five 2 dB intervals. For example, at 500 Hz, 58% of the subjects had acoustic-reflex thresholds that either were at the same level or were at levels <4 dB apart in the ears. The interaural acoustic-reflex thresholds differed by no more than 10 dB in 83 to 98% of the cases.

Whether true differences between ipsilateral and contralateral acoustic-reflex thresholds exist is uncertain. Figure 5.12 shows ipsilateral and contralateral reflex growth functions for a subject with normal hearing (Borg & Zakrisson, 1974). The data are plotted in percent of maximum impedance change. The ipsilateral growth function is steeper than the contralateral function, but the two functions converge on the same point at the origin. Applying a criterion for determining the reflex threshold (e.g., 10% on the vertical axis) results in a substantial difference between the ipsilateral and contralateral reflex thresholds. If the functions converge on a point at the origin, then no true difference between the reflex thresholds exists. The available data on ipsilateral and contralateral acoustic reflexes (e.g., Møller, 1962a) suggest that ipsilateral reflex thresholds are consistently 2 to 14 dB lower than contralateral thresholds. It is not clear that the threshold differences are due entirely to the differences in the slopes of the reflex growth functions. It is clear, however, that the more sensitive the measurement system is, the smaller the apparent differences are between reflex thresholds for ipsilateral and contralateral activator signals.

Lifespan Changes of the Acoustic Reflex

Little is known about the dynamic properties of acoustic reflexes in infants. The gross differences in middle-ear characteristics between infants and adults make quantitative

---

[4] Using the ANSI 1969 standard for a TDH-39 earphone, reflex thresholds for 500, 1000, and 2000 Hz are converted from hearing level to sound-pressure level by adding 11.5, 7.0, and 9.0 dB, respectively, to the threshold values expressed in hearing level.

TABLE 5.3 *Top panel:* The mean contralateral, acoustic-reflex thresholds (dB HL) for the left and right ears of 48 subjects. The absolute threshold differences (dB) also are listed as are the standard deviations (parentheses). *Bottom panel:* The cumulative percent of the 48 subjects for five 2 dB intervals of absolute reflex threshold differences. (Modified from Wilson, Shanks, & Velde, 1981)

CONDITION	LEFT EAR dB HL (SD)	RIGHT EAR dB HL (SD)	ABSOLUTE DIFFERENCE dB HL (SD)
500 Hz	87.1 (6.1)	86.4 (5.4)	3.4 (2.8)
1000 Hz	86.8 (5.1)	86.4 (6.0)	3.8 (2.9)
2000 Hz	85.4 (6.9)	85.7 (6.9)	4.5 (3.5)
Noise[a]	77.7 (9.0)	77.9 (10.5)	5.1 (4.7)

CONDITION	ABSOLUTE REFLEX THRESHOLD DIFFERENCE (dB)				
	<2	<4	<6	<8	<10
500 Hz	25	58	75	92	98
1000 Hz	27	54	73	85	98
2000 Hz	19	42	69	83	89
Noise	15	46	69	79	83

[a] Broadband noise thresholds (dB SPL)

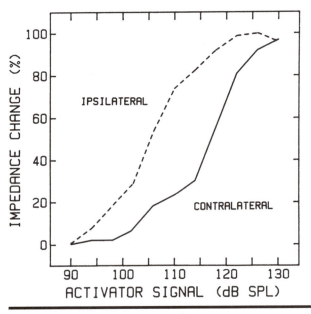

FIGURE 5.12 Ipsilateral (dashed line) and contralateral (solid line) acoustic reflex growth functions expressed as percentage of maximum impedance change. (From Borg & Zakrisson, 1974, with permission)

comparisons of acoustic-reflex magnitudes very difficult. Because the reflex-threshold measurement requires only the detection of a response and not a quantification of the response, reflex thresholds are easier to compare than are other reflex characteristics that require accurate determination of the response magnitude. Still, the changes in the levels of the reflex-activator signal that result from postnatal development of the external ear are problematic in making absolute comparisons of reflex thresholds across the lifespan. Despite the difficulties in comparing reflex thresholds among various age groups, a general description of lifespan changes in acoustic-reflex thresholds is possible.

Reflex Thresholds in Infants.   Because most commercially available aural acoustic immittance instruments offered only a low-frequency probe tone (220 or 226 Hz), early attempts to record acoustic reflexes in neonates employed only one probe frequency. Although there is some disagreement on the proportion of observable responses, the early reports indicated that acoustic reflexes were not observable in most neonates (Barajas, Olaizola, Tapia, Alarcon, & Alaminos, 1981; Bennett, 1975; Keith, 1975; Keith & Bench, 1978; Stream, Stream, Walker, & Breningstall, 1978). When acoustic conductance was monitored with a two-component admittance meter, the proportion of observable neonatal acoustic reflexes was higher (88%), but reflex thresholds were substantially elevated compared to older infants and adults (Himelfarb, Shanon, Popelka, & Margolis, 1978). Sprague, Wiley, and Goldstein (1985) reported that only 50% of their neonates had observable reflexes with a 220 Hz probe tone. Inexplicably, one study (Vincent & Gerber, 1987) reported a higher proportion of observable reflexes in neonates than previous investigators have reported. Vincent and Gerber reported that 92.5% of their 2-day-old neonates had observable acoustic reflexes at 220 Hz.

Investigators who used a probe frequency higher than 226 Hz were, in general, more successful in recording acoustic reflexes from neonates (Kankkunen & Lidén, 1984; Marchant, McMillan, Shurin, Johnson, Turczyk, Feinstein, & Panek, 1986; Margolis, 1993; McCandless & Allred, 1978; McMillan, Marchant, & Shurin, 1985; Sprague et al., 1985). Weatherby and Bennett (1980) explored most directly the effect of probe frequency on the measurement of acoustic reflexes in neonates and observed that as the probe frequency increased, the proportion of acoustic reflexes increased, and mean reflex threshold decreased. With a 600 Hz probe, 93.3% of the neonates had observable reflexes, whereas with an 800 Hz probe, 100% of the neonates had acoustic reflexes. In a subsequent investigation, Bennett and Weatherby (1982) used a 1200 Hz probe tone to measure reflex thresholds for tonal- and noise-activator signals

in 4- to 8-day-old infants (N = 28) and reported reflex thresholds that were similar to the reflex thresholds reported for normal adults.

In summary, the extant research on acoustic-reflex thresholds in neonates suggests that the acoustic reflex is fully developed at birth and that reflex thresholds in neonates are similar to the reflex thresholds observed with adults. Several reports presented reflex thresholds that are lower than the reflex thresholds of adults (e.g., Weatherby & Bennett, 1980), but these differences may be attributable to the use of standard calibration couplers (e.g., 2 cm^3 coupler) and the higher sound-pressure levels that are developed in the small external ear canal of the neonate (McMillan et al., 1985). The optimal probe frequency for reflex testing in neonates appears to be above 800 Hz. The differences between ipsilateral and contralateral reflex thresholds (McMillan et al., 1985; Sprague et al., 1985) are about the same as the differences between ipsilateral and contralateral reflexes that have been reported for adults.

Reflex Thresholds in Aging Adults.   There is some disagreement among investigators concerning acoustic-reflex thresholds in aging adults. Some studies suggest that reflex thresholds decrease with age (Jerger, Hayes, Anthony, & Mauldin, 1978; Jerger, Jerger, & Mauldin, 1972); some studies demonstrate no age-related change in the reflex threshold (Osterhammel & Osterhammel, 1979; Thompson, Sills, Recke, & Bui, 1980); some report an increase in reflex thresholds with aging (Wilson, 1981); and some report an increase in reflex thresholds for some activator signals but not other activators (Gelfand & Piper, 1981; Handler & Margolis, 1977; Silman, 1979; Silverman, Silman, & Miller, 1983). The disagreement can be attributed to the following four factors: (1) the reflex-threshold differences among age groups are small; (2) the measurement procedures used were not capable of resolving the small differences being studied; (3) the subject selection criteria were different in the various studies; and (4) the age groupings that were compared differed among studies.

A sensitive measurement system is needed to study the effects of age on the acoustic reflex. Figure 5.13 presents reflex growth functions for two age groups (<30 years and >50 years) from Wilson (1981). The growth functions for the two age groups differ in slope, with the >50-years group (triangles) exhibiting a more gradual increase in reflex amplitude than the <30-years group (circles). In general, the growth functions converge on the same point, suggesting minimal threshold differences between the groups. In contrast, applying an absolute criterion, such as the level producing an admittance change of 0.01 mmhos, produces 3 to 11 dB threshold differences. These threshold differences result from applying a criterion change to functions that differ in slope but not in origin. Because of the

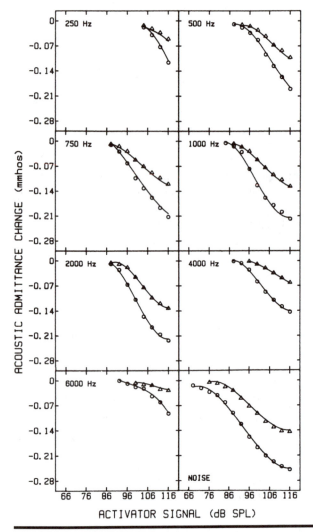

FIGURE 5.13. Acoustic reflex growth functions expressed as the change in admittance magnitude at 226 Hz for two groups of subjects, aged <30 years (circles) and >50 years (triangles). (From Wilson, 1981, with permission)

Piper, 1981; Handler & Margolis, 1977; Wilson, 1981). Other studies include subjects who had normal hearing for their age group (Osterhammel & Osterhammel, 1979). In all of the studies, sensitivity differences occurred among age groups, but the sensitivity differences were smaller in the studies that employed clinically normal subjects, as opposed to age-corrected norms. The technique of selecting clinically normal elderly subjects is useful for controlling the hearing sensitivity variable but may result in a biased control group of "supernormals," that is, a group that reflects the tail rather than the central tendency of the population represented.

With these considerations in mind, the following generalization can be drawn from studies that meet the procedural requirements of a sensitive measurement procedure. Reflex thresholds for tonal activator signals ≤2000 Hz do not change with age. Higher frequency activator signals and broadband noise produce small age-related elevations in reflex thresholds.

Abnormal Reflex Thresholds

An abnormality at any location in the acoustic-reflex arc can alter the characteristics of the acoustic reflex. Lesions in the afferent or input portion of the acoustic-reflex arc (namely, the middle ear, the cochlea, and CNVIII) produce either the absence of the acoustic reflex or the elevation of the acoustic-reflex threshold in the ear to which the reflex-activator signal is presented. The proportion of absent acoustic reflexes for patients with varying degrees of sensorineural hearing loss is illustrated in Figure 5.14.

slope differences in the reflex growth functions for different age groups, age-related reflex threshold differences are dependent on the criterion used to determine threshold. The reflex growth functions for tonal signals ≤2000 Hz appear to converge on the same point, suggesting that no age-related reflex threshold differences exist. With the three remaining activator signals (4000 Hz, 6000 Hz, and broadband noise), the growth functions for the two age groups converge on different origins, suggesting true reflex threshold differences for the two groups with the >50-years group having the higher reflex thresholds.

Another complicating factor in the study of age effects is subject selection criteria, particularly regarding auditory sensitivity. Some studies selected subjects in various age groups who had "clinically normal hearing" (Gelfand &

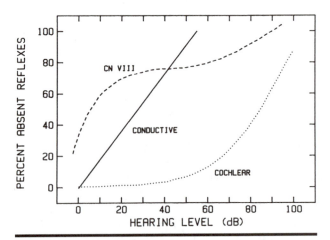

FIGURE 5.14 The percent of absent acoustic reflexes in the ear to which the reflex-activator signal is presented as a function of hearing threshold sensitivity (dB HL) for patients with CNVIII hearing loss (dashed line), with conductive hearing loss (solid line), and with cochlear hearing loss (dotted line). (From Jerger, Clemis, Harford, & Alford, 1974, with permission)

The percent of absent reflexes in patients with conductive hearing losses reflects the attenuation characteristics of the middle-ear lesion on the reflex-activator signal. If the level of the reflex-activator signal is high enough to overcome the amount of attenuation produced by the middle-ear lesion, then an acoustic reflex can be elicited in the opposite ear; the output limits of the instrumentation are the limiting factor. With a conductive hearing loss of 20 dB, 40% of the patients have no measurable acoustic reflex; with a 40 dB conductive loss, 80% of the patients have no measurable acoustic reflex (Jerger, Anthony, Jerger, & Mauldin, 1974). The acoustic reflex should be measurable with cochlear hearing losses to 40 dB HL (Jerger et al., 1972). With a 60 dB HL cochlear hearing loss, 15% of the patients do not have a measurable acoustic reflex. As the degree of cochlear hearing loss increases above 70 dB HL, the percent of absent reflexes increases rapidly. The picture is quite different for patients with CNVIII lesions. With 0 to 10 dB HL thresholds, as many as 50% of the patients with CNVIII lesions may have no measurable acoustic reflexes (Jerger, Clemis, Harford, & Alford, 1974). As the hearing loss increases above 10 dB HL, there is a corresponding increase in the percent of absent acoustic reflexes to 60 dB HL, at which level 80% of the patients have no measurable reflexes. Although the majority of cases in which there is no measurable acoustic reflex involve a pathological condition, a few people with apparent normal auditory systems have no measurable acoustic reflex. Jepsen (1951) reported the acoustic reflexes were not measurable in 1 of 182 subjects (<1%) who had normal auditory systems.

The relation between the degree of hearing loss and the acoustic-reflex threshold for pure tones is illustrated in the top panel of Figure 5.15. In the figure, the average acoustic-reflex threshold (in dB SPL) at 500, 1000, and 2000 Hz is shown as a function of the average behavioral pure-tone threshold (in dB HL) at 500, 1000, and 2000 Hz. The data are based on 355 ears with cochlear hearing loss (Popelka, 1981). The reflex threshold remains at normal levels until the hearing loss exceeds 40 dB HL. As hearing loss increases above 40 dB HL, there is an almost linear increase in the level of the acoustic-reflex threshold with a slope of ~0.38 dB/dB. This means that for each decibel increase in hearing loss above 40 dB HL, there is an increase of 0.38 dB in the acoustic-reflex threshold. As illustrated in the bottom panel of Figure 5.15, there is a somewhat different relation between the reflex threshold for a broadband noise activator and the degree of hearing loss. As hearing loss increases to about 50 dB HL, the reflex threshold for broadband noise increases linearly with a slope of 0.4 dB/dB. As the degree of hearing loss increases above 60 dB HL, there is no corresponding increase in the level of the reflex threshold for the broadband noise activator.

When the lesion is in the efferent or output portion of the acoustic-reflex arc (namely, CNVII, the stapedius nerve,

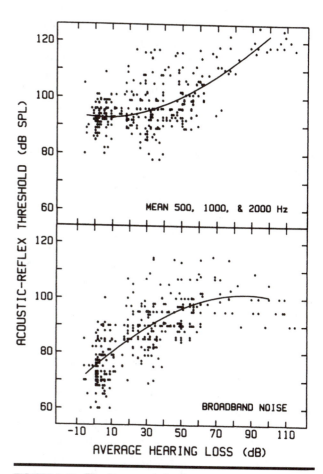

FIGURE 5.15 The top panel shows the mean acoustic-reflex thresholds (in dB SPL) for 500, 1000, and 2000 Hz activators depicted as a function of the mean hearing level (in dB HL, re: ANSI, 1969) for 355 ears at 500, 1000, and 2000 Hz. The solid line represents a best-fit, third-degree polynomial. The bottom panel shows the mean acoustic-reflex thresholds (in dB SPL) for broadband noise depicted as a function of the mean hearing level (in dB HL, re: ANSI, 1969) for 355 ears at 500, 1000, and 2000 Hz. The solid line represents a best-fit, third-degree polynomial. (From Popelka, 1981, with permission from W. B. Saunders)

the stapedius muscle, and the middle ear), the site of lesion, not the degree of hearing loss, is the primary determinant of the status of the acoustic reflex in the probe ear. In patients with a suspected CNVII lesion such as Bell's palsy or a facial nerve schwannoma, absent or elevated reflex thresholds suggest that the site of lesion is proximal to branching of the stapedius nerve from CNVII. Normal reflex thresholds suggest the site of lesion is distal to branching of the stapedius nerve from CNVII. Certain neuromuscular diseases such as myasthenia gravis physiologically render the stapedius muscle unable to contract normally, thereby altering the threshold and growth characteristics of the acoustic reflexes (Blom & Zakrisson, 1974).

A middle-ear abnormality in the probe ear usually precludes measurement of the acoustic reflex. In the presence of middle-ear disease, the stapedius muscle may contract but the contraction is not strong enough to alter the acoustic immittance characteristics of the middle ear. An ossicular discontinuity can produce a similar effect in which the stapedius muscle contracts, but because of a disruption in the ossicular chain, the change in acoustic immittance during the reflexive state is not measurable at the tympanic membrane.

There are some middle-ear disease processes, however, that do not obliterate measurement of the acoustic reflex in the probe ear. Examples of these disease processes are partial ossicular discontinuities including a fracture of the stapes crura central to insertion of the stapedius tendon (Jenkins, Morgan, & Miller, 1980), and congenital stapes anomaly (Shapiro, Canalis, Firemark, & Bahna, 1981). In these cases, the normal route of sound transmission through the middle ear is disrupted, but there is enough continuity of the middle-ear system to permit monitoring of the reflex. With some otosclerotic ears, the reflex is present with the probe in the affected ear but the response is diphasic. With the diphasic pattern, transient immittance changes occur at the onset and offset of the activator signal (Flottorp & Djupesland, 1970; Terkildsen, 1964; Terkildsen, Osterhammel, & Bretlau, 1973). Finally, the audiologist must be cautious in interpreting abnormal reflex data from the probe ear. The majority of patients with abnormal reflexes in the probe ear have middle-ear disorders, although less frequently the problem involves the stapedius muscle or CNVII.

ACOUSTIC-REFLEX ADAPTATION

During sustained activation of the acoustic reflex, the stapedius muscle begins to relax and the acoustic immittance of the middle-ear mechanism begins to return to the preactivator state. Relaxation of the stapedius muscle during presentation of a reflex-activator signal is called *acoustic-reflex adaptation* (or *decay*). [For a detailed review of acoustic-reflex adaptation see Wilson, Shanks, & Lilly (1984) and Fowler & Wilson (1984).] In the normal auditory system, the amount and rate of reflex adaptation is directly related to the frequency of the activator signal (Djupesland, Flottorp, & Winther, 1967; Johansson, Kylin, & Langfy, 1967) and is inversely related to the level of the activator signal, especially for levels near the acoustic-reflex threshold (Dallos, 1964).

Figure 5.16 illustrates the terminology that is used to describe reflex adaptation. The top tracing in the figure is an acoustic reflex (in acoustic mmhos, left ordinate; in percent of maximum, right ordinate) elicited by a 10.2 s, 4000 Hz activator signal (bottom tracing) presented 10 dB above the acoustic-reflex threshold of a young subject with normal hearing. The letters (*A-K*) are used to identify the various aspects of reflex adaptation. Point *B* denotes the onset of the reflex-activator signal. Segment *AB* defines the preactivator signal baseline of middle-ear activity (Y_{tm})

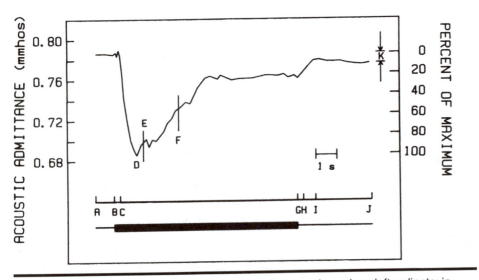

FIGURE 5.16   The top tracing is a reflex response (in acoustic mmhos, left ordinate; in percent of maximum, right ordinate) elicited by a 10.2 s, 4000 Hz activator signal (bottom tracing) presented 10 dB above the acoustic-reflex threshold of a young subject with normal hearing. See text for a discussion of letters *A-K*. (From Wilson, Shanks, & Lilly, 1984, with permission)

that corresponds to 0.79 acoustic mmhos or 0% of the maximum reflex amplitude. *C* is the time at which the reflex attained 10% of maximum amplitude (0.69 acoustic mmhos or 100% of maximum) that occurred at *D*. Point *E* is the time (1.6 s) at which the reflex adapted to 90% of the maximum reflex amplitude. Point *F* is the time (3.6 s) at which the reflex adapted to 50% of the maximum reflex amplitude. The time after onset of the activator signal at which the response adapts to 50% of maximum amplitude is called the *half-life time* and is the measure of reflex adaptation used clinically. The rate of reflex adaptation can be described as the slope of a line through 90% (point *E*) and 50% (point *F*). Thus, the slope of the adaptation function for the reflex shown in Figure 5.16 can be expressed as:

$$m = \Delta Y/\Delta t \qquad (5.13)$$

in which *m* is the slope, ΔY is the change in acoustic mmhos that occurred between the ordinal values at 90% (0.70 acoustic mmhos) and 50% (0.74 acoustic mmhos), and Δt is the change in seconds (s) that occurred between the abscissa values at 90% (1.6 s) and 50% (3.6 s). In this example, the rate of reflex adaptation in (mmhos/s) would be

$$m = -0.04 \text{ acoustic mmhos}/-2.0 \text{ s}$$
$$= 0.02 \text{ acoustic mmhos/s}$$

or the rate of reflex adaptation in percent/second would be

$$m = 40\%/-2.0 \text{ s}$$
$$= -20\%/\text{s}$$

At *G* in Figure 5.16 the activator signal ended, followed at *H* by the offset of the reflex. During segment *IJ*, the acoustic admittance of the middle ear approximated the pre-activator signal baseline value. In the example in Figure 5.16, however, the return to the preactivator signal baseline value is not complete, with *K* representing the difference between the pre- (0.79 acoustic mmhos) and postactivator signal (0.78 acoustic mmhos) baselines. This slight change in the acoustic admittance of the middle ear over 10 to 15 s is a common occurrence that reflects the slight but constantly changing air pressure in the middle ear (Tonndorf & Khanna, 1968; Wilson, McCullough, & Lilly, 1984; Wilson, Steckler, Jones & Margolis, 1978). When a large pre- and post-stimulus baseline acoustic immitance difference occurs, the adaptation measurement may be contaminated with the baseline shift and should be repeated.

The influence of the frequency of the reflex-activator signal on reflex adaptation is illustrated in Figure 5.17. No adaptation occurs for the 500 or 1000 Hz activator signals. With the 2000 Hz activator, adaptation to 90% of maximum is reached at 3.3 s, but adaptation to 50% is not attained over the duration of the activator signal. The reflex to the 4000 Hz activator, however, demonstrates adaptation both to 90% (1.1 s) and to 50% (2.2 s) of the maximum

acoustic admittance producing an adaptation slope of −36.4%/s. There is a direct relationship between the amount and rate of reflex adaptation and the frequency of the reflex-activator signal and an inverse relationship between the frequency of the activator signal and the half-life time, that is, the higher the frequency, the shorter the half-life time of the adaptation function.

The relation between reflex adaptation and the level of the reflex-activator signal is difficult to determine. As indicated earlier, at levels near the reflex threshold, the amount and rate of adaptation appears to be greater than at levels ≥10 dB above the reflex threshold (Dallos, 1964). This observation was confirmed by Djupesland and colleagues (1967), who observed with 250, 500, 1000, 3000, and 4000 Hz activators presented 2, 4, and 10 dB above the reflex threshold that the higher the activator level, the longer the reflex was maintained. In contrast, Wiley and Karlovich (1975) reported that as the level of a 500 Hz activator was increased from 5 to 15 dB above the reflex threshold, there was a corresponding increase in the amount of reflex adaptation; with a 4000 Hz activator, no change was noted in reflex adaptation as the level of the activator was increased. Kaplan, Gilman, and Dirks (1977) also reported that reflex adaptation at 500, 1000, 2000, 3000, and 4000 Hz was independent of the level of the activator signal (6, 12, and 18 dB above the reflex threshold). Data from three studies indicate that for activator signals <2000 Hz, reflex adaptation decreases as the level of the activator signal increases (Givens & Seidemann, 1979; Rosenhall, Lidén, & Nilsson,

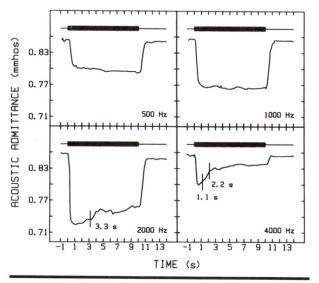

FIGURE 5.17 Acoustic-reflex adaptation functions elicited from a young adult with normal hearing by 500, 1000, 2000, and 4000 Hz activator signals presented for 10.2 s, 10 dB above the acoustic-reflex threshold. (From Wilson, Shanks, & Lilly, 1984, with permission)

TABLE 5.4 Half-life times (seconds) for acoustic-reflex adaptation in subjects with normal hearing from nine investigations (from Wilson, Shanks, & Lilly, 1984).

STUDY	REFLEX-ACTIVATOR SIGNAL				REFLEX-ACTIVATOR SIGNAL FREQUENCY (Hz)							
	Level	Duration (s)	Statistic	N	500	710	1000	1500	2000	3000	4000	6000
Anderson, Barr, & Wedenberg (1969)	+10 dB[a]	10	Median	50	>10.0		>10.0		14.0		7.0	
Cartwright & Lilly (1976)	+10 dB	30–40	Mean	15	>30.0		>30.0		21.0		5.0	
Chiveralls, FitzSimons, Beck, & Kernohan (1976)[b]	+10 dB	30	Mean	101–106	none		32.0		14.5		7.4	
			SD				(6.5)		(5.0)		(2.1)	
Habener & Snyder (1974)	+10 dB	10+	Mean	101–122	>10.0		>10.0		13.4		8.9	
Kaplan et al. (1977)	[c]	180	Model	6	240.0		158.0		25.0	13.0	7.2	
Lilly, Mekaru, & Chudnow (1983)[d]	+10 dB	120	Mean	12		78.4						
Tietze (1969)	[e]		Median	10	>100.0		>40.0	8.0	3.0	2.0	1.1	<1.0
Wilson et al. (1978)	96 dB SPL	180	Mean	7	76.6		20.8		6.2		3.5	
	104 dB SPL	180	Mean	7	141.6		41.1		16.9		4.7	
	116 dB SPL	180	Mean	7	145.3		55.9		12.5		4.4	
Wilson et al. (1984)	+10 dB	31	Mean	35	>31.0		>31.0	20.5	14.2	9.8	7.0	5.3
			SD					(10.5)	(7.4)	(7.4)	(6.2)	(4.3)

[a] Adaptation activator signal presented 10 dB above the acoustic-reflex threshold.
[b] Includes data from Chiveralls and FitzSimons (1973).
[c] Combined data for activator signals presented 6, 12, and 18 dB above the acoustic-reflex threshold.
[d] Personal communication.
[e] From the linear segment of the reflex growth function.

1979; Wilson et al., 1978). For reflex-activator signals >1000 Hz, there does not appear to be a systematic change in reflex adaptation as the activator level is increased (Givens & Seidemann, 1979; Wiley & Karlovich, 1975; Wilson et al., 1978). Procedural differences probably have lead to different conclusions.

The clinical use of reflex adaptation was suggested by the observation that patients with CNVIII lesions exhibit a high rate of adaptation (Anderson, Barr, & Wedenberg, 1969, 1970). Abnormal reflex adaptation was defined in the original reports as a half-life time <5 s for a reflex-activator signal presented 10 dB above the reflex threshold at 500 and 1000 Hz. In contrast to the patients with CNVIII lesions, Anderson and colleagues reported that patients with normal hearing or with cochlear hearing loss maintained the magnitude of the acoustic reflex over the duration of 10s, 500 or 1000 Hz activator signals. Table 5.4 presents a summary of the half-life times from nine investigations of reflex adaptation on subjects with normal hearing. With minor exceptions and considering the differences in experimental protocols, there is good agreement among the results of the studies indicating the frequency dependent nature of acoustic-reflex adaptation.

Of the original four test parameters employed by Anderson and colleagues, only the level of the reflex-activator signal (10 dB above the reflex threshold) and the half-life time measurement continue in common usage. The other two parameters (activator signal duration and frequency) vary from one investigation to another. Some investigators define adaptation over 10 s (Jerger, Clemis, et al., 1974b; Olsen, Stach, & Kurdziel, 1981). Other investigators define an abnormal response at either 500 or 1000 Hz. The following is a useful set of rules that can be applied to the interpretation of reflex adaptation data (Hirsch & Anderson, 1980a, 1980b):

1. RD[+++], if the reflex amplitude declines ≥50% within 5 s at 500 and 1000 Hz.
2. RD[++], if the reflex amplitude declines ≥50% within 5 s at 1000 Hz but not at 500 Hz.
3. RD[+], if the reflex amplitude declines <50% within 5 s at 500 and 1000 Hz.

RD[+++] is a positive sign of CNVIII disease, RD[++] is a questionable sign of CNVIII disease, and RD[+] is not a significant sign of CNVIII disease.

Anderson and colleagues (1969) in the original report on reflex adaptation noted that only 1% of 600 patients with cochlear hearing loss exhibited abnormal reflex adaptation. Subsequent investigations indicate substantially higher false-positive rates (i.e., abnormal reflex adaptation associated with cochlear hearing loss) than the 1% reported by Anderson and colleagues. This point is illustrated by the reflex adaptation functions shown in Figure 5.18 (Cartwright & Lilly, 1976). The data are from three groups of

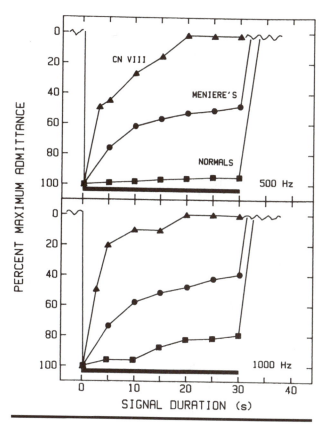

FIGURE 5.18 Acoustic-reflex adaptation data from three subject groups of 15 subjects each in response to 30 s, 500 Hz (top panel) and 1000 Hz (bottom panel) reflex-activator signals. (Adapted from Cartwright & Lilly, 1976)

15 subjects [normal hearing (squares), cochlear hearing loss from Ménière's disease (circles), and CNVIII hearing loss (triangles)] for 30 s, 500 Hz (top panel) and 1000 Hz (bottom panel) activator signals presented 10 dB above the reflex threshold. The functions in the figure illustrate that patients with cochlear hearing loss (Ménière's disease) exhibit reflex adaptation that is more than the adaptation shown by subjects with normal hearing, but less than the adaptation exhibited by patients with CNVIII lesions. Similar data from 100 ears with sensory hearing loss were reported by Olsen, Noffsinger, and Kurdziel (1975) in which abnormal reflex adaptation was demonstrated by one patient at 500 Hz and by 11 patients at 1000 Hz.

Finally, Mangham, Lindeman, and Dawson (1980) studied reflex adaptation as a function of activator level (5 to 25 dB above the reflex threshold) in patients with cochlear hearing loss and patients with CNVIII hearing loss. Mangham and colleagues observed that as the 500 Hz activator signal was presented at higher levels, there was a decrease in the amount of reflex adaptation for the patients with cochlear hearing loss, but there was an increase in the amount of reflex adaptation for patients with CNVIII lesions. These findings suggest that the use of multiple levels of the reflex-activator signal with reflex-adaptation measures may be useful in differentiating cochlear and CNVIII hearing losses.

Regardless of the method used clinically to define abnormal acoustic-reflex adaptation, that is, the 5 s or 10 s criteria at 500 and/or 1000 Hz, when abnormal adaptation is measured, the measurement should be repeated to demonstrate reliability. Additionally, when reflex adaptation is abnormal, it may be insightful to make adaptation measurements at multiple levels above the acoustic-reflex threshold.

OTHER SUPRA-THRESHOLD MEASURES OF THE ACOUSTIC REFLEX

Throughout the 1970s, measures of the acoustic-reflex threshold and acoustic-reflex adaptation were the primary parameters of the acoustic reflex that were used routinely in the differential diagnosis of auditory disorders. Since the early 1960s, other parameters of the acoustic reflex, namely, the temporal and magnitude characteristics, have been studied in animals and in young subjects with normal hearing. [Borg (1976) provides a good review of the dynamic characteristics of the acoustic reflex.]

The animal investigations with the acoustic reflex are exemplified by the work from two laboratories. Borg (1973) reported an increase in the latency of the rabbit stapedius reflex following the creation of a lesion at the level of the trapezoid body. Mangham and Miller (1979) developed an animal model with the macaque monkey that involved the surgical implantation of balloon catheters in the left internal auditory meatus of four monkeys. To mimic the effects of a retrocochlear lesion, pressure was exerted on CNVIII by inflating the implanted balloon with saline. During the experimental procedures, acoustic-reflex measurements were made (1) with the balloon deflated, (2) during a fifteen to thirty-minute period in which the balloon was inflated with volumes from 0.01 to 0.04 cm^3, and (3) following balloon deflation. Mangham and Miller reported that measures of reflex threshold and reflex adaptation were not as sensitive to pressure on CNVIII as were measures of reflex onset latency, onset rise, and amplitude.

The temporal (latency and rise) and amplitude characteristics of the acoustic reflex in subjects with normal auditory systems have been described in numerous studies (Dallos, 1964; Gorga & Stelmachowicz, 1983; McPherson & Thompson, 1977; Møller, 1962b; Overholt & Jerger, 1995; Sprague, Wiley, & Block, 1981; Wilson, 1979; Wilson & McBride, 1978). Clinically, the human investigations initially concentrated on the onset latency of the acoustic reflex with the most recent focus on the amplitude characteristics of the acoustic reflex.

Acoustic-Reflex Latency

The latency of the acoustic reflex is the time difference, Δt, between the onset of the reflex-activator signal and the onset of the acoustic reflex. Several variables, however, compound the measurement of reflex latency. First, the commercially available electroacoustic immittance instruments have various time constants (Jerger, Oliver, & Stach, 1986b; Lilly, 1984; Margolis & Gilman, 1977; Shanks, Wilson, & Jones, 1985). Second, the measurement of reflex latency is complicated by an imprecise definition of the onset of the acoustic reflex. Unlike the precise onset of an activator signal, the onset of the acoustic reflex can be monophasic or biphasic, making the reflex latency measurement difficult and arbitrary (Creten, Vanpeperstraete, Van Camp, & Doclo, 1976; Mangham, Burnett, & Lindeman, 1982, 1983; Van Camp, Vanpeperstraete, Creten, & Vanhuyse, 1975). Third, investigators use different onset landmarks to define onset of the acoustic reflex. Some investigations use the initial detectable acoustic immittance change whereas other investigations use a percentage of the maximum immittance change, which can be 10, 50, or 90% (Borg, 1982; Bosatra, Russolo, & Silverman, 1984; Lilly, 1984). Fourth, the latency of the acoustic reflex is inversely related to the level of the reflex-activator signal (Dallos, 1964; Hung & Dallos, 1972; Lilly, 1964; Møller, 1958; Ruth & Niswander, 1976; Terkildsen, 1960). Fifth, the latency of the acoustic reflex covaries with the frequency and level of the activator signal. Ruth and Niswander reported that the latency was shorter for a 3000 Hz activator than for a 500 Hz activator at levels ≤104 dB SPL, whereas at activator levels >104 dB SPL, the latencies for the two frequencies were the same.

Clinically, the Clemis and Sarno (1980a, 1980b) reports typify the implementation of acoustic-reflex latency as part of the differential diagnosis. One study (1980a) included 47 subjects with normal hearing, 12 patients with Ménière's disease, 16 patients with other types of cochlear hearing loss, and 16 patients with surgically confirmed CNVIII lesions. Reflex latency, which was measured 10 dB above the reflex threshold at 1000 and 2000 Hz, was defined as the time difference between onset of the activator signal and "the first detectable increase in acoustic impedance" as measured by a commercial electroacoustic device with the output displayed on a storage oscilloscope. As shown in the histograms in Figure 5.19, the absolute latency for the normals was longer for the 2000 Hz activator (105.3 ms) than for the 1000 Hz activator (93.0 ms). The reflex latencies for both cochlear hearing loss groups were about the same as the latencies measured for the normal subjects. Using the 95% confidence limit from the normal group as the normal range, 85 to 95% of the patients with cochlear hearing loss were classified as normal by Clemis and Sarno. The retrocochlear group had latencies of 181.5 ms

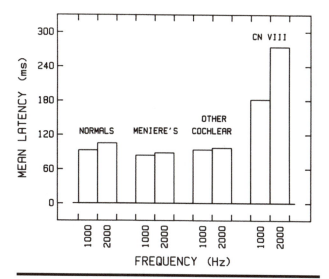

FIGURE 5.19 Histograms showing the mean reflex latencies (in ms) for 1000 and 2000 Hz activator signals for subjects with normal hearing (N = 47), patients with Ménière's disease (N = 12), patients with other cochlear hearing losses (N = 16), and patients with CNVIII lesions (N = 16). (Data from Clemis & Sarno, 1980a)

and 274.0 ms for 1000 and 2000 Hz, respectively, with no cases within the normal range. Interaural latency difference also was found to distinguish among the subject groups. The mean interaural latency difference was <25 ms for the normal subjects and the two groups with cochlear hearing loss and >90 ms for the patients with CNVIII lesions. Clemis and Sarno (1980a, 1980b), therefore, suggested that the latency of the acoustic reflex was useful in differentiating cochlear from retrocochlear disease.

In a subsequent investigation of reflex latency of four patients with confirmed CNVIII tumors, Jerger and Hayes (1983) reported that the reflex latencies for 500 to 2000 Hz activator signals presented at 100 dB SPL, which were measured on a laboratory constructed electroacoustic system, were two to nine times longer for the affected ear (mean = 184 ms; range 60 to 405 ms) than for the normal ear (mean = 40 ms; range, 30 to 45 ms).[5] Jerger and Hayes concluded that when the acoustic reflex was measurable with the activator signal presented to an ear with a CNVIII lesion, the acoustic reflex demonstrated a reduced maximum amplitude compared to the normal ear and was late with a slowly rising onset. From these observations and the measurement problems associated with the latency measure-

ments, Jerger and Hayes suggested that suprathreshold amplitude measures of the acoustic reflex provided essentially the same diagnostic information as provided by reflex latency data, and were easier to make than were the latency measurements.

Acoustic-Reflex Amplitude

The magnitude or amplitude of the acoustic-reflex is the difference between the immittance of the middle ear during the resting or quiescent state (baseline) and the immittance of the middle ear during the reflexive state (peak). During the past three decades, numerous investigations have explored the experimental parameters that affect the amplitude of the acoustic reflex, including the frequency, spectrum, level, and duration of the activator signal (Dallos, 1964; Djupesland & Zwislocki, 1971; Hung & Dallos, 1972; Metz, 1951; Møller, 1958, 1962a, 1962b; Peterson & Lidén, 1972; Silman, 1984; Wilson, 1979; Wilson & McBride, 1978). The common finding for all the investigations is the direct relation between the level of the activator signal and the amplitude of the acoustic reflex. Increases in the level of the activator signal produce increases in the amplitude of the reflex. Other observations include steeper reflex growth functions for mid-frequency activator signals than for low-frequency activators (Møller, 1961) and a hierarchy of reflex amplitudes in which binaural activator signals produce the largest reflex amplitudes, ipsilateral activator signals produce the second largest amplitudes, and contralateral activator signals produce the smallest reflex amplitudes (Møller, 1962a). The duration of the activator signal also influences the amplitude of the acoustic reflex (Djupesland, Sundby, & Flottorp, 1973; Djupesland & Zwislocki, 1971; Jerger, Mauldin, & Lewis, 1977). As duration increases to about 500 ms, reflex amplitude increases.

Several additional characteristics of contralateral acoustic-reflex amplitude are illustrated in Figure 5.20. In the top panel of the figure are reflex growth functions for broadband noise and for 250, 1000, and 4000 Hz signals obtained with a 678 Hz probe and a computer averaging technique from eight young adults with normal hearing (Wilson & McBride, 1978). The data were fit with third-degree polynomial functions, the first derivatives of which (slope functions) are illustrated in the bottom panel of Figure 5.20. The most obvious characteristic of the reflex growth functions is that increases in the level of the activator signal produce increases in the amplitude of the acoustic reflex. The growth functions are characterized by a relatively slow increase in amplitude of the reflex at low activator signal levels and at high activator levels, and by a more rapid, almost constant, increase in amplitude between the low and high activator signal levels. These two characteristics can be observed readily in "U-shaped" slope functions (mmhos/dB) in the bottom panel of Figure 5.20. The

---

[5] The latency difference between the 40 ms reported by Jerger and Hayes (1983) and the 93 to 105 ms latency reported by Clemis and Sarno (1980a) is attributable to different instrumentation and procedures. Jerger and Hayes did report a 78 ms latency for the normal ears when the measurements were made 10 dB above the reflex threshold.

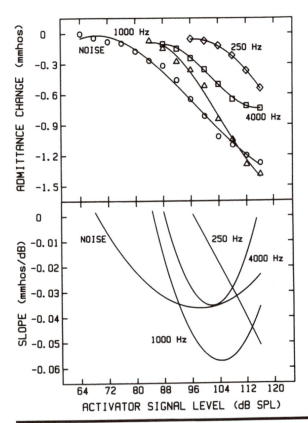

FIGURE 5.20 The top panel shows the mean (N = 8) reflex amplitude in admittance change (mmhos) shown as a function of the activator signal level (dB SPL). The data are modeled with best-fit, third-degree polynomials. The bottom panel shows the slope functions (mmhos/dB) calculated as the first derivatives of the polynomials used to fit the respective activator signal data. (Reprinted with permission from R. H. Wilson & L. M. McBride, "Threshold and growth of the acoustic reflex." *Journal of the Acoustical Society of America, 63*, 147–154. Copyright 1978 Acoustical Society of America.)

growth function for the 4000 Hz activator signal becomes asymptotic at the high signal levels indicating that the growth function is saturated, that is, further increases in the level of the activator signal do not produce further increases in the magnitude of the acoustic reflex. These characteristics of the 4000 Hz growth function (top panel) are reflected in the 4000 Hz slope function (bottom panel) in which (1) a slow change (0 to −0.02 mmhos/dB) occurs over the first few activator levels from 88 dB SPL, (2) the maximum slope (−0.035 mmhos/dB) occurs at 102 dB SPL, and (3) the slope becomes more gradual (−0.02 to 0 mmhos/dB) at higher levels where the function begins to saturate. The dynamic range of a reflex growth function is the signal level range between reflex threshold and saturation. According to the data in Figure 5.20, the dynamic ranges are >50 dB for broadband noise, >28 dB for 1000

Hz, 23 dB for 4000 Hz, and >16 dB for 250 Hz. Three of the four dynamic ranges are "greater than" because saturation was not attained by the growth function. Finally, the status of the ear in which the measurement probe is inserted also has an influence on the amplitude of the acoustic reflex. In general, subjects with higher peak compensated static immittance exhibit larger reflex amplitudes (Lutman & Martin, 1977; Wilson, 1979, Figures 7, 8, and 9).

There are several clinical reports in the literature that indicate that patients with ear pathology have reduced reflex amplitudes. An increased rise time and a decreased magnitude of the acoustic reflex was reported as characteristic of patients with multiple sclerosis (Colletti, 1975). Silman, Gelfand, and Chun (1978) reported acoustic-reflex growth data from a case with an acoustic neuroma in the left ear. With the 500 Hz activator signal presented to the unaffected, right ear, the amplitude of the reflex increased with increased activator level. With the 500 Hz activator signal presented to the affected left ear, however, the amplitude of the reflex did not increase with increases in the level of the activator signal. Ruth, Nilo, and Mravec (1978) reported that Bell's palsy patients have smaller contralateral reflex amplitudes with the measurement probe in the affected ear than with the probe in the unaffected ear. Alternatively, therefore, the reduced function of the acoustic reflex caused by the Bell's palsy, which would reduce the low-frequency attenuation characteristics of the reflex, could have permitted the 500 Hz activator signal to reach the cochlea of the affected ear at a higher than normal level, thereby increasing the amplitude of the acoustic reflex in the unaffected contralateral ear. To clarify this issue, the Ruth and colleagues study must be replicated with both ipsilateral and contralateral reflex growth functions. If the alternative hypothesis were true, then the contralateral reflex amplitude would be larger than the ipsilateral amplitude, which is a relation that is reversed in the normal auditory system. Finally, data from several studies indicate that there is a decrease in the magnitude of the acoustic reflex (and growth functions) with increasing age (Silman & Gelfand, 1981; Thompson et al., 1980; Wilson, 1981).

Jerger and his colleagues (Hayes & Jerger, 1982; Jerger et al., 1987; Jerger, Oliver, Rivera, & Stach, 1986a; Stach & Jerger, 1984) advocate the use of reflex amplitude measures as an indicator of auditory dysfunction. In this Jerger scheme, a probe assembly (270 Hz, 85 dB SPL probe tone) is sealed in each ear with the 500, 1000, or 2000 Hz activator tones (500 ms duration) presented at 110 dB SPL alternately between ears with a 1500 ms intersignal interval. The reflex to each activator signal is digitized, sorted, and averaged for the ipsilateral and the contralateral ear. Thus, four reflexes (right ipsilateral, right contralateral, left ipsilateral, and left contralateral) are obtained from 16 signal presentations. The amplitude of the reflex is the maximum decibel change (0.01 dB resolution) in the sound-pressure level of the probe tone following offset of the activator signal. The reflex amplitudes for the four response modes are combined in the following ways to produce three indices of reflex amplitude:

1. Afferent Index = $(\text{Right}_{ipsi} + \text{Right}_{contra}) - (\text{Left}_{ipsi} + \text{Left}_{contra})$
2. Efferent Index = $(\text{Right}_{ipsi} + \text{Left}_{contra}) - (\text{Left}_{ipsi} + \text{Right}_{contra})$
3. Central Index = $(\text{Right}_{ipsi} + \text{Left}_{ipsi}) - (\text{Right}_{contra} + \text{Left}_{contra})$

in which, Right_{ipsi} is the amplitude of the right ipsilateral acoustic reflex, Right_{contra} is the amplitude of the right contralateral acoustic reflex, Left_{ipsi} is the amplitude of the left ipsilateral acoustic reflex, and Left_{contra} is the amplitude of the left contralateral acoustic reflex. As Jerger and colleagues (1986a, p. 167) stated, "the index concept is used for two purposes: (1) to isolate the locus of reflex amplitude abnormality to (a) the probe ear, (b) the ear to which the signal is being presented, or (c) the central pathway of the crossed reflexes; and (2) to reduce the considerable intersubject variability of individual measures of acoustic reflex amplitudes." The Afferent Index is sensitive to abnormalities on the input side (stimulus ear) of the acoustic-reflex arc, that is, lesions that affect the input of the reflex-activator signal, for example, cochlear and CNVIII lesions. The Efferent Index is sensitive to abnormalities on the output side (probe ear) of the acoustic-reflex arc, that is, lesions that directly affect contraction of the stapedius muscle in the probe ear, for example, CNVII and middle-ear lesions. The Central Index is sensitive to abnormalities in the contralateral pathways of the acoustic-reflex arc. The reflex amplitudes from a subject with a normal auditory system are about the same for the left and right ears, therefore, the Afferent Index and the Efferent Index [6] are essentially the same or zero. Because the amplitude of the ipsilateral reflex is larger than the amplitude of the contralateral reflex, the Central Index on a subject with a normal auditory system is slightly greater than zero. As the instrumentation used by Jerger and his colleagues is unique to their facility, other clinics must establish equipment specific norms for the three indices that are based on immittance units or the sound-pressure level of the probe tone. Additionally, the approach may benefit by a method for quantifying reflex amplitude that is not sensitive to ear-canal volume (see Figure 5.10).

---

[6] The Efferent Index can be influenced by a difference between ears in ear-canal volume (see Figure 5.10). With the Afferent Index and the Central Index, ear differences owing to ear-canal volume differences or peak compensated static immittance differences do not influence the indices because the characteristics of both ears are present in the expressions on either side of the minus argument.

DETECTION OF HEARING LOSS FROM ACOUSTIC-REFLEX THRESHOLDS

Acoustic-reflex thresholds can provide information about hearing sensitivity (i.e., pure-tone behavioral thresholds). The use of acoustic-reflex thresholds to detect hearing loss or estimate hearing sensitivity is based on the following two relations: the relation between the acoustic-reflex thresholds and the bandwidth of the reflex-activator signal and the relation between the acoustic-reflex threshold and the degree of hearing loss. In this section these two relations will be described and applied to the detection of hearing loss. [Popelka (1981) presents a thorough review of this topic.]

Lüscher (1929) was the first to point out that complex signals are more effective in eliciting the acoustic reflex than are tonal signals. The effect of bandwidth on acoustic-reflex thresholds was initially explored by Flottorp, Djupesland, and Winther (1971) and later by several other investigators (Djupesland & Zwislocki, 1973; Green & Margolis, 1983; Margolis, Dubno, & Wilson, 1980; Popelka, Karlovich, & Wiley, 1974; Popelka, Margolis, & Wiley, 1976; Schwartz & Sanders, 1976). Figure 5.21 illustrates the influence of the reflex-activator signal bandwidth on the reflex thresholds of normal subjects. Reflex thresholds remain constant as the signal bandwidth is increased up to a "critical bandwidth," beyond which the reflex thresholds decrease. The bandwidth effect appears to be the same for ipsilateral and contralateral activator signals (Green & Margolis, 1983).

Thelin (1980) suggested that the logarithmic bandwidth axis in Figure 5.21 does not accurately reflect the frequency representation in the auditory system, and an octave scale better approximates the logarithmic frequency representation on the basilar membrane. In fact, if frequency is represented logarithmically in the auditory system as suggested by a considerable body of evidence (Zwislocki, 1965), then the log frequency axis in Figure 5.21 is not proportional to distance on the basilar membrane. Bandwidth measured in octaves, however, produces a measure that closely approximates the area of cochlear excitation (Green & Margolis, 1984). It is likely that the relatively flat portion of the acoustic-reflex threshold function in Figure 5.21 is flat because changes in the bandwidth of the reflex-activator signal in that frequency range produce very small differences in the area of excitation on the basilar membrane.

Figure 5.22 illustrates the effect of the reflex-activator signal bandwidth on acoustic-reflex thresholds plotted on an octave bandwidth axis. The effect of bandwidth on ipsilateral and contralateral acoustic-reflex thresholds are similar, that is, acoustic-reflex threshold decreases linearly with increases in activator signal bandwidth. The slope of the ipsilateral function may be slightly steeper than the slope

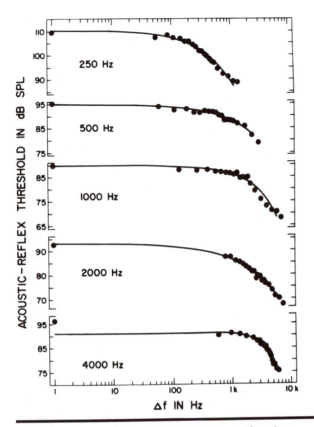

FIGURE 5.21 Acoustic-reflex thresholds as a function of reflex-activator signal bandwidth (Δf) in Hertz on a log frequency axis. The activator signals were tonal complexes, logarithmically centered around the indicated frequency. The left-most data point in each function is the reflex threshold for a tonal stimulus at the indicated frequency. Each point is the mean reflex threshold for 10 normal-hearing young-adult subjects. (Reprinted from G. R. Popelka, R. H. Margolis, & T. L. Wiley, "Effect of activating signal bandwidth on acoustic-reflex thresholds." *Journal of the Acoustical Society of America, 59*, 153–159. Copyright 1976 Acoustical Society of America.)

between sensitivity (behavioral) thresholds and acoustic-reflex thresholds. Metz (1946) stated that,

> With the exception of one ear a muscle contraction can be elicited in all the ears with unilateral perception deafness or completely deaf ears from the opposite normal ears. The conditions are a little more complicated in patients with bilateral perception deafness, as a muscle contraction can be elicited in many cases, in others not, without this definitely being dependent on the magnitude of the hearing loss. However, it is impossible to elicit a muscle contraction from any of the completely deaf ears. (p. 241)

The variability in reflex thresholds from patients with sensorineural hearing loss was illustrated earlier in Figure 5.15. Reflex thresholds for tones (Figure 5.15, top panel) tend to remain unchanged for hearing losses up to about 40 dB and then increase as the degree of hearing loss increases. Acoustic-reflex thresholds for noise activator signals (Figure 5.15, bottom panel) are elevated for mild hearing losses and stabilize for more severe hearing losses. It should be pointed out, however, that most patients with severe hearing losses do not exhibit acoustic reflexes, so that the function

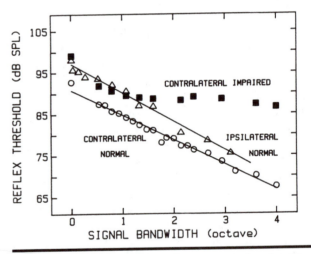

FIGURE 5.22 Acoustic-reflex thresholds as a function of the reflex-activator signal bandwidth (in octaves) for three subject groups. The center frequency was 2000 Hz and the left-most data point in each function is the reflex threshold for a 2000 Hz activator signal. The circles depict the contralateral reflex thresholds for normal-hearing young-adult subjects from Popelka and colleagues, 1976 (see Figure 5.21). The triangles represent ipsilateral reflex thresholds for normal-hearing young-adult subjects from Green and Margolis (1983). The squares represent the mean reflex thresholds for eight subjects with noise-induced, sensorineural hearing loss. (Reprinted from G. R. Popelka, R. H. Margolis, & T. L. Wiley, "Effect of activating signal bandwidth on acoustic-reflex thresholds." *Journal of the Acoustical Society of America, 59*, 153–159. Copyright 1976 Acoustical Society of America.)

of the contralateral function. The 5 to 6 dB differences in ipsilateral and contralateral acoustic-reflex thresholds may be entirely attributable to calibration differences between the two procedures (Green & Margolis, 1983). The relation illustrated in Figure 5.22 suggests a much simpler interpretation of the bandwidth effect than the "critical band" mechanism (e.g., Flottorp et al., 1971). That is, the acoustic-reflex threshold is linearly related to the area of excitation on the basilar membrane. A similar relationship has been found between loudness and signal bandwidth in octaves (Cacace & Margolis, 1985), suggesting that both loudness and acoustic-reflex threshold are linearly related to an area of excitation on the basilar membrane.

The effect of sensorineural hearing loss on acoustic-reflex thresholds was first explored by Metz who was perplexed by the extreme variability in the relationship

for broadband noise in the bottom panel of Figure 5.15 probably underestimates the acoustic-reflex thresholds for severe hearing losses. The variability evident in Figure 5.15 presents a challenge to the detection of hearing loss from acoustic-reflex thresholds. A similar effect of signal bandwidth is shown in Figure 5.22. The filled square symbols show the effect of reflex-activator signal bandwidth on acoustic-reflex thresholds for a group of patients with noise-induced sensorineural hearing loss. In comparison to the reflex thresholds from the subjects with normal hearing, the reflex thresholds from the hearing impaired group are only slightly elevated for narrowband activator signals but more significantly elevated for broadband activator signals.

Niemeyer and Sesterhenn (1974) were the first to use the relation between the reflex-activator signal bandwidth and the acoustic-reflex threshold to estimate the degree of hearing loss. This method for detecting hearing loss, which was dependent upon the relation between the reflex thresholds for pure-tone signals and noise signals, subsequently was modified by Jerger, Burney, Mauldin, and Crump (1974) and by Popelka and colleagues (1976). The detection methods are all based on the effect of hearing loss on the bandwidth effect in patients with sensorineural hearing loss. The various detection methods differ in the specificity of the outcome. Whereas the Niemeyer and Sesterhenn method estimates hearing loss in decibels hearing level, the Jerger and colleagues method classifies hearing loss into one of four severity categories. The bivariate plotting method (Figure 5.23) described by Popelka and colleagues (1976)

is the least ambitious of the sensitivity prediction methods in that it separates subjects into two groups—normal and impaired. An evaluation of the three methods suggested that the variability illustrated in Figure 5.15 does not allow the more specific predictions of the Niemeyer and Sesterhenn method and the Jerger and colleagues method to be made with acceptable error rates. The bivariate plotting method, by making a gross discrimination among subjects, accomplishes that goal with acceptable false positive and hit rates (Margolis & Fox, 1977). The appropriate use of the detection procedure is as a screening device that identifies patients who need further audiologic evaluation.

CASE STUDIES

This section contains cases that illustrate the use of acoustic-reflex data in the differential diagnosis of auditory disorders. Figures 5.24 to 5.33 contain simplified schematics of the acoustic-reflex arc (top panel) and pure-tone audiograms[7] for the left and right ears (bottom panel). The acoustic-reflex arc is represented by the middle ear, the cochlea, CNVIII, the brainstem, CNVII, the stapedius muscle, and the middle ear. The cases that follow introduce the various threshold response patterns associated with the four acoustic-reflex conditions, namely, left ipsilateral, right ipsilateral, left contralateral, and right contralateral. [See Jerger & Jerger (1981) for other case studies.]

Case 1

Case 1 (Figure 5.24) illustrates the acoustic-reflex arc and threshold data for a young adult subject with a normal auditory system. As with the behavioral pure-tone thresholds, the reflex thresholds are recorded on the audiogram that represents the ear to which the reflex-activator signal is presented. For example, if the activator signal is presented ipsilaterally to the right ear (probe and activator signal in the right ear), then the reflex threshold is recorded as a caret on the audiogram for the right ear. If the activator signal is presented contralaterally to the right ear (probe in the left ear and activator signal in the right ear), then the reflex threshold is recorded as a filled circle on the audiogram for the right ear. In the cases that follow, each audiogram should have both contralateral (250–4000 Hz) and ipsilateral (500–2000 Hz) reflex thresholds recorded; an

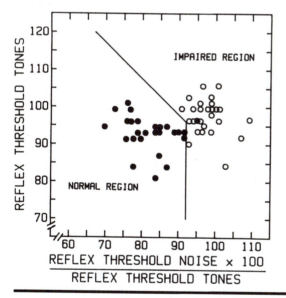

FIGURE 5.23 Bivariate plot of contralateral acoustic-reflex thresholds for subjects with normal hearing (filled circles) and patients with sensorineural hearing loss (open circles) exceeding 30 dB (mean at 500, 1000, and 2000 Hz). (Adapted from Margolis, Fox, Lilly, Silman, & Trumpf, 1981)

---

[7]Some examples also contain pure-tone, bone-conduction thresholds ([or]). For the air- or bone-conduction thresholds that required masking, the appropriate effective masking was used, but to maintain clarity, the effective masking levels were not recorded on the audiograms; this is true for all cases except the one depicted in Figure 5.33, which is a masking dilemma. The use of only the hearing sensitivity thresholds and the acoustic-reflex thresholds given with each case is for illustrative purposes only and is not intended to preclude the other auditory tests that are involved in the differential diagnosis of auditory disorders.

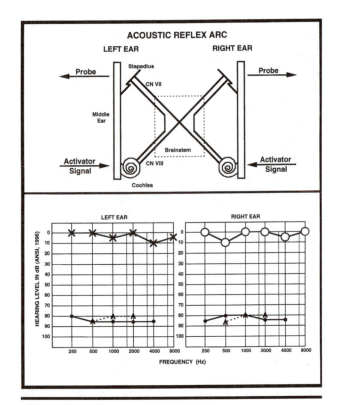

FIGURE 5.24 CASE 1. This case represents a young adult subject with a normal auditory system. *Top panel:* Schematic of the ipsilateral (uncrossed) and contralateral (crossed) auditory pathways of the acoustic-reflex arcs for the left and right ears. *Bottom panel:* Audiograms for the normal left and right ears on which the pure-tone sensitivity thresholds are plotted along with the ipsilateral (^) and contralateral (o) acoustic-reflex thresholds. The reflex thresholds are recorded on the audiogram for the ear to which the reflex-activator signal is presented.

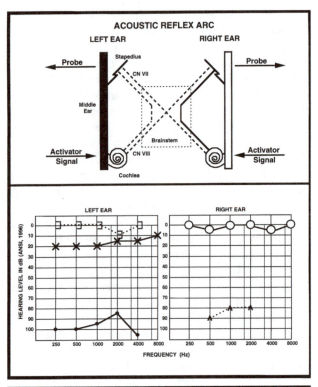

FIGURE 5.25 CASE 2. A left middle-ear lesion (filled rectangle in the top panel) that produced a mild conductive hearing loss and no measurable acoustic reflex with the probe in the left ear (activator signal in either the left or right ears) and elevated left contralateral reflex thresholds (activator signal in the left ear, probe in the right ear). The right ipsilateral reflex thresholds are normal. The dashed lines in the schematic of the reflex arc represent the pathways that are affected by the left middle-ear lesion.

absence of the reflex symbol on the audiogram indicates that an acoustic reflex was not measurable at that activator frequency. In Case 1, the acoustic-reflex thresholds are within normal limits, that is, ≤95 dB HL for activator signals below 4000 Hz and ≤100 to 105 dB HL for 4000 Hz. The acoustic-reflex arc for Case 1 is normal and, therefore, the ipsilateral auditory pathways are depicted as the solid lines between the cochlea and stapedius muscle on the same side, and the contralateral auditory pathways are shown as the solid lines between the cochlea and stapedius muscle on opposite sides. In the cases that follow, the site of lesion is indicated on the schematic of the acoustic-reflex arc by a filled rectangle, and disruption of an auditory pathway(s) is indicated by a dashed line.

Case 2

Case 2 (Figure 5.25) has otosclerosis in the left ear (filled rectangle) that produced a mild, conductive hearing loss (the bone thresholds on the left ear were masked appropriately); the right ear is normal. The acoustic reflexes are absent with the probe in the left (conductive) ear and present with the probe in the right ear. Reflexes are absent probe left (impaired left ipsilateral and right contralateral reflex pathways shown by the dashed lines) because the mechanical problem in the left middle ear prevented the stapedius contraction from changing the acoustic immittance of the middle-ear system. Except for 2000 Hz, the left contralateral reflex thresholds were elevated (i.e., >95 dB HL) (impaired left contralateral pathway shown by the

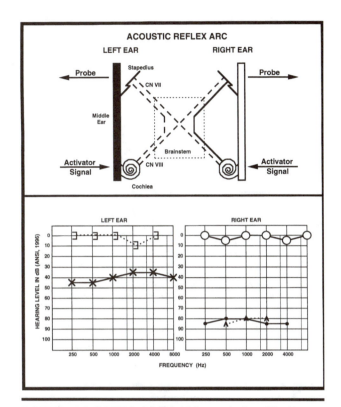

FIGURE 5.26 CASE 3. A left middle-ear lesion (filled rectangle) that produced a moderate conductive hearing loss. No acoustic reflex was measurable with the probe in the left ear (activator signal in either the right or left ear) or with the activator signal presented to the left ear. Hearing sensitivity and the ipsilateral reflex thresholds in the right ear are normal.

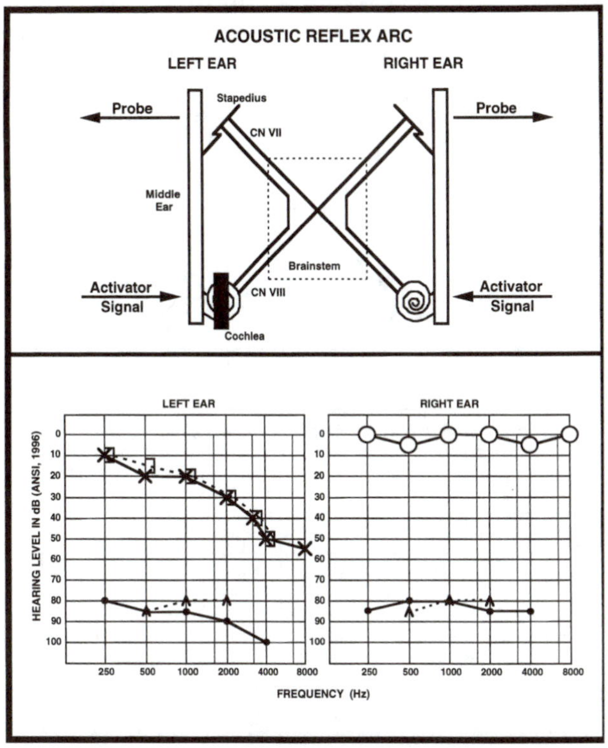

FIGURE 5.27 CASE 4. A left cochlear lesion that produced a mild-to-moderate high-frequency sensory (cochlear) hearing loss. The ipsilateral and contralateral reflex thresholds for the left ear are within the normal range as are the half-life times for reflex adaptation at 500 and 1000 Hz. Hearing sensitivity and the ipsilateral and contralateral reflex thresholds in the right ear are normal.

dashed line) because the left conductive component attenuated the level of the reflex-activator signal that reached the cochlea.

Case 3

This case (Figure 5.26) is identical to Case 2, except that the conductive hearing loss in the left ear of Case 3 is moderate (35 to 45 dB HL) instead of mild. The large conductive component in the left ear precludes measurement of the left contralateral acoustic reflex because the maximum output level of the reflex-activator signal does not overcome the attenuation of the activator signal produced by the conductive component.

Case 4

Case 4 (Figure 5.27) is a left cochlear hearing loss that produced a mild-to-moderate high-frequency hearing loss.

The right ear is normal. All acoustic reflexes are within the normal range. Although there is a hearing loss in the left ear, reflex thresholds are ≤95 dB HL for 250 through 2000 Hz and ≤100 to 105 dB HL for 4000 Hz. The half-life times of acoustic-reflex adaptation at 500 and 1000 Hz in the left ear were normal, both being >10 s. Because the acoustic-reflex data are normal, the auditory pathways in the reflex arc are not impaired and are therefore depicted as solid lines.

Case 5

This case (Figure 5.28) has a left cochlear lesion that produced a moderate-to-profound sensorineural hearing loss. The right ear is normal. The acoustic-reflex thresholds are normal with the activator signal presented to the right ear and abnormal with the activator signal presented to the left ear. In the left ear, only the left contralateral reflexes

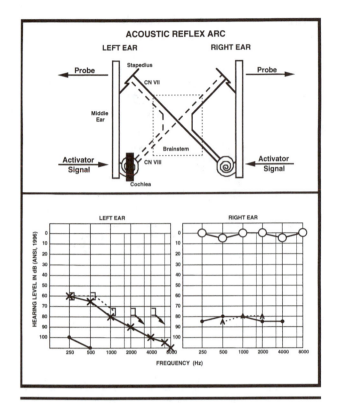

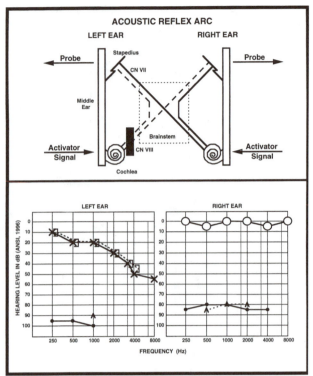

FIGURE 5.28   CASE 5. A left cochlear lesion that produced a moderate-to-profound sensorineural hearing loss. On the left ear, only left contralateral reflex thresholds at 250 and 500 Hz were recorded. Left ipsilateral reflexes are absent because they are beyond the output limits of the equipment. The right ipsilateral and contralateral reflex thresholds are present at normal levels.

FIGURE 5.29   CASE 6. A left CNVIII lesion that produced a mild-to-moderate sensorineural hearing loss. Although several reflex thresholds were measurable with the activator signal presented to the left ear, abnormal reflex adaptation (6 s and 3 s for 500 and 1000 Hz, respectively) was observed for the contralateral reflexes. The right ipsilateral and contralateral reflex thresholds are present at normal levels.

at 250 and 500 Hz are present at elevated levels. The degree of hearing loss in the mid- to high-frequencies precluded the measurement of the left contralateral acoustic reflexes at frequencies >500 Hz and of the left ipsilateral reflexes. Because of the high reflex threshold at 500 Hz (110 dB HL), reflex adaptation could not be measured in the left ear. These reflex findings for the left ear are reflected in the impaired ipsilateral and contralateral pathways of the acoustic-reflex arc (dashed lines). The reflex thresholds for the right ear are within normal limits. The normal right contralateral reflex thresholds (probe left) indicates a normal left middle ear, which substantiates the equality of air- and bone-conduction thresholds for the left ear.

Case 6

In Case 6 (Figure 5.29), a left CNVIII lesion produced a mild-to-moderate sensorineural hearing loss. The right ear

is normal. Again, the acoustic-reflex thresholds are normal with the activator signal presented to the right ear and abnormal with the activator signal presented to the left ear. The left contralateral acoustic-reflex thresholds were present at normal levels at 250 and 500 Hz, slightly elevated at 1000 Hz, and not measurable in the higher frequencies; the left ipsilateral reflex was present only at 1000 Hz. The half-life times for reflex adaptation in the left contralateral condition were abnormal, 4 s and 1.5 s for 500 and 1000 Hz, respectively. These reflex results from the left ear are represented as the impaired pathways (dashed lines) in the acoustic-reflex arc.

Case 7

With Case 7 (Figure 5.30), a left CNVIII lesion produced a mild-to-moderate sensorineural hearing loss. The right ear is normal. The acoustic-reflex thresholds are normal with the activator signal presented to the right ear and absent

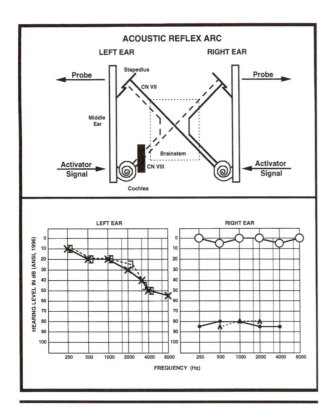

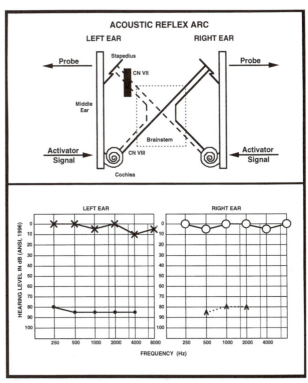

FIGURE 5.30 CASE 7. A left CNVIII lesion that produced a mild-to-moderate sensorineural hearing loss. No left ipsilateral or contralateral acoustic reflexes were measurable when the activator signal was presented to the left ear. The right ipsilateral and contralateral reflex thresholds are present at normal levels.

FIGURE 5.31 CASE 8. A left CNVII lesion (Bell's palsy) that produced no measurable acoustic reflexes when the probe was in the left ear (activator signal either ipsilateral left ear, or contralateral right ear). The reflexes were normal when the probe was in the right ear and the activator signal presented in either the right or left ears.

with the activator signal presented to the left ear. This case is identical to Case 6 except that there are no measurable acoustic reflexes when the reflex activator is presented to the left ear, a finding that is reflected in the impaired left ipsilateral and left contralateral pathways in the reflex arc (dashed lines).

Case 8

Case 8 (Figure 5.31) illustrates a left CNVII lesion (Bell's palsy) in which the behavioral pure-tone thresholds are within normal limits. The acoustic reflexes are absent with the probe in the left ear and present with the probe in the right ear. With the probe in the left ear, there were no measurable acoustic reflexes with the reflex-activator signal in the left or right ears (impaired left ipsilateral and right contralateral reflex pathways shown by the dashed lines) because the CNVII lesion inhibited innervation of the left stapedius muscle. The right ipsilateral and left contra-

lateral reflex thresholds are within normal limits because those pathways are not involved with the left CNVII lesion.

Case 9

This case (Figure 5.32) has an intra-axial brainstem lesion that is manifested by normal behavioral pure-tone thresholds. The acoustic-reflex thresholds are normal ipsilaterally and absent contralaterally. The left and right contralateral pathways are disrupted (dashed lines) by a lesion involving the auditory fibers that decussate.

Case 10

Case 10 (Figure 5.33) has a left ear with a moderate-to-severe sensory hearing loss, whereas the right ear has a moderate-to-severe conductive hearing loss. The unmasked bone-conduction thresholds are displayed on the left-ear

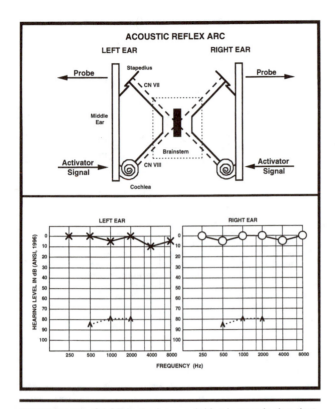

FIGURE 5.32 CASE 9. An intra-axial brainstem lesion that resulted in no measurable contralateral acoustic reflexes. The ipsilateral reflex thresholds in the left and right ears are present at normal levels.

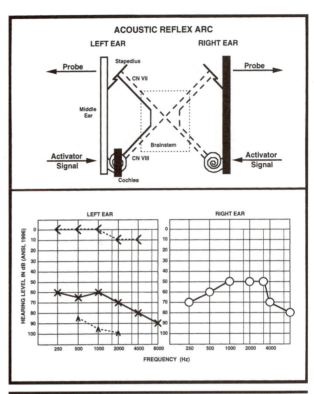

FIGURE 5.33 CASE 10. A left cochlear lesion that produced a moderate-to-severe sensory (cochlear) hearing loss and a right middle-ear lesion that produced a moderate-to-severe conductive hearing loss. Of the acoustic-reflex measures, only the ipsilateral acoustic reflexes in the left ear were measurable.

audiogram. Accurate masked bone conduction thresholds could not be obtained owing to the masking dilemma. The acoustic reflexes are present only for the left ipsilateral condition. With the probe in the right ear, there were no measurable acoustic reflexes, which is consistent with the disrupted left contralateral and right ipsilateral auditory pathways. The right stapedius muscle contracted when the activator signal was presented in the left contralateral condition, but the mechanical problem in the right middle ear prevented a change in the acoustic immittance of the right middle ear. The right ipsilateral reflexes were obscured by both the attenuation of the activator signal on the activator signal and the mechanical problems of the right middle-ear lesion. With the probe in the left ear, there were no measurable reflexes for the right contralateral condition, again because of the attenuation effects caused by the right middle-ear lesion. The left ipsilateral reflexes were present at normal limits. The presence of the left ipsilateral acoustic reflexes indicates that the left middle ear functions normally, and that the hearing loss in the left ear is cochlear.

One can infer that the unmasked bone-conduction thresholds originate from the right ear, which is consistent with a conductive hearing loss in the right ear.

CONCLUSIONS

Although this chapter reviewed in detail many of the subtle characteristics of the acoustic reflex, clinical implementation of acoustic-reflex measures is straightforward. First, acoustic reflex measures should be made at the air pressure that corresponds to the peak of the tympanogram. In some cases, more stable measures can be made with the air pressure slightly off the air pressure at the peak of the tympanogram. Second, because of time constraints acoustic reflex thresholds should be measured ipsilaterally with a 226 Hz probe and 500, 1000, and 2000 Hz activator signals. When acoustic reflexes are abnormal (i.e., either elevated or not measurable), especially in one ear, then contralateral acoustic reflexes should be measured. As demonstrated in the example case studies, the various ipsilateral and contralateral reflex threshold patterns are useful in determining the site of lesion in the auditory system. Third, the reference levels (i.e., hearing level or sound-pressure level) of the signals delivered ipsilaterally through the probe assembly should be known. Future probe assemblies should include a microphone that can monitor the sound-pressure level developed in the ear canal by either the probe signal or the reflex-activator signal. *Reflex-activator signals levels in excess of 110 dB SPL should not be used.* Fortunately, the characteristics of most probe assemblies preclude ipsilateral levels higher than 110 dB SPL, however, unfortunately, levels to 125 dB SPL can be achieved through supra-aural earphones. Fourth, the majority of acoustic-reflex adaptation data are based on activator signals presented continuously for 10 s or more. It is unclear (perhaps doubtful) that pulsed and continuous activator signals produce comparable acoustic-reflex adaptation characteristics.

REFERENCES

American National Standards Institute. (1969). *Specifications for Audiometers* (ANSI S3.6-1969). New York: Author.

Anderson, H., & Barr, B., & Wedenberg, E. (1969). Intra-aural reflexes in retrocochlear lesions. In C. A. Hamberger & J. Wersäll (Eds.), *Nobel Symposium 10, Disorders of the Skull Base Region* (pp. 48–54). Stockholm: Almqvist & Wikell.

Anderson, H., & Barr, B., & Wedenberg, E. (1970). Early diagnosis of VIIIth-nerve tumours by acoustic reflex tests. *Acta Otolaryngologica, 262,* 232–237.

Anderson, H., & Wedenberg, E. (1968). Audiometric identification of normal hearing carriers of genes for deafness. *Acta Otolaryngologica, 65,* 535–554.

Barajas, J. J., Olaizola, F., Tapia, M. C., Alarcon, J. L., & Alaminos, D. (1981). Audiometric study of the neonate: Impedance audiometry. Behavioral responses and brain stem audiometry. *Audiology, 20,* 41–52.

Beattie, R. C., & Leamy, D. P. (1975). Otoadmittance: Normative values, procedural variables, and reliability. *Journal of the American Auditory Society, 1,* 21–27.

Bennett, M. J. (1975). Acoustic impedance bridge measurement with the neonate. *British Journal of Audiology, 9,* 117–124.

Bennett, M. J., & Weatherby, L. A. (1982). Newborn acoustic reflexes to noise and pure-tone signals. *Journal of Speech and Hearing Research, 25,* 383–387.

Blom, S., & Zakrisson, J. E. (1974). The stapedius reflex in the diagnosis of myasthenia gravis. *Journal of the Neurological Sciences, 21,* 71–76.

Borg, E. (1973). On the neuronal organization of the acoustic middle ear reflex. A physiological and anatomical study. *Brain Research, 49,* 101–123.

Borg, E. (1976). Dynamic characteristics of the intra-aural muscle reflex. In A. Feldman & L. Wilber (Eds.), *Acoustic Impedance and Admittance, The Measurement of Middle Ear Function* (pp. 236–299). Baltimore: Williams & Wilkins.

Borg, E. (1982). Time course of the human acoustic stapedius reflex. *Scandinavian Audiology, 11,* 237–242.

Borg, E., Counter, S. A., & Rösler, G. (1984). Theories of middle-ear muscle function. In S. Silman (Ed.), *The Acoustic Reflex: Basic Principles and Clinical Applications* (pp. 63–99). Orlando, FL: Academic Press.

Borg, E., & Møller, A. (1975). Effect of central depressants on the acoustic middle ear reflex in rabbit. *Acta Physiologica Scandinavica, 94,* 327–338.

Borg, E., & Zakrisson, J-E. (1974). Stapedius reflex and monaural masking. *Acta Otolaryngologica, 78,* 155–161.

Bosatra, A., Russolo, M., & Silverman, C. A. (1984). Acoustic-reflex latency: State of the art. In S. Silman (Ed.), *The Acoustic Reflex: Basic Principles and Clinical Applications* (pp. 301–328). Orlando, FL: Academic Press.

Brask, T. (1978). Extratympanic manometry in man. Clinical and experimental investigation of the acoustic stapedius and tensor tympani contractions in normal subjects and in patients. *Scandinavian Audiology, Supplement 7,* 1–199.

Burke, K. S., & Herer, G. R. (1973). Impedance and admittance bridge differences in middle ear study. *Journal of Auditory Research, 13,* 251–256.

Cacace, A. T., & Margolis, R. H. (1985). On the loudness of complex stimuli and its relationship to cochlear excitation. *Journal of the Acoustical Society of America, 78,* 1568–1573.

Cartwright, D., & Lilly, D. (1976). *A Comparison of Acoustic-Reflex Decay Patterns for Patients with Cochlear and VIIIth-Nerve Disease.* Paper presented at the American Speech-Language-Hearing Association Convention, Houston.

Chiveralls, K. (1977). Further examination of the use of the stapedius reflex in the diagnosis of acoustic neuroma. *Audiology, 16,* 331–337.

Chiveralls, K., & FitzSimons, R. (1973). Stapedial reflex action in normal subjects. *British Journal of Audiology, 7,* 105–110.

Chiveralls, K., FitzSimons, R., Beck, G., & Kernohan, H. (1976). The diagnostic significance of the stapedius reflex. *British Journal of Audiology, 10,* 122–128.

Clemis, J. D., & Sarno, C. N. (1980a). Acoustic reflex latency test in the evaluation of nontumor patients with abnormal brainstem latencies. *Annals of Otology, Rhinology and Laryngology, 89,* 296–302.

Clemis, J. D., & Sarno, C. N. (1980b). The acoustic reflex latency test: Clinical application. *The Laryngoscope, 90,* 601–611.

Colletti, V. (1975). Stapedius reflex abnormalities in multiple sclerosis. *Audiology, 14,* 63–71.

Creten, W. L., Vanpeperstraete, P. M., Van Camp, K. J., & Doclo, J. R. (1976). An experimental study on diphasic acoustic reflex patterns in normal ears. *Scandinavian Audiology, 5,* 3–10.

Dallos, P. (1964). Dynamics of the acoustic reflex: Phenomenological aspects. *Journal of the Acoustical Society of America, 36,* 2175–2183.

Davis, R. C. (1948). Motor effects of strong auditory stimuli. *Journal of Experimental Psychology, 38,* 257–275.

Djupesland, G. (1965). Electromyography of the tympanic muscles in man. *International Audiology, 4,* 34–41.

Djupesland, G. (1976). Nonacoustic reflex measurement—Procedures, interpretations and variables. In A. Feldman & L. Wilber (Eds.), *Acoustic Impedance and Admittance, The Measurement of Middle Ear Function* (pp. 217–235). Baltimore: Williams & Wilkins.

Djupesland, G., Flottorp, G., & Winther, F. (1967). Size and duration of acoustically elicited impedance changes in man. *Acta Otolaryngologica, 224*, 220–228.

Djupesland, G., Sundby, A., & Flottorp, G. (1973). Temporal summation in the acoustic stapedius reflex mechanism. *Acta Otolaryngologica, 76*, 305–312.

Djupesland, G., & Zwislocki, J. J. (1971). Effect of temporal summation on the human stapedius reflex. *Acta Otolaryngologica, 71*, 262–265

Djupesland, G., & Zwislocki, J. J. (1973). On the critical band in the acoustic stapedius reflex. *Journal of the Acoustical Society of America, 54*, 1157–1159.

Flottorp, G., & Djupesland, G. (1970). Diphasic impedance change and its applicability in clinical work. *Acta Otolaryngologica, 263*, 200–204.

Flottorp, G., Djupesland, G., & Winther, F. (1971). The acoustic stapedius reflex in relation to critical bandwidth. *Journal of the Acoustical Society of America, 49*, 457–461.

Fowler, C. G., & Wilson, R. H. (1984). Adaptation of the acoustic reflex. *Ear and Hearing, 5*, 281–288.

Gelfand, S. A., & Piper, N. (1981). Acoustic reflex thresholds in young and elderly subjects with normal hearing. *Journal of the Acoustical Society of America, 69*, 295–297.

Givens, G., & Seidemann, M. (1979). A systematic investigation of measurement parameters of acoustic-reflex adaptation. *Journal of Speech and Hearing Disorders, 44*, 534–542.

Goodhill, V. (1981). *Ear Diseases, Deafness, and Dizziness.* New York: Harper & Row.

Gorga, M. P., & Stelmachowicz, P. G. (1983). Temporal characteristics of the acoustic reflex. *Audiology, 22*, 120–127.

Green, K. W., & Margolis, R. H. (1983). Detection of hearing loss with ipsilateral acoustic reflex thresholds. *Audiology, 22*, 471–479.

Green, K. W., & Margolis, R. H. (1984). The ipsilateral acoustic reflex. In S. Silman (Ed.), *The Acoustic Reflex: Basic Principles and Clinical Applications* (pp. 276–301). Orlando, FL: Academic Press.

Guinan, J. J. & McCue, M. P. (1987). Asymmetries in the acoustic reflexes of the cat stapedius muscle. *Hearing Research, 26*, 1–10.

Habener, S. A., & Snyder, J. M. (1974). Stapedius reflex amplitude and decay in normal hearing ears. *Archives of Otolaryngology, 100*, 294–297.

Hall, J. W. (1982). Quantification of the relationship between crossed and uncrossed acoustic reflex amplitude. *Ear and Hearing, 3*, 296–300.

Handler, S. D., & Margolis, R. H. (1977). Predicting hearing loss from stapedial reflex thresholds in patients with sensorineural impairment. *Transactions of the American Academy of Ophthalmology and Otology, 84*, 425–431.

Hayes, D., & Jerger, J. (1982). Signal averaging of the acoustic reflex: Diagnostic applications of amplitude characteristics. *Scandinavian Audiology, 17*, 31–36.

Hensen, V. (1878). Beobachtungen über die trommelfell-spanners bei hund und katze. *Archiv für Anatomie und Physiologie, Physiologische Abtheilung, 2*, 312–319.

Himelfarb, M. Z., Shanon, E., Popelka, G. R., & Margolis, R. H. (1978). Acoustic reflex evaluation in neonates. (pp. 109–123). In S. E. Gerber & G. T. Mencher (Eds.), *Early Diagnosis of Hearing Loss*. New York: Grune & Stratton.

Hirsch, A., & Anderson, H. (1980a). Elevated stapedius reflex threshold and pathologic reflex decay. *Acta Otolaryngologica, Supplement, 368*, 1–28.

Hirsch, A., & Anderson, H. (1980b). Audiologic test results in 96 patients with tumours affecting the eighth nerve. *Acta Otolaryngologica, 369*, 1–26.

Holst, H. E., Ingelstedt, S., & Örtegren, U. (1963). Ear drum movements following stimulation of the middle ear muscles. *Acta Otolaryngologica, 182*, 140–145.

Hung, I., & Dallos, P. (1972). Study of the acoustic reflex in human beings: I. Dynamic characteristics. *Journal of the Acoustical Society of America, 52*, 1168–1180.

International Standards Organization. (1964). *Standard Reference Zero for the Calibration of Pure-Tone Audiometers* (ISO Recommendation R 389). New York: Author.

Jenkins, H. A., Morgan, D. E., & Miller, R. H. (1980). Intact acoustic reflexes in the presence of ossicular disruption. *The Laryngoscope, 90*, 267–273.

Jepsen, O. (1951). The threshold of the reflexes of the intratympanic muscles in a normal material examined by means of the impedance method. *Acta Otolaryngologica, 39*, 406–408.

Jepsen, O. (1953). Intratympanic muscle reflexes in psychogenic deafness. *Acta Otolaryngologica, 109*, 61–69.

Jepsen, O. (1955). *Studies on the Acoustic Stapedius Reflex in Man. Measurements of the Acoustic Impedance of the Tympanic Membrane in Normal Individuals and in Patients with Peripheral Facial Palsy.* Unpublished doctoral thesis. University of Aarhus, Denmark.

Jepsen, O. (1963). Middle-ear muscle reflexes in man. In J. Jerger (Ed.), *Modern Developments in Audiology* (pp. 193–237). New York: Academic Press.

Jerger, J., Anthony, L., Jerger, S., & Mauldin, L. (1974). Studies in impedance audiometry III. Middle ear disorders. *Archives of Otolaryngology, 99*, 165–171.

Jerger, J., Burney, P., Mauldin, L., & Crump, B. (1974). Predicting hearing loss from the acoustic reflex. *Journal of Speech and Hearing Disorders, 39*, 11–22.

Jerger, J., Clemis, J., Harford, E., & Alford, B. (1974). The acoustic reflex in eighth nerve disorders. *Archives of Otolaryngology, 99*, 409–413.

Jerger, J., & Hayes, D. (1983). Latency of the acoustic reflex in eighth-nerve tumor. *Archives of Otolaryngology, 109*, 1–5.

Jerger, J., Hayes, D., Anthony, L., & Mauldin, L. (1978). Factors influencing prediction of hearing level from the acoustic reflex. *Monographs in Contemporary Audiology, 1*, 1–20.

Jerger, J., Jerger, S., & Mauldin, L. (1972). Studies in impedance audiometry: I. Normal and sensorineural ears. *Archives of Otolaryngology, 89*, 513–523.

Jerger, J., Mauldin, L., & Lewis, N. (1977). Temporal summation of the acoustic reflex. *Audiology, 16*, 177–200.

Jerger, J., Oliver, T. A., & Jenkins, H. (1987). Suprathreshold abnormalities of the stapedius reflex in acoustic tumor: A series of case reports. *Ear and Hearing, 8*, 131–139.

Jerger, J., Oliver, T. A., Rivera, V., & Stach, B. A. (1986a). Abnormalities of the acoustic reflex in multiple sclerosis. *American Journal of Otolaryngology, 7*, 163–176.

Jerger, J., Oliver, T. A., & Stach, B. (1986b). Problems in the clinical measurement of acoustic reflex latency. *Scandinavian Audiology, 15*, 31–40.

Jerger, S., & Jerger, J. (1977). Diagnostic value of crossed vs. uncrossed acoustic reflexes. *Archives of Otolaryngology, 103*, 445–453.

Jerger, S., & Jerger, J. (1981). *Auditory Disorders, A Manual for Clinical Evaluation*. Boston: Little, Brown & Company.

Johansson, B., Kylin, B., & Langfy, M. (1967). Acoustic reflex as a test of individual susceptibility to noise. *Acta Otolaryngologica, 64*, 256–262.

Joseph, M. P., Guinan, J. J., Jr., Fullerton, B. C., Norris, B. E., & Kiang, N. Y. S. (1985). Number and distribution of stapedius motoneurons in cats. *Journal of Comparative Neurology, 232*, 43–54.

Kankkunen, A., & Lidén, G. (1984). Ipsilateral acoustic reflex thresholds in neonates and in normal-hearing and hearing impaired pre-school children. *Scandinavian Audiology, 13*, 139–144.

Kaplan, H., Gilman, S., & Dirks, D. D. (1977). Properties of acoustic reflex adaptation. *Annals of Otology, Rhinology, and Laryngology, 86*, 348–356.

Kato, T. (1913). Zur physiologie der binnenmuskeln des ohres. *Pflüegers Archiv fuer die Gesamte Physiologie des Menschen und der Tiere, 150*, 569–625.

Keith, R. W. (1975). Middle ear function in neonates. *Archives of Otolaryngology, 101*, 376–379.

Keith, R. W., & Bench, R. J. (1978). Stapedial reflex in neonates. *Scandinavian Audiology, 7*, 187–191.

Kobler, J. B., Vacher, S. R., & Guinan, J. J., Jr. (1985). Acoustic response properties of motoneurons innervating the stapedius muscle of the cat. *Society of Neurosciences Abstracts, 11*, 288.

Kobler, J. B., Vacher, S. R., & Guinan, J. J., Jr. (1987). The recruitment order of stapedius motoneurons in the acoustic reflex varies with sound laterality. *Brain Research, 425*, 372–375.

Kobrak, H. G. (1948). Present status of objective hearing tests. *Annals of Otology, Rhinology and Laryngology, 57*, 1018–1026.

Kristensen, H. K., & Jepsen, O. (1952). Recruitment in otoneurological diagnostics. *Acta Otolaryngologica, 42*, 553–560.

Kunov, H. (1977). The "eardrum artifact" in ipsilateral reflex measurements. *Scandinavian Audiology, 6*, 163–166.

Lilly, D. J. (1964). *Some Properties of the Acoustic Reflex in Man*. Paper presented at the 68th meeting of the Acoustical Society of America, Austin, Texas [*Journal of the Acoustical Society of America, 36*, 2007].

Lilly, D. J. (1984). Evaluation of the response time of acoustic-immittance instruments. In S. Silman (Ed.), *The Acoustic Reflex: Basic Principles and Clinical Applications* (pp. 276–301). Orlando, FL: Academic Press.

Lilly, D. J., Mekaru, M., & Chudnow, S. (1983). Personal communication.

Lindsay, J. R., Kobrak, H., & Perlman, H. B. (1936). Relation of the stapedius reflex to hearing sensation in man. *Archives of Otolaryngology, 23*, 671–687.

Lorente de Nó, R. (1935). The function of the central acoustic nuclei examined by means of the acoustic reflexes. *The Laryngoscope, 45*, 573–595.

Lüscher, E. (1929). Die funktion des musculus stapedius beim menschen. *Z. Hals-Nasen-Ohrenheilkunde, 23*, 105–132.

Lutman, M., & Leis, B. R. (1980). Ipsilateral acoustic reflex artefacts measured in cadavers. *Scandinavian Audiology, 9*, 33–39.

Lutman, M., & Martin, A. (1977). The acoustic reflex threshold for impulses. *Journal of Sound and Vibration, 51*, 97–109.

Lyon, M. J. (1978). The central location of the motor neurons to the stapedius muscle in the cat. *Brain Research, 143*, 437–444.

Lyon, M. J. (1979). Peripheral innervation of the stapedius muscle in the cat: An electron microscopic study. *Experimental Neurology, 66*, 707–720.

Mangham, C. A., Burnett, P. A., & Lindeman, R. C. (1982). Standardization of acoustic reflex latency. A study in humans and nonhuman primates. *Annals of Otology, Rhinology and Laryngology, 91*, 169–174.

Mangham, C. A., Burnett, P. A., & Lindeman, R. C. (1983). Evaluation of tensor tympani muscle dominance in the biphasic acoustic reflex. *Audiology, 22*, 105–119.

Mangham, C. A., Lindeman, R. C., & Dawson, W. (1980). Stapedius reflex quantification in acoustic tumor patients. *The Laryngoscope, 90*, 242–250.

Mangham, C. A., & Miller, J. M. (1979). A case for further quantification of the stapedius reflex. *Archives of Otolaryngology, 105*, 593–596.

Marchant, C. D., McMillan, P. M., Shurin, P. A., Johnson, C. E., Turczyk, V. A., Feinstein, J. C., & Panek, D. M. (1986). Objective diagnosis of otitis media in early infancy by tympanometry and ipsilateral acoustic reflex thresholds. *Journal of Pediatrics, 109*, 590–595.

Margolis, R. H. (1993). Detection of hearing impairment with the acoustic stapedius reflex. *Ear and Hearing, 14*, 3–10.

Margolis, R. H., Dubno, J. R., & Wilson, R. H. (1980). Acoustic reflex thresholds for noise stimuli. *Journal of the Acoustical Society of America, 68*, 892–895.

Margolis, R. H., & Fox, C. M. (1977). A comparison of three methods for predicting hearing loss from acoustic reflex threshold. *Journal of Speech and Hearing Research, 20*, 241–253.

Margolis, R. H., Fox, C., Lilly, D. J., Popelka, G., Silman, S., & Trumpf, A. (1981). The bivariate plotting procedure for hearing assessment with acoustic-reflex threshold measures. In G. R. Popelka (Ed.), *Hearing Assessment with the Acoustic Reflex* (pp. 59–84). New York: Grune & Stratton.

Margolis, R. H., & Gilman, S. (1977). Methods for measuring the temporal characteristics and filter response of electroacoustic impedance instruments. *Journal of Speech and Hearing Research, 20*, 409–414.

McCandless, G. A., & Allred, P. L. (1978). Tympanometry and emergence of the acoustic reflex in infants. In E. R. Harford, F. H. Bess, C. D. Bluestone, et al. (Eds.), *Impedance Screening for Middle Ear Disease in Children* (pp. 57–67). New York: Grune & Stratton.

McCue, M. P., & Guinan, J. J. Jr. (1983). Functional segregation within the stapedius motoneuron pool. *Society of Neuroscience Abstracts, 19*, 1085.

McCue, M. P., & Guinan, J. J. Jr. (1988). Anatomical and functional segregation in the stapedius motoneuron pool of the cat. *Journal of Neurophysiology, 60*, 1160–1180.

McMillan, P. M., Marchant, C. D., & Shurin, P. A. (1985). Ipsilateral acoustic reflexes in infants. *Annals of Otology, Rhinology and Laryngology, 94*, 145–148.

McPherson, D. L., & Thompson, D. (1977). Quantification of the threshold and latency parameters of acoustic reflex in humans. *Acta Otolaryngologica, 353*, 1–37.

Metz, O. (1946). The acoustic impedance measured on normal and pathological ears. *Acta Otolaryngologica, 63*, 1–254.

Metz, O. (1951). Studies on the contraction of the tympanic muscles as indicated by changes in the impedance of the ear. *Acta Otolaryngologica, 39*, 397–405.

Metz, O. (1952). Threshold of reflex contractions of muscles of the middle ear and recruitment of loudness. *Archives of Otolaryngology, 55*, 536–543.

Møller, A. R. (1958). Intra-aural muscles contraction in man, examined by measuring acoustic impedance of the ear. *The Laryngoscope, 68*, 48–62.

Møller, A. R. (1961). Bilateral contraction of the tympanic muscles in man. *Annals of Otology, Rhinology and Laryngology, 70*, 735–752.

Møller, A. R. (1962a). Acoustic reflex in man. *Journal of the Acoustical Society of America, 34*, 1524–1534.

Møller, A. R. (1962b). The sensitivity of contraction of the tympanic muscles in man. *Annals of Otology, Rhinology and Laryngology, 71*, 86–95.

Møller, A. R. (1978). A comment on H. Kunov: The "eardrum artifact" in ipsilateral reflex measurements. *Scandinavian Audiology, 7*, 61–64.

Niemeyer, W., & Sesterhenn, G. (1974). Calculating the hearing threshold from the stapedius reflex thresholds for different sound stimuli. *Audiology, 13*, 421–427.

Olsen, W. O., Noffsinger, D., & Kurdziel, S. (1975). Acoustic reflex and reflex decay. *Archives of Otolaryngology, 101*, 622–625.

Olsen, W., Stach, B., & Kurdziel, S. (1981). Acoustic reflex decay in 10 seconds and in 5 seconds for Ménière's disease patients and for VIIIth nerve tumor patients. *Ear and Hearing, 2*, 180–181.

Osterhammel, D., & Osterhammel, P. (1979). Age and sex variations for the normal stapedial reflex thresholds and tympanometric compliance values. *Scandinavian Audiology, 8*, 153–158.

Overholt, S. M., & Jerger, J. (1995). Comparison of crossed and uncrossed acoustic reflex latencies. *Ear and Hearing, 16*, 295–298.

Perlman, H. B., & Case, T. J. (1939). Latent period of the crossed stapedius reflex in man. *Annals of Otology, Rhinology and Laryngology, 48*, 663–675.

Peterson, J. L., & Lidén, G. (1972). Some static characteristics of the stapedial muscle reflex. *Audiology, 11*, 97–114.

Popelka, G. R. (1981). The acoustic reflex in normal and pathologic ears. In G. R. Popelka (Ed.), *Hearing Assessment with the Acoustic Reflex* (pp. 5–21). New York: Grune & Stratton.

Popelka, G. R., & Dubno, J. R. (1978). Comments on the acoustic-reflex response for bone-conducted signals. *Acta Otolaryngologica, 86*, 64–70.

Popelka, G. R., Karlovich, R., & Wiley, T. L. (1974). Acoustic reflex and critical bandwidth. *Journal of the Acoustical Society of America, 55*, 883–885.

Popelka, G. R., Margolis, R. H., & Wiley, T. L. (1976). Effect of activating signal bandwidth on acoustic-reflex thresholds. *Journal of the Acoustical Society of America, 59*, 153–159.

Porter, T. A. (1972). Normative otoadmittance values for three populations. *Journal of Auditory Research, 12*, 53–58.

Potter, A. B. (1936). Function of the stapedius muscle. *Annals of Otology, Rhinology and Laryngology, 45*, 639–643.

Rabinowitz, W. M. (1977). *Acoustic-Reflex Effects on the Input Admittance and Transfer Characteristics of the Human Middle-Ear.* Unpublished doctoral dissertation, Massachusetts Institute of Technology, Cambridge.

Rosenhall, U., Lidén, G., & Nilsson, E. (1979). Stapedius reflex decay in normal hearing subjects. *Journal of the American Auditory Society, 4*, 157–163.

Ruth, R. A., Nilo, E. R., & Mravec, J. J. (1978). Consideration of acoustic reflex magnitude (ARM) in cases of idiopathic facial paralysis. *Archives of Otolaryngology, 86*, 215–220.

Ruth, R. A., & Niswander, P. S. (1976). Acoustic reflex latency as a function of frequency and intensity of eliciting stimulus. *Journal American Audiology Society, 2*, 54–60.

Salomon, G., & Starr, A. (1963). Electromyography of middle ear muscles in man during motor activities. *Acta Neurologica Scandinavica, 39*, 161–168.

Schwartz, D. M., & Sanders, J. W. (1976). Critical bandwidth and sensitivity prediction in the acoustic stapedial reflex. *Journal of Speech and Hearing Disorders, 41*, 244–255.

Shanks, J. E., Wilson, R. H., & Jones, H. C. (1985). Earphone-coupling technique for measuring the temporal characteristics of aural acoustic-immittance devices. *Journal of Speech and Hearing Research, 28*, 305–308.

Shapiro, I., Canalis, R. F., Firemark, R., & Bahna, M. (1981). Ossicular discontinuity with intact acoustic reflex. *Archives of Otolaryngology, 107*, 576–578.

Shaw, M. D., & Baker, R. (1983). The locations of stapedius and tensor tympani motoneurons in the cat. *Journal of Comparative Neurology, 216*, 10–19.

Silman, S. (1979). The effects of aging on the stapedius reflex thresholds. *Journal of the Acoustical Society of America, 66*, 735–738.

Silman, S. (1984). Magnitude and growth of the acoustic reflex. In S. Silman (Ed.), *The Acoustic Reflex: Basic Principles and Clinical Applications* (pp. 301–328). Orlando, FL: Academic Press.

Silman, S., & Gelfand, S. A. (1981). Effect of sensorineural hearing loss on the stapedius reflex growth function in the elderly. *Journal of the Acoustical Society of America, 69*, 1099–1106.

Silman, S., Gelfand, S. A., & Chun, T. (1978). Some observations in a case of acoustic neuroma. *Journal of Speech and Hearing Disorders, 43*, 459–466.

Silverman, C. A., Silman, S., & Miller, M. H. (1983). The acoustic reflex threshold in aging ears. *Journal of the Acoustical Society of America, 73*, 248–255.

Sprague, B. H., Wiley, T. L., & Block, M. G. (1981). Dynamics of acoustic reflex growth. *Audiology, 20*, 15–40.

Sprague, B. H., Wiley, T. L., & Goldstein, R. (1985). Tympanometric and acoustic-reflex studies in neonates. *Journal of Speech and Hearing Research, 28*, 265–272.

Stach, B., & Jerger, J. (1984). Acoustic reflex averaging. *Ear and Hearing, 5,* 289–296.

Stach, B. A., Jerger, J. F., & Jenkins, H. A. (1984). The human acoustic tensor tympani reflex. *Scandinavian Audiology, 13,* 93–99.

Stream, R. W., Stream, K. S., Walker, J. R., & Breningstall, G. (1978). Emerging characteristics of the acoustic reflex in infants. *Otolaryngology, 86,* 628–636.

Terkildsen, K. (1957). Movements of the eardrum following inter-aural muscle reflexes. *Archives of Otolaryngology, 66,* 484–488.

Terkildsen, K. (1960). The intra-aural muscle reflexes in normal persons and in workers exposed to intense industrial noise. *Acta Otolaryngologica, 52,* 384–396.

Terkildsen, K. (1964). Clinical application of impedance measurements with a fixed frequency technique. *International Audiology, 3,* 147–155.

Terkildsen, K., Osterhammel, P., & Bretlau, P. (1973). Acoustic middle ear muscle reflexes in patients with otosclerosis. *Archives of Otolaryngology, 98,* 152–155.

Terkildsen, K., & Scott-Nielsen, S. (1960). An electroacoustic impedance measuring bridge for clinical use. *Archives of Otolaryngology, 73,* 339–346.

Thelin, J. W. (1980). *Acoustic Reflex Summation in the Frequency Domain.* Unpublished doctoral dissertation, University of Iowa, Iowa City.

Thompson, D. J., Sills, J. A., Recke, K. S., & Bui, D. M. (1980). Acoustic reflex growth in the aging adult. *Journal of Speech and Hearing Research, 23,* 405–418.

Tietze, G. (1969). Zum zeitverhalten des akustischen reflexes bei reizung mit dauertönen. *Archiv fuer Klinische und Experimentelle Ohren-, Nasen-, und Kehlkopfheilkunde, 193,* 43–52.

Tonndorf, J., & Khanna, S. (1968). Submicroscopic displacement amplitudes of the tympanic membrane (cat) measured by a laser interferometer. *Journal of the Acoustical Society of America, 44,* 1546–1554.

Van Camp, K. J., Vanpeperstraete, P. M., Creten, W. L., & Vanhuyse, V. J. (1975). On irregular acoustic reflex patterns. *Scandinavian Audiology, 4,* 227–232.

Vincent, V. L., & Gerber, S. E. (1987). Early development of the acoustic reflex. *Audiology, 26,* 356–362.

Weatherby, L. A., & Bennett, M. J. (1980). The neonatal acoustic reflex. *Scandinavian Audiology, 9,* 103–110.

Wersäll, R. (1958). The tympanic muscles and their reflexes. *Acta Otolaryngologica, 139,* 1–112.

Wiley, T. L., & Block, M. G. (1984). Acoustic and nonacoustic reflex patterns in audiologic diagnosis. In S. Silman (Ed.), *The Acoustic Reflex: Basic Principles and Clinical Applications* (pp. 387–411). Orlando, FL: Academic Press.

Wiley, T. L., & Karlovich, R. S. (1975). Acoustic reflex response to sustained signals. *Journal of Speech and Hearing Research, 18,* 148–157.

Wilson, R. H. (1979). Factors influencing the acoustic-immittance characteristics of the acoustic reflex. *Journal of Speech and Hearing Research, 22,* 480–499.

Wilson, R. H. (1981). The effects of aging on the magnitude of the acoustic reflex. *Journal of Speech and Hearing Research, 24,* 406–414.

Wilson, R. H., & McBride, L. M. (1978). Threshold and growth of the acoustic reflex. *Journal of the Acoustical Society of America, 63,* 147–154.

Wilson, R. H., McCullough, J. K., & Lilly, D. J. (1984). Acoustic-reflex adaptation: Variability in subjects with normal hearing. *Journal of Speech and Hearing Research, 27,* 586–595.

Wilson, R. H., Morgan, D. E., & Dirks, D. D. (1972). *Relationships between the Acoustic Reflex and the Loudness Discomfort Level.* Paper presented at the meeting of the 11th International Congress of Audiology, Budapest, Hungary.

Wilson, R. H., Shanks, J. E., & Lilly, D. J. (1984). Acoustic-reflex adaptation. In S. Silman (Ed.), *The Acoustic Reflex: Basic Principles and Clinical Applications* (pp. 329–387). Orlando, FL: Academic Press.

Wilson, R. H., Shanks, J. E., & Velde, T. M. (1981). Aural acoustic-immittance measurements: Inter-aural differences. *Journal of Speech and Hearing Research, 46,* 413–421.

Wilson, R. H., Steckler, J. F., Jones, H. C., & Margolis, R. H. (1978). Adaptation of the acoustic reflex. *Journal of the Acoustical Society of America, 64,* 782–791.

Zakrisson, J-E., & Borg, E. (1974). Stapedius reflex and auditory fatigue. *Audiology, 13,* 231–235.

Zakrisson, J-E., Borg, E., & Blom, S. (1974). The acoustic impedance change as a measure of stapedius muscle activity in man. *Acta Otolaryngologica, 78,* 357–364.

Zwislocki, J. J. (1965). Analysis of some auditory characteristics. In R. D. Luce, R. B. Bush, & E. Galenter (Eds.), *Handbook of Mathematical Psychology, Vol. III* (pp. 1–97). New York: Wiley.

CHAPTER 6

OTOACOUSTIC EMISSIONS IN CLINICAL PRACTICE

BRENDA L. LONSBURY-MARTIN
GLEN K. MARTIN
FRED F. TELISCHI

Otoacoustic emissions (OAEs) offer the clinician a number of benefits as objective measures of the peripheral ear's ability to process sound. Over the past decade, a great many studies have demonstrated that evoked OAEs are useful in the differential diagnosis of sensorineural hearing loss, in the screening of cochlear function in infants and other difficult-to-test patients, and in the monitoring of outer hair cell (OHC) healthiness in patients either exposed to ototoxic drugs or suffering from certain progressive hearing ailments. The following discussion on the clinical applications of OAEs is divided into two main sections. The first part reviews our current knowledge about the biological basis of OAEs, which, in turn, is followed by a summary of the various types of OAEs and the methods used to measure them. The second section focuses on the primary features of evoked OAEs that make them a useful audiological test and summarizes the current applications of OAE testing in a number of distinct clinical settings. A number of examples exist in the literature of the various types of OAEs along with case-study illustrations of the adverse effects that many of the etiologies that cause hearing loss have on OAEs. Thus, to avoid overrepetition of familiar depictions in the present discussion, the reader will be referred to these well-known examples when appropriate.

BACKGROUND

Biological Basis of Otoacoustic Emissions

Sound stimuli result in vibration of the cochlear partition. Previously, it was thought that these movements were produced only by the energy in the acoustic stimulus, and that the sensory hair cells of the cochlea passively transduced the sound-induced vibrations into neural impulses. However, three major discoveries during the past twenty years brought a definite end to this view of "passive" cochlear function.

Acknowledgment: This work was supported by grants from the Public Health Service (DC00613, DC/ES03114).

The first notable discovery was that the normal cochleas of humans and other animals produce audio-frequency sounds, called *otoacoustic emissions* (OAEs), both spontaneously and in response to acoustic stimuli (Kemp, 1978, 1979). Otoacoustic emissions are diminished or abolished by manipulations that reduce or eliminate the metabolic energy supply to the cochlea. The existence of *spontaneous OAEs* (SOAEs), that is, sound energy produced by the ear in the absence of any deliberate sound input, also suggests that metabolic energy can be converted into sound energy within the cochlea. Thus, these observations provide evidence that the cochlea can use metabolic energy to influence the mechanical response of the organ of Corti to sound.

The second important breakthrough came from direct *in vivo* measurements of basilar-membrane motion in animal models. These studies showed that, in healthy ears—that is, ears with normal thresholds of sound-evoked auditory-nerve activity—there are two distinct components to sound-evoked basilar-membrane motion. One component behaves approximately as predicted by the passive models of cochlear mechanics, that is, by representations that assume that only the energy in the acoustic stimulus causes vibration of the cochlear partition. However, the other component of basilar-membrane vibration, which is elicited by sound stimuli at low and moderate stimulus levels, is largely restricted to a narrow region of the basilar membrane around the characteristic place for each stimulus frequency. This component is greatly reduced or abolished by manipulations that diminish or eliminate the metabolic energy supply to the cochlea. This result again indicates that a process involving metabolic energy influences the mechanical response of the cochlea to sound. Specifically, it appears that some cellular component(s) of the organ of Corti must convert metabolic energy into vibratory energy in such a way as to enhance the sound-induced motion of the basilar membrane, at low and moderate sound levels, around the characteristic place for each stimulus frequency.

The process responsible for the enhancement of basilar-membrane motion has been referred to as the "cochlear amplifier" (Davis, 1983). The properties of the metabolically dependent component of basilar-membrane motion suggest that the action of the cochlear amplifier involves a cycle-by-cycle—that is, audio-frequency—application of force to the cochlear partition. This conclusion is consistent with the existence of OAEs at audio frequencies.

The third major discovery was that OHCs isolated from the mammalian cochlea demonstrate electromotility—they change shape in response to electrical stimuli, on a cycle-by-cycle basis at audio frequencies (Brownell, Bader, Bertrand, & Ribaupierre, 1985). In the isolated OHC, changes in the voltage drop across the cell membrane cause the cell to change its shape. *In vivo* sound stimulation results in voltage changes across the OHC membrane, that is, generation of the hair-cell receptor potential, suggesting that OHCs produce a mechanical force on a cycle-by-cycle basis in response to sound stimuli *in vivo*. The audio-frequency electromotility of the OHCs is unique in nature. Thus, it appears probable that the *in vivo* cochlear process that produces the audio-frequency vibrations observed in the form of OAEs, and of enhancement of sound-evoked basilar-membrane motion, is based in OHC electromotility (Brownell, 1990; Brownell & Lue, 1996).

The result of these three breakthroughs is the present understanding that the normal cochlea actively processes sound, that is, anatomical structures within the cochlea utilize metabolic energy to enhance the sound-induced vibration of the basilar membrane and organ of Corti. The current consensus about the peripheral processing of sound is that the action of this active cochlear process results in the enhanced sensitivity and sharp frequency tuning of basilar-membrane vibration (Davis, 1983; Johnstone, Patuzzi, & Yates, 1986; Ruggero & Rich, 1991).

In this view of cochlear function, OHCs act primarily as motor elements, rather than sensory elements. A motor role for OHCs is consistent with the observation that, whereas there are approximately three times as many OHCs as inner hair cells (IHCs), OHCs have little afferent innervation, but a substantial efferent innervation (Spoendlin, 1988). Moreover, direct electrical stimulation of the efferent-nerve supply to the OHCs reduces sound-evoked basilar-membrane motion (LePage, 1989) and alters OAEs (Mountain, 1980; Siegel & Kim, 1982). It is the IHCs, which receive the great majority of the afferent innervation of the cochlea and transduce cochlear-partition vibrations to excite the auditory nerve endings, that represent the final output of the ear.

To summarize, the cochlear amplifier is a process that uses metabolic energy to enhance the passive sound-induced vibration of the cochlear partition at low and moderate levels, around the characteristic place for each stimulus frequency. The action of the cochlear amplifier is such that, at low and moderate stimulus levels, it enhances the amplitude and frequency selectivity of sound-induced vibration, at the input to the IHCs, around the characteristic place

along the basilar membrane for each stimulus frequency. Finally, the IHCs are thought to passively transduce their input to neural activity. Thus, it is the action of the cochlear amplifier that is responsible for the exceptional normal hearing sensitivity, frequency selectivity, and dynamic range of the cochlea.

The anatomical structures involved in the actions of the cochlear amplifier are not definitively known. However, it seems certain that the cochlear amplifier is based in the OHCs, that it presumably involves the electromotility of the OHCs, and that the source of metabolic energy utilized by the cochlear amplifier is, primarily, the endolymphatic potential (Ruggero & Rich, 1991), which is generated by the stria vascularis. It is also certain that other anatomical structures within the organ of Corti are necessary, perhaps in a more passive supporting role. Thus, the coupling of forces generated by the OHCs to the basilar membrane, and to IHC stereocilia, must be influenced by the mechanical properties of those structures immediately surrounding the OHCs, that is, the pillar cells and Dieters cells. Alteration of the physical properties of these cells likely alters the way in which force generated by the OHCs produces vibrations within the cochlear partition.

Hearing Loss and Otoacoustic Emissions

Within the framework of this view of cochlear function, some forms of sensorineural hearing loss result from a reduction of the action of the cochlear amplifier, which appears particularly vulnerable to physical and physiological traumas (Johnstone et al., 1986). When the cochlear amplifier is impaired, vibration of the cochlear partition at low and moderate sound levels is reduced. Consequently, a higher-level stimulus is required to reach the threshold of excitation of the IHCs and afferent neurons, that is, an elevation in hearing threshold occurs. Because the cochlear amplifier enhances cochlear-partition vibration only at low and moderate sound levels, threshold elevations resulting solely from reduced action of the cochlear amplifier are limited, but substantial. The maximum threshold elevation associated with complete loss of cochlear amplifier function is estimated to range from 30 to 55 dB SPL, depending on a number of factors (Harris & Probst, 1997).

The outcomes of a number of experimental studies of the cochlea have given rise to an assumption on which the interpretation of clinical OAE test results can be based. According to this notion, the cochlear amplifier acts to enhance the sound-induced motion of the cochlear partition at low stimulus levels. Diminished enhancement of cochlear-partition vibration, due to dysfunction of the cochlear amplifier, results in reduced stimulation of the IHCs and, thus, of the auditory afferent nerve fibers, resulting in a sensory hearing loss. Whereas the enhancement of basilar-membrane motion is thought to be carried out by the OHCs, and presumably involves the OHC electromotility demonstrated *in vitro*, the normal operation of this mechanism *in vivo* also appears to require the normal function of the stria vascularis, and, presumably, the structural integrity of other elements of the organ of Corti. Otoacoustic emissions appear to be produced by the cochlear amplifier, presumably as a by-product of the action of the mechanism that acts to enhance cochlear-partition vibration. Thus, reduced operation of the cochlear amplifier is reflected as both elevated hearing thresholds, and reduced OAE amplitudes. For this reason, OAEs can be used as an indicator of certain hearing losses.

This conceptualization of the relationship between emissions, cochlear function, and hearing threshold has the following implications for the clinical utility of OAEs: (1) Reduced OAEs are an indication of a specific sensory component of sensorineural hearing loss, that is, dysfunction of the cochlear amplifier, which is distinct from conductive, neural, or retrocochlear hearing losses, and from other possible sensory losses. It appears, however, that a considerable portion of the sensorineural hearing loss observed in the clinic is attributable to dysfunction of the cochlear amplifier; (2) because normal function of the cochlear amplifier appears to involve, or to depend on, several structures within the cochlea, including the OHCs and the stria vascularis, a reduction of OAEs could reflect trauma to any of these structures; and (3) dysfunction of elements within the cochlea that are not required for the normal operation of the cochlear amplifier, for example, the IHCs, may cause sensory hearing loss without reduced OAE levels. It is important to emphasize that many hearing losses involve dysfunction of both the cochlear amplifier, and other elements within the cochlea.

To summarize, OAEs are thought to be produced as a by-product of the action of the cochlear amplifier, that is, by the metabolically vulnerable cochlear process responsible for enhancing cochlear-partition vibration at low and moderate sound levels. Thus, within the present understanding of cochlear function, the clinical utility of OAEs is based on the fact that they can provide information concerning the status of the cochlear amplifier. Because dysfunction of the cochlear amplifier represents a specific type of sensory-based hearing loss, OAEs provide information concerning the presence or absence of this type of hearing loss, and do not provide information about hearing losses of other origin.

Types and Measurement of Otoacoustic Emissions

There are two general types of OAEs, the SOAEs described above and the evoked OAEs (transient-evoked, stimulus-frequency, and distortion-product OAEs). A number of examples of all the OAE forms are available in the literature (e.g., Lonsbury-Martin, Martin, & Balkany, 1994;

Martin, Probst, & Lonsbury-Martin, 1990; Probst, Lonsbury-Martin, & Martin, 1991; Whitehead, Lonsbury-Martin, Martin, & McCoy, 1996).

Typically, OAEs are measured using a system that is configured around a personal microcomputer (Whitehead, Stagner, Lonsbury-Martin, & Martin, 1994) like the one schematized in Figure 6.1. In this arrangement, the commercially available probe (e.g., Etymotic Research, ER-10B[+]) containing a sensitive miniature microphone is sealed securely into the outer ear canal with a soft-rubber eartip. The microphone output is directed via a preamplifier/amplifier (microphone amplifier) and analog-to-digital (A/D) converter to a digital-signal processor (DSP) mounted in the microcomputer. This hardware is all that is needed to detect SOAEs (Probst et al., 1991).

To allow measurement of the evoked OAEs, one or two loudspeakers can be used to deliver sound to the ear canal via tubes passing through the probe. Voltage commands for each speaker are generated by the DSP, and passed to each speaker via separate digital-to-analog (D/A) circuits, amplifiers, and impedance-matching devices (speaker drivers). To elicit transient-evoked (TEOAEs) or stimulus-frequency OAEs (SFOAEs), only one speaker is required to generate either brief acoustic stimuli, or continuous pure tones, respectively. For distortion-product OAEs (DPOAEs), two pure tones (f_1 and f_2) are presented, one over each speaker, in order to prevent artifactual distortion products from being produced by a single transducer being driven electrically by two sinusoids. Analysis of the microphone output typically involves spectral averaging (averaging of amplitude spectra obtained by fast-Fourier transformation [FFT] of samples of the microphone output) to detect SOAEs, conventional stimulus-locked averaging to detect TEOAEs, and conventional stimulus-locked averaging followed by FFT processing to reveal DPOAEs.

It is noteworthy that virtually all the commercially available instruments devised to measure OAEs are designed as described above (Decker, 1997). However, each device has its own particular selection of hardware/software components, with some instruments being equipped with both adult and neonatal acoustic probes. Additionally, although a few devices record only one type of evoked OAE (i.e., either the TEOAE or DPOAE), other instruments permit several types of OAEs to be measured (TEOAEs and DPOAEs, TEOAEs and SOAEs, DPOAEs and SOAEs). Indeed, several devices aimed at the newborn-hearing screening application permit the recording of one of the evoked OAEs (TEOAEs or DPOAEs) along with the auditory brainstem response (ABR).

Spontaneous Otoacoustic Emissions (SOAEs)

Spontaneous OAEs are tonal signals that are naturally emitted by the cochlea in the absence of deliberate acoustic

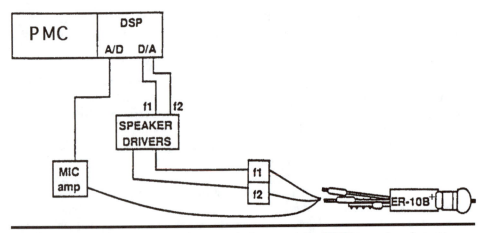

FIGURE 6.1 Schematic of a typical personal microcomputer (PMC) based equipment setup permitting measurement of any of the four types of OAEs. The commercially available probe (Etymotic Research, ER-10B+) contains a sensitive miniature microphone sealed into the ear canal with a rubber eartip. The microphone output is led via a preamplifier and amplifier (MIC amp) and analog-to-digital (A/D) converter to a digital-signal processor (DSP) on board the computer. This is all the hardware that is needed to detect SOAEs. To allow measurement of evoked OAEs, two loudspeakers (f_1, f_2) can be used to deliver stimuli to the ear canal via sound tubes passing through the probe. Voltage commands for each speaker are generated by the DSP and passed via separate digital-to-analog (D/A) circuits, amplifiers, and impedance-matching devices (SPEAKER DRIVERS) to each loudspeaker. To evoke TEOAEs by click or tonepip stimuli, or SFOAEs with a swept pure-tone stimulus, only one speaker is required. For eliciting DPOAEs, two pure tones are presented, one over each speaker to prevent generation of artifactual distortion products by a single speaker driven by two sinusoids. Analysis of the microphone output typically involves spectral averaging (i.e., averaging of spectra obtained by FFT processing of samples of the microphone output to detect SOAEs, conventional stimulus-locked averaging to detect TEOAEs, and conventional stimulus-locked averaging followed by FFT processing to reveal DPOAEs).

stimulation (Kemp, 1979). The SOAEs, which are detected at one or more discrete frequencies in approximately 70% of normal human ears (Penner, Glotzbach, & Huang, 1993; Talmadge, Long, Murphy, & Tubis, 1993), are more prevalent in females than males. Further, although the most common frequency range of SOAEs is between 1 and 3 kHz (Lonsbury-Martin, Harris, Stagner, Hawkins, & Martin, 1990b; Whitehead, Kamal, Lonsbury-Martin, & Martin, 1993; Wier, Norton, & Kincaid, 1984; Zurek, 1981), their precise frequencies, which typically vary by only a few Hertz, even over several years, are unique to each spontaneously emitting ear. For all these reasons, SOAEs have not been developed into a useful clinical test. However, several aspects of SOAEs impact the measurement of OAEs.

First, they influence the fine structure of the evoked OAEs. For example, that the frequencies of SOAEs are associated with the sharp peak frequencies sometimes exhibited by the TEOAE spectrum (Probst, Coats, Martin, & Lonsbury-Martin, 1986) helps to clarify peculiarities observed between the frequency/level patterns of different subjects. Second, SOAEs enhance the levels of the evoked OAEs so that they often are at the upper limits of their normal distribution range (Lonsbury-Martin et al., 1990b; Osterhammel, Rasmussen, Olsen, & Nielsen, 1996). Such knowledge helps explain the presence of uncommonly large evoked OAEs. Finally, Penner (1990) has established that tinnitus is SOAE-related in about 4% of patients with this complaint. That is, if the frequency of an SOAE corresponds to the tinnitus frequency, when the SOAE is suppressed by application of an external tone, the tinnitus disappears. Moreover, it appears that treatment with aspirin suppresses both the bothersome SOAE and the tinnitus (Penner, 1989). Thus, in patients who have tinnitus within a frequency range that is associated with reasonably normal hearing, it is beneficial to test for this relationship between the frequencies of an SOAE and tinnitus, in case the annoying perceptual symptom can be treated. Although SOAEs are typically present only in ears associated with normal hearing, it is important to emphasize that these emissions can be detected in ears exhibiting hearing loss, but only within the frequency regions in which relatively normal audiometric hearing remains.

There is a rare subtype of SOAE that differs in several respects from the SOAEs routinely observed in normal human ears (Mathis, Probst, De Min, & Hauser, 1991; Wilson & Sutton, 1983; Yamamoto, Takagi, Hirono, & Yagi, 1987). Specifically, these "atypical" SOAEs are: (1) much larger (up to 60 dB SPL) than normal SOAEs, which usually are ~0 dB SPL; (2) detected in a higher frequency range than the majority of SOAEs, which typically occur between 0.8 and 4 kHz; and (3) often associated with regions of audiometric abnormality. These atypical SOAEs also differ from most typical SOAEs in that they often demonstrate considerable short-term instability of frequency and level, and frequently they have broad multi-lobed, rather than sharp, single-lobed suppression contours (Wilson & Sutton, 1983). In fact, evidence from the experimental literature indicates that these abnormal SOAEs may be a form of objective tinnitus (Zurek & Clark, 1981).

Spontaneous OAEs are thought to be produced by the same process as TEOAEs and SFOAEs, which are described below, apparently as a result of feedback of the output of the TEOAE/SFOAE generator into its input (Kemp, 1981; Wilson & Sutton, 1981). At frequencies where this feedback is positive, self-sustaining oscillation will result, if the loop gain is sufficient, in a similar manner to the feedback "whistle" of hearing aids. This self-sustaining oscillation is observed in the ear canal as an SOAE. Thus, SOAEs can be thought of as continuously self-evoking evoked OAEs. Consistent with this view, as noted above, SOAEs are found especially in frequency regions of strong evoked response, that is, at 1 to 2 kHz, where the gain of the emission generator is presumably high (Kemp, 1981; Wilson, 1980a; Zwicker & Schloth, 1984), and rarely exceed 20 dB SPL, due to the compressive nonlinearity of the OAE generator.

Evoked Otoacoustic Emissions

The second general class of emissions is the evoked OAEs. Essentially, all normal human ears demonstrate evoked OAEs, which are grouped into three forms on the basis of the type of sound stimulus that is used to measure them: (1) TEOAEs are elicited by brief acoustic stimuli such as clicks or tonepips; (2) SFOAEs are evoked by a single, low-level, continuous pure tone; and, (3) DPOAEs are elicited by two simultaneously presented, long-duration pure tones of different, but related, frequencies.

Transient-Evoked Otoacoustic Emissions (TEOAEs). Figure 6.2A shows a click-evoked TEOAE measured from a representative normal adult ear with the commonly used ILO88 system (Otodynamics Ltd) in the standard "nonlinear" clinical mode. Essentially all the ears of normal-hearing humans exhibit TEOAEs (Bonfils, Uziel, & Pujol, 1988; Kemp, 1978; Kemp, Bray, Alexander, & Brown, 1986; Probst et al., 1986; Stevens, 1988). In general, in adult ears, TEOAE levels are greatest around 1 to 2 kHz and decline at both lower and higher frequencies, such that they are typically very small or immeasurable below 0.5 kHz and above 4.5 kHz. Presumably, the decline below 1 kHz is primarily due to middle-ear effects. The decrease at high frequencies may also be partially due to the filtering properties of the middle ear, but it also reflects other factors, including the effects of latency. The latency of the TEOAE, that is, the time between presentation of a tonepip stimulus and detection of the response, varies from <3 to 20 ms in humans, and, on average, decreases with increasing frequency (Kemp, 1978; Wilson, 1980a; Wit & Ritsma, 1980). Thus, at high frequencies that have very short latencies, it is difficult to separate TEOAE energy from the stimulus-induced ringing of the speakers and middle ear. For example, the ILO88 system loses some high-frequency TEOAE energy in windowing out the tail of the stimulus click (that is, the 2.5 ms "blank" time interval at the beginning of the response window) and shaping the onset of the response window. The dependence of latency on frequency is thought to arise, at least partially, from a progressively more apical origin of OAEs within the cochlea as frequency decreases.

Except at the lowest stimulus levels, growth of TEOAE amplitude with stimulus level is compressively nonlinear, that is, TEOAE amplitudes increase by less than 1 dB per dB increase of stimulus level, and they saturate at moderate stimulus levels such that click-evoked TEOAEs rarely exceed 15 to 20 dB SPL in magnitude. This saturation is consistent with the view that TEOAEs are generated by the action of the cochlear amplifier, because the action of the cochlear amplifier is also thought to saturate at moderate stimulus levels.

Within the 0.5 to 4.5 kHz frequency region in which TEOAEs are typically detected in normal adult ears, their levels vary across frequency—TEOAEs are strong, weak, or absent, at different frequencies, which are constant in any one ear in the absence of ear-related pathology, but vary greatly between individual ears. The cause of the unique spectral patterns observed for different ears, particularly in the absence of SOAEs, is obscure, especially because the action of the cochlear amplifier is thought to be quite uniform across the mid-frequency range. This observation suggests that factors in addition to the action of the cochlear amplifier influence the generation or expression of TEOAEs. In terms of the model of cochlear function described above, this observation infers that TEOAE level at any one frequency does not provide a perfect indication of the action of the cochlear amplifier.

Figure 6.2B shows a TEOAE from an infant obtained with the same equipment as that used to elicit the adult

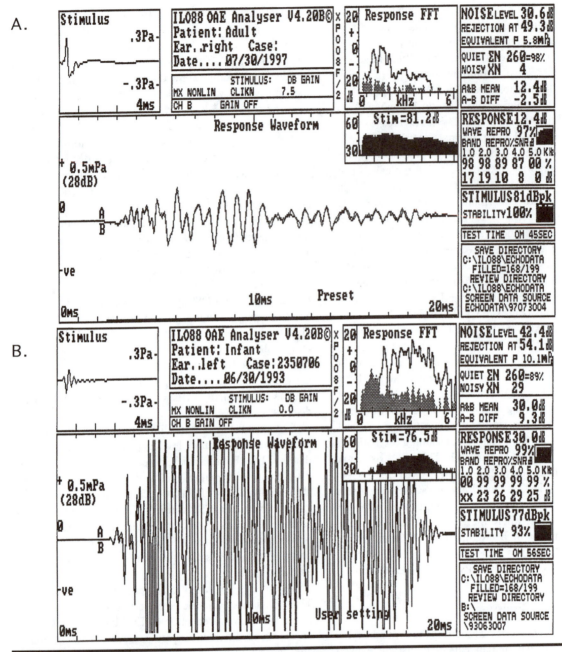

FIGURE 6.2 Measurement of TEOAEs. The large panels in the **A** and **B** portions of the figure labeled "Response Waveform" show the temporal waveform of a click-evoked TEOAE from normal human ears (**A** = 25-year-old adult; **B** = 2-day-old infant), collected with a commercially available device, the ILO88 (Otodynamics Ltd). Two independently averaged responses (A and B) are overplotted to show the extremely high repeatability of the emission (**A:** WAVE REPRO = 97%; **B** = 99%). A click stimulus (**A** = 81 dB$_{peak}$ SPL; **B** = 77 dB$_{peak}$ SPL) was presented at time zero. The initial 2.5 ms of the waveform has been blanked to remove the stimulus artifact. However, the click-stimulus waveform is shown on the same time scale, but a much compressed pressure scale, in the upper left plot ("Stimulus") of each portion of the figure. The frequency spectrum of the TEOAE response is indicated by the unshaded region in the upper right plot entitled "Response FFT," and the background noise of the measurement is indicated by the shaded area in this plot. The response signal-to-noise ratio ("BAND REPRO/SNR") is 8 to 19 dB (**A**) and 23 to 29 dB (**B**) over most of the range in which it is present. The small panel below the "Response FFT" plot shows the frequency spectrum of the stimulus click, for comparison. The set of panels to the right of each portion of the figure display information about the stimulus parameters, the TEOAE response and background noise, and also details concerning test parameters [see Robinette & Glattke (1997) for a detailed explanation of these measures and values].

response of Figure 6.2A, except that the ILO88's baby probe, rather than the adult probe, was used, which produces a less intense click. In babies and young children, although TEOAEs are generally similar to those in adults, their levels are greater and their high-frequency limit often extends up to 5 to 6 kHz. It is clear that infants and young children have smaller ear-canal volumes and, thus, their higher-level TEOAEs would be expected from the presumed enhancement of emission sound pressures in the child ear canal relative to the adult ear canal. The higher upper-frequency extent of TEOAEs in neonates and young children than in adults also likely results from the physical properties of the smaller ear canal, which favor a resonant frequency shift toward high frequencies.

Clinically, TEOAEs are typically measured with the ILO88 system developed by Bray and Kemp (1987), which is, to date, the only instrument in the United States approved for this purpose by the Federal Drug Administration (FDA). This equipment automatically determines and displays information that is important for establishing the presence or absence of a TEOAE. Such details, which are evident in the panels at the right of Figure 6.2, include information on the stimulus and response waveforms and their spectral counterparts, TEOAE level, noise levels and the selected noise-rejection criterion, and waveform reproducibility indicating how well two separately determined response waveforms (A and B) overlap. The latter factor includes information for the entire response as well as replicability outcomes for five frequency regions from 1 to 5 kHz. Finally, details about the stability of the stimulus during the test session, the elapsed time for data collection, and patient identification and disk-filing information are provided. A complete description of the ILO88 display and instrument details was presented recently by Glattke and Robinette (1997).

The presence of a TEOAE is typically determined by some commonly used criterion or set of criteria. For example, to ensure that a valid test was performed, stimulus stability should be at least 70% or greater. In addition, the peak stimulus level in adults should be around 82 ± 3 dB peSPL, and its spectrum should extend from 0.5 to 5 kHz at about 40 to 50 dB SPL, whereas the noise level in the ear canal should be 40 dB SPL or less. If the validity of the test is established, the response is usually defined as being present, if the TEOAE protrudes above the noise floor for the majority of frequencies between 0.5 to 4 kHz, that is, the signal-to-noise ratio (SNR) is >0 dB and typically ≥ 3 dB. Another frequently used index for determining the presence of a TEOAE is that the whole-wave reproducibility should be >50 to 70%. In screening applications in which pass/fail information is the goal of the test, it is often acceptable for the SNR to be >0 dB, or the reproducibility to be >50%, for a subset of frequency bands within the overall 1 to 5 kHz response range, rather than require these criteria be fulfilled over the entire frequency-test extent (Vohr & Maxon, 1996; Vohr, White, Maxon, & Johnson, 1993).

Stimulus-Frequency Otoacoustic Emissions (SFOAEs).

A stimulus-frequency OAE is a continuous, low-level signal at the frequency of a uninterrupted pure-tone stimulus, apparently generated by the same mechanism as that which produces TEOAEs in response to transient stimuli (Kemp & Chum, 1980; Long & Tubis, 1988; Wilson, 1980a; Zwicker & Schloth, 1984). The properties of SFOAEs are similar to those of TEOAEs, in that SFOAEs are present in nearly all normal ears, are robust at those frequencies where TEOAEs are strong, and demonstrate latencies and a compressive nonlinearity similar to those of TEOAEs (Dallmayr, 1987; Kemp & Brown, 1983; Kemp & Chum, 1980; Rutten & Buisman, 1983; Zwicker & Schloth, 1984). Thus, it appears that SFOAEs are the steady-state response, and TEOAEs the transient response, of a common emission-generator mechanism.

Because the stimulus is larger than the SFOAE in the ear canal, and it is present at the same time and frequency, SFOAEs are more difficult to measure than the other OAE phenomena. The existence of SFOAEs is revealed by slowly sweeping the frequency of the stimulus tone. The phase lag of the emission relative to the stimulus increases with increasing frequency, resulting in the physical interference of the stimulus and the emission in the sealed ear canal. Thus, regularly spaced ripples occur in the otherwise smooth frequency response of the ear-canal sound pressure as the stimulus and the SFOAE move alternately into and out of phase (Kemp & Chum, 1980; Wilson, 1980a). The frequency spacing of the maxima or minima of these ripples is inversely proportional to the latency of the SFOAE so that the peaks and valleys occur at greater frequency distances as frequency increases (Lonsbury-Martin et al., 1990b).

It is clear that the complicated interaction of the evoking stimulus and the emitted response makes the significance of common SFOAE properties including the peak/valley frequencies difficult to interpret. Further, because TEOAEs are much simpler to measure with commercially available devices, and because they appear to provide the same information about the status of the emission generator, SFOAEs have not been widely studied, and are not used clinically.

Distortion-Product Otoacoustic Emissions (DPOAEs).

The largest DPOAE in all mammalian species occurs at the $2f_1$-f_2 frequency, although, in ears with normal hearing, DPOAEs are often present at other distortion-product frequencies (e.g., $3f_1$-$2f_2$, $2f_2$-f_1, and f_2-f_1). The amplitude of the $2f_1$-f_2 DPOAE varies systematically with the parameters of the two stimulus tones or primaries, including the frequency (f_1, f_2), frequency separation or ratio (f_2/f_1), level (L_1, L_2), and level difference (L_1-L_2). For instance, the amplitude of the $2f_1$-f_2 DPOAE is greatest when f_2/f_1 is about 1.22 (Gaskill & Brown, 1990; Harris, Lonsbury-Martin, Stagner, Coats, & Martin, 1989), and when $L_1 - L_2$ = 0 dB at high (e.g., $L_1 = L_2 = 75$ dB SPL) stimulus levels, or when $L_1 - L_2$ = 10–15 dB at low (e.g., $L_1 = 60$, $L_2 = 50$ dB SPL) stimulus levels (Gaskill & Brown, 1990; Whitehead, Stagner, McCoy, Lonsbury-Martin, & Martin, 1995). The $2f_1$-f_2 DPOAE increases in amplitude with increasing $L_1 = L_2$ at a rate of ≤ 1 dB/dB and saturates above $L_1 = L_2 = 70$–75 dB SPL (Lonsbury-Martin, Harris, Hawkins, Stagner, & Martin, 1990a).

Whereas DPOAEs can be detected in essentially all normal human ears (Gaskill & Brown, 1990; Harris, 1990; Kemp et al., 1986; Lonsbury-Martin et al., 1990a), they are typically small, usually about 55 to 65 dB below equilevel ($L_1 = L_2$) stimulus tones. Although the absolute amplitudes of DPOAEs are somewhat larger in neonate than in adult ears (Kimberley, Brown, & Allen 1997; Lonsbury-Martin, Martin, McCoy, & Whitehead, 1994), this difference of about 5 dB, on average, is not as great as the 10 dB plus differences observed for TEOAEs.

The presence or absence of DPOAEs is commonly determined by comparing the level of the signal in the DPOAE-frequency FFT bin to the level of closely adjacent frequency bins, which contain only background noise. Typically, a DPOAE is assumed to be present, if the level of the DPOAE-frequency bin is greater than that of the noise-level estimate derived from the nearby bins by some criterion amount (e.g., by 3 or 6 dB, greater than the 90th percentile, or two standard deviations of noise-bin levels).

When illustrated in a graphics format, DPOAEs are typically plotted as a function of the primary-tone frequencies, rather than the DPOAE frequency, because research findings indicate that the $2f_1$-f_2 DPOAE is generated in the region of the cochlea that maximally responds to the primary tones (Brown & Kemp, 1984; Martin, Probst, Scheinin, Coats, & Lonsbury-Martin, 1987). Thus, the DPOAEs best reflect the status of OHC function in this frequency region. The reference frequency typically used is either f_2, or the geometric mean of the primary tones [i.e., the logarithmic mean of the two primary tones, which is computed by taking the square root of the product of the frequency of the lower-level primary times that of the higher-level primary: $(f_1 \times f_2)^{.5}$]. Current thinking concerning which frequency most accurately reflects the generation site is that the relationship is likely level-dependent, with lower-level tones best activating the frequency region nearest to f_2, and moderate- to higher-level primaries optimally stimulating the geometric-mean region.

The most commonly measured DPOAE feature is amplitude, which typically is plotted as a function of the frequency of the primary tones, across a range of frequencies, in response to constant-level primary tones (see example in Figure 6.3). Currently, such a DPOAE level/frequency plot is referred to as a DP-gram, rather than the "DP-audiogram" terminology used in the early literature, in order to avoid the inference that DPOAE threshold is being measured with this paradigm. A positive feature of the DP-gram is the detailed frequency configuration that can be obtained, which presumably specifies the pattern of remaining OHC function.

When DPOAE levels are measured in fine frequency intervals of <100 Hz, an irregular microstructure occurs consisting of peaks and valleys, which exhibit excursions that can be more than 10 dB (He & Schmeidt, 1993). In relating emission amplitude and hearing level, depending on the frequency at which the behavioral hearing threshold is measured, the DPOAE may be enhanced (peak) or reduced (valley). Thus, the existence of a DPOAE microstructure, which persists in the presence of damage-induced reductions in emissions levels (He & Schmeidt, 1996), likely contributes toward the difficulty in uncovering a strong correlation between hearing level and DPOAE magnitude.

Another DPOAE-level response form, which is less commonly used, assesses DPOAE amplitude at a particular frequency as a function of primary-tone level for a number of progressively increasing stimulus levels. This measure is known as the response/growth or input/output (I/O) function (Lonsbury-Martin et al., 1990a), and a set of these is usually obtained for several discrete frequencies, which are typically selected to complement the conventional audiometric-test frequencies. A major benefit of the I/O measure is that several properties of DPOAE activity including detection threshold, maximum output, and the slope of the function as a measure of response growth, can all be derived from the same function.

A notable feature of DPOAEs is the shape of certain I/O functions (Stover & Norton, 1993). In individual ears, the functions for some primary-tone frequencies, but not others, are non-monotonic, in that they demonstrate a minimum, or notch, at particular stimulus levels. However, the occurrence of notches is highly idiosyncratic in that the primary-tone frequency pairs that yield non-monotonic growth functions vary greatly across ears, and occur over a wide range of stimulus levels (Lonsbury-Martin, Whitehead, & Martin, 1993; Nelson & Kimberley, 1992; Stover & Norton, 1993), rather than only in a specific range of stimulus levels as exhibited by non-primate species (Whitehead, Lonsbury-Martin, & Martin, 1992a).

Detailed studies in rabbits and rodents strongly suggest that the growth-function minima, which occur in these animals with stimulus levels around 50 to 70 dB SPL, arise from a cancellation of out-of-phase components, indicating that the $2f_1$-f_2 DPOAE may actually consist of two discrete components, each of which has a differential dependence on stimulus parameters, and each of which dominates the total ear-canal $2f_1$-f_2 at different stimulus levels (Mills & Rubel, 1994; Whitehead, Lonsbury-Martin, & Martin, 1992b; Whitehead et al., 1992a). However, because of the different properties of the growth-function notches in humans, it is not clear whether the $2f_1$-f_2 DPOAE in humans consists of two discrete components, as appears to be the case in rabbits and rodents (Whitehead, Stagner, et al., 1995). It is possible that some of the non-monotonicities observed in DPOAE growth functions in humans reflect interactions of the DPOAEs with the mechanism that produces the tonally elicited SFOAEs, because, in humans, SFOAEs are much larger relative to DPOAEs than in animals.

As noted above, DPOAE levels depend systematically on the parameters of the f_1 and f_2 primary tones including their frequencies, levels, frequency separation, and level difference. Thus, a representative stimulus protocol used to examine an ear would include a frequency range from about 0.55 to 8.81 kHz with respect to f_2 (or 0.5 to 8 kHz re the geometric-mean frequency), along with an f_2/f_1 ratio of 1.22, a level difference of 10 dB, and absolute levels of $L_1 = 65$ dB and $L_2 = 55$ dB SPL (e.g., Gorga, Stover, Neely, & Montoya, 1996).

Relationships between the Various Emission Phenomena

The available evidence is consistent with the hypothesis that TEOAEs, SFOAEs, and the typical, low-level SOAEs, reflect the output of a common mechanism responding to different stimuli, that is, transient stimulation, tonal stimulation, and positive feedback of OAE energy into the OAE generator's input, respectively. The relationship of the extremely rare, high-level, atypical SOAEs observed in humans and other species, to the other OAE phenomena, is obscure. However, the atypical SOAEs tend to be associated with cochlear pathology, unlike TEOAEs, SFOAEs, and the common SOAEs, which tend to be reduced or absent in the presence of cochlear pathology.

The relationship of DPOAEs to TEOAEs and SFOAEs is less clear. The mechanism that produces TEOAEs and SFOAEs demonstrates a compressive nonlinearity of a form expected to produce distortion products upon stimulation with two tones. Thus, it would be parsimonious to assume that DPOAEs are produced by the same mechanism as TEOAEs and SFOAEs. However, as noted above, studies in rabbits and rodents indicate that DPOAEs consist of two distinct, and at least partially independent, components in these species (Mills, Norton, & Rubel, 1993; Mills & Rubel, 1994; Whitehead et al., 1992a, 1992b; Whitehead, Stagner, et al., 1995). If so, these two components must have somewhat different relationships to TEOAEs and SFOAEs. Moreover, our understanding of the relationship of DPOAEs

to TEOAEs and SFOAEs is further confounded by the large differences of the relative amplitudes of DPOAEs and TEOAEs/SFOAEs between humans and the common laboratory mammals and by the uncertainty regarding whether there are two distinct components of DPOAEs in human ears analogous to those in the rabbits and rodents.

CLINICAL APPLICATIONS OF EVOKED OTOACOUSTIC EMISSIONS

Of the four classes of evoked OAEs, the most widely utilized in applied settings are the TEOAEs and DPOAEs. The following discussion emphasizes how the advantageous features of evoked OAEs benefit the clinical examination of ears with hearing-related difficulties. It should be stressed, however, that many of these applications await large-scale, clinical trial investigations to substantiate the claims based on small, research-oriented studies that OAEs have truly made useful contributions to the diagnosis, treatment, and study of ear disease.

Beneficial Properties of Otoacoustic Emissions

The OAEs exhibit a number of properties that make them ideal for clinical testing. First, they are an objective measure that can be used to examine difficult-to-test patients, who are either noncommunicative (e.g., newborns and older infants, the critically ill, and the mentally or physically incompetent due to stroke or head injury) or noncooperative (e.g., young children, pseudohypacusics). The objectivity feature is also compatible with the computer control of the test procedure, which permits emissions testing to be conducted accurately and rapidly and in great detail with respect to stimulation level and frequency.

A second positive feature of evoked OAEs is that the test instrumentation is relatively inexpensive, mostly because the equipment is configured around an economical personal microcomputer system. Moreover, technical personnel who operate the test equipment do not require extensive education or training.

A third advantage of evoked-OAE testing is that the patient setup time is minimal, because emission measurements are noninvasive. All that is required is the insertion of the acoustic probe securely into the outer ear canal, which is a maneuver that can be performed quickly. This particular benefit is especially useful in examining very young patients, who often are restless and irritable.

A fourth positive characteristic is that evoked OAEs are present in the ears of nearly all normal-hearing individuals and are reduced or absent in ears exhibiting impairment caused by cochlear or middle-ear dysfunction. Moreover, a number of descriptions of normal response ranges are available in the literature, thus permitting the assessment of the healthiness of an unknown ear on the basis of comparisons of its properties to the database of normal responses.

A fifth advantageous feature of evoked OAEs is their presumed preneural origin in OHC activity. Thus, for the first time, OAE results provide specific information concerning the contribution that a major sensory-cell type of the organ of Corti, the OHC system, makes to a hearing impairment. In combination with the findings of other audiologic tests, knowledge about the functional status of the OHCs permits the unambiguous determination of the sensory component of a sensorineural hearing loss. Additionally, because of their OHC origin, OAEs are highly sensitive to a number of common forms of damage including the adverse effects of excessive sounds and ototoxic drugs, viral and bacterial pathogens, congenital factors, and genetic defects, as well as the more insidious consequences on hearing of the natural aging process.

Finally, a sixth beneficial property of evoked OAEs is that emissions are also sensitive to the onset stages of hearing problems, because they operate maximally in response to low to moderate levels of stimulation. Moreover, OAEs provide a direct measure of the nonlinear operations of the cochlea that are responsible for the normal ear's keen sensitivity and frequency-tuning abilities, and it is these listening qualities that are initially affected in the early stages of hearing impairment.

Clinical Utility of Evoked Otoacoustic Emissions

Based on the positive features reviewed above for evoked OAEs, a number of clinical applications are ideally suited for emissions testing including: (1) the differential diagnosis of hearing impairment, (2) hearing screening, (3) monitoring the progression of already established hearing ailments or of treatment effects, (4) testing the functional status of the cochlear-efferent system, and (5) identifying pseudohypacusics.

Both TEOAEs and DPOAEs have been used to describe the practical applications described above. However, in most cases, and particularly in the hearing screening and efferent-testing utilizations, DPOAEs have been used less frequently than TEOAEs, primarily because of the earlier availability of commercial instrumentation for measuring the latter type of emissions. However, as DPOAE equipment is becoming more available in the marketplace, published reports on DPOAEs with respect to the majority of these utilities are regularly appearing. However, before reviewing the particular applications of evoked OAEs noted above, the significant influence of the middle ear on emission properties will be considered.

Middle-Ear Influences on Otoacoustic Emissions

Because the stimuli and the emissions must both pass through the middle ear, OAEs are modified in cases of impaired sound conduction through the middle ear. The adverse effects of middle-ear dysfunction on the level and frequency attributes of OAEs have been demonstrated in human patient groups with various middle-ear disorders such as otosclerosis (Rossi, Solero, Rolando, & Olina, 1989) or middle-ear disease (Lonsbury-Martin, Martin, et al., 1994; Owens, McCoy, Lonsbury-Martin, & Martin, 1992, 1993), and by experimental manipulations of the middle ear in normal-hearing humans using postural adjustments (Johnsen & Elberling, 1982b), alterations in atmospheric pressure (Hauser, Probst, & Harris, 1993), or changes in ear-canal pressure (Marshall, Heller, & Westhusin, 1997; Naeve, Margolis, Levine, & Fournier, 1992). In addition, for the DPOAEs, which are measured in the presence of the primary tones, rather than occurring after a transient stimulus like TEOAEs, direct interactions between the stimulus and response occur both within the conduction apparatus and the cochlea, which further complicate the relationship of simple measurement parameters (e.g., amplitude) to cochlear status, especially under conditions of a poorly functioning middle ear.

Kemp (1980) originally devised a conceptual model describing the difference in OAE amplitude due to forward conduction, that is, stimulus travel to the cochlea, compared to backward transmission, that is, OAE travel out of the cochlea. This difference was estimated to be at least 12 to 16 dB within the most efficiently processed 0.8 to 2 kHz frequency region. Thus, before the OAE reaches the pick-up microphone in the ear canal, it has already undergone considerable reduction due to the forward and backward filtering properties of the conduction apparatus of the middle ear.

Middle-ear disease in the form of negative intratympanic pressure significantly reduces the levels of both TEOAEs and DPOAEs, particularly for the low to mid-frequencies (Lonsbury-Martin, Martin et al., 1994; Owens et al., 1992, 1993). Fortunately, according to the systematic study of Trine and associates (Margolis & Trine, 1997; Trine, Hirsch, & Margolis, 1993) on the effects of middle-ear pressure on TEOAEs, ear-canal pressure can be adjusted to compensate for negative intratympanic pressure conditions so that the overall emission amplitude is increased. This result is promising in terms of improving the outlook for successfully applying OAE testing to young children, who often exhibit middle-ear pathologies of this sort.

The effects of otitis media on OAE measurements are more controversial than the findings for the influence of negative middle-ear pressure. Owens and colleagues (1992) noted that the presence of any amount of middle-ear effusion, verified by myringotomy prior to inserting tympanostomy tubes, essentially made TEOAEs immeasurable, whereas larger volumes of fluid were necessary to reduce DPOAEs completely to noise-floor levels. In contrast, Amadee (1995) discovered that, if the viscosity of the fluid in the middle ear was not too great, TEOAEs were measurable in the presence of effusion. Margolis and Trine (1997) recently suggested that, in children with very mild hearing losses due to otitis media, it is likely that OAEs are measurable, whereas, if the effusion-induced hearing loss is substantial (i.e., resulting in hearing levels up to 50 dB), emissions are probably undetectable.

In summary, it is well established that if OAEs are to be used in clinical settings to assess cochlear status, normal middle-ear function is essential. Thus, to distinguish between the effects of middle-ear pathology and cochlear abnormalities on emitted responses, it is necessary to evaluate middle-ear function at the time of OAE testing (Kemp et al., 1986).

Specific Clinical Applications

Differential Diagnosis of Hearing Difficulties. One of the principal applications of evoked-OAE testing is in the differential diagnosis of a hearing problem. Based on their exceptional site-of-lesion testing ability, studies conducted in patient groups have shown that OAEs can be used in the clinic to detect sensorineural hearing losses resulting from such factors as administration of ototoxic drugs, exposure to excessive sounds, aging, Ménière's disease, sudden idiopathic sensorineural hearing loss, acoustic tumors, bacterial and viral infections, and congenital and hereditary hearing disorders. In the following discussion, the results of studies of a variety of traumas on OAEs in patient groups are reviewed in order to provide insight into the relationship of OAE-amplitude reductions to impairments of cochlear structure and function.

Retrocochlear Hearing Loss. In humans, SFOAEs can be detected at stimulus levels well below the threshold of hearing (Wilson, 1980b), and the TEOAE waveform shows precise inversion with stimulus polarity, and only slight adaptation (Anderson, 1980). These properties indicate that the evoked OAEs are produced without direct afferent neural involvement. Other studies of SOAEs and TEOAEs (Collet, Kemp, Veuillet, Duclaux, Moulin, & Morgon, 1990; Mott, Norton, Neely, & Warr, 1989) have suggested that the olivocochlear-efferent system, which innervates the OHCs preferentially, may influence OAEs, but these changes are typically small. Thus, OAEs may be expected to be essentially normal in cases of pure retrocochlear dysfunction.

Consistent with these findings is that TEOAEs and DPOAEs have been shown to be present in some ears with sensorineural hearing losses due to acoustic neuromas (Bonfils & Uziel, 1988; Robinette, 1992; Telischi, Roth, Lonsbury-Martin, & Balkany, 1995), or other retrocochlear or more central auditory-system disorders (Gravel & Stapells, 1993; Lutman, Mason, Sheppard, & Gibbin, 1989; Monroe, Krauth, Arenberg, Prenger, & Philpot, 1996; Prieve, Gorga, & Neely, 1991; Widen, Ferraro, & Trouba, 1995). However, both TEOAEs and DPOAEs have also been shown to be reduced in ears with acoustic neuromas

(Bonfils & Uziel, 1988; Kemp et al., 1986; Lonsbury-Martin & Martin, 1990; Martin, Probst, et al., 1990; Ohlms, Lonsbury-Martin, & Martin, 1991; Robinette, 1992). In fact, Telischi, Roth, and colleagues (1995) reported recently that of 44 patients diagnosed with surgically verified acoustic tumors, 31 (71%) showed reduced levels of TEOAEs and DPOAEs. These findings indicate that, in the majority of cases, OAEs are adversely affected by such retrocochlear pathologies as acoustic neuromas. It is probable that the reduction in OAE amplitude in these cases was due to cochlear injury resulting from the tumor, perhaps secondarily produced by the growth affecting mechanical pressure on the vascular supply to the cochlea. In support of this notion, direct mechanical pressure on the vascular supply to the cochlea has been shown in experimental animals to impair many measures of cochlear function including DPOAEs (Widick, Telischi, Lonsbury-Martin, & Stagner, 1994). In any case, it is clear that knowledge about the viability of OAEs, before surgical intervention, not only helps the surgeon in planning the most expedient anatomical approach to the tumor site (e.g., whether hearing-conservation surgery is a realistic option), but also provides the patient with a pragmatic appreciation of the potential of the procedure to improve hearing.

Cochlear Hearing Loss. One practical approach to distinguishing a cochlear hearing loss with OAE testing emphasizes the specific features of emissions that make them useful in the differential diagnosis of a sensorineural hearing loss. This strategy consists of a comparison of the outcomes of conventional audiometric testing, using the pure-tone audiogram, with the results of an emissions-test protocol for the same ear that establishes the frequency pattern of evoked-OAE levels as a function of a constant level of acoustic stimulation, that is, the spectral TEOAE plot and/or the DP-gram evaluation. Using such an analysis, the results of the two types of tests (audiogram versus pattern of emitted activity) can either agree or disagree. Further, assuming that the middle-ear conduction system is functioning normally, a disagreement between the two measures likely indicates one of three possibilities: (1) The primary site of pathology is located more proximal in the auditory pathway, that is, at the level of the IHCs, auditory nerve, or a more central auditory structure; (2) there is no pathology present, as would occur in pseudohypacusis; or, (3) the DPOAEs are capable of identifying OHC dysfunction before it is behaviorally apparent.

Cochlear Pathologies That Predominantly Target Outer Hair Cells

There are a number of hearing impairments in which the OHCs are the primary target of the damaging agent, particularly during the early stages, including noise-induced hearing loss (NIHL) and ototoxicity. Given the primary involvement of the OHC system in these pathologies, it is expected that good agreement should occur between the results of pure-tone testing in the form of the clinical audiogram and the frequency analysis performed by both the click-evoked TEOAE spectrum and the DP-gram.

It has long been known that exposure to intense acoustic stimuli can result in temporary or permanent behavioral threshold elevations in humans and other mammals, with the latter permanent hearing loss being associated with damage to the organ of Corti. Deliberate experimental sound exposures to human subjects that produced a temporary behavioral threshold shift also reduced the amplitudes of SOAEs (Kemp, 1981; Norton, Mott, & Champlin, 1989), TEOAEs (Kemp 1981, 1982; Zwicker, 1983), and DPOAEs (Engdahl, 1996; Engdahl & Kemp, 1996; Sutton, Lonsbury-Martin, Martin, & Whitehead 1994). These OAE-amplitude reductions were frequency specific and demonstrated a correlate of the psychophysical half-octave shift effect, that is, the maximum functional reduction tended to occur at a frequency approximately one-half octave above the exposure frequency. Additionally, the recovery of the post-exposure OAE level followed, in general, a time course similar to that of the behavioral threshold.

The experimental work on noise exposure in humans uncovered an important result showing that decreasing L_2 below L_1 increased the trauma-induced reductions in DPOAE levels (Sutton et al., 1994). This finding emphasizes the need to exercise care in the choice of stimuli to be used in detecting early changes in cochlear condition (Whitehead, McCoy, Lonsbury-Martin, & Martin, 1995).

In human patient groups, Probst, Lonsbury-Martin, Martin, and Coats (1987) determined that noise-induced high-frequency hearing loss was associated with a reduction in the number of prominent peaks in the spectra of TEOAEs. Frequency-specific reductions of $2f_1$-f_2 DPOAE amplitudes in frequency regions of behaviorally measured noise-induced hearing loss have also been demonstrated by Harris (1990), Lonsbury-Martin and Martin (1990), Martin and colleagues (1990), Balkany, Telischi, Lonsbury-Martin, and Martin (1994), and Lonsbury-Martin, Martin, and Balkany (1994).

It has also long been known that certain pharmacological agents can result in profound, permanent hearing losses. For example, cis-platinum is a known ototoxin used in anti-tumor therapy (Pasic & Dobie, 1991), and the literature contains a number of case-study examples of the reductions of TEOAEs (Zorowka, Schmitt, & Gutjahr, 1993) and DPOAEs (Balkany et al., 1994; Ozturan, Jerger, Lew, & Lynch, 1996) in patients undergoing cis-platinum treatment. In these patients, the OAE reductions tended to occur at high frequencies, corresponding to the cis-platinum induced hearing losses.

Other ototoxins that affect hearing include aspirin and aminoglycoside antibiotics. It is well known that oral aspirin (acetylsalicylic acid) administration can cause a reversible,

mild to moderate (≤ 40 dB) threshold elevation in humans, often associated with tinnitus (McFadden, Plattsmier, & Pasanen, 1984). Oral aspirin administration also temporarily reduces TEOAEs, SFOAEs, and SOAEs in humans (Johnsen & Elberling, 1982a; Long & Tubis, 1988; McFadden & Plattsmier, 1984). Wier, Pasanen, and McFadden (1988) found that aspirin had less effect on $2f_1$-f_2 DPOAEs evoked by low-level stimulus tones than on SOAEs at nearby frequencies in the same ears. Thus, it appears that salicylate reduces TEOAEs, SFOAEs, and SOAEs, but has relatively little effect on DPOAEs, even at quite low stimulus levels. This finding suggests at least a partial dissociation of the mechanism underlying low-level DPOAEs and the generation of TEOAEs, SFOAEs, and SOAEs. It is possible that the pattern of trauma-induced loss among the different types of OAEs may provide useful diagnostic information regarding the precise subcellular origin of certain cochlear injuries.

Chronic administration of some aminoglycoside antibiotics can produce permanent hearing loss in humans, particularly at high frequencies (Brummett & Fox, 1989; Govaerts, Claes, Van De Heyning, Jorens, Marquet, & De Broe, 1990; Rybak, 1986). Consistent with this finding are the results of histological studies in animal models, which have demonstrated damage at almost every level of the cochlea upon chronic aminoglycoside treatment, with basal OHCs being the most vulnerable cochlear element (Govaerts et al., 1990; Rybak, 1986). Hotz, Harris, and Probst (1994) studied the effects of aminoglycosides on OAEs in humans, and reported a small but significant reduction of TEOAEs in leukemia patients undergoing amikacin-sulfate therapy for more than 12 days.

Aminoglycoside antibiotics and loop diuretics administered in combination are known to have a powerful ototoxic effect in humans, which can result in a profound, permanent hearing loss (West, Brummett, & Himes, 1973). Although animal studies have demonstrated that acute administrations of these drugs in combination cause a reduction of DPOAEs at all stimulus levels measured up to $L_1 = L_2 = 75$ dB (Whitehead et al., 1992b), there are no reports in humans describing the combined effects of aminoglycoside antibiotics and loop diuretics.

Other drugs reported to reduce OAE amplitudes include quinine, which causes a reversible mild to moderate hearing loss through an unknown mechanism. In several studies using small numbers of normal volunteer subjects, quinine was found to reduce TEOAEs, SFOAEs, and DPOAEs in humans (Berninger, Karlsson, Hellgren, & Eskilsson, 1995; Karlsson, Berninger, & Alvan, 1991; McFadden & Pasanen, 1994). Karlsson and colleagues (1991) reported a good correlation between TEOAE-amplitude decrease and hearing-threshold elevation. However, this relationship was less clear in the data of McFadden and Pasanen (1994), although most of the quinine-induced hearing-threshold shifts were quite small in the latter study.

Because the OHCs are most vulnerable to insults to the inner ear by external agents such as sound overexposure or ototoxic agents, OAEs can be used to detect the initial signs of cochlear injury. In Figure 6.3, the ability of the two major types of evoked OAEs in the form of TEOAE spectra and the DP-gram to describe the configuration of a developing NIHL is illustrated. The 41-year-old female patient illustrated here had participated regularly in recreational rifle shooting for three years prior to OAE testing. Even though the patient claimed to wear hearing protection during this time, the right-shouldered shooter presented in the otology clinic with complaints of a decrease in hearing sensitivity, tinnitus, muffled hearing, and difficulty discerning speech in the presence of background noise. It is clear from the test results illustrated in Figure 6.3 that the magnitude and frequency extent of the TEOAEs bilaterally reflected the pattern of normal hearing depicted by the clinical audiogram. However, the DP-gram shown below clearly describes abnormal DPOAE activity with the right ear (open circles) showing below-average response levels above about 1 kHz, and the left ear (filled circles) exhibiting a significant reduction in emitted responses for frequencies >2 kHz. True to classic acoustical principles, the left ear, which was closer to the gun muzzle, went essentially unprotected by the head-shadow effect. This example of the ability of evoked OAEs to detect cochlear pathology caused by an agent that primarily targets the OHC system attests to the potential usefulness of emission tests in identifying early hearing problems in individuals regularly exposed to loud sounds.

In summary, past studies have demonstrated that evoked OAEs provide information regarding the frequency extent of NIHL and ototoxicity. Thus, noises and drugs producing predominantly mid- to high-frequency hearing loss also cause mainly mid- to high-frequency reductions in OAEs. Moreover, the ability of evoked OAEs to measure OHC activity, particularly over the higher-frequency test range, makes it an especially useful test for identifying the onset of either NIHL or ototoxicity, at an early stage of development. Other disorders in which the results of both the clinical audiogram and OAE testing tend to agree include many of the familial and congenital hearing losses and the hearing impairments caused by bacterial and viral infections. In patients with either autosomal dominant- or recessive-based hereditary hearing loss, OAEs have been shown to be reduced below population means, or absent (Lonsbury-Martin & Martin, 1990; Martin et al., 1990). Also, congenital hearing disorders such as cytomegalovirus (Owens et al., 1992) and hearing impairments caused by viral (Soucek & Michaels, 1996) or bacterial agents (Daya, Amedofu, Woodrow, Agranoff, Brobby, Agbenyega, & Krishna 1997; Fortnum, Farnsworth, & Davis, 1993)

also adversely affect OAEs in a manner that is consistent with the related hearing loss. Finally, TEOAEs, SOAEs, and DPOAEs decrease with age over about 40 to 50 years (Bonfils, 1989; Bonfils, Bertrand, & Uziel, 1988; Collet, Moulin, Gartner, & Morgon, 1990; Lonsbury-Martin, Cutler, & Martin, 1991; Stover & Norton, 1993), suggesting that OAEs represent an objective means of studying presbycusis.

Cochlear Pathologies That May or May Not Target Outer Hair Cells

There are several types of hearing impairments that, depending on the patient, produce conflicting results between the two types of functional tests consisting of behavioral and OAE measures. These categories of hearing loss represent, for the most part, the more puzzling ear diseases including Ménière's disease and sudden idiopathic sensorineural hearing loss (Lonsbury-Martin, McCoy, Whitehead, & Martin, 1993; Martin et al., 1990; Ohlms, Lonsbury-Martin, & Martin, 1990).

The exact mechanisms responsible for the fluctuating hearing loss observed in ears with Ménière's disease are unclear, as there are changes at many levels of the cochlea, including the hair cells, the cochlear innervation, and the chemical composition of the cochlear fluids (Nadol, 1989). Measurements of TEOAEs in human patient groups with sensorineural hearing losses of various etiologies have demonstrated that these emissions are typically absent in frequency regions in which the hearing level is greater than 25 to 30 dB (Kemp et al., 1986). This observation is also true for TEOAEs in some Ménière's ears. However, TEOAEs have been measured in Ménière's ears with corresponding hearing thresholds, at the time of measurement, exceeding 40 dB HL (Bonfils, Uziel, & Pujol, 1988; Harris & Probst, 1992). Similarly, in the majority of Ménière's ears, DPOAE levels are reduced below population averages at frequencies corresponding to those of behavioral-threshold increase, consistent with data obtained from ears with sensorineural hearing loss of other etiologies. However, in some patients DPOAE amplitudes are relatively normal in the presence of equally large behavioral-threshold increases (Lonsbury-Martin & Martin, 1990; Martin et al., 1990). One interpretation of these findings is that only in some cases of Ménière's disease, that is, those demonstrating reduced OAEs, is the motile action of OHCs compromised, and that in ears with normal emissions the hearing loss does not result from OHC pathology, but from dysfunction of other sensory or neural components of the cochlea.

Similarly, evoked OAEs have been shown to be either appropriately reduced or unexpectedly normal-like in cases of sudden idiopathic sensorineural hearing loss (Lonsbury-Martin, Martin, & Balkany, 1994; Ohlms et al., 1990;

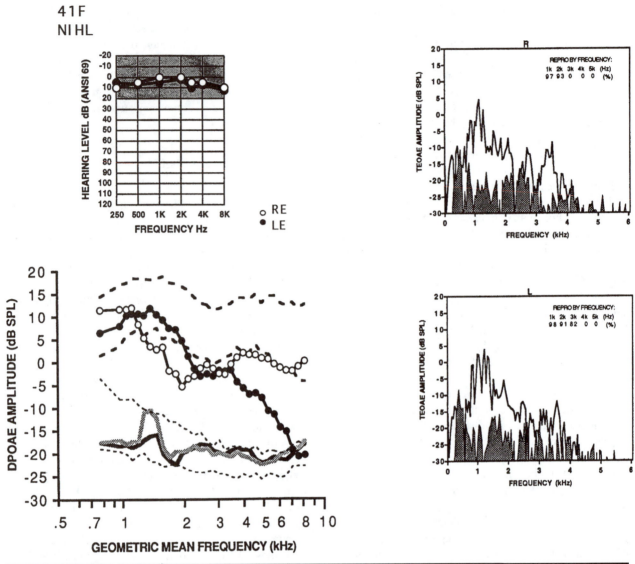

FIGURE 6.3 Hearing and evoked-OAE test results for both ears of a 41-year-old female patient complaining of hearing difficulties (see text). The top left plot shows the conventional behavioral audiogram obtained from the right (open circles) and left (filled circles) ears. The stippling indicates the region considered clinically normal, and for this patient, hearing was normal in both ears. The bottom left panel shows the DP-gram plot of DPOAE levels from the two ears measured as a function of the geometric-mean frequency of the primary tones, with $f_2/f_1 = 1.21$, and $L_1 = L_2 = 75$ dB SPL. The pair of bold dashed lines around 3 to 15 dB SPL shows the ±1 standard deviation (SD) of the mean DPOAEs levels measured with these stimulus parameters from 94 ears of normal-hearing adults, to indicate the expected DPOAE amplitudes. The lower pair of dashed lines show ±1 SD of the corresponding noise-floor levels. It is clear that DPOAE levels were within the normal range up to about 1.4 kHz for the right ear (open circles) and ~2.3 kHz for the left (filled circles) ear, but were mainly below the normal range above these cut-off frequencies. This pattern of DPOAE-amplitude reduction is in contrast to the normal hearing thresholds depicted in the behavioral audiograms. The lower hatched and dark lines indicate the noise floors associated with the right and left ears (open and filled symbols, respectively). The panels to the right show the spectra (right ear = top; left ear = bottom) of TEOAE responses evoked by click stimuli of approximately 80 dB_peak SPL, measured using the ILO88 device (see Figure 6.1). Robust TEOAE components (open area) were present above the background noise (filled area) between approximately 0.5 and 4 kHz in both ears, as expected for a normal adult ear. The percentage values ("REPRO BY FREQUENCY") given in each TEOAE panel are measures of the reproducibility of the TEOAE response, determined by cross-correlation of the two independently averaged TEOAE waveforms. In general, a reproducibility value greater than 50% indicates the presence of a genuine TEOAE response. Note that in the other examples of patient test results presented in the following figures, the stimuli used to evoke DPOAEs and TEOAEs are the same as in this figure.

Sakashita, Minowa, Hachikawa, Kubo, & Nakai, 1991; Truy, Veuillet, Collet, & Morgon, 1993). Additionally, to some extent, OAEs have been shown to be able to track the recovery of behavioral thresholds in sudden hearing loss cases (Gaskill & Brown, 1990; Lonsbury-Martin & Martin, 1990; Ohlms et al., 1990).

Besides Ménière's disease and sudden idiopathic sensorineural hearing loss, another example of how OAEs can help in better understanding the cochlear basis of a hearing problem comes from our own work on patients with Ushers syndrome. There is no question that in Ushers type 1, the most severe form of the disorder, which results in a profound hearing loss, OAEs are completely obliterated. However, Ushers type 2, which is associated with a relatively more moderate impairment, appears to be comprised of several subtype variants. Whereas, as in the type 1 condition, OAEs are typically immeasurable in the majority of Ushers type 2 patients, in some cases, relatively normal OAEs can be observed in frequency regions in which hearing sensitivities of 60 to 70 dB HL are not compatible with the generation of OAEs. An example of this variant of Ushers type 2 is shown in Figure 6.4 for a 39-year-old female patient. Note that the DPOAEs are reduced almost to noise floor levels by about 2 kHz, but return toward the normal range, particularly in the right ear (open circles), over the frequency region where corresponding hearing levels are 50 dB HL or greater.

At present, the clinical meaningfulness of the subvariant type of information for any of these cochlear pathologies is unclear. However, one potential use might be the planning of some more rationally grounded treatment regimens based on knowing the precise location of the primary lesion site. For example, in Ménière's disease, if healthy OHC activity is detectable in the presence of poor hearing ability, medical therapy in the form of diuretic-drug treatment and a low-salt diet might be more logical than surgical therapy consisting of an endolymphatic-shunt procedure, which might lead to the eradication of all remaining OHCs. The principal rationale here is that healthy OHCs could contribute more effectively to normal hearing behavior, if the presumed dilated endolymphatic space was reduced pharmacologically in order that the organ of Corti become more optimally positioned in order to permit maximal stimulus transduction.

Similarly, the outcome of OAE testing can also provide potentially useful information to the clinician with respect to sudden hearing loss. For example, from our own work, it appears that healthy OHC function along with poor hearing is a poor indicator of any treatment-related recovery of hearing ability, possibly caused by a persistent lesion located more proximally to the OHC system. With the information provided by the presence or absence of OAEs, the clinician can, at least, counsel patients concerning their expectations for the likely outcome of a particular treatment.

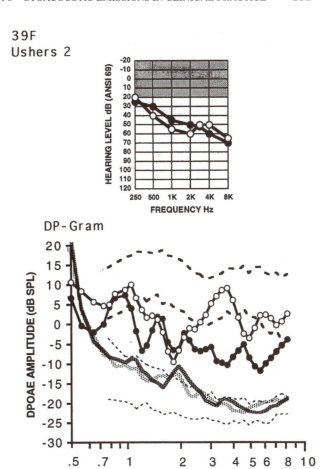

FIGURE 6.4 Hearing and evoked-OAE findings for the left (filled circles) and right (open circles) ears of a 39-year-old female with Ushers syndrome type 2. The top plot shows the results of the behavioral audiogram. Note the similar pattern of hearing loss at and above about 500 Hz. Also note that the DPOAE responses below are inconsistent with the behavioral hearing thresholds in that as hearing sensitivity worsens to hearing levels >45 dB, the emissions remain detectable (left ear) or become more normal-like (right ear).

Other Useful Applications of Site-of-Lesion Testing with Otoacoustic Emissions

In addition to confirming the primary site of pathology, OAE testing can be used in certain types of hereditary disorders (e.g., Waardenburg's syndrome, Ushers syndrome) to identify the carrier status of family members who are not overtly affected by the familial-related pathology (Liu & Newton, 1997; Meredith, Stephens, Sirimanna, Meyer-Bisch, & Reardon, 1992). Work in our own laboratory on TEOAEs and DPOAEs in the near relatives of patients with Ushers syndrome is finding that the evoked OAEs appear to exhibit pathological features in the absence of significant abnormalities in hearing ability. This outcome of OAE testing is apparent in the form of early aging and advanced NIHL patterns of emitted activity, in particular, which are not reflected in the clinical audiogram. It is clear that information concerning the presence of subclinical signs of hearing deficiency can potentially contribute towards the optimal genetic counseling of such affected individuals.

One important application of the site-of-lesion confirmation ability of OAE testing is in the assessment of patients who qualify as candidates for a cochlear implant. At first glance, it may seem excessive to perform OAE testing on such patients, who typically have a profound bilateral hearing loss consisting of essentially no audiometric hearing as well as absent ABRs. However, case-study examples of such candidate patients who display evoked OAEs, and thus present a dilemma to the clinician, have been reported (Robinette & Durrant, 1997). One example of such a perplexing case from our own work is shown in Figure 6.5 for the right ear of a 12-year-old male, who was hospitalized three times for meningitis induced by different head traumas that eventually led to bilateral deafness. In cochlear-implant candidate cases like these who exhibit robust OAEs, the mere presence of emissions indicates that the profound hearing loss is due primarily to a retrocochlear pathology. Thus, a cochlear implant would be unwarranted, because such a retrocochlear impairment would also affect the viable function of the implant device, that is, the neural activity generated by the implant's artificial electrical impulses also would be unlikely to activate more central auditory structures given that the neural impulses elicited by normal hair cell responses are incapable of functioning normally.

Finally, the ability of evoked OAEs to describe precisely the frequency extent of remaining OHCs in pathologies known to mainly affect this most prevalent receptor type promises to provide an objective method for determining the appropriate amplification features of, for example, digital hearing aids that can be specifically adjusted according to an individual patient's needs. In Figure 6.6, an example is provided of the potential utility of OAE testing in the fitting of hearing aids. In this case, the 59-year-old female patient, who had been receiving cis-platinum regularly for treatment of an ovarian carcinoma, had requested a hearing aid in order to remedy the hearing difficulties she was experiencing in terms of muffled speech and an inability to converse in the presence of background noises. Although the configuration of the patient's audiometric hearing suggested that amplified hearing would not be useful to her, the DP-gram, in particular, indicated that OHC activity was abnormally low across the entire frequency-test range. In fact, once fitted with a conventional hearing aid, the patient reported a marked improvement in her hearing ability.

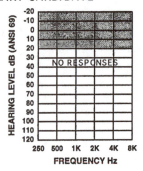

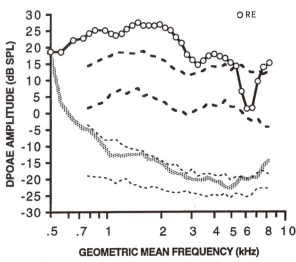

FIGURE 6.5 Hearing and evoked-OAE results for a 12-year-old male with meningitis-induced deafness, who was undergoing testing to determine his eligibility for a cochlear implant. Although no hearing was measurable bilaterally (shown here for the right ear), note the robust DPOAEs displayed in the DP-gram below.

Hearing Screening

Newborns.   One of the most widely used applications of evoked OAEs is in newborn-hearing screening. It is well-established that about 0.1% of newborns are born with a profound hearing loss. Unfortunately, the average age for identifying a hearing loss can be up to 2 to 3 years of age (American Academy of Otolaryngology—Head and Neck Surgery, 1990), because of the difficulties in detecting these infants at a young age with existing audiometric tests. Because early identification and habilitation are directly linked to the successful development of the language and speech skills of a hearing-impaired child, a reliable method for identifying newborn hearing loss is essential. Previous attempts to use testing methods that focus on behavioral activity have not been shown to be efficient and effective. Other work using an objective electrophysiological measure such as the ABR has been shown to be reliable, but it

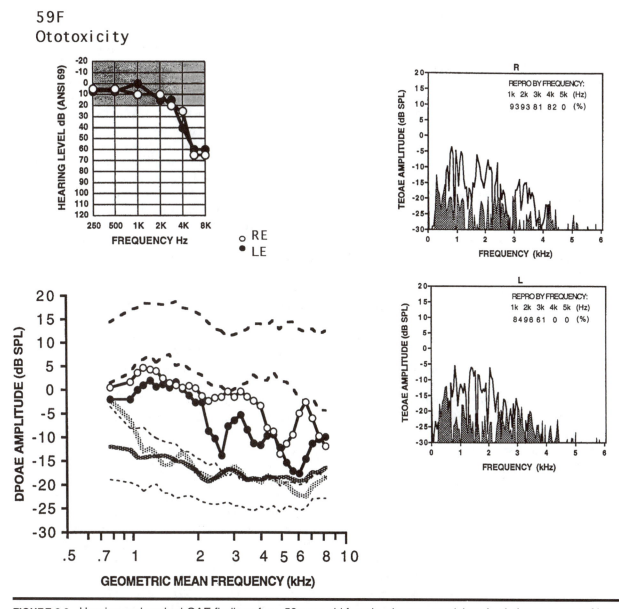

FIGURE 6.6 Hearing and evoked-OAE findings for a 59-year-old female who was receiving cis-platinum as part of her antitumor therapy. Note the symmetrical high-frequency hearing loss associated with ototoxicity shown at the top left. The DP-gram below indicates that DPOAE levels were abnormally low across the entire test range with the left ear (filled circles) exhibiting lower levels than the right (open circles). This asymmetry is also reflected in the TEOAE plots at the right in that the frequency extent for the left ear (lower right) extends only to about 3 kHz, whereas the right ear (upper right) exhibits responses up to about 4 kHz.

is also time-consuming and relatively expensive considering the costs of training highly skilled personnel to both administer and interpret the test. Thus, rather than being used as a universal newborn screener, the ABR has been traditionally used to screen infants identified as being "at-risk" for hearing loss. Although at-risk infants typically comprise about 10% of all newborns, Bess (1993) estimated that only about one-third of these actually undergo ABR testing. In addition, high-risk registers developed to detect

the neonates who are most likely to be susceptible to hereditary-, congenital-, or perinatal-related hearing loss identify, at most, only one-half of the children eventually proven to have significant sensorineural hearing loss (Mauk, White, Mortensen, & Behrens, 1991).

These disheartening facts have, in recent years, led to the proposed strategy of using TEOAEs to test all newborns. In this manner, a rapid pass/fail decision can be achieved that reveals whether the threshold of hearing is less than, or greater than about 30 dB HL, respectively (Bray & Kemp, 1987; Hurley & Musiek, 1994). Indeed, TEOAEs are being used in a number of settings as an indicator of hearing difficulties in newborns (Decreton, Hanssens, & De Sloovere, 1991; Doyle, Burggraaff, Fujikawa, Kim, & MacArthur, 1997; Elrefaie, Parker, & Bamford, 1996; Francois, Bonfils, & Narcy, 1995; Giebel & Redemann, 1992; Grandori & Lutman, 1996; Hunter, Kimm, Dees, Kennedy, & Thornton, 1994; Huynh, Pollack, & Cunningham, 1996; Kemp & Ryan, 1991, 1993; Kemp, Ryan, & Bray, 1990; McNellis & Klein, 1997; Meredith, Stephens, Hogan, Cartilidge, & Drayton, 1994; Norton, 1994; Oudesluys-Murphy, Vanstraaten, Bholasingh, & Vanzanten, 1996; Plinkert, Sesterhenn, Anold, & Zenner, 1990; Richardson, Williamson, Lenton, Tarlow, & Rudd, 1995; Solomon, Groth, & Anthonisen, 1993; Schorn, 1993; Watkin, 1996a, 1996b).

In the United States, over the past decade, one program in particular, the Rhode Island Hearing Assessment Project, has been instrumental in conducting a clinical-trials study on applying TEOAEs to newborn-hearing screening (Clarkson, Vohr, Blackwell, & White, 1994; Johnson, Maxon, White, & Vohr, 1993; Maxon, White, Behrens, & Vohr, 1995; Vohr & Maxon, 1996; White, 1996; White & Behrens, 1993; White, Maxon, Behrens, Blackwell, & Vohr, 1992; White, Maxon, Vohr, & Behrens, 1993b; White, Vohr, & Behrens, 1993a; White, Vohr, Maxon, Behrens, McPherson, & Mauk, 1994). The Rhode Island program uses TEOAEs for the initial screening, followed by a second-stage TEOAE rescreen for failures and ABR testing for those who again fail the TEOAE. In addition to establishing the feasibility of using TEOAEs as a universal screener for newborns, that is, regardless of whether neonates are classified as being at risk or being healthy, other useful information on emissions screening has been obtained by the Rhode Island project. This beneficial knowledge includes devising probe-fit strategies to ensure valid TEOAE measurements by clearing the outer ear canal of debris before seating the acoustic probe (Chang, Vohr, Norton, & Lekas, 1993). Additional useful information concerns calculating the cost efficiency of operating a TEOAE-screening program (Maxon et al., 1995) and establishing the validity of using special-purpose TEOAE devices (Maxon, Vohr, & White, 1996), or customized versions of the standard adult protocol, such as the Quickscreen test option (Vohr et al., 1993), to screen infant hearing. Finally, the Rhode Island newborn-screening program has been a leader in developing new approaches that integrate screening with database management strategies (Culpepper, 1997).

Another large newborn hearing screening program that uses TEOAEs is the Concerted Action on Otoacoustic Emissions project sponsored by the European Community (EC). By combining the expertise of researchers, engineers, and clinicians, the goal of the EC program is "to promote the development and application of otoemissions in monitoring, prevention and follow-up of hearing handicaps" (Grandori, 1994a). Although the EC consortium is investigating the general application of OAEs to audiological problems, a major goal of the project is to develop recording methods and perform clinical trials investigating the utility of TEOAEs as a newborn hearing screening test (Grandori & Lutman, 1996). Thus, a great deal of useful information on this application and related issues is emerging in the literature due to the efforts of the various investigators involved in the European Concerted Action project (Grandori, 1994b; Thornton & Grandori, 1994).

Although TEOAEs have been used much more extensively than DPOAEs in newborn-hearing screening, as DPOAE instrumentation has become more readily available, these bitonally elicited emissions are becoming an acceptable applied test of the status of the peripheral-auditory processor in newborns and older infants (Bergman, Gorga, Neely, Kaminski, Beauchaine, & Peters, 1995; Lonsbury-Martin, Martin, McCoy, & Whitehead, 1996). It is anticipated that they will be used more often for this screening application when specially designed DPOAE instruments and software are developed to more deliberately focus on this practical application (Sheppard, Brown, & Russell, 1996).

Given the steady advances in our knowledge base about OAEs, and the rapid improvements in technology, instrumentation, and software development, it is clear that newborn hearing screening using evoked OAEs will become even more commonplace in the years to come. For example, one encouraging technique that makes use of the maximum length sequence (MLS) approach to effect rapid click-stimulus presentation rates promises to make the administration of an OAE screening test a matter of seconds rather than the few minutes it currently takes to perform (Hine & Thornton, 1997; Picton, Kellett, Vezseny, & Rabinovitch, 1993; Thornton, Folkard, & Chambers, 1994). Recently, Culpepper (1997) assembled a comprehensive and helpful review of the clinical, practical, and logistical issues that are involved in establishing an evoked OAE-based neonatal hearing-screening program.

Noise-Exposed Workers, School Children, and the Elderly. The objective and rapid test-administration properties of evoked OAEs also make this an ideal procedure for hearing screening in large numbers of military personnel or industrial workers, who are exposed to high levels of environmental sound, school children, and oldsters living under long-term care conditions. There are a few studies in the literature on screening for hearing problems using evoked OAEs in military personnel (Engdahl, Woxen, Arnesen, & Mair, 1996; Hotz, Probst, Harris, & Hauser, 1993), industrial workers (Kvaerner, Engdahl, Arnesen, & Mair, 1995; Lucertini, Bergamaschi, & Urbani, 1996), and school children (Nozza & Sabo, 1992; Nozza, Sabo, & Mandel,

1997). However, to our knowledge, there is no published work on the worthwhile applications of using emissions to screen for hearing impairment in the elderly.

Monitoring Changes in Hearing

Tracking Dynamic Changes. One advantageous feature of evoked OAE testing is the ability of emissions to actively track changes in the status of cochlear function. There are a number of examples of useful applications of this attribute of OAEs in the literature including the documentation of natural fluctuations in cochlear activity that sometimes occur between examination sessions in patients in the early stages of Ménière's disease (Lonsbury-Martin, McCoy, et al., 1993). Other examples of the ability of OAEs to document dynamic changes in the condition of the OHC system include monitoring the recovery sometimes associated with sudden idiopathic sensorineural hearing loss as noted above. In addition, the administration of glycerol or urea, hyperosmotic agents, which often produce a temporary improvement of hearing sensitivity in Ménière's ears, have also been shown using baseline compared to post-ingestion measures to increase both TEOAE (Bonfils, Uziel, & Pujol, 1988) and DPOAE (Lonsbury-Martin & Martin, 1990; Martin et al., 1990) levels. Other pre/post testing of treatment effects from our own work include documenting the aftereffects of cerebellopontine angle (CPA) surgery for acoustic neuroma removal, intratympanic gentamicin or dexamethasone application for vertigo, endolymphatic-sac surgery for Ménière's disease, insertion of tympanostomy tubes for middle-ear effusion, and pharmacological agent administration (systemic and topical) for middle-ear disease. Together, these data indicate that OAEs can be used to dynamically track temporal changes in cochlear condition.

It is interesting to note that evoked-OAE testing is also being used as an intraoperative monitoring procedure due to its faithful and immediate sensitivity to cochlear malfunction, and its ability to be measured quite rapidly in what is essentially real time. In this manner, neurotological surgeons are depending on the timely feedback from either TEOAE (Cane, O'Donoghue, & Lutman, 1992) or DPOAE (Telischi, Widick, Lonsbury-Martin, & McCoy, 1995) recordings to ensure hearing preservation during CPA surgery. However, it is important to note that often eustachian-tube function is impaired during anesthesia, which results in a buildup of negative pressure in the middle ear. As noted above, negative middle-ear pressure reduces or eliminates OAEs, particularly over the low- to mid-frequency range, even when the cochlea is normal. Interestingly, decrements in OAE levels in humans have been reported during general anesthesia and appear to be primarily due to middle-ear factors (Hauser, Probst, Harris, & Frei, 1992). However, in the majority of cases, anesthetic-induced negative pressure in the middle ear does not appear to have an adverse influence on the monitoring of OAEs during CPA surgery (Telischi, Widick, et al., 1995).

Tracking Progressive Changes. Other applications of the temporal-tracking features of evoked OAEs include confirming the development of more progressive disorders such as inherited disorders or presbycusis (Lonsbury-Martin, Whitehead, & Martin, 1991). In individuals like these, it is straightforward to regularly monitor cochlear function in order to detect any unexpected reductions in OHC-related activity that may require habilitative intervention.

In combination with the accurate tracking properties of evoked OAEs, their unique ability to specifically measure the effects of stimulus transduction by the OHCs can be used for the purpose of monitoring the effects of ototoxic drugs on the ears of patients who are receiving regular doses as part of their treatment regimen. Because of this latter attribute, OAEs can delineate quite precisely the frequency boundary between normally functioning cochlear regions and those impaired by the administration of ototoxic antibiotics or chemotherapeutic drugs. As noted above, there are a number of examples in the literature of the adverse consequences on evoked OAEs of treatment with, in particular, the antitumor agent, cis-platinum. However, to date, to our knowledge, no reports have been published describing the serial measurement of OAEs in an ototoxicity monitoring program.

The plots of Figure 6.7 illustrate the objective OAE serial testing in the right ear of a patient receiving a moderately high dose of cis-platinum (100 mg/M^2) for the treatment of a lung malignancy. It is clear from the baseline audiograms (filled circles), TEOAE spectrum (top right), and DP-gram (hashed line beginning on the *y*-axis at about 20 dB SPL) that this 59-year-old female patient showed some prior signs of presbycusis in the form of a mild audiometric hearing loss and low-normal levels of DPOAE activity for frequencies above about 3 kHz. Following the first dose of cis-platinum, audiometric hearing thresholds (open circles) were elevated further for both conventional and ultra-high frequency test tones, and DPOAEs (open circles) were more reduced. Finally, after the second cis-platinum treatment (open triangles), although audiometric hearing was not additionally affected, both the TEOAEs and DPOAEs showed further reductions in their levels, particularly for frequencies >2 kHz.

Thus, serial OAE testing provides a simple, objective, and accurate measure of drug-induced hearing loss that can even be used at the bedside for critically ill patients. Using OAEs to identify the early stages of such sensorineural hearing losses can provide the clinician with the opportunity to reestablish informed consent with patients and families regarding the ototoxic consequences of certain medications. Moreover, treatment regimens can be changed in certain cases in which ototoxicity is demonstrable, or

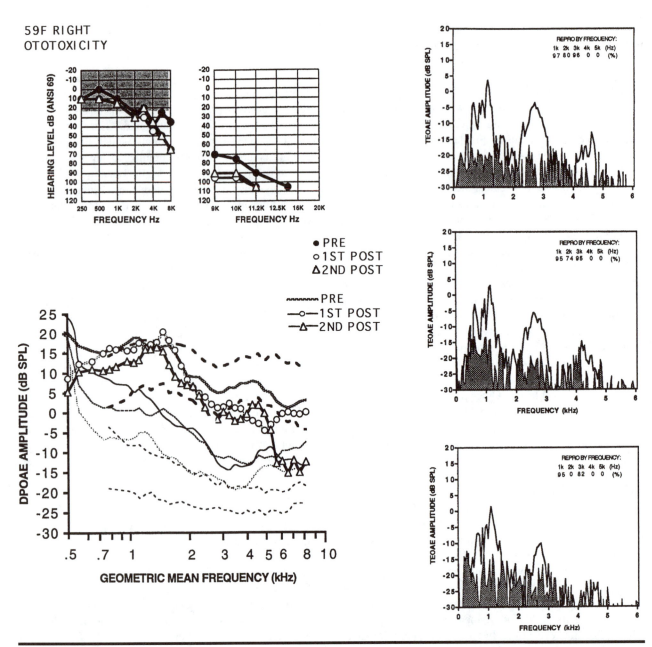

FIGURE 6.7   Hearing and evoked-OAE results for both ears of a 59-year-old female with a lung carcinoma. Data were obtained before (PRE) and following two drug treatments (1ST and 2ND POST) with the anti-neoplastic agent cis-platinum. The plots at the top left show the conventional and ultra-high frequency behavioral audiograms obtained pre-(filled symbols) and post-treatment (open symbols) for the right ear. Before treatment (filled circles), hearing was normal up to about 2 kHz, above which a mild hearing loss, likely associated with presbycusis, was observed over the higher-frequency range. The DP-gram below indicates that before treatment (hatched line), DPOAE levels were essentially within normal limits for this ear. Three weeks following the initial treatment (open circles), hearing thresholds above 3 kHz were elevated to 45 dB HL or greater. The corresponding DP-gram below shows DPOAE levels also decreased at frequencies >1 kHz following the first drug treatment (open circles). The TEOAE plots at the right show little change between the baseline (top) and first-treatment (middle) records. After the second treatment (open triangles), there was, in essence, no change in behavioral hearing. However, DPOAEs continued to decrease for frequencies above about 1 kHz, and showed a precipitous drop to noise-floor levels for test frequencies above about 5 kHz. The TEOAE plot at the bottom right also shows lower levels for emissions greater than about 1 kHz.

the rate of administration can be slowed to control the magnitude of the ototoxic reaction. Thus, specific therapeutic interventions can be recommended based on the outcome of OAE testing.

Cochlear-Efferent System Testing.   Anatomical data indicate that the majority of medial olivocochlear efferent fibers cross below the floor of the fourth ventricle so that they form axosomatic synapses along the base and lateral aspects of the OHCs of the ipsilateral cochlea. Thus, the OHCs receive descending input directly and mainly from contralateral auditory brainstem structures. The contralateral acoustic stimulation (CAS) method developed by Collet and his colleagues (Collet, Kemp, et al., 1990) using a broadband noise 15 dB above the perceptual threshold and evoked OAEs take advantage of this anatomical arrangement in order to noninvasively assess the status of efferent-system function in human ears. The underlying assumption of comparing OAE levels in the presence and absence of a CAS is that the emitted responses provide the most direct means of observing overall efferent effects on OHC activity. Contralateral sound stimulation has been shown to induce a reduction in the levels of both TEOAEs (Collet, Kemp, et al., 1990; Veuillet, Collet, & Duclaux, 1991) and DPOAEs (Chery-Croze, Moulin, & Collet, 1993; Moulin, Collet, & Duclaux, 1993). The suppression effect of about 0.5 to 1 dB of the overall emission level has been demonstrated to be almost entirely due to the olivocochlear-efferent system (Collet, Veuillet, Bene, & Morgon, 1992).

Berlin and his colleagues (Berlin, Hood, Wen, Szabo, Cecola, Rigby, & Jackson, 1993) modified the CAS technique in order to uncover a larger suppression of TEOAE levels. Toward this end, they focused on a temporal interval between about 12 and 14 ms, which emphasizes the contribution of mid-frequency cochlear regions to the overall emission level. Using this approach and correlating response levels, phase, and timing delays between TEOAE waveforms collected in the presence and absence of CAS, these investigators identified efferent-reducing effects of up to 7 dB, in specific cases. Further refinements of the CAS-induced reductions in evoked OAEs have used ipsilateral and binaural stimulation methods compared to the contralateral strategy in order to show the greater suppression effects of binaurally applied suppressors (Berlin, Hood, Hurley, Wen, & Kemp, 1995).

Using the temporal-windowing CAS strategy, Berlin, Hood, Hurley, and Wen (1994) uncovered an interesting group of neurologically impaired patients who exhibited robust TEOAEs, no CAS-suppression effect, abnormal or absent ABRs, and no masking level-difference effects. These findings suggest that the CAS-efferent test is sensitive to abnormalities in auditory-brainstem pathways that include the descending cochlear-efferent system.

Other collaborative research between our own colleagues and those of Axelsson in Sweden (Eliasson, Magnusson, Anari, Lonsbury-Martin, & Axelsson, in press) demonstrated in patients complaining of hyperacusis the ability of CAS to suppress to a greater degree DPOAEs in the ipsilateral test ear than in a group of normal hearing individuals. These results suggest that abnormal levels of efferent activity may contribute to the difficulties that patients with hyperacusis experience in appreciating acoustic-stimulus levels in a normal manner.

Certainly, work aimed at uncovering the clinical usefulness of evoked OAEs as part of a test battery for examining auditory efferent-system function is only in its beginning stages. Based on the interesting findings of the few studies that have examined efferent function, to date, in select patient populations, it seems likely that efferent testing using evoked OAEs will eventually become an important part of the assessment of central auditory processing disorders.

Identifying Pseudohypacusics.   The term pseudohypacusis specifies a hearing loss that is greater than can be explained by a pathology of the auditory system. Nonorganic hearing loss can exist as a psychogenic deafness or as intentional malingering. Traditionally, establishing a diagnosis of a functional hearing loss has been time consuming in that typically the examiner needs to identify some discrepancy in the results of a set of audiological tests. Because evoked-OAE testing requires minimal patient compliance, it has been used successfully to detect pseudohypacusis in several patient populations consisting of either adults in which there is a suspicion on account of monetary compensation for a trauma-induced hearing loss, or children anticipating the possibility of secondary gains due to having a hearing disorder (Durrant, Kesterson, & Kamerer, 1997; Kvaerner, Engdahl, Aursnes, Arnesen, & Mair, 1996; Musiek, Bornstein, & Rintelmann, 1995). In Figure 6.8, the results of both audiometric and OAE testing are shown for a 35-year-old male patient who claimed that a fall on the waxy floor of a municipal airport caused deafness in his left ear (filled circles). Although the profound hearing loss exhibited by the clinical audiogram appeared to support his claim for economic compensation, the healthy and bilaterally symmetrical DPOAE activity indicated that the cochlea was essentially unharmed by the mishap. These data suggested the appropriateness of a subsequent ABR test to rule out a retrocochlear pathology. However, in this case, the bilaterally normal ABRs indicated the absence of a retrocochlear pathology, too. Thus, together, the outcome of the audiometric evaluations implied that the patient was most likely not fully compliant during the behavioral-hearing assessment. (See Chapter 14 for further discussion of pseudohypacusis).

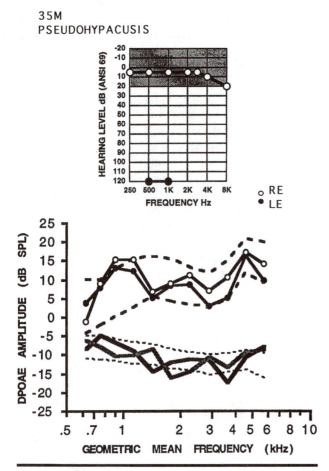

FIGURE 6.8 Hearing and evoked-OAE findings for both ears of a 35-year-old male complaining of an injury-related hearing loss in his left (filled circles) ear. Although hearing thresholds were immeasurable for this ear, DPOAEs were present bilaterally within normal limits.

FINAL CONSIDERATIONS

The relationship between evoked-OAE amplitude reduction and hearing-threshold elevation depends on stimulus parameters, particularly with respect to DPOAEs. Thus, the L_1 and L_2 stimulus levels, L_1-L_2, and f_2/f_1 may all vary how much DPOAE amplitude reduction will be associated with a given threshold elevation. It has been shown in humans that DPOAE amplitudes are reduced by approximately 0.4 dB per 1 dB elevation of hearing threshold in subjects with sensorineural hearing losses (Whitehead, McCoy, Martin, & Lonsbury-Martin, 1993). However, this slope presumably increases with decreasing frequency. Also, decreasing L_2 below L_1 increases the degree of DPOAE-amplitude reduction for a given threshold elevation (Sutton et al., 1994; Whitehead, McCoy, et al., 1995).

Further, over a wide variety of cochlear traumas, there is often more behavioral or evoked-potential threshold elevation than OAE-amplitude reduction. In general, this finding is to be expected, because OAEs are thought to reflect only those hearing losses arising from dysfunction of the cochlear amplifier, whereas behavioral or evoked-potential thresholds will reflect dysfunction of other components of the cochlea, or at the neural level, in addition to dysfunction of the cochlear amplifier. However, although there is often substantial variability of the relationship between OAE-level reduction and hearing-threshold elevation, there does not appear to be any consistent evidence for greater reductions in emission amplitude than expected on the basis of the associated hearing or evoked-potential threshold elevations.

In patient groups, most sensory hearing loss appears to occur in the high frequencies associated with the basal turn, and this is associated with a high frequency loss of OAEs. Presumably, these phenomena reflect trauma to OHCs, which appears to be greatest in the basal turn. It also appears that OAEs are reduced by very minor hearing losses, and that such a hearing loss is often associated with dysfunction of OHCs, which are the first components of the ear to reflect many cochlear traumas.

CONCLUSIONS

Findings showing that there is no direct afferent neural involvement in the generation of OAEs, and that OAEs are influenced by stimulation of the olivocochlear-efferent system, which preferentially innervates the OHCs, are consistent with the proposed involvement of OHC electromotility in the generation of OAEs. Together, these observations support the assumption that OAEs are particularly valuable as specific indicators of the status of the sensory component of the hearing process. Thus, findings from clinical studies indicate that OAEs can help differentiate cochlear from retrocochlear losses, and further, to specifically detect a particular sensory component of hearing loss. Clearly, therefore, OAEs represent a valuable differential diagnostic tool for use in the hearing clinic. However, the significant dependence of OAE levels in the ear canal upon the status of the middle ear indicates that the use of OAEs in clinical tests must be combined with assessment of middle-ear function.

In general, the results of studies in human patient groups are highly consistent. Factors known to cause both temporary and permanent sensorineural hearing loss have been found to reduce or abolish all OAE types in humans. Those traumas that result primarily in damage to the OHC system (i.e., ototoxins, noise overexposure) tend to demonstrate a greater correlation of OAE reductions with behavioral or electrophysiological measures of hearing impairment, whereas this correlation is less clear in the more complicated pathologies involving Ménière's disease, sudden hearing loss, and acoustic neuroma.

Animal experiments indicate that DPOAEs elicited by high-level stimuli, that is, above 65 to 70 dB SPL, do not appear to reflect the action of the cochlear amplifier or the integrity of OHCs. However, it is not clear to what extent, or over what range of stimulus levels, this situation also applies in humans. In human patients with sensorineural hearing loss, on average, TEOAEs appear to show a similar amplitude reduction with hearing-threshold elevation as do DPOAEs evoked at moderate levels. Certainly, in human patients, even DPOAEs at high stimulus levels ($L_1 = L_2 = 75$ dB SPL) are affected by cochlear traumas. In clinical practice, stimulus levels of 60 to 75 dB SPL are commonly used and appear to perform well in the detection of hearing loss. In fact, for screening tests that aim to detect early-loss conditions (e.g., screening in a hearing-conservation program), offset-level primary-tone conditions, such as $L_1 = 65$ dB and $L_2 = 55$ dB SPL, may be the stimulus parameters most sensitive to early changes in cochlear function (e.g., Sutton et al., 1994).

Thus, because experimental manipulations like the deliberate administration of loop diuretics or an induced temporary anoxia cannot be used in human subjects due to ethical considerations and because of the different parametric properties of DPOAEs in humans than in other mammalian species, it is not clear whether there are distinct low- and high-level DPOAE components in humans as in other species. Interestingly, in salicylate-treated humans, it was found to be possible to eliminate SOAEs without reducing DPOAEs evoked by low primary-tone levels. This suggests at least partially separate generation processes of DPOAEs and the other OAEs in humans. Clearly, the relationship of the DPOAE generator to the TEOAE/SFOAE generator in humans requires further study.

In humans, otherwise normal ears are sometimes encountered in which either TEOAEs and/or DPOAEs are very small or absent in quite wide frequency regions. To date, it is not clear whether this phenomenon reflects the low-end of the range of normal variability of OAE levels in normal ears, or whether OAEs are sometimes reduced or absent in the presence of normal hearing thresholds. This is a critical issue for the clinical utility of OAEs. If OAEs are reduced in the absence of hearing threshold elevation, then false positive errors will occur. However, if OAEs begin to decrease before hearing threshold increases, then it is possible that OAEs may allow us to predict future hearing loss, which would be of great value. However, there is no clear evidence for or against this alternative yet, other than a few case studies like those presented above in Figure 6.2. Along this line, it is possible that OAE reductions may be detected before threshold elevations, even when the sensitivity to trauma is similar, because they are typically measured in much finer resolution (e.g., fractions of a dB relative to the ±5 dB used to test hearing). However, establishing whether OAEs have the ability to detect the onset

of cochlear pathologies prior to existing audiometric tests can only be accomplished with careful and systematic studies. Such studies may involve longitudinal measurements of OAEs in combination with hearing thresholds in new workers in noisy industrial environments, or normal-hearing patients about to undergo therapy with ototoxic drugs.

Both TEOAEs and DPOAEs are capable of providing information regarding the frequency extent and time course of sensorineural hearing losses of various etiologies in human ears. However, it appears that TEOAEs and DPOAEs may be influenced in different ways by various traumas. Evidence from human studies suggests that aspirin has less effect on DPOAEs than on TEOAEs and the other OAE types. Some sort of differentiation of TEOAEs from DPOAEs is also suggested by the different relative amplitudes of these emission types in humans and the small laboratory mammals. These findings suggest that DPOAEs may be generated by a partially independent mechanism to TEOAEs. Furthermore, experimental studies in animal models have clearly demonstrated that the sensitivity of DPOAEs to cochlear traumas (e.g., anoxia, acute administration of loop diuretics, and chronic aminoglycoside poisoning) is dependent on the level of the f_1 and f_2 stimulus tones. This suggests that separate mechanisms are responsible for the generation of $2f_1-f_2$ DPOAEs at low- and high-stimulus levels. The results of experimental studies suggest that the low-level DPOAE component depends upon the integrity both of the energy supply to the organ of Corti and of the OHCs. The high-level DPOAEs appear relatively independent of these factors, although they, too, can be reduced by trauma.

Because of the differences between DPOAEs in humans and the small mammals, in particular the large difference in the absolute amplitude of $2f_1-f_2$ DPOAEs over much of the frequency range, it is not clear that there are two distinct components of $2f_1-f_2$ DPOAEs in humans, as appears to be the case in small mammals. This issue clearly needs to be resolved. If humans also possess discrete low-level more vulnerable and high-level less vulnerable DPOAE components, then careful attention must be paid to the stimulus parameters to be used in clinical tests utilizing DPOAEs, as lower-level stimuli would be expected to be more faithful indicators of cochlear condition. If humans do not possess distinct DPOAE components, this may limit the relevance of studies of DPOAEs in animal models to the human situation.

In summary, there is a great deal of evidence suggesting that OAEs are produced by the action of the cochlear amplifier. However, the evidence suggesting that OAEs are produced by precisely the same mechanism as the cochlear amplifier (i.e., the enhancement of cochlear partition vibration presumably by the actions of electromotile OHCs), while consistent, is not absolute, because: (1) Many cochlear manipulations in animal models, and etiologies of hearing loss in humans, involve trauma to several components of the cochlea; and (2) there appears to be great variability of the relationship of OAEs to cochlear dysfunction. This may arise from a number of different reasons, many of which are being addressed in both basic and clinical studies.

Despite our incomplete understanding of the generation processes underlying the production of OAEs and the exact relationship of OAE features to measures of hearing ability, emissions are being used in a number of distinct applications in various clinical settings. The major applications include: (1) the differential diagnosis of hearing difficulties to assist in determining the primary site of the problem; (2) serial monitoring in potential ototoxicity and intraoperative procedures, tracking progressive disorders, and determining the efficacy of medical/surgical treatments by making pre- versus post-comparisons; (3) hearing screening in difficult-to-test patients including newborns, multiply handicapped persons, school children, the elderly, workers participating in hearing-conservation programs and so on; (4) cochlear-efferent system testing; and (5) identifying pseudohypacusics. As both our experience with OAE testing and our knowledge of their biological basis continue to grow, otoacoustic emissions promise to become an even more important component of the routine audiological test battery.

REFERENCES

Amadee, R. G. (1995). The effects of chronic otitis media with effusion on the measurement of transiently evoked otoacoustic emissions. *Laryngoscope, 105*, 589–595.

American Academy of Otolaryngology—Head and Neck Surgery (1990). Infant hearing screening program launched. *Bulletin of the American Academy of Otolaryngology—Head and Neck Surgery, 9*, 46–47.

Anderson, S. D. (1980). Some ECMR properties in relation to other signals from the auditory periphery. *Hearing Research, 2*, 273–296.

Balkany, T. J., Telischi, F. F., Lonsbury-Martin, B. L., & Martin, G. K. (1994). Otoacoustic emissions in clinical practice. *American Journal of Otology, 15, Supplement 1*, 29–38.

Bergman, B., Gorga, M., Neely, S., Kaminski, J., Beauchaine, K., & Peters, J. (1995). Preliminary descriptions of transient evoked and distortion product otoacoustic emissions from graduates of an intensive care nursery. *Journal of the American Academy of Audiology, 6*, 150–162.

Berlin, C. I., Hood, L. J., Hurley, A., & Wen, H. (1994). Contralateral suppression of otoacoustic emissions: An index of the function of the medial olivocochlear system. *Otolaryngology—Head and Neck Surgery, 110*, 3–21.

Berlin, C. I., Hood, L. J., Hurley, A. E., Wen, H., & Kemp, D. T. (1995). Binaural noise suppresses linear click-evoked otoacoustic emissions more than ipsilateral or contralateral noise. *Hearing Research, 87*, 96–103.

Berlin, C. I., Hood, L. J., Wen, H., Szabo, P., Cecola, R. P., Rigby, P., & Jackson, D. F. (1993). Contralateral suppression of nonlinear click-evoked otoacoustic emissions. *Hearing Research, 71*, 1–11.

Berninger, E., Karlsson, K. K., Hellgren, U., & Eskilsson, G. (1995). Magnitude changes in transient evoked otoacoustic emissions and high-level $2f_1$-f_2 distortion products in man during quinine administration. *Scandinavian Audiology, 24*, 27–32.

Bess, F. H. (1993). Early identification of hearing loss: The whys, hows, and whens. *The Hearing Journal, 46*, 22–25.

Bonfils, P. (1989). Spontaneous otoacoustic emissions: Clinical interest. *Laryngoscope, 99*, 752–756.

Bonfils, P., Bertrand, Y., & Uziel, A. (1988). Evoked otoacoustic emissions: Normative data and presbycusis. *Audiology, 27*, 27–35.

Bonfils, P., & Uziel, A. (1988). Evoked otoacoustic emissions in patients with acoustic neuromas. *American Journal of Otology, 9*, 412–417.

Bonfils, P., Uziel, A., & Pujol, R. (1988). Evoked otoacoustic emissions from adults and infants: Clinical applications. *Acta Otolaryngologica, 105*, 445–449.

Bray, P., & Kemp, D. T. (1987). An advanced cochlear echo technique suitable for infant screening. *British Journal of Audiology, 21*, 191–204.

Brown, A. M., & Kemp, D. T. (1984). Suppressibility of the $2f_1$-f_2 stimulated acoustic emissions in gerbil and man. *Hearing Research, 13*, 29–37.

Brownell, W. E. (1990): Outer hair cell electromotility and otoacoustic emissions. *Ear and Hearing, 11*, 82–92.

Brownell, W. E., Bader, C. R., Bertrand, D., & Ribaupierre, Y. (1985). Evoked mechanical responses of isolated outer hair cells. *Science, 227*, 194–196.

Brownell, W. E., & Lue, A. J. C. (1996). Hair cell motility. *Current Opinions in Otolaryngology—Head and Neck Surgery, 4*, 289–293.

Brummett, R. E., & Fox, K. E. (1989). Aminoglycoside-induced hearing loss in humans. *Antimicrobial Agents and Chemotherapy, 33*, 797–800.

Cane, M. A., O'Donoghue, G. M., & Lutman, M. E. (1992). The feasibility of using oto-acoustic emissions to monitor cochlear function during acoustic neuroma surgery. *Scandinavian Audiology, 21*, 131–141.

Chang, K. W., Vohr, B. R., Norton, S. J., & Lekas, M. D. (1993). External and middle ear status related to evoked otoacoustic emission in neonates. *Archives of Otolaryngology—Head and Neck Surgery, 119*, 276–282.

Chery-Croze, S., Moulin, A., & Collet, L. (1993). Effect of contralateral sound stimulation on the distortion product $2f_1$-f_2 in humans: Evidence of a frequency specificity. *Hearing Research, 68*, 53–58.

Clarkson, R. L., Vohr, B. R., Blackwell, P. M., & White, K. R. (1994). Universal infant hearing screening and intervention: The Rhode Island Program. *Infants and Young Children, 6*, 65–74.

Collet, L., Kemp, D. T., Veuillet, E., Duclaux, R., Moulin, A., & Morgon, A. (1990). Effect of contralateral auditory stimuli on active cochlear micro-mechanical properties in human subjects. *Hearing Research, 43*, 251–262.

Collet, L., Moulin, M., Gartner, M., & Morgon, A. (1990). Age-related changes in evoked otoacoustic emissions. *Annals of Otology, Rhinology and Laryngology, 99*, 993–997.

Collet, L., Veuillet, E., Bene, J., & Morgon, A. (1992). Effects of contralateral white noise on click-evoked emissions in normal and sensorineural ears: Towards an exploration of the medial olivocochlear system. *Audiology, 31*, 1–7.

Culpepper, N. B. (1997). Neonatal screening via evoked otoacoustic emissions. In M. S. Robinette, & T. J. Glattke (Eds.), *Otoacoustic Emissions: Clinical Applications* (pp. 233–270). New York: Thieme.

Dallmayr, C. (1987). Stationary and dynamical properties of simultaneous evoked otoacoustic emissions (SEOAE). *Acustica, 63*, 243–255.

Davis, H. (1983). An active process in cochlear mechanics. *Hearing Research, 9*, 79–90.

Daya, H., Amedofu, G., Woodrow, C. J., Agranoff, D., Brobby, G., Agbenyega, T., & Krishna, S. (1997). Assessment of cochlear damage after pneumococcal meningitis using otoacoustic emissions. *Transactions of the Royal Society of Tropical Medical Hygiene, 91*, 248–249.

Decker, T. N. (1997). General recording considerations and clinical instrument options. In M. S. Robinette & T. J. Glattke (Eds.), *Otoacoustic Emissions: Clinical Applications* (pp. 307–332). New York: Thieme.

Decreton, S. J. R. C., Hanssens, K., & De Sloovere, M. (1991). Evoked otoacoustic emissions in infant hearing screening. *International Journal of Pediatric Otorhinolaryngology, 21*, 235–247.

Doyle, K. J. O., Burggraaff, B., Fujikawa, S., Kim, J. U., & MacArthur, C. J. (1997). Neonatal hearing screening with otoscopy, auditory brain stem response, and otoacoustic emissions. *Otolaryngology—Head and Neck Surgery, 116*, 597–603.

Durrant, J. D., Kesterson, R. K., & Kamerer, D. B. (1997). Evaluation of the nonorganic hearing loss suspect. *American Journal of Otology, 18*, 361–367.

Eliasson, A., Magnusson, L., Anari, M., Lonsbury-Martin, B. L., & Axelsson, A. (in press). Effects of contralateral acoustic stimulation on distortion-product otoacoustic emissions in patients with hyperacusis. *Scandinavian Audiology*.

Elrefaie, A., Parker, D. J., & Bamford, J. M. (1996). Otoacoustic emission versus ABR screening: The effect of external and middle ear abnormalities in a group of SCBU neonates. *British Journal of Audiology, 30*, 3–8.

Engdahl, B. (1996). Effects of noise and exercise on distortion product otoacoustic emissions. *Hearing Research, 93*, 72–82.

Engdahl, B., & Kemp, D. T. (1996). The effect of noise exposure on the details of distortion product otoacoustic emissions in humans. *Journal of the Acoustical Society of America, 99*, 1573–1587.

Engdahl, B., Woxen, O., Arnesen, A. R., & Mair, I. W. S. (1996). Transient evoked otoacoustic emissions as screening for hearing losses at the school for military training. *Scandinavian Audiology, 25*, 71–78.

Fortnum, H., Farnsworth, A., & Davis, A. (1993). The feasibility of evoked otoacoustic emissions as an in-patient hearing check after meningitis. *British Journal of Audiology, 27*, 227–231.

Francois, M., Bonfils, P., & Narcy, P. (1995). Screening for neonatal and infant deafness in Europe in 1992. *International Journal of Pediatric Otolaryngology, 31*, 175–182.

Gaskill, S. A., & Brown, A. M. (1990). The behavior of the acoustic distortion product, $2f_1-f_2$, from the human ear and its relation to auditory sensitivity. *Journal Acoustical Society of America, 88*, 821–839.

Giebel, A., & Redemann, E. (1992). Screening infants and children by means of TEOAE. *The Hearing Journal, 45*, 25–28.

Glattke, T. J., & Robinette, M. S. (1997). Transient evoked otoacoustic emissions. In M. S. Robinette & T. J. Glattke (Eds.), *Otoacoustic Emissions: Clinical Applications* (pp. 63–82). New York: Thieme.

Gorga, M. P., Stover, L., Neely, S. T., & Montoya, D. (1996). The use of cumulative distributions to determine critical values and levels of confidence for clinical distortion product otoacoustic emission measurements. *Journal of the Acoustical Society of America, 100*, 968–977.

Govaerts, P. J., Claes, J., Van De Heyning, P. H., Jorens, Ph. G., Marquet, J., & De Broe, M. E. (1990). Aminoglycoside-induced ototoxicity. *Toxicology Letter, 52*, 227–251.

Grandori, F. (1994a). The European Concerted Action on otoacoustic emissions. In F. Grandori (Ed.), *Advances In Otoacoustic Emissions, vol 1, Fundamental and Clinical Applications* (pp. v–vii). Brussels: Commission of the European Communities.

Grandori, F. (1994b). *Advances in Otoacoustic Emissions, vol 1, Fundamental and Clinical Applications* (pp. 1–164). Brussels: Commission of the European Communities.

Grandori, F., & Lutman, M. E. (1996). Neonatal screening programs in Europe: Towards a consensus development conference. *Audiology, 35*, 291–295.

Gravel, J. S., & Stapells, D. R. (1993). Behavioral, electrophysiologic, and otoacoustic measures from a child with auditory processing dysfunction: Case report. *Journal of the American Academy of Audiology, 4*, 441–419.

Harris, F. P. (1990). Distortion-product otoacoustic emissions in humans with high frequency sensorineural hearing loss. *Journal of Speech Hearing Research, 33*, 594–600.

Harris, F. P., Lonsbury-Martin, B. L., Stagner, B. B., Coats, A. C., & Martin, G. K. (1989). Acoustic distortion products in humans: Systematic changes in amplitude as a function of f_2/f_1 ratio. *Journal of the Acoustical Society of America, 85*, 220–229.

Harris, F. P., & Probst, R. (1992). Transiently evoked otoacoustic emissions in patients with Ménière's disease. *Acta Otolaryngologica, 112*, 36–44.

Harris, F. P., & Probst, R. (1997). Otoacoustic emissions and audiometric outcomes. In M. S. Robinette & T. J. Glattke (Eds.), *Otoacoustic Emissions: Clinical Applications* (pp. 151–180). New York: Thieme.

Hauser, R., Probst, R., & Harris, F. P. (1993). Effects of atmospheric pressure variation on spontaneous, transiently evoked, and distortion product otoacoustic emissions in normal human ears. *Hearing Research, 69*, 133–145.

Hauser, R., Probst, R., Harris, F. P., & Frei, F. (1992). Influence of general anesthesia on transiently evoked otoacoustic emissions in humans. *Annals of Otology, Rhinology and Laryngology, 101*, 994–999.

He, N-J., & Schmiedt, R. A. (1993). Fine structure of the $2f_1-f_2$ acoustic distortion product: Changes with primary level. *Journal of the Acoustical Society of America, 94*, 2659–2669.

He, N-J., & Schmiedt, R. A. (1996). Effects of aging on the fine structure of $2f_1-f_2$ acoustic distortion product. *Journal of the Acoustical Society of America, 99*, 1002–1015.

Hine, J. E., & Thornton, A. R. D. (1997). Transient evoked otoacoustic emissions recorded using maximum length sequences as a function of stimulus rate and level. *Ear and Hearing, 18*, 121–128.

Hotz, M. A., Harris, F. P., & Probst, R. (1994). Otoacoustic emissions: An approach for monitoring aminoglycoside-induced ototoxicity. *Laryngoscope, 14*, 1130–1134.

Hotz, M. A., Probst, R., Harris, F. P., & Hauser, R. (1993). Monitoring the effects of noise exposure using transiently evoked otoacoustic emissions. *Acta Otolaryngologica, 113*, 478–482.

Hunter, M. F., Kimm, L., Dees, D. C., Kennedy, C. R., & Thornton, A. R. D. (1994). Feasibility of otoacoustic emission detection followed by ABR as a universal neonatal screening test for hearing impairment. *British Journal of Audiology, 28*, 47–51.

Hurley, R. M., & Musiek, F. E. (1994). Effectiveness of transient-evoked otoacoustic emissions (TEOAEs) in predicting hearing level. *Journal of the American Academy of Audiology, 5*, 195–203.

Huynh, M. T., Pollack, R. A., & Cunningham, R. A. J. (1996). Universal newborn hearing screening: Feasibility in a community hospital. *Journal of Family Practice, 42*, 487–490.

Johnsen, N. J., & Elberling, C. (1982a). Evoked acoustic emissions from the human ear. I. Equipment and response parameters. *Scandinavian Audiology, 11*, 3–12.

Johnsen, N. J., & Elberling, C. (1982b). Evoked acoustic emissions from the human ear. II. Normative data from young adults and influence of posture. *Scandinavian Audiology, 11*, 69–77.

Johnson, M. J., Maxon, A. B., White, K. R., & Vohr, B. R. (1993). Operating a hospital-based universal newborn hearing screening program using transient evoked otoacoustic emissions. *Seminars in Hearing, 14*, 46–56.

Johnstone, B. M., Patuzzi, R., & Yates, G. K. (1986). Basilar membrane measurements and the travelling wave. *Hearing Research, 22*, 147–153.

Karlsson, K. K., Berninger, E., & Alvan, G. (1991). The effect of quinine on psychoacoustic tuning curves, stapedius reflexes and evoked otoacoustic emissions in healthy volunteers. *Scandinavian Audiology, 20*, 83–90.

Kemp, D. T. (1978). Stimulated acoustic emissions from within the human auditory system. *Journal of the Acoustical Society of America, 64*, 1386–1391.

Kemp, D. T. (1979). Evidence of mechanical nonlinearity and frequency selective wave amplification in the cochlea. *Archives of Otorhinolaryngology, 224*, 37–45.

Kemp, D. T. (1980). Towards a model for the origin of cochlear echoes. *Hearing Research, 2*, 533–548.

Kemp, D. T. (1981). Physiologically active cochlear micromechanics—one source of tinnitus. In D. Evered & G. Lawrenson (Eds.), *Tinnitus* (pp. 54–81). London: Pitman Books Ltd.

Kemp, D. T. (1982). Cochlear echoes: Implications for noise-induced hearing loss. In R. P. Hamernik, D. Henderson, &

R. Salvi (Eds.), *New Perspectives on Noise-Induced Hearing Loss* (pp. 189–207). New York: Raven Press.

Kemp, D. T., Bray, P., Alexander, L., & Brown, A. M. (1986). Acoustic emission cochleography—practical aspects. In G. Cianfrone & F. Grandori (Eds.), *Cochlear Mechanics and Otoacoustic Emissions, Scandinavian Audiology, Supplement 25*, 71–96.

Kemp, D. T., & Brown, A. M. (1983). A comparison of mechanical nonlinearities in the cochleae of man and gerbil from ear canal measurements. In R. Klinke, & R. Hartmann (Eds.), *Hearing—Physiological Bases and Psychophysics* (pp. 82–88). Berlin: Springer-Verlag.

Kemp, D. T., & Chum, R. (1980). Observations on the generator mechanism of stimulus frequency acoustic emissions, two-tone suppression. In G. van den Brink, & F. A. Bilsen (Eds.), *Psychophysical, Physiological and Behavioural Studies in Hearing* (pp. 34–41). Delft: Delft Univ Press.

Kemp, D. T., & Ryan, S. (1991). Otoacoustic emission tests in neonatal screening programmes. *Acta Otolaryngologica, Supplement 482*, 73–84.

Kemp, D. T., & Ryan, S. (1993). The use of transient evoked otoacoustic emissions in neonatal hearing screening program. *Seminars in Hearing, 14*, 30–45.

Kemp, D. T., Ryan, S., & Bray, P. (1990). A guide to the effective use of otoacoustic emissions. *Ear and Hearing, 11*, 93–105.

Kimberley, B. P., Brown, D. K., & Allen, J. B. (1997). Distortion product otoacoustic emissions and sensorineural hearing loss. In M. S. Robinette, & T. J. Glattke (Eds.), *Otoacoustic Emissions: Clinical Applications* (pp. 181–204). New York: Thieme.

Kvaerner, K. J., Engdahl, B., Arnesen, A. R., & Mair, I. W. S. (1995). Temporary threshold shift and otoacoustic emissions after industrial noise exposure. *Scandinavian Audiology, 24*, 137–141.

Kvaerner, K. J., Engdahl, B., Aursnes, J., Arnesen, A. R., & Mair, I. W. S. (1996). Transient-evoked otoacoustic emissions—Helpful tool in the detection of pseudohypacusis. *Scandinavian Audiology, 25*, 173–177.

LePage, E. L. (1989). Functional role of the olivo-cochlear bundle: A motor unit control system in the mammalian cochlea. *Hearing Research, 38*, 177–198.

Liu, X. Z., & Newton, V. E. (1997). Distortion product emissions in normal-hearing and low-frequency hearing loss carriers of genes for Waardenburg's syndrome. *Annals of Otology, Rhinology and Laryngology, 106*, 220–225.

Long, G. R., & Tubis, A. (1988). Modification of spontaneous and evoked otoacoustic emissions and associated psychoacoustic microstructure by aspirin consumption. *Journal of the Acoustical Society of America, 84*, 1343–1353.

Lonsbury-Martin, B. L., Cutler, W. M., & Martin, G. K. (1991). Evidence for the influence of aging on distortion-product otoacoustic emissions in humans. *Journal of the Acoustical Society of America, 89*, 1749–1759.

Lonsbury-Martin, B. L., Harris, F. P., Hawkins, M. D., Stagner, B. B., & Martin, G. K. (1990a). Distortion-product emissions in humans: I. Basic properties in normally hearing subjects. *Annals of Otology, Rhinology and Laryngology, Supplement 236*, 3–13.

Lonsbury-Martin, B. L., Harris, F. P., Stagner, B. B., Hawkins, M. D., & Martin, G. K. (1990b). Distortion-product emissions in humans: II. Relations to stimulated and spontaneous emissions and acoustic immittance in normally hearing subjects. *Annals of Otology, Rhinology and Laryngology, Supplement 236,* 14–28.

Lonsbury-Martin, B. L., & Martin, G. K. (1990). The clinical utility of distortion-product otoacoustic emissions. *Ear and Hearing, 11,* 90–99.

Lonsbury-Martin, B. L., Martin, G. K., & Balkany, T. (1994). Clinical applications of otoacoustic emissions. In F. E. Lucente (Ed.), *Highlights of the Instructional Courses—1994* (pp. 343–355). Alexandria VA: American Academy of Otolaryngology—Head and Neck Surgery.

Lonsbury-Martin, B. L., Martin, G. K., McCoy, M. J., & White-head, M. L. (1994). Testing young children with otoacoustic emissions: Middle-ear influences. *American Journal of Otology, 15, Supplement 1,* 13–20.

Lonsbury-Martin, B. L., Martin, G. K., McCoy, M. J., & White-head, M. L. (1996). Testing newborns, infants, toddlers, and children with otoacoustic emissions. In S. E. Gerber (Ed.), *Handbook of Pediatric Audiology* (pp. 173–205). Washington: Gallaudet University Press.

Lonsbury-Martin, B. L., McCoy, M. J., Whitehead, M. L., & Martin, G. K. (1993). Clinical testing of distortion-product otoacoustic emissions. *Ear and Hearing, 14,* 11–22.

Lonsbury-Martin, B. L., Whitehead, M. L., & Martin, G. K. (1991). Clinical applications of otoacoustic emissions. *Journal of Speech and Hearing Research, 34,* 964–981.

Lonsbury-Martin, B. L., Whitehead, M. L., & Martin, G. K. (1993). Distortion product otoacoustic emissions in normal and impaired ears: Insights into generation processes. In J. H. J. Allum, D. J. Mecklenburg, & R. Probst (Eds.), *Natural and Artificial Nervous Control of Hearing and Balance, Progress in Brain Research, 97,* 77–90.

Lucertini, M., Bergamaschi, A., & Urbani, L. (1996). Transient evoked otoacoustic emissions in occupational medicine as an auditory screening test for employment. *British Journal of Audiology, 30,* 79–88.

Lutman, M. E., Mason, S. M., Sheppard, S., & Gibbin, K. P. (1989). Differential diagnostic potential of otoacoustic emissions: A case study. *Audiology, 28,* 205–210.

Margolis, R. H., & Trine, M. B. (1997). Influence of middle-ear disease on otoacoustic emissions. In M. S. Robinette & T. J. Glattke (Eds.), *Otoacoustic Emissions: Clinical Applications* (pp. 130–150). New York: Thieme.

Marshall, L., Heller, L. M., & Westhusin, L. J. (1997). Effect of negative middle-ear pressure on transient-evoked otoacoustic emissions. *Ear and Hearing, 18,* 218–226.

Martin, G. K., Franklin, D. J., Harris, F. P., Ohlms, L. A., & Lonsbury-Martin, B. L. (1990). Distortion-product emissions in humans: III. Influence of hearing pathology. *Annals of Otology, Rhinology and Laryngology, Supplement 236,* 29–44.

Martin, G. K., Probst, R., & Lonsbury-Martin, B. L. (1990). Otoacoustic emissions in human ears: Normative findings. *Ear and Hearing, 11,* 106–120.

Martin, G. K., Probst, R., Scheinin, S. A., Coats, A. C., & Lonsbury-Martin, B. L. (1987). Acoustic distortion products in rabbits. II. Sites of origin revealed by suppression and pure-tone exposures. *Hearing Research, 28,* 191–208.

Mathis, A., Probst, R., De Min, N., & Hauser, R. (1991). A child with an unusually high-level spontaneous otoacoustic emission. *Archives of Otolaryngology—Head and Neck Surgery, 117,* 674–676.

Mauk, G. W., White, K. R., Mortensen, L. B., & Behrens, T. R. (1991). The effectiveness of screening programs based on high-risk characteristics in early identification of hearing impairment. *Ear and Hearing, 12,* 312–319.

Maxon, A. B., Vohr, B. R., & White, K. R. (1996). Newborn hearing screening: Comparison of a simplified otoacoustic emissions device (ILO1088) with the ILO88. *Early Human Development, 45,* 171–178.

Maxon, A. B., White, K. R., Behrens, T. R., & Vohr, B. R. (1995). Referral rates and cost efficiency in a universal newborn hearing screening program using transient evoked otoacoustic emissions. *Journal of the American Academy of Audiology, 6,* 271–277.

McFadden, D., & Pasanen, E. G. (1994). Otoacoustic emissions and quinine sulfate. *Journal of the Acoustical Society of America, 95,* 3460–3474.

McFadden, D., & Plattsmier, H. S. (1984). Aspirin abolishes spontaneous oto-acoustic emissions. *Journal of the Acoustical Society of America, 76,* 443–448.

McFadden, D., Plattsmier, H. S., & Pasanen, E. G. (1984). Aspirin-induced hearing loss as a model of sensorineural hearing loss. *Hearing Research, 16,* 251–260.

McNellis, E. L., & Klein, A. J. (1997). Pass/fail rates for repeated click-evoked otoacoustic emission and auditory brain stem response screening in newborns. *American Academy of Otolaryngology—Head and Neck Surgery, 116,* 431–437.

Meredith, R., Stephens, D., Hogan, S., Cartilidge, P. H. T., & Drayton, M. (1994). Screening for hearing loss in an at-risk neonatal population using evoked otoacoustic emissions. *Scandinavian Audiology, 23,* 187–193.

Meredith, R., Stephens, D., Sirimanna, T., Meyer-Bisch, C., & Reardon, W. (1992). Audiometric detection of carrier of Ushers syndrome type II. *Journal of Audiological Medicine, 1,* 11–19.

Mills, D. M., & Rubel, E. W. (1994). Variation of distortion product otoacoustic emissions with furosemide injection. *Hearing Research, 77,* 183–199.

Mills, D. M., Norton, S. J., & Rubel, E. W. (1993). Vulnerability and adaptation of distortion-product otoacoustic emissions to endocochlear potential variation. *Journal of the Acoustical Society of America, 94,* 2108–2122.

Monroe, J. A. B., Krauth, L., Arenberg, I. K., Prenger, E., & Philpot, P. (1996). Normal evoked otoacoustic emissions with a profound hearing loss due to a juvenile pilocytic astrocytoma. *American Journal of Otology, 17,* 639–642.

Mott, J. B., Norton, S. J., Neely, S. T., & Warr, W. B. (1989). Changes in spontaneous otoacoustic emissions produced by acoustic stimulation of the contralateral ear. *Hearing Research, 38,* 229–242.

Moulin, A., Collet, L., & Duclaux, R. (1993). Contralateral auditory stimulation alters acoustic distortion products in humans. *Hearing Research, 65,* 193–210.

Mountain, D. C. (1980). Changes in endolymphatic potential and crossed olivocochlear bundle stimulation alter cochlear mechanics. *Science, 210,* 71–72.

Musiek, F. E., Bornstein, S. P., & Rintelmann, W. F. (1995). Transient evoked otoacoustic emissions and pseudohypacusis. *Journal of the American Academy of Audiology, 6,* 293–301.

Nadol, J. B. (1989). *Ménière's Disease: Pathogenesis, Pathophysiology, Diagnosis and Treatment.* Amsterdam: Kugler and Ghedini Publications.

Naeve, S. L., Margolis, R. H., Levine, S. C., & Fournier, E. M. (1992). Effect of ear-canal air pressure on evoked otoacoustic emissions. *Journal of the Acoustical Society of America, 91,* 2091–2095.

Nelson, D. A., & Kimberley, B. P. (1992). Distortion-product emissions and auditory sensitivity in human ears with normal hearing and cochlear hearing loss. *Journal of Speech and Hearing Research, 35,* 1142–1159.

Norton, S. J. (1994). The emerging role of evoked otoacoustic emissions in neonatal hearing screening. *American Journal of Otology, 15, Supplement 1,* 4–12.

Norton, S. J., Mott, J. B., & Champlin, C. A. (1989). Behavior of spontaneous otoacoustic emissions following intense ipsilateral acoustic stimulation. *Hearing Research, 38,* 243–258.

Nozza, R. J., & Sabo, D. L. (1992). Transiently evoked OAE for screening school-age children. *The Hearing Journal, 45,* 29–31.

Nozza, R. J., Sabo, D. L., & Mandel, E. M. (1997). A role for otoacoustic emissions in screening for hearing impairment and middle ear disorders in school-age children. *Ear and Hearing, 18,* 227–239.

Ohlms, L. A., Lonsbury-Martin, B. L., & Martin, G. K. (1990). The clinical application of acoustic distortion products. *Otolaryngology—Head and Neck Surgery, 102,* 315–322.

Ohlms, L. A., Lonsbury-Martin, B. L., & Martin, G. K. (1991). Acoustic-distortion products: Separation of sensory from neural dysfunction in sensorineural hearing loss in humans and rabbits. *Archives of Otolaryngology—Head and Neck Surgery, 104,* 159–174.

Osterhammel, P. A., Rasmussen, A. N., Olsen, S. O., & Nielsen, L. H. (1996). The influence of spontaneous otoacoustic emissions on the amplitude of transient-evoked emissions. *Scandinavian Audiology, 25,* 187–192.

Oudesluys-Murphy, A. M., Vanstraaten, H. L. M., Bholasingh, R., & Vanzanten, G. A. (1996). Neonatal hearing screening. *European Journal of Pediatrics, 155,* 429–435.

Owens, J. J., McCoy, M. J., Lonsbury-Martin, B. L., & Martin, G. K. (1992). Influence of otitis media on evoked otoacoustic emissions in children. *Seminars in Hearing, 13,* 53–66.

Owens, J. J., McCoy, M. J., Lonsbury-Martin, B. L., & Martin, G. K. (1993). Otoacoustic emissions in children with normal ears, middle-ear dysfunction, and ventilating tubes. *American Journal of Otology, 14,* 34–40.

Ozturan, O., Jerger, J., Lew, H., & Lynch, G. R. (1996). Monitoring of cisplatin ototoxicity by distortion-product otoacoustic emissions. *Auris Nasus Larynx, 23,* 147–151.

Pasic, T. R., & Dobie, R. A. (1991). Cis-platinum ototoxicity in children. *Laryngoscope, 101,* 985–991.

Penner, M. J. (1989). Aspirin abolishes tinnitus caused by spontaneous otoacoustic emissions: A case study. *Archives of Otolaryngology—Head and Neck Surgery, 115,* 871–875.

Penner, M. J. (1990). An estimate of the prevalence of tinnitus caused by spontaneous otoacoustic emissions. *Archives of Otolaryngology—Head and Neck Surgery, 116,* 418–423.

Penner, M. J., Glotzbach, L., & Huang, T. (1993). Spontaneous otoacoustic emissions: Measurement and data. *Hearing Research, 68,* 229–237.

Picton, T. W., Kellett, A. J. C., Vezseny, M., & Rabinovitch, D. E. (1993). Otoacoustic emissions recorded at rapid stimulus rates. *Ear and Hearing, 14,* 299–314.

Plinkert, P. K., Sesterhenn, G., Anold, R., & Zenner, H. P. (1990). Evaluation of otoacoustic emissions in high-risk infants by using an easy and rapid objective auditory screening method. *European Archives of Otorhinolaryngology, 247,* 356–360.

Prieve, B. A., Gorga, M. P., & Neely, S. T. (1991). Otoacoustic emissions in an adult with severe hearing loss. *Journal of Speech and Hearing Research, 34,* 379–385.

Probst, R., Lonsbury-Martin, B. L., & Martin, G. K. (1991). A review of otoacoustic emissions. *Journal of the Acoustical Society of America, 89,* 2027–2067.

Probst, R., Coats, A. C., Martin, G. K., & Lonsbury-Martin, B. L. (1986). Spontaneous, click- and toneburst-evoked otoacoustic emissions from normal ears. *Hearing Research, 21,* 261–275.

Probst, R., Lonsbury-Martin, B. L., Martin, G. K., & Coats, A. C. (1987). Otoacoustic emissions in ears with hearing loss. *American Journal of Otology, 8,* 73–81.

Richardson, M. P., Williamson, T. J., Lenton, S. W., Tarlow, M. J., & Rudd, P. T. (1995). Otoacoustic emissions as a screening test for hearing impairment in children. *Archives of Disease in Childhood, 72,* 294–297.

Robinette, M. (1992). Clinical observations with transient evoked otoacoustic emissions with adults. *Seminars in Hearing, 13,* 23–35.

Robinette, M. S., & Durrant, J. D. (1997). Contributions of evoked otoacoustic emissions in differential diagnosis of retrocochlear disorders. In M. S. Robinette & T. J. Glattke (Eds.), *Otoacoustic Emissions: Clinical Applications* (pp. 205–232). New York: Thieme.

Robinette, M. S., & Glattke, T. J. (1997). *Otoacoustic Emissions: Clinical Applications.* New York: Thieme.

Rossi, G., Solero, P., Rolando, M., & Olina, M. (1989). Delayed oto-acoustic emissions evoked by bone-conduction stimulation: Experimental data on their origin, characteristics and transfer to the external ear in man. *Scandinavian Audiology, Supplement 29,* 1–24.

Ruggero, M. A., & Rich, N. C. (1991). Furosemide alters organ of Corti mechanics: Evidence for feedback of outer hair cells upon the basilar membrane. *Journal of Neuroscience, 11,* 1057–1067.

Rutten, W. L. C., & Buisman, H. P. (1983). Critical behaviour of auditory oscillators near feedback phase transitions. In E. de Boer & M. A. Viergever (Eds.), *Mechanics of Hearing* (pp. 91–99). Delft: Delft University Press.

Rybak, L. P. (1986). Drug ototoxicity. *Annual Review of Pharmacology and Toxicology, 26,* 79–99.

Sakashita, T., Minowa, Y., Hachikawa, K., Kubo, T., & Nakai, Y. (1991). Evoked otoacoustic emissions from ears with idiopathic sudden deafness. *Acta Otolaryngologica, Supplement 486*, 66–72.

Schorn, K. (1993). The Munich screening programme in neonates. *British Journal of Audiology, 27*, 143–148.

Sheppard, S. L., Brown, A. M., & Russell, P. T. (1996). Feasibility of acoustic distortion product testing in newborns. *British Journal of Audiology, 30*, 261–274.

Siegel, J. H., & Kim, D. O. (1982). Efferent neural control of cochlear mechanics? Olivocochlear bundle stimulation affects cochlear biomechanical nonlinearity. *Hearing Research, 6*, 171–182.

Solomon, G., Groth, J., & Anthonisen, B. (1993). Preliminary results and considerations in hearing screening of newborns based on otoacoustic emissions. *British Journal of Audiology, 27*, 139–141.

Soucek, S., & Michaels, L. (1996). The ear in the acquired immunodeficiency syndrome: 2. Clinical and audiologic investigation. *American Journal of Otology, 17*, 35–39.

Spoendlin, H. H. (1988). Neural anatomy of the inner ear. In A. F. Jahn & J. Santos-Sacchi (Eds.), *Physiology of the Ear* (pp. 201–219). New York: Raven Press.

Stevens, J. C. (1988): Click-evoked oto-acoustic emissions in normal and hearing impaired adults. *British Journal of Audiology, 22*, 45–49.

Stover, L., & Norton, S. J. (1993): The effects of aging on otoacoustic emissions. *Journal of the Acoustical Society of America, 94*, 2670–2681.

Sutton, L. A., Lonsbury-Martin, B. L., Martin, G. K., & Whitehead, M. L. (1994). Sensitivity of distortion-product otoacoustic emissions in humans to tonal over-exposure: Time course of recovery and effects of lowering L_2. *Hearing Research, 75*, 161–174.

Talmadge, C. L., Long, G. R., Murphy, W. J., & Tubis, A. (1993). New off-line method for detecting spontaneous otoacoustic emissions in human subjects. *Hearing Research, 71*, 170–182.

Telischi, F. F., Roth, J., Lonsbury-Martin, B. L., & Balkany, T. J. (1995). Patterns of evoked otoacoustic emissions associated with acoustic neuromas. *Laryngoscope, 105*, 675–682.

Telischi, F. F., Widick, M. P., Lonsbury-Martin, B. L., & McCoy, M. J. (1995). Monitoring cochlear function intraoperatively using distortion-product otoacoustic emissions. *American Journal of Otology, 16*, 597–608.

Thornton, A. R. D., Folkard, T. J., & Chambers, J. D. (1994). Technical aspects of recording evoked otoacoustic emissions using maximum length sequences. *Scandinavian Audiology, 23*, 225–231.

Thornton, A. R. D., & Grandori, F. (1994). *Advances in Otoacoustic Emissions, vol 2, Recording Techniques for Otoacoustic Emissions* (pp. 1–67). Brussels: Commission of the European Communities.

Trine, M. B., Hirsch, J. E., & Margolis, R. H. (1993). The effect of middle ear pressure on transient evoked otoacoustic emissions. *Ear and Hearing, 14*, 401–407.

Truy, E., Veuillet, E., Collet, L., & Morgon, A. (1993). Characteristics of transient otoacoustic emissions in patients with sudden idiopathic hearing loss. *British Journal of Audiology, 27*, 379–385.

Veuillet, E., Collet, L., & Duclaux, R. (1991). Effect of contralateral acoustic stimulation on active cochlear micromechanical properties in human subjects—Dependence on stimulus variables. *Journal of Neurophysiology, 65*, 724–735.

Vohr, B. R., & Maxon, A. B. (1996). Screening infants for hearing impairment. *Journal of Pediatrics, 128*, 710–714.

Vohr, B. R., White, K. R., Maxon, A. B., & Johnson, M. J. (1993). Factors affecting the interpretation of transient evoked otoacoustic emission results in neonatal hearing screening. *Seminars in Hearing, 14*, 57–72.

Watkin, P. M. (1996a). Neonatal otoacoustic emission screening and the identification of deafness. *Archives of Disease in Childhood, 74*, F16–25.

Watkin, P. M. (1996b). Outcomes of neonatal screening for hearing loss by otoacoustic emission. *Archives of Disease in Childhood, 75*, F158–168.

West, B. A., Brummett, R. E., & Himes, D. L. (1973). Interaction of kanamycin and ethacrynic acid. *Archives of Otolaryngology, 98*, 32–37.

White, K. R. (1996). Universal newborn hearing screening using transient evoked otoacoustic emissions: Past, present, and future. *Seminars in Hearing, 17*, 171–184.

White, K. R., & Behrens, T. R. (1993). The Rhode Island Hearing Assessment Project: Implications for universal newborn hearing screening. *Seminars in Hearing, 14*, 1–119.

White, K. R., Maxon, A. B., Behrens, T. R., Blackwell, P. M., & Vohr, B. R. (1992): Neonatal screening using evoked otoacoustic emissions: The Rhode Island Hearing Assessment Project. In F. H. Bess & J. W. Hall III (Eds.), *Screening Children for Auditory Function* (pp. 207–239). Nashville: Bill Wilkerson Center Press.

White, K. R., Maxon, A. B., Vohr, B. R., & Behrens, T. R. (1993b): Using transient evoked otoacoustic emissions for neonatal hearing screening. *British Journal of Audiology, 27*, 149–153.

White, K. R., Vohr, B. R., & Behrens, T. R. (1993a). Universal newborn hearing screening using transient evoked otoacoustic emissions: Results of the Rhode Island Hearing Assessment Project. *Seminars in Hearing, 14*, 18–29.

White, K. R., Vohr, B. R., Maxon, A. B., Behrens, T. R., McPherson, M. G., & Mauk, G. W. (1994), Screening all newborns for hearing loss using transient evoked otoacoustic emissions. *International Journal of Pediatric Otorhinolaryngology, 29*, 203–217.

Whitehead, M. L., Kamal, N., Lonsbury-Martin, B. L., & Martin, G. K. (1993). Spontaneous otoacoustic emissions in different racial groups. *Scandinavian Audiology, 22*, 3–10.

Whitehead, M. L., Lonsbury-Martin, B. L., & Martin, G. K. (1992a). Evidence for two discrete sources of $2f_1$-f_2 distortion-product otoacoustic emission in rabbit: I. Differential dependence on stimulus parameters. *Journal of the Acoustical Society of America, 91*, 1587–1607.

Whitehead, M. L., Lonsbury-Martin, B. L., & Martin, G. K. (1992b): Evidence for two discrete sources of $2f_1$-f_2 distortion-product otoacoustic emission in rabbit: II. Differential physiological vulnerability. *Journal of the Acoustical Society of America, 92*, 2662–2682.

Whitehead M. L., Lonsbury-Martin, B. L., Martin, G. K., & McCoy, M. J. (1996). Otoacoustic emissions: Animal models and clinical observations. In T. R. Van De Water, A. H. Popper, & R. R. Fay (Eds.), *Clinical Aspects of Hearing, vol 6, Springer Series in Auditory Research* (pp. 199–257). New York: Springer-Verlag.

Whitehead, M. L., McCoy, M. J., Lonsbury-Martin, B. L., & Martin, G. K. (1995). Dependence of distortion-product otoacoustic emissions on primary levels in normal and impaired ears: I. Effects of decreasing L_2 below L_1. *Journal of the Acoustical Society of America, 97*, 2346–2358.

Whitehead, M. L., McCoy, M. J., Martin, G. K., & Lonsbury-Martin, B. L. (1993). Click-evoked and distortion-product otoacoustic emissions in adults: Detection of high-frequency sensorineural hearing loss. *Association for Research in Otolaryngology Abstracts, 16*, 100.

Whitehead, M. L., Stagner, B. B., Lonsbury-Martin, B. L., & Martin, G. K. (1994). Measurement of otoacoustic emissions for hearing assessment. In O. Ozdamar (Ed.), *Hearing and Speech, International Electronics Engineering and Electrical Engineering in Medicine and Biology, 13*, 210–226.

Whitehead, M. L., Stagner, B. B., McCoy, M. J., Lonsbury-Martin, B. L., & Martin, G. K. (1995). Dependence of distortion-product otoacoustic emissions on primary levels in normal and impaired ears: II. Asymmetry in L_1,L_2 space. *Journal of the Acoustical Society of America, 97*, 2359–2377.

Widen, J. E., Ferraro, J. A., & Trouba, S. E. (1995). Progressive neural hearing impairment: Case report. *Journal of the American Academy of Audiology, 6*, 217–224.

Widick, M. P., Telischi, F. F., Lonsbury-Martin, B. L., & Stagner, B. F. (1994). Early effects of cerebellopontine angle compression on rabbit distortion-product otoacoustic emissions: A model for monitoring cochlear function during acoustic neuroma surgery. *Otolaryngology—Head and Neck Surgery, 111*, 407–416.

Wier, C. C., Norton, S. J., & Kincaid, G. E. (1984). Spontaneous narrow-band oto-acoustic signals emitted by human ears: A replication. *Journal of the Acoustical Society of America, 76*, 1248–1250.

Wier, C. C., Pasanen, E. G., & McFadden, D. (1988). Partial dissociation of spontaneous otoacoustic emissions and distortion products during aspirin use in humans. *Journal of the Acoustical Society of America, 84*, 230–237.

Wilson, J. P. (1980a). Evidence for a cochlear origin for acoustic re-emissions, threshold fine-structure and tonal tinnitus. *Hearing Research, 2*, 233–252.

Wilson, J. P. (1980b). Subthreshold mechanical activity within the cochlea. *Journal of Physiology, 298*, 32P–33P.

Wilson, J. P., & Sutton, G. J. (1981). Acoustic correlates of tonal tinnitus. In D. Evered & G. Lawrenson (Eds.), *Tinnitus* (pp. 82–107). London: Pitman Books Ltd.

Wilson, J. P., & Sutton, G. J. (1983). "A family with high-tonal objective tinnitus"—An update. In R. Klinke & R. Hartmann (Eds.), *Hearing—Physiological Bases and Psychophysics* (pp. 97–103). Berlin: Springer-Verlag.

Wit, H. P., & Ritsma, R. J. (1980). Evoked acoustical responses from the human ear: Some experimental results. *Hearing Research, 2*, 253–261.

Yamamoto, E., Takagi, A., Hirono, Y., & Yagi, N. (1987). A case of "spontaneous otoacoustic emission." *Archives of Otolaryngology—Head and Neck Surgery, 113*, 1316–1318.

Zorowka, P. G., Schmitt, H. J., & Gutjahr, P. (1993). Evoked otoacoustic emissions and pure tone threshold audiometry in patients receiving cisplatinum therapy. *International Journal of Pediatric Otorhinolaryngology, 25*, 73–80.

Zurek, P. M. (1981). Spontaneous narrowband acoustic signals emitted by human ears. *Journal of the Acoustical Society of America, 62*, 514–523.

Zurek, P. M., & Clark, W. W. (1981). Narrow-band acoustic signals emitted by chinchilla ears after noise exposure. *Journal of the Acoustical Society of America, 70*, 446–450.

Zwicker, E. (1983). On peripheral processing in normal hearing. In R. Klinke, & R. Hartmann (Eds.), *Hearing-Physiological Bases and Psychophysics* (pp. 104–110). Berlin: Springer-Verlag.

Zwicker, E., & Schloth, E. (1984). Interrelation of different otoacoustic emissions. *Journal of the Acoustical Society of America, 75*, 1148–1154.

CHAPTER 7

SHORT-LATENCY AUDITORY EVOKED POTENTIALS
ELECTROCOCHLEOGRAPHY & AUDITORY BRAINSTEM RESPONSE

JOHN D. DURRANT
JOHN A. FERRARO

Noninvasive electrophysiology and the measurement of evoked sensory potentials have assumed increasing importance in clinical audiology, including applications in differential diagnostics, estimation of hearing sensitivity, newborn screening, and intraoperative monitoring. Thanks to modern technology, the instrumentation necessary to perform evoked potential examinations has become cost-effective for such broad applications. As a result, evaluations of auditory evoked potentials (AEPs) have become routine services performed by audiologists, whether in private practice or university/hospital centers.

The AEP is computer-extracted from the ongoing bioelectric activity recorded from the surface of the scalp and related sites following the presentation of acoustic stimuli. The resultant waveforms represent stimulus-evoked voltage changes of the auditory nerve, brainstem, and cortex. Depending on the level of the nervous system where the response is generated as well as the nature of the stimulus, AEPs can last anywhere from a few to several hundred milliseconds (Figure 7.1). It is impossible within the confines of a textbook chapter to do justice to any single component of the AEP, let alone the entire family, considering the voluminous literature in all areas of interest and the variety of clinical applications reported. Emphasis here will be upon the short-latency responses, which include the auditory brainstem response (ABR) and those potentials recorded from the inner ear and auditory nerve via electro-

cochleography (ECochG). These responses are the most popular clinically in the audiology and otolaryngology settings, both for purposes of otoneurologic evaluation and estimation of hearing sensitivity.

This chapter is intended to serve as an overview of the basic aspects of AEP recording and the specific measurement and applications of ECochG and the ABR, primarily in differential diagnosis. Other applications (e.g., intraoperative monitoring) and related phenomena (e.g., longer-latency potentials and otoacoustic emissions) are covered elsewhere in this book (see Chapters 6, 8, and 9). The objective here will be to develop general concepts and principles that the authors have found valuable in pursuing both clinical and research interests and to provide useful references to serve the reader interested in more in-depth coverage, both directly and via the references contained therein. The interested reader also is referred to texts by Jacobson (1994) and Hall (1992) who have provided comprehensive/in-depth treatments of this subject.

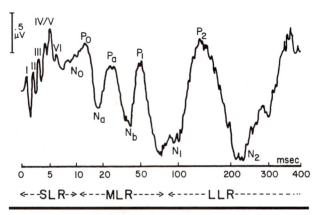

FIGURE 7.1 Auditory evoked potential: time windows of short- (SLR), middle- (MLR), and long- (LLR) latency responses (logarithmic time base). (Based on figure from Michelini, Arslan, Prosser, & Pedrielli, 1982; from ASHA, 1988, with permission)

Acknowledgments: This chapter was developed in part from a draft of "The Short Latency Auditory Evoked Potentials," a tutorial document developed by the Working Group on Auditory Evoked Potential Measurement of the American Speech-Language-Hearing Association, on which the authors served (JDD, chair). The authors, therefore, wish to acknowledge the efforts and contributions of members of the Committee on Audiologic Evaluation and peer reviewers, too numerous to mention, and, especially, those of their fellow working group members, Drs. Cynthia Fowler, Richard Folsom, Kenneth Wolf, and Bruce Weber. Dr. Wolf also contributed substantially to the adaptation of the Working Group's document to the previous edition of this chapter in the second edition of *Hearing Assessment*.

RUDIMENTS OF INSTRUMENTATION FOR AEP MEASUREMENT

Electrical Interface to the Subject

The nervous system is constantly active and generating electrical potentials that are conducted to the body's surface, where they can be recorded with electrodes. These voltage changes are minute (e.g., microvolts or less, where 1 microvolt = 1/1,000,000 volt) and buried in a background of electrical noise, often many times greater in magnitude. Additionally, the skin is electrically insulative, particularly the corneum stratum (the outermost dead-skin layer). There is also a fundamental difference between bioelectricity (ion-mediated current) and physical electricity (electron-mediated current). Therefore, applying an electrode (i.e., a metal conductor) to the skin to record neural potentials constitutes a barrier over which there can be no net charge transfer. Such an interface thus opposes current flow, and the interface (contact) can be characterized by its impedance (Geddes, 1972).

Electrode impedance is determined by the electrode characteristics (i.e., surface area and electrode and application materials), the tissue to which it is interfaced (e.g., skin, muscle, etc.) and anything in between (e.g., oil, dirt, fluid, etc.). Silver, gold, and platinum have relatively low impedances in this application and are widely used in clinical electrophysiology. Additionally, silver is useful because it can be plated with salt, forming a silver-silver-chloride (Ag-AgCl) electrode. This further lowers impedance and forms a reversible or nonpolarized electrode, making it possible to record very low-frequency potentials (i.e., approaching dc). Impedance is also lowest when the electrode makes direct contact with body fluids, for example, just under the skin's surface. This can be accomplished with needle electrodes, but this approach is unattractive for clinical work. In addition, the small surface area of the needle tip may counter any advantage due to direct contact with body fluid. Good electrical contact for surface electrodes, however, can be obtained by cleansing the skin thoroughly and applying an electrolyte gel, paste, or cream. The latter improves conductivity of the dead-skin layer, gives contact stability, and effectively increases the electrode-surface area. Various methods for obtaining low electrode impedances may be found in electroencephalography texts (e.g., Binnie, Rowan & Gutter, 1982). Electrode impedance should be measured routinely and, as a rule, should not exceed 5 kohms (measured in the vicinity of 15 Hz). In addition, interelectrode impedances (i.e., the difference between impedances for electrode pairs) should be balanced to optimize common-mode rejection of noise (see Amplification, below). Again, as a rule, interelectrode impedances ideally should not exceed 2 kohms.

Bioelectric Signal Conditioning

Amplification. The purpose of amplification is twofold. The first is to magnify the recorded signal (which contains both the AEP and background noise) to bring it within the range of amplitude resolution of the analog-to-digital (A-D) converter. The second purpose is to optimize the voltage sampling for the desired potential while, as much as possible, rejecting unwanted signals. This is possible by using an amplifier with a balanced input to perform a differential recording. The differential amplifier thus amplifies the difference in voltage sampled by its two inputs. Consequently, one input is negative and inverts the signal, whereas the other is positive and is noninverting. A connection also is made between the subject and the electrical ground, that is, the chassis, of the amplifier. Unwanted signals or noise common to the two inputs (A_{noise}) are seen in the same phase and will tend to be canceled by the amplifier. Complete cancellation occurs when the common-mode noise is of precisely equal amplitude and phase at the two inputs. The signal or response of interest (A_{signal}), on the other hand, is seen in opposite phase by the two electrodes and thus will be enhanced via differential amplification. In short, $(+A_{signal} + A_{noise}) - (-A_{signal} + A_{noise}) = (+A_{signal} - -A_{signal}) + (A_{noise} - A_{noise}) = 2 A_{signal} - 0$. In practice, the signal will not actually be doubled in most cases since the recording electrodes will not likely sample the generator of a given potential at exactly opposite poles and/or distances. Similarly, noises are rarely precisely of equal phase and amplitude. Further complications of real-world recordings are that desired signals may be canceled, at least partially, if less than optimal sites of recording are used/available. Conversely, some noises may be sampled out of phase at the two inputs, thus enhancing them. Nevertheless, differential amplification generally is quite effective in making the biologic recording workable, even under less-than-ideal conditions.

What the caveats at the end of the above paragraph reveal is the importance of the judicious choice of recording electrode montage. For AEP measurement, the three electrodes required—connected to the inverting and non-inverting inputs and ground—are placed typically on the head. Most myogenic artifacts and extraneous electrical noises of concern, indeed, will appear at the two electrode sites with nearly equal amplitudes and phases, and an improvement of signal-to-noise ratio (SNR) will be realized via common-mode rejection. Signals not common to the two inputs (which still contain background noise in addition to the AEP) thus will be amplified, as desired. In reality, the resultant waveform (e.g., ABR) will derive from two notably different signals sampled by the inverting and noninverting amplifier inputs (Figure 7.2).

The required gain of amplification depends upon the AEP being sought but typically ranges from 10,000, for

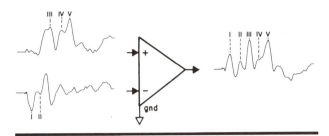

FIGURE 7.2 Derivation of the ABR via differential amplifier from pick-ups at the vertex (+) and mastoid (−). (From ASHA, 1988, with permission)

the longest-latency (and largest amplitude) potentials, to 500,000 (for the shortest-latency potentials). The amount of gain also will depend upon the location of the electrodes with respect to the generators. Recording short-latency potentials from the surface of the scalp (far-field), amplification in the range of 100,000 to 500,000 is typically needed. Recording nearer the generators (i.e., near-field), as in transtympanic electrocochleography (see below) gains as low as 10,000 to 20,000 may be adequate. Finally, within the various ranges specified above the determining variable will be the input sensitivity and range of the signal averaging instrument, that is, by the analog-digital converter, as discussed below.

Filtering. Considerable background noise actually can be removed via filtering since the noise generally has a much broader spectrum than the desired AEP component. This can be done before and/or after signal averaging, but some prefiltering usually is desirable. High-pass filtering is used to eliminate very low-frequency and dc potentials so that baseline drift and the effects of low-frequency artifact are minimized. Low-pass filtering is used to reject signals of frequencies beyond the sampling limits of the A-D conversion process, plus high frequency noise. In general, the better the SNR is before averaging, the more efficient the averaging process will be. However, analog filtering introduces phase shifts that become increasingly severe as the filter cut-off frequencies are approached. In addition, the filter may ring and otherwise color the response by its own characteristics. Because they have different spectra, different AEP components will not be affected in the same manner by a given filter. Therefore, analog filtering using extremely narrow bandwidths and/or steep filter skirts generally is avoided.

Signal Processing

As mentioned earlier, the desired signal (i.e., the AEP) is buried in a background of physical and biological electrical noise. The SNR can be improved substantially via computer-based, time-ensemble averaging (Figure 7.3). The recorded signal and noise are continuous functions in time that must be sampled in discrete pieces, as illustrated in Figure 7.4A. This is accomplished through A-D conversion wherein the amplitude of the signal (over a given interval of time) is translated into a binary value for computations by the computer. The more points that can be sampled in the waveform, the more accuracy with which it can be can be represented in the computer's memory (Figure 7.4B). The sampling rate of the A-D conversion process thus determines the temporal resolution of the waveform (i.e., the number of data points per cycle). There also

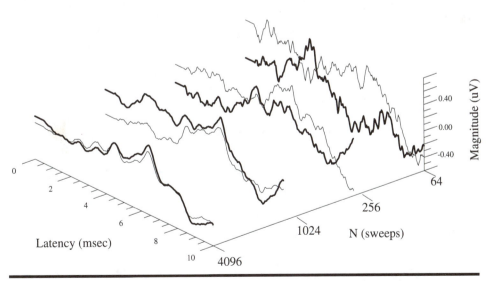

FIGURE 7.3 Increased reproducibility of test and retest tracings for ABR that are averages for the indicated number of sweeps.

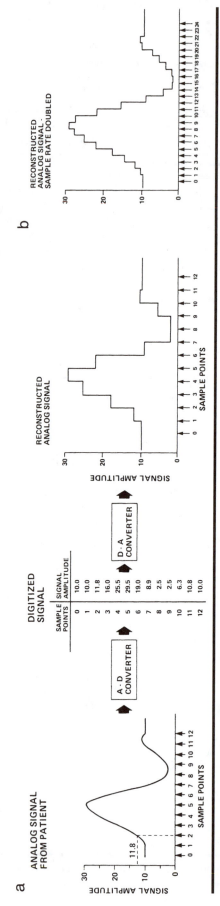

FIGURE 7.4 (A) Digital sampling and reconstruction of an analog signal. (B) Reconstructed signal sampled at twice the rate as in A. (Adapted from Coats, 1983, with permission from Grune & Stratton, Inc.)

is a limit to the resolution of the signal's amplitude. Amplitude resolution depends upon the numeric precision of the A-D converter, that is, the number of bits representing full-scale. Manufactured evoked potential test equipment typically provides temporal resolution of at least 40 microseconds per data point and 8 to 12 bit resolution of amplitude ($1/256$–$1/4096$ volts). With amplitude resolution in the thousands of microvolts and recorded signals in the microvolt or submicrovolt range, the recorded potentials must be amplified prior to signal averaging, as discussed earlier.

The basis for the SNR improvement due to signal averaging is that the noise is not time-locked with the stimulus and is likely to be canceled over time. Synchronous signals will be preserved. The improvement in the SNR is proportional to the square root of the number (N) of samples that are averaged (Picton & Hink, 1974). For example, increasing N by a factor of 4 will increase the SNR by a factor of 2. As a more practical example, increasing the number of samples from 2000 to 4000 (which also doubles the testing time) will improve the SNR by a factor of only 1.4. The recording of reproducible AEPs typically requires Ns of hundreds (longer-latency potentials) to thousands (shorter-latency potentials).

Additional digital processing of the signal may be applied to further enhance the SNR of the response and, thus, wave identification (e.g., see Lettrem & Laukli, 1995). Approaches are varied and numerous, but include so-called smoothing and other forms of filtering. Unlike analog filters, digital filters do not introduce the above-mentioned filtering artifacts, most notably latency effects (Boston & Ainslie, 1980; Domico & Kavanaugh, 1986). This is because digital filtering or smoothing is accomplished computationally by the computer after signal averaging and therefore does not shift the phase of the response. Most currently available instruments utilize a combination of analog (pre-)filtering, smoothing, and digital (post hoc) filtering, that is, band-pass filtering at the amplifier stage with, at least, low-pass digital filtering available to effect smoothing of the waveform.

Additional Noise and Artifact Rejection Strategies

Even with analog prefiltering and post hoc digital smoothing/filtering, it is likely that a noise artifact will occur during the sampling epoch that may not be canceled by averaging within a practical time period of signal analysis. For example, an incidental swallow can create a large electromyogenic artifact that never may be averaged out completely. Such artifacts often are much greater in magnitude than the desired potential, so they usually can be detected and excluded on the basis of their amplitude. Most commercially available test systems provide control

of the permissible amplitude limits or automatically reject overscale signals. In the case of the latter, control of the maximal permissible amplitude is tied to the gain setting. Amplitude artifact rejection (AR) generally involves the detection of any instant of overscale voltage within the sampling epoch or a specified portion thereof. Any time an artifact of this magnitude occurs, the entire sweep is excluded from the average. It is important to recognize that there is a cost in efficiency of data collection, and amplitude AR is most effective in eliminating samples containing incidental voltage spikes in otherwise quiet recordings. AR is not a very effective means of dealing with overall noisy subjects, and its usage does not diminish the need for careful electrode application, cooperation of the subject (if not sedated), and appropriate filtering.

The tremendous amplification required for extracting AEPs makes the recordings susceptible to the pickup of extraneous electrical noises via electrostatic and/or electromagnetic coupling. Typical noise sources include electric (especially fluorescent) lights and other electrical devices and wiring that produce 60 Hz noise, radiation from power transformers and electrical machinery, and stimulus artifact radiation from the earphone. Sixty-Hertz noise (and harmonics and related artifacts thereof) generally are substantially reduced by the signal averaging process itself, if the sampling epoch is not synchronized with the noise. The phase of the noise will vary randomly within the sampling epoch and (largely) be canceled. Nevertheless, various precautions are worthwhile for optimal noise reduction, such as proper shielding of equipment and, perhaps, the subject (i.e., using a shielded test suite). Proper grounding also is important for minimizing 60 Hz artifact via ground loops (Pfeiffer, 1974), as well as ensuring proper electrical safety for patient and examiner (Binnie et al., 1982). It also is helpful to dress the electrode leads close to the subject's body, braiding and/or shielding excess leads, and making the leads as short as practical. Stimulus artifact can be minimized by electromagnetically shielding the earphone (Elberling & Solomon, 1973). Another way to minimize contamination of the desired response due to stimulus artifacts was described by Sohmer and Pratt (1976), who used a tube to couple the earphone to the subject's ear. This approach introduces an acoustic delay that helps to separate stimulus artifact from the onset of the response. This may now be accomplished through the use of tubal insert earphones (Clemis, Ballad, & Killion, 1986). Some evoked response test instruments also permit the zeroing of samples over a specified interval. For instance, the first 1 msec may be used to blank out the stimulus artifact, without interfering much with the acquisition of the desired response. Lastly, alternating stimulus polarity (see below) can be used to minimize stimulus artifact via phase cancellation.

Advanced Analysis Techniques

Numerous methods have been described and tested over the history of AEPs, especially the ABR, wherein the computer is "asked" to go beyond the basic averaging process, simple artifact rejection paradigm, and digital smoothing/filtering, namely to assist the examiner to carry out more efficient tests and make decisions. Gabriel, Durrant, and colleagues (1980) described some time ago a reasonably reliable "peak picking" program for the ABR. More sophisticated programs have since been described that employ so-called expert systems. The ABR expert endeavors to define the rules of interpretation, or even diagnoses, and the programmer endeavors to implement an adaptive decision matrix that functions somewhat like the expert thinks (e.g., see Brai, Vibert, & Koutlidis, 1994). (Another term in vogue at one time, but a misnomer, is "artificial intelligence.") Even more advanced and/or current endeavors approach the task via so-called neural networks (e.g., see Habraken, van Gils, & Cluitmans, 1993), a virtual, brain-like learning process implemented in the computer. Perhaps because of the potential liabilities perceived by instrument manufacturers, such methods remain in the laboratory, despite the time savings and practicality of even primitive methods of peak identification. However, for addressing the inherently poor SNR attendant to recording the ABR and helping the examiner to automate intelligently the threshold search paradigm, a highly promising technique has emerged—F_{sp} ("F" for the underlying probability distribution of the measure and "sp" for the single point used to estimate background variance [i.e. noise]; see Elberling & Don, 1984).

The F_{sp} approach utilizes a software routine to compare the overall variance through the response epoch (akin to determining the root-mean-square magnitude) to the single-point variance calculated across sweeps (i.e., the epochs averaged to form the [averaged] evoked response). These measures of variance permit the calculation of an F-ratio, as one would do in the statistical test called analysis of variance. Consequently, F_{sp} serves as a test of the significance of the SNR, can be calculated "on the fly" (i.e., continuously updated by the computer) and set to a predetermined level to automatically stop the acquisition/averaging process. If the criterion is not reached by, say, 10,000 sweeps, the system also stops, assuming no response to be measurable. In other words, this technique terminates the averaging process dynamically, not according to a preset number of sweeps; if 200 sweeps yield a significant response, then averaging is suspended. But, if the SNR is much poorer (say, after having lowered the stimulus intensity 20 dB in search of the limit of detection of the response), then the process might proceed for some 4000 sweeps. The result is that time is focused on conditions requiring the greatest SNR enhancement, not conditions

for which SNR is inherently more robust. In addition, the F_{sp} algorithm assigns weightings to the blocks of sweeps according to their noise levels, which minimizes the effects of large, transient fluctuations (much like conventional artifact rejection routines; Elberling & Wahlgreen, 1985). In contrast, the noisy sweeps are not merely discarded from the averaging process as done by the inherently inefficient artifact-rejection algorithm, thus helping to further minimize test time. Consequently, the procedure saves valuable test time, especially for "difficult-to-test" populations and provides a uniform basis for deciding when there is no response (Sininger, 1993). A high degree of correlation between behavioral and ABR-F_{sp} thresholds has been reported for this method (Sininger, 1993; Sininger & Don, 1989), and the algorithm is beginning to be supplied on commercially available instruments, although not widely distributed at the time of this writing.

Sound Stimulation

Spectral and Temporal Factors. As a general rule, the more concise the stimulus, temporally, the better synchronized the neural discharges elicited and the more robust the evoked potentials. The broadband click (BBC), a sound obtained by applying a dc pulse to an earphone, loudspeaker, or bone vibrator, provides an excellent stimulus for eliciting AEPs. The BBC's brief duration minimizes stimulus artifact while providing a broad spectrum stimulus (Figure 7.5A); the result is the excitation of many nerve fibers with excellent synchronization. Earphones, however, do not perfectly reproduce the spectrum of a dc pulse (Figure 7.5A.2), and the auditory system itself filters the stimulus. Therefore, frequency limits are imposed upon BBC stimulation (Durrant, 1983).

Frequency specificity (at least to some extent) can be obtained via sinusoidal pulses (tonepips or bursts) or band-pass-filtered clicks (e.g., ringing a filter with a dc pulse). Such stimuli are transients, so they have continuous (Figure 7.5B) rather than discrete spectra, as in the case of pure tones. The energy in their spectra is concentrated around a central frequency (Figure 7.5B), and the use of sinusoidal pulses has been shown to produce even short-latency potentials whose latencies vary as a function of frequency (for a given intensity). Thus, traveling-wave propagation time in the cochlea is somewhat reflected under these conditions. (Naunton & Zerlin, 1976). Further details of such relationships for other AEPs are discussed in sections to follow.

There also are various temporal parameters associated with stimulation, which in turn affect the spectrum of the stimulus. However, they also may have effects more or less specific to the temporal parameter, such as plateau duration, rise/fall duration, and the gating function by which the amplitude envelope of the sinusoid is shaped (e.g., rectangular, cosine, etc.). The AEPs are relatively insensitive

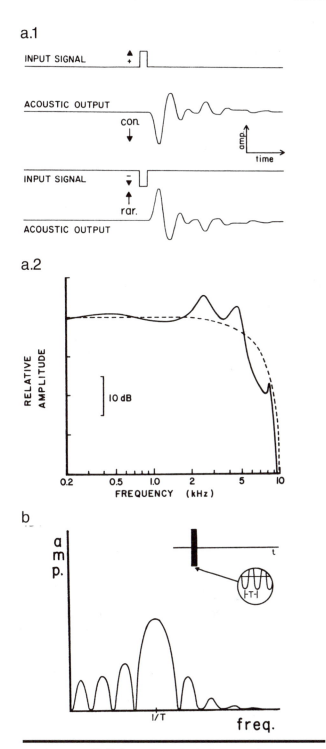

to plateau duration of the stimulus since they are largely onset responses. Rise-fall duration, however, is influential. In general, the slower the rise time, the less the amplitude and the longer will be the latency of the evoked potential (see below). Stimulus repetition rate is another important parameter. The repetition rate of the stimulus must be slow enough to avoid neural adaptation but high enough for efficient data collection (particularly important in testing newborns/infants; see Chapter 11). Typical rates range from 1/sec or less to 50/sec or more, depending upon AEP component of interest and/or purpose of the AEP evaluation. The precise rate, however, should be chosen so as not to be an integer submultiple of 60 Hz (e.g., 1/6—10, 1/3—20, and 1/2—30/sec) to avoid synchronizing the response sampling to this source of interference (see Hyde, 1994).

Stimulus Calibration. Evoked response evaluation requires calibration of the test stimulus, as with other audiometric procedures. The intensity of the click stimulus frequently is reported in terms of dB above the behavioral threshold of a group of normal listeners and referred to as nHL. Regretably, there currently are no hearing level standards for BBCs and other brief transients. Existing audiometric calibration procedures are not applicable, and sound level meters typically used for audiometric calibration require long duration signals for accurate measurement. A popular method of physical calibration of AEP test equipment is to determine the peak-equivalent sound pressure level (peSPL). This measurement is obtained by using an oscilloscope to match the amplitude of a sine wave (e.g., 1000 Hz pure tone) with the peak amplitude of the click stimulus. The SPL of the long duration pure tone can then be measured on a sound level meter, and this value becomes the peSPL of the click. The behavioral threshold of the BBC for normal listeners has been found to be approximately 30 dB peSPL (Stapells, Picton, & Smith, 1982).

Cann and Knott (1979) also have described a method of determining the starting phase of the acoustic signal relative to the polarity or starting phase of the signal driving the transducer. However, stimulus polarity (or phase) determined in a cavity, or for that matter by real-ear measurement, may not adequately characterize the effective phase of the stimulus at the level of the organ of Corti. This is because the overall phase response of the ear canal, middle ear, and cochlea differs among individuals. This issue is rendered noncritical, however, if both stimulus polarities are employed in the evaluation of the response in the first place (see below).

When determining hearing levels, the psychophysical method for threshold measurement and number and rate of stimulus presentations are important factors. The integrity of the hearing of the normative group sample must be affirmed. For more in-depth discussions of these and other

FIGURE 7.5 (A.1) Acoustic output of an earphone (Telephonics TDH 39) in response to direct current pulses (input signal), producing clicks (acoustic output) of condensation (con.) or rarefaction (rar.) polarities. (A.2) Spectrum of the click (solid line) versus the electrical pulse (dashed line). (From J. D. Durrant, *Bases of Auditory Brain-Stem Evoked Responses*, p. 31, 1983, with permission of Grune & Stratton, Inc.) (B) Spectrum of a brief tone burst. (From ASHA, 1988, with permission)

aspects of stimulus calibration (e.g., choice and effect of pulse duration for click stimulation), the reader is referred to Durrant (1983), Gorga, Abbas, and Worthington (1985), and Yost and Klein (1979).

ELECTROCOCHLEOGRAPHY

Historical Perspective

The recording of stimulus-related potentials from the cochlea and eighth nerve is called electrocochleography (ECochG), and the record of the recorded potentials is the electrocochleogram (ECochGm). Efforts to perform ECochG date back to the 1930s and 1940s, when several investigators recorded the cochlear microphonic (CM) from humans following its discovery in the cat by Wever and Bray in 1930 (e.g., Fromm, Nylen, & Zotterman, 1935; Lempert, Wever, & Lawrence, 1947; Perlman & Case, 1941). The first recording of the human eighth-nerve action potential (AP) is credited to Dr. Robert Ruben and his co-workers, who performed their measurements intraoperatively. However, what ultimately made routine clinical evaluations of auditory evoked responses possible was the application of signal (time-ensemble) averaging of the recorded potentials and the great improvement of signal-to-noise ratio made possible by this relatively simple and straightforward mathematical "trick."

The summating potential (SP), first reported by Davis, Fernandez, & McAuliffe (1950) and von Bekesy (1950), received relatively little attention in comparison to the CM and AP until the early 1980s. At this time, the ABR was emerging as a clinical tool, and this stimulated renewed attention to all AEPs, including ECochG. Currently, the most popular clinical applications for ECochG include (but are not limited to) the diagnosis, assessment, and monitoring of Ménière's disease/endolymphatic hydrops; the enhancement of Wave I of the ABR in patients with hearing loss or under difficult recording conditions; and intraoperative monitoring of cochlear and auditory nerve status (Ferraro & Ruth, 1994; Ruth, Lambert, & Ferraro, 1988).

Response Morphology

When elicited by a transient stimulus such as a click, the SP appears as a brief deflection or a shoulder on the leading edge of the superimposed AP waveform (as shown in Figure 7.6 below, from Coats, 1981). However, in the click-evoked ECochGm obtained via noninvasive recordings, the first negative peak of the AP (i.e., the N1 component) is the most salient feature of the response in humans (Coats, 1974). (For a more extensive overview of these potentials see Durrant & Lovrinic, 1995.)

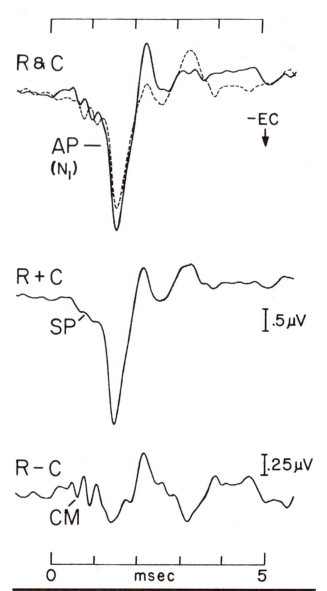

FIGURE 7.6 Component potentials of the (human) electrocochleogram recorded from the ear canal using condensation (C) and rarefaction (R) clicks; action potential (AP); cochlear microphonic (CM); summating potential (SP). The CM and SP can be selectively enhanced by manipulating the R and C responses, as indicated. Ear-canal negative (−EC) potentials are plotted as downward deflections. (Based on figure by Coats, 1981, from ASHA, 1988, with permission)

Generators

The ECochGm, again, consists of several potentials (Figure 7.6): the CM and the SP, which are generated by the hair cells (i.e., prior to excitation of the auditory nerve); and the whole-nerve AP, which represents the summed response of numerous, even thousands, synchronous discharges of the eighth nerve. The CM has much the same waveform as the stimulus. For example, a sinusoidal voltage is recorded in response to a pure tone burst. However, the CM often is observed to be asymmetrical about the zero axis, due to the presence of the SP. The SP, in turn, can be isolated via low-pass filtering or phase cancellation of the CM (Coats, 1981; Dallos, 1973). Depending upon the combination of stimulus parameters and recording site and method, the SP may be of either positive or negative polarity. This is because the SP reverses in polarity in reference to the best frequency of the recording site (Dallos, 1973), namely when frequency is increased such that the recording effectively sees activity on the apicalward, versus basalward, slope of the traveling wave. The frequency of reversal also is level dependent. Polarity—and, thus, the effects of other stimulus parameters—also may be biased mechanically by another stimulus (Durrant & Dallos, 1974) or perhaps pathological conditions like hydrops (e.g., see Eggermont, 1976b).

Recording/Interface Methods

ECochG recording approaches can be either invasive or noninvasive. The invasive transtympanic approach involves placing a needle electrode through the tympanic membrane to rest on the cochlear promontory (e.g., see Aran, Portmann, Portmann, et al., 1972; Yoshie & Ohashi, 1969). Promontory recordings offer the advantage of being near-field. Thus, relatively few signal averages can produce responses with very large amplitudes. Although widely practiced in other countries, transtympanic ECochG has not been well-accepted in the United States. The reasons for this center around the invasiveness of the approach. For example, recordings are not accomplished without some degree of patient discomfort, most patients have a negative attiude about puncturing their eardrums, and a physician is needed to insert the electrode under topical/local anesthesia. Thus, this latter aspect limits the practice of transtympanic ECochG to medical settings and precludes nonmedical personnel (i.e., audiologists) from performing the examination independently.

The above concerns regarding invasive ECochG have facilitated the development of noninvasive recording approaches that are now widely used in the United States. Noninvasive approaches may be classified as extratympanic (Cullen, Ellis, Berlin, & Lousteau, 1972; Ferraro & Ferguson, 1989; Stypulkowski & Staller, 1987) or ear canal (Coats, 1974; Durrant, 1977, 1986; Ferraro, Murphy, & Ruth, 1986). The method devised by Cullen and his associates involved the use of a silver wire electrode wrapped in a saline-soaked cotton pledget, placed against the tympanic membrane. Interest in this method recently has been rekindled by a new electrode, designed by Stypulkowski,

that uses a very flexible Silastic tube to hold the wire and a foam-rubber electrolyte-impregnated tip (Durrant & Ferraro, 1991; Ferraro & Ferguson, 1989; Ruth, Lambert, & Ferraro, 1988; Stypulkowski & Staller, 1987). In contrast, Coats' (1974) and similar designs (e.g., Durrant, 1977, 1986) employ a light springy "clip" to hold a small electrode against the canal wall near (but not touching) the eardrum. These types of electrode assemblies generally are tolerated well by subjects, even while wearing earphones. They are capable of providing recordings of the AP traceable to or close to the perceptual limits of the stimulus (Figure 7.7). However, there is a considerable amount of variability in extratympanic or ear canal ECochG (Durrant, 1986), which may lead to much less successful recordings in some subjects, although this appears to be less of a problem with the Stypulkowski design (Stypulkowski & Staller, 1987).

Other ear-canal electrode designs have been described wherein the electrode is placed much less deep in the ear canal (e.g., Whitaker, 1986; Yanz & Dodds, 1985). There also now are earplug-type ear canal electrodes available commercially (Nicolet, tiptrodes) that replace the tips and are used with the drivers of tubal insert earphones. Such shallow ear-canal electrodes compare favorably in performance with electrodes of the Coats type when the latter is placed laterally in the ear canal (Ferraro et al., 1986). These more recent designs have substantially reduced the inherent impedance problem of ear canal electrodes. Still, as demonstrated by Coats (1974), a price is paid in that the farther out in the canal the recording is made, the smaller the recorded potential.

As in all AEP measurements, differential recording of ECochG requires two electrode leads besides ground. The

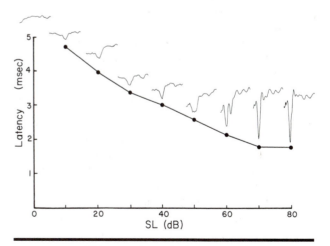

FIGURE 7.7 AP latency-intensity function and corresponding ECochG tracings (recorded via an ear-canal electrode). (From ASHA, 1988, with permission)

second electrode (sometimes referred to as the reference) is usually a disk EEG-type recording electrode, and its site is no less important than that of the ear-canal electrode. At first glance, the ipsilateral earlobe or mastoid might seem most appropriate for ECochG. However, these are not inactive sites (see section on ABRs). Preferable sites are the nasion or contralateral earlobe/mastoid, which are relatively inactive for the ECochGm. Durrant (1977; see also Durrant, 1986) also suggested recording between the ear canal and the vertex or forehead to provide simultaneous pickup of the eighth nerve and brainstem components (Figure 7.8).

Stimulus Variables

Clicks. The AP, like all compound nerve potentials, grows in proportion to the strength of the stimulus, but equally remarkable is the concomitant decrease in its latency. Latency is the time interval between stimulus onset and onset or peak of the response. Because the latency of the occurrence of the peak of the AP (i.e., N1) is easier to measure, it is the preferred measure, at least for clinical purposes. The typical graph of AP (peak) latency versus stimulus level was shown in Figure 7.7; in general, such graphs are called latency-intensity functions. The basis of this phenomenon is evident from the recordings presented in Figure 7.9, wherein broadband and derived narrowband click elicited APs are shown. These data show that the high-level response reflects more basalward (i.e., high-frequency) contributions of eighth nerve fibers in the cochlea, whereas the contributions from lower-frequency regions tend to cancel one another (Eggermont, 1976a). The latencies and broader waveforms of low-level responses (Figure 7.9A) correspond more to responses generated by lower frequency bands, namely around 2 kHz (Figure 7.9B), consistent with the greater sensitivity of the 2 kHz region near threshold. The latency-intensity shift largely reflects the time required for the traveling wave to propagate between the corresponding places along the basilar membrane.

Tone Bursts. The BBC has been the most popular stimulus for ECochG, especially for evoking the AP. However, the transient nature of the click makes it less than ideal for studying cochlear potentials such as the CM and SP whose durations are stimulus-dependent. Figure 7.10 displays a synthetic SP superimposed on a real AP to illustrate this condition (Durrant & Ferraro, 1991). As shown, the click-evoked SP extends into the timeframe of the AP and is thus abbreviated when both potentials are displayed together (as is usually the case in clinical recordings). To address this problem, tone-burst stimuli can be applied to make the stimulus last longer than the AP (see Dallos,

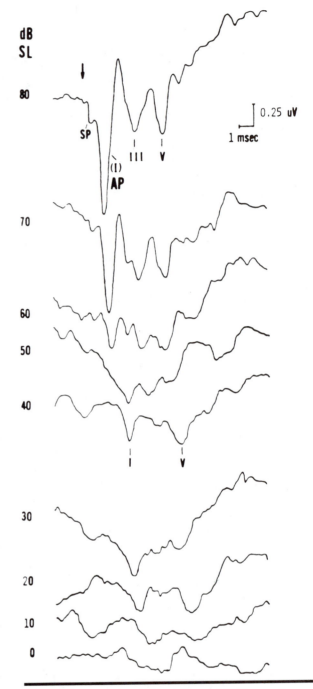

FIGURE 7.8 Combined ECochGm and ABR recording at different sensation levels of the click stimulus, obtained by differential recording between the forehead at hairline (inverted input) and the ear canal (noninverted input). Using this montage and configuration of inputs to the recording amplitude, both ear-canal negative and forehead/vertex positive potentials are plotted as downward deflections. (From J. D. Durrant, "Observation on combined noninvasive electrocochleography." *Seminars in Hearing*, Volume 7, Number 3, New York, 1986, Thieme Medical Publishers, Inc. Reprinted by permission.)

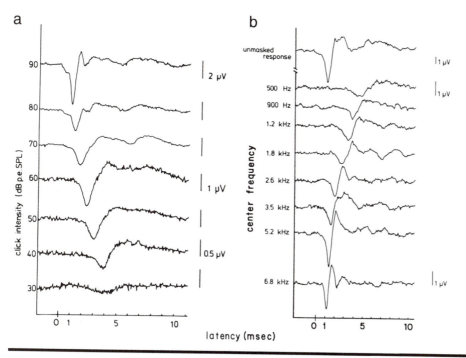

FIGURE 7.9 (A) Wide-band click-evoked APs. (Adapted from Eggermont, Odenthal, Schmidt, & Spoor, 1974.) (B) Derived narrowband responses with click stimulus presented at 90 dB peSPL. (From J. J. Eggermont, *Clinical and Special Topics*, pp. 625–705, 1976a, with permission from Springer-Verlag.) Both sets of recordings are from the promontory via a transtympanic electrode.

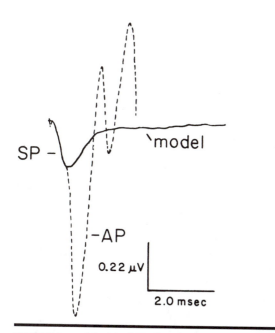

FIGURE 7.10 Model of SP produced by click stimulus, overlaid on actual recording of human ECochGm. (From J. D. Durrant & J. A. Ferraro, "Analog model of human click-elicited SP and effects of high-pass filtering." *Ear and Hearing, 12*, 144–148. Reprinted by permission of Williams & Wilkins.)

1973; Eggermont, 1976b). Figure 7.11 illustrates a normal ECochGm in response to a 2000 Hz tone burst (1 ms rise/fall, 5 ms plateau). In addition to extending the duration of the SP, tone-burst stimuli permit the examination of the response at specific frequencies (see Ferraro, Blackwell, Mediavilla, & Thedinger, 1994).

Signal Conditioning and Processing—Parameters

As described earlier, ECochG recording procedures may be either invasive or noninvasive. Recording parameters are virtually identical regardless of procedure, with the exceptions that transtympanic measurements generally require less amplification and fewer signal averages than extratympanic ECochG.

Analog filter settings for ECochG are fairly wide-band so that both dc (i.e., the SP) and ac (the AP) components are allowed to pass with minimum distortion of the waveform. In reality, the click-evoked SP is not a true dc potential, and a low frequency cut-off as high as 30 Hz may be acceptable (Durrant & Ferraro, 1991). A high-pass setting of 1 to 5 Hz and a 3000 Hz low-pass setting are common for routine ECochG applications and can subserve tests employing either clicks or tone bursts of several milliseconds' duration. A lower frequency cut-off is required

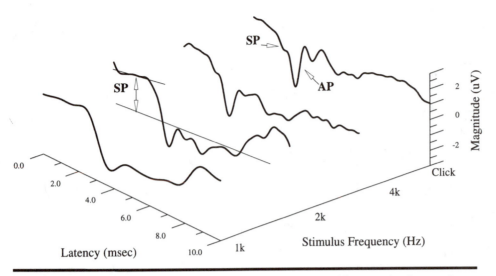

FIGURE 7.11 SP elicited by click versus tone bursts of indicated frequencies (tympanic-membrane electrode; EAR 3A earphone; click presented at 90 dB nHL; tone bursts presented at 105 dB HL).

the longer the duration of this tone burst. This is because the waveform of the SP follows the envelope of the stimulus, thereby representing a direct-current pulse that will be greatly distorted if the cut-off frequency is set too high (i.e., effecting too short of a time constant), leading to a gross underestimation of the SP's magnitude.

The averaging window for ECochG must be long enough to accommodate the duration of the response envelope. Thus, this window can be relatively short when BBCs are used as stimuli, since the SP and AP will generally occur within 5 ms of stimulus onset. A 10 ms window is a popular choice because this also allows for visualization of ABR components. For tone bursts, a good guideline is to use a window twice as long as the stimulus envelope so that the entire SP can be visualized.

Nonpathologic Variables

As noted earlier, considerable variability between subjects often is observed in the amplitude of the ECochGm. This, however, appears to be inherent to the pickup of the AP at extracochlear sites and not necessarily to the method of recording. For instance, transtympanic recordings from the promontory using needle electrodes produce on the order of 10 times larger signals than extratympanic/ear canal recordings but can yield a range of AP amplitudes as much as 20:1 (e.g., see data of Eggermont, 1976b). This range exceeds the range of amplitudes recorded with noninvasive methods (Durrant, 1986). The main difficulty with the extratympanic methods, compared to the transtympanic, is a matter of SNR, that is, the more remote the site of recording, the poorer the SNR. This is because the signal, the AP,

gets smaller while the noise remains essentially constant. In contrast to amplitude, the variability of latency is much less and is relatively independent of recording technique (Durrant, 1986). In general, standard deviations are typically less than 0.2 msec for the AP recorded from normal-hearing subjects.

Pathologic Variables and Differential Diagnostic Applications of ECochG

Diagnosis of Ménière's Disease. One of the two primary categories of clinical utility for AEP evaluations is in otoneurologic/differential diagnostics. Noninvasive ECochG has not proven too valuable for threshold estimation and is not considered as reliable as transtympanic ECochG (Probst, 1983) or even the ABR. In differential diagnoses, most clinical interest in ECochG has been directed toward the identification, assessment, and monitoring of Ménière's disease or hydrops. Advances in this area stem largely from the work of Coats (1981, 1986; see also Ferraro, Arenberg, & Hassanein, 1985; Staller, 1986), following observations of Eggermont (1976b) and Gibson, Moffat, and Ramsden (1977). Namely, many patients with Ménière's disease demonstrate amplitude-enhanced SPs, as illustrated in Figure 7.12. Such enhancement of the SP is rarely, if ever, seen in cases of pure retrocochlear lesions and is seen only infrequently in other cochlear disorders.

The major deficiency of ECochG in this application is that, while it is a highly specific test, it suffers in test sensitivity (e.g., see Pou, Hirsch, Durrant, Gold, & Kamerer, 1996). Specificity has generally been found to exceed 90%, but sensitivity may barely exceed 50%. False positives,

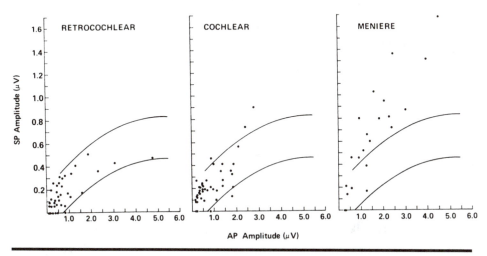

FIGURE 7.12 Scatterplots of SP versus AP amplitudes for three groups of pathologic ears. The curves represent best-fit estimates of ±2 standard deviations for responses obtained from normal ears. Recordings from ear canal. (Based on figure by Coats, 1981, from ASHA, 1988, with permission.)

however, are not entirely illogical; in the series of Pou and co-workers (1996), these included a perilymphatic fistula, which Campbell and Abbas (1993; 1994) had previously demonstrated to be possible. From the perspective of a hydromechanical model of hydrops (i.e., mechanical biasing of the motion of the basilar membrane), anomalous SP behavior in the case of perilymphatic fistula is not surprising. The poor sensitivity, on the other hand, may be accounted for by a variety of contingencies, albeit incompletely so. Ferraro and co-workers (1985) have reported on the degree to which positive ECochG findings depend upon active presentation of the classical symptoms of the disorder. Indeed, their observations raise the question as to whether ECochG is even worthwhile. That is, is it necessary to have a test to corroborate what the patient is reporting? The answer is affirmative. Symptoms, in the final analysis, are subjective by nature and not all patients are good historians. Therefore, it is compelling to have objective confirmation of symptoms. The high specificity of the findings certainly justify this application.

There also is the very real possibility that the sensitivity of ECochG in detecting Ménière's disease is underestimated as an artifact of methods. The click-evoked ECochGm was popularized effectively by noninvasive ECochG by virtue of the desire to minimize possible contamination of stimulus artifact. The inherent brevity of this stimulus makes it quite attractive for any AEP applications, because the stimulus artifact is generally over before the AEP of interest is elicited (i.e., due to ear-canal- and traveling-wave-based propagation delays and synaptic delays).

However, as described previously, the SP traditionally is defined and the response is more completely characterized by tone burst-elicited responses (see Dallos, 1973 for overview). Several transtympanic electrocochleographers faithfully honored this tradition (e.g., see Dauman, Aran, Charlet de Sauvage, & Portmann, 1988; Eggermont, 1976b; Gibson, 1993), and this technique has enjoyed recent growth of interest in the noninvasive recording area (Ferraro et al., 1994; Ferraro, Thedinger, Mediavilla, & Blackwell, 1994; Levine, Margolis, Fournier, & Winzenburg, 1992; Margolis, Levine, Fournier, Hunter, Smith, & Lilly, 1992). Since the click is broad spectrum, there is the possibility that the click could stimulate both positive and negative SP components. Both components could be enhanced, yet the net potential might be of unremarkable magnitude. This, however, is much less likely using a transducer like the Eartone 3A due to its TDH-39-like roll-off in frequency response above 4 kHz (i.e., much less sound pressure to evoke a positive component). [Note: Transtympanic methods traditionally have relied upon sound-field stimulation using transducers that, in turn, are capable of producing substantial SPLs at high frequencies. More recently, procedures for using the tubal insert type earphone have emerged (e.g., see Schwaber & Hall, 1990).] Still, cases will occasionally be encountered (see Figure 7.13) that show enhancement of SP to tone bursts wherein the click-evoked SP was only marginally or negligibly enhanced. In any event, the authors routinely include tone bursts to corroborate the click-response findings. Margolis and co-workers (Margolis, Rieks, Fournier, & Levine, 1995) have also suggested the use of both stimulus polarities and careful scrutiny of interpolarity latency differences, which apparently can be exaggerated by Ménière's. The success of recordings with tone

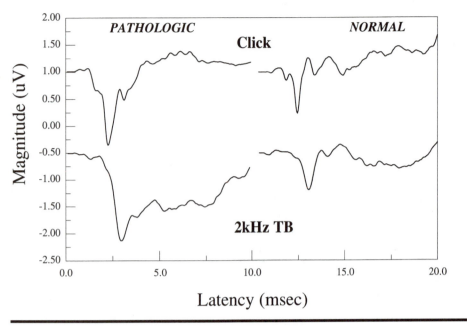

FIGURE 7.13 SP evoked by 2 kHz tone burst and enhanced in symptomatic ear of Ménière's patient in a case wherein results obtained with clicks were not positive. (Recording methods and parameters as in Figure 7.11)

bursts requires, again, appropriate recording parameters and meticulous technique—low low-frequency cut-offs of the preamplifier filter, consistent electrode placement, transducers (ideally shielded) that radiate minimal artifact, and judicious routing and/or shielding of electrode leads and leads to the transducers.

Finally, there is a technical limitation of trying to assess sensitivity/specificity of ECochG in detection of Ménière's disease. Namely, there is no true "gold standard" for the disease, despite efforts of the American Academy of Otolaryngology—Head and Neck Surgery to establish strict guidelines for the diagnosis (see Alford, 1972; Pearson & Brackmann, 1985). While the concurrent presentation of the full triad of symptoms is compelling, the symptoms clearly are not unique to this disorder.

Hearing Loss and ABR-Wave-I Enhancement. The major application of noninvasive ECochG to differential diagnostic testing, otherwise, is the facilitation of the ABR evaluation, that is, to improve detection and definition of the AP (ABR Wave I) and thereby provide information important to the interpretation of the ABR (discussed below). As illustrated in Figure 7.14, cochlear and more peripheral pathologies can be reflected in the latency-intensity functions of the AP. Latency shifts of the AP will be echoed by the latency-intensity functions of the later waves of the AEP, especially the ABR (Davis, 1976). Additionally, as shown previously in Figures 7.7 and 7.8,

ECochG can provide measurable APs at levels approaching the perceptual limits of the stimulus. Thus, measurable APs can be obtained in cases with peripheral hearing losses (Stypulkowski & Staller, 1987) for whom even high levels of stimulation will still represent relatively low sensation levels of stimulation. Consequently, the contribution of peripheral components to observed prolongations of later waves of the AEP can be more critically assessed when supplemented by ECochG techniques (Ferraro & Ferguson, 1989).

Threshold Estimation. Historically, the second major clinical application of ECochG was threshold estimation. Indeed, before the ABR, transtymanic ECochG was well on its way to becoming established as the objective method of choice (e.g., see Naunton & Zerlin, 1978), especially in Europe and elsewhere outside of the United States. However, in the American system with its growing audiology profession, a noninvasive method was more attractive. The extratymanic methods of the day seemed inadequately reliable, so the ABR soon completely captured clinical interest. Still, there continues to be interest in this application of ECochG, namely in accuracy of audiometric predictions of transtympanic ECochG and comparisons among results obtained via transtympanic ECochG, extratympanic ECochG, and surface-recorded ABR (e.g., Bellman, Barnard, & Beagley, 1984; Schoonhoven, Prijs, & Grote, 1996). The transtympanic method tends to win out when it

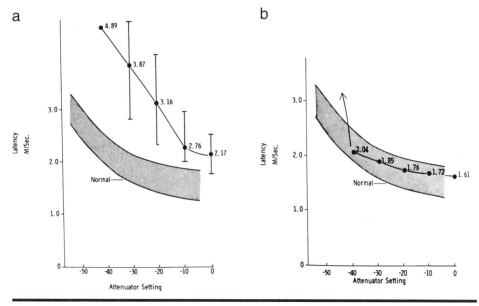

FIGURE 7.14 AP latency-intensity functions for group of patients with (A) mild-to-moderate conductive and (B) sloping sensorineural hearing loss. (Data from recordings from surface of the eardrum; adapted from Berlin, Cullen, Ellis, Lousteau, Yarbrough, & Lyons, 1974, with permission from *Otolaryngology—Head and Neck Surgery Journal*.)

comes to evaluating the profound loss, but the gains are lost in the shadow of the technical nuances of the method, most critically the need to examine the difficult-to-test patient under general anesthesia. At the same time, the occasional study of extratympanic ECochG in this application (e.g., see Laureano, McGrady, & Campbell, 1995) fails to garner much enthusiasm for even noninvasive ECochG, in comparison to ABR testing (the more accurate of the two).

Intraoperative Monitoring. The last major clinical application for ECochG involves monitoring of cochlear and eighth-nerve responses during otologic/otoneurologic surgery. As discussed in depth in Chapter 9, the short-latency potentials are inherently attractive for intraoperative monitoring because of their endurance across stages of sedation or anesthesia. Although still in its infancy, intraoperative ECochG monitoring is generally applied to help protect and/or preserve hearing during the surgical process (e.g., Ruth et al., 1988), assist the surgeon in identifying anatomical landmarks (e.g., Arenberg, Obert, & Gibson, 1991; Gibson, 1991), and help predict surgical outcome (e.g., Arenberg, Kobayashi, Obert, & Gibson, 1993, Arenburg et al., 1991).

The features of the ECochGm monitored during surgery may include the SP and AP amplitudes and the SP/AP amplitude ratio. For example, changes in the SP amplitude have been observed from probing the endolymphatic sac.

This finding, in turn, is used to help identify the sac from surrounding tissue for placement of an endolymphatic-mastoid shunt tube (Arenberg et al., 1991; Bojrab, Bhansali & Andreozzi, 1994). Improvement (i.e., reductions) in the SP/AP amplitude ratio following decompression of the sac and/or placement of a shunt tube have been interpreted to indicate a successful surgical outcome (Arenberg et al., 1993). However, long-term follow-up studies on the relationship between peri-operative changes in the ECochGm and patient outcome are needed to verify this finding.

Changes in the AP-N1 amplitude and absolute latency may be a harbinger of either good or bad surgical outcomes. For example, if the morphology of the AP improves and/or its latency shortens (e.g., after removal of an acoustic tumor), this may indicate an improvement in hearing status, or at least that hearing has been preserved during surgery. On the other hand, if AP morphology begins to worsen and/or N1 latency increases, this should serve as a warning that hearing status is being threatened. If the AP disappears and does not return, it is likely that hearing has not been preserved in that ear (Ruth et al., 1988). A potential, but as yet underexplored, application for intraoperative ECochG is in surgeries involving the middle ear (e.g., tympanic membrane/ossicular chain repair/replacement). It has long been known that the measurement of cochlear potentials (such as the CM) at the round window is sensitive to middle ear status (Gerhardt, Melnick, & Ferraro, 1979). This may prove useful for monitoring the effects of surgical repair of middle ear structures while the patient is still under anesthesia.

MEASUREMENT OF AUDITORY BRAINSTEM EVOKED POTENTIALS

Historical Perspective

Shown in Figure 7.15 is the typical ABR, as obtained in a normally hearing and neurologically intact subject, using moderately high levels of click stimulation and recording between vertex and the ipsilateral earlobe/mastoid with surface (disc) electrodes. This ostensibly yields the same short latency AEP as reported by Jewett, Romano, and Williston (1970). From another perspective, this is simply another method of noninvasive ECochG. Indeed, using this recording montage, but connecting the earlobe lead to the noninverting input of the differential amplifier (i.e., rather than the vertex lead, as in Figure 7.15), Sohmer and Feinmesser (1967; see also Sohmer & Feinmesser, 1973) earlier described a potential that proved to contain not only the AP, but up to seven component waves (see peak labels in Figure 7.15 in parentheses; Sohmer, Feinmesser, & Szabo, 1974). Of course, the peaks of their recorded response were negative, rather than positive as in Figure 7.15, but it was Jewett and Williston's (1971) polarity convention and peak labeling scheme that subsequently prevailed as the most widely accepted representation of the ABR.

Generators

Far more important than the vertex positive-versus-negative convention was the revelation that what Sohmer and Jewett had recorded independently were potentials containing both eighth nerve and brainstem potentials (Jewett, 1970).

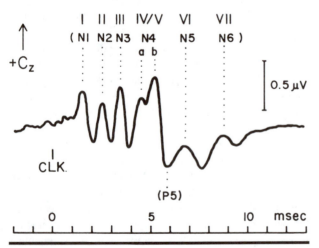

FIGURE 7.15 Auditory brainstem response. Onset of click (CLK) stimulus and vertex positive deflection (+Cz) as indicated. (From ASHA, 1988, with permission)

Therefore, Wave I of the auditory brainstem potential actually arises from the auditory nerve (Buchwald & Huang, 1975; Sohmer et al., 1974) and is none other than the N1 component of the AP. Furthermore, Wave II of the human ABR now is attributed predominantly to the eighth nerve (Martin, Pratt & Schwegler, 1995; Møller & Janetta, 1982). Only the waves beyond II (or N2) appear to arise from brainstem level generators per se. Consequently, Waves I, II, and III arise from structures ipsilateral to the side of stimulation, whereas later waves may come from structures that receive ipsilateral, contralateral, or bilateral inputs from the auditory periphery (Achor & Starr, 1980a, 1980b; Buchwald & Huang, 1975; Møller, Jannetta, Bennett, & Møller, 1981; Wada & Starr, 1983a, 1983b, 1983c), although the most recent studies suggest a predominantly crossed pathway for components arising rostrally (Durrant, Martin, Hirsch, & Schwegler, 1994; Levine, Gardner, Stufflebeam, Fullerton, Carlisle, Furst, Rosen, & Kiang, 1993b). However, although the details continue to be debated (e.g., see reviews by Legatt, Arezzo, & Vaughan, 1988; Møller, 1994; Moore, 1987), the IV/V complex would appear to arise predominantly from the lateral lemniscus with Wave V predominantly deriving from excitation of crossed pathways and a generator site at the rostral extreme of this tract, if not at the inferior colliculus (Durrant & Lovrinic, 1995; Møller, Jho, Yokota, & Jannetta, 1995; Møller, Jannetta & Jho, 1994). Finally, although a given level of the auditory pathway may dominate the contribution to a given peak (e.g., along the lines of Moore, 1987), a more realistic model (e.g., Scherg & Von Cramon, 1985) may be one wherein each level contributes a poliphasic potential. The overall ABR recorded thus would be the phasor summation of these complex waves.

Wave Morphology and Measures

Frequently measured parameters of the ABR waveform are illustrated in Figure 7.16. The amplitude measures commonly used are peak-to-peak, that is, the voltage difference between the designated positive peak and the subsequent negative peak/trough. This avoids the difficulty of determining the true baseline of the potential; however, this parameter may compound effectively amplitude measures of potentials actually arising from separate generators (Hughes, Fino, & Hart, 1985; Moore, 1987; Wada & Starr, 1983a, 1983b, 1983c). Relative amplitude measures also have been employed, namely the ratio of the Wave V to Wave I amplitudes. However, by far the most extensively used measures for clinical purposes are those of latency. As defined earlier, the (absolute) latency is the time difference between the onset of the stimulus to the peak of the wave (Figure 7.16). Relative latency measures also are of keen interest and are referred to as interwave latencies or interpeak intervals, namely the differences between

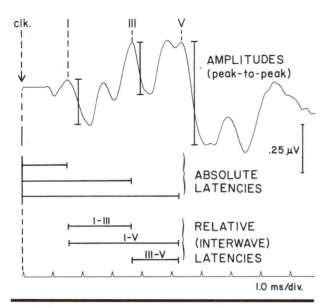

FIGURE 7.16 Fundamental measures of amplitude and latency of the ABR. (From ASHA, 1988, with permission)

absolute latencies of two peaks (e.g., I-V). By convention, the ABR evaluation favors the vertex-positive peaks of the waveform, but this may not be entirely justified from the perspective of assessment of all generators (Hughes et al., 1985) and/or the fact that the negative peaks can provide useful alternative measures (e.g., if residual noise has obscured a positive peak).

Recording/Interface Methods

Because the generators of the ABR are located at appreciable distances from the recording electrodes, small variations in electrode placement are not critical (Martin & Moore, 1977). An electrode in the vicinity of an imaginary line drawn between vertex or forehead at hairline picks up the primary brainstem waves as positive potentials relative to ground, and this zone provides optimal pickup of the brainstem potentials (Beattie, Beguwala, Mills, & Boyd, 1986; Van Olphen, Rodenburg, & Verway, 1978). However, the area of the earlobe or mastoid, while providing optimal pickup of the eighth nerve response (via surface recording methods), is not totally inactive for the brainstem potentials (Terkildsen, Osterhammel, & Huis int Veld, 1974). Still, recording between vertex/forehead to earlobe/mastoid is the most widely used recording montage because it does provide pickup of eighth nerve and brainstem components simultaneously and is inherently less noisy than recordings between vertex and a noncephalic reverence.

Two- or multichannel recordings have also gained popularity for clinical purposes, most commonly utilizing the ipsilateral and contralateral recording montages. The vertex/forehead inputs are tied together and leads from each

earlobe/mastoid are connected to a separate channel. As shown in Figure 7.17, Wave I is attenuated/negligible in the contralateral recording, and there are other morphological differences between the ABRs recorded via the two channels. These differences are largely attributable to the difference in "view" of the generators provided by the two channels (Durrant, Boston, & Martin, 1990). Analyses of three-dimensional voltage space (bearing in mind that the head is a solid conductor) have shown that each ABR wave has an associated voltage plane of particular orientation (Pratt, Martin, Bleich, Kaminer, & Har'El, 1987; Williston, Jewett, & Martin, 1981). Consequently, as one moves about the head and alters the axis of orientation of the bipolar electrode pair (like turning the "rabbit ears" type of indoor television antenna), more or less different wave morphologies should be observed. Consequently, both amplitude and latency differences will be observed (e.g., see Creel, Garber, King, & Witkop, 1980; Stockard, Stockard, & Sharbrough, 1978). As illustrated in Figure 7.17, the second channel may resolve the peaks of the IV/V complex better, thereby ensuring the proper labeling of the Wave V peak (although they typically do not have identical latencies). Corroboration of the interpretation of the ipsilaterally recorded ABR perhaps represents the broadest clinical usage of two-channel recordings currently, although multichannel recordings may enhance the detection of pathology, per

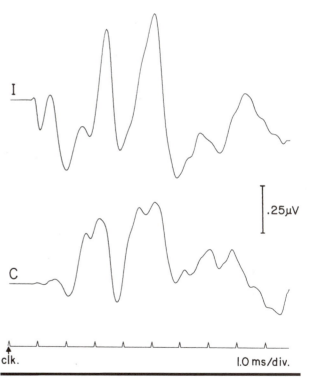

FIGURE 7.17 Ipsilateral (I) versus contralateral (C) recordings of the ABR. (From ASHA, 1988, with permission)

se (e.g., see Hammond & Yiannikas, 1987; Hashimoto, Ishiyama, & Tozuka, 1979).

Stimulus Parameters

Intensity. The effects of (click) stimulus level and typical latency-intensity functions of major components of the ABR are shown in Figure 7.18. Naturally, the amplitude of the response diminishes with decreasing intensity but more notable is the tendency for the earliest waves to disappear in the noise floor of the recording. Otherwise, the latency-intensity functions of the brainstem components roughly parallel those of Wave I, that is the AP (N1). The basis for the latency-intensity shift, again, is attributed primarily to the basalward spread of excitation with increasing intensity. This has been demonstrated for the ABR by Don and Eggermont (1978), as illustrated in Figure 7.19.

Spectrum. The fact that the abrupt onset and broad spectrum of a click synchronizes and excites a broad population of neuronal discharges also makes the click a very effective stimulus for the ABR, indeed for most AEPs. The click also can provide general high-frequency threshold information (Don, Eggermont, & Brackmann, 1979), although brief tone bursts and similar transients and related

methods are essential for more frequency-specific information (Stapells, Picton, Perez-Abalo, Read, & Smith, 1985). Again, stimulus frequency specificity is not compatible with stimulus brevity, so there is a spread of energy around the central frequency and, with increasing stimulus intensity, a basalward spread of excitation (Folsom, 1984). Low-frequency sinusoidal pulses also have, effectively, longer rise times than high-frequency pulses, which adds to the propagation delay in the cochlea, causing longer ABR latencies. There also is a concomitant reduction of synchrony so that low-frequency stimuli are not nearly as reliable as high-frequency stimuli for eliciting the ABR. Still, the ABR can be evoked by stimuli with spectral lobes centered at frequencies of 500 Hz or lower (Stapells & Picton, 1981; Suzuki, Hirai, & Horiuchi, 1977). With the use of such stimuli, Wave V often may be tracked down to the limits of visual detection of the response, with observed stimulus levels within 10 dB of behavioral thresholds at corresponding audiometric frequencies, at least down to 500 Hz (Suzuki & Yamane, 1982). Indeed, Stapells, Gravel, and Martin (1995), using tone pips in notch-band noise, found a high correlation overall between behavioral auditory thresholds in young children (0.94) over the range of 500 to 4000 Hz with nearly all ABR-derived thresholds falling within 30 dB (98%), and the vast majority within 15 dB (80%). However, in normally or impaired hearing subjects, the accuracy of prediction of behavioral thresholds via ABR testing is not constant across frequency that is decreasing with decreasing frequency (Beattie, Garcia & Johnson, 1996; Stapells, Gravel, & Martin, 1995).

The opposite end of the spectrum, toward the upper-frequency limit of hearing, presents significant technical challenges as well, including the production of adequately clean signals. Any sound energy below the intended frequency range of interest easily could become the effective stimulus, since hearing sensitivity decreases so dramatically above the conventional audiometric range (i.e., above 8 kHz). This frequency range is important for possible applications of ABR testing to the screening/monitoring of ototoxicity in patients too ill to participate in behavioral testing. Despite the technical problems, Fausti and coworkers (Fausti, Mitchell, Frey, Henry, & O'Connor, 1995) have recently suggested a practical and efficient method of high-frequency ABR testing.

Duration/Gating Function. The ABR is relatively insensitive to the stimulus duration (Gorga, Beauchine, Reiland, Worthington, & Javel, 1984) but quite dependent on the rise/fall times (Kodera, Marsh, Suzuki, & Suzuki, 1983). The more gradual the rise-fall time is, the lower the amplitude and the longer the latencies of the waves will be, with Wave V being the least sensitive to this stimulus parameter (Hecox, Squires, & Galambos, 1976). The gating function itself also is important, since it is what mainly determines

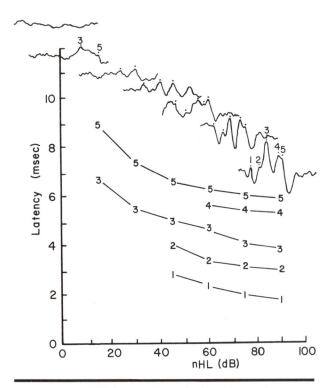

FIGURE 7.18 ABR latency-intensity functions and corresponding waveforms. (From ASHA, 1988, with permission)

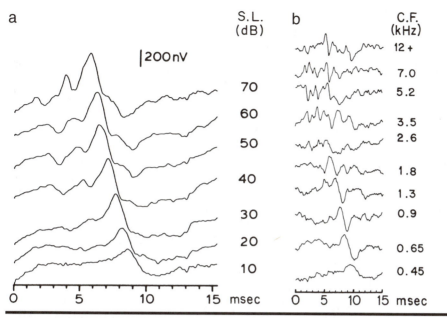

FIGURE 7.19 (A) Broadband click-elicited ABRs. (From M. Don, J. J. Eggermont, & D. E. Brackmann, "Reconstruction of the audiogram using brain-stem responses and high-pass noise masking." *Annals of Otology, Rhinology and Laryngology, 88* [Supplement 5]), 1–20, 1979. Reprinted with permission of Annals Publishing Company.) (B) Derived narrowband responses. (Adapted from Don & Eggermont, 1978)

the spectrum. Various functions are available to minimize spectral splatter (Durrant & Lovrinic, 1995; Gorga, Abbas, & Worthington, 1985), although stop-band masking may be added to further ensure frequency specificity (Picton, Ouellette, Hamel, & Smith, 1979; Stapells et al., 1985). Another method for obtaining frequency-specific information, albeit more time consuming, is the "subtractive" masking method originally described by Teas, Eldridge, and Davis (1962). It is this method that was used by Don, Eggermont, and Brackmann (1979) to derive the narrowband ABRs shown in Figure 7.19B, as well as the narrowband APs shown previously in Figure 7.9 (Eggermont, 1976a).

Repetition Rate. Since signal averaging requires many repetitions of the stimulus, the efficiency of data collection is directly dependent upon stimulus repetition rate. However, due to adaptation, the ABR is sensitive to this feature (Fowler & Noffsinger, 1983; Picton, Stapells, & Campbell, 1981). As shown in Figure 7.20, the latencies of the waves are prolonged and amplitudes are decreased as stimulus repetition rate increases. Rates of 10/sec or less are necessary for maximal definition of all the waves, although rates up to 20/sec may be used with little compromise. Rates of 30/sec or higher may be used if only Wave V definition is essential. Such high stimulus rates are particularly attractive for deriving thresholds in newborns and difficult-to-test subjects wherein time is of the essence. High stimulus

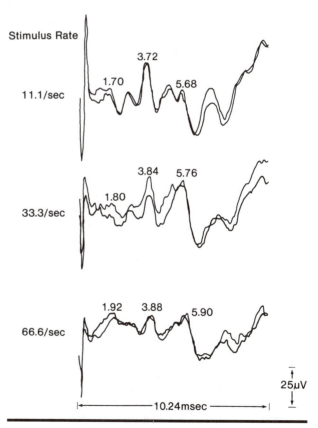

FIGURE 7.20 Effect of click repetition rate on the ABR. (From ASHA, 1988, with permission)

rates also are used by some clinicians as a way of stressing the system and, perhaps, exaggerating an otherwise marginal abnormality in the response, that is, by (presumably) adapting the system (e.g., see Tanaka, Komatsuzaki, & Hentona, 1996). However, high repetition rates may not involve adaptation alone (Durrant, 1986), and the adaptation effects may not be uniform over the entire train of stimuli presented, that is, from the first to the last (Lasky, Maier, & Hecox, 1996). Consequently, interpretation of the results of increasing repetition rate ("positive" or "negative") should be tempered accordingly.

Polarity. Although not affecting the spectrum of the stimulus and imperceptible to the listener, polarity or starting phase of the stimulus often affects the detailed morphology of the ABR waveform. For example, condensation and rarefaction clicks frequently are observed to differentially affect the amplitudes, latencies, and/or resolution of some peaks of the ABR (Figure 7.21). Although still a relatively minor effect, the underlying mechanisms are intriguing and the examiner's choices important for the clearest interpretation. The effects of polarity, first, tend to be variable across subjects. In most subjects the rarefaction phase leads to the shortest latency, but the condensation phase elicits the earlier responses in others (Orlando & Folsom, 1995). Latency differences usually amount to no more than 0.1 to 0.2 msec in normal listeners. However, a sloping high-

frequency hearing loss can lead to more dramatic effects of stimulus polarity (Coats & Martin, 1977; Sand & Saunte, 1994). These effects depend largely upon the low-frequency components of the stimulus (e.g., see Deltenre & Mansbach, 1995; Don, Vermiglio, Ponton, Eggermont, & Masuda, 1996; Fowler & Swanson, 1988; Orlando & Folsom, 1995; Salt & Thornton, 1983), since the auditory neurons are most capable of preserving phase information for low frequency stimuli. For humans, relative to the polarity effect in the ABR, "low" frequencies appear to be delimited by 1000 Hz (Deltenre & Mansbach, 1995). That phase should affect, particularly, the latency of the ABR's wave components is not surprising from principles of cochlear physiology, that is, given that hair cells respond directionally to shearing displacements of their hairs with displacements of the organ of Corti toward scala vestibuli being excitatory, and toward scala tympani, inhibitory (see Durrant & Lovrinic, 1995, for review).

Contrary to expectations, however, the interpolarity latency differences do not necessarily correspond to a half-cycle difference for a given frequency and are subject to inherent variability of neural timing (Don et al., 1996). Dallos and Wang (1974), however, suggested some time ago that since the cochlear hair cell system responds to both displacement and velocity, then movement—not merely displacement—toward scala vestibuli is excitatory. Consequently, a latency difference corresponding to only a quarter-cycle difference would be expected, as observed in the results of their study of the whole-nerve action potential in the guinea pig. The polarity effect also appears to be negligible at low intensities (namely, below 30 to 55 dB), and the combination of limiting frequency and intensity of stimulation for a given frequency has been suggested to be associated with the break point on the low-frequency skirts of tuning curve of the corresponding primary auditory neurons (Deltenre & Mansbach, 1995).

Although use of alternating stimulus polarity offers the advantage of canceling stimulus artifact, it thus is preferable to separately collect responses to each phase, at least for otoneurologic applications wherein details of the waveform are important. This precaution avoids the muddling of polarity effects on the waveform and the uncertainties thereof. Should it be desired/necessary, the responses to each polarity stimulus can be combined later in the computer memory to derive the alternating polarity response.

Bone-Conduction Stimuli

Regardless of application, conductive pathology is likely to be encountered in routine ABR testing. This variable may be addressed on the test administration side or on the interpretation side. The latter is handled later in this chapter. The former is addressed at this juncture because an obvious

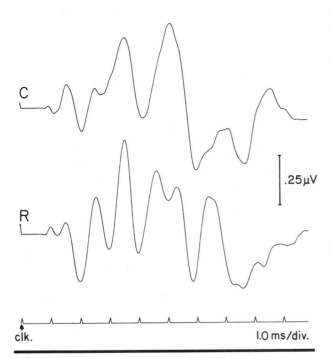

FIGURE 7.21 Effects of click polarity on the ABR: (C) condensation; (R) rarefaction. (From ASHA, 1988, with permission)

approach from an audiologist's perspective, of course, is to invoke the use of bone-conduction stimulation. Evaluation of the auditory brainstem response (ABR) using bone-conducted stimulation has met with guarded interest. The major concern has been generated seemingly by the observation that, except in very young children (discussed below), the ABR elicited by bone-conduction (BC) clicks tends to have a longer latency than the ABR elicited by clicks produced by conventional audiometric earphones (Cornacchia, Martini & Morra, 1983; Kavanaugh & Beardsley, 1979; Mauldin & Jerger, 1979; Weber, 1983). Until recently, it was assumed that the BC click appears to be a low-pass-filtered version of the air-conduction (AC) click and, therefore, that ABR latency differences between modes of stimulation are entirely attributable to spectral differences in these stimuli.

The "low-pass" concept seems consistent with measured frequency response of bone vibrators versus earphones on their respective calibration couplers and even by casual listening to broadband stimuli (white noise or clicks) via the two transducers. Gorga and Thornton (1989) were the first to question inadequate high-frequency output as the main/only factor in the BC-evoked response. A subsequent study of the effective frequency response of the Telephonics TDH-39 versus the Radioear B71 bone vibrator, using an adaptation of the sensorineural acuity level (SAL) test, demonstrated, indeed, that the artificial mastoid appreciably underestimates the efficiency of high-frequency output of the bone vibrator, although the bone vibrator is more variable than the earphone (Durrant & Hyre, 1993b). Previous research in BC, however, had suggested yet another factor. Bekesy (1960) used a wire model to show how the skull is probably set into modal vibration, and, indeed, Boezeman and co-workers (Boezeman, Bronkhurst, Kapteyn, Houffelaar, & Shel, 1984) concluded that there are significant propagation delays in the plates of the skull. In a follow-up study, real-head accelerometer measurements were made in normal adults and yielded results suggesting that the ABRs elicited by BC reflect the influence primarily of propagational delays, which are most acute for forehead vibrator placement (in addition to the well-known decrease in stimulator efficiency at this site [Durrant & Hyre, 1993a]). Nevertheless, some low-pass filtering also was evident.

These results are gratifying in the backdrop of observations of BC stimulation in premature and newborn infants— shorter latencies for BC than AC clicks with mastoid placement (e.g., see Hooks & Weber, 1984; Mauldin & Jerger, 1979; Yang, Rupert, & Moushegian, 1987). This suggests that the effects of vibratory nuances of the skull, varies over ontogeny.

With matching of sensation levels of BC (mastoid placement) and AC clicks, Durrant and Hyre (1993a) suggested

that, at least in some subjects, very comparable ABRs are recordable in adults, but such matching clearly is a luxury in many applications. The point becomes moot, however, if the differences are accepted for what they are, technical differences in mode of stimulation, just as the differences between tubal insert and supra-aural earphones have been accepted. Then one simply develops normative data for the given transducer. And, if there remains anxiety that the AC and BC click may not be identical in every subject, there is always frequency-specific stimuli, which Stapells and his co-workers (e.g., see Foxe & Stapells, 1993) have employed effectively in pediatric applications. Still other researchers have demonstrated utility of the SAL procedure (Ysunza & Cone-Wesson, 1997). Admittedly, estimation of the air-bone gap via any of these methods may be less than perfect, but then such is the case in conventional audiometry.

There are, nevertheless, substantial technical difficulties in BC testing. Due to some 40 dB less sensitivity, there is the dual problem of reduced maximum output (which also plagues conventional audiometry) and increased stimulus artifact, further enhanced by the proximity of the transducer to the skin and the impossibility of effectively shielding it. Still, these problems are manageable, and BC stimulation can be effectively employed to resolve issues of conductive involvement.

Masking

There still is considerable debate as to whether masking is ever needed for ABR testing. First, at least for clicks, there appears to be greater transcranial attenuation than encountered in pure tone audiometry (Finitzo-Hieber, Hecox, & Cone, 1979). Additional transcranial attenuation can be realized through the use of tubal insert earphones (Clemis et al., 1986). Second, in terms of determining the possibility of retrocochlear pathology, a response to crossover stimuli would be so delayed as to raise as much suspicion as an absent response. Nevertheless, in the audiologic-oriented evaluation, much the same consideration for masking must be given as in behavioral audiometry.

Monaural versus Binaural Stimulation

Binaural stimulation greatly enhances the amplitude of the response. Were the central pathways conveying right- and left-eared information totally separately, it might be expected that the binaurally stimulated ABR would be twice as large as the monaurally elicited response. As illustrated by Figure 7.22, the binaural ABR does approach the sum of the monaural ABRs, but not quite (Dobie & Norton, 1980). The difference between the binaural and summed monaural ABRs yields the binaural interaction (BI) potential (Dobie & Berlin, 1979; Dobie & Norton, 1980). This

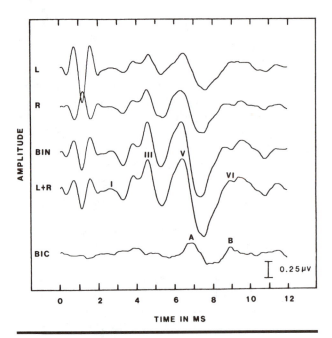

FIGURE 7.22 Binaural (BIN) versus monaural ABRs (L and R) and the derivation (i.e., BIN – [L+R]) of the binaural interaction component (BIC, demarked by peaks A and B). (From ASHA, 1988, with permission)

high-intensity stimuli comprises frequencies between 50 and 1000 Hz (Kevanishvili & Aponchenko, 1979), with a shift toward lower-frequency content at low-stimulus levels (Elberling, 1979). Nevertheless, current practices deemphasize the low-frequency content, since emphasis is placed upon the peak latencies. The peaks themselves represent relatively high-frequency features of the ABR. Therefore, typical bandpasses employed clinically in analog prefiltering are 100 to 3000 Hz (6 dB/oct roll-offs). In signal averaging, sampling epochs of 10 to 15 msec are typical for broadband click stimuli. However, such parameters are nominal and assume recordings of responses primarily from older children and adults and the use of clicks presented at moderately high level stimuli, that is, conditions more typical of otoneurologic diagnostic applications. In young children and even adults, particularly with an interest in estimating hearing thresholds, a lower low-frequency cut-off may be preferable (Sininger, 1995; Spivak, 1993). A lower cut-off, as well as windows (epochs) of 20 msec certainly are desirable when recording responses to low-frequency and/or longer duration stimuli (Suzuki & Horiuchi, 1977).

potential is most prominent in the Wave V-VII time frame and is attributed to neurons that are shared by the left and right brainstem auditory pathways. Indeed, recent work applying sophisticated three-dimensional analyses to the BI potential (i.e., 3-channel Lissajous trajectories) appear to validate it as a true manifestation of binaural processing, specifically auditory neural activity subserving binaural lateralization/localization (Polyakov & Pratt, 1994, 1996). Still, perhaps because the binaural interaction potential is small and intimately depends upon the nuances of the morphology of the monaural ABRs, its clinical utility has yet to be established (Fowler & Swanson, 1988). Emerging methods, namely involving analyses designed in deference to the inherently poor signal-to-noise ratio of the BI potential (Stollman, Snik, Hombergen, Nieuwenhys, & ten Koppel, 1996), hold promise in this area.

Signal Conditioning and Processing— Parameters

Because the amplitudes of its component waves fall in the submicrovolt range and the background noise is in the tens of microvolts, the ABR usually requires amplifier gains of 100,000 to 500,000 and Ns of 500 to 2000, or more. Again, some analog prefiltering is helpful in improving the SNR, even with signal averaging. The normal ABR elicited by

Nonpathologic Variables

Beside stimulus parameters, there are various nonpathologic or subject variables that are worth considering to fully appreciate the clinical utility, limitations, and interpretation of the ABR evaluation. First, the widespread popularity of ABR measurement for clinical purposes is owed partly to the fact that the ABR is relatively unaffected by changes in subject state, including natural and sedated sleep (Amadeo & Shagass, 1973; Sohmer, Gafni, & Chisin, 1978) and attention (Picton & Hillyard, 1974). Sedation often is required for ABR evaluations in young children and other uncooperative subjects to obtain acceptable background noise and allow for adequate time to collect data. Newborns usually are testable under natural sleep (Fria, 1980; see also Chapter 10), but noisy recordings can lead to ABR misinterpretations even in this population (McCall & Ferraro, 1991). In some cases and for other purposes (e.g., intraoperative monitoring), examination of patients under heavy sedation or anesthesia may be required. While various anesthesthetic agents and/or strong sedatives may be used with negligible effects on the latencies or amplitudes of the ABR (see Hall, 1992, for review), care must be taken to maintain the core temperature of the body or to account for the effects thereof. A reduction in core temperature prolongs the latency of the ABR and can be substantive for temperatures below 33°C (Stockard, Sharbrough, & Tinker, 1978).

Substantial maturational changes occur in the ABR during early life, both in terms of waveform morphology

(Figure 7.23A) and latencies (Figure 7.23B) (Cevette, 1984; Fria, 1980; Salamy, Fenn, & Bronshvag, 1979; Salamy & McKean, 1976; Starr, Amlie, Martin, & Sanders, 1977; see also Chapter 10). Interpeak intervals ostensibly reflect neuronal conduction velocities (determined by axonal diameter and myelinization) and lengths of paths (Moore, Ponton, Eggermont, Wu, & Huang, 1996; Ponton, Moore & Eggermont, 1996). This necessitates the use of age-adjusted norms for the interpretation of ABR evaluations in premature infants and newborns. Failure to account for the maturation variable also can lead to substantial errors in estimation of hearing level (Klein, 1984).

The early maturational changes of the ABR are ostensibly complete within two years (chronological age) in normally hearing children. Adult-like latencies are reached by this time, with only modest changes throughout early childhood thereafter (Jiang, 1996). In adolescence, males begin to develop slightly longer latencies than females. By adulthood, the gender difference amounts to approximately 0.2 msec in absolute Wave V latency on average (Jerger & Hall, 1980; Rowe, 1978). Separate norms are thus preferred for the most critical interpretation of the ABR in males versus females. As adults age, latencies of all the waves may again increase, especially over the age of 50, but this issue continues to be debated. Indeed, age-related changes may be potentiated/confounded by the presence of hearing loss (Watson, 1996), and it may be that ABRs recorded in older subjects are simply more variable (Jerger & Hall, 1980; Spivak, 1993). Nevertheless, separate norms may be desirable for older subjects.

Pathologic Variables and Differential Diagnostic Applications of ABR—Cochlear and More Peripheral Hearing Loss

It should be evident from the latency-intensity function (Figures 7.18 and 7.19) that whenever the level of the stimulus is either directly or effectively reduced, the latency, if not the waveform, of the ABR is affected. The impact upon the ABR, as manifested by latency-intensity functions, is much as demonstrated earlier for the AP (Figure 7.14), but is worth repeating and elaborating here. Since conductive hearing losses cause sound energy to be attenuated, the latency-intensity function is shifted along the intensity axis by essentially the amount of the conductive hearing loss (Figure 7.24). The I-V interpeak interval is altered little (Mendelson, Salamy, Lenoir, & McKean, 1979; see also review by Fria, 1980), but the waves prior to Wave V may be lost at low-levels and impede this measurement. However, the shift of the latency-intensity function may not be parallel if the loss involved has a sloping configuration (Gorga, Reiland, & Beauchaine, 1985). Cochlear hearing losses also effectively reduce the sensation level and cause

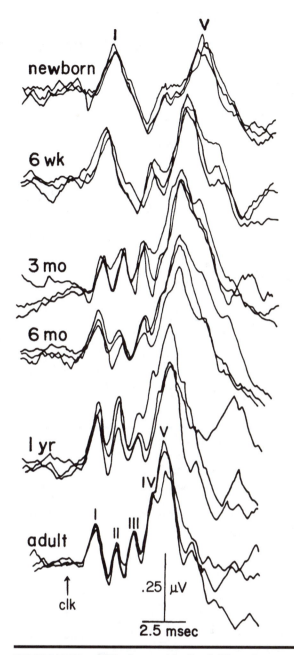

FIGURE 7.23A ABRs from subjects of different ages, as indicated. (Adapted from A. Salamy & C. M. McKean, "Postnatal development of human brainstem potentials during the first year of life." *Electroencephalography and Clinical Neurophysiology, 40,* 418–426, 1976, with permission from Elsevier Scientific Publishers Ireland, Ltd.)

shifts in the latency-intensity function (Figure 7.25), but the results are more complex. The overall effect is dependent upon the severity and configuration of the loss (Bauch & Olsen, 1988, 1989) and the frequency composition of

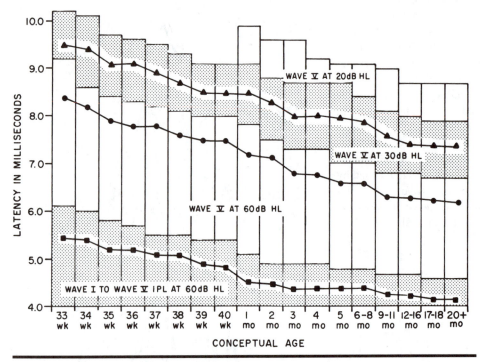

Primary Children's Medical Center
Auditory Brainstem Response Normative Data
(N=580)

FIGURE 7.23B ABR Wave V latencies and I–V interpeak latencies at indicated nHLs versus conceptual age. Conceptual ages in months (mo) are actually 44 weeks (wk) + the indicated number of months. Horizontal bars above each data point demark latencies that are 2 standard deviations (s.d.) above the means (N = 580 newborns). (Adapted from M. J. Cevette, "Auditory brainstem response testing in the intensive care unit." *Seminars in Hearing, 5,* 57–68, with permission from Thieme Medical Publishers, Inc.)

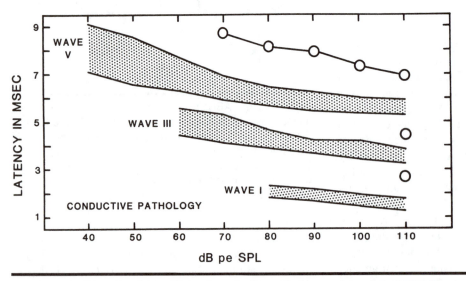

FIGURE 7.24 Example of the effects of conductive pathology on latencies of ABR Waves I, III, V. Stippled area represents ±2 standard deviations of latencies for normal-hearing subjects. (From ASHA, 1988, with permission)

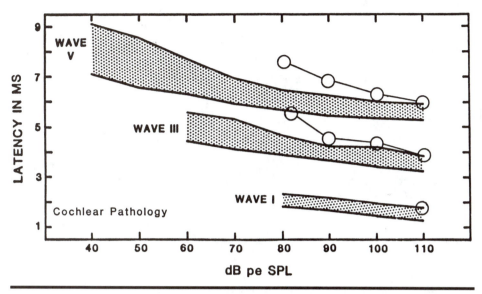

FIGURE 7.25 Example of the effects of cochlear pathology on latencies of ABR Waves I, III, V. Stippled area represents ±2 standard deviations of latencies for normal-hearing subjects (From ASHA, 1988, with permission)

the stimulus. It thus is essential to account for cochlear and more peripheral hearing loss in the interpretation of the ABR.

Dealing with Cochlear and More Peripheral Losses—Conceptual Bases and Strategy. The complications of lesions peripheral to the auditory nerve are common in routine practice, and the proper accounting for this factor is of utmost importance to the interpretation of the ABR. The approach to dealing with the potential confounds of such losses, in the final analysis, is a matter of strategy (Durrant & Fowler, 1996). This, in turn, is a dynamic decision process that is not readily supplanted by mere correction factors or any monolithic "game plan." Such a strategy is particularly important in the approach to diagnostic testing in patients with asymmetric hearing loss, since it is this symptom that is so common in lesions of the auditory nerve and lower auditory brainstem pathways, for example, acoustic tumors. As will be emphasized later, interaural latency differences (ILDs) in latency measures are important parameters in assessing the possibility of retrocochlear pathology. However, ILDs are not necessarily the most sensitive detectors of retrocochlear pathology, nor are they equally sensitive across pathologies (Musiek, Johnson, Gollegly, Josey, & Glasscock, 1989). Of all the latency measures, interpeak intervals provide some of the most compelling information by which to differentiate between retrocochlear and cochlear/more peripheral pathologies, and among sites of retrocochlear lesions. Still, no parameter by itself can be expected to provide adequate sensitivity in all cases (Musiek & Lee,

1995). It thus is critical to have as clear of a picture of the patient's ABR as possible.

Pathology peripheral to the eighth nerve, unfortunately, tends to compromise the definition of the earlier waves of the ABR, due to the effective reduction of sensation level and/or filtering effects of the hearing-loss configuration (as discussed in more detail below). Consequently, the principal strategy in such cases is to set the stimulus level high enough to obviate, as much as possible, the effects of peripheral hearing loss. Nevertheless, the combination of the hearing loss degree and configuration and the spectrum and level of the stimulus determine the effective sensation level of the stimulus (Lightfoot, 1993), so a variety of approaches are needed to handle the gamut of cases encountered clinically.

The discussion, for the moment, will focus on responses elicited by clicks, since the BBC is the most widely used stimulus for otoneurologic-oriented evaluations. Furthermore, the focus here will be on high-frequency hearing loss since low-frequency hearing losses, in general, have little or no affect on the click-elicited ABR (see Figure 7.26, *ULF* data) (Fowler & Durrant, 1994; Rosenhamer, Lindstrom, & Lundborg, 1981). Now, in cases of pure cochlear lesions, the stated goal of effectively bypassing the cochlear pathology is potentially achievable because of recruitment-like characteristics in the ABR latency-intensity (L-I) function, as described earlier (Figure 7.25). These characteristics are attributed to a combination of basalward spread of excitation in the cochlea and recruitment of neural fibers. In other words, the underlying mechanisms are themselves cochlear. Basalward spread of

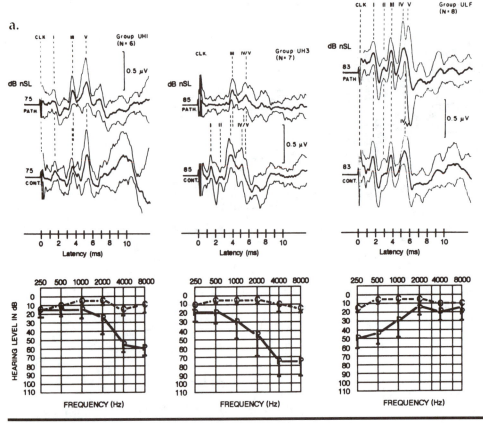

FIGURE 7.26 In each panel, ABRs in heavy lines are grand averages of ABRs for pathologic (P) and control (C) ears of three groups of subjects with hearing losses indicated by audiometric data below. (From C. G. Fowler & J. D. Durrant, "The effects of peripheral hearing loss on the auditory brainstem response." In J. T. Jacobson, Ed., *Principles and Applications in Auditory Evoked Potentials*, pp. 237–250. Boston: Allyn & Bacon, 1994, with permission.)

excitation, again, accounts for much of the latency-intensity (L-I) function measured in normal ears. From the principles of cochlear mechanics (see Durrant & Lovrinic, 1995, for more extensive review), the traveling wave progresses systematically from base to apex. As the stimulus level is increased, the basalward excitation becomes increasingly dominant. At the basal end of the cochlea, the phase of the vibration is least variable with distance along the basilar membrane and wave velocity is highest. Consequently, synchronization of neural excitation is superior at the base.

In contrast, wave propagation toward the apex is increasingly slower, and activity from adjacent regions along the basilar membrane cancel due to phase dispersion (i.e., phase changes rapidly over distance). This is the "norm" and explains why the normal click-evoked ABR is dominated by the frequencies between 2 and 4 kHz at moderately high levels of stimulation. It is the absolute level of the stimulus, not the sensation level, that determines the stimulation pattern on the basilar membrane and, consequently, the latency of the ABR. Near threshold, however, relatively few neurons are excited. With increasing stimulus levels, more

and more neurons are activated and already active neurons respond more vigorously. Consequently, the near-threshold levels of activity become insignificant. By the same token, if there is pathology of the hearing organ that decreases sensitivity, the associated "loss" of activity becomes insignificant with increasing levels of stimulation. The effects of cochlear hearing loss thus are more evident at low stimulus levels than at high levels. Consequently, obstensibly normal ABRs are recordable when the degree of loss in the vicinity of 4000 Hz is no worse than mild to moderate (see Figure 7.26, *UH1* data) (Rosenhamer et al., 1981; Selters & Brackmann, 1977). Latency-intensity functions in such cases converge upon the normative functions at high stimulus levels, as illustrated by Figure 7.25. [Note: This particular case demonstrated a fairly flat hearing loss of moderate degree.]

Precipitously sloping high-frequency losses of moderate or worse severity, on the other hand, cause increased latencies (Coats & Martin, 1977; Gorga et al., 1985; Gorga, Worthington, Reiland, Beauchaine, & Goldgar, 1985). Although a converging pattern in the latency-intensity function may still be evident, even at high stimulus levels, the latencies are less likely to fall within normal ranges. The ABR waveform also is likely to be degraded, with the detection of the earlier waves being most vulnerable (see Figure 7.26, *UH3* data). The reason for this is that an impaired cochlea causing high-frequency hearing loss has its most sensitive regions located apically. The traveling wave then has further to travel to reach a portion of the cochlea that is sufficiently intact to allow effective stimulation. Thus, the ABR latencies at low stimulus levels are longer than normal.

Cochlear hearing loss thus acts essentially as a filter for the stimulus. The hearing loss may prevent effective stimulation in regions in the impaired cochlea, as compared to the normal cochlea. Whether the latencies attain normal values with increasing stimulus level depends upon the extent and configuration/slope of the high-frequency hearing loss (Bauch & Olsen, 1988; Lightfoot, 1993; see also Fowler & Durrant, 1994 for more detailed consideration of these effects). Experience dictates that 20 dB or more "overhead" is needed typically in the 2 to 4 kHz region for the recruitment effect to be robust enough to overcome the effects of the hearing loss or asymmetry thereof. That is, the stimulus level needs to be >20 dB over audiometric thresholds in this frequency region for essentially normal latencies to be produced. With progressively more involvement of frequencies below 4 kHz, even more overhead may be needed.

If it is not feasible to stimulate ≥20 dB over the threshold at 4000 Hz, namely due to the degree of the loss, the latencies may not attain normal values (compare *UH1* and *UH3* data in Figure 7.26). The likely question at this juncture is, Why not start stimulating at, say, 85 to 90 dB nHL in the first place? The fact is that if the hearing loss at 4 kHz is already around 70 dB HL, this precisely is what should be done. Otherwise, there is a wealth of data in the literature that defines "normal" ABRs based upon data obtained with stimuli at 60 to 70 dB nHL. Consequently, it seems most prudent to consider an unqualified "normal" interpretation as the results that fall within the clinic's norms at this level. Thereafter, the strategy can be structured to see what other parameters fall into place. First, if the recruitment effect is incomplete, the L-I function, again, is expected to converge toward the normal function, barring conductive involvement (see below). This does not necessarily require detailed tracing of the L-I function. A two-point function using, say 70 and 90 dB nHL, generally is adequate. However, at the higher level, it is highly desirable to witness a full complement of waves (at least I, III, and V). If the interpeak intervals are reasonably symmetric and within the norms, it is safe to consider the lesion to be cochlear, regardless of the absolute latency values.

To reiterate, it is only in the cochlear case that this convergence toward the norm presumably can happen. Unfortunately, as cochlear hearing loss increases, the ABR deteriorates. Particularly vulnerable is the definition of Wave I. It might be tempting to increase the level even further and the authors have gone as high as 105 dB nHL to resolve the issue in some cases. Still, few test systems are capable of such levels. Furthermore, increasing stimulus level increases risk of patient discomfort, auditory fatigue, tinnitus, and temporary or (ultimately) permanent threshold shifts. It must be borne in mind that peak-equivalent SPL is over 30 dB higher than the specified nHL. Thus, at 90 dB nHL, the dB peSPL is over 120! Besides, there are more palatable solutions. The most compelling is to use electrocochleography to pull out Wave I.

Alternative Approaches.   Another approach is to use a brief tone burst at, say, 1 kHz, where thresholds are likely to be more symmetrical between ears (Telian & Kileny, 1989). As reported by others (Campbell & Brady, 1995), the authors have had only limited success with this approach. As suggested earlier, a full complement of waves is not typical with this stimulus, and symmetry of the ABR may still not be achieved if there is a steeply sloping configuration just above the test frequency. There also is a question of the degree to which a retrocochlear lesion differentially affects high and low frequency fibers and, consequently, if the sensitivity and specificity of the ABR are compromised.

If the above approaches fail or are not convenient, this is where, at last, the latency correction approach (see Hall, 1992 for an in-depth discussion of such strategies) seems most useful and most valid. The Selters and Brackmann (1977) approach is attractive for its simplicity, namely allowing 0.1 msec for each 10 dB that the hearing loss at 4 kHz exceeds 50 dB HL. Admittedly, this is only a crude correction with the potential for a large amount of variation among individual patients, and it certainly underestimates the impact of peripheral loss when there is much additional loss below 4 kHz or excessive hearing loss in general (e.g., over 90 dB at 4 kHz). In a retrospective study of a very large clinical cohort (1539 patients), the false positive rate was reduced by a half with the correction applied, but at the cost of more than doubling false negatives (Cashman, Stanton, Sagle, & Barber, 1993). Such a correction factor, thus, must be applied judiciously (i.e., in deference to the qualifiers noted above). In any event, if there are reasonable absolute latencies and interaural latency differences for the degree of hearing loss, it seems safe to render a "cochlear" interpretation.

When all of the forgoing efforts fail and all nonpathologic variables are fully accounted for—as inevitably will occur with enough hearing loss—the strongest conclusion simply is that a retrocochlear component cannot be ruled out. It then is left to the referring professional to pursue the case more aggressively (e.g., via imaging) or simply to follow the patient for three to six months to look for progression of the symptoms.

Conductive Pathology and Test Strategy. Returning to the conductive case, it is now possible to appreciate how different are the effects of this versus cochlear pathology. Again, the point of departure of the strategy described in the forgoing paragraphs is observation (or not) of at least a trend of "recruitment" behavior in the L-I functions, an effect firmly seated in cochlear encoding mechanisms. As noted earlier (see Figure 7.24), the L-I functions tend not to converge in the case of conductive pathology. Still, if the stimulus level can be increased enough, it should be possible to elicit a response with a reasonably full set of waves, permitting measurement of the I-V interval (Figure 7.27). The conductive loss thus acts primarily as a sound attenuator that is countered by correspondingly increased stimulus level (assuming a fairly flat or rising configuration). If the I-V interval can be measured and is within normal limits, then presumably nerve action potentials are propagating through the auditory nerve and brainstem with normal timing. The possibility of a retrocochlear lesion is thereby excluded.

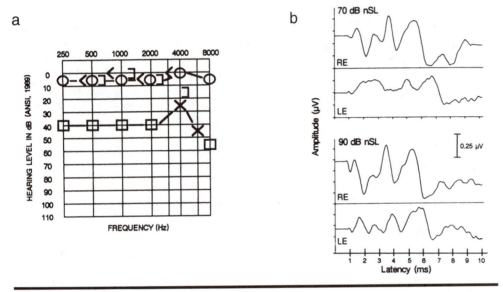

FIGURE 7.27 Case of conductive hearing loss due to glomus tumor, evaluated preoperatively. (From C. G. Fowler & J. D. Durrant, "The effects of peripheral hearing loss on the auditory brainstem response." In J. T. Jacobson, Ed., *Principles and Applications in Auditory Evoked Potentials*, pp. 237–250. Boston: Allyn & Bacon, 199, with permission.)

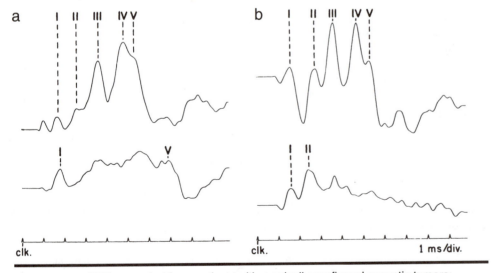

FIGURE 7.28 ABRs recorded from patients with surgically confirmed acoustic tumors: (A) neuroma; (B) meningioma in the cerebellopontine angle. Upper trace: normal ear response; lower trace: pathological ear response. (From ASHA, 1988, with permission)

Conductive lesions are particularly problematic, however, as an overlay to sensorineural loss, since they can completely sabotage the observation of neural recruitment under any stimulus conditions. As demonstrated earlier, decreased stimulus intensity, or the equivalent thereof (i.e., conductive lesions), degrades the ABR wave morphology and increases latencies. This too is what is expected of retrocochlear lesions, as discussed in the section to follow, so it is a good policy to avoid the confounds of conductive lesion to whatever extent possible (e.g., by waiting until a middle ear infection has been treated and cleared up). Since, however, the examiner is not likely to have any control over this, then it is prudent to characterize the nature and extent of the conductive lesion (i.e., via other tests at the audiologist's disposal) as completely as possible via conventional audiologic analysis, including immittance testing, to provide at least the best basis for interpreting the ABR findings.

Differential Diagnosis—Retrocochlear Pathology

Effects of Retrocochlear Pathology (General). It is not practical here to delve extensively into the effects of all the various known retrocochlear pathologies; rather, the focus here will be upon the principal effects of retrocochlear pathology on the ABR and characteristic examples. The most rudimentary concept is that any pathology that effectively blocks the conduction of action potentials is likely to cause dysynchrony of neural discharges, reduce the available neuronal pool, and/or alter the orientation of the generators, leading to abnormalities in the ABR waveform. Some retrocochlear lesions cause relatively straightforward effects on the ABR, such as that of a tumor affecting the eighth nerve (Figure 7.28). It is well established that such a lesion, if not so severe as to greatly disrupt cochlear blood supply (see below), will cause abnormalities in the ABR limited to waves following Wave I (Starr & Achor, 1975). The ABR, indeed, has been demonstrated to have exquisite sensitivity to acoustic tumors, a case in point being presented in Figure 7.29. This patient, in whom completely normal hearing was demonstrated (with excellent word recognition ability), presented to the otolaryngology clinic with complaints of sinus problems. The ABR is clearly abnormal and a small tumor of the eighth nerve was ultimately discovered and removed surgically.

Studies of the ABR in cases of acoustic tumor suggest sensitivity and specificity at the 90% level or better (e.g., Eggermont, 1984; see Figure 7.30). More recent studies continue to demonstrate relatively high sensitivities (Chandrasekhar, Brackmann, & Devgan, 1995), especially when hearing loss is taken into account (Stanton & Cashman, 1996). On the other hand, the more recent reports (e.g., see Chandrasekhar et al., 1995; Gordon & Cohen, 1995; Ruckenstein, Cueva, Morrison, & Press, 1996) have

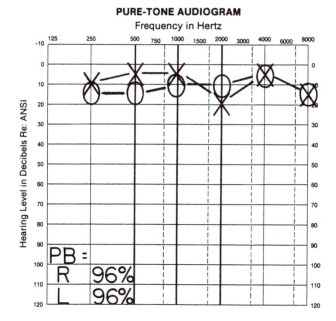

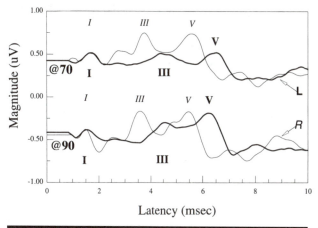

FIGURE 7.29 Results from a patient presenting originally in the ear, nose, and throat clinic with the complaint of sinus problems, but subsequently found to have an acoustic tumor.

suggested poorer performance of the ABR test, at least for the smallest tumors, doubtlessly due to the improvement in imaging techniques that now permit detection of quite small tumors (i.e., as small as 3 mm). Consequently, MRI with gadolinium is expected to be able to detect virtually all acoustic tumors (Ferguson, Smith, Lutman, Mason, Coles, & Gibbin, 1996). Still, such imaging may not be available to all clinicians, or not available in an acceptably timely manner. Also, some cases may be at less risk, practically, for life-threatening and/or other serious consequences of tumors of such a small size as to be missed by the ABR exam, for example, patients of advanced age. And, just as technological advances have improved MRI, advances in ABR testing reasonably may be expected, resulting in

a

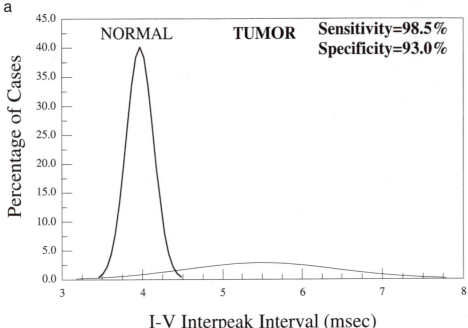

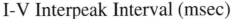

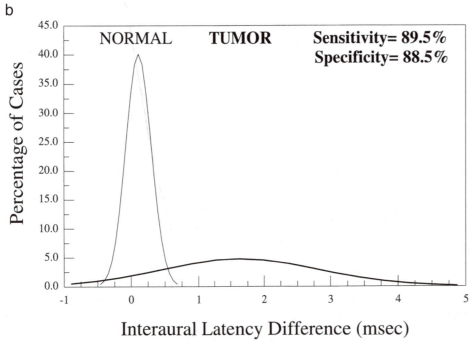

b

FIGURE 7.30   Relative performance of ABR analysis, using interaural latency differences of (a) Wave V and (b) Wave I-V interpeak intervals. (Normal distributions fitted to data of Eggermont, 1984)

enhanced sensitivity. Therefore, it seems ill-advised, and certainly premature, to retire ABR testing in the management of suspect cases of acoustic tumor (Jacobson, 1994). Even more fundamental, however, is the logical issue that ruling out an acoustic tumor does not completely rule out retrocochlear pathology.

It is important to bear in mind at all times that what is being sampled via the ABR evaluation is not etiology, but rather the functional impact of the lesion. There is no precise coupling between a given etiology and ABR waveform abnormalities. Various pathologies can cause similar patterns of findings, namely when they affect the same

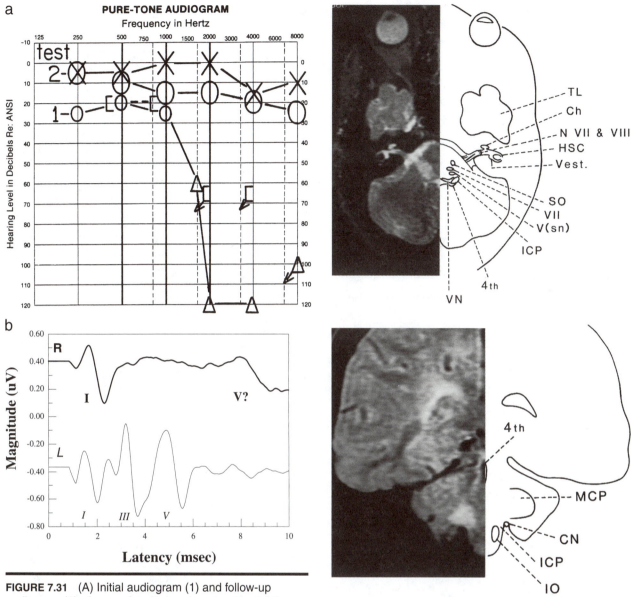

FIGURE 7.31   (A) Initial audiogram (1) and follow-up audiogram (2) of case of multiple sclerosis with eighth-nerve-root entry involvement (see Figure 7.32 for imaging findings). (B) ABR findings. (From J. M. R. Furman, J. D. Durrant, & W. L. Hirsch, "Eighth nerve signs in a case of multiple sclerosis." *American Journal of Otolaryngology, 10,* 376–381, 1989, with permission.)

FIGURE 7.32   Magnetic resonant images for case presented in Figure 7.31. (From J. M. R. Furman, J. D. Durrant, & W. L. Hirsch, "Eighth nerve signs in a case of multiple sclerosis." *American Journal of Otolaryngology, 10,* 376–381, 1989, with permission.)

function and level of the system. For example, as illustrated in Figures 7.31 and 7.32, a focus of multiple sclerosis (MS) in the cochlear nucleus can mimic a tumor in the cerebellopontine angle (Furman, Durrant, & Hirsch, 1989). The audiogram in Figure 7.31A looks much like the "classical" acoustic tumor case, showing a unilateral high-frequency sensorineural loss and poor word recognition ability in the involved ear. The catch is that this loss of sensitivity (but not other retrocochlear signs) virtually disappeared over the next several weeks (Figure 7.31A), hardly

characteristic of acoustic tumors. Imaging (Figure 7.32) demonstrated root-entry involvement, thus apparently causing a nerve-conduction block functionally similar to a cerebellopontine-angle space-occupying lesion. While root-entry lesions of this type are perhaps unusual for the eighth nerve, they are not so uncommon for the central nervous system overall (see review in Furman et al., 1989). Indeed, even distal nerve involvement, evidenced by ABR and MRI abnormalities, has been observed in MS (Bergamaschi, Romani, Zappoli, Versino, & Cosi, 1997).

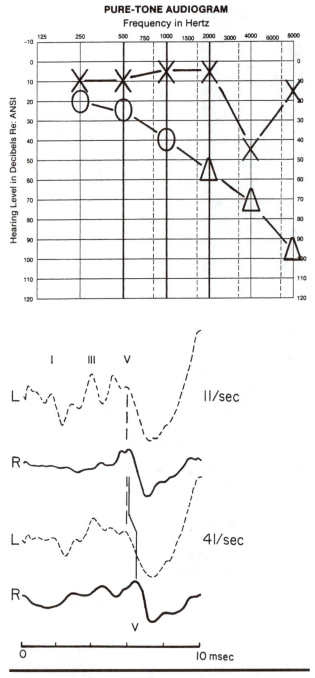

FIGURE 7.33 Case presenting much as a cochlear high-frequency loss, including ABRs tested at a routine stimulus rate (11/s) with latencies and interaural latency differences not inconsistent with the audiogram. However, at a high stimulation rate (41/s), the ILD is clearly significant. (Courtesy of Dr. J. K. Shallop, Mayo Clinic)

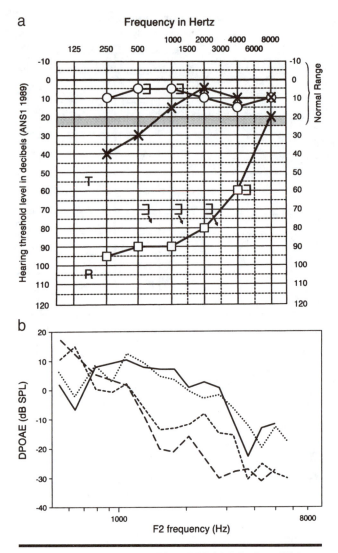

FIGURE 7.34 Audiometric (A) and DPOAE findings (B) in case of viral neuritis of the eighth nerve secondary to HIV+. Hearing decreased dramatically in the left ear over a period of weeks (compare test [T] and retest [R] audiograms), but the DPOAEs (measured at time of retest [R] audiogram) were symmetric. (DPOAEs measured at 65 dB SPL with $f_1 = f_2$; solid line indicates right-ear data; dotted line, left ear; heavy and light dashed lines, respective noise floors.) (From M. S. Robinette & J. D. Durrant, "Contributions of evoked otoacoustic emissions in differential diagnosis of retrocochlear disorders." In M. S. Robinette & T. J. Glattke, Eds., *Clinical Applications*, pp. 205–232. New York: Thieme Medical Publishers, Inc., with permission; adapted from Hirsch, Durrant, Yetiser, Kamerer, & Martin, 1996.)

acteristic, in cases of acoutic tumor. They also serve as a reminder of the prevalence of substantial hearing loss in many such cases that, in turn, clouds the interpretation. Here, the interaural difference of Wave V, as measured using the typical and (nominally) nonadapting repetition rate, cannot be interpreted unequivocally. However, in this case, the use of a high stimulus rate did exaggerate the interaural

There are yet other peripheral nerve pathologies, such as vasocompression of the eighth nerve, that can have similar affects on the ABR (see Hall, 1992, for review). The results shown in Figure 7.33 are instructive in this regard. These are not unlikely results, although not the most char-

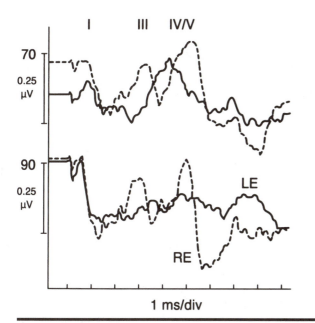

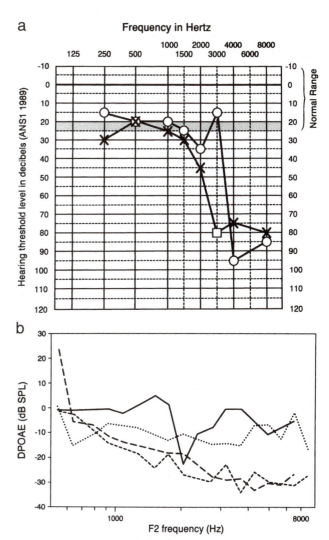

FIGURE 7.35 ABR data for case in Figure 7.34. (From M. S. Robinette & J. D. Durrant, "Contributions of evoked otoacoustic emissions in differential diagnosis of retrocochlear disorders." In M. S. Robinette & T. J. Glattke, Eds., *Clinical Applications*, pp. 205–232. New York: Thieme Medical Publishers, Inc., with permission; adapted from Hirsch, Durrant, Yetiser, Kamerer, & Martin, 1996.)

FIGURE 7.36 A case of "auditory neuropathy"? This unusual hearing loss (A) observed in a 9-year-old boy was congenital, but the DPOAEs (B) were fairly robust over the frequency ranges of greatest loss, bilaterally. (From M. S. Robinette & J. D. Durrant, "Contributions of evoked otoacoustic emissions in differential diagnosis of retrocochlear disorders." In M. S. Robinette & T. J. Glattke, Eds., *Clinical Applications*, pp. 205–232. New York: Thieme Medical Publishers, Inc., with permission; adapted from Hirsch, Durrant, Yetiser, Kamerer, & Martin, 1996)

difference. A retrocochlear interpretation was rendered, and a vascular loop was subsequently surgically confirmed and treated.

Another instructive case is illustrated by the data presented in Figures 7.34 and 7.35; here, neural conduction of the eighth nerve was effectively blocked by a viral neuritis secondary to HIV+, which ultimately effected a complete disconnect of the nerve (Hirsch et al., 1996). Cochlear function appeared to be preserved completely, as demonstrated using otoacoustic emissions (OAEs) and electrocochleography. The distortion-product OAEs and electrocochleograms were essentially symmetrical between ears (Figure 7.34b). Indeed, OAE analysis can enhance the differential diagnosis (Durrant, Kamerer, & Chen, 1993; Robinette & Durrant, 1997). This case reminds one of a variety of possible neuropathies of the auditory nerve that include a presumptive congenital defect recently coined "auditory neuropathy" (Starr, Picton, Sininger, Hood, & Berlin, 1996). As illustrated in Figures 7.36 and 7.37, combined OAE, ECochG, ABR, and other AEP testing can be quite useful in detecting and/or comprehensively defining the nature of the functional lesion in such cases.

While not the focus of this chapter (see Chapter 6 for a more in-depth treatment of OAEs), the contrast of several cases of combined OAE and ABR testing is useful here. The data in Figure 7.38 were obtained in a patient with an acoustic tumor confirmed by magnetic resonance imaging

(MRI) and surgery ultimately. The right ear, with substantial hearing loss (bottom, lower panel), demonstrated an abnormal ABR (top panel; clicks presented at 90 db nHL) showing prolongation of the I-III and I-V interpeak intervals, but a normal III-V. This is consistent with a conduction block along the nerve. The distortion product OAEs (DPOAEs—top, bottom panel) were not measurable above the noise floor at high frequencies in the involved ear, much as would be observed in cases of comparable cochlear hearing loss, thus demonstrating hair cell damage associated

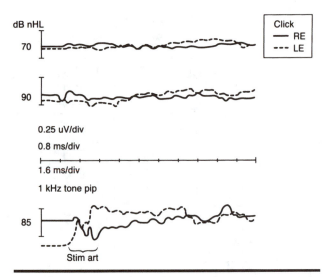

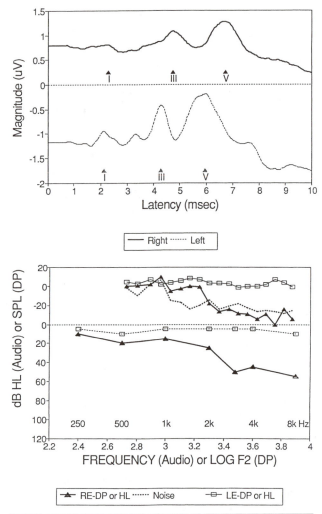

FIGURE 7.37 ABR data for case in Figure 7.36 suggest little or no synchronized response of the eighth nerve, even with stimuli at a frequency within the range of essentially normal sensitivity. (From M. S. Robinette & J. D. Durrant, "Contributions of evoked otoacoustic emissions in differential diagnosis of retrocochlear disorders." In M. S. Robinette & T. J. Glattke, Eds., *Clinical Applications*, pp. 205–232. New York: Thieme Medical Publishers, Inc., with permission; adapted from Hirsch, Durrant, Yetiser, Kamerer, & Martin, 1996.)

FIGURE 7.38 Case of acoustic tumor confirmed by magnetic resonance imaging and, subsequently, surgery. ABR (top panel) and combined audio- and DP-grams (bottom panel). (Dashed line in DP-gram [distortion product output versus frequency] represents noise floor of the recording [poorer ear]; f_1 presented at 65 dB, f_2 at 55 dB SPL; $f_2/f_1 = 1.2$.)

with this presumptive pure "neural" lesion! The etiology of the secondary end-organ lesion is assumed to be compression of the cochlear artery (Durrant et al., 1993; Telischi, Roth, Stagner, Lonsbury-Martin, & Balkany, 1995) and such end-organ involvement in cases of acoustic tumor appears to be the rule, not the exception (Robinette & Durrant, 1997). In contrast is the case illustrated by Figure 7.39. This case presented with essentially symmetrical "DP-grams," despite asymmetrical audiometric configurations and ABRs. This patient did not have an acoustic tumor or any other obvious eighth nerve lesion, since the I-III intervals were essentially symmetric. Rather, she was the victim of repeated strokes, including one just days after examination. She thus had extensive cerebral vascular disease. Although discrete lesions of the brainstem were not evident upon MRI, the examining radiologist concurred with interpretation of the combined ABR and OAE findings—namely the involvement of brainstem-level dysfunction. These results were particularly of interest to speech pathology colleagues who had diagnosed and were treating the patient for a swallowing, as well as a communication, disorder.

It thus is important to use and interpret the ABR evaluation for what it is—a neurologic screening test—albeit a powerful test for such purposes. The ABR abnormalities reflect functional impact of disease, can distinguish among gross differences in site of lesion, but are not specific to etiology. Indeed, lesions at a particular site along the auditory

nerve, or pathway in general, but due to different etiologies, will not have necessarily the same impact on the ABR. The detailed underlying pathophysiologies must be considered, which, in turn, may have differential potencies of effects. For instance, demyelinization may more often cause ABR abnormalities than axonal neuropathies (Pareyson, Scaioli, Berta, & Sghirlanzoni, 1995). Furthermore, not all retrocochlear lesions demonstrate results consistent with the presumptive site of lesion (e.g., site of putative conduction block). The results presented in Figure 7.40, at first glance, seem to be characteristic of a cochlear lesion. However, the latency delay and degree of degradation of the response are at odds with the results of the audiologic analysis, demon-

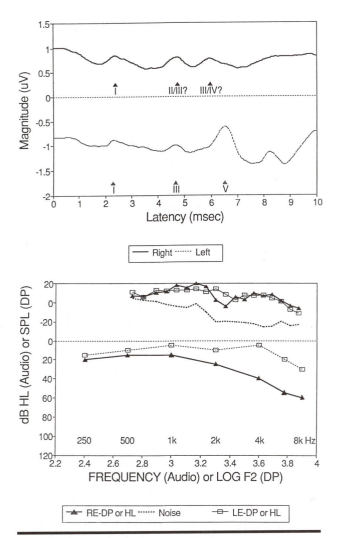

FIGURE 7.39 Case of stroke and widespread cerebral vascular disease confirmed by magnetic resonance imaging. (Dashed line in DP-gram [distortion product output versus frequency] represents noise floor of the recording [poorer ear]; f_1 presented at 65 dB, f_2 at 55 dB SPL; f_2/f_1 = 1.2.)

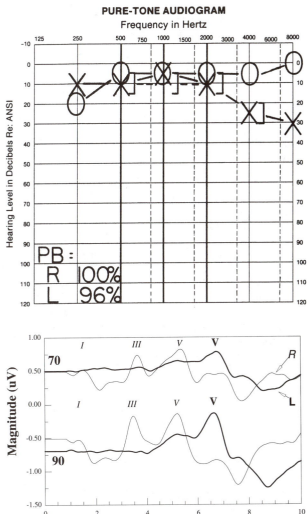

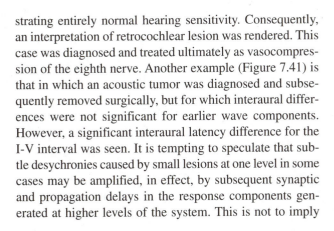

FIGURE 7.40 Another case of vasocompression of the eighth nerve, in this example with degraded ABR not unlike cases of cochlear hearing loss. However, hearing sensitivity was clearly within normal limits.

strating entirely normal hearing sensitivity. Consequently, an interpretation of retrocochlear lesion was rendered. This case was diagnosed and treated ultimately as vasocompression of the eighth nerve. Another example (Figure 7.41) is that in which an acoustic tumor was diagnosed and subsequently removed surgically, but for which interaural differences were not significant for earlier wave components. However, a significant interaural latency difference for the I-V interval was seen. It is tempting to speculate that subtle desychronies caused by small lesions at one level in some cases may be amplified, in effect, by subsequent synaptic and propagation delays in the response components generated at higher levels of the system. This is not to imply

that the longer latency AEPs will act in the same manner. In the MS case described above (Figures 7.31 and 7.32), the middle latency response subsequently was found to be abnormal, but not the long-latency potential. However, the wiring of the auditory pathways clearly is complex, with more than one path by which signals may reach the cortices (Hendler, Squires, Moore, & Coyle, 1996). It is also possible to have prolongation of the I-III interval without proglongation of the I-V interval, as observed, for example, in a case of cerebellar astrocytoma reported by Sostarich, Ferraro, and Karlsen (1993). While not necessarily compromising site-of-lesion interpretation in this case, such results potentially suggest the generation of the components of the

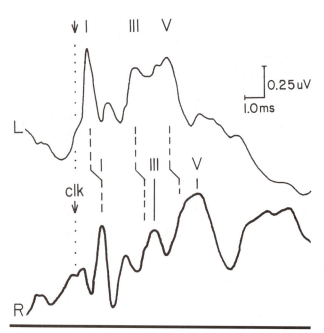

FIGURE 7.41 Combined electrocochleography and ABR measurements in the case of confirmed acoustic tumor in the left/pathological (Path) ear.

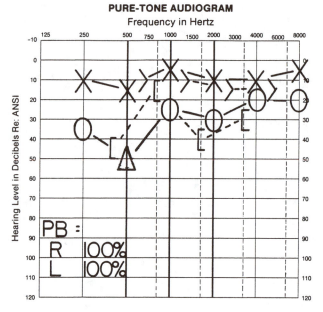

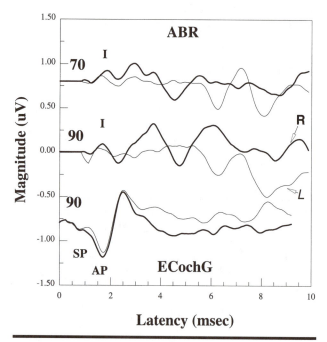

FIGURE 7.42 Audiogram and ABR findings in a case of multiple sclerosis with pontine-level (i.e., intra-axial) lesion. Electrocochleography is also shown to more clearly demonstrate normality and symmetry of whole-nerve action potentials, performed to help rule out possible concurrent hydrops.

ABR to not be sequential and somewhat more complicated that the unique association of a given wave component with a level of the system (as discussed earlier).

Multiple sclerosis is a diagnostic group of obvious interest in the neurodiagnostic applications of the ABR, both from practical and theoretical perspectives. While the case discussed earlier is perhaps not characteristic, it reflects certain aspects of findings that may be expected in this population, one directly and the other indirectly. The direct implication is that the earlier the ABR wave(s) are involved, the more lateralized the effects. This seems to be a general rule (Hendler et al., 1996). What is suggested indirectly is perhaps all too obvious, but bears iteration: An abnormality of the ABR in the MS patient is likely only if there is a focus of demyelinization. When such lesions in the (pontine) brainstem are evident in the MRI, then abnormalities of the ABR are observed faithfully (Hendler et al., 1996). However, by the same token, the ABR exam is not a good screening test for MS, per se. Rather, by virtue of its keen sensitivity to such lesions, the ABR is useful in helping to characterize the specific effects of the disease on the individual MS patient. Also in contrast to the case discussed above, MS can cause intra-axial brainstem and/or more central lesions (e.g., see Levine, et al., 1993a). Exemplary data are shown in Figure 7.42.

The nature of MS, in the final analysis, precludes a set pattern of findings. The only consistent ABR and other auditory-test findings in MS perhaps is variability itself.

Nevertheless, Levine and co-workers (1993a, 1993b) have demonstrated the potential to better detect and characterize the extent of MS brainstem lesions by combining ABR testing and MRI with a sound lateralization (psychoacoustic)

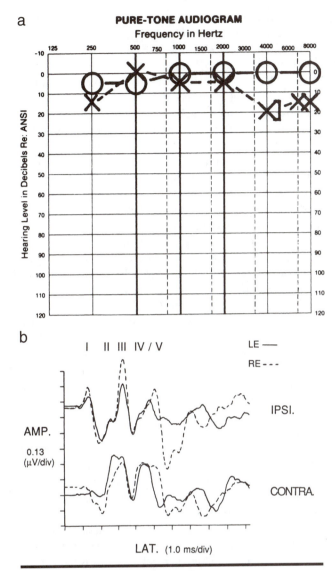

a

PURE-TONE AUDIOGRAM
Frequency in Hertz

b

I   II III IV / V   LE ——
                                RE - - -

                                IPSI.

AMP.

0.13
(μV/div)

                                CONTRA.

LAT. (1.0 ms/div)

FIGURE 7.43   Case of lesion of the right inferior colliculus, secondary to radiosurgery of a cerebellar arteriovenous malformation. Audiometric (A) and ABR findings (B), showing both ipsilateral and contralateral recording. (From B. E. Hirsch, J. D. Durrant, S. Yetiser, D. B. Kamerer, & W. H. Martin, "Localizing retrocochlear hearing loss." *American Journal of Otology, 17*, 537–546, 1996, with permission.)

a focal lesion of the brainstem secondary to radio surgery of a cerebellar lesion (Figures 7.43 and 7.44). This lesion caused loss of the right inferior colliculus, apparently in its entirety, but with minimal involvement of the lateral lemniscus below. The patient offered complaints not unlike those of unilaterally hearing impaired cases involving cochlear lesions, but experienced only minor loss of hearing sensitivity as demonstrated by pure tone audiometry (Figure 7.43A). However, the ABR (Figure 7.43B) demonstrated a clear abnormality, namely complete loss of Wave V, verified, as shown in Figure 7.45, by analysis of three-channel Lissajous trajectories (3CLTs, an analysis of the three dimensional voltage space; Durrant et al., 1994).

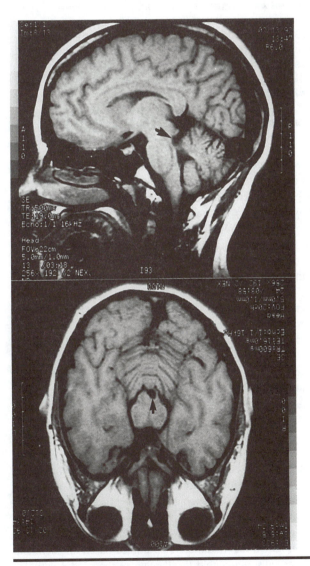

FIGURE 7.44   Magnetic resonance images for case in Figure 7.43. (From B. E. Hirsch, J. D. Durrant, S. Yetiser, D. B. Kamerer, & W. H. Martin, "Localizing retrocochlear hearing loss." *American Journal of Otology, 17*, 537–546, 1996, with permission.)

paradigm. Just noticeable differences are determined for interaural time and level using high- and low-pass noise bursts. Resulting patterns of results provide insight into the relationships among psychoacoustic performance, ABR parameters, and neuroanatomic findings (via imaging).

Various other intra- and extra-axial tumors have been studied using the ABR. A particularly intriguing case has been described by Durrant and colleagues (1994) and Hirsch and colleagues (1996) wherein the patient suffered

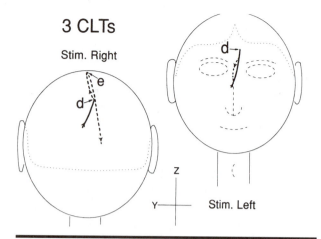

3 CLTs

Stim. Right

Stim. Left

FIGURE 7.45 Three-channel Lissajous trajectories (limited to timeframe of IV-V complex of conventional ABR). Schematic views of head oriented to permit direct comparison of right- (from behind) and left-ear-stimulated responses (face on). (From B. E. Hirsch, J. D. Durrant, S. Yetiser, D. B. Kamerer, & W. H. Martin, "Localizing retrocochlear hearing loss." *American Journal of Otology,* *17*, 537–546, 1996, with permission; based on analyses from Durrant et al., 1994.)

The Retrocochlear Interpretation. The actual detection of an abnormality and arriving at an interpretation suggesting the presence of retrocochlear pathology depend upon the criteria for normalcy of the ABR and the parameters employed. There are no firmly established rules for which of the various parameters are best suited to this task. Each parameter has its strengths and weaknesses, and a multiparameter approach, as alluded to earlier, provides a diagnostic advantage (Musiek & Lee, 1995). Like multiple tests, however, it should be borne in mind that not all ABR measures have the same sensitivity and specificity, nor are they independent from one another. These factors influence the sensitivity and specificity of the overall test "battery" (Turner, Frazer & Shepard, 1984; Turner & Nielsen, 1984; Turner, Shepard & Frazer, 1984; see also Chapter 15). Furthermore, sensitivity and specificity themselves are established assuming a gold standard, for instance, magnetic resonance imaging or surgical confirmation, or both. The problem is that not all possible retrocochlear lesions lend themselves to equally accurate detection/confirmation even by surgical confirmation (e.g., vasocompression of the eighth nerve and degenerative disease processes). So, while acoustic tumors offer a convenient and well-defined test of the ability of ABR to detect retrocochlear lesions, it cannot be assumed that parameters optimized based on such data are equally applicable to all other retrocochlear pathologies. In any event, the predictive values will not be the same (i.e., since, a priori, the different etiologies have different incidences), nor are the risk-benefit ratios expected to be constant across etiologies.

The weakest measure of the ABR for diagnostic purposes tends to be amplitude, again due to its high variability (Thornton, 1975). The use of relative amplitudes, particularly the ratio between Wave V (or IV/V) and Wave I has been suggested as an alternative (Starr & Achor, 1975), but in practice the V:I ratio does not improve precision of measurement beyond that of the absolute measures (Durrant, 1986). Still, the consistent observation of a relatively small Wave V compared to Wave I may warrant followup. An important point to keep in mind regarding this aspect is that the V/I amplitude ratio will be sensitive to electrode montage. That is, ABR amplitudes (especially Wave V) will vary depending on whether the vertex or high forehead was used as the positive (noninverting) site. Thus, separate norms for the V/I ratio will need to be established for different electrode configurations.

Certainly, the most basic approach to ABR evaluation is that based upon the absolute latencies. This, however, tends to be the approach most subject to interpretational error due to the influence of the various nonpathological and pathological variables, as noted above. Some of these variables are circumvented by reliance upon interpeak intervals. Prolongation of these intervals is presumed to reflect increased time required for peripheral nerve and/or central propagation of nerve impulses (Starr & Achor, 1975) and is strongly suggestive of retrocochlear pathology (e.g., see Figure 7.29). Therefore, lesion of the eighth nerve generally leads to prolongation of the I-III interval and lesions of the brainstem to III-V prolongation, although the more peripheral lesions may lead to too much desynchrony of the brainstem waves for the former to be seen clearly (see Figure 7.28). It also may take the entire I-V interval for the effects of the more peripheral lesion to lead to a significant deviation from the norm. The limitation of interpretation based upon interpeak intervals is the vulnerability of the ABR to the effects of peripheral hearing loss—the inadequate definition of the earlier waves. It should be noted that the impact of high-frequency hearing loss is not necessarily the same for all ABR waves; consequently, the interpeak intervals may be altered (Coats & Martin, 1977; Fowler & Noffsinger, 1983; Keith & Greville, 1987).

In the neurologically intact, normal-hearing subject, the ABRs recorded with each ear of stimulation differ only slightly (Starr & Achor, 1975), that is, 0.2 msec or less in most cases. This provides the basis for a sensitive test of abnormality, since the subject is his or her own control. Interaural latency comparisons are applied primarily to absolute Wave V latencies (Clemis & McGee, 1979; Selters & Brackmann, 1977) but also can be applied to interpeak intervals. Here again, hearing loss, particularly unilateral/asymmetrical types, can be an obstacle to correct interpretation, especially regarding interaural differences in absolute latencies.

The most clear-cut ABR indicator of pathology, when observed, is the absence of waves (Figure 7.28). As a general rule, the absence of waves prior to V, while being a confounding variable for interpretation, tends to occur due to nonpathologic and (peripheral) pathologic factors, such as hearing loss. The absence of waves after Wave I, however, strongly suggests pathology of the auditory nerve and/or lower brainstem-auditory pathways. Similarly, the absence of waves following III may be suggestive of pathology affecting pontine level, presumably at or above the superior olivary complex (as in the case illustrated in Figure 7.43 above). Even here, the rules are not rigorous, and the functional nature of the test as well as the unclear relationship between ABR components and their generators must be borne in mind. Thus, if an eighth-nerve tumor or vasocompression, for instance, restricts or cuts off the cochlear blood supply, then a normal Wave I is not likely. That many cases of acoustic tumor, like the case discussed above, involve concomitant cochlear damage (again, presumably due to secondary constriction of cochlear blood supply) is suggested by observed abnormalities of otoacoustic emissions (Durrant et al., 1993; Robinette & Durrant, 1997; Telischi et al., 1995). Lastly, the presence/absence of the ABR waves, just as normalcy of the ABR waveform itself, is inherently a subjective matter, and this judgment too can be biased by the various variables discussed above.

Advanced Techniques and Final Considerations

ABR measurement and ECochG are useful points of departure for any treatment of auditory evoked potentials and objective audiometry. The extent to which the generators of the short-latency AEPs are known and understood, even if incomplete, make the test objectives clear and interpretation of results comprehensible. The underlying principles of instrumentation transcend evoked potential components in other timeframes and sensory modalities. An understanding of the characteristics of the short-latency potentials and their dynamics is fundamental to full comprehension of the later responses. The short-latency potentials, finally, enjoy a broad range of applications, from diagnostics to intraoperative monitoring, to estimation of hearing sensitivity. Any of the numerous subtopics covered in this chapter are capable of being developed into whole chapters (e.g., see Chapters 9, 10, and 11 of this book). Furthermore, various other topics could have been added. First, there are other response components of interest falling within the short-latency timeframe, with substantive literatures of their own—the frequency following response (FFR) and the slow negative wave (SN10). There are nonpathologic variables that certainly have commanded much more attention than reflected herein and continue to be debated, such as the gender differences and the bases

thereof. Then, there are other applications of significance. Short-latency evoked potential and related measurements have been explored in recipients with cochlear implants and are receiving increasing use in the verification of function of the device in these patients. Tinnitus, of course, commands attention from all sectors and, as expected, efforts have been made in evoked potential testing to help define/objectify the phenomenon. And, the ABR especially has been examined virtually in every clinical population involving the slightest suggestion of concommitant peripheral nerve and/or brainstem involvement (e.g., Alzheimer's disease, diabetes, panic disorder, etc.). Finally, the technical aspects themselves continue to evolve and garner bursts of enthusiasm that are not trivial, although not yet integrated in the main-stream, such as the high-speed response acquisition method of minimum length sequences.

In each area of interest there also is ample room for further study, development, and refinement. With the advent of today's high-resolution MRIs, and the emerging functional MRI of the future, however, it is tempting to wonder if such advancements might prove to be for naught. Even within the field of auditory evoked potential measurement the "sailing" has been less than smooth, nor has the course been chartered. When the ABR itself was introduced, the audiology community all but abandoned the other AEPs, but thankfully not all. Witness over the past several years the enormous renewal of interest in the middle- and long-latency responses, giving rise to relative newcomers like the mismatched negativity (see Chapter 8). And as far as the "threat" to AEPs from the advancement of imaging techniques, the simple fact is that, even when one can see the circuit (like opening up the back of a computer), one still has to test it to see if it really works!

The real threat to the longevity and advancement of short-latency AEPs, rather, is completely from within. Various advanced techniques, at least, have been touched upon in this chapter and, again, still numerous others could have been. Most have yet to be implemented in instrumentation at the disposal of the clinician, or even the researcher. The examiner is often burdened with redundant tasks, such a picking peaks, which could be entrusted largely to the computer. Unfortunately, given our current "time-is-money" environment of managed health care, the examiner may overlook or not have the time to do what he or she does better than the computer—think. To think about which response components are most relevant. To think about what strategy would be most appropriate or which procedures to apply. To think about what is the diagnostic question. Consequently, ABR examinations remain highly time-consuming and routine. Yet, methods like analysis of three-channel Lissajous trajectory (3CLT; discussed briefly above) or dipole modeling effectively remain prisoners of only the more specialized research laboratories. Such techniques take into account the orientation of the ABR wave generators and do not assume all activity and/or changes in the waves to be effectively limited to the coronal plane, as do conventional techniques. Such three-dimensional analysis techniques are *already* known to be capable of demonstrating subtleties of the response that escape conventional recordings (e.g., see Pratt, Har'el, & Golos, 1983; Pratt et al., 1987).

Advancement of short-latency AEPs also has been hampered by the inevitable reinventing of the wheel that goes on in the publish-or-perish-driven literature. In review of the literature for this chapter, it was striking to note how few net gains were evident in this area, and also how unaware the more recent authors were of basic and applied research that had gone before. There also are inevitably perpetuated misconceptions. Good taste precludes specific references, but an example is the apparent promulgation of the illusion that, just because one places electrodes on one side of the head versus the other, this yields information necessarily unique to one side of the brainstem or the other. Similarly, one encounters the attitude of more-channels-are-better when, in fact, more than three channels for the ABR are truly redundant. In fact, if not appropriately configured and analyzed (3CLT analysis, for example), even three-channel recordings offer little substantive gains over the conventional two-channel approach.

Consequently, it may be tempting to wonder if the subjects of this chapter—the ECochGm and ABR—will have interest/value in the next edition of this textbook, or will they go the way of a number of other auditory tests in the past (e.g., the short-increment-sensitivity index). The answer is, "Only if we let them." Having helped to breathe life back into clinical electrocochleography, the authors, for their part, remain optimistic for the future of the short-latency potentials in differential diagnosis and hearing assessment.

REFERENCES

Achor, L. J., & Starr, A. (1980a). Auditory brain stem responses in the cat I: Intracranial and extracranial recordings. *Electroencephalography and Clinical Neurophysiology, 48,* 154–173.

Achor, L. J., & Starr, A. (1980b). Auditory brain stem responses in the cat II: Effects of lesions. *Electroencephalography and Clinical Neurophysiology, 48,* 174–190.

Alford, B. R. (1972). Ménière's disease: Criteria for diagnosis and evaluation of therapy for reporting. *Transactions of the American Academy of Ophthalmology and Otolaryngology, 76,* 1462–1464.

Amadeo, M., & Shagass, C. (1973). Brief latency click-evoked potentials during waking and sleep in man. *Psychophysiology, 10,* 244–250.

American Speech-Language-Hearing Association (ASHA). (1988). *The Short Latency Auditory Evoked Potentials: A Tutorial Paper by the Working Group on Auditory Evoked Potential Measurements of the Committee on Audiologic Evaluation.* Rockville, MD: American Speech-Language-Hearing Association.

Aran, J. M., Portmann, M., & Portmann, C., et al. (1972). Electrocochleography in adults and children: Electrophysiological study of the peripheral receptor. *Audiology, 11,* 77–89.

Arenberg, I. K., Kobayashi, H., Obert, A. D., & Gibson, W. P. (1993). Intraoperative electrocochleography of endolymphatic hydrops surgery using clicks and tone bursts. *Acta Otolaryngologica, Supplement 504,* 58–67.

Arenberg, I. K., Obert, A. D., & Gibson, W. P. (1991). Intraoperative electrocochleographic monitoring of inner ear surgery for endolymphatic hydrops. A review of cases. *Acta Otolaryngologica, Supplement 485,* 53–64.

Bauch, C. D., & Olsen, W. O. (1988). Auditory brainstem responses as a function of average hearing sensitivity for 2000–4000 Hz. *Audiology, 27,* 156–163.

Bauch, C. D., & Olsen, W. O. (1989). Wave V interaural latency differences as a function of asymmetry in 2000–4000 Hz hearing sensitivity. *American Journal of Otology, 10,* 389–392.

Beattie, R. C., Beguwala, F. E., Mills, D. M., & Boyd, R. L. (1986). Latency and amplitude effects of electrode placement on the early auditory evoked response. *Journal of Speech and Hearing Disorders, 51,* 63–70.

Beattie, R. C., Garcia, E., & Johnson, A. (1996). Frequency-specific auditory brainstem responses in adults with sensorineural hearing loss. *Audiology, 35,* 194–203.

Bekesy, G. v. (1950). DC potentials and energy balance of the cochlear partition. *Journal of the Acoustical Society, 22,* 576–582.

Bekesy, G. v. (1960). *Experiments in Hearing* (Tr. and Ed. E. G. Wever). New York: McGraw-Hill.

Bellman, S., Barnard, S., & Beagley, H. A. (1984). A nine-year review of 841 children tested by transtympanic electrocochleography. *Journal of Laryngology and Otology, 98,* 1–9.

Bergamaschi, R., Romani, A., Zappoli, F., Versino, M., & Cosi, V. (1997). MRI and brainstem auditory evoked potential evidence of eighth cranial nerve involvement in multiple sclerosis. *Neurology, 48,* 270–272

Berlin, C. I., Cullen, J. K., Ellis, M. S., Lousteau, R. J., Yarbrough, W. M., & Lyons, G. D. (1974). Clinical application of recording human VIIIth nerve action potentials from the tympanic membrane. *Transactions of the American Academy of Ophthalmology and Otolaryngology, 78,* 401–410.

Binnie, C. D., Rowan, A. J., & Gutter, T. (1982). *A Manual of Electroencephalographic Technology.* Cambridge, England: Cambridge University Press.

Boezeman, E. H. J. F., Bronkhorst, A. W., Kapteyn, T. S., Houffelaar, A., & Snel, A. M. (1984). Phase relationship between bone and air conducted impulse signals in the human head. *Journal of the Acoustical Society of America, 76,* 111–115.

Bojrab, D. I., Bhansali, S. A., & Andreozzi, M. P. (1994). Intraoperative electrocochleography during endolymphatic sac surgery: Clinical results. *Otolaryngology—Head and Neck Surgery, 111,* 478–484.

Boston, J. R., & Ainslie, P. J. (1980). Effects of analog and digital filtering on brain stem evoked potentials. *Electroencephalography and Clinical Neurophysiology, 48,* 361–364.

Brai, A., Vibert, J. F., & Koutlidis, R. (1994). An expert system for the analysis and interpretation of evoked potentials based on fuzzy classification: Application to brainstem auditory evoked potentials. *Computers and Biomedical Research, 27,* 351–366.

Buchwald, J. S., & Huang, C. M. (1975). Far-field acoustic response: Origins in the cat. *Science, 189,* 382–384.

Campbell, K. C., & Abbas, P. J. (1993). Electrocochleography with postural changes in perilymphatic fistula and Ménière's disease: Case reports. *Journal of the American Academy of Audiology, 4,* 376–383.

Campbell, K. C., & Abbas, P. J. (1994). Electrocochleography with postural changes in perilymphatic fistula: Animal studies. *Annals of Otology, Rhinology and Laryngology, 103,* 474–482.

Campbell, K. C. M., & Brady, B. A. (1995). Comparison of 1000-Hz tone burst and click stimuli in otoneurologic ABR. *American Journal of Audiology, 4,* 55–60.

Cann, J., & Knott, J. (1979). Polarity of acoustic click stimuli for eliciting brain-stem auditory evoked responses: A proposed standard. *American Journal of Electroencephalography and Technology, 19,* 125–132.

Cashman, M. Z., Stanton, S. G., Sagle, C., & Barber, H. O. (1993). The effect of hearing loss on ABR interpretation: Use of a correction factor. *Scandinavian Audiology, 22,* 153–158.

Cevette, M. J. (1984). Auditory brainstem response testing in the intensive care unit. *Seminars in Hearing, 5,* 57–68.

Chandrasekhar, S. S., Brackmann, D. E., & Devgan, K. K. (1995). Utility of auditory brainstem response audiometry in diagnosis of acoustic neuromas. *American Journal of Otology, 16,* 63–67.

Clemis, J. D., & McGee, T. (1979). Brain stem electric response audiometry in the differential diagnosis of acoustic tumors. *Laryngoscope, 89,* 31–42.

Clemis, J. D., Ballad, W. J., & Killion, M. C. (1986). Clinical use of an insert earphone. *Annals of Otology, Rhinology and Laryngology, 95,* 520–524.

Coats, A. C. (1974). On electrocochleographic electrode design. *Journal of the Acoustical Society of America, 56,* 708–711.

Coats, A. C. (1981). The summating potential and Ménière's disease. *Archives of Otolaryngology, 107,* 199–208.

Coats, A. C. (1983). Instrumentation. In E. J. Moore (Ed.), *Bases of Auditory Brain Stem Evoked Responses* (pp. 197–220). New York: Grune and Stratton.

Coats, A. C. (1986). Electrocochleography: Recording techniques and clinical applications. *Seminars in Hearing (Electrocochleography), 7,* 247–266.

Coats, A. C., & Martin, J. L. (1977). Human auditory nerve action potentials and brainstem evoked responses. *Archives of Otolaryngology, 103,* 605–622.

Cornacchia, L., Martini, A., & Morra, B. (1983). Air and bone conduction brain stem responses in adults and infants. *Audiology, 22,* 430–437.

Creel, D., Garber, S. R., King, R. A., & Witkop, C. J., Jr. (1980). Auditory brainstem anomalies in human albinos. *Science, 209,* 1253–1255.

Cullen, J. K., Jr., Ellis, M. S., Berlin, C. I., & Lousteau, R. J. (1972). Human acoustic nerve action potential recordings from the tympanic membrane without anesthesia. *Acta Otolaryngologica, 74,* 15–22.

Dallos, P. (1973). *The Auditory Periphery.* New York: Academic.

Dallos, P., & Wang, C. Y. (1974). Bioelectric correlates of kanamycin intoxication. *Audiology, 13,* 277–289.

Dauman, R., Aran, J. M., Charlet de Sauvage, R., & Portmann, M. (1988). Clinical significance of the summating potential in Ménière's disease. *American Journal of Otology, 9,* 31–38.

Davis, H. (1976). Principles of electric response audiometry. *Annals of Otology, Rhinology, and Otolaryngology, 85 (Supplement 28),* 1–96.

Davis, H., Fernandez, C., and McAuliffe, D. R. (1950). The excitatory process in the cochlea. *Proceedings of the National Academy of Science U.S., 36,* 580–587.

Deltenre, P., & Mansbach, A. L. (1995). Effects of click polarity on brainstem auditory-evoked potentials in cochlear hearing loss: A working hypothesis. *Audiology, 34,* 17–35.

Dobie, R. A., & Berlin, C. I. (1979). Binaural interaction in brainstem-evoked responses. *Archives of Otolaryngology, 105,* 391–398.

Dobie, R. A., & Norton, S. J. (1980). Binaural interaction in human auditory evoked potentials. *Electroencephalography and Clinical Neurophysiology, 49,* 303–313.

Domico, W. D., & Kavanaugh, K. T. (1986). Analog and zero phase-shift digital filtering of the auditory brain stem response waveform. *Ear and Hearing, 7,* 377–382.

Don, M., & Eggermont, J. J. (1978). Analysis of the click-evoked brain stem potentials in man using high-pass noise masking. *Journal of the Acoustical Society of America, 63,* 1084–1092.

Don, M., Eggermont, J. J., & Brackmann, D. E. (1979). Reconstruction of the audiogram using brain-stem responses and high-pass noise masking. *Annals of Otology, Rhinology and Laryngology, 88 (Supplement 57),* 1–20.

Don, M., Vermiglio, A. J., Ponton, C. W., Eggermont, J. J., & Masuda, A. (1996). Variable effects of click polarity on auditory brain-stem response latencies: Analyses of narrow-band ABRs suggest possible explanations. *Journal of the Acoustical Society of America, 100,* 458–472.

Durrant, J. D. (1977). Study of a combined noninvasive-ECochG and BSER recording technique. *Journal of the Acoustical Society of America, 62,* S87.

Durrant, J. D. (1983). Fundamentals of sound generation. In E. J. Moore (Ed.), *Bases of Auditory Brain Stem Evoked Responses* (pp. 15–49). New York: Grune and Stratton.

Durrant, J. D. (1986). Combined EcochG-ABR versus conventional ABR recordings. *Seminars in Hearing (Electrocochleography), 7,* 289–305.

Durrant, J. D., Boston, J. R., & Martin, W. H. (1990). Correlation study of two-channel recordings of the brain-stem auditory evoked potentials. *Ear and Hearing, 11,* 215–221.

Durrant, J. D., & Dallos, P. (1974). Modification of DIF summating potential components by stimulus biasing. *Journal of the Acoustical Society of America, 56,* 562–570.

Durrant, J. D., & Ferraro, J. A. (1991). Analog model of human click-elicited SP and effects of high-pass filtering. *Ear and Hearing, 12,* 144–148.

Durrant, J. D., & Fowler, C. G. (1996). ABR protocols for dealing with asymmetric hearing loss. *American Journal of Audiology, 5,* 5–6.

Durrant, J. D., & Hyre, R. (1993a). Observations on temporal aspects of bone conduction clicks: Real head measurements. *Journal of the American Academy of Audiology, 4,* 213–219.

Durrant, J. D., & Hyre, R. (1993b). Relative effective frequency response of bone versus air conduction stimulation examined via masking. *Audiology, 32,* 175–184.

Durrant, J. D., Kamerer, D. B., & Chen, D. (1993). Combined OAE and ABR studies in acoustic tumor patients. In D. Hoehmann (Ed.), *ECoG, OAE and Intraoperative Monitoring* (pp. 231–239). Amsterdam: Kugler.

Durrant, J. D., & Lovrinic, J. H. (1995). *Bases of Hearing Science* (3rd ed.). Baltimore: Williams and Wilkins.

Durrant, J. D., Martin, W. H., Hirsch, B., & Schwegler, J. (1994). 3CLT ABR analyses in a human subject with unilateral extirpation of the inferior colliculus. *Hearing Research, 72,* 99–107.

Eggermont, J. J. (1976a). Analysis of compound action potential responses to tone bursts in the human and guinea pig cochlea. *Journal of the Acoustical Society of America, 60,* 1132–1139.

Eggermont, J. J. (1976b). Electrocochleography. In W. D. Keidel & W. D. Neff (Eds.), *Handbook of Sensory Physiology, Vol. V/3: Auditory System—Clinical and Special Topics* (pp. 625–705). Berlin: Springer-Verlag.

Eggermont, J. J. (1984). Use of electrocochleography and brain stem auditory evoked potentials in the diagnosis of cerebellopontine angle pathology. *Advances in Otology-Rhinology-Laryngology, 34,* 47–56.

Eggermont, J. J., Odenthal, D. W., Schmidt, P. H., & Spoor, A. (1974). Electrocochleography: Basic principles and clinical application. *Acta Otolaryngologica, Supplement 316,* 1–84.

Elberling, C. (1979). Auditory electrophysiology: Spectral analysis of cochlear and brainstem evoked potentials. *Scandinavian Audiology, 8,* 57–64.

Elberling, C., & Don, M. (1984). Quality estimation of averaged auditory brainstem response. *Scandinavian Audiology, 13,* 187–197.

Elberling, C., & Solomon, G. (1973). Cochlear microphonics recorded from the ear canal in man. *Acta Otolaryngologica, 75,* 489–495.

Elberling, C., & Wahlgreen, R. (1985). Estimation of auditory brainstem responses, ABR, by means of Bayesian Reference. *Scandinavian Audiology, 14,* 89–96.

Fausti, S. A., Mitchell, C. R., Frey, R. H., Henry, J. A., & O'Connor J. L. (1995). Reliability of auditory brainstem responses from sequenced high-frequency (> or = 8 kHz) tonebursts. *Audiology, 34,* 177–188.

Ferguson, M. A., Smith, P. A., Lutman, M. E., Mason, S. M., Coles, R. R., & Gibbin, K. P. (1996). Efficiency of tests used to screen for cerebello-pontine angle tumours: a prospective study. *British Journal of Audiology, 30,* 159–176.

Ferraro, J. A., Arenberg, I. K., & Hassanein, R. S. (1985). Electrocochleography and symptoms of inner ear dysfunction. *Archives of Otolaryngology, 111,* 71.

Ferraro, J. A., Blackwell, W. L. Mediavilla, S. J., & Thedinger, B. S. (1994). Normal summating potential to tone bursts recorded from the tympanic membrane in humans. *Journal of the American Academy of Audiology, 5,* 17–23.

Ferraro, J. A., & Ferguson, R. (1989). Tympanic ECochG and conventional ABR: A combined approach for the identification of Wave I and the I-V interwave interval. *Ear and Hearing, 10,* 161–166.

Ferraro, J. A., Murphy, G. B., & Ruth, R. A. (1986). A comparative study of primary electrodes used in extratympanic electrocochleography. *Seminars in Hearing, 7,* 279–287.

Ferraro, J. A., & Ruth, R. A. (1994). Electrocochleography. In J. T. Jacobson (Ed.), *Principles and Applications in Auditory Evoked Potentials* (pp. 101–122). Boston: Allyn & Bacon.

Ferraro, J. A., Thedinger, B. S., Mediavilla, S. J., & Blackwell, W. L. (1994). Human summating potential to tone bursts: Observations on tympanic membrane versus promontory recordings in the same patients. *Journal of the American Academy of Audiology, 5,* 24–29.

Finitzo-Hieber, T., Hecox, K., & Cone, B. (1979). Brain stem auditory evoked potentials in patients with congenital atresia. *Laryngoscope, 89,* 1151–1158.

Folsom, R. C. (1984). Frequency specificity of human auditory brainstem responses as revealed by pure-tone masking profiles. *Journal of the Acoustical Society of America, 66,* 919–924.

Fowler, C. G., & Durrant, J. D. (1994). The effects of peripheral hearing loss on the auditory brainstem response. In J. T. Jacobson (Ed.), *Principles and Applications in Auditory Evoked Potentials* (pp. 237–250). Boston: Allyn & Bacon.

Fowler, C. G., & Noffsinger, D. (1983). The effects of stimulus repetition rate and frequency on the auditory brainstem response in normal, cochlear-impaired, and VIII nerve/brainstem-impaired subjects. *Journal of Speech and Hearing Research, 26,* 560–567.

Fowler, C. G., & Swanson, M. R. (1988). Validation of addition and subtraction of ABR waveforms. *Scandinavian Audiology, 17,* 195–199.

Foxe, J. J., & Stapells, D. R. (1993). Normal infant and adult auditory brainstem responses to bone-conducted tones. *Audiology, 32,* 95–109.

Fria, T. J. (1980). The auditory brain stem response: Background and clinical applications. *Monographs in Contemporary Audiology, 2,* 1–44.

Fromm, B., Nylen, C. O., & Zotterman, Y. (1935). Studies in the mechanism of the Wever and Bray effect. *Acta Otolaryngologica, 22,* 477–486.

Furman, J. M. R., Durrant, J. D., & Hirsch, W. L. (1989). Eighth nerve signs in a case of multiple sclerosis. *American Journal of Otolaryngology, 10,* 376–381.

Gabriel, S., Durrant, J. D., et al. (1980). Computer identification of waves in the auditory brain stem evoked potentials. *Electroencephalography and Clinical Neurophysiology, 49,* 421–423.

Geddes, L. A. (1972). *Electrodes and the Measurement of Bioelectric Events.* New York: Wiley-Interscience.

Gerhardt, K. J., Melnick, W., & Ferraro, J. A. (1979). Reflex threshold shift in chinchillas following a prolonged exposure to noise. *Journal of Speech and Hearing Research, 22,* 63–72.

Gibson, W. P. R. (1991). The use of intraoperative electrocochleography in Ménière's surgery. *Acta Otolaryngologica, Supplement 485,* 65–73.

Gibson, W. P. R. (1993). A comparison of clicks versus tone bursts in the diagnosis of endolymphatic hydrops. In D. Hoehmann (Ed.), *ECoG, OAE and Intraoperative Monitoring* (pp. 55–59). Amsterdam: Kugler.

Gibson, W. P. R., Moffat, D. A., & Ramsden, R. T. (1977). Clinical electrocochleography in the diagnosis and management of Ménière's disorder. *Audiology, 16,* 389–401.

Gordon, M. L., & Cohen, N. L. (1995). Efficacy of auditory brainstem response as a screening test for small acoustic neuromas. *American Journal of Otology, 16,* 136–139.

Gorga, M. P., Abbas, P. J., & Worthington, D. W. (1985). Stimulus calibration in ABR measurements. In J. T. Jacobson (Ed.), *The Auditory Brainstem Response* (pp. 49–62). San Diego: College-Hill.

Gorga, M. P., Beauchaine, K. A., Reiland, J. K., Worthington, D. W., & Javel, E. (1984). The effects of stimulus duration on ABR and behavioral thresholds. *Journal of the Acoustical Society of America, 76,* 616–619.

Gorga, M. P., Reiland, J. K., & Beauchaine, K. A. (1985). Auditory brainstem responses in a case of high-frequency conductive hearing loss. *Journal of Speech and Hearing Disorders, 50,* 346–350.

Gorga, M. P., & Thornton, A. R. (1989). The choice of stimuli for ABR measurements. *Ear and Hearing, 10,* 217–230.

Gorga, M. P., Worthington, D. W., Reiland, J. K., Beauchaine, K. A., & Goldgar, D. E. (1985). Some comparisons between auditory brain stem response thresholds, latencies, and the pure-tone audiogram. *Ear and Hearing, 6,* 105–112.

Habraken, J. B., van Gils, M. J., & Cluitmans, P. J. (1993). Identification of peak V in brainstem auditory evoked potentials with neural networks. *Computers in Biology and Medicine, 23,* 369–380.

Hall, J. W. III. (1992). *Handbook of Auditory Evoked Responses.* Boston: Allyn & Bacon.

Hammond, S. R., & Yiannikas, C. (1987). The relevance of contralateral recordings and patient disability to assessment of brain-stem auditory evoked potential abnormalities in multiple sclerosis. *Archives of Neurology, 44,* 382–387.

Hashimoto, I., Ishiyama, Y., & Tozuka, G. (1979). Bilaterally recorded brain stem auditory evoked responses. Their asymmetric abnormalities and lesions of the brain stem. *Archives of Neurology, 36,* 161–167.

Hecox, K., Squires, N., & Galambos, R. (1976). Brainstem auditory evoked responses in man. I. Effect of stimulus rise-fall time and duration. *Journal of the Acoustical Society of America, 60,* 1187–1192.

Hendler, T., Squires, N. K., Moore, J. K., & Coyle, P. K. (1996). Auditory evoked potentials in multiple sclerosis: Correlation with magnetic resonance imaging. *Journal of Basic and Clinical Physiology and Pharmacology, 7,* 245–278.

Hirsch, B. E., Durrant, J. D., Yetiser, S., Kamerer, D. B., & Martin, W. H. (1996). Localizing retrocochlear hearing loss. *American Journal of Otology, 17,* 537–546.

Hooks, R. G., & Weber, B. A. (1984). Auditory brain stem responses of premature infants to bone-conducted stimuli: A feasibility study. *Ear and Hearing, 5,* 42–46.

Hughes, J. R., Fino, J. J., & Hart, L. A. (1985). The significance of the negativities in the brainstem auditory evoked potential (BAEP). *International Journal of Neuroscience, 28,* 111–118.

Hyde, M. L. (1994). Signal processing and analysis. In J. T. Jacobson (Ed.), *Principles and Applications in Auditory Evoked Potentials* (pp. 47–83). Boston: Allyn & Bacon.

Jacobson, J. T. (Ed.). (1994). *Principles and Applications in Auditory Evoked Potentials.* Boston: Allyn & Bacon.

Jerger, J., & Hall, J. (1980). Effects of age and sex on auditory brainstem response. *Archives of Otolaryngology, 106,* 387–391.

Jewett, D. L. (1970). Volume-conducted potentials in response to auditory stimuli as detected by averaging in the cat. *Electroencephalography and Clinical Neurophysiology, 28,* 609–618.

Jewett, D. L., & Williston, J. S. (1971). Auditory-evoked far fields averaged from the scalp of humans. *Brain, 94,* 681–696.

Jewett, D. L., Romano, M. N., & Williston, J. S. (1970). Human auditory evoked potentials: Possible brain-stem components detected on the scalp. *Science, 167,* 1517–1518.

Jiang, Z. D. (1996). Binaural interaction and the effects of stimulus intensity and repetition rate in human auditory brain-stem. *Electroencephalography and Clinical Neurophysiology, 100,* 505–516, 1996.

Kavanaugh, K. T., & Beardsley, J. V. (1979). Brain stem auditory evoked response: III. Clinical uses of bone conduction in the evaluation of otologic disease. *Annals of Otology, Rhinology and Laryngology, 88,* 22–28.

Kevanishvili, Z., & Aponchenko, V. (1979). Frequency composition of brain-stem auditory evoked potentials. *Scandinavian Audiology, 8,* 51–55.

Keith, W. J., & Greville, K. A. (1987). Effects of audiometric configuration on the auditory brain stem response. *Ear and Hearing, 8,* 49–55.

Klein, A. J. (1984). Frequency and age-dependent auditory evoked thresholds in infants. *Hearing Research, 16,* 291–297.

Kodera, K., Marsh, R. R., Suzuki, M., & Suzuki, J. (1983). Portions of tone pips contributing to frequency-selective auditory brain stem responses. *Audiology, 22,* 209–218.

Lasky, R. E., Maier, M. M., & Hecox, K. (1996). Auditory evoked brain stem responses to trains of stimuli in human adults. *Ear and Hearing, 17,* 544–551.

Laureano, A. N., McGrady, M. D., & Campbell, K. C. (1995). Comparison of tympanic membrane-recorded electrocochleography and the auditory brainstem response in threshold determination. *American Journal of Otology, 16,* 209–215.

Lempert, J., Wever, E. G., & Lawrence, M. (1959). The cochleogram and its clinical application: A preliminary report. *Archives of Otolaryngology, 45,* 61–67.

Lettrem, I., & Laukli, E. (1995). Analog and digital filtering of ABR: Ipsi- and contralateral derivations. *Ear and Hearing, 16,* 508–514.

Legatt, A. D., Arezzo, J. C., & Vaughan, H. G. (1988). The anatomic and physiologic bases of brain stem auditory evoked potentials. *Neurologic Clinics, 6,* 681–704.

Levine, R. A., Gardner, J. C., Stufflebeam, S. M., Fullerton, B. C., Carlisle, E. W., Furst, M., Rosen, B. R., & Kiang, N. Y. (1993a). Binaural auditory processing in multiple sclerosis subjects. *Hearing Research, 68,* 59–72.

Levine, R. A., Gardner, J. C., Fullerton, B. C., Stufflebeam, S. M., Carlisle, E. W., Furst, M., Rosen, B. R., & Kiang, N. Y. (1993b). Effects of multiple sclerosis brainstem lesions on sound lateralization and brainstem auditory evoked potentials. *Hearing Research, 68,* 73–88.

Levine, S. C., Margolis, R. H., Fournier, E. M., & Winzenburg, S. M. (1992). Tympanic electrocochleography for evaluation of endolymphatic hydrops. *Laryngoscope, 102,* 614–622.

Lightfoot, G. R. (1993). Correcting for factors affecting ABR Wave V latency. *British Journal of Audiology, 27,* 211–220.

Margolis, R. H., Levine, S. C., Fournier, E. M., Hunter, L. L., Smith, S. L., & Lilly, D. J. (1992). Tympanic electrocochleography: Normal and abnormal patterns of response. *Audiology, 31,* 8–24.

Margolis, R. H., Rieks, D., Fournier, E. M., & Levine, S. C. (1995). Tympanic electrocochleography for diagnosis of Ménière's disease. *Archives of Otolaryngology—Head and Neck Surgery, 121,* 44–55.

Martin, M. E., & Moore, E. J. (1977). Scalp distribution of early (0 to 10 msec) auditory evoked responses. *Archives of Otolaryngology, 103,* 326–328.

Martin, W. H., Pratt, H., & Schwegler, J. W. (1995). The origin of the human auditory brain-stem response Wave II. *Electroencephalography and Clinical Neurophysiology, 96,* 357–370.

Mauldin, L., & Jerger, J. (1979). Auditory brain stem evoked responses to bone-conducted signals. *Archives of Otolaryngology, 105,* 656–661.

McCall, S., & Ferraro, J. A. (1991). Pediatric ABR screening: Pass-fail rates in awake versus asleep neonates. *Journal of the American Academy of Audiology, 2,* 18–23.

Mendelson, T., Salamy, A., Lenoir, M., & McKean, C. (1979). Brain stem evoked potential findings in children with otitis media. *Electroencephalography and Clinical Neurophysiology, 105,* 17–20.

Michelini, S., Arslan, E., Prosser, S., & Pedrielli, F. (1982). Logarithmic display of auditory evoked potentials. *Journal of Biomedical Engineering, 4,* 62–64.

Møller, A. R. (1994). Neural generators of auditory evoked potentials. In J. T. Jacobson (Ed.), *Principles and Applications in Auditory Evoked Potentials* (pp. 23–46). Boston: Allyn & Bacon.

Møller, A. R., & Jannetta, P. J. (1982). Comparison between intracranially recorded potentials from the human auditory nerve and scalp recorded auditory brainstem responses (ABR). *Scandinavian Audiology, 11,* 33–40.

Møller, A. R., Jannetta, P. J., Bennett, M., & Møller, M. B. (1981). Intracranially recorded responses from the human auditory nerve: New insights into the origin of brainstem evoked potentials (BSEP). *Electroencephalography and Clinical Neurophysiology, 52,* 18–27.

Møller, A. R., Jannetta, P. J., & Jho, H. D. (1994). Click-evoked responses from the cochlear nucleus: A study in humans. *Electroencephalography and Clinical Neurophysiology, 92,* 215–224.

Møller, A. R., Jho, H. D., Yokota, M., & Jannetta, P. J. (1995). Contribution from crossed and uncrossed brainstem structures to the brainstem auditory evoked potentials: A study in humans. *Laryngoscope, 105,* 596–605.

Moore, J. K. (1987). The human auditory brain stem as a generator of auditory evoked potentials. *Hearing Research, 29,* 33–43.

Moore, J. K., Ponton, C. W., Eggermont, J. J., Wu, B. J., & Huang, J. Q. (1996). Perinatal maturation of the auditory brain stem response: Changes in path length and conduction velocity. *Ear and Hearing, 17,* 411–418.

Musiek, F. E., Johnson, G. D., Gollegly, K. M., Josey, A. F., & Glasscock, M. E. III. (1989). The auditory brain stem response interaural latency difference (ILD) in patients with brain stem lesions. *Ear and Hearing, 10,* 131–134.

Musiek, F. E., & Lee, W. W. (1995). The auditory brain stem response in patients with brain stem or cochlear pathology. *Ear and Hearing, 16,* 631–636.

Naunton, R. F., & Zerlin, S. S. (1976). Basis and some diagnostic implications of electrocochleography. *Laryngoscope, 86,* 475–482.

Naunton, R. F., & Zerlin, S. S. (1978). Electrocochleography: Behavioral threshold comparisons. In R. F. Naunton & C. Fernandez (Eds.), *Evoked Electrical Activity in the Auditory Nervous System* (pp. 221–236). New York: Academic.

Orlando, M. S. & Folsom, R. C. (1995). The effects of reversing the polarity of frequency-limited single-cycle stimuli on the human auditory brain stem response. *Ear and Hearing, 16,* 311–320.

Pareyson, D., Scaioli, V., Berta, E., & Sghirlanzoni, A. (1995). Acoustic nerve in peripheral neuropathy: A BAEP study. Brainstem Auditory Evoked Potentials. *Electromyography and Clinical Neurophysiology, 35,* 359–364.

Pearson, B. W., & Brackmann, D. E. (1985). Committee on hearing and equilibrium guidelines for reporting treatment results in Ménière's disease. *Otolaryngology—Head and Neck Surgery, 93,* 579–581.

Perlman, H. B., & Case, T. J. (1941). Electrical phenomena of the cochlea in man. *Archives of Otolaryngology, 34,* 710–718.

Pfeiffer, R. R. (1974). Consideration of the acoustic stimulus. In W. D. Keidel & W. D. Neff (Eds.), *Handbook of Sensory physiology, Vol. V/1: Auditory System—Anatomy and Physiology (Ear)* (pp. 9–38). Berlin: Springer-Verlag.

Picton, T. W., & Hillyard, S. A. (1974). Human auditory evoked potentials. II: Effects of attention. *Electroencephalography and Clinical Neurophysiology, 36,* 191–199.

Picton, T. W., & Hink, R. F. (1974). Evoked potentials: How? What? and Why? *American Journal of EEG Technology, 14,* 9–44.

Picton, T. W., Ouellette, J., Hamel, G., & Smith, A. D. (1979). Brainstem evoked potentials to tonepips in notched noise. *Journal of Otolaryngology 8,* 289–314.

Picton, T. W., Stapells, D. R., & Campbell, K. B. (1981). Auditory evoked potentials from the human cochlea and brainstem. *Journal of Otolaryngology, 10* (Supplement 9), 1–41.

Polyakov, A., & Pratt, H. (1994). Three-channel Lissajous' trajectory of the binaural interaction components in human auditory brain-stem evoked potentials. *Electroencephalography and Clinical Neurophysiology. 92,* 396–404.

Polyakov, A., & Pratt, H. (1995). The effect of broad-band noise on the binaural interaction components of human auditory brainstem-evoked potentials. *Audiology, 34,* 36–46.

Polyakov, A., & Pratt, H. (1996). Evidence of spatio-topic organization of binaural processing in the human brainstem. *Hearing Research, 94,* 107–115.

Ponton, C. W., Moore, J. K., & Eggermont, J. J. (1996). Auditory brain stem response generation by parallel pathways: Differential maturation of axonal conduction time and synaptic transmission. *Ear and Hearing, 17,* 402–10.

Pou, A. M., Hirsch, B. E., Durrant, J. D., Gold, S. R., & Kamerer, D. B. (1996). Efficacy of tympanic electrocochleography in the diagnosis of endolymphatic hydrops. *American Journal of Otology, 17,* 607–611.

Pratt, H., Har'el, Z., & Golos, E. (1983). Geometrical analysis of human three-channel Lissajous' trajectory of auditory brainstem evoked potentials. *Electroencephalography and Clinical Neurophysiology, 56,* 682–688.

Pratt, H., Martin, W. H., Bleich, N., Kaminer, M., & Har'El, Z. (1987). Application of the three-channel Lissajous trajectory of auditory brainstem-evoked potentials to the question of generators. *Audiology, 26,* 188–196.

Probst, R. (1983). Electrocochleography: Using extratympanic or transtympanic methods? *ORL—Journal of Otorhinolaryngology and Related Specialties, 45,* 322–329.

Robinette, M. S., & Durrant, J. D. (1997). Contributions of evoked otoacoustic emissions in differential diagnosis of retrocochlear disorders. In M. S. Robinette & T. J. Glattke (Eds.), *Otoacoustic Emissions: Clinical Applications* (pp. 205–232). New York: Theime.

Rosenhamer, H. J., Lindstrom, B., & Lundborg, T. (1981). On the use of click-evoked electric brainstem responses in audiological diagnosis. III. Latencies in cochlear hearing loss. *Scandinavian Audiology, 10,* 3–11.

Rowe, M. J. (1978). Normal variability of the brain stem auditory evoked response in young and old adult subjects. *Electroencephalography and Clinical Neurophysiology, 44,* 459–470.

Ruckenstein, M. J., Cueva, R. A., Morrison, D. H., & Press, G. (1996). A prospective study of ABR and MRI in the screening for vestibular schwannomas. *American Journal of Otology, 17,* 317–320.

Ruth, R. A., Lambert, P. R., Ferraro, J. A. (1988). Electrocochleography: Methods and clinical applications. *American Journal of Otology, 9 (Supplement),* 1–11.

Salamy, A., & McKean, C. M. (1976). Postnatal development of human brainstem potentials during the first year of life. *Electroencephalography and Clinical Neurophysiology, 40,* 418–426.

Salamy, A., Fenn, E., & Bronshvag, M. (1979). Ontogenesis of human auditory brainstem evoked potential amplitude. *Developmental Psychology, 12,* 519–526.

Salt, A. N., & Thornton, A. R. (1983). The effects of stimulus rise-time and polarity on the auditory brainstem responses. *Scandinavian Audiology, 13,* 119–127.

Sand, T., & Saunte, C. (1994). ABR amplitude and dispersion variables. Relation to audiogram shape and click polarity. *Scandinavian Audiology, 23,* 7–12.

Scherg, M., & Von Cramon, D. (1985). A new interpretation of the generators of BAEP Waves I-V: Results of a spatio-temporal dipole model. *Electroencephalography and Clinical Neurophysiology, 62,* 290–299.

Schoonhoven, R., Prijs, V. F., & Grote, J. J. (1996). Response thresholds in electrocochleography and their relation to the pure tone audiogram. *Ear and Hearing, 17,* 266–275.

Schwaber, M. K., & Hall, J. W. III. (1990). A simplified approach for transtympanic electrocochleography. *American Journal of Otology, 11,* 260–265.

Selters, W. A., & Brackmann, D. E. (1977). Acoustic tumor detection with brain stem electric response audiometry. *Archives of Otolaryngology, 103,* 181–187.

Sininger, Y. (1993). Auditory brainstem responses for objective measures of hearing. *Ear and Hearing, 14,* 23–29.

Sininger, Y. S. (1995). Filtering and spectral characteristics of averaged auditory brain-stem response and background noise in infants. *Journal of the Acoustical Society of America, 98,* 2048–2055.

Sininger, Y., & Don, M. (1989). Effects of click rate and electrode orientation on the threshold detectability of the ABR. *Journal of Speech and Hearing Research, 32,* 880–886.

Sohmer, H., & Feinmesser, M. (1967). Cochlear action potentials recorded from the external ear in man. *Annals of Otology, Rhinology and Laryngology, 76,* 427–435.

Sohmer, H., & Feinmesser, M. (1973). Routine use of electrocochleography (cochlear audiometry) on human subjects. *Audiology, 12,* 167–173.

Sohmer, H., Feinmesser, M., & Szabo, G. (1974). Electrococh-leographic (auditory nerve and brain-stem auditory nuclei) responses to sound stimuli in patients with brain damage. *Electroencephalography and Clinical Neurophysiology, 37,* 663–669.

Sohmer, H., Gafni, M., & Chisin, R. (1978). Auditory nerve and brain stem responses: Comparison in awake and unconscious subjects. *Archives of Neurology, 35,* 228–230.

Sohmer, H., & Pratt, H. (1976). Recording of the cochlear microphonic potential with surface electrodes. *Electroencephalography and Clinical Neurophysiology, 40,* 253–260.

Sostarich, M. E., Ferraro, J. A., & Karlsen, E. A. (1993). Prolonged I-III interwave interval in cerebellar astrocytoma. *Journal of the American Academy of Audiology, 4,* 269–271.

Spivak, L. G. (1993). Spectral composition of infant auditory brainstem responses: Implications for filtering. *Audiology, 32,* 185–194.

Staller, S. (1986). Electrocochleography in the diagnosis and management of Ménière's disease. *Seminars in Hearing (Electrocochleography), 7,* 267–277.

Stanton, S. G., & Cashman, M. Z. (1996). Auditory brainstem response. A comparison of different interpretation strategies for detection of cerebellopontine angle tumors. *Scandinavian Audiology, 25,* 109–120.

Stapells, D. R., Gravel, J. S., & Martin B. A. (1995). Thresholds for auditory brain stem responses to tones in notched noise from infants and young children with normal hearing or sensorineural hearing loss. *Ear and Hearing, 16,* 361–371.

Stapells, D. R., & Picton, T. W. (1981). Technical aspects of brainstem evoked potential audiometry using tones. *Ear and Hearing, 2,* 20–29.

Stapells, D. R., Picton, T. W., Perez-Abalo, M., Read, D., & Smith, A. (1985). Frequency specificity in evoked potential audiometry. In J. T. Jacobson (Ed.), *The Auditory Brainstem Response* (pp. 147–177). San Diego: College-Hill.

Stapells, D. R., Picton, T. W., & Smith, A. D. (1982). Normal hearing thresholds for clicks. *Journal of the Acoustical Society of America, 72,* 74–79.

Starr, A., & Achor, L. J. (1975). Auditory brain stem responses in neurological disease. *Archives of Neurology, 32,* 761–768.

Starr, A., Amlie, R. N., Martin, W. H., & Sanders, S. (1977). Development of auditory function in newborn infants revealed by auditory brainstem potentials. *Pediatrics, 60,* 831–839.

Starr, A., Picton, T. W., Sininger, Y., Hood, L. J., & Berlin, C. I. (1996). Auditory neuropathy. *Brain, 119,* 741–753.

Stockard, J. J., Sharbrough, F. W., & Tinker, J. A. (1978). Effects of hypothermia on the human brainstem auditory response. *Annals of Neurology, 3,* 368–370.

Stockard, J. J., Stockard, J. E., & Sharbrough, F. W. (1978). Nonpathologic factors influencing brainstem auditory evoked potentials. *American Journal of Electroencephalogram Technology, 18,* 177–209.

Stollman, M. H., Snik, A. F., Hombergen, G. C., Nieuwenhuys, R., & ten Koppel, P. (1996). Detection of the binaural interaction component in the auditory brainstem response. *British Journal of Audiology, 30,* 227–232.

Stypulkowski, P. H., & Staller, S. J. (1987). Clinical evaluation of a new ECocG recording electrode. *Ear and Hearing, 8,* 304–310.

Suzuki, J. I., & Yamane, H. (1982). The choice of stimulus in the auditory brainstem response test for neurological and audiological examinations. *Annals of the New York Academy of Sciences, 388,* 731–736.

Suzuki, T., & Horiuchi, K. (1977). Effect of high-pass filter on auditory brainstem responses to tone pips. *Scandinavian Audiology, 6,* 123–126.

Suzuki, T., Hirai, Y., & Horiuchi, K. (1977). Auditory brainstem responses to pure tone stimuli. *Scandinavian Audiology, 6,* 51–56.

Tanaka, H., Komatsuzaki, A., & Hentona, H. (1996). Usefulness of auditory brainstem responses at high stimulus rates in the diagnosis of acoustic neuroma. *Journal of Oto-Rhino-Laryngology and Its Related Specialties, 58,* 224–228.

Teas, D. C., Eldridge, D. H., & Davis, H. (1962). Cochlear responses to acoustic transients and interpretation of the whole nerve action potentials. *Journal of the Acoustical Society of America, 34,* 1438–1459.

Telian, S. A., & Kileny, P. R. (1989). Usefulness of 1000 Hz tone-burst-evoked responses in the diagnoses of acoustic neuroma. *Otolaryngology—Head and Neck Surgery, 101,* 466–471.

Telischi, F. F., Roth, J., Stagner, B. B., Lonsbury-Martin, B. L., & Balkany, T. J. (1995). Patterns of evoked otoacoustic emissions associated with acoustic neuromas. *Laryngoscope, 105,* 675–682.

Terkildsen, K., Osterhammel, P., & Huis int Veld, F. (1974). Far field electrocochleography, electrode positions. *Scandinavian Audiology, 3,* 123–129.

Thornton, A. R. D. (1975). Statistical properties of surface-recorded electrocochleographic responses. *Scandinavian Audiology, 4,* 91–102.

Turner, R. G., Frazer, G. J., & Shepard, N. T. (1984). Formulating and evaluating audiological test protocols. *Ear and Hearing, 5,* 321–330.

Turner, R. G., & Nielsen, D. W. (1984). Application of clinical decision analysis to audiological tests. *Ear and Hearing, 5,* 125–133.

Turner, R. G., Shepard, N. T., & Frazer, G. J. (1984). Clinical performance of audiological and related diagnostic tests. *Ear and Hearing, 5,* 187–194.

Van Olphen, A. F., Rodenburg, M., & Verway, C. (1978). Distribution of brain stem responses to acoustic stimuli over the human scalp. *Audiology, 17,* 511–578.

Wada, S-I., & Starr, A. (1983a). Generation of auditory brain stem responses (ABRs). I. Effects of injection of a local anesthetic (procaine HCL) into the trapezoid body of guinea pigs and cat. *Electroencephalography and Clinical Neurophysiology, 56,* 326–339.

Wada, S-I., & Starr, A. (1983b). Generation of auditory brain stem responses (ABRs). II. Effects of surgical section of the trapezoid body on the ABR in guinea pigs and cat. *Electroencephalography and Clinical Neurophysiology, 56,* 340–351.

Wada, S-I., & Starr, A. (1983c). Generation of the auditory brain stem responses (ABRs). III. Effects of lesions of the superior olive, lateral lemniscus and inferior colliculus on the ABR in guinea pig. *Electroencephalography and Clinical Neurophysiology, 56,* 352–366.

Watson, D. R. (1996). The effects of cochlear hearing loss, age and sex on the auditory brainstem response. *Audiology, 35,* 246–258.

Weber, B. A. (1983). Masking and bone conduction testing in brainstem response audiometry. *Seminars in Hearing, 4,* 343–352.

Whitaker, S. R. (1986). Sequential electrocochleography and auditory dehydration testing in patients with Ménière's disease. *Seminars in Hearing (Electrocochleography), 7,* 329–336.

Williston, J. S., Jewett, D. L., Martin, W. H. (1981). Planar curve analysis of three-channel auditory brain stem responses: A preliminary report. *Brain Research, 223,* 181–184.

Yang, E. Y., Rupert, A. L., & Moushegian, G. (1987). A developmental study of bone conduction auditory brain stem response in infants. *Ear and Hearing, 8,* 244–251.

Yanz, J. L., & Dodds, H. J. (1985). An ear-canal electrode for the measurement of the human auditory brain stem response. *Ear and Hearing, 6,* 98–104.

Yoshie, N., & Ohashi, T. (1969). Clinical use of cochlear nerve action potential responses in man for differential diagnosis of hearing losses. *Acta Otolaryngologica, Supplement 252,* 71–87.

Yost, W. A., & Klein, A. J. (1979). Thresholds of filtered transients. *Audiology, 18,* 17–23.

Ysunza, A., & Cone-Wesson, B. (1987). Bone conduction masking for brainstem auditory-evoked potentials (BAEP) in pediatric audiological evaluations. Validation of the test. *International Journal of Pediatric Otorhinolaryngology, 12,* 291–302.

CHAPTER 8

AUDITORY MIDDLE AND LATE POTENTIALS

FRANK MUSIEK
WEI WEI LEE

INTRODUCTION AND WAVEFORM DESCRIPTIONS

This chapter presents information on the auditory middle and late evoked potentials (EPs). We will not discuss all auditory EPs in these categories. Rather, we will focus only on the middle latency response (MLR), MLR steady state or 40 Hz potential, N1 and P2 late potentials, P300, and the mismatched negativity (MMN) response.

The MLR, first reported by Geisler, Frishkopf, and Rosenblith (1958), consists of a series of positive and negative waves that follow the ABR in time and extend into the range of 60 to 80 msec (post stimulus) (Figure 8.1). The initial MLR wave is Na, followed by Pa, Nb, Pb, and at times Nc and Pc. In some cases, a Po wave may be recorded preceding the Na response, but this is not a consistent response (Musiek, 1991; Musiek, Geurkink, Weider, & Donnelly, 1984). The Na-Pa waveform is the most consistent, most often used, and most researched waveform. The MLR 40 Hz response, sometimes called a *steady-state response* (Figure 8.2), is obtained at a high presentation rate of approximately 40 stimuli per second. This rate results in an overlapping of responses in time, which enhances the amplitude of the response. These four waves of the 40 Hz potential usually occur at intervals of 25 msec.

The N1 and P2 were first reported by Davis (1939). These large responses are obtained easily with a variety of acoustic stimuli. The N1 exists commonly between 80 and 110 msec, while the P2 usually exists between 150 and 200 msec (Figure 8.3).

The P3 or P300, first reported by Sutton, Braren, Zubin, and John (1965), is larger than the P2 and occurs at approximately 300 msec post stimulus. This potential is a result of the subject attending to a target stimulus within an *oddball paradigm*. This paradigm has a series of stimuli that are occasionally different. For example, an oddball paradigm could be a series of tones as follows: 1 kHz, 1 kHz, 1 kHz, 2 kHz, 1 kHz, 1 kHz, 2 kHz, 1 kHz, 1 kHz, 1 kHz.

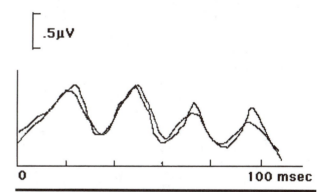

FIGURE 8.2 Example of auditory 40 Hz response waveforms (steady state response).

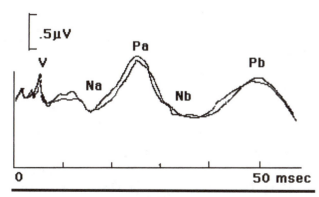

FIGURE 8.1 Example of MLR with ABR Wave V from a normal subject.

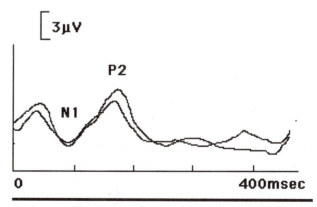

FIGURE 8.3 Example of N1 and P2 response waveforms.

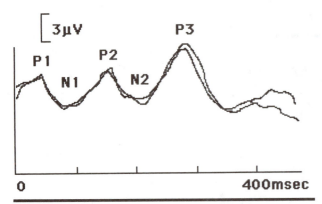

FIGURE 8.4 Example of P300 including N1 and P2 in response to the target stimuli within an oddball paradigm.

The 2 kHz tones would be the target or "rare" stimuli, while the 1 kHz tones would be the nontarget or "frequent" stimuli. The different—or target—stimuli occur at a rate of approximately 20%, and the subject must identify (usually by counting) when these stimuli occur (Figure 8.4). When the subject selectively attends to the target stimulus, the P300 results. Two averages exist for the P300. One average is for the electrical response to the target stimuli, which include the N1, P2, and P300; the second average is for the nontarget stimuli, which yield only an N1 and a P2 complex. Subtracting the waveform of the nontarget stimuli from the waveform of the targeted stimuli should provide a waveform of only the P300.

The MMN is a negative deflection that occurs after the P2 response. This negative potential is a result of a change in the stimulus within an oddball paradigm. This change in the stimulus, often called the deviant stimulus, does not have to be attended to as in the P300. Small changes in the stimulus train in either frequency, intensity or phonetic character of speech stimuli can result in the MMN.

GENERATORS AND MATURATION OF THE MIDDLE AND LATE POTENTIALS

MLR

The MLR seems to have multiple generators: Major contributions come from the thalamocortical pathway, and to a lesser degree from the inferior colliculus and the (mesencephalic) reticular formation (Kraus, Kileny, & McGee, 1994). In adults a deep subcortical origin of Na was revealed by magnetic studies (Makela, Hamalainen, Hari, & McEvoy, 1994). Minimal effect on Na was found in patients with cortical lesions (Kaseda, Tobimatsu, Morioko, & Kato, 1991). In addition, significant reduction was observed in Na in a patient with lesion of the inferior colliculus and medial geniculate body of the thalamus (Fischer, Bognar, Turjman,

& Lapras, 1995). A large negativity corresponding to Na at the level of inferior colliculus was found in intracranial recordings (Hashimoto, 1982).

Studies have also shown a critical role of the auditory reception area of the temporal lobe in the Na response. A wave at the latency of Na obtained from human intracranial recording seemed to originate at the medial tip of Heschl's gyrus (Liegeois-Chauvel, Musolino, Badier, Marquis, & Chauvel, 1994), and it is consistent with magnetic findings reported by Kuriki, Nogai, and Hirata (1995). From studies of scalp topography and magnetic response patterns, and from results in adult patients with cortical lesions, hypotheses regarding a temporal lobe origin for wave Pa have been derived. Major dipole sources underlying Pa and Pb were shown in the temporal lobes by theoretical analyses of topography with the agreement of intracranial recordings (Liegeois-Chauvel et al., 1994). A medial-to-lateral progression across Heschl's gyrus was observed for Na, Pa, Pb, and N1 (McGee & Kraus, 1996). An asymmetry of Pa amplitude or absent response on the affected side was the most consistent finding from patients with temporal lobe lesions (Kraus, Ozdamar, Hier, & Stein, 1982; Scherg & Von Cramon, 1986). However, a possible subcortical generator—a thalamic generator or generation from the thalamocortical projections (McGee & Kraus, 1996)—is indicated by the bilaterally disrupted but persistence of Pa after bilateral temporal lobe lesions (Graham, Greenwood, & Lecky, 1980; Ozdamar, Kraus, & Curry, 1983; Parving, Solomon, Elbering, Larsen, & Lassen, 1980; Peronnet & Michel, 1977), and the finding that only lesions of the thalamocortical pathway produced Pa abnormalities (Woods, Clayworth, Knight, Simpson, & Naeser, 1987). Therefore, two generators for Pa, one cortical and one subcortical, were proposed (Jacobson, Newman, Privitera, & Grayson, 1991; Polyakov & Pratt, 1994). For wave Pb, the temporal lobe generator and the reticular formation contribute (Buchwald, Erwin, Read, Van Lancker, & Cummings, 1989; Buchwald, Erwin, Van Lancker, Schwafer, & Tanguay, 1992).

In children Na is reliably apparent at birth. In contrast, wave Pa is affected by arousal state and thus is tied by inference into the reticular formation (Collett, Duclaux, Challamel, & Revol, 1988; Kraus, McGee, & Comperatore, 1989; Osterhammel, Shllop, & Terkildsen, 1985). In children this system is only partially developed and does not reach maturity until puberty. Evidence shows that myelinization of the human thalamocortical pathway and sensory cortex continues until puberty (Kraus, Kileny, & McGee, 1994; Yakovlev & Lecours, 1967; reviewed by Courchesne, 1990). The systematic development of MLR components observed in humans is consistent with such a maturational process. From infancy to adolescence, the ability of Pa to be detected and recorded during sleep increases monotonically from 20% in infancy to 90% at 12 years of age (Kraus, Smith, Reed, Stein, & Cartee, 1985). Therefore, development of the temporal lobe and the auditory thalamocortical pathway may account for increases with age in the ability of Pa to be detected.

Development patterns in animals were recorded from gerbils aged 11 to 90 days (Kraus & McGee, 1995; Kraus, Smith, & McGee, 1988). Results showed the following: The midline responses developed early, wave C (second peak) is evident early but has a longer developmental time course, and temporal lobe wave A (first peak) is not detected at early ages. The later developing waves have been linked closely to the thalamocortical pathway. The early developing waves have been linked to the function of the reticular formation (Kraus, McGee, Littman, & Nicol, 1992; Kraus et al., 1988). It may also be important to consider that the generators of the MLR in animals could be different from those in humans.

Based on the results of human and animal studies, McGee and Kraus (1996) infer the following points. Two generator systems are involved in human wave Pa: One develops early and is a part of the nonprimary auditory pathway, while the second has a longer course of development and is a part of the primary auditory pathway. The MLR in young children is the more labile nonprimary component, has an early development, and is state-dependent. It is related to the function of the reticular formation. Therefore, the robustness of Pa in children would be related to depth of sleep or to sleep state. The development of primary cortical generator varies among individuals but is well developed by age 10 to 12 years. Pb is likely a cortical response with nonprimary characteristics, possibly originating in association areas. The nonprimary cortical generator may not be fully developed until early adulthood.

N1, P2

The scalp distribution of the auditory N1, the magnetic fields recorded at the same latency as the N1, and the effects of cerebral lesions on the N1 suggest three different components contributing to this scalp-recorded wave (reviewed by Naatanen & Picton, 1987). The first component is a frontocentral negativity generated by bilateral vertically oriented dipole planes in the auditory cortices on the superior aspect of the temporal lobe (Scherg & Von Cramon, 1986; Vaughan & Ritter, 1970). The second component is the T-complex with a positive wave at 100 msec and a negative wave at 150 msec (Wolpaw & Penry, 1975). The third component generates a negative wave at the vertex with a latency of 100 msec (Hari, Kaila, Katila, Tuomisto, & Varpula, 1982; Velasco & Velasco, 1986; Velasco, Velasco, & Olvera, 1985).

The generators of these obligatory potentials are controversial, but these EPs are now recognized as complex potentials that are generated mainly within the primary and secondary auditory cortex in the superior and lateral surface of the superior temporal gyrus (reviewed by Steinschneider, Kurtzberg, & Vaughan, 1992). This conclusion is supported by converging sources of evidence from human EP topography (Peronnet, Michel, Echallier, & Girod, 1974; Scherg, Vajar, & Picton, 1989; Scherg & von Cramon, 1986; Vaughan & Ritter, 1970; Wood & Wolpaw, 1982), event-related magnetic field recordings (Hari, Aittonie, Jarvinen, Katila, & Varpula, 1980; Sams, Hamalainen, Antervo, Kaukoranta, Reinikainen, & Hari, 1985), and intracerebral recordings in primates (Arezzo, Pickoff, & Vaughan, 1975; Arezzo, Vaughan, Kraut, Steinschneider, & Legatt, 1986). The P2 appears to have major generators within the auditory cortex (Elberling, Bak, Kofoed, Lebech, & Saermark, 1982; Hari et al., 1980; Vaughan & Ritter, 1970). Other studies suggest that the P2 occurs in the primary auditory cortex, along the sylvian fissure on the side contralateral to stimulation (Baumann, Rogers, Papanicolaou, & Saydjari, 1990).

It appears that the N1 and P2 have a long maturational course, and they change in latency, amplitude, and general morphology from infancy through the elementary school years (Musiek, Verkest, & Gollegly, 1988). These EPs in newborns and young infants can be classified into five maturational levels on the basis of their polarity over the frontocentral and lateral temporal regions. These developmental stages include the following: (1) an immature phase with negative waves at both midline and lateral scalp sites, (2) a sequence of intermediate stages with ill-defined midline and negative lateral EPs, (3) positive midline and negative lateral EPs, (4) positive midline and ill-defined lateral EPs, and (5) a mature stage with positive midline and lateral EPs (Kurtzberg, Hipert, Kreuzer, & Vaughan, 1984; Novak, Kurtzberg, Kreuzer, & Vaughan, 1989; Weitzman & Graziani, 1968). Approximately 90% of normal-term infants display EPs with maturational stages of 3 to 5 at birth. By age 3 months nearly all normal infants display the mature stage-5 EPs (Kurtzberg et al., 1984). The components recorded over the midline represent activity generated predominantly by primary auditory cortex located on the superior surface of the superior temporal gyrus, whereas lateral sites record activity mainly from secondary auditory cortex located on the lateral surface of the superior temporal gyrus (Steinschneider et al., 1992). The maturation of the N1, P2 continues through the first years of life at both the midline and lateral temporal recording sites. The changes include complex alterations in response morphology, amplitude, and timing that likely reflect the maturation of neural elements and synaptic connections within auditory cortical areas (Vaughan & Kurtzberg, in press). Moreover, the development of N1 and P2 waves appears to continue beyond the first ten years of life (reviewed by

Kraus & McGee, 1994), but this finding can be affected by electrode montage and stimulus characteristics.

P300

In humans intracranial recordings of P3 suggest that its generation involves multiple subcortical sites (Wood, Allison, Goff, Williamson, & Spencer, 1980). Regions of the limbic system, particularly the hippocampus, have been postulated as generators both on the basis of surface electromagnetic recordings (Okada, Kaufman & Williamson, 1983) and intracranial recordings (Halgren, Squires, Wilson, Rohrbaugh, Babb, & Crandall, 1980; McCarthy, Wood, Allison, Goff, Williamson, & Spencer, 1982; Squires, Halgren, Wilson, & Crandall, 1983).

Thalamic contributions to P3 have been proposed based on intracranial recordings in humans (Wood et al., 1980). Pathways involving the mesencephalic reticular formation, medial thalamus, and prefrontal cortex are thought to contribute to the P3 due to the role of these structures in the regulation of selective attention (Yingling & Hosobuchi, 1984; Yingling & Skinner, 1977). Topographic mapping, intracranial recordings, and neuromagnetic field data indicate that contributors to the P3 include the frontal cortex (Courchesne, 1978; Desmedt & Debecker, 1979), centroparietal cortex (Goff, Allison, & Vaughan, 1978; Pritchard, 1981; Simson, Vaughan & Ritter, 1977a, 1977b; Vaughan & Ritter, 1970) and the auditory cortex (Richer, Johnson, & Beatty, 1983).

Topographic patterns suggest a major right centroparietal P3 generator (Sangal & Sangal, 1996). Decreased regional cerebral blood flow in the right cerebral hemisphere, especially the frontal lobe and/or thalamus, is associated with prolonged P3 latency, suggesting that the right cerebral hemisphere is important in human cognitive processes (Kuwata, Funahashi, Maeshima, Ogura, Hyotani, et al., 1993). The concordance between magnetoencephalography and brain electric sources analysis localization results supports the notion of generators in temporal and hippocampal areas for the P3 component (Tarkka, Stokic, Basile, & Papanicolaou, 1995). Magnetoencephalography findings also support the idea that the source of the P3 is in either the temporal cortex or the hippocampus (Gordon, Rennie, & Collins, 1990). However, the idea that the origin of the P3 is in the temporal lobe has been disputed using animal models. P3 responses were recorded following bilateral lesions in the medial temporal lobe in monkeys (Paller, Zola, Squire, & Hillyard, 1988). Similar findings of an intact P3 were revealed when the association cortex in cats was ablated (Harrison, Dickerson, Song, & Buchwald, 1990).

There is evidence that the temporal-parietal junction is important to the generation of the P3 in humans. The P3 was recorded in patients with extensive lateral parietal cortical lesions, although the P3 was absent in patients with unilateral lesions centered in the posterior superior temporal plane (Knight, Scabini, Woods, & Clayworth, 1989). A biphasic potential similar to the P3 was observed in epileptic patients who had electrodes implanted in the frontal, temporal, and parietal regions (Richer, Alain, Achim, Bouvier, & Saint, 1989). The potential completed a 180-degree phase shift from the posterior temporal area to the frontal area; therefore, the investigators suggested a dorsofrontal-oriented posterior temporal generator for the P3. In addition, results obtained from a different group of epileptic patients also implanted with subdural electrodes suggest that P3 is a complex arising from multifactorial generator sources, including the mid-temporal and inferior frontal area (Neshige & Luders, 1992). The idea that the P3 has initial generators in the temporal lobe (hippocampus) is also supported by a investigation of various forms of epilepsy (focal cortical epilepsy of the frontal or of the temporal lobe) (Psatta & Matei, 1995).

The exact generator sites of the P3 are unknown, but it is evident that the P3 is not mature until the teenage years (Buchwald, 1990). During age 6 years to late adolescence, P3 latency decreases, amplitude increases, and morphology improves (Courchesne, 1978; Goodin, Squires, Henderson, & Starr, 1978a; Polich, Howard, & Starr, 1985a; Squires & Hecox, 1983). However, waveforms do not generally reach adult values until age 17 years (Buchwald, 1990). There is a significant negative correlation between age and P3 latency. The relation between age and latency was defined by a P3 latency/age slope of -19 msec/year up to age 15 years (Martin, Barajas, & Fernandez, 1988). The P3 reaches its shortest latency between ages 18 to 24 years (Barajas, 1990). A distinct P3 response to speech sounds in newborns and changes in response morphology with development have been reported (Kurtzberg, 1989). P3 amplitude was smaller and its peak latency longer for infants as compared to adults. Also, its measures remained stable across stimulus trials, indicating that ERP habituation did not occur (McIsaac & Polich, 1992). This provides clues to the ontogeny of the developing brain for cognitive versus sensory brain system. Investigators reported cases of the absence of sensory components of auditory EP (short, middle, and long latency) with the presence of the cognitive component P3 (Sininger, Norton, Starr, & Ponton, 1993; Starr, McPherson, Patterson, Don, Luxford, et al., 1991). The P3, well within normal limits, was recorded from a young adult with congenital absence of the left temporal lobe (Allen, Cranford, & Pay, 1996).

MMN

Information provided by magnetic recording has localized MMN generators to the vicinity of the primary auditory cortex (Sams et al., 1985). Using dipole analysis of scalp-recorded ERPs, investigators concluded that the generators of the MMN were either in the primary or immediately adjacent auditory cortex (Kaukoranta, Sams, Hari, Hamalainen, & Naatanen, 1989; Scherg et al., 1989). An intensity-specific MMN generator that is mediated by N-methyl-D-aspartate receptor mechanisms has been identified in the primary auditory cortex of the monkey (Javitt, Schroeder, Arezzo, & Vaughan, 1991). Intracranial electrical recordings in cats (Csepe, Karmos, & Molnar, 1987) and monkeys (Javitt, Schroeder, Steinschneider, Arezzo, & Vaughan, 1992) have localized the MMN in the primary auditory cortex (obtained in experimental paradigms similar to those used with human subjects). Studies using intensity changes as the deviant feature confirm that the primary auditory cortex contributes greatly to the surface-recorded MMN (Javitt, Schroeder, Steinschneider, Arezzo, & Vaughan, 1995). Consistent with this conclusion, the MMN in scalp-recorded ERPs is largest frontocentrally and inverts in polarity at the mastoids (Alho, Paavilainen, Reinikainen, Sams, & Naatanen, 1986; Novak, Ritter, Vaughan, & Wiznitzer, 1990). The specific generator sites and mechanisms for the various human MMNs are unknown. It is clear, however, that the short latency, automatic preattentive characteristics and their localization within the auditory fields of the superior temporal plane implicate the MMN in early stages of auditory cortical processing (reviewed by Steinschneider et al., 1992).

The MMN response is present early in life and reaches adult-like values in early school-age years (Kraus & McGee, 1994). Little information is available on how the MMN is influenced by age. It is remarkable to note that the MMNs in newborns and 8-year-old children are similar under the same experimental conditions (750 msec interstimulus interval [ISI], oddball paradigm). The scalp current density topography of the MMN at each age is also similar, leaving little doubt that these potentials represent the same phenomena. Investigators have concluded that the MMN represents similar cortical processes from birth to adulthood, despite large developmental changes in other aspects of the cortical response characteristics. Presumably the underlying physiology of the MMN reflects an early developing, stable cortical processing mechanism (Kurtzberg, Vaughan, Kreuzer, & Fliegler, 1995).

In view of the fact that the MMN can be elicited in early life, the characteristics of the MMN waveform itself might differ from that of adults. A negativity potential resembling the MMN recorded in adults was elicited in sleeping newborns (Alho, Sainio, Sajaniemi, Reinikainen, & Naatanen, 1990; Cheour-Luhtanen, Alho, Kujala, Sainio, Reinikainen, et al., 1995). Some indication of negativity was present in 75% of subjects in a group of twenty-five quiet, awake healthy newborns (Kurtzberg et al., 1995). In contrast, responses to a deviant stimulus, consisting of a positivity that peaked at 250 to 300 msec, were recorded from fourteen awake infants (seven normal full-term, seven prematurely born) at ages 4 to 7 months, with a preterm group exhibiting a significantly larger positive deflection than a full-term group (Alho, Sajaniemi, Niittyvuopio, Sainio, & Naatanen, 1990).

In healthy children aged 3 years or older, the MMN can be elicited without exception, and its peak latency shortens with increasing age (Korpilahti & Lang, 1994). Recently, the MMN has been shown to be robust in school-age children and to occur at adult latencies; the MMN magnitude is generally larger in children than in adults (Csepe, Dieckmann, Hoke, & Ross, 1992; Kraus, McGee, Micco, Sharma, Carrell, & Nicol, 1993; Kraus, McGee, Sharma, Carrell, & Nicol, 1992). High-amplitude MMNs were also elicited by both speech and nonspeech deviations in children ages 8 to 10 years (Csepe, Molnar, Winkler, Osman-Sagi & Karmos, unpublished data, 1995). In addition, Kurtzberg and colleagues (1995) were able to identify clear MMNs in the grand mean responses of approximately two-thirds of their subjects (ages 4 to 10 years); however, in one-third of these children a clear MMN was not present, even with the presence of robust obligatory response to both the standard and deviant tones. Kurtzberg and colleagues reported that the mean MMN in newborns peaked at 241 msec and was -2.0 ± 1.3 μV in amplitude, while the mean MMN in the 8-year-olds peaked at 207 msec at an amplitude of -1.7 ± 1.03 μV. In adults, MMN latencies under similar conditions peak at approximately 140 msec. The MMN may represent similar cortical processes from birth to adulthood. (Kurtzberg et al., 1995).

METHODOLOGICAL CONSIDERATIONS AND BACKGROUND

Several factors can influence findings when using the auditory EP to assess the CANS or estimate hearing sensitivity. If the clinician is not aware of these factors, poor, contaminated, or diminished waveforms may lead to misinterpretation.

MLR and CNS Assessment

The recording of the MLR for central auditory assessment requires the placement of multiple electrodes. A clinically feasible and diagnostically useful electrode array is placement at C3, C4, and Cz (noninverting electrode) (Pool, Finitzo, Hong, Rogers, & Pickett, 1989). This allows for the comparison of amplitudes and latencies for each hemisphere and midline. The inverting electrode can be placed at the earlobe, ipsilateral and or contralateral to the ear stimulated, or at the nape of the neck (noncephalic) with the ground electrode on the forehead (Hall, 1992).

Three additional noninverting electrode sites best suited for MLR recording are designated by a 10–20 International

Electrode System. The 10–20 system correlates to definite anatomical locations on the head so that electrodes can be placed at particular sites. The most anterior site is the nasion or bridge of the nose; the most posterior site is the inion (lower back midline of head). The distance between the nasion and inion is divided into 10% and 20% increments to define particular sites; hence, the 10–20 system (see Hall, 1992 for review). A Fz (forehead) electrode revealed a response with comparable latency and amplitude characteristics as the response recorded from Cz. The other two noninverting electrodes are C5 and C6, which are located over the left and right temporoparietal regions. The average amplitude of the Pa component obtained from C5 and C6 is larger (0.90 to 1.0 μV) than the one recorded from C3 and C4 (0.60 to 0.80 μV) (Hall, 1992).

The MLR may be recorded ipsilateral or contralateral to the ear of stimulation without substantially affecting the MLR in adults (Peters & Mendel, 1974), but it seems that only the ipsilateral recorded MLR can be demonstrated reliably in the neonate (Wolf & Goldstein, 1978, 1980).

A common difficulty in recording the MLR is that scalp muscle reflexes occur at the same latency as the cerebral EP (Bickford, 1972; Picton, Hillyard, Krausz, & Galambos, 1974). At high stimulus intensities, several reflexes originating from scalp musculature occur within a poststimulus latency range of 7 to 50 msec (Picton et al., 1974). These include the postauricular reflex, temporalis reflex, and inion and frontalis reflexes. The postauricular muscle reflex is the most common contaminant and usually occurs from 14 to 19 msec post stimulus.

MLR and Hearing Sensitivity Assessment

For the assessment of hearing sensitivity, the MLR and ABR can be recorded simultaneously using Cz as the noninverting electrode, the mastoid or earlobe ipsilateral to the stimulating ear as an inverting electrode placement, and a ground electrode on the forehead.

An online measure indicating favorable periods for recording MLR during sleep is important for interpreting absent potentials (McGee, Kraus, Killion, Rosenberg, & King, 1993). Ongoing EEG can be recorded from locations C3-A2, Cz-A2, and Oz-A2. Bipolar recordings of muscle (chin-A2) and eye activity (right outer cathus-A1 and left outer cathus-A2) should be monitored. Newborns (1 to 15 days) spend up to 50% of total sleep time in REM sleep (Roffwarg, Muzio, & Dement, 1966). Thus, it is likely that the MLR can be obtained in this population, even without sleep-stage monitoring. However, from age 6 to 12 months stage-4 sleep has developed and the proportion of time spent in REM sleep time drops to 30%. By age 2 years, 46% of total sleep time is spent in stage 4, while total time in REM sleep time remains at 25% (Roffwarg et al., 1966). Thus, monitoring EEG delta activity for children who are

ages 6 to 24 months will allow reliable testing of the MLR in clinical situations (McGee et al., 1993).

MLR

The effects of arousal and attention on the MLR are controversial. The influence of sleep is a main consideration when using the MLR in CAPD evaluation or hearing-sensitivity assessment. Although some latency and amplitude changes with sleep state may be observed in adults (Okitzu, 1984; Osterhammel et al., 1985), sleep does not impede MLR recording in adults as it does in children (Kraus, Kileny, & McGee, 1994). In adults the amplitude of the MLR waves are attenuated as a function of the stage of sleep (Okitzu, 1984; Osterhammel et al., 1985), whereas the Pa amplitude is largest during REM sleep and smallest during sleep stages 3 and 4. Furthermore, the relationship between stimulus rate, sleep state, and Pa amplitude has been shown. At 1 click-per-second Pa amplitude is stable in all sleep states (Erwin & Buchwald, 1986). At 20 clicks per second significant amplitude fluctuations are observed during sleep (Osterhammel et al., 1985). At 40 clicks per second the amplitude declines with sleep by 50% to 70% (Jerger, Chmeil, Frost, & Coker, 1986; reviewed by McGee & Kraus, 1996). In children, a different effect of sleep (Kraus, McGee, & Comperatore, 1989) occurs. In stages 1, 2, and REM sleep the Pa wave is often recordable. In stage-3 sleep the Pa wave can be recorded only occasionally, and in stage-4 sleep it is absent or seldom recordable.

A recent study demonstrated that the absence of the Pa wave shows a relationship with the presence of delta activity. With increased delta activity, Pa amplitude decreased (McGee et al., 1993). However, the MLR may be altered by attention in some tasks (McCallum, Curry, Cooper, Pocock, & Pakakostopoulos, 1983; Woldorff, Hansen, & Hillyard, 1987) but not in others (Picton et al., 1974). A recent study examined the relationship between the Na and Pa components of the MLRs and the performance of different tasks. At Cz, the Na and Pa components decreased significantly for all tasks other than pegging with the right hand, while at Fz these components decreased significantly for all tasks. The Na and Pa components decreased when various tasks were performed while the subjects were concentrating (Nishihira, Araki, Ishihara, Funase, Nagas, & Kinjo, 1994).

Although sleep stage influences the detectability of the MLR waves in children, maturation of the CNS may also play a role (Kraus et al., 1985; Musiek et al., 1984). The Na is apparent and reliable at birth (McGee & Kraus, 1996), but age influences the MLR significantly. The incidence of recognizable Na and Pa waves increases with increasing age (Kraus et al., 1985; Okitzu, 1984). From infancy to adolescence the detectability of MLR waves recorded during sleep increases monotonically, from 20%

at age 1 to 6 months to 90% at age 12 years. The MLR wave can be delayed or absent in normal children younger than 10 years, and thus maturation should be considered as a factor in using this test for central or peripheral assessments. In children under age 10 years the MLR may be used for monitoring the maturation of the CANS. Recordings from children contain greater amounts of background noise, but digital filters can eliminate much of this low-frequency noise without distorting the MLR (Kraus et al., 1985; Suzuki, Hirabayashi, & Kobayashi, 1984). Another difficulty may be that the MLR of young subjects is susceptible to rapid stimulus rates. At stimulus rates of 1 to 2.5/second, it is possible to record in neonates a positive wave at 50 msec (Jerger, Chmiel, Glaze, & Frost, 1987), whereas the newborn may not show any MLR at stimulus rates near 10/second.

The Pa wave becomes significantly later and larger in elderly subjects (Woods & Clayworth, 1986). Distinct MLR deterioration and latency shift in advanced aging was found by Lenzi, Chiarelli, and Sambataro (1989). The absolute and peak-to-peak amplitudes of Pa and Pb were significantly larger for the older subjects at all stimulus rates (Chambers, 1992). Furthermore, a linear relationship between the amplitude of Na-Pa and Pa-Nb components and aging was observed, although there was no correlation between aging and the latency of Na, Pa, and Nb. The increases in the amplitudes of Na-Pa and Pa-Nb components might reflect the age-related change of auditory responses (Azumi, Nakasgima, & Takahashi, 1995). Although MLR components tend to be shorter in latency and larger in amplitude in females than in males (Palaskas, Wilson, & Dobie, 1989), there is either no significant latency difference between males and females (Stewart, Jerger, & Lew, 1993), or the differences do not always reach statistical significance (Ozdamar & Kraus, 1983; reviewed by Hall, 1992).

The filtering of the MLR is another important factor in the use of this test. Analog filtering with narrow band and sharp rolloffs can result in phase shifting or the ringing of filters (Musiek et al., 1984; Scherg, 1982). A response filter bandpass of less than 10 Hz to 300 Hz will cause distortion, amplitude reduction, and latency shifts (Kavanaugh & Domico, 1987; McGee, Krause, & Manfredi, 1988). This in turn may provide a waveform that could be misinterpreted. Wider filtering bands, such as 20 Hz (children) or 30 Hz to 1500 Hz with 6 to 12 dB per octave rolloffs, will curb distortions of the waveform. These wider filtering bands result in noisy waveforms but allow simultaneous recording of the ABR. Digital filtering prevents many distortion problems encountered with the MLR. Furthermore, post hoc digital filtering can reduce noisy effects on the waveforms, aiding accurate interpretation of results (Musiek & Lee, 1997).

The MLR (P1) may be affected by handedness (Hood, Martin, & Berlin, 1990). The peaks Po, Na, Pa, Nb, and Pb showed progressive, statistically significant latency increase in left-handed subjects when compared with right-handed subjects (Stewart, Jerger, & Lew, 1993). This may suggest a modulatory influence from the cortex (Kraus, Kileny, & McGee, 1994).

A distinct increase in amplitude and a small increase in latency as rise/fall time was lengthened from 3 to 5 to 10 msec has been observed in tonal MLR recordings (Vivion, Hirsch, Frye-Osier, & Goldstein, 1980). As click-stimulus intensity level increases from behavioral threshold (for the click) up to approximately 40 to 50 dB SL, latency systematically decreases. For higher intensity levels latency remains relatively constant (Goldstein & Rodman, 1967; Madell & Goldstein, 1972; Mendel & Goldstein, 1969a, 1969b; Thornton, Mendel, & Anderson, 1977). Amplitude, in contrast, increases steadily from over the intensity range of 0 to 70 dB SL, but the amplitude-intensity function is not linear (reviewed by Hall, 1992). However, Madell and Goldstein (1972) found a high linear correlation between MLR amplitude, especially of the Pa-Na components and loudness.

In general, amplitude for the MLR Pa component is smaller for true binaural recording than for the sum of monaural responses (Dobie & Norton, 1980; Kelly-Ballweber & Dobie, 1984; Ozdamar, Kraus, & Grossmann, 1986; Peters & Mendel, 1974; Woods & Clayworth, 1985; reviewed by Hall, 1992). Binaural interaction has been observed in MLRs at a latency of approximately 20 to 40 msec (Anslie & Boston, 1980; Berlin, Hood, & Allen, 1984; Dobie & Norton, 1980). Binaural interaction of the MLR was greatest at N20 in term infants and was maximal at P39.6 msec in adults. The binaural interaction takes the form of a reduction of amplitude of the binaural EP relative to the sum of the monaural responses, which suggests that inhibitory processes are represented in the binaural interaction using EPs (McPherson & Starr, 1993; McPherson, Tures, & Starr, 1989). The magnitude of binaural interaction was observed largest in Pa-Nb (smallest in ABR I-V) in both waking and sleeping states. Binaural interaction values for the peak-to-peak amplitudes in MLR (and ABR) were significantly lower in the sleeping state than in the waking state (Suzuki, Kobayashi, Aoki, & Umegaki, 1992).

N1, P2

The N1 and P2 potentials used for central auditory assessment should be recorded from C3, C4, and Cz sites. This allows comparisons between ears and electrode sites. In using the oddball paradigm for the P3, the N1 and P2 can also be recorded, which provides a variety of potentials for analysis with little additional time commitment (Chermak & Musiek, 1997). If estimates of threshold are the purpose, then recording from Cz should be sufficient, as this site generally provides the largest amplitude for the N1, P2 (Hall, 1992).

Sleep and sedation are well known to affect N1, P2 by causing poor repeatability and attenuation of the amplitude of the waveforms (Rapin, Schimmel, & Cohen, 1972). In sleep, for example, latency increases, the intensity at which the N1, P2 is first observed in normal-hearing people is elevated by approximately 20 to 30 dB (Cody, Klass, & Bickford, 1967; Mendel, Hosick, Windman, Davis, Hirsh, & Dinges, 1975; Osterhammel, Davis, Wier, & Hirsh, 1973), and amplitude becomes more variable (Rapin et al., 1972; Weitzman & Kremen, 1965). During sedation with chloral hydrate, as with natural sleep (Hosick & Mendel, 1975; Skinner & Antinoro, 1969; Skinner & Shimota, 1975), or with secobarbital-induced sleep (Mendel et al., 1975) the variability in the N1, P2 increases and, in turn, auditory threshold estimation is less accurate. Curiously, sleep differentially affects late components. The amplitude of the N2 increases markedly during sleep (Ornitz, Ritvo, Carr, Panman, & Walter, 1967; Picton & Hillyard, 1974; Williams, Tepas, & Morlock, 1962) while the amplitude of N1 decreases (Anch, 1977; Kevanishvili & von Specht, 1979).

The N1 and P2 are also influenced by the degree of attention to the stimulus. If the stimulus is ignored, the waveforms are attenuated and possibly delayed. The N1 and P2 components are larger when the subject pays close attention to the stimulus or listens for a change in some aspect of the stimulus. This effect is especially prominent for N1 amplitude, which increases up to 50% (reviewed by Hall, 1992). Attention may be accompanied by a general and nonspecific increase in cerebral excitability, which might increase the amplitude of the N1 wave (Naatanen & Picton, 1987). Later studies show that in most conditions auditory selective attention causes the superimposition on the N1 wave of a processing negativity, consisting of two components that overlap the true N1 components (reviewed by Naatanen & Picton, 1987). It is possible that under certain conditions attention may selectively enhance a true N1 component, as suggested by Hillyard and colleagues (Hillyard, Hink, Schwent, & Picton, 1973). In that case, this enhanced component would probably be the supratemporal component (component 1) (Naatanen & Picton, 1987).

States of arousal and levels of performance are additional factors influencing the auditory late response. The N1 evoked by unattended auditory stimuli is larger at higher levels of alertness (Fruhstorfer & Bergstrom, 1969). Studies suggest that the N1 amplitude recorded during wakefulness correlates with task performance (reviewed by Naatanen & Picton, 1987). Increasing motivation by making the amount of monetary reward dependent on performance (Wilkinson & Morlock, 1966) has resulted in enhanced N1 amplitudes and better performance. However,

it is not possible to conclude with certainty that increased arousal consistently enhanced the N1 amplitude (Naatanen & Picton, 1987).

The N1, P2 components are assumed to represent exogenic responses; therefore, they are influenced by stimulus characteristics such as intensity, frequency, type of stimulus (click, tone, or speech), and interstimulus interval (ISI). The amplitudes of N1 and P2 increase with an increasing ISI (Davis, 1976; Naatanen & Picton, 1987; Picton, Woods, Baribeau-Braun, & Healey, 1977). As stimulus intensity increases, the amplitudes of N1 and P2 increase. The increase in N1-P2 amplitude saturates at higher intensities, particularly at shorter ISI (Picton, Goodman, & Bryce, 1970). The latencies of the N1 and P2 peaks increase with decreasing stimulus intensity (Picton et al., 1977). The amplitude of the responses increases with stimulus duration of up to 30 msec and decreases if the rise time of the tonal stimulus exceeds 30 msec (Onishi & Davis, 1968). The amplitude of the response is smaller for tones of higher frequency, even when the subjective loudness of the tones is controlled (Picton, Woods, & Proulx, 1978). Higher frequency stimuli result in shorter latency of the components (Jacobson et al., 1991).

Ocular artifacts can severely contaminate the scalp-recorded late potentials (reviewed by Picton, 1990). Several techniques such as artifact rejection, filtering, and visual fixation can help remove (or reduce) ocular artifacts from the recording (Gratton, Coles, & Donchin, 1983; Picton, 1987).

In general, auditory late potential amplitude tends to be larger and the amplitude-versus-intensity function steeper for females than for males (Onishi & Davis, 1968). Shucard and colleagues showed that in verbal and nonverbal stimulus conditions females produced higher amplitude responses from the left hemisphere than did male subjects, while males showed higher amplitude responses from the right hemisphere than did females (Shucard, Shucard, & Cummins, 1981; Shucard, Shucard, & Thomas, 1977).

Monaural acoustic stimulation produces an N1 component that is consistently shorter in latency (up to 8 msec) when recorded from the hemisphere contralateral to the stimulus, in comparison to the ipsilaterally recorded response (Butler, Keidel, & Spreng, 1969). Early studies show that the amplitude of the long latency response was greater for binaural than for monaural stimulation (Butler et al., 1969; Davis & Zerlin, 1966; Davis, Zerlin, Bowers, & Spoor, 1968). Berlin and colleagues (Berlin et al., 1984) reported the presence of binaural interaction in the long-latency auditory EP. The extent of binaural interaction in the long-latency potentials is approximately 40% in regard to binaural amplitude versus the two monaural amplitudes summed. (McPherson & Starr, 1993).

P300

The P3 is generally recorded from Fez, Cz, and Paz. However, if one wishes to also look at the N1, P2, and P3, it may be useful to use a C3, C4, and Cz montage. If one has the option of using more recording channels, Fez, Cz, Paz, C3, and C4 can be used. The reference electrode can be linked from the ear lobes or positioned at the midline (Chermak & Musiek, 1997).

The N1, P2, and P3 can be recorded reliably with a non-inverting electrode located anywhere over the frontal portion of the scalp of the head, especially in the midline; it usually has maximum amplitude with a vertex site. The waveform recorded with electrodes over temporal regions (T3 and T4) have smaller amplitude. The amplitudes of the N1 and P2 also were greater when recorded contralateral to the stimulus, and they were greater for T4 than for T3 (reviewed by Hall, 1992). Thus, one should take into account the effects of these variations when using T3 and T4 electrode placement and contralateral stimulation.

The P3 latency increases with age (Picton, Stapells, Perrault, Baribeau-Braun, & Stuss, 1984). A latency increase of 1.8 msec/year between the ages of 15 and 76 years was first reported by Goodin, Squires, Henderson, and Starr (1978b). This has been confirmed by many other investigators (Hillyard & Picton, 1987; Picton & Hillyard, 1988; Picton, Stuss, Champagne, & Nelson, 1984), and most findings show a linear increase with age of 1 to 2 msec/year, while amplitude decreases at the average rate of 0.2 μV/year (Goodin et al., 1978b).

Larger P3 amplitude in adult females compared to males has been shown (Martin et al., 1988; Niwa & Hayashida, 1993), but with no gender differences in P3 for young subjects under age 15 years (Martin et al., 1988). Other studies found no significant effect of gender on either latency (Niwa & Hayashida, 1993; Polich, 1986; Sangal & Sangal, 1996) or amplitude (Polich, 1986; Sangal & Sangal, 1996) responses. Significantly shorter latency of P3 was reported in gifted children at Cz (Martin, Delpont, Suisse, Richelme, & Dolisi, 1993).

A recent study found hemispheric asymmetries of the P3 recordings (Alexander, Bauer, Kupernan, Morzorati, O'Connor, et al., 1996). P3 amplitude was larger over the right hemisphere versus the left hemisphere electrode sites (F3/4, C3/4) for both target and standard stimuli in a group of right-handed male subjects.

Various states of arousal, alertness, and psychological status will affect the P3 where attention is key (Hall, 1992; McPherson, 1995). The P3 may be viewed in attentive (oddball paradigm), passive, and ignore conditions. The most robust P3 with the greatest amplitude and shortest latency is in the attentive condition. In the ignore condition the P3 is either greatly reduced or absent. The amplitude of the P3 is reduced in the passive condition (Pfefferbaum, Ford,

Weller, & Kopell, 1985). However, Iwanami, Kamijima, and Yoshizawa (1996) found no significant correlation between either the P3 latency or the amplitude in the oddball task and the two kinds of passive tasks (a sequence task and a novel task). Furthermore, an active task such as a go/no go paradigm increases the amplitude of the P3 over active or passive attention (McPherson, 1995; Pfefferbaum et al., 1985). Also, with the P3 the difficulty of the task can affect the waveform with complex tasks, yielding a greater latency and smaller amplitude (Polich, 1987).

Although a prominent P3 wave was elicited by deviant stimuli during presleep, this presleep P3 was delayed and reduced relative to values obtained during full wakefulness. There was no P3 elicited by the frequent tone during the presleep waking stage. A progressive attenuation and delay of the P3 in response to deviant stimuli without major changes in morphology, as compared with the waking state, was observed from waking to sleep stage 1. During sleep stages 2, 3, and 4 the brain seems able to detect both frequent and deviant stimuli; however, the responses to rare stimuli were four to five times larger than responses to frequent tones. During paradoxical sleep the P3 morphology again became comparable to that of wakefulness and the P3 appeared in response to deviant stimuli exclusively. Thus, only during stage-1 and paradoxical sleep were the electrophysiological counterparts of deviance detection comparable to those of the waking state (Bastuji, Garcia-Larrea, Franc, & Mauguiere, 1995). Effects of night work on the P3 are greater for elderly than for young workers (Yasukouchi, Wada, Urasaki, & Yokota, 1995). In addition to the attention factor, alertness plays a important role on the P3. Evidence showed that electrophysiological brain function differs in the light drowsy and awake states. With light drowsiness P3 increased in latency and decreased in amplitude, but the counts of infrequent tones remained correct nevertheless (Koshino, Nishio, Murata, Omori, Murata, et al., 1993). Significant decreases in P3 amplitude and increases in latency were also found during sleep deprivation, and these changes correlated with body temperature and fatigue (Morris, So, Lee, Lash, & Becker, 1992). P3 and individual difference regarding morning/evening activity preference, food, and time of day were described by Geisler and Polich (1992). They suggested that the P3 component is sensitive to physiological and psychological changes originating from individual differences related to bodily state, which perhaps stem from individual differences in arousal level.

The P3 is an endogenous potential, along with the selective attention factor, but is virtually inseparable from stimulus factors. Auditory stimuli parameters influence P3 measures, which are apparently different for young versus elderly subjects. With equal intensity perception, younger subjects demonstrated larger P3 amplitudes and shorter latencies than did elderly subjects. Low-intensity stimuli yielded small P3 amplitudes and longer peak latencies as compared with high-intensity stimulus tones (Vesco, Bone, Ryan, & Polich, 1993). For the target stimuli, intensity increases produced reliable increases in P3 amplitude and decreases in peak latency. Using the lowest intensity level, the P3 latency was marginally longer for the low-frequency condition. For the standard stimuli, P3 amplitude increased as intensity level increased, and low-frequency stimuli yielded smaller components; P3 latency increased as intensity level decreased, and the low-frequency tone produced longer latencies than high-frequency stimuli (Sugg & Polich, 1995). Optimally, P3 is recorded with a relatively long ISI. Amplitudes of the P3 components decrease as stimulus rate increases above 1 or 0.5 stimulus/sec (Hall, 1992). The P3 is not elicited if the frequency difference for rare versus frequent stimuli is smaller than the threshold for discrimination (Hall, 1992). However, peripheral hearing loss can affect the latency of P3 indirectly, as N1 and P2 waves are often shifted in latency (resulting in a shift of the P300) in hearing-loss conditions. Differences in hearing threshold levels at the two frequencies, as in some elderly subjects, must be considered for P3 interpretation (Pollock & Schneider, 1989). Prolonged P3 latency for a 2000 Hz rare stimulus frequency was evident in older subjects with age-related hearing deficits (Pollock & Schneider, 1989). Using speech stimuli, including a subject's own name in two passive conditions, Berlad and Pratt (1995) found that P3 amplitude was larger in response to the name, as compared with the other word in the two-word paradigm. It was also larger than either of the other two words in the three-word paradigm, suggesting that stimulus relevance has an additional effect on P3 amplitude beyond rarity. The effect of different high-pass filters (0.25 Hz and 1.0 Hz) has been investigated. Using either filter, well-formed and reproducible responses were obtained, although the latency was slightly shorter when the 1.0 Hz filter was used (Goodin, Aminoff, & Chequer, 1992).

Test-retest variability of the P3 was analyzed from a group of young adults (ages 17 to 37 years) who were tested during two sessions scheduled 1 to 2 weeks apart. There was no evidence of systematic age-related change of component latencies and amplitudes between subjects. Within subjects, there were no statistically significant changes of component latencies and amplitudes between test and retest, although the latency of the P3 tended to be reduced on retest (Kileny & Kripal, 1987). Reliability of the probability effect on P3 during repeated testing was reported recently by Kinoshita and colleagues (Kinoshita, Maeda, Nakamura, Kodama, & Morita, 1995). There was no significant difference in the P3 measures during the eight sessions over 7 to 10 days. Their findings indicated that the P3 amplitude calculated from the difference waveforms may be the most stable marker for the between-session

reliability. Significant trait stability was also reported for P3 amplitude and latency among a group of adolescents during a 22-month period, supporting the P3 as a reliable measure (Segalowitz & Barnes, 1993). However, Ivey and Schmidt (1993) reported habituation due to repeated stimulation resulted in decreased P3 amplitude. Lew and Polich (1993) found that response mode is one factor responsible for the habituation. The count task demonstrated less habituation than the button-press task, with a strong interaction obtained between response mode and trial block. Lew and Polich suggested that habituation of P3 amplitude is sensitive to the amount of attention resources allocated to the processing of target stimuli, with more resources required for a count task and fewer needed for a button-press response.

The effects of the natural state (circadian, ultradian, seasonal, menstrual) and the environmentally induced state (exercise, fatigue, drugs) can produce variations of the P3 (Polich & Kok, 1995). Operant conditioning may increase the P3 component above a level obtained without contingent training (Sommer & Scheinberger, 1992).

Random and or rapid eye movements can contaminate the P300 response; hence, the subject should focus on a target during testing.

MMN

Most psychophysiological MMN studies have used three midline electrodes (Fz, Cz, Pz), referred to the linked ear or mastoid electrodes, plus two extraocular electrodes.

The scalp location of the MMN maximum amplitude seems to center more often parasagittally than the midline. Furthermore, the diagnostic sensitivity of the MMN appears to increase if the electrode yielding the largest amplitude is used. Therefore, it is beneficial to use at least seven scalp electrodes (Fpz, F4, Fz, F3, C4, Cz, and C3) plus the reference and extraocular electrodes (Lang, Eerola, Korpilahti, Holopaien, Salo, & Aaltonen, 1995). M1 and M2 are also recommended in order to satisfy one criterion (mastoid inversion) for the identification of MMN (Alho et al., 1986; Kurtzberg et al., 1995; Novak et al., 1990).

MMN-to-frequency deviation (Alho, Sainio, et al., 1990), and deviation to synthesized vowels (Cheour-Luhtanen et al., 1995) has been obtained in sleeping newborns and in adults (Nielsen-Bohlman, Knight, Woods, & Woodward, 1991). In addition, intracranial recordings from anesthetized cats (Csepe, Karmos, & Molnar, 1989) and guinea pigs (Kraus, McGee, Carrell, King, Littman, & Nicol, 1994; Kraus, McGee, Littman, Nicol, & King, 1994) provide evidence for the occurrence of the MMN even during sleep or under anesthesia. However, not all studies found a MMN in sleep (Paavilainen, Tiitinen, Alho, & Naatanen, 1987). The MMN can disappear in sleep, although some minor responses similar to the MMN have been elicited in early morning recordings (Campbell, Bell, & Bastien, 1991). The

MMN varies strongly with alertness, even if the subject is not allowed to fall asleep. In different states of vigilance, the MMN amplitude and latency behaved in various ways. In the beginning, both the MMN latency and amplitude increased as the subject felt drowsy. When slow eye movements began to occur at the S1 sleep stage, the MMN amplitude began to decrease while the latency continued to increase (Lang, Mikola, & Eerola, unpublished data, 1995; reviewed by Lang, Eerola, Korpilahti, Holopaien, Salo, & Aaltonen, 1995a). It is possible that just before a subject falls asleep the MMN latency fluctuates strongly. This partially explains the fall of the MMN amplitude in stage-1 sleep. In deeper sleep other mechanisms may also cause attenuation of the MMN (Lang, Eerola, Korpilahti, et al., 1995). Moreover, Winter, Kok, Kenemans, and Elton (1995) detected no separate mismatch negativity during drowsiness, but the variant tone evoked a broad frontocentral early negative deflection, suggesting an overlap of N1 and MMN.

The MMN is an attention-independent potential, but it is influenced greatly by stimulus characteristics such as ISI, probability of the stimulus, and other factors. If simple stimuli are used, MMN amplitude increases when the ISI is shortened (Naatanen, Paavilainen, Alho, Reinikainen, & Sams, 1987). Aging did not affect frequency or duration of MMN with the 0.5 second ISI (Pekkonen, Rinne, Reinikainen, Kujala, Alho, & Naatanen, 1996). Moreover, the amplitude of the MMN did not change as a function of ISI (800, 2400, or 7200 msec). However, amplitude was larger in younger individuals (Czigler, Csibra, & Csontos, 1992). The MMN amplitude decreases with increasing age, especially if a long ISI between the standard stimuli is used. Furthermore, the number of biphasic responses increases and the signal-to-noise ratio deteriorates with age (Lang, Portin, & Rinne, 1995; Pekkonen, Jousmaki, Reinikainen, & Partanen, 1995; Woods, 1992). Pekkonen and colleagues (Pekkonen, Jousmaki, Partanen, & Karhu, 1993; Pekkonen et al., 1996) showed that the MMN is stable regardless of age when short (1 second) ISIs are used. However, with longer (3 seconds) ISIs the MMN amplitude was considerably more attenuated in older than in young subjects. When using ISIs of 0.5 and 1.5 seconds in young subjects, the amplitude of the duration MMN showed significant individual test-retest stability between two sessions separated by 1 month (Pekkonen, Rinne, & Naatanen, 1995). Synthesized and naturally produced speech stimuli appear to be viable for eliciting the MMN (Sandridge & Boothroyd, 1996).

The MMN amplitude is also affected by the probability of deviants in the stimulus sequence. When the probability is lower, the MMN amplitude increases. However, the total time of recording increases, which again reduces the quality of the response (Lang, Eerola, Korpilanti, et al., 1995). Moreover, the MMN amplitude decreased significantly without preceding sleep deprivation when a monotonous recording session had lasted 1 to 1.5 hours, although individual variation was great. Even in young adults, the MMN amplitude begins to attenuate after 1 to 2 hours on average (Lang, Eerola, & Aaltonen, 1995). The MMN did not vary significantly with changes of intensity over a 40 dB range (Schroger, 1994). However, the latency of the MMN to infrequent changes in intensity and duration was prolonged by increasing the ISI from 400 msec to 4 seconds (Schroger & Winkler, 1995). Furthermore, using a one-dimensional deviant (one frequency and one location) versus a two-dimensional deviant (both frequency and location), the MMN was enhanced by the two-dimensional deviant under the ignore condition (Schroger, 1995). With deviants that are difficult to detect, MMN amplitudes were enlarged under attentive conditions, but there was no change in amplitudes to easy-to-detect deviants (Woods, Alho, & Algazi, 1992).

One should note that even in a normal-hearing population there is a group of individuals (23% of subjects) who show a poor auditory discrimination of frequency differences (Lang, Nyrke, Ek, Aaltonen, Raimo, & Naatanen, 1990). The variation in the MMN waveforms was studied in 139 healthy subjects, aged 20 to 82 years. Waveforms were categorized into three classes according to response quality. Class 1 (excellent signal-to-noise ratio) consisted of 37 subjects, class 2 (less favorable SNR but signal clearly recognizable) consisted of 53 subjects, and class 3 (poor SNR, signal not recognizable in analogue curves) consisted of 46 subjects. The amplitude of the responses of subjects in classes 2 and 3 was smaller and the onset latency longer than the responses of those in class 1 (Lang, Portin, & Rinne, 1995).

Gender also has an influence on the MMN latency. With complex stimuli, the MMN latency is significantly longer in females than in males (Aaltonen, Eerola, Lang, Uusipaikka, & Tuomainen, 1994).

There was a significant change in MMN distribution with age: The MMN was reported to be larger over the right hemisphere for middle-aged subjects but larger over the left hemisphere for elderly subjects (Woods, 1992). The MMN also elicited by pure-tone and vowel deviants appeared with frontocentral maximum and showed a slight right hemisphere preponderance in school-age children (Csepe et al., 1995) and adults (Paavilainen, Alho, Reinikainen, Sams, & Naatanen, 1991). However, Remijn and Sugita (1996) found the amplitude of the negativity wave to be larger over the left hemisphere than over the right hemisphere in a tone experiment by continuously ascending frequency or ascending intensity, with a tone repeated occasionally. In contrast, no interhemispheric asymmetries were demonstrated under a dichotic oddball paradigm (Praamstra & Stegeman, 1992).

It appears that auditory frequency is fully analyzed even in the absence of attention. Under dichotic conditions, even in the attentive conditions with very strong focus, the MMN was elicited by the slight deviants in the unattended input stream (Paavilainen et al., 1993), and its amplitude was similar to the MMN elicited by equivalent deviant stimuli in the attended input stream. In contrast, the MMN-to-intensity deviation was clearly attenuated in the absence of attention (Naatanen, Paavilainen, Tiitinen, Jiang, & Alho, 1993). In an attentive condition, older subjects showed a significant decline in hit rate and reduction in MMN amplitude in response to a dichotic presentation (Karayanidis, Andrews, Ward, & Michie, 1995). The MMN amplitude attenuated significantly when contralateral masking was used. However, the latencies were not affected by white noise masking (Salo, Lang, & Salmivalli, 1995).

The acute effect of low doses of alcohol on the MMN has been shown. This effect was stronger when stimulus deviation was smaller (Jaaskelainen, Pekkonen, Alho, Sinclair, Sillanuakee, & Naatanen, 1995), when amplitude was diminished significantly, and when latency was increased significantly (Jaaskelainen, Lehtokoski, Alho, Kujala, Pekkonen, et al., 1995b).

A frequency band of 0.1 to 30 Hz is sufficient for the MMN recordings. AC-power frequency can be further filtered by using a 50 Hz notch filter, although it is preferable to eliminate noise with shielding in case there are sources of noise in the vicinity (Lang, Eerola, Korpilahti, et al., 1995).

APPLICATIONS

Auditory EP are sensitive indicators of the physiological integrity of the afferent auditory sensory pathway. They provide a unique objective capability for evaluating infants, young children, and other patients whose cognitive or physical status precludes accurate behavioral audiometry or other conventional clinical techniques.

Middle Latency Evoked Response (MLR)

Estimates of Hearing Sensitivity and Related Issues. The MLR is used clinically for electrophysiologically determining hearing thresholds in the low-frequency range, assessing cochlear implant function, assessing auditory pathway function, localizing auditory pathway lesions, and for intraoperative applications (reviewed by Kraus, Kileny, & McGee, 1994).

Longer duration and low-frequency stimuli can be used to elicit the MLR, allowing for more frequency-specific evaluation of low-frequency auditory thresholds (reviewed by Stapells & Kurtzberg, 1991). Several studies in adults have demonstrated reasonable threshold accuracy using the MLR (Musiek & Geurkink, 1981; Musiek et al., 1988; Palaskas et al., 1989) (Figure 8.5). It has also been shown in adults that the MLR will accurately reflect low-frequency hearing thresholds (Scherg & Volk, 1983; Zerlin & Naun-

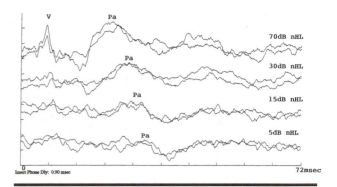

FIGURE 8.5 MLR intensity (70, 30, 15, & 5 dB nHL) function recorded from Cz electrode placement on a young woman with normal hearing.

ton, 1974). Other studies indicate that the MLR is susceptible to patient electrophysiologic artifact (Stapells & Kurtzberg, 1991). Furthermore, thresholds were more variable than those obtained using the ABR (Stapells, 1984).

Assessing threshold when neural synchrony is marginally impaired is one advantage of the MLR over the ABR. The MLR is less dependent on neural synchrony than is the ABR. The MLR can often be recorded in patients sustaining diffuse neurologic damage as a consequence of perinatal asphyxia, hyperbilirubinemia, or head trauma when the ABR was abnormal or absent (Kraus, Ozdamar, Stein, & Reed, 1984; Worthington & Peters, 1980). Furthermore, the click-evoked MLR can reflect the patient's audiologic threshold when an absent ABR was reported (Kavanaugh, Gould, McCormick, & Frank, 1989). These results indicate that the MLR provides information about hearing sensitivity at all frequencies important for understanding speech, although the peripheral hearing mechanism or the brainstem pathway may have been deficient in the synchrony necessary to produce an ABR (reviewed by Kraus, Kileny, & McGee, 1994).

The MLR has been obtained with tone bursts at or near threshold in a group of subjects with known conductive, sensorineural, or mixed hearing loss (McFarland, Vivion, & Goldstein, 1977). Note that in many cases peripheral or brainstem dysfunction will compromise the MLR.

The steady-state MLR (often referred to as the 40 Hz potential) has been reported as more effective than the transient MLR in evaluating auditory thresholds (Picton, 1990). Most studies have shown that in the waking adult the 40 Hz potential can be recorded to within 10 dB of behavioral thresholds (Dauman, Szyfter, Charlet de Sauvage, & Cazals, 1984; Rodriguez, Picton, Linden, Hamel, & Laframboise, 1986; Szyfter, Dauman, & Charlet de Sauvage, 1984). In sleep the response is smaller and the threshold may be elevated by 10 to 20 dB above that found with the subject awake (Picton, Vajar, Rodriquez, & Campbell, 1987).

The clinical use of the MLR in evaluating auditory thresholds and central function in children is limited by its variability. It is recorded inconsistently in infants and children under age 5 years (Kileny, 1983; Kraus et al., 1985; Kurtzberg, Stapells, & Wallace, 1988; Stapells, Galambos, Costello, et al., 1988). Recent work shows that MLRs are recorded reliably in children (ages 4 to 9 years) during wakefulness, stage-1, and REM sleep (Kraus et al., 1989). Because of the technical difficulty of recording from awake infants and young children, MLRs are not often used to evaluate auditory system integrity or to estimate hearing threshold in pediatric patients. Nevertheless, if MLR components are present, they provide a measure of hearing sensitivity and evidence for integrity of the auditory pathways at the initial stages of cortical processing. Their absence, however, must be interpreted with caution because this may not indicate lack of hearing sensitivity or central dysfunction in children under age 10 years.

Those who use cochlear implants can be monitored preoperatively and postoperatively with the MLR. The MLR has at least two advantages over the ABR. The first advantage is the remote time frame of wave Pa from the onset of the electrical artifact when compared to the relevant component of the ABR. This means that the MLR is far less likely to be contaminated and distorted by the spread of the electrical artifact than is the ABR (Kileny & Kemink, 1987; Kileny, Kemink, & Miller, 1989; reviewed by Kraus, Kileny, & McGee, 1994). The second advantage is the possibility of eliciting the MLR with relatively long-duration pulses, resulting in the use of a lower current level to elicit a response (Kraus, Kileny, & McGee, 1994). In threshold determination investigators found that MLR thresholds closely approximated behavioral thresholds in most cases (Kraus, Kileny, & McGee, 1994).

Pseudohypacusis. The tone-burst-elicited MLR also has potential for the evaluation of pseudohypacusis and the determination of organic hearing loss (Musiek et al., 1984; Musiek & Donnelly, 1983) (see Chapter 14).

Neurodiagnostic Applications: MLR Indices and Interpretation. There is much interest in the use of and research on the MLR in measuring central auditory function or dysfunction. In using the MLR for central auditory assessment, several measurements or indices can be used to determine the normality or abnormality of the MLR. Generally, only the Na and Pa waves are used to determine the appropriateness of the response. The other waves of the MLR (Nb, Pb, Nc, Pc) are not reliable enough for clinical use. Both amplitude and latency indices can be used for MLR interpretation, but the latency measures are not as sensitive as the amplitude indices (Kraus et al., 1982; Musiek & Lee, 1997; Scherg & Von Cramon, 1986).

A key factor in the diagnostic use of the MLR is that the intersubject variability for amplitude indices is too great for clinical use (Musiek et al., 1984). However, for older children and adults the MLR should be present, and its absence is cause for concern. One excellent index is the comparison of amplitudes obtained for electrodes placed over each hemisphere. Often the electrode closest to the area of the lesion will be compromised in regard to amplitude. Thus, there will be a difference when comparing amplitude measures for the electrodes over each hemisphere. This difference is called the *electrode effect* (Musiek, Baran, & Pinheiro, 1994). Studies show the value of comparing MLR amplitudes across electrodes (Kileny, Paccioretti, & Wilson, 1987; Kraus et al., 1982; Scherg & Von Cramon, 1986). It is uncertain, however, how much of an amplitude difference across electrodes is significant. A 50% difference in amplitude has been used to indicate potential dysfunction (Musiek et al., 1994), but recent research indicates that less of a difference could be diagnostically significant (Kelly, Lee, Charrette, & Musiek, 1996).

Ear effects are another index used in MLR interpretation (and also the late potentials). This is when one ear, regardless of electrode site, consistently shows reduced amplitudes (Figure 8.6). Again, a 50% difference in amplitude is considered important; however, diagnostically this measure is less valuable than are electrode measures (Kelly et al., 1996; Musiek et al., 1994; Shehata-Dieler, Shimizu, Soliman, & Tusa, 1991).

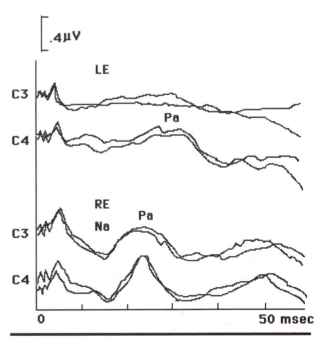

FIGURE 8.6 Abnormal ear effect (left ear) of MLR waveforms obtained from C3 and C4 electrode placements on a neurologically (left temporal stroke) involved subject.

Although Na and Pa latencies can be delayed in CANS disorders, latency indices have not proved valuable (Kileny et al., 1987; Shehata-Dieler et al., 1991).

The application of MLRs in subjects with central auditory involvement is a new and partially experimental procedure. There is little information on the sensitivity and specificity of the MLR in this context, but further research is underway. The following studies reveal the MLR's value in CANS involvement. Kraus and colleagues (1982) studied 24 patients with central lesions in the auditory areas. Of this group, approximately 50% had normal MLRs. Of the patients who had abnormal MLRs, the most telling index was Na-Pa amplitude for the electrode over the involved hemisphere. Kileny and colleagues (1987) tested 11 patients with temporal lobe involvement and compared the results to a control group of normal patients and patients with other brain lesions. The MLR demonstrated significantly reduced amplitudes when comparing left and right hemisphere electrode sites. Ibanez, Deiber, and Fischer (1989) reported significant electrode effects in 11 of 21 patients (52% sensitivity) who had cortical or subcortical lesions. Woods, Clayworth, and Knight (1985) evaluated 9 patients with unilateral cortical lesions, and 6 showed abnormal ear or electrode effects. Also studied were 9 patients with subcortical lesions, all of whom revealed ear and/or electrode effects. Shehata-Dieler and colleagues (1991) showed an electrode effect in 8 of 9 patients tested with the MLR (2 patients had large myogenic responses). Statistically, the recordings from the side of the lesions were significantly smaller than those from the intact side. By comparison, a group of patients with nonauditory lesions of the temporal lobe did not show this trend.

A recent study investigating MLR with 30 patients with multiple sclerosis showed abnormal findings in 22 patients (73.3%). The most common abnormality was absent Na and Pa waves (Celebisoy, Ayogdu, Ekmekci, & Akurekliet, 1996). A study on children with learning disabilities showed differences in the latencies of the MLR when compared to children with no learning problems (Arehole, Augustine, & Simhadri, 1995). This study reported extended latencies of the Pa wave in 5 of 11 children with learning disabilities; only 1 child of 11 in the control group demonstrated an increased Pa latency. There are other reports of children with learning disabilities who yielded abnormal MLRs upon testing (Jerger, Johnson, Jerger, Coker, Pirozzolo, & Gray, 1991; Jerger & Jerger, 1985). Conversely, Kraus and colleagues (1985) reported no significant difference in MLRs between children with learning disabilities and control patients.

Abnormal wave P1 (which has been considered the MLR Pb wave per a different recording condition) has been associated with Alzheimer's disease (Buchwald et al., 1989), autism (Buchwald et al., 1992), schizophrenia (Erwin, Mauhinney-Hec, & Gur, 1988) and stuttering (Hood, Martin, & Berlin, 1990).

Late Auditory Evoked Potentials (N1, P2)

Estimates of Hearing Sensitivity.   Before the discovery of the ABR, late auditory evoked potentials (LAEP) were used for an objective evaluation of hearing threshold (Barnet & Lodge, 1966; Davis, Hirsh, Shelnutt, & Bowers, 1967; Rapin, Ruben, & Lyttle, 1970; Rapin, Schimmel, Tourk, Krasnegor, & Pollack, 1966; Suzuki & Taguchi, 1965; Taguchi, Picton, Orpin, & Goodman, 1969). The N1 and P2 responses could be obtained using tonal stimuli for a wide range of frequencies, making it valuable in estimating frequency-specific hearing sensitivity. However, attempts to use LAEP for threshold estimation were not entirely successful because the LAEP is more variable than the ABR, is sensitive to the sleep state of the patient, and is elicited less reliably near threshold (reviewed by Stapells & Kurtzburg, 1991). However, in cases where the ABR is elevated in threshold or absent due to brainstem dysfunction (Kraus et al., 1984; Worthington & Peters, 1980), the late potentials can still provide a valuable measure of hearing threshold (Gravel, Kurtzberg, Stapells, Vaughan, & Wallace, 1989). However, its usefulness under sedation is tentative and it is not often used to assess hearing sensitivity in infants or young children.

It has also been shown that the LAEP derived from tone bursts can be used to assess threshold levels in pseudohypacusic patients (McCandless & Lentz, 1968; Rintelmann & Schwan, 1991). It has long been used in Canada as an adjunct to the hearing assessment of compensation cases for occupational hearing loss (Hyde, Matsumoto, Alberti, & Li, 1986, reviewed by Durrant and Wolf, 1991) (see Chapter 14).

Assessment of Higher Auditory Status.   As with the MLR, the LAEP is increasingly under study more as an indicator of central auditory function (Figure 8.7). In principle, the N1 and P2 can be used to examine higher level auditory cortical processing, including the ability to discriminate sounds on the basis of their acoustic or phonetic properties. Even in newborns the obligatory N1 and P2 potentials to consonant-vowel syllables exhibit differences in waveshape and/or topography in response to stimuli that differ in their place of articulation (Kurtzberg, Stone, & Vaughan, 1986; Molfese & Molfese, 1979, 1985) or in voice onset time (Kurtzberg at al., 1986). These late potentials appear to be potentially valuable in assessing central auditory integrity.

Ear effects and a complete lack of response (with adequate hearing) can indicate CANS abnormality. Extended latencies of N1 and/or P2 can also be used as an index of central auditory dysfunction (Musiek, Baran, & Pinheiro, 1994).

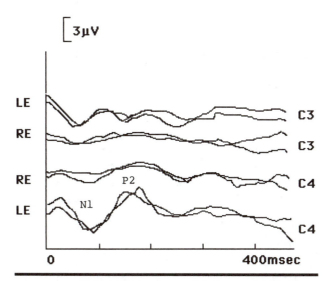

FIGURE 8.7 N1 and P2 late potentials in an adult patient with a left temporal lobe lesion.

Little information exists on the sensitivity and specificity of the late potentials for central auditory processing disorders. With recent cases added to our 1992 study, sensitivity and specificity rates of approximately 70% were computed for the N1 and P2 responses (Chermak & Musiek, 1997; Musiek, Baran, & Pinheiro, 1992). It is clear from this study that the P300 was more effective diagnostically than were the N1 and P2 potentials for central auditory disorders. Knight, Hillyard, Woods, and Neville (1980) showed that the N1 is more sensitive than the P2 to focal brain lesions in the temporoparietal region. A strong electrode effect has been shown for the N1 and P2 potentials in patients with lesions limited to one hemisphere (Peronnet & Mickel, 1977) (Figure 8.7).

In cases with bitemporal lesions, the N1 and P2 have been essentially absent or the latencies were extended and amplitudes decreased (Musiek, 1991; Woods et al., 1987). In a review by Woods and colleagues (1987), with additional cases by Musiek (1991), 19 (73%) of 26 patients with bitemporal lesions demonstrated abnormal N1-P2 potentials. Twelve of the 19 patients had an absence of responses, while the remaining patients had latency or amplitude abnormalities. Knight and colleagues (Knight, Scabini, Woods, & Clayworth, 1988) studied a normal control group, 9 patients with lesions of the superior temporal gyrus (STG) and 6 patients with inferior parietal lesions. They found that the amplitude of the N1 was significantly reduced for the STG group, as compared with the control group and the group with inferior parietal lesions. The STG group had a definite electrode effect for N1 that was not noted for the other comparison groups of patients. Interestingly, no significant difference was shown between these three groups for P2 amplitude and latency characteristics. Jirsa and Clontz

(1990) showed increased latencies of the N1 and P2 in children with CAPD when compared to a control group of children. Tonnquist-Uhlen (1996) showed that language-impaired subjects had increased latency of N1 and P2, as compared with controls.

Abnormal LAEP have also been observed in patients with psychiatric disorders such as schizophrenia (Hink, Hillyard, & Benson, 1978). Distinctive EPs have been reported in autistic children (Martineau, Garreau, Barthelemy, Callaway, & Lelord, 1981; Novick, Vaughan, Kurtzberg, & Simson, 1980). Deficits of selective attention such as hyperactivity and autism also are reflected in EP changes (Ciesielki, Courchesne, & Elmasian, 1990; Loiselle, Stamm, Maitinsky, & Whipple, 1980; Satterfield, Schell, & Backs, 1987). Children with Down syndrome showed longer N1 latency (Squires, Galbraith, & Aine, 1979) and higher amplitude P2 than did control subjects (Dustman & Callner, 1979).

Developmental status of the LAEP can provide a direct and noninvasive assessment of auditory cortical maturation. The LAEP can be used to evaluate the maturation of auditory cortical function, which can be readily quantified in terms of changes in component latency, amplitude and topography. The establishment of age-specific norms for LAEP may make it possible to identify infants with deviant auditory cortical physiology who are thus at increased risk for later language dysfunction (Kurtzberg et al., 1988).

Because late components need not depend on intact earlier potentials in some cases, late potentials have been observed when ABRs are absent or very abnormal in patients with neurologic disease (Satya-Murti, Wolpaw, Cacace, & Schaffer, 1983; Squires & Hecox, 1983). This could help in the evaluation of patients with severe peripheral involvement and higher auditory dysfunction, or even in the assessment of patients with cochlear implants (Kileny, 1991; Kraus, McGee, Ferre, Hoeppner, Carrell, Sharma, & Nicol, 1993b; Oviatt & Kileny, 1981).

P300. Historically, the first processing contingent potential described was the prominent positive component P3, which follows the obligatory N1 and P2 when stimuli are presented in an unpredictable sequence (Sutton et al., 1965). Since its discovery, the P3 has been the most frequently reported ERP component in studies of cognitive dysfunction and dementia.

The P300 does not appear to provide the laterality information seen with the MLR or N1 and P2 (Knight et al., 1989; Musiek et al., 1992). However, the P300 will occasionally show an electrode effect in unilateral disease (Musiek et al., 1992). Nonetheless, the convention is to use Fz, Cz, and Pz (midline) electrode sites. With these electrode sites the P300 latencies and/or absence of the P300 can indicate abnormality. The amplitude measure with the

P300 is highly variable, which makes the effectiveness of this index uncertain. Latency measures must be adjusted for age because the P300 begins to increase in latency in the second or third decade of life (Polich, Howard, & Starr, 1985a).

In adults the P3 has been studied in patients with cerebrovascular lesions, head trauma, brain tumors (Figure 8.8) (Ebner, Haas, Lucking, Schily, Wallesch, & Zimmerman, 1986; Michaelewski, Rosenberg, & Starr, 1986; Musiek et al., 1992), senile dementia (Goodin et al., 1978a, 1978b; Pfefferbaum, Ford, Roth, & Kopell, 1980), schizophrenia (Baribeau-Braun, Picton, & Gosselin, 1983; Roth, Horvath, Pfefferbaum, & Kopell, 1980), aphasia (Selinger & Prescott, 1989), chronic renal failure (Cohen, Syndulko, Rever, Kraut, Coburn, & Tourtellotte, 1983), and chronic alcoholism (Pfefferbaum, Horvath, Roth, & Kopell, 1979). The P3 is delayed in a variety of cortical and subcortical dementias (Goodin, 1986; Johnson, 1992; Michaelewski et al., 1986; Squires, Chipperdale, Wrege, Goodin, & Starr, 1980). Moreover, P3 latency has correlated with cognitive decline as evidenced by selective neuropsychological test scores in the elderly (Polich, Ehlers, Otis, Mandell, & Bloom, 1986) and in patients with multiple sclerosis (Giesser, Schroeder, LaRocca, Ritter, Scheinberg, & Vaughan, 1992), Parkinson's disease (Hansch, Syndulko, Cohen, Goldberg, Potvin, & Tourtellotte, 1982; O'Donnell, Squires, Martx, Chen, & Phay, 1987), Huntington's disease (Homberg, Hefter, Granseyer, Strauss, Lange, & Hennerici, 1986), progressive supranuclear palsy (Johnson, Litvan, & Grafman, 1991), and AIDS dementia complex (ADC) (Handelsman, Horvath, Aronson, Schroeder, et al., 1992; Messenbeimer, Robertson, Wilins, Kalkowski, & Hall, 1992). In recent studies

(Goodin, Aminoff, Chernoff, & Hollander, 1990; Schroeder, Handelsman, Torres, Dorfman, Rinaldi, et al., 1994) P3 peak latency was significantly delayed and P3 amplitudes were significantly reduced for all HIV-1 seropositives, including asymptomatics, when compared to parenteral drug users and seronegative controls. The study suggested that the P3 is sensitive to early stages of HIV-1 infection, possibly because of its dependence on higher order processes of attention and memory, which are vulnerable early in ADC. Amplitude reductions and prolonged latencies have also been observed in patients with Alzheimer's disease (Brown, Marsh, & Larue, 1982; Chayasirisobhon, Brinkman, Gerganoff, Gershon, Pomara, & Green, 1984; Goodin et al., 1978b; Syndulko, Hansch, Cohen, Pearce, Goldberg, et al., 1982).

Knight and colleagues (1989) compared six patients with lesions of the temporal-parietal junction to six patients with parietal lesions. For the P300 amplitude index, the temporal group showed markedly reduced waves, as compared with the parietal group, which yielded results similar to the normal control subjects. Knight and colleagues (1989) also used a P300 paradigm involving novel stimuli (stimuli that change in character to keep the subjects' attention) rather than targets, and the results comparing the two groups (temporal and parietal) were similar to those obtained using the standard P300 paradigm. Knight and colleagues (1980, 1988) found no laterality effect on the patients or normal control subjects. Other studies show increased latencies and/or decreased amplitudes of the P300 in focal brain lesions, most of which involved the auditory areas of the cerebrum. Based on statistical comparisons to various control groups, the P300 was sensitive to either cognitive impairment or focal brain lesions (Ebner et al., 1986; Knight, 1990; Musiek et al., 1992).

Studies have also examined diffuse lesions of the cerebrum or lesions at various sites in the cerebrum. Obert and Cranford (1990) used the P300 to test 10 patients with neocortical lesions of various sites and reported that in 53% of the experimental conditions the patients had absent or delayed waveforms. Significantly delayed P300s also have been noted in patients with traumatic brain injury (Rappaport & Clifford, 1994).

Kutus, Hillyard, Volpe, and colleagues (1990) measured the P300 after commissurotomy in 5 patients, and concluded that the corpus callosum was not needed for the generation of the P300. However, in these commissurotomy patients a larger response occurred over the right hemisphere. Because of this, one cannot rule out the possibility of the contribution of the corpus callosum to the P300. Certainly this asymmetry could also be a result of other kinds of brain dysfunction in this population.

The P300 has also been measured in learning disabled populations. Jirsa and Clontz (1990) used the P300 in a

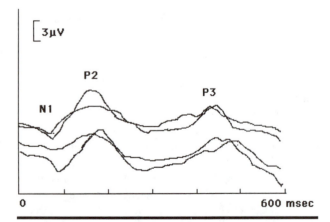

FIGURE 8.8 An example of a delayed P300 recorded from the right ear of an adult patient who suffered bilateral, subdural hematomas after a head injury. The top two traces are from electrodes placed at C3; the bottom traces are from C4.

population of normal school-aged children and children who had CAPD. The CAPD group had significantly delayed latencies, but there was no significant difference in the P300 amplitude between the two groups. Squires and Hecox (1983) demonstrated P300 abnormalities and subtle auditory discrimination problems in children with receptive and expressive language disorders. Low-amplitude P3s have been linked to hyperactivity, schizophrenia, autism, and reading disability with few changes in P3 latency (Ciesielki et al., 1990; Squires et al., 1983). Loiselle and colleagues (1980) used a dichotic P300 paradigm with 11 boys classified as hyperactive; 15 boys comprised a control group. When each group was asked to attend to stimuli in one ear over the other, a latency difference was found between the control and hyperactive groups. However, when this selective listening task was not used no latency differences were found between groups.

Abnormal P3s have also been linked to Down syndrome (Lincoln, Courchesne, Kilman, & Galambos, 1985) and psychiatric disorders in children (Diner, Holcomb, & Dykman, 1985). The use of P3 to differentiate functional from organic cognitive disorders in children has been reported by Finley and colleagues (Finley, Faux, Hutcheson, & Amstutz, 1985).

The late potentials, especially the P300, offer advantages to the professional interested in auditory diagnostics, but in order to use these potentials to define central auditory lesions, patients must be selected carefully. The clinician must be sure the patient has no other nonauditory disorders, such as parkinsonism, or many of the disorders just mentioned which could result in abnormal late potentials. If other factors have been excluded, an abnormal late potential can be linked to an auditory problem with greater certainty, especially if the patient has a history consistent with auditory problems. If a patient has a diagnosed nonauditory disorder known to affect the P300, one must consider the disorder as the reason for the abnormal P300. Conversely, patients with known nonauditory disorders and abnormal late potentials could have a concomitant peripheral or central auditory problem. In these complex situations, the use of other auditory tests may prove helpful in defining an auditory disorder.

MMN.   Some promising applications of ERP involve the study of potentials associated with perceptual and cognitive operations. These perceptual and cognitive potentials include both automatic and voluntary cortical discriminative responses such as the MMN. The MMN reflects central processing of very fine differences in acoustic stimuli (Figure 8.9). It also appears that the MMN reflects a neuronal representation of the discrimination of numerous auditory stimulus attributes (reviewed by Kraus & McGee, 1994). The MMN is elicited passively and does not require attention (Naatanen, 1992) or a behavioral response (re-

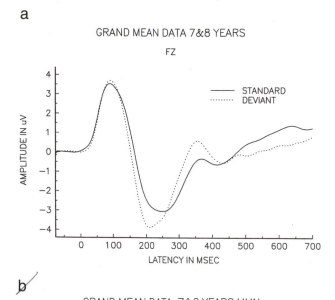

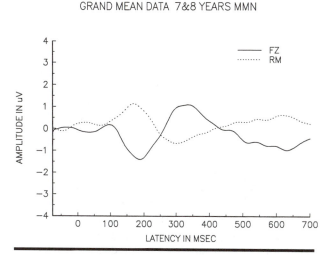

FIGURE 8.9   (A) Grand mean of the standard and deviant responses recorded from Fz from 15 subjects (ages 7 and 8 years). The standard stimulus was a 1000 Hz tone and the deviant stimulus was a 1200 Hz tone. (B) MMN was derived from data above with right mastoid (RM) inversion. (Courtesy of D. Kurtzberg)

viewed by Kraus & McGee, 1994). It has been obtained in sleeping infants (Alho, Sainio, et al., 1990) and adults (Nielsen-Bohlman et al., 1991), and in animals during sleep and under barbiturate anesthesia (Csepe, Karmos, & Molnar, 1987). Because the MMN is an automatic response that is not influenced significantly by attention, it may provide an ideal probe of auditory sensory memory and discrimination in infants and young children, and in the clinical assessment of auditory processing disorders in the pediatric population (reviewed by Steinschneider et al., 1992). It could also be used for those in whom communication is difficult or compromised, or for whom auditory discrimination is in question, such as adults with aphasia or dementia (Korpilahti, Ek, & Lang, 1992; Naatanen, 1992). Consequently, it may permit an objective analysis of sensory processing and discrimination (reviewed by Kraus & McGee, 1994).

In terms of auditory memory, the MMN may be useful for examining the properties, not only of the literal and long-term aspects of sensory memory (Cowan, 1988, 1991), but of factors that influence the incorporation of sensory information into longer-term storage. Thus, the MMN provides a powerful objective tool to clarify issues related to the processing and storage of sensory information (Ritter, Deacon, Gomes, Javitt, & Vaughan, 1995).

The use of the MMN in defining central auditory deficits is in its early stages. Kraus and colleagues (1993) have shown deficits correlated to an abnormal MMN in patients with CAPD and specific auditory discrimination problems. A recent study on patients with frontal cortex lesions demonstrated that the MMN amplitude was diminished, most notably over the lesioned hemisphere and from the ear ipsilateral to the lesioned hemisphere (Alho, Woods, Algazi, Knight, & Naatanen, 1994).

The MMN may be a useful tool for assessing the discrimination ability of electrical stimulation patterns produced by a cochlear implant. Recent studies show that the MMN can be elicited by differences in speech (Kraus, McGee, Sharma, Carrell, & Nicol, 1993a) and by physical differences in stimulus train duration and pitch (Ponton & Don, 1995) when presented through a cochlear implant. However, the MMN may be elicited in individuals with cochlear implants by differences in the location of stimulated electrode pairs along the implant array.

Because durational differences and site of activation differences along the implant array produce an MMN component in the cortical potentials of cochlear implant users, it may be possible to use this neurophysiological response for both clinical and theoretical evaluation of implant function (Ponton & Don, 1995).

CONCLUSION

The auditory middle and late potentials can provide the audiologist with an electrophysiologic method for assessing the integrity of the higher central auditory system and for estimating audiometric threshold. Presently, these evoked potentials do not have the clinical value of the better known ABR procedure. They also require detailed knowledge of their limitations and strengths in order to be applied optimally. However, if applied carefully, the middle and late potentials can supplement the audiologist's diagnostic test battery. These potentials can help provide an objective measurement for central auditory function, which will allow the clinician to make a more comprehensive evaluation of the entire auditory system. Procedures such as the P300 and MMN have the additional capability of assessing particular processes of higher auditory function, which should lead to information about how the CANS functions. Taken with their strengths and limitations, the middle and late evoked potentials provide a challenging but rewarding area of endeavor for audiologists.

REFERENCES

Aaltonen, O., Eerola, O., Lang, A. H., Uusipaikka, E., & Tuomainen, J. (1994). Automatic discrimination of phonetically relevant and irrelevant vowel parameters as reflected by mismatch negativity. *Journal of the Acoustical Society of America, 96,* 1489–1493.

Alexander, J., Bauer, L., Kuperman, S., Morzorati, S., O'Connor, S., Rohrbaugh, J., Porjesz, B., Begleiter, H., & Polich, J. (1996). Hemispheric differences for P300 amplitude from an auditory oddball task. *International Journal of Psychophysiology, 21,* 189–196.

Alho, K., Paavilainen, P., Reinikainen, K., Sams, M., & Naatanen, R. (1986). Separability of different negative components associated with auditory stimulus processing. *Psychophysiology, 23,* 613–624.

Alho, K., Sainio, K., Sajaniemi, N., Reinikainen, K., & Naatanen, R. (1990). ERBPs of human newborns to pitch change of an acoustic stimulus. *Electroencephalography and Clinical Neurophysiology, 77,* 151–155.

Alho, K., Sajaniemi, N., Niittyvuopio, T., Sainio, K, & Naatanen, R. (1990). ERPs to an auditory stimulus change in pre-term and full-term infants. In C. Brunia, A. Gaillard, A. Kok (Eds.), *Psychophysiological Brain Research* (pp. 139–142). Tilburg: Tilburg University Press.

Alho, K., Woods, D., Algazi, A., Knight, R., & Naatanen, R. (1994). Lesions of the frontal cortex diminish the auditory mismatch negativity. *Electroencephalography and Clinical Neurophysiology, 91,* 353–362.

Allen, R., Cranford, J., & Pay, N. (1996). Central auditory processing in an adult with congenital absence of left temporal lobe. *Journal of the American Academy of Audiology, 7,* 282–288.

Altman, J., & Vaitulevich, S. (1990). Auditory image movement in evoked potentials. *Electroencephalography and Clinical Neurophysiology, 75,* 323–333.

Anch, M. (1977). The auditory evoked brain response during adult human sleep. *Waking and Sleeping, 1,* 189–194.

Anslie, J., & Boston, J. (1980). Comparison of brain stem auditory evoked potentials or monaural and binaural stimuli. *Electroencephalography and Clinical Neurophysiology, 49,* 291–302.

Arehole, S., Augustine, L., & Simhadri, R. (1995). Middle latency response in children with learning disabilities: Preliminary findings. *Journal of Communication Disorders, 28,* 21–38.

Arezzo, J., Pickoff, A., & Vaughan, H. Jr. (1975). The sources and intracerebral distribution of auditory evoked potentials in the alert rhesus monkey. *Brain Research, 90,* 57–73.

Arezzo, J., Vaughan, H. Jr., Kraut, M., Steinschneider, M., & Legatt, A. (1986). Intracranial generators of event-related potentials in monkey. In R. Cracco & I. Bodis-Wollner (Eds.), *Frontiers of Clinical Neuroscience, Vol. 3, Evoked Potentials* (pp. 174–189). New York: Alan Liss.

Azumi, T., Nakasgima, K., & Takahashi, K. (1995). Aging effects on auditory middle latency responses. *Electromyography and Clinical Neurophysiology, 35,* 397–401.

Barajas, J. (1990). The effects of age on human P3 latency. *Acta Otolaryngologica, Supplement 476,* 157–160.

Baribeau-Braun, J., Picton., T., & Gosselin, J-Y. (1983). A neurophysiological evaluation of abnormal information processing. *Science, 219,* 874–876.

Barnet, A., & Lodge, A. (1966). Diagnosis of deafness in infants with the use of computer averaged electroencephalographic responses to sound. *Journal of Pediatrics, 69,* 753–758.

Bastuji, H., Garcia-Larrea, L., Franc, C., & Mauguiere, F. (1995). Brain processing of stimulus deviance during slow-wave and paradoxical sleep: A study of human auditory evoked responses using the oddball paradigm. *Journal of Clinical Neurophysiology, 12,* 155–167.

Baumann, S., Rogers, R., Papanicolaou, A., & Saydjari, C. (1990). Intersession replicability of dipole parameters in three components of the auditory evoked magnetic field. *Brain Topography, 3,* 311–319.

Berlad, I., & Pratt, H. (1995). P300 in response to the subject's own name. *Electroencephalography and Clinical Neurophysiology, 96,* 472–474.

Berlin, C., Hood, L., & Allen, P. (1984). Asymmetries in evoked potentials. In C. Berlin (Ed.), *Hearing Science: Recent Advances* (pp. 461–477). San Diego: College-Hill.

Bickford, R. (1972). Physiological and clinical studies of microflexes. *Electroencephalography and Clinical Neurophysiology, Supplement 31,* 93–108.

Brown, W., Marsh, J., & Larue, A. (1982). Event-related potentials in psychiatry: Differentiating depression and dementia in the elderly. *Bulletin of the LA Neurological Society, 47,* 91–107.

Buchwald, J. (1990). Comparison of plasticity in sensory and cognitive processing systems. *Clinical Perinatology, 17,* 57–66.

Buchwald, J., Erwin, R., Read, S., Van Lancker, D., & Cummings, J. (1989). Midlatency auditory evoked response: Differential abnormality of P1 in Alzheimer's disease. *Electroencephalography and Clinical Neurophysiology, 74,* 378–384.

Buchwald, J., Erwin, R., Van Lancker, D., Schwafel, T., & Tanguay, P. (1992). Midlatency auditory evoked responses: P1 abnormalities in adult autistic subjects. *Electroencephalography and Clinical Neurophysiology, 84,* 164–171.

Butler, R., Keidel, W., & Spreng, M. (1969). An investigation of the human cortical evoked potential under conditions of monaural and binaural stimulation. *Acta Otolaryngologica, 68,* 317–326.

Callaway, E. (1975). *Brain Electrical Potentials and Individual Psychological Differences.* New York: Grune & Stratton.

Callaway, E. & Halliday, R. (1973). Evoked potential variability: Effects of age, amplitude and methods of measurement. *Electroencephalography and Clinical Neurophysiology, 34,* 125–133.

Campbell, K., Bell, I., & Bastien, C. (1991). Evoked potential measures of information processing during natural sleep. In R. Broughton & R. Ogilvie (Eds.), *Sleep, Arousal and Performance* (pp. 88–116). Boston: Birkhauser.

Celebisoy, N., Aydogdu, I., Ekmekci, O., & Akurekli, O. (1996). Middle latency auditory evoked potentials (MLAEPs) in MS. *Acta Neurologica Scand, 93,* 318–321.

Chambers, R. (1992). Differential age effects for components of the adult auditory middle latency response. *Hearing Research, 58,* 123–131.

Chayasirisobhon, S., Brinkman, S., Gerganoff, S., Gershon, S., Pomara, N., & Green, V. (1984). Event-related potential in Alzheimer's disease. *Clinical Electroencephalography, 16,* 48–53.

Cheour-Luhtanen, M., Alho, K., Kujala, T., Sainio, K., Reinikainen, K., Renlung, M., Aaltonen, O., Eerola, O., & Naatanen, R. (1995). Mismatch negativity indicates vowel discrimination in newborns. *Hearing Research, 82,* 53–58.

Chermak, G., & Musiek, F. (1997). *Central Auditory Processing Disorders.* San Diego: Singular Publishing.

Ciesielki, K., Courchesne, E., & Elmasian, R. (1990). Effects of focused selective attention tasks on event-related potentials in autistic and normal individuals. *Electroencephalography and Clinical Neurophysiology, 75,* 207–220.

Cody, D., Klass, D., & Bickford, R. (1967). Cortical audiometry: An objective method of evaluating auditory function in awake and sleep man. *Transactions of the American Academy of Ophthalmology and Otolaryngology, 19,* 81–91.

Cohen, M. (1982). Coronal topography of the middle latency auditory evoled potential in man. *Electroencephalography and Clinical Neurophysiology, 53,* 231–236.

Cohen, S., Syndulko, K., Rever, B., Kraut, J., Coburn, J., & Tourtellotte, W. (1983). Visual evoked potentials and long latency event-related potnetials in chronic renal failure. *Neurology, 33,* 1219–1222.

Collett, L., Duclaux, R., Challamel, M., & Revol, M. (1988). Effect of sleep on middle latency response (MLR) in infants. *Brain and Development, 10,* 169–173.

Courchesne, E. (1978). Neurophysiological correlates of cognitive development: Changes in long-latency event-related potentials from childhood to adulthood. *Electroencephalography and Clinical Neurophysiology, 45,* 468–482.

Courchesne, E. (1990). Chronology of postnatal human brain development: Event related potential, positron emission tomography, myelinogenesis, and synaptogenesis studies. In J. Rohrbaugh, R. Parasuraman, & R. Johnson (Eds.), *Event-Related Brain Potentials* (pp. 210–241). New York: Oxford University Press.

Cowan, N. (1988). On short and long auditory stores. *Psychological Bulletin, 96,* 341–370.

Cowan, N. (1991). Sensory memory and its role in information processing. *Proceedings of the 10th International Conference of Event-Related Potentials of the Brain.* Eger, Hungary.

Csepe, V. (1995). On the origin and development of the mismatch negativity. *Ear and Hearing, 16,* 91–104.

Csepe, V., Dieckmann, B., Hoke, M., & Ross, B. (1992). Mismatch negativity to pitch change of acoustic stimuli in preschool and school-age children. *EPIC X Abstract.*

Csepe, V., Karmos, D., & Molnar, M. (1987). Evoked potential correlates of stimulus deviance during wakefulness and sleep in cat-animal model of mismatch negativity. *Electroencephalography and Clinical Neurophysiology, 66,* 571–578.

Csepe, V., Karmos, D., & Molnar, M. (1989). Subcortical evoked potential correlates of early information processing: Mismatch negativity in cats. In E. Basar & T. Bullock (Eds.), *Springer Series in Brain Dynamics 2* (pp. 278–289). Berlin: Springer Verlag.

Csepe, V., Molnar, M., Winkler, I., Osman-Sagi, J., & Karmos, G. (1995). Mismatch negativity to deviating speech stimuli in school-age children: Hierarchy in development of ERP waves? Unpublished data.

Czigler, I., Csibra, G., & Csontos, A. (1992). Age and interstimulus interval effects on event-related potentials to frequent and infrequent auditory stimuli. *Biological Psychology, 33,* 195–206.

Dauman, R., Szyfter, W., Charlet de Sauvage, R., & Cazals, Y. (1984). Low frequency thresholds assessed with 40 Hz MLR in adults with impaired hearing. *Archives of Otorhinolaryngology, 240,* 85–89.

Davis, H. (1976). Principles of electric response audiometry. *Annals of Otology, Rhinology and Laryngology (Supplement), 28,* 1–96.

Davis, H., Hirsh, S., Shelnutt, J., & Bowers, C. (1967). Further validation of evoked response audiometry (ERA). *Journal of Speech and Hearing Research, 10,* 717–732.

Davis, H., & Zerlin, S. (1966). Acoustic relations of the human vertex potential. *Journal of the Acoustical Society of America, 39,* 109–116.

Davis, H., Zerlin, S., Bowers, C., & Spoor, A. (1968). Some interaction of the vertex potentials. *Electroencephalography and Clinical Neurophysiology, 24,* 285.

Davis, P. (1939). Effects of acoustic stimuli on the waking human brain. *Journal of Neurophysiology, 2,* 494–499.

Desmedt, J., & Debecker, J. (1979). Wave form and neural mechanism of the decision P350 elicited without pre-stimulus CNV or readiness potential in random sequences of near threshold auditory clicks and finger stimuli. *Electroencephalography and Clinical Neurophysiology, 47,* 648–670.

Diner, B., Holcomb, P., & Dykman, R. (1985). P-300 in a major depressive disorder. *Psychiatric Research, 15,* 175–185.

Dobie, R., & Norton, S. (1980). Binaural interaction in human auditory evoked potentials. *Electroencephalography and Clinical Neurophysiology, 49,* 303–313.

Durrant, J., & Wolf, K. (1991). Auditory evoked potentials: Basic aspects. In W. Rintelmann (Ed.), *Hearing Assessment* (2nd ed.). Boston: Allyn & Bacon.

Dustman, R., & Callner, D. (1979). Cortical evoked responses and responses decrement in nonretarded and Down's syndrome individuals. *American Journal of Mental Deficiency, 83,* 391–397.

Ebner, A., Haas, J., Lucking, C., Schily, M., Wallesch, C., & Zimmerman, P. (1986). Event-related brain potentials (P300) and neuropsychological deficit in patients with focal brain lesions. *Neuroscience Letters, 64,* 330–334.

Elberling, C., Bak, C., Kofoed, B., Lebech, J., & Saermark, K. (1982). Auditory magnetic fields from the human cerebral cortex: Location and strength of an equivalent current dipole. *Acta Neurologica Scandinavia, 65,* 553–569.

Erwin, R., & Buchwald, J. (1986). Midlatency auditory evoked responses: Differential effects of sleep in the human. *Electroencephalography and Clinical Neurophysiology, 65,* 383–392.

Erwin, R., Mauhinney-Hec, M., & Gur, R. (1988). Milatency auditory evoked responses in schizophrenics. *Neuroscience, 14,* 339 (Abstract).

Finley, W., Faux, S., Hutcheson, J., & Amstutz, L. (1985). Long-latency event-related potentials in the evaluation of cognitive function in children. *Neurology, 35,* 323–327.

Fischer, C., Bognar, L., Turjman, F., & Lapras, C. (1995). Auditory evoked potentials in a patient with a unilateral lesion of the inferior colliculus, and medial geniculate body. *Electroencephalography and Clinical Neurophysiology, 96,* 261–267.

Fruhstorfer, H., & Bergstrom, R. (1969). Human vigilance and auditory evoked responses. *Electroencephalography and Clinical Neurophysiology, 27,* 346–355.

Fuchigami, T., Okubo, O., Ejiri, K., Fujita, Y., Kohira, R., Noguchi, Y., Fuchigami, S., Hiyoshi, K., Nishimura, A., & Harada, K. (1995). Developmental changes in P300 wave elicited during two different experimental conditions. *Pediatric Neurology, 13,* 25–28.

Geisler, C., Frishkopf, L., & Rosenblith, W. (1958). Extra cranial responses to acoustic clicks in man. *Science, 128,* 1210–1211.

Geisler, M., & Polich, J. (1992). P300 and individual differences: Morning/evening activity preference, food, and time-of-day. *Psychophysiology, 29,* 86–94.

Giesser, B., Schroeder, M., LaRocca, N., Ritter, W., Scheinberg, L., & Vaughan, H. Jr. (1992). Endogenous event-related potentials correlate with dementia in multiple sclerosis patients. *Journal of Electroencephalography and Clinical Neurophysiology, 82,* 320–329.

Goff, E., Allison, T., & Vaughan, H. Jr. (1978). The functional neuroanatomy of event-related potentials in man. In E. Callway, P. Tueting, & S. Koslow (Eds.), *Event-Related Potentials in Man* (pp. 1–79). New York: Academic Press.

Goldstein, R., & Rodman, L. (1967). Early components of averaged evoked responses to rapidly repeated auditory stimuli. *Journal of Speech and Hearing Research, 10,* 697–705.

Goodin, D. (1986). Event-related (endogenous) potentials. In M. Aminoff (Ed.), *Electrodiagnosis in Clinical Neurology* (pp. 575–595). New York: Churchill Livingstone.

Goodin, D., Aminoff, M., & Chequer, R. (1992). Effect of different high-pass filters on the long-latency event-related auditory evoked potentials in normal human immunodeficiency virus. *Journal of Clinical Neurophysiology, 9,* 97–104.

Goodin, D., Aminoff, M., Chernoff, D., & Hollander, H. (1990). Long latency event-related potentials in patients infected with human immunodeficiency virus. *Annals of Neurology, 27,* 414–420.

Goodin, D., Squires, K., Henderson, B., & Starr, A. (1978a). Age-related variations in evoked potentials to auditory stimuli in normal human subjects. *Electroencephalography and Clinical Neurophysiology, 44,* 447–458.

Goodin, D., Squires, K., Henderson, B., & Starr, A. (1978b). An early event-related cortical potential. *Psychophysiology, 15,* 360–365.

Goodin, D., Squires, K., & Starr, A. (1978). Long latency event-related components of the auditory evoked potentials in dementia. *Brain, 101,* 635–648.

Gordon, E., Rennie, C., & Collins, L. (1990). Magnetoencephalography and late component ERPs. *Clinical and Experimental Neurology, 27,* 113–120.

Graham, J., Greenwood, R., & Lecky, B. (1980). Cortical deafness: Case report and review of the literature. *Journal of Neurological Science, 48,* 35–49.

Gratton, G., Coles, M., & Donchin, E. (1983). A new method for off-line removal of ocular artifacts. *Electroencephalography and Clinical Neurophysiology, 55,*468–484.

Gravel, J., Kurtzberg, D., Stapells, D., Vaughan, H., & Wallace, I. (1989). Case studies. *Seminars in Hearing, 10,* 272–287.

Halgren, E., Squires, N., Wilson, C., Rohrbaugh, J., Babb, T., & Crandall, P. (1980). Endogenous potentials generated in the human hippocampal formation and amygdala by infrequent events. *Science, 210,* 803–805.

Hall, J. (1992). *Handbook of Auditory Evoked Responses.* Boston: Allyn & Bacon.

Handelsman, L., Horvath, T., Aronson, M., Schroeder, M., et al. (1992). Auditory event-related potentials in HIV-1 infection: A study in the drug user risk group. *Journal of Neuropsychiatric Clinical Neuroscience, 4,* 294–302.

Hansch, E., Syndulko, K., Cohen, S., Goldberg, Z., Potvin, A., & Tourtellotte, W. (1982). Cognition in Parkinson's disease: An event-related potential perspective. *Annals of Neurology, 11,* 599–607.

Hari, R., Aittonie, K., Jarvinen, M., Katila, T., & Varpula, T. (1980). Auditory evoked transient and sustained magnetic fields of the human brain. *Experimental Brain Research, 40,* 237–240.

Hari, R., Kaila, K., Katila, T., Tuomisto, T., & Varpula, T. (1982). Interstimulus interval dependence of the auditory vertex response and its magnetic counterpart: Implications for their neural generation. *Electroencephalography and Clinical Neurophysiology, 54,* 561–569.

Harrison, J., Dickerson, L., Song, S., & Buchwald, J. (1990). Cat-P300 present after association cortex ablation. *Brain Research Bulletin, 24,* 551–560.

Hashimoto, I. (1982). Auditory evoked potentials from the human midbrain: Slow brain stem responses. *Electroencephalography and Clinical Neurophysiology, 53,* 652–657.

Hillyard, S., Hink, R., Schwent, V., & Picton, T. (1973). Electrical signs of selective attention in the human brain. *Science, 182,* 177–180.

Hillyard, S., & Picton, T. (1987). Electrophysiology of cognition. In F. Plum (Ed.), *Handbook of Physiology, Vol. V, Higher Functions of the Nervous System* (pp. 519–584). Bethesda: American Physiological Society.

Hink, R., Hillyard, S., & Benson, P. (1978). Electrophysiological measures of attentional processes in man as related to the study of schizophrenia. *Journal of Psychiatric Research, 14,* 155–165.

Homberg, V., Hefter, H., Granseyer, G., Strauss, W., Lange, A., & Hennerici, M. (1986). Event-related potentials in patients with Huntington's disease and relatives at risk in relation to detailed psychometry. *Electroencephalography and Clinical Neurophysiology, 63,* 552–569.

Hood, L., Martin, D., & Berlin, C. (1990). Auditory evoked potentials differ at 50 milliseconds in right- and left-handed listeners. *Hearing Research, 45,* 115–122.

Hosick, E., & Mendel, M. (1975). Effects of secobarbital on the late components of the auditory evoked potentials. *Revue de Laryngologie Otologie Rhinologie (Bordeaux), 96,* 185–191.

Hyde, M., Matsumoto, N., Alberti, P., & Li, Y. (1986). Auditory evoked potentials in audiometric assessment of compensarion and medicolegal patients. *Annals of Otology, Rhinology and Laryngology, 95,* 514–519.

Ibanez, V., Deiber, P., & Fischer, C. (1989). Middle latency auditory evoked potentials and cortical lesions: Criteria of interhemispheric asymmetry. *Archives of Neurology, 46,* 1325–1332.

Ivey, R., & Schmidt, H. (1993). P300 response: Habituation. *Journal of the American Academy of Audiology, 4,* 182–188.

Iwanami, A., Kamijima, K., & Yoshizawa, J. (1996). P300 component of event-related potentials in passive tasks. *International Journal of Neuroscience, 84,* 121–126.

Jaaskelainen, I., Lehtokoski, A., Alho, K., Kujala, T., Pekkonen, E., Sinclair, J. D., Naatanen, R., & Sillanaukee, P. (1995). Low dose of ethanol suppresses mismatch negativity of auditory event-related potentials. *Alcoholism, Clinical and Experimental Research, 19,* 607–610.

Jaaskelainen, I., Pekkonen, E., Alho, K., Sinclair, J., Sillanaukee, P., & Naatanen, R. (1995). Dose-related effect of alcohol on mismatch negativity and reaction time performance. *Alcohol, 12,* 491–495.

Jacobson, G., Newman, C., Privitera, M., & Grayson, A. (1991). Differences in superficial and deep source contributions to middle latency auditory evoked potential Pa component in normal subjects, and patients with neurologic disease. *Journal of the American Academy of Audiology, 2,* 7–17.

Javitt, D., Schroeder, C., Arezzo, J., & Vaughan, H. (1991). Selective inhibition of processing-contingent auditory event-related potentials by the phencyclidine (PCP)-like agent MK-801. *Electroencephalography and Clinical Neurophysiology, 79,* 65P.

Javitt, D., Schroeder, C., Steinschneider, M., Arezzo, J. & Vaughan, H. Jr. (1992). Demonstration of mismatch negativity in the monkey. *Electroencephalography and Clinical Neurophysiology, 83,* 87–90.

Javitt, D., Schroeder, C., Steinschneider, M., Arezzo, J., & Vaughan, H. Jr. (1995). Cognitive event-related potentials in human and non-human primates: Implications for the PCP/NMDA model of schizophrenia. *Electroencephalography and Clinical Neurophysiology, 44,* 161–175.

Jerger, J., Chmeil, R., Frost, J. D., & Coker, N. (1986). Effect of sleep on auditory steady state evoked potential. *Ear and Hearing, 7,* 240–245.

Jerger, J., Chmiel, R., Glaze, D., & Frost, J. (1987). Rate and filter dependence of the middle-latency response. *Audiology, 26,* 269–283.

Jerger, J., Johnson, K., Jerger, S., Coker, N., Pirozzolo, F., & Gray, L. (1991). Central auditory processing disorder: A case study. *Journal of the American Academy of Audiology, 2,* 36–54.

Jerger, S., & Jerger, J. (1985). Audiological application of early, middle and late auditory evoked potentials. *Hearing Journal, 38,* 31–36.

Jirsa, R., & Clontz, K. (1990). A long latency auditory event-related potentials from children with auditory processing disorders. *Ear and Hearing, 11,* 222–232.

Johnson, R. (1992). Invited commentary on the neural generators of the P300 component of the event-related potential. *Psychophysiology, 30,* 94–101.

Johnson, R., Litvan, I., & Grafman, J. (1991). Progressive supranuclear palsy: Altered sensory processing leads to degraded cognition. *Neurology, 41,* 1257–1262.

Karayanidis, F., Andrews, S., Ward, P., & Michie, P. (1995). ERP indices of auditory selective attention in aging and Parkinson's disease. *Psychophysiology, 32,* 335–350.

Kaseda, Y., Tobimatsu, S., Morioko, T., & Kato, M. (1991). Auditory middle-latency responses in patients with localized and non-localized lesions of the central nervous system. *Journal of Neurology, 238,* 427–432.

Kaukoranta, E., Sams, M., Hari, R., Hamalainen, M., & Naatanen, R. (1989). Reactions of human auditory cortex to a change in tone duration. *Hearing Research, 41,* 15–21.

Kavanaugh, K., & Domico, W. (1987). High pass digital and analog filtering of the middle latency response. *Ear and Hearing, 8,* 101–109.

Kavanaugh, K., Gould, H., McCormick, G., & Frank, R. (1989). Comparison of the identifiability of the low intensity ABR and MLR in the mentally handicapped patient. *Ear and Hearing, 10,* 124–130.

Kelly, T., Lee, W., Charrette, L., & Musiek, F. (1996). Middle latency evoked response sensitivity and specificity. *Proceedings of the American Auditory Society Annual Meeting,* Salt Lake City, April 21.

Kelly-Ballweber, D., & Dobie, R. (1984). Binaural interaction measured behaviorally and electrophysiologically in young and old adults. *Audiology, 23,* 181–194.

Kevanishvili, Z., & von Specht, H. (1979). Human slow auditory evoked potentials during natural and drug-induced sleep. *Electroencephalography and Clinical Neurophysiology, 47,* 280–288.

Kileny, P. (1983). Auditory evoked middle latency responses: Current issues. *Seminars in Hearing, 4,* 403–413.

Kileny, P. (1991). Use of electrophysiologic measures in the management of children with cochlear implants: Brainstem, middle latency and cognitive (P300) responses. *American Journal of Otology, 12,* 37–42.

Kileny, P., Dodson, D., & Gelfand, E. (1983). Middle-latency auditory evoked responses during open-heart surgery with hypothermia. *Electroencephalography and Clinical Neurophysiology, 55,* 268–276.

Kileny, P., & Kemink, J. (1987). Electrically evoked middle-latency auditory potentials in cochlear implant candidates. *Archives of Otolaryngology—Head and Neck Surgery, 113,* 1072–1077.

Kileny, P., Kemink, J., & Miller, J. (1989). An intrasubject comparison of electric and acoustic middle latency responses. *American Journal of Otology, 10,* 23–27.

Kileny, P., & Kripal, J. (1987). Test-retest variability of auditory event-related potentials. *Ear and Hearing, 8,* 110–114.

Kileny, P., Paccioretti, D., & Wilson, A. (1987). Effects of cortical lesions on middle latency auditory evoked response (MLR). *Electroencephalography and Clinical Neurophysiology, 66,* 108–120.

Kinoshita, S., Maeda, H., Nakamura, J., Kodama, E., & Morita, K. (1995). Reliability of the probability effect on event-related potentials during repeated testing. *Kurume Medical Journal, 42,* 199–210.

Knight, R. (1990). Neuromechanisms of event-related potentials: Evidence from human lesion studies. In J. Roharbaugh, R. Parasuraman, & R. Johnson (Eds.), *Event-Related Potentials: Basic Issues in Applications* (pp. 3–18). New York: Oxford University Press.

Knight, R., Hillyard, S., Woods, D., & Neville, H. (1980). The effects of frontal and temporal-parietal lesions on the auditory evoked potential in man. *Electroencephalography and Clinical Neurophysiology, 50,* 112–124.

Knight, R., Scabini, D., Woods, D., & Clayworth, C. (1988). The effects of lesions of the superior temporal gyrus and inferior parietal lobe on temporal and vertex components of the human AEP. *Electroencephalography and Clinical Neurophysiology, 70,* 499–509.

Knight, R., Scabini, D., Woods, D., & Clayworth, C. (1989). Contributions of temporal-parietal junction to the human auditory P3. *Brain Research, 502,* 109–116.

Korpilahti, P., & Lang, A. (1994). Auditory ERP components and MMN in dysphasic children. *Electroencephalography and Clinical Neurophysiology, 91,* 256–264.

Korpilahti, P., Ek, M., & Lang, A. (1992). The defect of "pitch MMN" in dysphasic children. *EPIC X Abstract 82.*

Koshino, Y., Nishio, M., Murata, T., Omori, M., Murata, I., Sakamoto, M., & Isaki, K. (1993). The influence of light drowsiness on the latency and amplitude of P300. *Clinical Electroencephalography, 24,* 110–113.

Kraus, N., Kileny, P., & McGee, T. (1994). Middle latency auditory evoked potentials. In J. Katz (Ed.), *Handbook of Clinical Audiology* (4th ed.). Baltimore: Williams & Wilkins.

Kraus, N., & McGee, T. (1988). Color imaging of the human middle latency response. *Ear and Hearing, 9,* 159–167.

Kraus, N., & McGee, T. (1994). Auditory event-related potentials. In J. Katz (Ed.), *Handbook of Clinical Audiology* (4th ed.). Baltimore: Williams & Wilkins.

Kraus, N., & McGee, T. (1995). The middle latency response generating system. *Electroencephalography and Clinical Neurophysiology, 44* (Suppl.), 93–101.

Kraus, N., McGee, T., Carrell, T., King, C., Littman, T., & Nicol, T. (1994). Discrimination of speech-like contrasts in the auditory thalamus and cortex. *Journal of the Acoustical Society of America, 96,* 2758–2768.

Kraus, N., McGee, T., & Comperatore, C. (1989). MLRs in children are consistently present during wakefulness, stage 1 and REM sleep. *Ear and Hearing, 10,* 339–345.

Kraus, N., McGee, T., Ferre, J., Hoeppner, J., Carrell, T., Sharma, A., & Nicol, T. (1993b). Mismatch negativity in the neurophysiologic/behavioral evaluation of auditory processing deficits: A case study. *Ear and Hearing, 14,* 223–234.

Kraus, N., McGee, T., Littman, T., & Nicol, T. (1992). Reticular formation influences on primary and non-primary auditory pathway as reflected by the middle latency responses. *Brain Research, 587,* 186–294.

Kraus, N., McGee, T., Littman, T., Nicol, T., & King, C. (1994). Non-primary auditory thalamic representation of acoustic change. *Journal of Neurophysiology, 72,* 1270–1277.

Kraus, N., McGee, T., Micco, A., Sharma, A., Carrell, T., & Nicol, T. (1993). Mismatch negativity in school-age children to speech stimuli that are just perceptibly different. *Electroencephalography and Clinical Neurophysiology, 88,* 123–130.

Kraus, N., McGee, T., Sharma, A., Carrell, T., & Nicol, T. (1992). Mismatch negativity event-related potential to speech stimuli. *Ear and Hearing, 13,* 158–164.

Kraus, N., McGee, T., Sharma., A., Carrell, T., & Nicol, T. (1993a). Mismatch negativity in school-age children to speech stimuli that are just perceptibly defferent. *Electroencephalography and Clinical Neurophysiology, 88,* 123–130.

Kraus, N., Micco, A., Koch, D., McGee, T., Carrell, T., Wiet, R., Weingarten, C., & Sharma, A. (1993). The mismatch negativity cortical evoked potential elicited by speech in cochlear-implant users. *Hearing Research, 65,* 118–124.

Kraus, N., Ozdamar, O., Hier, D., & Stein, L. (1982). Auditory middle latency response in patients with cortical lesions. *Electroencephalography and Clinical Neurophysiology, 5,* 247–287.

Kraus, N., Ozdamar, O., Stein, L., & Reed, N. (1984). Absent auditory brain stem response: Peripheral hearing loss or brain stem dysfunction? *Laryngoscope, 94,* 400–406.

Kraus, N., Smith, D., & McGee, T. (1988). Midline and temporal lobe MLRs in the guinea pig originate from different generator systems: A conceptual framwork for new and existing data. *Electroencephalography and Clinical Neurophysiology, 71,* 541–558.

Kraus, N., Smith, D., Reed, N., Stein, L., & Cartee, C. (1985). Auditory middle latency responses in children: Effects of age and diagnostic category. *Electroencephalography and Clinical Neurophysiology, 62,* 343–351.

Kuriki, S., Nogai, T., & Hirata, Y. (1995). Cortical sources of middle latency responses of auditory evoked magnetic field. *Hearing Research, 92,* 47–51.

Kurtzberg, D. (1989). Cortical event-related potential assessment of auditory system function. *Seminars in Hearing, 10,* 252–261.

Kurtzberg, D., Hipert, P., Kreuzer, J., & Vaughan, H. Jr. (1984). Differential maturation of cortical auditory evoked potentials to speech sounds in normal fullterm and very low-birth-weight infants. *Developmental Medicine and Child Neurology, 26,* 466–475.

Kurtzberg, D., Stapells, D., & Wallace, I. (1988). Event-related potential assessment of auditory system integrity: Implications for language development. In P. Vietze & H. Vaughan, Jr. (Eds.), *Early Identification of Infants with Developmental Disabilities* (pp. 161–180). Philadelphia: Grune & Stratton.

Kurtzberg, D., Stone, C. Jr., & Vaughan, H. Jr. (1986). Cortical responses to speech sounds in the infant. In R. Cracco & I. Bodis-Wollner (Eds.), *Frontiers of Clinical Neuroscience, Vol 3—Evoked Potentials* (pp. 513–520). New York: Alan R. Liss.

Kurtzberg, D., Vaughan, H., Kreuzer, J., & Fliegler, K. (1995). Developmental studies and clinical applications of mismatch negativity: Problems and prospects. *Ear and Hearing, 16,* 105–117.

Kutus, M., Hillyard, S., Volpe, B., et al. (1990). Late positive event-related potentials after commissural section in humans. *Journal of Cognitive Neuroscience, 2,* 258–271.

Kuwata, T., Funahashi, K., Maeshima, S., Ogura, M., Hyotani, G., Terada, T., Itakura, T., Hayashi, S., & Komai, N. (1993). Influence of regional cerebral blood flow on event-related potential (P300). *Neurologia Medico-Chirurgica, 33,* 146–151.

Lang, A. H., Eerola, O., & Aaltonen, O. (1995). Intra-individual variation of the mismatch negativity. Unpublished data.

Lang, A., Eerola, O., Korpilahti, P., Holopaien, I., Salo, S., & Aaltonen, O. (1995). Practical issues in the clinical application of mismatch negativity. *Ear and Hearing, 16,* 118–129.

Lang, A. H., Mikola, H., & Eerola, O. (1995). [Slight variations of vigilance affect the mismatch negativity]. Unpublished data.

Lang, A. H., Nyrke, T., Ek, M., Aaltonen, O., Raimo, I., & Naatanen, R. (1990). Pitch discrimination performance and auditive event-related potentials. In C. Brunia, A. Gaillard, & A. Kok (Eds.), *Psychophysiological Brain Research* (pp. 294–298). Tilburg, Netherlands: Tilburg University Press.

Lang, A. H., Portin, R., & Rinne, J. (1995). [Inter-individual variation of mismatch negativity]. Unpublished data.

Lenzi, A., Chiarelli, G., & Sambataro, A. (1989). Comparative study of middle-latency responses and auditory brainstem responses in elderly subjects. *Audiology, 28,* 144–151.

Lew, G., & Polich, J. (1993). P300, habituation, and response mode. *Physiology and Behavior, 53,* 111–117.

Liegeois-Chauvel, C., Musolino, A., Badier, J., Marquis, P., & Chauvel, P. (1994). Evoked potentials recorded from the auditory cortex in human: Evaluation and topography of the middle latency components. *Electroencephalography and Clinical Neurophysiology, 92,* 204–214.

Lincoln, A., Courchesne, E., Kilman, B., & Galambos, R. (1985). Neuropsychological correlates of information processing by children with Down's syndrome. *American Journal of Mental Deficiency, 89,* 403–414.

Loiselle, D., Stamm, J., Maitinsky, S., & Whipple, S. (1980). Evoked potential and behavioral signs of attention dysfunction in hyperactive boys. *Psychophysiology, 17,* 193–201.

Madell, J., & Goldstein, R. (1972). Relation between loudness and the amplitude of the early components of the averaged electroencephalic response. *Journal of Speech and Hearing Research, 15,* 134–141.

Makela, J., Hamalainen, M., Hari, R., & McEvoy, L. (1994). Whole-head mapping of middle-latency auditory evoked magnetic fields. *Electroencephalography and Clinical Neurophysiology, 92,* 414–421.

Martin, F., Delpont, E., Suisse, G., Richelme, C., & Dolisi, C. (1993). Long latency event-related potentials (P300) in gifted children. *Brain and Development, 15,* 173–177.

Martin, L., Barajas, J., & Fernandez, R. (1988). Auditory P3 development in childhood. *Scandinavian Audiology (Supplement), 30,* 105–109.

Martin, L., Barajas, J., Fernandez, R., & Torres, E. (1988). Auditory event-related potentials in well-characterized group of children. *Electroencephalography and Clinical Neurophysiology, 17,* 375–381.

Martineau, J., Garreau, B., Barthelemy, C., Callaway, E., & Lelord, G. (1981). Effects of vitamin B6 on averaged evoked potentials in infantile autism. *Biological Psychiatry, 16,* 625–639.

McCallum, W., Curry, S., Cooper, R., Pocock, P., & Pakakostopoulos, D. (1983). Brain event-related potentials as indicators of early selective processes in auditory target localization. *Psychophysiology, 20,* 1–17.

McCandless, G., & Lentz, W. (1968). Amplitude and latency characteristics of the auditory evoked response at low sensation levels. *Journal of Auditory Research, 8,* 273–282.

McCarthy, G., Wood, C., Allison, T., Goff, W., Williamson, P., & Spencer, D. (1982). Intracranial recordings of event-related potentials in humans engaged in cognitive tasks. *Society of Neuroscience Abstracts, 8,* 976.

McFarland, W., Vivion, M., & Goldstein, R. (1977). Middle components of the AEP to tone-pips in normal-hearing and hearing-impaired subjects. *Journal of Speech and Hearing Research, 20,* 781–798.

McGee, T., & Kraus, N. (1996). Auditory development reflected by middle latency response. *Ear and Hearing, 17,* 419–429.

McGee, T., Kraus, N., Killion, M., Rosenberg, R., & King, C. (1993). Improving the reliability of the auditory middle latency response by monitoring EEG delta activity. *Ear and Hearing, 14,* 76–84.

McGee, T., Kraus, N., & Manfredi, C. (1988). Toward a strategy for analyzing the human MLR waveform. *Audiology, 27,* 119–130.

McIsaac, H., & Polich, J. (1992). Comparison of infant and adult P300 from auditory stimuli. *Journal of Experimental Child Psychology, 53,* 115–128.

McPherson, D. (1995). *Late Potentials of the Auditory System* (pp. 75–100). San Diego: Singular.

McPherson, D., & Starr, A. (1993). Binaural interaction in auditory evoked potentials: Brainstem, middle- and long-latency components. *Hearing Research, 66,* 91–98.

McPherson, D., Tures, C., & Starr, A. (1989). Binaural interaction of the auditory brainstem potentials and middle latency auditory evoked potentials in infants and adults. *Electroencephalography and Clinical Neurophysiology, 74,* 124–130.

Mendel, M., & Goldstein, R. (1969a). Stability of the early components of the averaged electroencephalic response. *Journal of Speech and Hearing Research, 12,* 351–361.

Mendel, M., & Goldstein, R. (1969b). The effect of test conditions on the early components of the averaged electroencephalic response. *Journal of Speech and Hearing Research, 12,* 344–350.

Mendel, M., Hosick, E., Windman, T., Davis, H., Hirsh, S., & Dinges, D. (1975). Audiometric comparison of the middle and late components of the adult auditory evoked potentials awake and sleep. *Electroencephalography and Clinical Neurophysiology, 38,* 27–33.

Messenbeimer, J., Robertson, K., Wilins, J., Kalkowski, J., & Hall, C. (1992). Event-related potentials in human immunodeficiency virus infection: A prospective study. *Archives of Neurology, 49,* 396–400.

Michaelewski, H., Rosenberg, C., & Starr, A. (1986). Event related potentials in dementia. In R. Cracco & I. Bodis-Wollner (Eds.), *Evoked Potentials* (pp. 521–528). New York: Alan Liss.

Molfese, D., & Molfese, V. (1979). Hemisphere and stimulus differences as reflected in the cortical responses of newborn infants to speech stimuli. *Developmental Psychology, 15,* 505–511.

Molfese, D., & Molfese, V. (1985). Electrophysiological indices of auditory discrimination in newborn infants: The basis for predicting later language development? *Infant Behavior and Development, 8,* 197–211.

Morris, A., So, Y., Lee, K., Lash, A., & Becker, C. (1992). The P300 event-related potential: Effects of sleep deprivation. *Journal of Occupational Medicine, 34,* 1143–1152.

Musiek, F. (1991). Auditory evoked responses in site of lesion assessment. In W. Rintelmann (Ed.), *Hearing Assessment* (2nd ed.). Boston: Allyn & Bacon.

Musiek, F., Baran, J., & Pinheiro, M. (1992). P300 results in patients with lesions of the auditory areas of the cerebrum. *Journal of the American Academy of Audiology, 3,* 5–15.

Musiek, F., Baran, J., & Pinheiro, M. (1994). *Neuroaudiology: Case Studies.* San Diego: Singular.

Musiek, F., & Donnelly, K. (1983). Clinical applications of the (auditory) middle latency response—An overview. *Seminars in Hearing, 4,* 391–401.

Musiek, F., & Geurkink, N. (1981). Auditory brainstem and middle latency evoked response sensitivity near threshold. *Annals of Otology, Rhinology and Laryngology, 90,* 236–240.

Musiek, F., Geurkink, N., Weider, D., & Donnelly, K. (1984). Past, present and future applications of the auditory middle latency response. *Laryngoscope, 94,* 1545–1552.

Musiek, F., & Lee, W. (1997). Conventional and maximum length sequences middle latency response in patients with central nervous system lesions. *Journal of the American Academy of Audiology.*

Musiek, F., Verkest, S., Gollegly, K. (1988). Effects of neuromaturation of auditory evoked potentials. *Seminars in Hearing, 9,* 1–13.

Naatanen, R. (1992). *Attention and Brain Function.* Hillsdale, NJ: Lawrence Erlbaum.

Naatanen, R., Paavilainen, P., Alho, K., Reinikainen, K., & Sams, M. (1987). Interstimulus interval and the mismatch negativity. In C. Barber & T. Blum (Eds.), Evoked potentials III. *The Third International Evoked Potentials Symposium.*

Naatanen, R., Paavilainen, P., Tiitinen, H., Jiang, D., & Alho, K. (1993). Attention and mismatch negativity. *Psychophysiology, 30,* 436–450.

Naatanen, R., & Picton, T. (1987). The N1 wave of the human electric and magnetic response to sound: A review and an analysis of the component structure. *Psychophysiology, 24,* 375–425.

Neshige, R., & Luders, H. (1992). Recording of event-related potentials (P300) from human cortex. *Journal of Clinical Neurophysiology, 9,* 294–298.

Nielsen-Bohlman, L., Knight, R., Woods, D., & Woodward, K. (1991). Differential processing of auditory stimuli continues during sleep. *Electroencephalography and Clinical Neurophysiology, 79,* 281–290.

Nishihira, Y., Araki, H., Ishihara, A., Funase, K., Nagao, T., & Kinjo, S. (1994). Auditory middle latency responses under different task conditions. *Electromyography and Clinical Neurophysiology, 34,* 409–414

Niwa, S., & Hayashida, S. (1993). Nd and P300 in healthy volunteers. *Environmental Research, 62,* 283–288.

Novak, G. Kurtzberg, D., Kreuzer, J., & Vaughan, H. Jr. (1989). Cortical responses to speech sounds and their formants in normal infants: Maturational sequence and spatiotemporal analysis. *Electroencephalography and Clinical Neurophysiology, 73,* 295–305.

Novak, G., Ritter, W., Vaughan, H. Jr., & Wiznitzer, M. (1990). Differentiation of negative event-related potentials in an auditory discrimination task. *Electroencephalography and Clinical Neurophysiology, 75,* 255–275.

Novick, B., Vaughan, H. Jr., Kurtzberg, D., & Simson, R. (1980). An electrophysiologic indication of auditory processing defects in autism. *Psychiatry Research, 3,* 107–114.

Obert, A., & Cranford, J. (1990). Effects of neocortical lesions on the P300 component of the auditory evoked response. *American Journal of Otology, 11,* 447–453.

O'Donnell, B., Squires, N., Martx, M., Chen, J., & Phay, A. (1987). Evoked potential changes and neuropsychological performance in Parkinson's disease. *Biological Psychology, 24,* 23–37.

Ohlrich, E., Barnet, A., Weiss, I., & Shanks, B. (1978). Auditory evoked potential development in early childhood: A longitudinal study. *Electroencephalography and Clinical Neurophysiology, 44,* 411–423.

Okada, Y., Kaufman, L., & Williamson, S. (1983). The hippocampal formation as a source of the slow endogenous potentials. *Electroencephalography and Clinical Neurophysiology, 55,* 417–426.

Okitzu, T. (1984). Middle components of auditory evoked response in young children. *Scandinavian Audiology, 13,* 83–86.

Onishi, S., & Davis, H. (1968). Effects of duration and rise time of tonebursts on evoked V-potentials. *Journal of the Acoustical Society of America, 44,* 582–591.

Ornitz, E., Ritvo, E., Carr, E., Panman, L., & Walter, R. (1967). The variability of the auditory averaged evoked response during sleep and dreaming in children and adults. *Electroencephalography and Clinical Neurophysiology, 22,* 514–524.

Osterhammel, P., Davis, H., Wier, C., & Hirsh, S. (1973). Adult auditory evoked vertex potentials in sleep. *Audiology, 12,* 116–128.

Osterhammel, P., Shllop, J., & Terkildsen, K. (1985). The effect of sleep on the auditory brainstem response (ABR) and middle latency response (MLR). *Scandinavian Audiology, 14,* 47–50.

Oviatt, D., & Kileny, P. (1981). Auditory event-related potentials elicited from cochlear implant recipients and hearing subjects. *American Journal of Audiology, 1,* 48–55.

Ozdamar, O., & Kraus, N. (1983). Auditory middle latency responses in humans. *Audiology, 22,* 34–49.

Ozdamar, O., Kraus, N., & Curry, F. (1983). Auditory brainstem, and middle latency responses in a patient with cortical deafness. *Electroencephalography and Clinical Neurophysiology, 53,* 275–287.

Ozdamar, O., Kraus, N., & Grossmann, J. (1986). Binaural interaction in the auditory middle latency response of the guinea pig. *Electroencephalography and Clinical Neurophysiology, 63,* 476–483.

Paavilainen, P., Alho, K., Reinikainen, K., Sams, M., & Naatanen, R. (1991). Right-hemisphere dominance of different mismatch negativities. *Electroencephalography and Clinical Neurophysiology, 78,* 466–479.

Paavilainen, P., Cammann, R., Alho, K., Reinikainen, K., Sams, M., & Naatanen, R. (1987). Event-related potentials to pitch change in an auditory stimulus sequence during sleep. In R. Johnson & J. Rohrbaugh (Eds.), Current trends in event-related potential research. *Electroencephalography and Clinical Neurophysiology (Supplement), 40,* 246–255.

Paavilainen, P., Tiitinen, H., Alho, K., & Naatanen, R. (1993). Mismatch negativity to slight pitch changes outside strong attentional focus. *Biological Psychology, 37,* 23–41.

Palaskas, C., Wilson, M., & Dobie, R. (1989). Electrophysiologic assessment of low-frequency hearing: Sedation effects. *Otolaryngology—Head and Neck Surgery, 101,* 434–441.

Paller, K., Zola, M., Squire, L., & Hillyard, S. (1988). P3-like brain waves in normal monkeys and in monkeys with medial temporal lesions. *Behavioral Neuroscience, 102,* 714–725.

Parving, A., Solomon, G., Elbering, C., Larsen, B., & Lassen, N. (1980). Middle components of the auditory evoked response in bilateral temporal lobe lesions. *Scandinavian Audiology, 9,* 161–167.

Pekkonen, E., Jousmaki, V., Partanen, J., & Karhu, J. (1993). Mismatch negativity area and age-related auditory memory. *Electroencephalography and Clinical Neurophysiology, 87,* 321–325.

Pekkonen, E., Jousmaki, V., Reinikainen, K., & Partanen, J. (1995). Automatic auditory discrimination is impaired in Parkinson's disease. *Electroencephalography and Clinical Neurophysiology, 95,* 47–52.

Pekkonen, E., Rinne, T., & Naatanen, R. (1995). Variability and replicability of the mismatch negativity. *Electroencephalography and Clinical Neurophysiology, 96,* 546–554.

Pekkonen, E., Rinne, T., Reinikainen, K., Kujala, T., Alho, K., & Naatanen, R. (1996). Aging effects on auditory processing: An event-related potential study. *Experimental Aging Research, 22,* 171–184.

Peronnet, F., & Michel, F. (1977). The asymmetry of the auditory evoked potentials in normal man and in patients with brain lesions. In J. Desmedt (Ed.), *Auditory Evoked Potentials in Man: Psychopharmacology Correlates of ERPS. Vol 2* (pp. 130–141). Basel, Switzerland: Karger.

Peronnet, F., Michel, F., Echallier, J., & Girod, J. (1974). Coronal topography of human auditory evoked responses. *Electroencephalography and Clinical Neurophysiology, 37,* 225–230.

Peters, J., & Mendel, M. (1974). Early components of the averaged electroencephalic response to monaural and binaural stimulation. *Audiology, 13,* 195–204.

Pfefferbaum, A., Ford, J., Roth, W., & Kopell, B. (1980). Age-related changes in auditory event-related potentials. *Electroencephalography and Clinical Neurophysiology, 49,* 266–276.

Pfefferbaum, A., Ford, J., Weller, B., & Kopell, B. (1985). ERPs to response production and inhibition. *Electroencephalography and Clinical Neurophysiology, 60,* 423–434.

Pfefferbaum, A., Horvath, T., Roth, W., & Kopell, B. (1979). Event related potential changes in chronic alcoholics. *Electroencephalography and Clinical Neurophysiology, 47,* 637–647.

Picton, T. (1987). The recording and measurement of evoked potentials. In A. M. Halliday, S. Butler, & R. Paul (Eds.), *Textbook of Clinical Neurophysiology* (pp. 23–40). Chichester, England: John Wiley & Sons.

Picton, T. (1990). Auditory evoked potentials. In D. Daly, & T. Pedley (Eds.), *Current Practice of Clinical Electroencephalography* (2nd ed., pp. 623–678). New York: Raven Press.

Picton, T., Goodman, W., & Bryce, D. (1970). Amplitude of evoked responses to tones of high intensity. *Acta Otolaryngologica, 79,* 77–82.

Picton, T., & Hillyard, S. (1974). Human auditory evoked potentials: Effects of attention. *Electroencephalography and Clinical Neurophysiology, 36,* 191–199.

Picton, T., & Hillyard, S. (1988). Endogenous event-related potentials. In T. Picton (Ed.), *Handbook of Electroencephalography and Clinical Neurophysiology, Vol. 3* (pp. 361–426). Amsterdam: Elsevier.

Picton, T., Hillyard, S., Krausz, H., & Galambos, R. (1974). Human auditory potentials. I. Evaluation of components. *Electroencephalography and Clinical Neurophysiology, 36,* 179–190.

Picton, T., Stapells, D., Perrault, N., Baribeau-Braun, J., & Stuss, D. (1984). Human event-related potentials: Current perspectives. In R. Nodar & C. Barber (Eds.), *Evoked Potentials II* (pp. 3–16). Boston: Butterworths.

Picton, T., Stuss, D., Champagne, S., & Nelson, R. (1984). The effects of age on human event-related potentials. *Psychophysiology, 21,* 312–325.

Picton, T., Vajar, J., Rodriguez, R., & Campbell, K. (1987). Reliability estimates for steady state evoked potentials. *Electroencephalography and Clinical Neurophysiology, 68,* 119–131.

Picton, T., Woods, D., Baribeau-Braun, J., & Healey, T. (1977). Evoked potential audiometry. *Journal of Otolaryngology, 6,* 90–119.

Picton, T., Woods, D., & Proulx, G. (1978). Human auditory sustained potentials. II. Stimulus relationships. *Electroencephalography and Clinical Neurophysiology, 45,* 198–210.

Polich, J. (1986). Normal variation of P300 from auditory stimuli. *Electroencephalography and Clinical Neurophysiology, 65,* 236–240.

Polich, J. (1987). Task difficulty, probability and interstimulus interval as determinants of P300 from auditory stimuli. *Electroencephalography and Clinical Neurophysiology, 68,* 311–320.

Polich, J., Ehlers, C., Otis, S., Mandell, A., & Bloom, F. (1986). P300 latency reflects the degree of cognitive decline in dementing illness. *Electroencephalography and Clinical Neurophysiology, 63,* 138–144.

Polich, J., Howard, L., & Starr, A. (1985a). Aging effects on the P300 component of the event-related potential from auditory stimuli: Peak definition, variation and measurement. *Journal of Gerontology, 40,* 721–726.

Polich, J., Howard, L., & Starr, A. (1985b). Stimulus frequency and masking as determinants of P300 latency in event-related potentials from auditory stimuli. *Biological Psychology, 21,* 309–318.

Polich, J., & Kok, A. (1995). Cognitive and biological determinants of P300: An integrative review. *Biological Psychology, 41,* 103–146.

Pollock, V., & Schneider, L. (1989). Effects of tone stimulus frequency on late positive component activity (P3) among normal elderly subjects. *International Journal of Neuroscience, 45,* 127–132.

Polyakov, A., & Pratt, H. (1994). Three-channel Lissajous' trajectory of human middle latency auditory evoked potentials. *Ear and Hearing, 15,* 390–399.

Ponton, C., & Don, M. (1995). The mismatch negativity in cochlear implant users. *Ear and Hearing, 16,* 131–146.

Ponton, C., Don, M., Eggermont, J., Waring, M., & Masuda, A. (1996). Maturation of human cortical auditory function: Differences between normal-hearing children and children with cochlear implants. *Ear and Hearing, 17,* 432–437.

Pool, K., Finitzo, T., Hong, C., Rogers, J., & Pickett, R. (1989). Infarction of the superior temporal gyrus: A description of auditory evoked potential latency and amplitude topology. *Ear and Hearing, 10,* 144–152.

Praamstra, P., & Stegeman, D. (1992). On the possibility of independent activation of bilateral mismatch negativity (MMN) generators. *Electroencephalography and Clinical Neurophysiology, 82,* 67–80.

Pritchard, W. (1981). Psychophysiology of P300. *Psychological Bulletin, 89,* 506–540.

Psatta, D., & Matei, M. (1995). Investigation of P300 in various forms of epilepsy. *Romanian Journal of Neurology & Psychiatry, 33,* 183–202.

Rapin, I., Ruben, R., & Lyttle, M. (1970). Diagnosis of hearing loss in infants using auditory evoked responses. *Laryngoscope, 80,* 712–722.

Rapin, I., Schimmel, H., & Cohen, M. (1972). Reliability in detecting the auditory evoked response (AEP) for audiometry in sleep subjects. *Electroencephalography and Clinical Neurophysiology, 32,* 521–528.

Rapin, I., Schimmel, H., Tourk, L., Krasnegor, N., & Pollack, C. (1966). Evoked responses to clicks and tones of varying intensity in waking adults. *Electroencephalography and Clinical Neurophysiology, 21,* 335–344.

Rappaport, M., & Clifford, J. (1994). Comparison of passive P300 brain evoked potentials in normal and severely traumatically brain-injured subjects. *Journal of Head Trauma and Rehabilitation, 9,* 94–104.

Remijn, G., & Sugita, Y. (1996). Mismatch between anticipated and actually presented sound stimuli in human. *Neuroscience Letters, 202,* 169–172.

Richer, F., Alain, C., Achim, A., Bouvier, G., & Saint, H. (1989). Intracerebral amplitude distributions of the auditory evoked potential. *Electroencephalography and Clinical Neurophysiology, 74,* 202–208.

Richer, F., Johnson, R., & Beatty, J. (1983). Sources of late components of the brain magnetic response. *Society of Neuroscience Abstracts, 9,* 656.

Rintelmann, W., & Schwan, S. (1991). Pseudohypacusis. In W. Rintelmann (Ed.), *Hearing Assessment* (2nd ed., pp. 603–652). Boston: Allyn & Bacon.

Ritter, W., Deacon, D., Gomes, H., Javitt, D., & Vaughan, H. Jr. (1995). The mismatch negativity of event-related potentials as a probe of transient auditory memory: A review. *Ear and Hearing, 16,* 52–67.

Rodriguez, R., Picton, T., Linden, R., Hamel, G., & Laframboise, G. (1986). Human auditory steady state responses: Effects of intensity and frequency. *Ear and Hearing, 7,* 300–313.

Roffwarg, H., Muzio, N., & Dement, W. (1966). Ontogenetic development of the human sleep-dream cycle. *Science, 152,* 604–619.

Roth, W., Horvath, T., Pfefferbaum, A., & Kopell, B. (1980). Event-related potentials. *Electroencephalography and Clinical Neurophysiology, 48,* 127–139.

Sallinen, M., Kaartinen, J., & Lyytinen, H. (1994). Is the appearance of mismatch negativity during stage 2 sleep related to the elicitation of K-complex? *Electroencephalography and Clinical Neurophysiology, 91,* 140–148.

Salo, S., Lang, A., & Salmivalli, A. (1995). Effect of contralateral white noise masking on the mismatch negativity. *Scandinavian Audiology, 24,* 165–173.

Sams, M., Hamalainen, M., Antervo, A., Kaukoranta, E., Reinikainen, K., & Hari, R. (1985). Cerebral neuromagnetic responses evoked by short auditory stimuli. *Electroencephalography and Clinical Neurophysiology, 61,* 254–266.

Sandridge, S., & Boothroyd, A. (1996). Using naturally produced speech to elicit the mismatch negativity. *Journal of the American Academy of Audiology, 7,* 105–112.

Sangal, R., & Sangal, J. (1996). Topography of auditory and visual P300 in normal children. *Clinical Electroencephalography, 27,* 46–51.

Satterfield, J., Schell, A., & Backs, R. (1987). Longitudinal study of AERPs in hyperactive and normal children: Relationship to antisocial behavior. *Electroencephalography and Clinical Neurophysiology, 67,* 531–536.

Satya-Murti, S., Wolpaw, J., Cacace, A., & Schaffer, C. (1983). Late auditory evoked potentials can occur without brain stem potentials. *Electroencephalography and Clinical Neurophysiology, 56,* 304–308.

Scherg, M. (1982). Distortion of the middle latency auditory response produced by analog filtering. *Scandinavian Audiology, 11,* 57–69.

Scherg, M., Vajar, J., & Picton, T. (1989). A source analysis of the late human auditory evoked potentials. *Journal of Cognitive Neuroscience, 1,* 336–355.

Scherg, M., & Volk, S. (1983). Frequency specificity of simultaneously recorded early and middle latency auditory evoked potentials. *Electroencephalography and Clinical Neurophysiology, 56,* 443–452.

Scherg, M., & Von Cramon, D. (1986). Evoked dipole source potentials of the human auditory cortex. *Electroencephalography and Clinical Neurophysiology, 65,* 344–360.

Schroeder, M., Handelsman, L., Torres, L., Dorfman, D., Rinaldi, P., Jacobson, J., Wiener, J., & Ritter, W. (1994). Early and late cognitive event-related potentials mark stages of HIV-1 infection in the drug-user risk group. *Biological Psychiatry, 35,* 54–69.

Schroger, E. (1994). Automatic detection of frequency change is invariant over a large intensity range. *Neuroreport, 5,* 825–828.

Schroger, E. (1995). Processing of psychology deviants with changes in one versus two stimulus dimensions. *Psychophysiology, 32,* 55–65.

Schroger, E., & Winkler, I. (1995). Presentation rate and magnitude of stimulus deviance effects on human pre-attentive change detection. *Neuroscience Letters, 193,* 169–172.

Segalowitz, S., & Barnes, K. (1993). The reliability of ERP components in the auditory oddball paradigm. *Psychophysiology, 30,* 451–459.

Selinger, M., & Prescott, T. (1989). Auditory event-related potentials probes and behavioral measures of aphasia. *Brain and Language, 36,* 377–390.

Shehata-Dieler, W., Shimizu, H., Soliman, S., & Tusa, R. (1991). Middle latency auditory evoked potentials in temporal lobe disorders. *Ear and Hearing, 12,* 377–388.

Shucard, D., Shucard, J., & Thomas, D. (1977). Auditory evoked potentials as probes of hemispheric differences in cognitive processing. *Science, 197,* 1295–1298.

Shucard, J., Shucard, D., & Cummins, K. (1981). Auditory evoked potentials and sex-related differences in brain development. *Brain and Language, 13,* 91–102.

Simson, R., Vaughan, H. Jr., & Ritter, W. (1977a). The scalp topography of potentials in auditory and visual go/no go tasks. *Electroencephalography and Clinical Neurophysiology, 43,* 864–875.

Simson, R., Vaughan, H. Jr., & Ritter, W. (1977b). The scalp topography of potentials in auditory and visual discrimination tasks. *Electroencephalography and Clinical Neurophysiology, 42,* 528–535.

Sininger, Y., Norton, S., Starr, A., & Ponton, C. (1993). Auditory neural synchrony disorders in children. *Asha, 35,* 231.

Skinner, P., & Antinoro, F. (1969). Auditory evoked responses in normal hearing adults and children before and during sedation. *Journal of Speech and Hearing Research, 12,* 394–401.

Skinner, P,. & Shimota, J. (1975). A comparison of the effects of sedatives on the auditory evoked cortical response. *Journal of the American Auditory Society, 1,* 71–78.

Sommer, W., & Scheinberger, S. (1992). Operant conditioning of P300. *Biological Psychology, 33,* 37–49.

Spink, U., Johannsen, H., & Pirsig, W. (1979). Acoustically evoked potential: Dependence upon age. *Scandinavian Audiology, 8,* 11–14.

Squires, K., Chipperdale, T., Wrege, K., Goodin, D., & Starr, A. (1980). Electrophysiological assessment of mental function in aging and dementia. In L. Poon (Ed), *Aging in the 1980s: Selected Contemporary Issues in the Psychology of Aging* (pp. 125–134). Washington, DC: American Psychological Press.

Squires, N., Galbraith, G., & Aine, C. (1979). Event-related potential assessment of sensory and cognitive deficits in the mentally retarded. In D. Lehmann & E. Callaway (Eds.), *Human Evoked Potentials: Applications and Problems* (pp. 397–413). New York: Plenum Press.

Squires, N., Halgren, E., Wilson, C., & Crandall, P. (1983). Human endogenous limbic potentials: Cross-modality and depth/surface comparisons in epileptic subjects. In A. Gaillard & W. Rittaer (Eds.), *Tutorials in ERP Research: Endogenous Components* (pp. 217–232). Amsterdam: North-Holland.

Squires, K., & Hecox, K. (1983). Electrophysiological evaluation of higher level auditory processing. *Seminars in Hearing, 4,* 415–433.

Stapells, D. (1984). Studies in evoked potential audiometry. Doctoral dissertation, University of Ottawa, Ottawa, CA.

Stapells, D., & Kurtzberg, D. (1991). Evoked potential assessment of auditory system integrity in infants. *Clinics in Perinatology, 18,* 497–518.

Stapells, D., Galambos, R., Costello, J., et al. (1988). Inconsistency of auditory middle latency and steady-state response in infants. *Electroencephalography and Clinical Neurophysiology, 71,* 289.

Starr, A., McPherson, D., Patterson, J., Don, M., Luxford, W., Shannon, R., Sininger, Y., Tonakawa, L., & Waring, M. (1991). Absence of both auditory evoked potentials and auditory percepts dependent on timing cues. *Brain, 114,* 1157–1180.

Steinschneider, M., Kurtzberg, D., & Vaughan, H. Jr. (1992). Event-related potentials in developmental neuropsychology. In I. Rapin & S. Segalowitz (Eds.), *Handbook of Neuropsychology, Vol. 6, Child Neuropsychology* (pp. 239–299). Amsterdam: Elsevier.

Stewart, M., Jerger, J., & Lew, H. (1993). Effect of handedness on the middle latency auditory evoked potential. *American Journal of Otology, 14,* 595–600.

Sugg, M., & Polich, J. (1995). P300 from auditory stimuli: Intensity and frequency effects. *Biological Psychology, 41,* 255–269.

Sutton, S., Braren, M., Zubin, J., & John, E. (1965). Evoked potential correlates of stimulus uncertainty. *Science, 150,* 1187–1188.

Suzuki, T., Hirabayashi, M., & Kobayashi, K. (1984). Effects of analog and digital filtering on auditory middle latency responses in adults and young children. *Annals of Otology, Rhinology and Laryngology, 93,* 267–270.

Suzuki, T., Kobayashi, K., Aoki, K., & Umegaki, Y. (1992). Effect of sleep on binaural interaction in auditory brainstem response and middle latency response. *Audiology, 31,* 25–30.

Suzuki, T., & Taguchi, K. (1965). Cerebral evoked response to auditory stimuli in waking man. *Annals of Otology, Rhinology and Laryngology, 74,* 128–139.

Syndulko, K., Hansch, M., Cohen, S., Pearce, J. Goldberg, Z., Montan, B., Tourtellotte, W., & Potvin, A. (1982). Long-latency event-related potentials in normal aging and dementia. In J. Courjon & F. Mauguiere (Eds.), *Clinical Applications of Evoked Potentials in Neurology* (pp. 279–285). New York: Raven Press.

Szyfter, W., Dauman, R., & Charlet de Sauvage, R. (1984). 40-Hz middle latency responses to low-frequency tone pips in normally hearing adults. *Journal of Otolaryngology, 13,* 275–280.

Taguchi, K., Picton, T., Orpin, J., & Goodman, J. (1969). Evoked response audiometry in newborn infants. *Acta Otolaryngologica (Stockholm), Supplement 252,* 5–17.

Tarkka, I., Stokic, D., Basile, L., & Papanicolaou, A. (1995). Electric source localization of the auditory P300 agrees with magnetic source localization. *Electroencephalography and Clinical Neurophysiology, 96,* 538–545.

Thornton, A., Mendel, M., & Anderson, C. (1977). Effect of stimulus frequency and intensity on the middle components of the averaged auditory electroencephalic response. *Journal of Speech and Hearing Research, 20,* 81–94.

Tonnquist-Uhlen, I., Borg, E., & Spens, K. (1995). Topography of auditory evoked long-latency potentials in normal children with particular reference to the N1 component. *Electroencephalography and Clinical Neurophysiology, 95,* 34–41.

Tonnquist-Uhlen, U. (1996). Topography of auditory-evoked cortical potentials in children with severe language impairment. *Scandinavian Audiology, Supplement, 44.*

Ungan, P., Sahinoglu, B., & Utkucal, R. (1989). Human laterality reversal auditory evoked potentials: Stimulation by reversing the interaural delay of dichotically presented continuous click trains. *Electroencephalography and Clinical Neurophysiology, 73,* 306–321.

Vaughan, H. Jr., & Kurtzberg, D. (in press). Electrophysiologic indices of human brain maturation and cognitive development. In M. Gunnar & C. Nelson (Eds.), *Minnesota Symposia on Child Psychology, V. 24.*

Vaughan, H., & Ritter, W. (1970). The sources of auditory evoked responses recorded from the human scalp. *Electroencephalography and Clinical Neurophysiology, 28,* 360–367.

Velasco, M., & Velasco, F. (1986). Subcortical correlates of the somatic, auditory and visual vertex activities. Referential EEG responses. *Electroencephalography and Clinical Neurophysiology, 63,* 62–67.

Velasco, M., Velasco, F., & Olvera, A. (1985). Subcortical correlates of the somatic, auditory and visual vertex activities in man. Bipolar EEG responses and electrical stimulation. *Electroencephalography and Clinical Neurophysiology, 61,* 519–529.

Vesco, K., Bone, R., Ryan, J., & Polich, J. (1993). P300 in young and elderly subjects: Auditory frequency and intensity effects. *Electroencephalography and Clinical Neurophysiology, 88,* 302–308.

Vivion, M., Hirsch, J., Frye-Osier, J., & Goldstein, R. (1980). Effects of stimulus rise fall time and equivalent duration on middle components of AER. *Scandinavian Audiology, 9,* 223–232.

Weitzman, E., & Graziani, L. (1968). Maturation and topography of the auditory evoked response of the prematurely born infant. *Developmental Psychobiology, 1,* 79–89.

Weitzman, E., & Kremen, H. (1965). Auditory evoked responses during different stages of sleep in man. *Electroencephalography and Clinical Neurophysiology, 18,* 65–70.

Wilkinson, R., & Morlock, H. (1966). Auditory evoked response and reaction time. *Electroencephalography and Clinical Neurophysiology, 23,* 50–56.

Williams, H., Tepas, D., & Morlock, H. (1962). Evoked responses to clicks and electroencephalography stages of sleep in human. *Science, 138,* 685–686.

Winter, O., Kok, A., Kenemans, J., & Elton, M. (1995). Auditory event-related potentials to deviant stimuli during drowsiness and stage 2 sleep. *Electroencephalography and Clinical Neurophysiology, 96,* 398–412.

Woldorff, M., Hansen, J., & Hillyard, S. (1987). Evidence for effects of selective attention in the mid-latency range of the human auditory event-related potential. In R. Johnson, J. Rohrbaugh, & R. Parasuraman (Eds.), *Current Trends in Event-Related Potential Research* (pp. 146–154). Amsterdam: Elsevier.

Wolf, K., & Goldstein, R. (1978). Middle component AERs to tonal stimuli from normal neonates. *Archives of Otolaryngology, 104,* 508–513.

Wolf, K., & Goldstein, R. (1980). Middle component AERs from neonates to low-level tonal stimuli. *Journal of Speech and Hearing Research, 23,* 185–201.

Wolpaw, J., & Penry, J. (1975). A temporal component of the auditory evoked response. *Electroencephalography and Clinical Neurophysiology, 39,* 609–620.

Wood, C. Allison, T., Goff, W., Williamson, P., & Spencer, D. (1980). On the neural origin of P300 in man. In H. Kornhuber & L. Deecke (Eds.), *Motivation, Motor and Sensory Processes of the Brain: Progress in Brain Research, Vol. 54* (pp. 51–56). Amsterdam: Elsevier.

Wood, C., & Wolpaw, J. (1982). Scalp distribution of human auditory evoked potentials. II. Evidence for overlapping sources and involvement of auditory cortex. *Electroencephalography and Clinical Neurophysiology, 54,* 25–38.

Woods, D. (1992). Auditory selective attention in middle-aged and elderly subjects: An event-related brain potential study. *Electroencephalography and Clinical Neurophysiology, 84,* 456–468.

Woods, D., Alho, K., & Algazi, A. (1992). Intermodal selective attention. I. Effects on event-related potentials to lateralized auditory and visual stimuli. *Electroencephalography and Clinical Neurophysiology, 82,* 341–355.

Woods, D., & Clayworth, C. (1985). Click spatial position influences middle latency auditory evoked potentials (MAEPs) in humans. *Electroencephalography and Clinical Neurophysiology, 60,* 122–129.

Woods, D., & Clayworth, C. (1986). Age-related changes in human middle latency auditory evoked potentials. *Electroencephalography and Clinical Neurophysiology, 65,* 297–303.

Woods, D., Clayworth, C., & Knight, R. (1985). Middle latency auditory evoked potentials following cortical and subcortical lesions. *Electroencephalography and Clinical Neurophysiology, 61,* 55.

Woods, D., Clayworth, C., Knight, R., Simpson, G., & Naeser, A. (1987). Generators of middle and long latency auditory evoked potentials: Implications from studies of patients with bitemporal lesions. *Electroencephalography and Clinical Neurophysiology, 68,* 132–148.

Worthington, D., & Peters, J. (1980). Quantifiable hearing and no ABR: Paradox or error? *Ear and Hearing, 5,* 281–285.

Yakovlev, P., & Lecours, A. (1967). The myelogenetic cycles of the regional maturation of the brain. In A. Minkowski (Ed.), *Regional Development of the Brain in Early Life* (pp. 3–70). Philadelphia: F. A. Davis.

Yasukouchi, H., Wada, S., Urasaki, E., & Yokota, A. (1995). Effects of night work on the cognitive function in young and elderly subjects with specific reference to the auditory P300. *Sangyo Ika Daigaku Zasshi, 17,* 229–246.

Yingling, C., & Hosobuchi, Y. (1984). A subcortical correlate of P300 in man. *Electroencephalography and Clinical Neurophysiology, 59,* 72–76.

Yingling, C., & Skinner, J. (1977). Gating of thalamic input to cerebral cortex by nucleus reticularis thalami. In J. Desmedt (Ed.), Attention, voluntary contraction and event-related cerebral potentials. *Progressive Clinical Neurophysiology, Vol. 1* (pp. 70–96). Basel: Karger.

Zerlin, S., & Naunton, R. (1974). Early and late average electroencephalic responses to low sensation levels. *Audiology, 13,* 366–378.

CHAPTER 9

INTRAOPERATIVE MONITORING (IOM)

GARY P. JACOBSON

OVERVIEW

Over the past twenty years there has been growing interest among audiologists in the development of skills that would enable them to evaluate central and peripheral nervous system function in the critical care unit and operating room. Due to the efforts of a number of forward-thinking audiologists, intraoperative monitoring (IOM) has been included in the audiology scope of practice (ASHA, 1996). Additionally, there now exists a national organization (the American Society of Neurophysiological Monitoring, ASNM) designed to foster and disseminate information about IOM. Finally, with the advent of improved techniques for neuroimaging and with the emerging popularity of otoacoustic emissions as a technique for screening auditory function, auditory evoked potentials are being employed less frequently in neurodiagnostics and infant hearing screening applications. In the future, it is likely that the demand for the auditory brainstem response (ABR) in the clinic will decrease, and the demand for neurophysiological testing in the operating room will increase.

The history of audiology and IOM is interesting. The initial clinical applications for evoked potentials were for the identification of both demyelinating disorders (e.g., multiple sclerosis, MS) and posterior fossa tumors (e.g., meningiomas, vestibular schwannomas). Thus, it was not unusual for the audiologist to be the first hospital professional to have an evoked potential machine. When the first papers were published that described methods for spinal cord monitoring and the efficacy of same, it was the audiologist (who had possession of the evoked potential system) who was called upon by the orthopedic surgeon, or neurosurgeon, to bring evoked potential testing into the operating room. It was a natural progression for audiologists to be the first health professionals to monitor auditory function during surgical procedures that placed the cochlea and VIIIn at risk.

Objectives of Monitoring

The purpose of IOM is to preserve the functional integrity of nervous system structures that are at risk due to the surgical procedure. The aim of auditory system monitoring is to preserve the functional integrity of the cochlea, VIIIn,

and central auditory pathways and to not only preserve auditory sensitivity (i.e., pure tone sensitivity) but to preserve useful (functional) hearing. For facial nerve monitoring the aim is to preserve the facial nerve anatomically and functionally. There is no reason to attempt neurophysiological monitoring if it is impossible to alter the surgical procedure once changes in function are observed (Grundy, Jannetta, Procopio, Lina, Boston, & Doyle, 1982).

At first glance, IOM using evoked potential techniques appears to be a simple issue of carrying out the same procedures in a different environment. There are, however, a number of challenges to IOM that one does not find in the outpatient clinic setting. Negative intraoperative events occur quickly, and signal averaging (when employed) requires time. Thus, it is possible for changes in the function of the auditory system to occur during the signal averaging process that go undetected until the next signal average. Also, the signal-to-noise ratio in the operating room is adverse to the goal of recording and measuring submicrovolt or microvolt level far-field signals. Optimal use of bandpass filtering and signal averaging are employed to extract these signals from the noise background. However, signal averaging may be too slow to permit the detection of changes in evoked potentials until it is too late for a surgeon to intervene. These time constraints, coupled with the low amplitudes of far-field recorded signals, have driven those involved in monitoring to place electrodes as close as possible to generators of the evoked responses. Near-field recorded evoked responses are often one to two orders of magnitude larger than far-field responses. Finally, the modality of interest may be unavailable due to the disease process. An example would be the desire to use the ABR to monitor the removal of a vestibular schwannoma (VS, also referred to as acoustic neuroma). It may well be the absence of the ABR past Wave I that led to the identification of the tumor. Thus, use of the ABR to monitor auditory function might provide little benefit.

There are a number of surgical procedures where auditory system monitoring has proven useful. A partial listing of these surgical procedures includes: endolymphatic sac decompression (shunt placement); vestibular neurectomy;

removal of VS; removal of other masses in the cerebello-pontine angle, including meningiomas, neurofibromas, and epidermoid tumors; neurovascular decompression of cranial nerves V, VII, and VIII; correction of brainstem vascular disorders (e.g., aneurysms and arteriovenous malformations); and cochlear implantation. Monitoring of the facial nerve often is conducted concurrently for most of the surgical procedures described above.

This chapter will focus on techniques used to monitor the function of both the auditory system and facial nerve (VIIn). These are the two most common types of monitoring conducted by audiologists. It should be understood, however, that the field of neurophysiological monitoring is quite broad. At this time it is possible to monitor the function of most sensory and motor cranial and peripheral nerves. The functional status of the sensory and motor tracts in the spinal cord can be monitored using somatosensory and motor tract evoked potential techniques. Additionally, it is possible to evaluate brain perfusion with evoked potentials (i.e., somatosensory evoked responses), electroencephalography (EEG), and transcranial doppler (TCD) techniques. It is possible to perform extraoperative identification of eloquent cortex using both evoked potential techniques and direct brain stimulation. Evoked potential and EMG techniques can be used to map motor pathways in the brainstem. Finally, neurophysiological monitoring techniques are being used to help guide surgeons in the stereotaxic ablation of structures in the basal ganglia in Parkinson's disease. Readers who are interested in obtaining a more complete understanding of the breadth of monitoring techniques are directed to two reviews published in the *Journal of Clinical Neurophysiology* (Fisher, Raudzens, & Nunemacher, 1995; Jacobson & Tew, 1987) and a number of textbooks that have been published on the topic of IOM (Møller, 1989; Nuwer, 1986). It is a small group of audiologists with highly advanced skills and training who are capable of performing full-scale IOM services.

Team Approach to Monitoring

A number of people who work in the operating room directly or indirectly influence the success of our monitoring efforts. The monitorist must be highly technically skilled. Further, it is critical that those engaged in neurotologic monitoring have a good working knowledge of the gross anatomy of the head and neck, auditory system, and general neuroanatomy and neurophysiology. It is not enough to inform the surgical team that an event has occurred that has changed the performance characteristics of a given monitoring modality. The monitorist must have the expertise to estimate (given what has transpired during the surgical procedure) what has triggered the negative event. Finally, the monitorist has the responsibility of understanding the

surgical procedure that is being performed. The anesthesiologist and certified registered nurse anesthetist (CRNA) control the consciousness and muscle relaxation of the patient. They have the capability of keeping the patient in a constant neurophysiological state that is conducive to the recording of the specific evoked response of interest. The operating room (OR) nurse coordinator has the ability to make certain that expendable supplies (such as specialized electrodes) are available for each case. The surgeon must be aware of monitoring constraints, that is, what information monitoring is, and alternately is not, capable of providing. Ultimately, it is the surgeon (not the monitoring team) who interprets the data provided by the monitoring team. That is, it is the surgeon who decides whether the change in function reported by the monitorist warrants some form of surgical intervention.

Issues in Monitoring

General. The signal-to-noise ratio in the operating room is quite different than that found in the clinic. In the clinic setting the greatest source of electrical interference comes from the patient and consists of electromyographic (EMG) interference. Additionally, in the clinical setting it is assumed that the patient has sustained an injury to the system being evaluated (due to a disease process). We do not expect the performance characteristics of the patient's auditory system to change as the evoked potential is being acquired. In the OR the greatest source of electrical interference comes from the environment. In the operating room there are a number of electrical devices including cautery systems, microscopes, blood warmers, heating pads, electronic operating tables, and anesthesia machines that require electricity to function and accordingly may emit electrical fields that can link magnetically with electrode wires that have been placed on the patient. Also, whereas the patient's neurophysiological state in the clinic is assumed to be relatively static, in the operating room the patient's neurophysiological state may be quite dynamic (due to the effects of surgery and anesthesia). For these reasons it has become critical to develop methods of data acquisition that reduce greatly the time required to acquire and interpret data. These methods have included online digital filtering, pseudorecursive averaging, and near-field recording techniques.

Technical. The single critical phase in neurophysiological monitoring occurs with the placement of recording electrodes, ground electrodes, and stimulators on or in the patient. If stimulators and recording electrodes (and grounds) are applied in a meticulous manner, any problems that arise during IOM will likely be caused by the efforts of the surgical team and/or anesthesia. Additionally, the location of recording equipment and staff in the operating room (OR) is important. The evoked potential instrumentation should be placed as close to the patient as possible. Also, electrode cabling should be kept as far away from sources that emit electrical fields. Finally, as mentioned previously, vigilance must be directed toward electrical activity emitted by all devices in the OR. These competing electrical signals serve to degrade the signal-to-noise ratio and prolong the process of data acquisition.

AUDITORY SYSTEM MONITORING

Modalities for Auditory System Monitoring

A number of modalities are available for use in intraoperative monitoring of the auditory system. These modalities include tympanic or transtympanic electrocochleography (ECochG), ABR, and direct recorded VIIIn compound action potentials (CAPs). It is noteworthy that recently (Cane, O'Donoghue, & Lutman, 1992; Telischi, Widick, Lonsbury-Martin, & McCoy, 1995) there have been reports suggesting that otoacoustic emissions (OAEs) might be useful for the instantaneous monitoring of cochlear function. Each of these modalities has merits and drawbacks for monitoring auditory function. The "art" of neurophysiological monitoring is knowing how to choose the best modalities to monitor auditory function.

OAE. The OAE (discussed in detail in Chapter 6) is generated by outer hair cells and therefore represents an indicator of outer hair cell integrity. Acquisition of OAEs can be accomplished quickly, and thus may provide an online metric of peripheral auditory function. Attempts to record both transient click-evoked OAEs (TOAEs; Cane et al., 1992) and distortion product OAEs (DPOAEs; Telischi et al., 1995) have been reported. As might be expected, acoustical noise in the OR was a potent contaminant complicating greatly the ability to record OAEs at certain stages of

surgery (e.g., during bone drilling). Both sets of investigators reported changes in OAEs associated with intraoperative events. It should be noted that there are a small number of patients (Cacace, Parnes, Lovely, & Kalathia, 1994) with tumors in the cerebellopontine angle who do not have measurable hearing but do have preserved OAEs (it is not clear how many of these patients have preserved ECochGs). In these instances it has been hypothesized that compression of the tumor on the VIIIn has impaired neural transmission to the brainstem, but the compression has not been great enough to have forced the cochlea into a permanent ischemic state. For these patients, monitoring the OAE (either TEOAE or DPOAE) has the advantage of providing fast continuous information about vascular function of the cochlea. However, it must be understood that the OAE is a *preneural* response. That is, measurement of OAEs is useful only if it is suspected that a given surgery will result in compromised vascular perfusion of the cochlea. Most neurotologic or neurosurgical procedures occur proximal to the brainstem where the VIIIn is placed at risk for injury. The OAE suffers from the shortcoming of being a low amplitude acoustical event (as opposed to an electrical potential). Therefore, ambient noise in the operating room which can be excessive (Hickey & Fitzgerald O'Connor, 1991; Jacobson & Balzer, 1992) can serve to "mask" this evoked acoustical response (see Table 9.1). Adequately sealing the external auditory canal with acoustical damping material appears to make it possible to limit the amount of ambient interference "leaking" into the ear canal. It is not clear what added advantage the OAE provides over electrocochleographic (ECochG) recordings for providing fast information specific to cochlear function. Finally, at the time of this writing there is no commercially available machine that will permit the simultaneous recording of OAEs and ABR (both ECochG and ABR may be recorded with all multichannel evoked potential systems).

TABLE 9.1 Sound levels (specified in dBA) generated by several surgical tools and measured at the level of the ear of the surgeon and monitoring person during surgery.

	LOCATION OF SOUND LEVEL METER		
SURGICAL TOOL	*Monitorist's Ear*	*Surgeon's Ear*	*Tool*
Pneumatic drill	78 dBA	83 dBA	85 dBA
CUSA*	73 dBA	73 dBA	78 dBA
CO2 laser	74 dBA	71 dBA	79 dBA
PD** + CUSA	79 dBA	85 dBA	—
CUSA + laser	80 dBA	86 dBA	—

(From Jacobson & Balzer, 1992).

 *CUSA = Cavitron Ultrasonic Surgical Aspirator

**PD = Pneumatic drill

ECochG. The electrocochleogram (ECochG) elicited by tone bursts or clicks is a near-field indicator of the integrity of the basal cochlea (the ECochG is discussed in detail in Chapter 7). The ECochG consists of both pre-neural responses (i.e., the cochlear microphonic [CM] and summating potentials [SP]) and a neural response (i.e., N1). The N1 is believed to represent the depolarization of the distal VIIIn afferents, possibly within the osseous spiral lamina. The advantage of recording this near-field response is that it is quite large in magnitude and may exceed 10 to 20 μV when recorded from the promontory of the cochlea. Thus, little signal averaging is required (the signal-to-noise ratio is optimal; large signal, low noise). The fact that the ECochG represents a combination of pre-neural and primary neural activity means that fast stimulation rates may be employed, and accordingly, the surgeon may be updated quickly. The disadvantage of monitoring only the ECochG is that most neurotologic surgeries occur more proximal to the central auditory nervous system. Accordingly, preservation of the CM and N1 in the absence of the ABR is not compatible with preserved auditory function. In fact, it is possible for the cochlear microphonic to be preserved for up to 72 hours after the VIIIn has been sectioned where the cochlear blood supply has been preserved (Ruben, Hudson, & Chiong, 1963). Despite the availability of this information, many respected groups (e.g., Nedzelski, Chiong, Cashman, Stanton, & Rowed, 1994; Symon, Sabin, Bentivoglio, Cheesman, Prasher, & Barratt, 1988) have recommended the use of ECochG in isolation for monitoring auditory system function during the resection of acoustic neuromas. It is not surprising that these same investigators have reported instances where hearing was lost but cochlear potentials were preserved at the end of surgery.

ABR. The auditory brainstem response (ABR) is a volume-conducted, far-field recorded, auditory evoked response (see detailed discussion of the ABR in Chapter 7). The ABR cannot be generated if the cochlea is profoundly damaged. It is a neural response consisting of potentials whose sources may be found in the VIIIn and pontine brainstem. Wave I occurs at roughly the same latency as the N1 of the ECochG and probably emanates as a depolarization of distal VIIIn afferents. Wave II appears to be generated from two sources, one representing the change in tissue impedance as the VIIIn exits the porus acousticus, and the second coming from the cochlear nucleus. The remaining ABR components are believed to represent an admixture of electrical fields generated by auditory pathway structures in the pons. Being a far-field response, the ABR is small (often less than 0.5 μV in amplitude) and may require much signal averaging to resolve an interpretable waveform. This means that time between updates can be quite long.

Direct VIIIn Recordings. Direct, near-field compound action potentials may be recorded once the skull has been opened and the VIIIn exposed. These responses are large (like promontory ECochG) and require little, if any, signal averaging to be observed. A drawback is that they can be recorded only after the skull has been opened. It should be noted that preservation of the direct recorded N1 with an absent ABR beyond Wave II usually is not compatible with preserved functional hearing sensitivity. Thus, it is possible to record successfully direct VIIIn action potentials at a location distal to the root entry zone (REZ) of the VIIIn, for the patient to have sustained an injury at the REZ intra-operatively, and for the patient to be profoundly deaf upon awakening.

As the reader might surmise, in most instances it is in the monitorist's (and patient's) best interest to employ two or more of the above techniques when monitoring auditory system function (e.g., ECochG + ABR, or, ECochG + ABR + direct VIIIn response).

Mechanisms of Intraoperative Damage

In most cases it is the cochlea, VIIIn, and/or REZ of the VIIIn that is imperiled during neurotologic surgery. In few instances is the auditory brainstem at risk of direct injury during neurosurgery. There are a number of types of injury that may affect the auditory system intraoperatively. The VIIIn may be stretched beyond its tolerance (traction injury). The VIIIn may be compressed by surgical instrumentation (compression injury). Various intraoperative events (compression and/or traction) may result in a decrease in blood perfusion to the cochlea (ischemic injury). That is, traction applied to the nerve could result in a reduction in the internal diameter of the artery supplying blood to both nerve and cochlea. Compression of the nerve also could result in decreases in perfusion of the nerve and cochlea. In this regard, Sekiya and Møller (1987a) have reported that the external diameter of the internal auditory artery (IAA) that branches from the anterior inferior cerebellar artery (AICA) averages 0.16 mm (range 0.1–0.25 mm). Given this information, one can envision how a small amount of stretch applied to the IAA could place the cochlea in an ischemic state. Finally, the VIIIn may be unintentionally interrupted (e.g., nerve transection or mechanical trauma injury).

We have good understanding now of how damage occurs intraoperatively to auditory system structures due to the marriage of applied and basic science. By way of example, Friedman and colleagues (Friedman, Kaplan, Gravenstein, & Rhoton, 1985) studied systematically the auditory brainstem response (ABR) in neurovascular decompression surgeries for the correction of hemifacial spasm (HFS). The Wave V absolute latency and amplitude was recorded during surgery as was the Wave I–V interwave interval.

These values were tabulated for each stage of the surgery (e.g., incision, bone drilling, dura opening, retraction of cerebellum, placement of teflon felt, and closing). The investigators reported that, although there was a gradual increase in Wave V latency and in the Wave I–V interwave interval throughout the surgical case, the greatest changes occurred during and following retraction of the cerebellum. During cerebellar retraction there were large increases in the latency of Wave V and there was a lengthening of the Wave I–V interwave interval. A loss of all ABR components happened on occasion. This finding usually was associated with irreparable damage to the auditory system (deafness).

This was a key paper in the development of monitoring practices because it represented a first attempt to evaluate in a systematic manner the effects of a surgical procedure on neural function. Specifically, the investigators divided the neurovascular decompression (NVD) procedure into steps and evaluated the effects of perioperative manipulations on auditory neurophysiology. The results validated the empirical observation that changes in ABR latency and amplitude could be predicted to occur at a particular point within a surgical procedure (i.e., retraction of the cerebellum in this case). The value of this information was that it served as a first stage in the study of a surgical procedure. The second stage was to develop an animal model of the procedure, to impose the same surgical manipulations as conducted intraoperatively and observe the effects of these manipulations neurophysiologically and histologically.

Such a study was conducted by Sekiya and Møller (1987b). The product of their research has helped us understand much about the microstructure of intraoperative changes in auditory evoked responses. The investigators recorded VIIIn CAPs and ABR from 10 adult mongrel dogs during cerebellopontine angle manipulations. These manipulations included medial retraction of the cerebellar hemisphere, and caudal-rostral retraction of the VIIIn. Thirty minutes following the manipulations the animals were perfused with fixative and their VIIIn's and brainstems prepared for histology. The results indicated that:

1. Cerebellar retraction resulted in stretching of the VIIIn that could cause irreparable damage to the myelin sheath, petechial hemorrhages to the nerve, and thromboses to the vascular supply to the nerve (vasa nervorum).
2. Manipulations resulting in latency and amplitude changes in both N1 and N2, or N2 only, might normalize when the manipulations were discontinued. However, histology showed significant morphological changes in the VIIIn (e.g., petechial hemorrhages).
3. Abrupt decrease in the amplitude of N2 (generator source believed to be cochlear nucleus in small animals) indicated avulsion of VIIIn at the Obersteiner-Redlich zone (i.e., the point at which peripheral and central myelin join in the VIIIn).

4. Lateral-to-medial retraction of the cerebellum was more traumatic to the VIIIn than caudal-to-rostral retraction.
5. Epiarachnoid retraction of VIIIn resulted in less dramatic changes in the CAP than subarachnoid retraction.

More recently, Levine and colleagues (Levine, Bu-Saba, & Brown, 1993) have conducted laser-doppler flow recordings in guinea pigs undergoing cerebellopontine angle manipulations similar to those a surgeon might impose on a human patient. The authors found that when the VIIIn complex was compressed, the laser-doppler measurements changed abruptly. Cochlear potentials also decreased in amplitude with a delay of 10 to 50 seconds (relative to the onset of change in laser-doppler measures). When compression was released, the laser-doppler measures returned and these were followed by a return of the cochlear potentials.

The value of these investigations to our understanding of perioperative changes in the CAP and ABR is obvious. The authors explained clearly the source of the evoked potential changes that were reported by Friedman and colleagues (1985). Additionally, Sekiya and Møller (1987a, 1987b) made it possible for those engaged in the monitoring of these (and other related) procedures to offer explanations for evoked potential abnormalities that are observed perioperatively. Specifically, it is most likely that lateral-medial retraction of the cerebellar hemisphere results in the delay in Wave V latency. When these changes are rapid and when the CAP and ABR are lost, the cause may be avulsion of the VIIIn at the REZ, or sudden ischemic events affecting the cochlea and/or VIIIn. When latency increases and amplitude reductions are observed during cerebellar retraction, it is incumbent upon the monitorist to inform the surgical team immediately. The corrective action would appear to be a lessening of retraction of the cerebellum and the VIIIn and a suspension the surgical procedure until it can be assessed whether overretraction was the source of the evoked potential aberrations (i.e., wait for normalization of the evoked response). Indeed, when changes occur and time is permitted for recovery, the evoked potentials usually normalize. Further, the investigators underscored the statement that preservation of Wave I in the absence of direct VIIIn recorded N2 or Waves II–V of the ABR does not portend preserved auditory function.

Technical Issues

Transducers. Transducers for auditory system monitoring may be either acoustical or mechanical (i.e., bone-conduction vibratory transducers). Historically, the first auditory transducers were hearing aid button receivers connected to stock soft earmolds. These transducers were secured in the pinna and ear canal with tape (i.e., the entire stimulus system was taped into place). In more recent times practitioners have used either "ear buds" or mini-earphones that have been taped into the ear canal. However, it is likely that the most common auditory transducers found in the OR are the ubiquitous Etymotic ER3A earphones. The soft earplug delivery system may be inserted deeply into the ear canal and retained by sealing the earplug in the ear canal with tape or bone wax.

Electrodes. Although conventional nondisposable EEG surface electrodes were used for many years to record auditory potentials in the operating room, their drawbacks outweighed their benefits. Time constraints usually dictated that these electrodes be applied prior to entry of the patient into the operating room. Also, they had to be applied to the scalp with collodion (an adhesive liquid with an ether base) to ensure that they would be retained over time. Even under the best of circumstances it was not unusual for these electrodes to be poorly retained on skin or scalp or for interelectrode impedances to be unbalanced. These shortcomings have driven most monitorists to the use 9–10mm platinum or stainless steel, presterilized, prepackaged needle electrodes. The application of these electrodes is straightforward. The skin is cleansed with rubbing alcohol at the point of electrode insertion. The electrodes are inserted subdermally on an angle and taped into place. We have found that overtaping the electrodes with small (2″ × 3″), moisture vapor permeable, hypoallergenic, transparent dressings (Bioclusive, Johnson and Johnson, Medical, Inc. Arlington, TX) has improved the retention of these electrodes in the skin. Once the electrode has been applied, a half-loop of electrode wire at the electrode hub is taped over the electrode as a means of strain-relief should forces attempt to pull the electrode out of the skin. For patients with excessively oily or hairy skin we have found that the application of Tincoben (Ferndale Laboratories, Inc., Ferndale, MI) to skin surrounding the puncture site improves significantly the adhesive properties of all tapes.

For ECochG recordings the same subdermal electrode used for scalp recordings may be inserted into skin on the floor of the external auditory canal (EAC) through the eardrum to rest on the promontory of the cochlea (Schwaber & Hall, 1990). To improve retention, a 27-gauge, 45 mm (instead of 9–10 mm) Teflon-coated monopolar needle electrode may be passed through the pretragal crease in a manner such that the needle exits the external auditory canal along the anterior wall. This electrode is advanced through the posterior inferior quadrant of the tympanic membrane midway between the umbo and fibrous annulus until it comes to rest on the promontory of the cochlea (Prass, Kinney, & Luders, 1987a).

There are a number of special purpose electrodes that may be used to record cochlear and auditory nerve potentials. The TIPtrode consists of an ER3A eartip that has been shrink-wrapped with conducting gold foil. A clip connects to the gold foil and an electrode wire is attached to the clip.

The ear canal is cleansed with alcohol and abraded lightly. An oily, liquid conductant is applied to the foil and the electrode-earplug assembly is compressed between the fingers and placed deeply into the ear canal, held in place, and allowed to expand. Care must be taken to ensure that no conductant occludes the sound delivery port and this can be ascertained only during the recording of baseline AEPs. The electrode must be sealed into place securely (some clinicians use bone wax for this purpose) to ensure retention. The TIPtrode has been shown to improve the recording of Wave I amplitude by 30% on average.

We recommend that eartips of the auditory stimulators and TIPtrode electrodes be inserted following induction of anesthesia prior to positioning of the patient on the operating table (i.e., while the patient is supine) to improve the access to both ears. Needle electrodes are best inserted once the patient has been positioned on the operating table and the head has been stabilized (e.g., in a head holder).

There are a number of types of "wick" electrodes that may be used to record electrical responses from the tympanic membrane (ECochG) or VIIIn. In its simplest form the wick electrode consists of a teflon-coated silver wire with a piece of sterile cotton on the end. The teflon is stripped from the last 3–4 mm of the tip of the electrode wire. The bare silver wire is threaded through the cotton and then twist-tied around itself. An electrode pin jack must be soldered to the other end of the wire so that the electrode may be connected to the electrode junction box of the evoked potential machine. This electrode may be soaked with conductant and placed on the tympanic membrane under direct visualization (for ECochG recordings). Alternately, once the skull has been opened, this same electrode may be soaked in physiological saline and placed on the exposed VIIIn (for direct VIIIn recordings) or brainstem (for direct auditory brainstem recordings; Møller, Jho, & Jannetta, 1994a, 1994b). Most recently, AD-TECH Medical Instrument Company (Racine, WI) has introduced an electrode that may be placed atraumatically on the exposed VIIIn (Cueva Cranial Nerve Electrode). The manufacturer contends that the electrode has superior retention properties (i.e., conventional wick electrodes often become dislodged from the VIIIn throughout the course of surgery).

Recording Techniques

Stimulating and data acquisition parameters for intraoperative ECochG and ABR are identical to those used for clinical recordings with few exceptions. Characteristic stimulating and recording parameters for ECochG and ABR (or direct VIIIn responses) have been discussed elsewhere in this text (see Chapter 7 for stimulation and recording parameters for ECochG and ABR). Note that for ABR recordings it is possible to reduce the low pass filter to

TABLE 9.2 Examples of ABR warning criteria (upper limits of change) that have been reported.

Wave I Latency Increase
1.5 msec (Nuwer, 1986)
Absolute latency Wave I = 2.0 msec (Fisher, Ibanez, & Mauguiere, 1985)

Wave V Latency Increase
1.0 msec (Friedman et al., 1985; Radke & Erwin, 1988; Slavit, Harner, Harper, & Beatty, 1991)
2.0 msec (Kemink, La Rouere, Kileny, Telian, & Hoff, 1990)
2.0 msec (Kileny, Kemink, Tucci, & Hoff, 1992)
Absence (Friedman et al., 1985)

Rate of Wave V Latency Increase
.07 msec/min. (Grundy et al., 1982)
.10 msec/min. (Radke & Erwin, 1988)

Wave I–Wave V Latency Increase
.50 msec (Little, Lesser, Lueders, & Furlan, 1983)
1.0 msec (Friedman et al., 1985)
Absolute wave I–V greater than 4.5 msec (Fisher et al., 1985)

Wave V Amplitude Decrease
50% (Radke & Erwin, 1988; Schramm, Mosrusch, Fahlbusch, & Hochsletter, 1988; Slavit et al., 1991)
80% (Nuwer, 1986)
Absence (Friedman et al., 1985; Schramm et al., 1988)

TABLE 9.3 Examples of ABR intraoperative events that have been reported to be associated with unfavorable outcomes (monitoring auditory system function during vestibular schwannoma removal).

Decrease in Wave I–Wave V interwave interval (Jacobson & Yeh, 1985)
Loss of all components beyond Wave I or Waves I and II (Kileny et al., 1992; Levine, Ojemann, Montgomery, & McGaffigan, 1984; Stanton, Cashman, Harrison, Nedzelski, & Rowed, 1989)
50% or more loss of any ABR component amplitude (Schramm et al., 1988)
Loss of any ABR component (Schramm et al., 1988)
Loss of ABR (Friedman et al., 1985)
Abrupt loss of ABR (Slavit et al., 1991)
Worsening of promontory recorded action potential threshold (Stanton et al., 1989)

TABLE 9.4 Examples of ABR intraoperative events that have been reported to be associated with favorable outcomes (monitoring auditory system function during vestibular schwannoma removal).

Unchanged ABR over baseline levels (amplitude and latency)
AP thresholds unchanged over baseline values (Stanton et al., 1989)
Intraoperative appearance of ABR peak not detectable in preoperative recordings (Schramm et al., 1988)
Less than 2.0 msec increase in Wave V latency (Kileny et al., 1992)
Preservation of CM and AP at end of surgery (Ojemann, Levine, Montgomery, & McGaffigan, 1984)

1500–2000 Hz to lower the level of extraneous electrical interference. Further, note that faster stimulation rates than used in the clinic may be used for intraoperative ABR recordings if the signal-to-noise ratio permits. That is, because muscle relaxation agents often are administered by anesthesia that reduce spontaneous EMG activity, often it is possible to record high quality ABR using stimulation rates of 30 to 60 clicks/sec.

Anesthetic Constraints

Neither the ECochG nor the ABR is affected significantly by commonly used anesthetic agents. Further, if facial nerve monitoring is not being performed concurrently, long-acting muscle relaxant medications may be administered by anesthesiology. Anesthetic constraints for EMG monitoring are discussed later in this chapter.

Interpretation of AEPs (Warning Criteria)

Perhaps the question most frequently asked of those engaged in monitoring is "How much change is too much change?" in the amplitude or latency of an evoked potential variable. In most cases the honest answer is "We don't really know." A number of critical differences have evolved over the years for various evoked potentials. For instance, a 50% decrease in the amplitude and/or a 3 msec increase in the latency (with reference to post-induction control records) of the tibial nerve cortically evoked somatosensory evoked potential P40 component was offered by Brown and colleagues (Brown, Nash, Berilla, & Amaddio, 1984). However these values were derived empirically, that is, patients whose data did not exceed these values fared well postoperatively. In a recent survey of critical "warning" criteria for the ABR, Jacobson (unpublished observations) reported that the range of published warning criteria was quite broad for Wave V amplitude, Wave V latency, Wave I latency, Wave I amplitude, interear Wave I–V difference and rate of Wave V latency change (see Tables 9.2 through 9.4).

In fact, whereas some practitioners have suggested that the surgical team be continuously apprised of any change in the evoked response that is larger than the random variations normally seen (Møller, 1989), others have suggested that warnings occur only in instances where the evoked response is absent (Friedman et al., 1985). The latter suggestion was offered based upon the investigator's observation that short of complete absence of the ABR, patients fared quite well postoperatively. It should be noted that Friedman and colleagues (1985) offered no audiometric data whereby residual auditory function could be assessed.

One method of determining warning criteria would be to observe changes in monitoring variables without warning the surgical team that a change has occurred. The patients would be evaluated postoperatively. Intraoperative changes in neurophysiological testing would be correlated with clinical outcome. However, we are in the unique position of having created a "perceived need" in the absence of controlled studies to prove that the need exists. In this regard, within the American Academy of Neurology (AAN) Assessment of Intraoperative Neurophysiology, it is stated that:

There has never been a double-blind prospective study of any surgical monitoring procedure in humans. This problem cannot be resolved because of ethical problems in carrying out the needed study. In the absence of such a definitive study, judgment regarding the efficacy of monitoring must be based on animal experimentation, uncontrolled human studies and general experience in applying these tools to humans. (American Academy of Neurology, 1990, p. 1645).

The issue of developing warning criteria is not an easy one. The easiest way to establish warning criteria would be to measure the amplitude and latency of a series of waveforms following induction of anesthesia. The mean amplitude (and/or latency) would be calculated, as well as 2 to 3 standard deviations above the mean. This would provide upper limits representing 95% to 99% ends of the distribution. There are problems with this technique. First, whereas the patient's neurophysiological status usually (but not always) is stable during the early stages of surgery, this status may change dramatically as time goes on. The question becomes, "Is the patient lying on the table at +6 hours into surgery the same patient who was lying on the table whose baseline traces were obtained at +30 minutes into surgery?" The answer is "no" in all but the best of operating rooms where anesthesia is tailored to suit the monitoring technique. Also, the use of standard deviations presumes that randomly sampled latency and amplitude measures are normally distributed. In practice, the latencies tend to be longer more often than earlier as surgery progresses.

It is clear that the best measure of neurophysiological function is the one associated with the lowest variability (i.e., least trial-to-trial fluctuation in amplitude and latency). For evoked potentials, near-field recorded responses from peripheral and cranial nerves, spinal cord, and brainstem are extremely consistent, high amplitude, highly reproducible responses requiring minimal signal averaging. It is likely that in the future statistically based techniques will be developed upon which warnings will be based. At present it is important to understand that, for the most part, current warning criteria are based upon empirical observations, not values derived from conventional scientific investigational techniques. Thus, there is no "law" to suggest that

a warning criterion of >3/8 amplitude decrease is any less sensitive that a >1/2 amplitude decrease for the detection of neurophysiological compromise of the spinal cord (or auditory system for that matter). In fact, York and colleagues (York, Chabot, & Gaines, 1987) have reported that fluctuations of up to 15% in the latency and 50% in amplitude of the cortical SEP P40 component occurred routinely in their recordings. These SEP changes were not associated with negative postoperative outcomes. Also, these warning criteria may change not only by monitoring modality (ABR, SEP, SSEP, VEP), but by the type of surgical procedure as we understand more about the tolerances of the nervous system based upon the necessary animal studies.

Finally, as suggested by Møller (1989), it is probably prudent to advise the surgical team about any negative trends, regardless of their magnitude. That is, for example, if on four consecutive measures an evoked potential is increasing in latency or decreasing in amplitude, the trend should be reported regardless of the magnitude of change. Perhaps, at present, this is more important than the imposition of more or less arbitrary warning criteria that have undergone little (if any) rigorous scientific testing.

Common Applications of Auditory System Monitoring

Surgery Affecting the Auditory and Vestibular End Organs

Endolymphatic Sac Surgery. Ménière's disease (MD) is believed to originate as either an overproduction or underresorption of endolymph. The audiometric profile of Ménière's disease is well known. The ECochG and ABR findings in MD also have been described in great detail. It is characteristic for the patient with mild-moderate flat sensorineural hearing loss to demonstrate an ABR at greatly reduced sensation levels that appears indistinguishable from that of a normal hearing individual obtained at equivalent HLs. This finding has been interpreted by many as an electrophysiological indicator of neural recruitment. The electrocochleographic characteristics of MD also have been described in detail. Abnormalities in ECochG for patients with MD have included: an increased SP/AP amplitude ratio (as a result of either increased amplitude SP or reduced amplitude AP; Eggermont, 1979; Gibson, 1991), enhanced SP to tone burst stimulation (Dauman, Aran, Savage, & Portmann, 1988; Gibson, 1991; Levine, Margolis, Fournier, & Winzenburg, 1992), and a latency difference in the AP recorded for condensation and rarefaction clicks separately (Levine et al., 1992; Margolis, Rieks, Fournier, & Levine, 1995).

Given the occurrence of a stereotypical pattern of ECochG findings, it would seem a natural next step to carry this technique into the operating room. Thus, it might be possible to document normalization of ECochG abnormalities during surgical procedures designed to correct the process underlying MD. A number of investigators have reported SP/AP amplitude ratio changes during endolymphatic sac surgery. For example, Arenberg and colleagues (Arenberg, Obert, & Gibson, 1991) reported their experience monitoring 62 patients (transtympanic ECochG) during endolymphatic sac surgery. The authors compared SP/AP ratios obtained at baseline to those at the end of surgery. They found statistically significant differences (a change in SP/AP ratio equal to or exceeding 7%) for those patients who demonstrated abnormal SP/AP ratios preoperatively (defined as SP/AP ratio greater than 35%). For patients with normal SP/AP ratios preoperatively a nonsignificant pre-postoperative difference in SP/AP ratio was observed. The authors reported that the improvements in SP/AP ratio occurred during drilling of the mastoid and endolymphatic sac opening and decompression. In another report (Arenberg, Kobayashi, Obert, & Gibson, 1993) the same investigators reported their experience recording the ECochG to both click and tone burst stimulation from 37 ears during placement of a valved shunt. The authors reported that 70% of the ears had abnormal absolute SP amplitudes at baseline and these reverted to normal at the end of surgery. It was the authors' view that the addition of tone burst derived SP data added significantly to information about cochlear function during endolymphatic shunt placement. In an outcome-based investigation Bojrab and colleagues (Bojrab, Bhansali, & Andreozzi, 1994) reported their observations of 38 patients undergoing endolymphatic shunt surgery. The investigators measured the SP/AP amplitude ratio during decompression and the mean follow-up period was four years. Of their sample 42% showed an improvement in the SP/AP ratio intraoperatively, the remainder either showed no change or worsening of the ratio. Improvement in hearing was reported in 11% and a worsening of hearing was reported in 32% of their patients. Interestingly, there was no predictable relationship noted between improvements in the SP/AP ratio and control of dizziness postoperatively. Alternately, there was a direct relationship between improvements in hearing sensitivity and improvements in the SP/AP ratio. Thus, intraoperative ECochG might serve as a prognosticator of quality of postoperative hearing sensitivity. Figure 9.1 illustrates improvement in the SP/AP ratio of a patient who underwent endolymphatic sac decompression. It can be see that improvements in the SP/AP ratio occurred during both mastoidectomy and decompression stages of the procedure.

Chemical Ablation of Vestibular End Organ.   At the Henry Ford Hospital, Detroit, MI, we have participated in a multisite study to help determine the efficacy of streptomycin infusion (chemical labyrinthectomy) into the vestibular end organ for relief of MD (Monsell & Shelton, 1992). In this technique a labyrinthotomy is created at the ampulated end

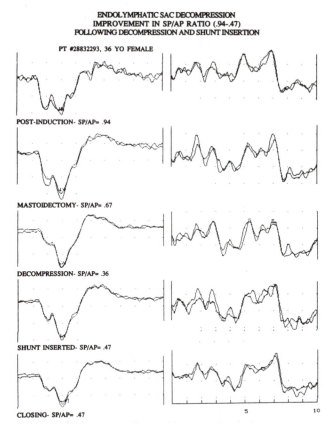

ENDOLYMPHATIC SAC DECOMPRESSION
IMPROVEMENT IN SP/AP RATIO (.94-.47)
FOLLOWING DECOMPRESSION AND SHUNT INSERTION

PT #28832293, 36 YO FEMALE

POST-INDUCTION- SP/AP= .94

MASTOIDECTOMY- SP/AP= .67

DECOMPRESSION- SP/AP= .36

SHUNT INSERTED- SP/AP= .47

CLOSING- SP/AP= .47

FIGURE 9.1   Tympanic ECochG and ABR recordings during endolymphatic sac decompression surgery for intractable vertigo. Note that at the beginning of surgery the SP/AP ratio was 0.94. Following mastoidectomy the SP/AP ratio was 0.67, and following decompression the ratio was 0.36. This patient was vertigo-free at follow-up.

of the horizontal semicircular canal. A small amount of streptomycin (2.5–25 μg in lactated Ringer's solution) is infused into the canal with a 27-gauge needle. The desired effect of the streptomycin infusion is to destroy hair cells and dark cells of the sensory epithelium of the vestibular labyrinth without affecting the cochlear labyrinth. Tympanic ECochG was recorded during this procedure. Our observations were that in every case there were significant changes in the SP/AP ratio (usually manifested as a decrease in the AP amplitude) during and following the labyrinthotomy. Characteristic changes are illustrated in Figures 9.2 and 9.3. In most cases, these changes were associated with significant postoperative (usually high-frequency) hearing loss. The preliminary results of a multicenter investigation of the efficacy of streptomycin infusion indicated that worsening of hearing loss postoperatively occurred in 68% of the patients (Monsell & Shelton, 1992). For 57% the hearing loss was severe to profound in degree. It is unclear whether the hearing losses occurred due to the direct

STREPTOMYCIN INFUSION FOR INTRACTABLE VERTIGO
SP/AP RATIO CHANGE FROM .41–1.0
NOT ASSOCIATED WITH CHANGE IN WAVE V LATENCY
NO SIGNIFICANT CHANGE IN PRE VERSUS POST-OP AUDIOMETRY

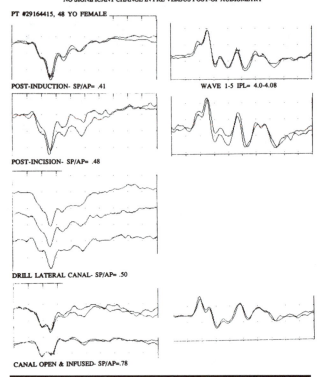

SIGNIFICANT CHANGES IN SP/AP RATIO OBSERVED FOLLOWING
OPENING OF LATERAL SEMICIRCULAR CANAL AND
FOLLOWING INFUSION

68 YO F #26470825

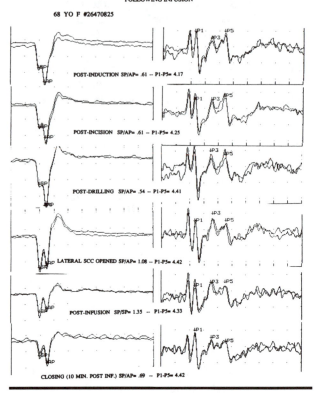

FIGURE 9.2   Tympanic ECochG recordings from a patient undergoing streptomycin infusion for intractable vertigo. Notice that following infusion the AP amplitude decreases. This patient did not demonstrate new hearing loss postoperatively.

FIGURE 9.3   Tympanic ECochG recordings from a patient undergoing streptomycin infusion for intractable vertigo. Notice that following labyrinthotomy the AP amplitude decreases and the SP amplitude increases. At closing both SP and AP are markedly decreased in amplitude. This is associated with a modest 0.25 msec increase in the ABR Wave I–V interwave interval. This patient demonstrated new hearing loss postoperatively.

effects of streptomycin or the process of exposing the labyrinth for the infusion. For these reasons, the streptomycin infusion procedure is not being performed at our site. However, this is a excellent example of a situation where a monitoring modality (ECochG) has provided information to surgeons (i.e., the effect that opening the endolymphatic space has on postoperative hearing sensitivity) that has affected their future behavior (i.e., the decision not to perform the streptomycin infusion procedure).

Surgery Affecting the VIIIn and Auditory Brainstem

Vestibular Schwannoma-VS (and Other Posterior Fossa Tumor) Surgery.   There are a number of tumors that grow in the cerebellopontine angle and compress the VIIIn. These tumors include vestibular schwannomas (VSs; acoustic neuromas), meningiomas, epidermoid tumors, and neurofibromas. The most common tumor growing in the cerebellopontine angle is the VS. The VS usually originates from

the Schwann cell sheath of the VIIIn and expands to fill the internal auditory canal. As it fills the IAC, it compresses the VIIIn. In early stages the tumor may not impair neuronal conduction to the extent that the ABR demonstrates deficits in transmission of coded neural activity. For this reason, there have been numerous reports of false negative findings in ABR testing of patients with confirmed VSs (Jacobson, Newman, Monsell, & Wharton, 1993; Telian, Kileny, Niparko, Kemink, & Graham, 1989). Further growth of the tumor will be reflected in various degrees of abnormality of the ABR. In the extreme, compression of the VIIIn by VS will result in reduced or absent blood perfusion of the VIIIn and cochlea. Definitive identification of VS is accomplished through gadolinium-enhanced MRI scanning. This test, which has the ability to detect tumors that are less than .5 cm in size, has become the "gold standard" in tumor detection. It is common for patients with VSs to present with continuous, high-pitched, unilateral tinnitus. Patients may or may not present with high- or low-frequency hearing loss and varying degrees of audiometric abnormalities. Finally, it is common for patients with VS to complain of intermittent dizziness and/or unsteadiness.

The removal of VS may be accomplished through a number of surgical approaches. A complete discussion of the surgical approaches to VS goes beyond the scope of the present review. However, the interested reader is directed to the excellent text by Jackler and Brackmann (1994) and, in particular, the chapter authored by Jackler (1994) in the above text. A translabyrinthine approach to tumor removal often is chosen for patients who have poor residual hearing, large tumors, and/or where preservation of facial nerve function is of paramount concern. The translabyrinthine surgical approach sacrifices residual hearing sensitivity for the ability to identify the facial nerve early and follow it as it courses through the porus acousticus. For these patients auditory system monitoring is not performed.

For those patients who have smaller tumors (usually less than 1.5 cm) and good residual auditory function, a number of surgical approaches including the suboccipital, middle fossa (for removal of intracanalicular tumors), and retrosigmoid (for removal of small tumors extending into the cerebellopontine angle) approaches have been developed that optimize preservation of the facial nerve while affording the surgeon access to the VIIIn, VIIn, and the VS. It is for these patients that a number of monitoring modalities have been developed in an attempt to improve the likelihood that useful, functional hearing will be preserved.

The degree to which monitoring has contributed to positive postoperative outcomes is colored somewhat by the criteria used by surgeons to select candidates for hearing preservation surgical procedures and the criteria that are used to define "preserved hearing." For example, some outcome studies have failed to disclose preoperative and postoperative audiometric data (e.g., either or both pure tone sensitivity and word recognition test findings). These investigators have tended to classify hearing preservation as *any* residual hearing sensitivity. It should be obvious that hearing-sparing surgical procedures are of little benefit if they do not result in the preservation of *useful* or *functional* hearing ability. For example, Wade and House (1984) conducted hearing-sparing procedures only if tumors were smaller than 1.5 cm, speech reception thresholds (SRTs) were better than 30 dB, and word recognition scores (WRSs) were better than 70%. Tator and Nedzelski (1985) reported their experience in hearing-sparing procedures for patients with tumors less than 2.5 cm in size, where SRTs were less than 50 dB, and WRSs were better than 60%. Cohen and colleagues (Cohen, Hammerschlag, Berg, & Ransohoff, 1986) invoked the 50/50 rule. That is, candidates for surgery had to demonstrate an SRT better than 50 dB and WRS better than 50%. Kileny and colleagues (1992) reported their experience preserving auditory function in patients with tumors less than 1.5 cm and where patients demonstrated SRTs of better than 30 dB and WRSs better than 70%.

The experiences of many appear to support the contention that the probability of preserving useful hearing is much poorer when the size of the VS exceeds 1.5 cm. Ojemann and colleagues (1984) reported that 75% of patients with 1 cm tumors had WRSs better than 35% postoperatively compared with 25% of patients with tumors greater than 3 cm. Abramson and colleagues (Abramson, Stein, Pedley, Emerson, & Wazen, 1985) reported their experience with removal of 20 VSs, 14 of which were greater than 3 cm in size. Whereas the authors reported functional hearing preserved in 100% of patients with tumors .5 to 1.0 cm in size, functional hearing was not preserved in any patients with tumors 3 cm or larger. Kemink and colleagues (1990) reported that no patients with tumors larger than 1.5 cm had serviceable hearing when a total resection of the tumor was performed. Slavit and colleagues (1991) reported that hearing was preserved in 82% of monitored cases where patients had tumors smaller than 1 cm and 0% of the time for patients with tumors exceeding 3 cm. Silverstein and colleagues (Silverstein, McDaniel, Norrell, & Heberkamp, 1986) reported preservation of hearing in 33% of patients with tumors less than 1.5 cm. It is interesting that the authors developed a grading system for audiometric outcome (see Table 9.5).

Nadol and colleagues (Nadol, Levine, Ojemann, Martuza, et al., 1987) reported that they were able to preserve useful hearing (defined as SRT no poorer than 70 dB and WRS no poorer than 15%) in 75% of patients with no greater than 0.5 cm extension of the tumor into the posterior fossa. Conversely, they were able to preserve useful hearing in only 22% of cases where extension of the tumor into the posterior fossa was greater than 2.5 cm. It is arguable whether a 15% WRS is compatible with useful residual hearing. Kanzaki and colleagues (Kanzaki, Ogawa, Shiobara, & Toya, 1989) reported their experience monitoring 30 cases of VS where tumors extended into the posterior fossa 2.0 cm or less. The authors reported that for 15 patients with SRT 50 dB or better and WRS 50% or better they were able to preserve hearing in 60% of the cases. The authors monitored auditory function with the combined approach of ABR, ECochG, and direct VIIIn CAP. Nedzelski and colleagues (1994) reported their experience monitoring the

TABLE 9.5 Grading system for audiometric outcome.

	HEARING	PTAdB	SPEECH DISCRIMINATION (%)
Class I	Good to excellent	0–30	70–100
Class II	Serviceable	35–50	50–65
Class III	Nonserviceable	55–75	25–45
Class IV	Poor	80–100	0–20
Class V	No measureable hearing	—	0

From Silverstein et al., 1986, p. 288.

cochlear CAP (round window electrode) in VS surgery. The authors reported that serviceable hearing was preserved in 38% of the monitored group and 15% of the unmonitored group. Finally, Harner and colleagues (Harner, Harper, Beatty, Litchy, & Ebersold, 1996) reported their experience monitoring auditory function for 144 consecutive patients with VS. The authors reported that hearing preservation occurred rarely for tumors greater than 2.5 cm. Additionally, they reported that the presence of Wave V at the end of surgery did not ensure preserved hearing was useful hearing. Further, of 5 patients who had normal hearing postoperatively, 3 had tumors less than 1 cm in size, 1 patient had a tumor between 1 and 2 cm and the final patient had a tumor between 2 and 3 cm in size. Interestingly, 3 patients had only Wave V present at the end of surgery and 2 patients demonstrated only Wave I. Of their sample who had normal hearing preoperatively, small tumors, and ABR Wave V present, 3 had normal hearing, 3 had poor hearing, and 3 had no hearing postoperatively. Figure 9.4 shows the pre- and postoperative audiometry, the preoperative ABR, and intraoperative ABR recordings for a patient with a small VS on the left side. As may be seen, hearing preservation was successful for this patient.

Despite the knowledge that irreparable damage to the auditory system may occur central to the VIIIn in the cerebellopontine angle, it is surprising to read of investigators

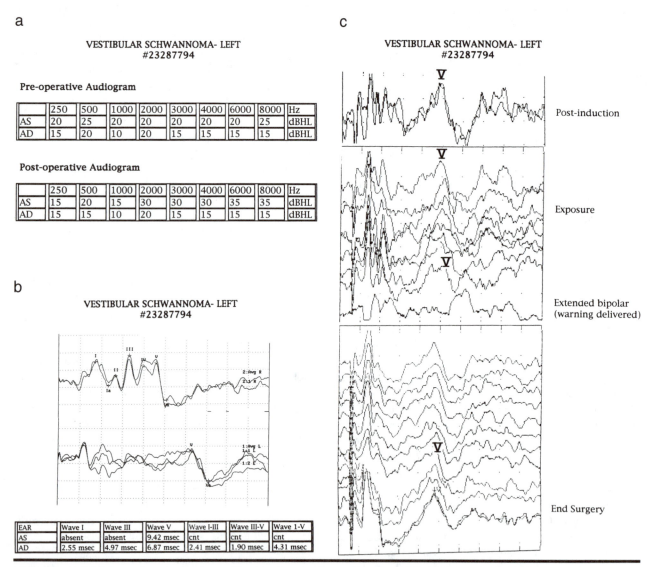

FIGURE 9.4 (A) Pre- and postoperative audiometry for a patient with a small VS. (B) Pre-operative ABR examination showing a normal ABR on the right side and a Wave V prolongation on the affected side. (C) Intraoperative ABR record showing Wave V present throughout the case. Notice that Wave V disappears following extended bipolar cautery probably due to the distributed effects of heat. Surgery was stopped and the ABR was observed for 10 minutes. Wave V returned and surgery proceeded to completion.

advocating the use of electrocochleography and/or the recording of direct CAPs in isolation to monitor auditory system function during VS surgery (Colletti & Fiorino, 1994; Kveton, 1990; Symon et al., 1988). For example, Symon and colleagues (1988) reported 37% of their patients had some residual hearing at the end of surgery. They reported that 2 of these patients had intact ECochG at the end of surgery and were found to be profoundly deaf. In this regard, Sabin and colleagues (Sabin, Prasher, Bentivoglio, & Symon, 1987) presented a case report of a patient with ECochG waves N1 and N2 present at the end of surgery but with profound hearing loss. Subsequently the patient was retested at 15 months post surgery and found to have only a CM and SP. The N1 and N2 were now absent. It is known that cochlear potentials can remain following sectioning of the VIIIn if blood supply to the cochlea has been preserved (Ruben et al., 1963). Undoubtedly in this instance perfusion of the cochlea was not affected by the maximum functional damage to the VIIIn. (The authors conjectured this damage represented a disconnection of the peripheral and central myelinated segments of the VIIIn at the Obersteiner-Redlich zone due to excessive traction.) In the same vein, investigators have documented the persistence of cochlear potentials for periods of up to 25 minutes following cochlear nerve section (Silverstein, McDaniel, & Norrell, 1985a) and up to 80 days in the presence of total deafness following VS surgery (Levine et al., 1984).

Despite the strong evidence that it is possible to preserve useful hearing with a combination of auditory system monitoring techniques, there are some who have suggested that the intraoperatively recorded ABR has contributed little to reducing auditory morbidity. Kveton (1990) reported his limited experience (N = 16, 7 patients unmonitored and 9 patients monitored) using ABR monitoring. With one exception (2.0 cm tumor) all patients had tumors less than 1.5 cm in diameter. The author reported that 57% of unmonitored and 44% of monitored patients demonstrated preserved serviceable hearing (defined as WRS of better than 50%).

Finally, it is noteworthy that Mustain and colleagues (Mustain, Al-Mefty, & Anand, 1992) have reported an unusual instance where all components beyond Wave I were lost during resection of an epidermoid tumor the right petrous apex. Loss of components beyond Wave I normally is associated with total deafness. The patient was found to have a mild flat conductive hearing loss postoperatively with excellent WRS. Once the conductive deficit cleared, an ABR was performed that revealed a reappearance of Waves I, III, and V with a nonsignificant Wave I–V interaural interear latency difference.

The success that any given investigator has experienced with preservation of auditory function in resection of VS is affected somewhat by a number of factors including but not limited to: the pre-morbid status of the patients, differences in the surgical approach to the tumors, the degree of cooperation among members of the surgical/monitoring team, tumor resection technique (use of lasers, ultrasonic aspirators, bipolar forceps), skill of surgeons (amount of experience), skill of monitoring team (amount of experience), technical abilities of monitoring team, signal-to-noise ratio found in each operating room, and differences in how each group classifies residual auditory function (pure tone thresholds or word recognition ability).

Vestibular Neurectomy. Vestibular neurectomy is the last resort surgical treatment for patients who have intractable vertigo and good auditory function. A craniotomy is performed and the VIIn/VIIIn complex is exposed. During exposure the cerebellum may be retracted and the VIIIn may be stretched to its neurophysiological limits. Additionally, at the time of sectioning it is critical for the surgeon to have the ability to identify accurately the auditory and vestibular divisions of the VIIIn. One method of accomplishing this goal is to place a fine bipolar recording electrode on what is felt to be the auditory division of the VIIIn. This electrode can be as simple as two strands of teflon coated silver wire (Medwire AG10T) that have been twined together and bared only at the tips (tips separated by 1–2 mm). We have found that folding over the bared ends of the silver wire ends creates a smooth (as opposed to a sharp) recording surface. The ear is stimulated simultaneously with unfiltered click stimuli. If the bipolar recording electrode has been placed on the vestibular division of the VIIIn, either no or a very small direct compound action potential will be recorded. Alternately, if the electrode has been placed on the auditory division of the VIIIn, a large triphasic potential will be recorded. This technique is quite sensitive (Colletti & Fiorino, 1993; Silverstein, McDaniel, Wazen, & Norrell, 1985b). Once the auditory division of the VIIIn has been identified, the vestibular division is sectioned. McDaniel and colleagues (McDaniel, Silverstein, & Norrell, 1985) reported that, using direct VIIIn monitoring techniques, they were able to maintain hearing (defined by pure tone average) within 20 dB of baseline levels in 83% of their patients. Additionally, they were able to maintain word recognition scores (word lists unreported) to within 20% of baseline levels in 83% of their patients. Figure 9.5 shows intraoperative tympanic ECochG, ABR, and direct VIIIn CAP recordings from a patient undergoing retromastoid vestibular neurectomy. There was no significant change in hearing postoperatively.

Neurovascular Decompression (NVD) Surgery. There are a number of diseases that are felt to occur as a result of compression of cranial nerves by redundant vessels or arteries. These diseases include trigeminal neuralgia (decompression of Vn), hemifacial spasm (decompression of VIIn), disabling positional vertigo (decompression of

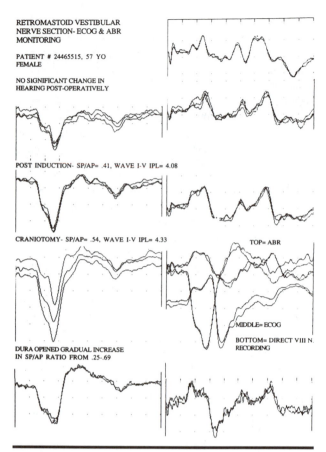

RETROMASTOID VESTIBULAR NERVE SECTION- ECOG & ABR MONITORING

PATIENT # 24465515, 57 YO FEMALE

NO SIGNIFICANT CHANGE IN HEARING POST-OPERATIVELY

POST INDUCTION- SP/AP= .41, WAVE I-V IPL= 4.08

CRANIOTOMY- SP/AP= .54, WAVE I-V IPL= 4.33

TOP= ABR

MIDDLE= ECOG

BOTTOM= DIRECT VIII N. RECORDING

DURA OPENED GRADUAL INCREASE IN SP/AP RATIO FROM .25-.69

FIGURE 9.5 Intraoperative tympanic ECochG, ABR, and direct VIIIn CAP from a patient undergoing vestibular neurectomy for intractable vertigo.

VIIIn), and intractable tinnitus. The most common applications of NVD are for the treatment of trigeminal neuralgia and hemifacial spasm (HFS). To accomplish an NVD for HFS, a suboccipital craniotomy usually is performed, the cerebellum is retracted, and the cerebellopontine angle is explored. The VIIn cranial nerve is then identified. Attempts are made to determine whether cross-compression of the VIIn is occurring at its REZ at the brainstem. It is common for compression to be caused by the anterior inferior cerebellar artery (AICA). At times the VIIn may be indented by the vessel or artery, and in these cases identification of source of compression is straightforward. Once the offending vasculature has been identified, a piece of teflon felt (a cushion) is interposed between the vasculature and the nerve. Unfortunately, this surgical procedure is associated with a risk of significant postoperative hearing impairment that ranges from 0.7 to 2.8% (Møller & Møller, 1985; Møller & Møller, 1989) to 15% (Auger, Peipgras, & Laws, 1986). Irreparable damage to the auditory system can occur quickly, and thus one might predict that monitoring auditory system function intraoperatively might be a method of

reducing postoperative morbidity. As noted previously, Friedman and colleagues (1985) evaluated systematically the NVD procedure to determine if it was possible to determine during what stage of the surgical procedure the auditory system was placed at greatest risk. They observed that abrupt changes in Wave V latency and Wave I–V interpeak latencies began once the cerebellar retractor had been placed. These latency prolongations worsened during the period when the sponge was placed and began to normalize (with reference to post induction values) once the cerebellar retractor had been removed. Since that report, the ABR coupled with recording of VIIIn action potentials directly from the exposed VIIIn have been conducted by most investigators in an attempt to decrease the likelihood of significant postoperative hearing impairment. By way of example, Møller & Møller (1989) have reported their experiences monitoring 140 NVD surgeries. The authors reported that word recognition scores were poorer in 7 patients by 15% or more and better in 6 patients by as much as 52% postoperatively. Nine patients demonstrated a worsening of PTA by 11 dB or more 4 to 5 days after surgery and 8 of these patients showed evidence of middle ear effusion. High-frequency hearing loss (hearing loss at 4000 Hz and/or 8000 Hz) occurred in approximately 15 to 20% of the cases. Radtke and colleagues (Radtke, Erwin, & Wilkins, 1989) reported a 6.6% prevalence of profound hearing loss in 152 patients not monitored with ABR. Alternately, none of the 70 patients in a monitored group suffered a profound hearing loss. In a separate investigation Sindou, Fobe, Cirano, and Fischer (1992) reported their findings monitoring 34 cases of NVD for HFS using ABR only. They reported transient hearing loss postoperatively in almost half of their patients. Changes in the ABR correctly predicted postoperative deafness in 1 patient. Changes in the ABR were observed in an additional 5 patients. These changes had not normalized at the end of surgery and were associated with transient hearing losses. Finally, recently Møller and colleagues (Møller, Møller, Jannetta, Jho, & Sekhar, 1993) have reported their successes monitoring auditory function (using ABR) during 254 NVD surgeries for disabling positional vertigo and disabling intractable tinnitus. The authors reported marked hearing loss in only 1.6% of their patients monitored with ABR.

In the author's experience, the NVD procedure always is associated with change in auditory evoked potentials. These changes can be abrupt (implicating vascular mechanisms) or can accumulate over minutes. The changes begin invariably with a broadening of the CAP (shown in Figures 9.6 and 9.7) that is accompanied with prolongations in the Wave I–V interwave interval (shown in Figures 9.8 and 9.9). Wave V may be prolonged 1 to 3 msec beyond post-induction baseline values. These changes begin usually (as reported by Friedman et al., 1985) at the onset of cerebellar retraction. It is common for these changes not to resolve

HEMIFACIAL SPASM

DIRECT AUDITORY NERVE RECORDINGS

S#23137185, 42YO FEMALE
LEFT HEMIFACIAL SPASM

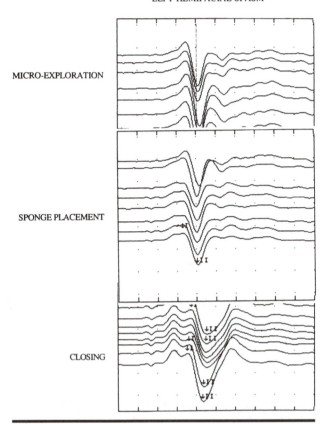

HEMIFACIAL SPASM

DIRECT AUDITORY NERVE RECORDINGS

S#08817451, 68 YO MALE
LEFT HEMIFACIAL SPASM

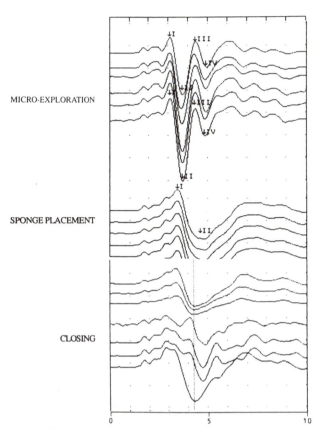

FIGURE 9.6   Direct CAP recordings from a patient with HFS who was undergoing an NVD procedure. Note that during placement of the Teflon felt ("sponge placement") the CAP broadens and increases in latency. These changes begin to normalize once retractors have been withdrawn from the surgical field (see bottom of figure). These changes in the CAP may be correlated with changes in the ABR from the same patient (see Figure 9.8).

FIGURE 9.7   From a different patient the same changes in the CAP may be observed during placement of Teflon felt. These changes begin to normalize at the end of the case once retractors have been removed. These changes may be correlated with the intraoperative ABR obtained from the same patient (see Figure 9.9).

completely at the end of surgery. Postoperatively often these patients demonstrate high-frequency hearing loss and tinnitus. The tinnitus and hearing loss resolve usually over the 4 to 6 weeks between discharge and their follow-up appointment. This application of monitoring is quite rewarding because changes always occur and in a predictable sequence. It is undoubted that neurophysiological monitoring techniques pioneered by Møller and his colleagues at the University of Pittsburgh have contributed to improved surgical outcomes of this patient population.

Brainstem Perfusion (Correction of Brainstem Arteriovenous Malformations and Aneurysms).   There are a variety of neurosurgical procedures involving correction of vascular

malformations that place the brainstem at risk for hypoperfusion (as a function of either ischemia or hemorrhage). These disorders include correction of arteriovenous malformations (AVMs) and aneurysms affecting the posterior blood supply (e.g., basilar arteries). A consideration in the monitoring of these procedures is that blood flow must be reduced beyond some critical level before brainstem evoked responses are affected. Specifically, as regards brainstem somatosensory evoked potentials (SEPs), local cerebral blood flow in the brainstem must be reduced to beyond 10 ml/100gm/min before brainstem SEPs show changes in latency and amplitude (Branston, Ladds, Symon, & Wang, 1984). This level is perilously close to the threshold of tissue infarction (i.e., irreparable damage). The fact that these

HEMIFACIAL SPASM

SCALP RECORDED BAEP

S#23137185, 42YO FEMALE
LEFT HEMIFACIAL SPASM

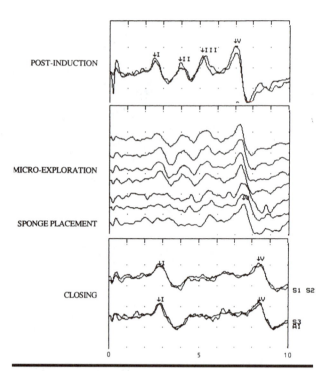

FIGURE 9.8   ABR recorded simultaneously with CAP from same patient as in Figure 9.6. Note shift in Wave V latency that occurs during placement of "sponge" when cerebellar retraction was greatest. Also, note that at closing the ABR is quite delayed with reference to baseline although the CAP has begun to normalize.

HEMIFACIAL SPASM

SCALP RECORDED BAEP

S#08817451, 68 YO MALE
LEFT HEMIFACIAL SPASM

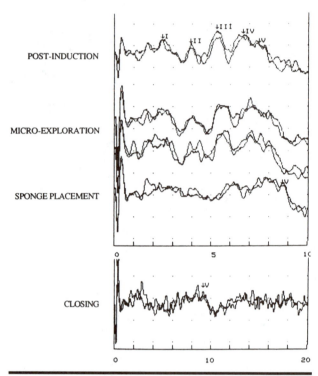

FIGURE 9.9   ABR recorded simultaneously with CAP from same patient as in Figure 9.7. Again, note shift in Wave V latency that occurs during placement of "sponge" when cerebellar retraction was greatest.

threshold blood flow levels are so close may explain why brainstem auditory evoked potentials have been found to be of questionable benefit for monitoring of brainstem perfusion. In this regard, Little and colleagues (1983) reported their observations of the sensitivity of ABR for the identification of impending neurological deficits in 10 patients who went to surgery for correction of vascular disorders affecting posterior circulation. In three cases the ABR was lost and all three patients died. In some cases the insensitivity of the ABR for the detection of impending neurological events may be linked to the limited portion of the neuraxis that may be evaluated with the ABR. Piatt, Radtke, and Erwin (1985) reported their observations of a single patient who was taken to surgery for treatment of trigeminal neuralgia. During surgery Wave V disappeared but reappeared and normalized following replacement of a retractor. However, upon awakening the patient was found to have neurological deficits outside the auditory system. A

somatosensory evoked potential examination was conducted that was abnormal. A CT scan was conducted and revealed evidence of infraction of the midbrain tegmentum and middle cerebellar peduncle. Thus, the authors reasoned that had they recorded brainstem somatosensory evoked potentials intraoperatively, they might have been able to identify the evolving somesthetic pathway deficit. This case report underscored the importance of evaluating more than one sensory modality intraoperatively in instances where the global status of brainstem function is in question. Finally, a report by Schwartz and colleagues (Schwartz, Gennarelli, Young, Fedder, & Schwinn, 1989) demonstrated the usefulness of monitoring ABR to document improvement in neural transmission during the emergent treatment of a hematoma at the cerebellar vermis. The investigators documented improvement in the ABR (rarely observed intraoperatively) following decompression of the vascular disorder.

Less Common Applications of Auditory System Monitoring

Intraoperative Evaluation of Pediatric Patient Candidates Undergoing Cochlear Implantation. Auditory evoked potential recordings may assist in the verification that there are enough viable nerve fibers in the spiral ganglion to support cochlear implantation in pediatric patients. For adults the preoperative behavioral determination of auditory threshold to promontory stimulation provides a good estimate of postoperative excitability of the peripheral auditory system following cochlear implantation. However, while these behavioral measurements have been reported to be stable in individuals older than 10 years of age (Kileny, Zwolan, Zimmerman-Phillips, & Telian, 1994), they cannot be made in young children. That is why it is vital for clinicians to have some semi-objective method for estimating how effectively the auditory system can be stimulated. A number of investigators have reported their experiences with recording electrically evoked auditory evoked potentials from pediatric cochlear implant candidates. The evoked potential of choice has been the electrically evoked auditory brainstem response (EABR); however, investigators also have recorded middle latency auditory evoked potentials following electrical stimulation of the auditory system (e.g., Kileny & Kemink, 1987). With electrical stimulation current pulses are delivered through either a bipolar needle electrode applied to the promontory of the cochlea or through the cochlear implant itself. For promontory stimulation, balanced biphasic constant current pulses (200–400 μsec/phase) are presented at up to 1 mA intensity at a rate of about 5/sec (Kileny et al., 1994). The noninverting electrode location is usually Fpz and the inverting electrode may be placed on the contralateral mastoid or high cervical area (above the C7 vertebral prominence for example). Standard ABR recording parameters may be used; however, the first 1 to 2 msec of the recording may be blocked to eliminate the stimulus artifact. If first-order cochlear afferents are viable, electrical stimulation will result in direct activation of the distal (cochlear) portion of the auditory nerve. ABR components are recorded with a latency shortened by the absence of traveling wave time (since the stimulus is delivered directly to neural elements). Wave V thresholds of 406.4 μA have been reported by Kileny and colleagues (1994).

The use of an electrical stimulus produces a number of unique challenges that must be overcome to make it possible to record evoked potentials. These challenges include the shunting of stimulus current from the promontory source through the head to the recording electrodes (creating a large stimulus artifact) and the inadvertent spread of stimulus current to the facial nerve, resulting in the triggering of evoked facial nerve (and facial muscle) activity. A number of solutions to these problems have been suggested, including the careful choice of inverting electrode locations,

alternating the onset phase of the balanced biphasic pulses, and the use of adequate levels of muscle relaxants by anesthesiology (Kileny et al., 1994).

Other intraoperative uses of the EABR in implantation of auditory prostheses have included: (1) the assessment of whether the implant is functioning properly, (2) the prediction of how successful the patient will be in discriminating speech, and (3) assisting in the determination of the most useful speech coding paradigm.

EABR measurement parameters have included Wave V threshold, Wave V input/output, and recovery (rate) functions. Gantz and colleagues (Gantz, Brown, & Abbas, 1994) demonstrated a modest correlation (r = 0.25–0.50) between EAP growth and recovery functions for subjects (pediatric-Nucleus Mini-22; and adult-Clarion and Nucleus).

Waring (1992) recorded the EABR (consisting of Wave V) from the scalp surface following direct electrical stimulation of the cochlear nucleus implant from a patient who had bilateral VIIIn tumors removed and was bilaterally deaf. The patient had received the brainstem implant 8.6 years earlier. This patient was taken to surgery for removal of a VIIn tumor. The ability to record EABR intraoperatively and compare this data to recordings made at the time of implantation made it possible to verify that the implant had not been harmed in the process of removing the VIIn tumor.

Assessing Level of Consciousness during Surgery. A more esoteric application of auditory evoked potential monitoring has been the assessment of level of consciousness during surgery. In particular, there has been a surprisingly high incidence of awareness of patients undergoing cardiac surgery (Schwender, Kaiser, Klasing, Peter, & Poppel, 1994). This includes awareness of voices and events prior to and during surgical procedures. It is interesting that, under general anesthesia, the auditory modality seems to be the most receptive sensory channel for perception. It has been the interest of several investigators to know whether auditory evoked potentials can be used to predict level of consciousness. Additionally, it has been an objective to know which anesthetic agents most effectively suppress both explicit (i.e., conscious recognition of a previous episode) and implicit memory (expressed as a change in task performance that may be attributed to the subconscious acquisition of information). Armed with this information anesthesiologists could deliver anesthesia more effectively. In this regard, Schwender and colleagues (1994) have evaluated awareness during anesthesia using middle latency auditory evoked potentials (MLAEPs). As discussed in Chapter 8, MLAEPs probably represent the admixture of (primarily) cortically generated potentials that occur in the 15 to 60 msec time period. Schwender and colleagues (1994) evaluated changes in MLAEPs and implicit memory of an audiotape presentation for 45 patients undergoing elective cardiac surgery. The authors reported that for patients under anesthesia without implicit memory the MLAEP showed either marked decreases in amplitude and increases in latency or was completely suppressed. For most anesthetized patients with implicit memory, the Pa component increased in latency <12 msec. The authors reported that the criterion of a shift of 12 msec or less in Pa latency from baseline levels had a 100% sensitivity and 77% specificity for separating patients with and without implicit memory.

FACIAL NERVE MONITORING (MOTOR CRANIAL NERVE MONITORING)

Monitoring of motor cranial nerve function, and specifically facial nerve function, has become one of the few applications of intraoperative monitoring that has gained widespread support in the clinical community. Conclusions and recommendations of the NIH Consensus Development Conference for Acoustic Neuroma (1991) includes the statement that "the benefits of routine intraoperative monitoring of the facial nerve have been clearly established. This technique should be included in surgical therapy for vestibular schwannoma. Routine monitoring of other cranial nerves should be considered" (p. 19). Additionally, parameters recommended for acquisition and interpretation of facial nerve data have been offered by national and international bodies (American Electroencephalographic Society, 1994; International Federation of Clinical Monitoring, in Nuwer, Daube, Fischer, Scramm, & Yingling, 1993). It should be noted that despite the widespread belief that facial nerve monitoring contributes significantly to a reduction in postoperative morbidity in resection of acoustic neuroma, there exists controversy as to whether facial nerve monitoring techniques should be applied as a standard of practice in routine otologic surgery (Jackler & Selesnick, 1994; Roland & Meyerhoff, 1994).

There exists an expanding body of literature attesting to the efficacy of facial nerve monitoring in resection of vestibular schwannoma (e.g., Benecke, Calder, & Chadwick, 1987; Esses, LaRouere, & Graham, 1994; Hammerschlag & Cohen, 1990; Harner, Daube, Beatty, & Ebersold, 1988; Jellinek, Tan, & Symon, 1991; Kirkpatrick, Tierney, Gleeson, & Strong, 1993; Kwartler, Luxford, Atkins, & Shelton, 1991; Lalwani, Yuan-Shin Butt, Jackler, Pitts, & Yingling, 1994; Nadol, Chiong, Ojemann, McKenna, et al., 1992; Prasad, Hirsch, Kamerer, Durrant, & Sekhar, 1993; Selesnick, Carew, Victor, Heise, & Levine, 1996; Uziel, Benezech, & Frerebeau, 1993), glomus jugulare tumors (Green, Brackmann, Nguyen, Arriaga, Telischi, & de la Cruz, 1994), correction of congenital atresia where the location of the facial nerve often is unknown (Chandrasekhar, de la Cruz, & Garrido, 1985; Jahrsdoerfer, 1995; Lambert, 1988; Linstrom & Meiteles, 1993; Molony &

de la Cruz, 1990) and in surgery for neurovascular decompression of the facial nerve (Møller & Jannetta, 1985a). Further, the techniques that will be described herein for facial nerve monitoring are generalizable to monitoring of other motor cranial nerves (e.g., Maloney, Murcek, Steehler, Sibly, & Maloney, 1994; Rice & Cone-Wesson, 1990; Yingling, 1994).

Background/Technique

In facial nerve monitoring we record motor unit activity from muscles innervated by the facial nerve. A motor unit consists of the nerve cell body (the alpha motor neuron), the motor nerve axon, and the terminal branches of the axon and muscle fibers supplied by these branches. When a motor neuron is depolarized electrically (e.g., with an electrical probe) a traveling wave is initiated that ends at the junction of the nerve and muscle (i.e., the myoneural junction). It is important to note that not all nerve fibers respond to the same electrical stimulus. That is, nerve fibers that are heavily myelinated have low thresholds to electrical stimulation and conduct quickly, whereas nerve fibers that are less well myelinated have higher thresholds to electrical stimulation and conduct more slowly. The magnitude of electrical stimulation that defines the point at which all neurons are responding is called "supramaximal stimulation."

A motor unit action potential (MUAP) occurs when the action potential reaches the myoneural junction. This results in a brief (1–4 msec) contraction of the muscle fiber followed by a relaxation phase. When all of the muscle fibers are depolarized, a compound muscle action potential (CMAP) can be recorded from the skin overlying the muscle. At supramaximal stimulation levels not all muscle fibers of a given muscle innervated by a motor cranial nerve contract simultaneously (due to the differing fiber diameters and conduction velocities of the various nerve fibers comprising the motor nerve). Therefore, the duration of a CMAP may be 5 to 12 msec in duration. There are a number of parameters that one may use to quantify the MUAP or CMAP, including latency of onset and area under the curve. However, the amplitude of the response is the metric most often employed to evaluate facial nerve function. The amplitude of the CMAP is related to the number of viable nerve fibers and their conduction velocities (i.e., the larger the number of synchronized nerve fibers, the larger the number of MUAPs responding per unit time, which results in a larger CMAP amplitude).

It is important to be aware that like sensory nerves, motor nerves may be stimulated along their course. Thus, if a motor cranial nerve is stimulated midway along its course, an action potential will be propagated both back to the brainstem (antidromic conduction) and toward the muscle (orthodromic conduction). It is possible for a nerve to be depolarized electrically (i.e., with an electrical probe), thermically (i.e., increasing or decreasing depolarization threshold by increasing or decreasing temperature of the nerve), or mechanically (i.e., with a surgical instrument). Therefore, it might be expected (and it is true) that it is possible to record evoked muscle contractions to each of these modes of stimulation.

The goal of the surgeon who resects tumors in the posterior fossa is to remove the tumor and leave the motor nerve both anatomically and physiologically intact. There are two purposes for facial nerve monitoring. The first objective is to identify the facial nerve in the surgical field. Often tumors overlie and compress the facial nerve to the point where it is flattened ("splayed out") and appears similar in color and substance to the tumor. Additionally, tumors may grow into and/or become adherent to the facial nerve. Thus, it becomes essential for a surgeon to have the ability to identify all that *is*, and alternately, to identify all that *is not* the facial nerve. The application of a pulsed current to what might be nerve and the recording of electrical activity from muscles innervated by that nerve is an effective method of mapping the location of the motor nerve. This makes it possible to resect all tissue that does not activate muscles innervated by the cranial nerve of interest.

A second purpose of facial nerve monitoring is to identify impending facial nerve injury. In the process of tumor resection, it is possible for the VIIn to be stretched, compressed, scraped, burned, and transected. Each of these events can result in depolarization of the facial nerve along its course. The traveling wave resulting from this surgically induced depolarization propagates to muscles innervated by the VIIn. Therefore, it is possible to monitor not only stimulus-evoked muscle activity, but also spontaneous electromyographic activity as a method of determining whether injury to the facial nerve is imminent. The process of functional mapping of the facial nerve during VS surgery was discussed first by Møller and Jannetta (1985b).

Techniques for Facial Nerve Monitoring

Historically, monitoring of the facial nerve fell under the domain of the anesthesiologist. In the early years, monitoring consisted of the anesthesiologist either peering at or feeling the patient's face under the surgical drape when the surgeon stimulated the facial nerve with an electrical probe. The disadvantage of this technique (in addition to the logistical nightmare) was that if current from the electrical source spread to the motor division of the trigeminal nerve, contraction of the masseter muscle might have been misinterpreted as a contraction of one of the muscles innervated by the facial nerve.

There have been principally two methods offered to monitor facial nerve function. Both methods involved attempts to depolarize the facial nerve in the surgical field and record evidence of facial nerve depolarization (i.e., facial muscle contractions) distal to the site of stimulation. The first technique (and the one that will be emphasized in this section) involves the recording of EMG activity emanating from muscles innervated by the VIIn (both spontaneous and electrically evoked muscle activity). Delgado and colleagues (Delgado, Bucheit, Rosenholtz, & Chrissian, 1979) were the first to report a method of recording evoked facial EMG with conventional EMG instrumentation. A pair of surface-recording electrodes were placed over the frontalis muscle. A ground electrode was placed in front of the ear. The stimulator, resembling a bayonet forcep, served as the cathode. A needle electrode embedded in the surgical wound served as the anode for the stimulator. With few modifications this technique is still being applied to the identification of all motor nerves. The technical variables have centered around whether a monopolar or bipolar stimulating electrode should be employed and whether the electrical source should provide a constant current or voltage level.

The clinician must be aware of potential problems associated with both monopolar and bipolar stimulators. It would be catastrophic if: (1) a piece of questionable tissue were to be electrically stimulated and identified as not being the facial nerve, the tissue was to be removed and later it was discovered that the tissue was the facial nerve, or (2) a piece of stimulated tissue was identified as being the facial nerve, was later found to be tumor, and had been left in the head to grow. One potential danger in monopolar stimulation is that current flows from the cathode of the electrical stimulator to the anode. Normally, in monopolar stimulation the cathode of an electrical stimulator is placed on the tissue of interest (nerve) and the anode is placed distally in the wound. If the facial nerve was to be located between the anode and cathode, and if the current level was great enough, then it is possible that the facial nerve would be stimulated and that the tumor being touched by the cathode would be identified as nerve. The possibility of this type of error has led many clinicians to use bipolar electrical stimulation, in which the distance between the anode and cathode is less than a millimeter. It is generally accepted that monopolar stimulators (i.e., a stimulator with the electrical signal leaving the tip and returning to an electrode placed distant from the stimulator in the wound) are best used for gross nerve identification (i.e., to determine whether the VIIn is in the near vicinity of the stimulating electrode). Alternately, a bipolar stimulator (i.e., stimulator where both cathode and anode are contained at the tip) is best used when great sensitivity is required to determine whether individual strands of tissue are tumor or nerve. The present author published a photograph of a "homemade" bipolar stimulator in 1987 (Jacobson & Tew, 1987). Many investigators have developed and patented versions of both monopolar and bipolar stimulators and these are available commercially.

It is noteworthy that controversy has surrounded the use of constant voltage versus constant current stimulators for facial nerve identification. Møller and Jannetta (1984a) have advocated the use of a monopolar constant voltage stimulator. Their rationale was that the effectiveness of constant current stimulation varies as a function of the degree of electrical shunting caused by cerebrospinal fluid (CSF). The level of current needed to effectively stimulate a nerve must be increased if a large amount of the current is shunted to the CSF. If the current is increased and the shunting of current were to decrease suddenly, then the effective electrical current applied to the nerve might be of a sufficient magnitude to cause it permanent damage. However, Kartush and colleagues (Kartush, Niparko, Bledsoe, Graham, & Kemink, 1985) reported that insulating stimulating electrodes down to the tip (tips left uninsulated) prevented shunting of current to the cerebrospinal fluid. Yokoyama, Uemura, and Ryn (1991) demonstrated that the spread of current (0.5–0.6 mA, .1 msec duration) from an insulated *monopolar* electrode was approximately 1 mm. Under these conditions constant current stimulation was as effective as constant voltage stimulation.

In practice, electrode wires (either standard, sterilized EEG needle electrodes or hook wire electrodes) are placed in at least two locations representing muscles innervated by two differing divisions of the facial nerve. The orbicularis oculi and the orbicularis oris muscles represent two sphincter muscles that easily are accessible. Although hook wire electrodes have been recommended by some, our recommendation is the use of paired, prepackaged, sterile, disposable, platinum EEG needle electrodes inserted into each of the facial muscles. An interelectrode distance of 1 to 2 cm is recommended. The electrodes should be secured with tape. The constant current electrical stimulus for monopolar stimulation should not exceed 1 mA. When a bipolar stimulator is used (i.e., the facial nerve is identified and there is little if any tissue interposed between the nerve and stimulator), constant current stimulation levels of .1 to .25 mA should not be exceeded. The stimulation rates are typically in the range of 2 to 5 Hz. The EMG signals are amplified ($\times$ 10,000) and filtered 10 or 100 Hz to 5000–10,000 Hz. The amplified signal may be routed either to an oscilloscope screen and/or routed to an audio amplifier so that the EMG signal can be made audible for the surgeon.

A second technique for facial nerve monitoring was developed by Silverstein and colleagues (Silverstein, Smouha, & Jones, 1988a, 1988b; Silverstein Nerve Stimulator Monitor) and involves the application of a strain-gauge sensor to the corner of the patient's mouth (corner consistent with the side of surgery). Application of electrical pulses to the facial nerve or inadvertent mechanical stimulation of the facial nerve results in facial muscle contractions (orbicularis oris muscle) and an audible warning signal emitted by the device. The reported advantage of this device is that electrical artifacts mimicking EMG activity caused by metal contacting metal in the surgical field do not serve as a contaminant for motion detectors.

A third technique not often used and first reported by Richmond and Mahla (1985) represents an attempt to assess the conductivity of the facial nerve through antidromic stimulation. In this technique the facial nerve is stimulated in the periphery (e.g., at the stylomastoid foramen) and the antidromically propagated action potential is recorded directly from the facial nerve proximal to the brainstem. This near-field technique should make it possible to evaluate the conductivity of the facial nerve in the presence of complete muscle paralysis. However, this technique has not received widespread use. It is likely that problems retaining the recording electrode in the surgical field during aggressive resection of tumor coupled with stimulus artifact contamination has made this technique unpracticeable.

Effects of Anesthetic Agents

It has been felt widely that for facial nerve monitoring to be successful patients had to be completely unparalyzed. That is, it was believed that the use of even small amounts of muscle relaxant medications would create a situation where direct intracranial stimulation of the facial nerve would not result in evoked EMG activity. The level of paralysis is assessed by the anesthesiologist with the aid of an electrical stimulator that usually is applied over the ulnar nerve. A train of four electrical pulses is delivered to the nerve superficially and the number of resulting twitches of the hypothenar muscle are counted. The finding of zero twitches out of four delivered normally is felt to represent complete muscle paralysis. The results of two recent publications have challenged the belief that no muscle depolarizing medications could be tolerated. Both Lennon and colleagues (Lennon, Hosking, Daube, & Welna, 1992) and Blair and colleagues (Blair, Teeple, Sutherland, Shih, & Chen, 1994) have reported that stimulus evoked EMG activity (i.e., elicited by an electrical probe) could be elicited at even 75% attenuation of the EMG response elicited by peripheral nerve stimulation (ulnar nerve and sciatic nerve). The differential effect of muscle relaxant medications on musculature innervated by peripheral nerves was explained as occurring because of the larger motor units and or the increased number of neuromuscular junctions for muscles of facial expression.

Representative Findings (Interpretation)

Stimulus-Evoked EMG. Four methods have been described to quantify and prognosticate quality of function of the facial nerve following surgery. All four methods are based upon the concept that if the facial nerve is intact functionally, stimulation of the nerve at the brainstem at a given stimulus intensity will evoke the same magnitude of EMG activity as stimulation of the nerve distal to the site of surgery. The four methods that have been described include: (1) stimulation of the proximal (brainstem) segment of the VIIn with a fixed amplitude current pulse (0.05 mA). If the evoked EMG response is equal to or greater than 500 µV, the prognosis is good that the VIIn will function postoperatively (Beck, Atkins, Benecke, & Brackman, 1991). (2) Stimulation of the nerve at a fixed supramaximal level at distal and proximal points and measuring the *absolute amplitude* of evoked EMG activity obtained at each location (Nuwer et al., 1993; Prass, Kinney, Hardy, Hahn, & Luders, 1987b). (3) Assessment of evoked EMG stimulus *thresholds* at the distal and proximal sites ([0.2 mA or 0.2 V threshold shows the best correlation with good facial function postoperatively] Prasad et al., 1993; Selesnick et al., 1996); and (4) stimulation of both distal and proximal sites at supramaximal intensities and creating a ratio of distal/proximal evoked EMG amplitudes (see Figure 9.10; *relative amplitude*) (Jacobson, unpublished observation).

Spontaneous EMG. A series of three reports published in the late 1980s by Prass and colleagues (Prass & Luders, 1986; Prass et al., 1987a, 1987b) served to describe types of spontaneous EMG activity and the significance of each as a portent of surgical outcomes. The types of EMG discharges were well known to electromyographers but had not been described in the context of surgical monitoring in

FACIAL NERVE MONITORING
PROXIMAL STIMULATION OF VII N. IS EQUAL TO DISTAL STIMULATION

38 YO FEMALE, #18095239
LEFT 1 CM INTRACANALICULAR ACOUSTIC NEUROMA

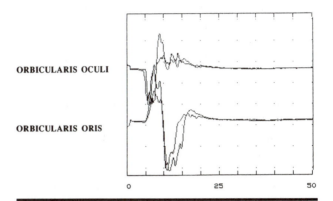

FIGURE 9.10 Stimulus-triggered EMG from orbicularis oculi and orbicularis oris muscles following bipolar stimulation of the distal (at the porus acousticus) and proximal (at brainstem) parts of the VIIn. Note that absolute amplitudes are identical. This patient awoke from surgery with intact facial motor function.

otology. The most common types of spontaneous motor responses are termed "bursts" and "trains." Burst activity (see Figure 9.11) was described by the authors as synchronous nonrepetitive discharges lasting less than one second

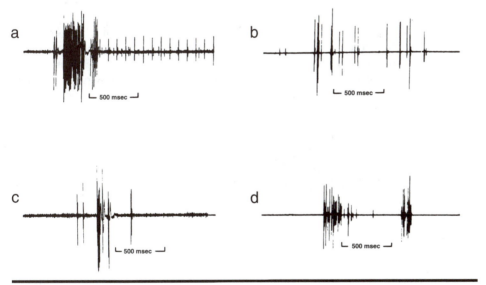

FIGURE 9.11 Various types of burst EMG activity following skeletonization of the internal auditory canal dura over the facial nerve. (A) Burst activity elicited by "limited nerve crush" by an elevating instrument. (B) Burst activity elicited by blunt facial nerve dissection at the brain stem. (C) and (D) Burst activity evoked by squirts of Ringer's solution into the surgical field. Figure from R. L. Prass and H. Luders (1986) Acoustic (loudspeaker) facial electromyographic monitoring: Part 1. *Neurosurgery, 19*: 392–400. Permission provided by Williams and Wilkins, Baltimore, MD.

(usually up to a few hundred msec) and associated in close temporal association with intraoperative triggers (e.g., direct manipulation of the nerve, free irrigation). It is interesting that mechanical stimulation of the nerve (via distortion of the nerve membrane) can result in increases in membrane permeability and the same type of synchronized motor unit activity as electrical stimulation. Sometimes bursts of EMG activity were associated with periods of sustained periodic discharges that could last up to 30 seconds. The authors observed that previously damaged facial nerves were more likely to exhibit burst activity. Burst activity probably represented the synchronized firing of motor unit potentials to single discharge of facial nerve axons. This type of spontaneous activity in isolation was not associated with permanent nerve injury and often was a precursor to trains of EMG discharges.

EMG trains (also called neurotonic discharge) were described by Prass and colleagues (Prass & Luders, 1986; Prass et al., 1987a, 1987b) as repetitive discharges of up to 100Hz with varying latency (with respect to the triggering event) and amplitude (see Figure 9.12). The entrained activity could last up to several minutes. Train activity occurred often with traction of the facial nerve in a lateral to medial direction. The delay between the trigger and the discharges could be as brief as a few seconds and as long as 2 to 3 minutes. The activity might end after retraction was lessened but could take as long as a few minutes. The train activity probably occurred as a function of repetitive firing of one or more motor units. The repetitive firing occurred due to the maintenance of the axonal membrane potential above that of the action potential threshold (due to traction injury). Frequent and extended neurotonic discharges often are associated with permanent nerve injury. In the present author's experience there have been at least two instances where neurotonic discharges occurred for periods in excess

of 30 minutes where patients awoke with a fully functional VIIn. However, this occurs seldom, and in most cases neurotonia is a portent of poor postoperative facial nerve function.

Common Applications of Facial Nerve Monitoring

Vestibular Schwannoma Surgery.   There have been a plethora of papers that have accumulated over the years attesting to the efficacy of facial nerve monitoring for preservation of function during removal of VS. Generally, these investigations have compared the outcomes of patients undergoing surgery for VS either with or without the benefit of facial nerve monitoring. The quality of facial nerve outcome has been evaluated using the House-Brackmann scale (Table 9.6). The results of these investigations have led to unanimity of support for facial nerve monitoring in surgery for removal of VS (NIH Consensus Development Conference, 1991). For example, Benecke and colleagues (1987) reported their experiences monitoring 18 consecutive VSs removed through the translabyrinthine technique. Of this sample 17 had House grade I or II. Harner and colleagues (1988) evaluated the quality of outcomes of two groups of patients undergoing a total of 264 excisions. The facial nerve was preserved in 92% of monitored and 84% of unmonitored patients. Furthermore, the facial nerve was preserved in 100% of patients with small tumors (regardless of whether they underwent facial nerve monitoring), 95% and 90% of monitored and unmonitored patients respectively with medium-sized tumors, and, 71% versus 41% of monitored versus unmonitored patients respectively with large tumors. Hammerschlag and Cohen (1990) estimated the prevalence in their practice of facial nerve weakness postoperatively prior to (207 surgeries) compared with after the advent of (111 surgeries) facial nerve monitoring.

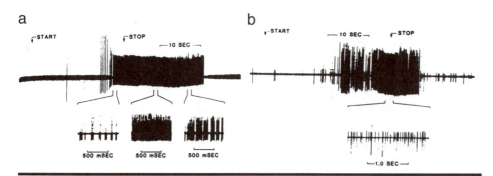

FIGURE 9.12   Two different types of acoustical train-type EMG activity (referred to as "bomber" [A] and "popcorn" [B] patterns by the authors). These EMG trains were observed during lateral-to-medial traction applied to the VIIn during tumor debulking with a Cavitron Ultrasonic Surgical Aspirator (CUSA). (From R. L. Prass and H. Luders (1986), Acoustic (loudspeaker) facial electromyographic monitoring: Part 1. *Neurosurgery, 19*: 392–400. Permission granted by Williams and Wilkins, Baltimore, MD.)

TABLE 9.6 House-Brackmann system of grading facial nerve function.

Grade I: **Normal**
Normal facial function in all areas.

Grade II: **Mild Dysfunction**
Gross: Slight weakness noticeable on close inspection. May have slight synkinesis. At rest, normal symmetry and tone.
Motion: Forehead, moderate-to-good function. Eye, complete closure with minimal effort. Mouth slight asymmetry.

Grade III: **Moderate Dysfunction**
Gross: Obvious but not disfiguring difference between two sides. Noticeable but not severe synkinesis, contracture or hemifacial spasm, or both. At rest, normal symmetry and tone.
Motion: Forehead, slight-to-moderate movement. Eye, complete closure with effort. Mouth, slightly weak with maximum effort.

Grade IV: **Moderately Severe Dysfunction**
Gross: Obvious weakness or disfiguring asymmetry, or both. At rest, normal symmetry and tone.
Motion: Forehead, none. Eye, incomplete closure. Mouth, asymmetric with maximum effort.

Grade V: **Severe Dysfunction**
Gross: Only barely perceptible motion. At rest, asymmetry.
Motion: Forehead, none. Eye, incomplete closure. Mouth, slight movement.

Grade VI: **Total Paralysis**
No movement.

From House & Brackmann, 1985.

Results indicated that the prevalence of paralysis was 14.5% prior to and 3.6% following the implementation of cranial nerve monitoring techniques. Kwartler and colleagues (1991) compared outcomes in 89 monitored compared with 155 unmonitored VS removals. The investigators evaluated facial function in the immediate postoperative period, at the time of discharge, and at one year postoperatively. Facial nerve function was better overall in the monitored group but not significantly so one year after surgery. It is worthy of noting that delayed facial nerve weakness or paralysis in the first few postoperative days has been reported in as many as 41% of patients undergoing resection of VS (Lalwani, Yuan-Shin Butt, Jackler, Pitts, &

1995). Lalwani and colleagues (1994) reported that 98% of patients with facial nerve EMG thresholds of 0.2 V or less at the end of surgery had House-Brackmann grades I or II facial function at one year postoperatively. Jellinek and co-workers (1991) reported their experience with continuous facial nerve monitoring. In their series, 94% of facial nerves were preserved anatomically in the monitored group compared with 64% in the unmonitored group. Where the facial nerve was anatomically preserved (n = 33) 64% had function in the postoperative period. Further, they reported that functional preservation was achieved in only 39% of anatomically preserved facial nerves prior to the implementation of facial monitoring.

Neurovascular Decompression (NVD). The second common type of facial nerve monitoring is associated with the correction of neurovascular compression of cranial nerves (described earlier). The theory behind the disorder is that the process of aging results in the elongation of arteries and sagging of the brain. The redundancy of arterial loops can cause cross compression of cranial nerves at their REZs. Local irritation caused by the pressure of the artery or vessels coupled with persistent pulsation of the vasculature on the nerve leads to focal demyelination. It is believed that cross compression of the VIIn results in hemifacial spasm (i.e., the face spasms with each pulsation of the vessel or artery). There are two theories as to how compression of the facial nerve at the REZ results in hemifacial spasm (HFS). Nielsen (1986) has hypothesized that HFS is caused by ectopic excitation and ephaptic transmission. In this theory cross compression of the nerve results in focal demyelination at the site of compression. The demyelination acts to lower the calcium level in the perinodal medium, making it possible for extracellular currents to flow during the passage of impulses in adjacent nerve fibers. This results in the initiation of impulses in affected nerve fibers by impulses traveling in adjacent nerve fibers. These false synapses are referred to as ephapses.

A second theory has been offered by Møller and Jannetta (1985b). These investigators suggested that the focal demyelination caused by the cross compression results in reverberant activity in the facial motor nucleus akin to kindling in epilepsy. In this manner facial nerve damage results in retrograde degeneration to the motor nucleus with resulting synaptic reorganization (i.e., a change occurs in the neuronal connections). Focal irritation caused by cross compression results in increased spontaneous activity in the most affected compressed nerve fibers. This increased spontaneous activity is carried back to the facial motor nucleus and the outflow from this nucleus (due to the synaptic reorganization) spreads like epileptiform activity to facial motor neurons that innervate other muscles. Support for this theory may be found in knowledge that antiseizure medications may serve

HEMIFACIAL SPASM

STIMULATING MARGINAL MANDIBULAR BRANCH OF VII
RECORDING FROM ORBICULARIS OCULI M.

S#08817451, 68 YO MALE
LEFT HEMIFACIAL SPASM

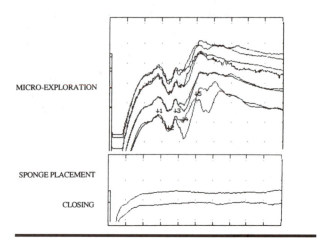

FIGURE 9.13 Electrical evidence of synkinesis disappears following NVD for this patient with HFS. Stimuli were 0.2 msec duration, 5 mA rectangular pulses delivered to the marginal mandibular nerve at a rate of 0.3/sec. Filter bandpass was 30–3000 Hz.

monitoring. As has been described by Møller and Jannetta (1984b, 1985a) the marginal mandibular branch (for example) can be stimulated with electrical pulses at sufficiently long interstimulus intervals (.5 Hz–.3 Hz), and evoked EMG responses may be recorded from the orbicularis oculi muscles (innervated by the zygomatic division of the facial nerve). When decompression has been accomplished, electrophysiological evidence of HFH (i.e., the facial synkinesis due to lateral spread of facial nerve activity) disappears (see Figures 9.13 and 9.14). It has been reported that there is a direct relationship between the success of the NVD procedure and the loss of lateral spread activity as evidenced in evoked EMG recordings (Haines & Torres, 1991; Isu, Kamada, Mabuchi, Kitaoka, Ito, Koiwa, & Abe, 1996). An example of a case where the hemifacial spasm was not completely controlled is shown in Figure 9.15. As noted previously, it is common to monitor ephaptic conduction,

to reduce the severity of HFS. Further support of this theory has been obtained from a comparison of intra- and extracranial measures of VIIn conduction times by Møller and Jannetta (1984b).

Surgery for correction of HFS has been associated with a risk of hearing loss that has ranged from approximately 2.8% to 15%. This risk is due primarily to retraction of the cerebellum to gain adequate visualization of the VIIn and the arterial and venous structures in the posterior fossa. It also is significant to note that incomplete decompression of the VIIn may occur as much as 10% of the time. In these circumstances, patients awaken with a HFS that is decreased in severity somewhat compared with their preoperative function.

The patient with hemifacial spasm generally is elderly and presents with a face that goes in and out of spasm. The spasms increase during emotional stress. The surgical "cure" for hemifacial spasm is the removal of the source of pressure (the arterial loop) from the facial nerve (hence the NVD). One manifestation of HFS (i.e., regardless of the mechanism of disease) is that stimulation of one branch of the facial nerve (e.g., the maxillary branch) in the periphery results in contraction of muscles innervated by a spatially separate branch of the facial nerve (e.g., the mandibular branch). It might be expected that removing the aberrant arterial loop abolishes the lateral spread of EMG activity and it does. This information can be used for purposes of

HEMIFACIAL SPASM

STIMULATING MARGINAL MANDIBULAR BRANCH OF VII
RECORDING FROM ORBICULARIS OCULI M.

S#27684689, 64 YO MALE
RIGHT HEMIFACIAL SPASM

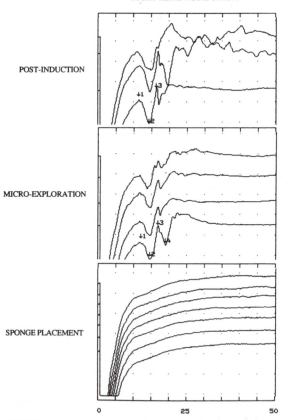

FIGURE 9.14 Electrical evidence of synkinesis disappears following NVD for another patient with HFS. Stimulating and recording parameters as reported in Figure 9.13.

HEMIFACIAL SPASM

STIMULATING MARGINAL MANDIBULAR BRANCH OF VII
RECORDING FROM ORBICULARIS OCULI M.

S#23137185, 42YO FEMALE
LEFT HEMIFACIAL SPASM

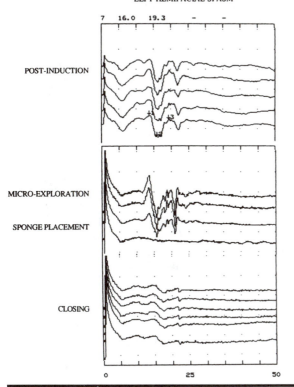

FIGURE 9.15 Patient for whom NVD did not result in a complete loss of HFS. Note small residual electrical evidence of synkinesis at the end of surgery (bottom of figure). Stimulation and recording parameters as reported in Figure 9.13.

ABR, and direct recorded CAP during NVD, and an example of this is shown in Figure 9.16.

OTHER ISSUES

On Site versus Remote Monitoring/Attended versus Nonattended Monitoring

There are a number of philosophical issues associated with neurophysiological monitoring. There are monitorists who support the use of devices (notably facial nerve monitoring devices) that do not require that sophisticated personnel be in attendance to interpret the data. Two devices of this type include the Nerve Integrity Monitor II (NIM II Xomed-Treace) and the Silverstein Nerve Stimulator Monitor. To operate these devices one need only apply subdermal needle electrodes (for the NIM II) or a strain gauge device to the corner of the mouth (for the Silverstein Nerve Stimulator Monitor). Depolarization of the facial nerve is associated with EMG activity that activates a warning tone. The advantage of these devices is that monitorists are not required for the interpretation of either evoked or spontaneous EMG activity over the course of the resection of a tumor. The disadvantage of these automated devices is that electrical artifacts can occur (e.g., metal instruments striking one another) that initiate electrical potentials not associated with EMG activity. If the artifactual electrical activity is not identified as such by the surgeon, it is possible that the surgical technique might be altered inappropriately (i.e., the surgeon may falsely think that the facial nerve is imperiled).

A second philosophical issue is whether it is necessary for a supervising monitorist to be in attendance during intraoperative monitoring. That is, is it possible (or ethical) for a supervising monitorist to place technologists in an operating room in one hospital to monitor a case and for the monitorist to be physically in another building (city, or state) observing the case through remote methods. Current technologies permit almost online transmission of evoked potential data through modem communications. It is my feeling that the monitoring staff places themselves and the patient at jeopardy by not being physically present during every procedure. At the very least the monitorist should be within 1 or 2 minutes access to the technologist support staff.

Documentation in Monitoring

Every person who performs an extended service in the operating room is obligated to generate a summary report at the end of the surgical procedure. The report can range from brief to extended narrative summaries of the monitoring activities that occurred during the procedure. The monitoring report has assumed greater importance as health financing issues surrounding reimbursement for monitoring and medicolegal issues associated with monitoring become more pressing. Like the anesthesia record, a dictated summary report with the monitoring record (i.e., the table containing latency and amplitude values associated with intraoperative events) should be entered into the patient's hospital chart. The monitoring record should include: (1) all of the patient identification data; (2) the name of the surgeon/s and anesthesia personnel; (3) the time the recordings began; (4) the side of stimulation (where appropriate); (5) the numeric data, including amplitude and latencies of the pertinent evoked potential peaks throughout surgery; (6) the surgical activities that occurred during the interval when the data was collected; (7) the esophageal temperature; (8) the names of the anesthetics that were being used at the time the data was collected, their concentrations, and their mode of administration (IV drip versus bolus injection); and (9) any additional useful data.

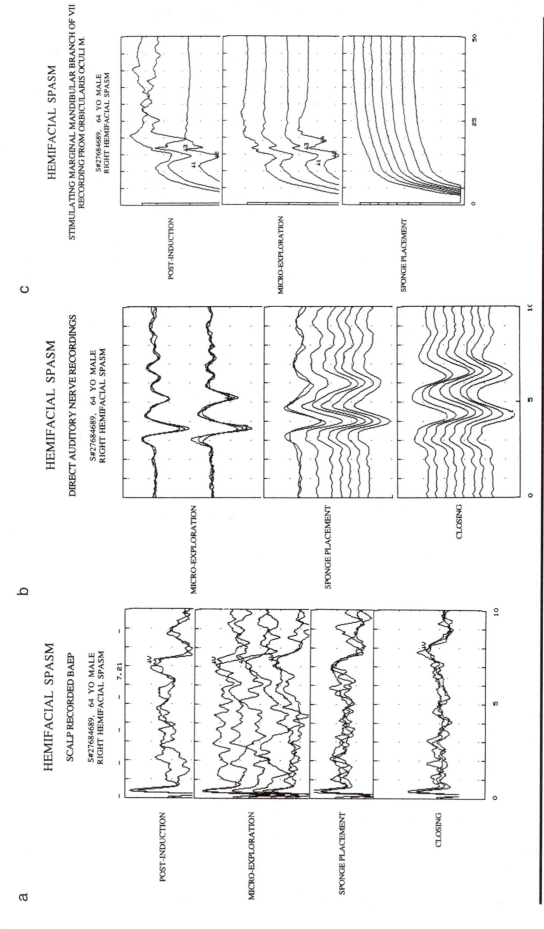

FIGURE 9.16 ABR (A), direct VIIIn CAP (B), and evoked facial EMG (C; ephaptic transmission) obtained from a patient undergoing NVD for HFS. Note that at the point of sponge placement the CAP broadens and there is a concomitant increase in Wave V latency (between sponge placement and closing). This patient had no significant change in his preoperative audiogram.

Credentialing for Providing IOM Services

In 1990 the Report of the Therapeutics and Technology Assessment Subcommittee of the American Academy of Neurology reported their assessment of intraoperative neurophysiology. In this statement the Committee stated that a "well-trained physician-neurophysiologist needs to provide or supervise monitoring" (p. 1644). Further, they stated that "Experience to date in both humans and controlled animal studies substantiates that several electrophysiology tests and monitoring techniques are safe and efficacious, to a variable degree, as commonly applied in the operating room . . . (including) . . . BAEP and cranial nerve EMG monitoring during posterior fossa procedures" (p. 1645). These statements on the one hand provide support that ABR and facial nerve monitoring are efficacious, but on the other hand support the belief that only a physician may supervise and provide these services. It is beliefs such as these by our physician colleagues that has led to the current state where only physicians may be reimbursed for professional components of monitoring services.

It is the present author's view that the future of neurophysiological monitoring will be bright as long as surgeons feel that monitoring nervous system function during surgery is essential. The sensitivity of imaging techniques has improved to the extent that evoked potentials are in danger of becoming redundant for the detection of tumors and demyelinating lesions. However, electrophysiological recordings are the only good method of measuring in a continuous manner the functional integrity of the nervous system during surgery. Those who have attempted to develop monitoring programs in major hospitals may have encountered resistance from their neurology colleagues. In fact, as a general statement, physician clinical neurophysiologists (e.g., electromyographers and electroencephalographers) are much better prepared to provide full-scale intraoperative evaluations of nervous system function than are nonphysician health professionals. Alternately, audiologists (for the most part) are better prepared to monitor auditory system function than are their physician colleagues. The audiologist who wishes to compete with the neurologist must acknowledge that EEG, EMG, and (for the most part) multimodality evoked potentials are the neurologists' "turf." If we are to compete with physicians to provide monitoring services, it is incumbent for all audiologists to become highly skilled in this area. It is by becoming highly skilled and respected by physicians and surgeons that we gain entry to the operating room.

There exists at this time a problem for non-physicians who wish to practice intraoperative monitoring. Specifically, there is not a means by which non-physicians can become credentialed to perform monitoring. This credentialing issue has acted as an impediment for non-physicians to bill and collect payment for professional services. Physician neurologists may become certified to perform neurodiagnostic testing through examinations administered under the auspices of the American Society of Electrodiagnostic Medicine and the American Board of Psychiatry and Neurology. Additionally, electroneurodiagnostic technologists through their membership in the American Society of Electroneurodiagnostic Technologists may obtain CNIM certification (Certification in Neurophysiological Intraoperative Monitoring), if they pass an examination sanctioned by the American Board of Registry for Electroneurodiagnostic Technologists (ABRET). However, technologists by their Code of Ethics cannot interpret the data they acquire. Therefore, although IOM falls within the audiologist's scope of practice (according to the American Academy of Audiology and the American Speech-Language-Hearing Association), only physicians may bill and collect for the professional components of monitoring services. It is our hope that speciality recognition (or credentialing) through our national organizations may make it possible in the future for audiologists to bill for professional services.

REFERENCES

Abramson, M., Stein, B. M., Pedley, T. A., Emerson, R. G., & Wazen, J. J. (1985). Intraoperative BAER monitoring and hearing preservation in the treatment of acoustic neuromas. *Laryngoscope, 95,* 1318–1321.

American Academy of Neurology. (1990). Report of the Therapeutics and Technology Assessment Subcommittee. Assessment: Intraoperative neurophysiology. *Neurology, 40,* 1644–1646.

American Electroencephalographic Society. (1994). Guideline eleven: Guidelines for intraoperative monitoring. *Journal of Clinical Neurophysiology, 11,* 77–87.

American Speech-Language-Hearing Association. (1996, Spring). Scope of practice in audiology. *Asha, 38* (Supplement), 16.

Arenberg, I. K., Obert, A. D., & Gibson, W. P. R. (1991). Intraoperative electrocochleographic monitoring of inner ear surgery for endolymphatic hydrops. *Acta Otolaryngologica, Supplement 485,* 53–64.

Arenberg, I. K., Kobayashi, H., Obert, A. D., & Gibson, W. P. R. (1993). Intraoperative electrocochleography of endolymphatic hydrops surgery using clicks and tone bursts. *Acta Otolaryngologica, Supplement 504,* 58–67.

Auger, R. G., Peipgras, D. G., & Laws, E. R. (1986). Hemifacial spasm: Results of microvascular decompression of the facial nerve in 54 patients. *Mayo Clinical Proceedings, 61,* 640–644.

Beck, D. L., Atkins, J. S., Benecke, J. E., & Brackmann, D. E. (1991). Intraoperative facial nerve monitoring: Prognostic aspects during acoustic tumor removal. *Archives of Otolaryngology—Head and Neck Surgery, 104,* 780–782.

Benecke, J. E., Calder, H. B., & Chadwick, G. (1987). Facial nerve monitoring during acoustic tumor removal. *Laryngoscope, 97,* 697–700.

Blair, E. A., Teeple, E. Jr., Sutherland, R. M., Shih, T., & Chen, D. (1994). Effect of neuromuscular blockade on facial nerve monitoring. *American Journal of Otology, 15,* 161–167.

Bojrab, D. I., Bhansali, S. A., & Andreozzi, M. P. (1994). Intraoperative electrocochleography during endolymphatic sac surgery: Clinical results. *Archives of Otolaryngology—Head and Neck Surgery, 111,* 478–484.

Branston, N. M., Ladds, A., Symon, L., & Wang, A. D. (1984). Comparison of the effects of ischaemia on early components of the somatosensory evoked potential in brainstem, thalamus, and cerebral cortex. *Journal of Cerebral Blood Flow and Metabolism, 4,* 68–81.

Brown, R. H., Nash, C. L., Berilla, J. A., & Amaddio, M. D. (1984). Cortical evoked potential monitoring. A system for intraoperative monitoring of spinal cord function. *Spine, 9,* 256–261.

Cacace, A. T., Parnes, S. M., Lovely, T. J., & Kalathia, A. (1994). The disconnected ear: Phenomenological effects of a large acoustic tumor. *Ear and Hearing, 15,* 287–298.

Cane, M. A., O'Donoghue, G. M., & Lutman, M. E. (1992). The feasibility of using oto-acoustic emissions to monitor cochlear function during acoustic neuroma surgery. *Scandinavian Audiology, 21,* 173–176.

Chandrasekhar, S. S., de la Cruz, A., & Garrido, E. (1995). Surgery of congenital aural atresia. *American Journal of Otology, 16,* 713–717.

Cohen, N. L., Hammerschlag, P., Berg, H., & Ransohoff, J. (1986). Acoustic neuroma surgery: An eclectic approach with emphasis on preservation of hearing. The New York University—Bellevue experience. *Annals of Otology, Rhinology and Laryngology, 95,* 21–27.

Colletti, V., & Fiorino, F. G. (1993). Electrophysiologic identification of the cochlear nerve fibers during cerebello-pontine angle surgery. *Acta Otolaryngologica, 113,* 746–754.

Colletti, V., & Fiorino, F. G. (1994). Vulnerability of hearing function during acoustic neuroma surgery. *Acta Otolaryngologica, 114,* 264–270.

Dauman, R., Aran J., Savage, R., & Portmann, M. (1988). Clinical significance of the summating potential in Ménière's disease. *American Journal of Otology, 9,* 31–38.

Delgado, T. E., Bucheit, W. A., Rosenholtz, H. R., & Chrissian, S. (1979). Intraoperative monitoring of facial muscle evoked responses obtained by intracranial stimulation of the facial nerve: A more accurate technique for facial nerve dissection. *Neurosurgery, 4,* 418–421.

Eggermont, J. J. (1979). Summating potentials in Ménière's disease. *Otolaryngology, 222,* 63–75.

Esses, B. A., LaRouere, M. J., & Graham, M. D. (1994). Facial nerve outcome in acoustic tumor surgery. *American Journal of Otology, 15,* 810–812.

Fisher, C., Ibanez, V., & Mauguiere, F. (1985). Monitorage peroperatoire des potentials evokques auditifs precoces. *Presse Medicale, 14,* 1914–1918.

Fisher, R. S., Raudzens, P., & Nunemacher, M. (1995). Efficacy of intraoperative neurophysiological monitoring. *Journal of Clinical Neurophysiology, 12,* 97–109.

Friedman, W. A., Kaplan, B. J., Gravenstein, D., & Rhoton, A. L. (1985). Intraoperative brain-stem auditory evoked potentials during posterior fossa microvascular decompression. *Journal of Neurosurgery, 62,* 552–557.

Gantz, B. J., Brown, C., & Abbas, P. J. (1994). Intraoperative measures of electrically evoked auditory nerve compound action potential. *American Journal of Otology, 15,* 137–144.

Gibson, W. P. R. (1991). The use of electrocochleography in the diagnosis of Ménière's disease. *Acta Otolaryngologica, 273 (Supplement 485),* 46–52.

Grabb, P. A., Albright, A. L., Sclabassi, R. J. & Pollack, I. F. (1997). Continuous intraoperative electromyographic monitoring of cranial nerves during resection of fourth ventricular tumors in children. *Journal of Neurosurgery, 86,* 1–4.

Green, J. D., Brackmann, D. E., Nguyen, C. D., Arriaga, M. A., Telischi, F. F., & de la Cruz, A. (1994). Surgical management of previously untreated glomus jugulare tumors. *Laryngoscope, 104,* 917–921.

Grundy, B. L., Jannetta, P. J., Procopio, P. T., Lina, A., Boston, J. R., & Doyle, E. (1982). Intraoperative monitoring of brainstem auditory evoked potentials. *Journal of Neurosurgery, 57,* 674–681.

Haines, S. J., & Torres, F. (1991). Intraoperative monitoring of the facial nerve during decompression surgery for hemifacial spasm. *Journal of Neurosurgery, 74,* 254–257.

Hammerschlag, P. E., & Cohen, N. L. (1990). Intraoperative monitoring of facial nerve function in cerebellopontine angle surgery. *Archives of Otolaryngology—Head and Neck Surgery, 103,* 681–684.

Harner, S. G., Daube, J. R., Beatty, C. W., & Ebersold, M. J. (1988). Intraoperative monitoring of the facial nerve. *Laryngoscope, 98,* 209–212.

Harner, S. G., Harper, C. M., Beatty, C. W., Litchy, W. J. & Ebersold, M. J. (1996). Far-field auditory brainstem response in neurotologic surgery. *American Journal of Otology, 17,* 150–153.

Hickey, S. A., & Fitzgerald O'Connor, A. F. (1991). Measurement of drill-generated noise levels during ear surgery. *Journal of Laryngology and Otology, 105,* 732–735.

House, J. W., & Brackmann, D. E. (1985). Facial nerve grading system. *Archives of Otolaryngology—Head and Neck Surgery, 93,* 146–147.

Isu, T., Kamada, K., Mabuchi, S., Kitaoka, A., Ito, T., Koiwa, M., & Abe, H. (1996). Intra-operative monitoring by facial electromyographic responses during microvascular decompressive surgery for hemifacial spasm. *Acta Neurochirogia, 138,* 19–23.

Jackler, R. K. (1994). Overview of surgical neurotology. In R. K. Jackler & D. E. Brackmann (Eds.), *Neurotology* (pp. 651–684). St. Louis: Mosby.

Jackler, R. K., & Brackmann, D. E. (1994). *Neurotology.* St. Louis: Mosby.

Jackler, R. K., & Selesnick, S. H. (1994). Indications for cranial nerve monitoring during otologic and neurotologic surgery. Synopsis of a panel held at the annual meeting of the American Otological Society, Los Angeles, California, April 1993. *American Journal of Otology, 15,* 611–613.

Jacobson, G. P., & Balzer, G. (1992). Basic considerations in intraoperative monitoring. In J. M. Kartush & K. R. Bouchard (Eds.), *Neuromonitoring in Otology and Head and Neck Surgery* (pp. 21–60). Raven Press: New York.

Jacobson, G. P., Newman, C. W., Monsell, E., & Wharton, J. A. (1993). False negative auditory brainstem response findings in vestibular schwannoma: Case reports. *Journal of the American Academy of Audiology, 4,* 355–359.

Jacobson, G. P., & Tew, J. M. (1987). Intraoperative evoked potential monitoring. *Journal of Clinical Neurophysiology, 4,* 145–176.

Jacobson, G. P., & Yeh, H. S. (1985). The auditory brainstem response in surgical monitoring: the pathological significance of a reduced P1-P5 interwave interval. *Clinical Electroencephalography, 16*, 83–87.

Jahrsdoerfer, R. A. (1995). Transposition of the facial nerve in congenital aural atresia. *American Journal of Otolology, 16*, 290–294.

Jellinek, D. A., Tan, L. C., & Symon, L. (1991). The impact of continuous electrophysiological monitoring on preservation of the facial nerve during acoustic tumour surgery. *British Journal of Neurosurgery, 5*, 19–24.

Kanzaki, J., Ogawa, K., Shiobara, R., & Toya, S. (1989). Hearing preservation in acoustic neuroma surgery and postoperative audiological findings. *Acta Otolaryngologica, 107*, 474–478.

Kartush, J. M., Niparko, J. K., Bledsoe, S. C., Graham, M. D., & Kemink, J. L. (1985). Intraoperative facial nerve monitoring: A comparison of stimulating electrodes. *Laryngoscope, 95*, 1536–1540.

Kemink, J. L., LaRouere, M. J., Kileny, P. R., Telian, S. A., & Hoff, J. T. (1990). Hearing preservation following suboccipital removal of acoustic neuromas. *Laryngoscope, 100*, 597–602.

Kileny, P. R., & Kemink, J. L. (1987). Electrically evoked middle-latency auditory potentials in cochlear implant candidates. *Archives of Otolaryngology—Head and Neck Surgery, 113*, 1072–1077.

Kileny, P. R., Kemink, J. L., Tucci, D. L., & Hoff, J. T. (1992). Neurophysiologic intraoperative facial and auditory function monitoring in acoustic neuroma surgery. In M. Tos & J. Thomsen (Eds.), *Proceedings of the First International Conference on Acoustic Neuroma* (pp. 569–574). Copenhagen, Denmark, August 25–29. New York: Kugler.

Kileny, P. R., Zwolan, T. A., Zimmerman-Phillips, S., & Telian, S. A. (1994). Electrically evoked auditory brain-stem response in pediatric patients with cochlear implants. *Archives of Otolaryngology—Head and Neck Surgery, 120*, 1083–1090.

Kirkpatrick, P. J., Tierney, P., Gleeson, M. J., & Strong, A. J. (1993). Acoustic tumor volume and prediction of facial nerve functional outcome from intraoperative monitoring. *British Journal of Neurosurgery, 7*, 657–664.

Kveton, J. F. (1990). The efficacy of brainstem auditory evoked potentials in acoustic tumor surgery. *Laryngoscope, 100*, 1171–1173.

Kwartler, J. A., Luxford, W. M., Atkins, J., & Shelton, C. (1991). Facial nerve monitoring in acoustic tumor surgery. *Archives of Otolaryngology—Head and Neck Surgery, 104*, 814–817.

Lalwani, A. K., Yuan-Shin Butt, F., Jackler, R. K., Pitts, L. H., & Yingling, C. D. (1994). Facial nerve outcome after acoustic neuroma surgery: A study from the era of cranial nerve monitoring. *Archives of Otolaryngology—Head and Neck Surgery, 111*, 561–570.

Lalwani, A. K., Yuan-Shin Butt, F., Jackler, R. K., Pitts, L. H., & Yingling, C. D. (1995). Delayed onset facial nerve dysfunction following acoustic neuroma surgery. *American Journal of Otology, 16*, 758–764.

Lambert, P. R. (1988). Major congenital ear malformations: Surgical management and results. *Annals of Otology, Rhinology and Laryngology, 97*, 641–649.

Lennon, R. L., Hosking, M. P., Daube, J. R., & Welna, J. O. (1992). Effect of partial neuromuscular blockage on intraoperative electromyography in patients undergoing resection of acoustic neuromas. *Anesthesia and Analgesia, 75*, 729–733.

Levine, R. A., Bu-Saba, N., & Brown, M. C. (1993). Laser-doppler measurements and electrocochleography during ischemia of the guinea pig cochlea: Implications for hearing preservation in acoustic neuroma surgery. *Annals of Otology, Rhinology and Laryngology, 102*, 127–136.

Levine, R. A., Ojemann, R. G., Montgomery, W. W., & McGaffigan, P. M. (1984). Monitoring auditory evoked potentials during acoustic neuroma surgery. Insights into the mechanism of hearing loss. *Annals of Otology, Rhinology and Laryngology, 93*, 116–123.

Levine, S. C., Margolis, R. H., Fournier, E. M., & Winzenburg, S. M. (1992). Tympanic electrocochleography for evaluation of endolymphatic hydrops. *Laryngoscope, 102*, 614–622.

Linstrom, C. J., & Meiteles, L. Z. (1993). Facial nerve monitoring in surgery or congenital auricular atresia. *Laryngoscope, 103*, 406–415.

Little, J. R., Lesser, R. P., Lueders, H., & Furlan, A. T. (1983). Brainstem auditory evoked potentials in posterior circulation surgery. *Neurosurgery, 12*, 496–502.

Maloney, R. W., Murcek, B. W., Steehler, K. W., Sibly, D., & Maloney, R. E. (1994). A new method for intraoperative recurrent laryngeal nerve monitoring. *ENT Journal, 73*, 30–33.

Margolis, R. H., Rieks, D., Fournier, E. M., & Levine, S. C. (1995). Tympanic electrocochleography for diagnosis of Ménière's disease. *Archives of Otolaryngology—Head and Neck Surgery, 121*, 44–55.

McDaniel, A. B., Silverstein, H., & Norrell, H. (1985). Retrolabyrinthine vestibular neurectomy with and without monitoring of eighth nerve potentials. *American Journal of Otology (Supplement)*, 23–25.

Møller, A. R. (1989). *Evoked Potentials in Intraoperative Monitoring*. Baltimore: Williams and Wilkins.

Møller, A. R., & Jannetta, P. J. (1984a). Preservation of facial nerve function during removal of acoustic neuromas. Use of monopolar constant-voltage stimulation and EMG. *Journal of Neurosurgery, 61*, 757–760.

Møller, A. R., & Jannetta, P. J. (1984b). On the origin of synkinesis in hemifacial spasm: Results of intracranial recordings. *Journal of Neurosurgery, 61*, 569–576.

Møller, A. R., & Jannetta, P. J. (1985a). Microvascular decompression in hemifacial spasm: Intraoperative electrophysiological observations. *Neurosurgery, 16*, 612–618.

Møller, A. R., & Jannetta, P. J. (1985b). Monitoring of facial nerve function during removal of acoustic tumor. *American Journal of Otology (Supplement)*, 27–29.

Møller, A. R., Jannetta, P. J., & Jho, H. D. (1994a). Click-evoked responses from the cochlear nucleus: A study in humans. *Electroencephalography and Clinical Neurophysiology, 92*, 215–224.

Møller, A. R., Jho, H. D., & Jannetta, P. J. (1994b). Preservation of hearing in operations on acoustic tumors: An alternative to recording brain stem auditory evoked potentials. *Neurosurgery, 34*, 688–693.

Møller, A. R., & Møller, M. B. (1989). Does intraoperative monitoring of auditory evoked potentials reduce incidence of hearing loss as a complication of microvascular decompression of cranial nerves? *Neurosurgery, 24,* 257–263.

Møller, M. B., & Møller, A. R. (1985). Loss of auditory function in microvascular decompression for hemifacial spasm: Results in 143 consecutive cases. *Journal of Neurosurgery, 63,* 17–20.

Møller, M. B., Møller, A. R., Jannetta, P. J., Jho, H. D., & Sekhar, L. N. (1993). Microvascular decompression of the eighth nerve in patients with disabling positional vertigo: Selection criteria and operative results in 207 patients. *Acta Neurochirurgica, 125,* 75–82.

Molony, T. B., & de la Cruz, A. (1990). Surgical approaches to congenital atresia of the external auditory canal. *Archives of Otolaryngology—Head and Neck Surgery, 103,* 991–1001.

Monsell, E. M., & Shelton, C. (1992). Labyrinthotomy with streptomycin infusion: Early results of a multicenter study. *American Journal of Otology, 13,* 416–422.

Mustain, W. D., Al-Mefty, O., & Anand, V. K. (1992). Inconsistencies in the correlation between loss of brain stem auditory evoked response waves and postoperative deafness. *Journal of Clinical Monitoring, 8,* 231–235.

Nadol, J. B., Levine, R., Ojemann, R. G., Martuza, R. L., Montgomery, W. W., & Klevens de Sandoval, P. (1987). Preservation of hearing in surgical removal of acoustic neuromas of the internal auditory canal and cerebellar pontine angle. *Laryngoscope, 97,* 1287–1294.

Nadol, J. B., Chiong, C. M., Ojemann, R. G., McKenna, M. J., Martuza, R. L., Montgomery, W. W., Levine, R. A., Ronner, S. F., & Glynn, R. J. (1992). Preservation of hearing and facial nerve function in resection of acoustic neuroma. *Laryngoscope, 102,* 1153–1158.

Nedzelski, J. M., Chiong, C. M., Cashman, M. Z., Stanton, S. G., & Rowed, D. W. (1994). Hearing preservation in acoustic neuroma surgery: Value of monitoring cochlear nerve action potentials. *Archives of Otolaryngology—Head and Neck Surgery, 111,* 703–709.

Nielsen, V. K. (1986). Electrophysiology of hemifacial spasm. In M. May (Ed.), *The Facial Nerve* (pp. 487–497). New York: Thieme.

NIH Consensus Development Conference (1991). *Consensus Statement: Acoustic Neuroma, 9,* 1–24.

Nuwer, M. R. (1986). *Evoked Potentials in the Operating Room.* New York: Raven Press

Nuwer, M. R., Daube, J., Fischer, C., Schramm, J., & Yingling, C. D. (1993). Neuromonitoring during surgery. Report of an IFCN committee. *Electroencephalography and Clinical Neurophysiology, 87,* 263–276.

Ojemann, R. G., Levine, R. A., Montgomery, W. W., & McGaffigan, P. (1984). Use of intraoperative auditory evoked potentials to preserve hearing in unilateral acoustic neuromal removal. *Journal of Neurosurgery, 61,* 938–948.

Piatt, J. H., Radke, R. A., & Erwin, C. W. (1985). Limitations of brain stem auditory evoked potentials for intraoperative monitoring during a posterior fossa operation: Case report and technical note. *Neurosurgery, 16,* 818–821.

Prasad, S., Hirsch, B. E., Kamerer, D. B., Durrant, J., & Sekhar, L. N. (1993). Facial nerve function following cerebello-

pontine angle surgery: Prognostic value of intraoperative thresholds. *American Journal of Otology, 14,* 330–333.

Prass, R. L., & Luders, H. (1986). Acoustic (loudspeaker) facial electromyography monitoring: Part 1: Evoked electromyographic activity during acoustic neuroma resection. *Neurosurgery, 19,* 392–400.

Prass, R. L., Kinney, S. E., & Luders, H. (1987a). Transtragal, transtympanic electrode placement for intraoperative electrocochleographic monitoring. *Archives of Otolaryngology—Head and Neck Surgery 97,* 343–350.

Prass, R. L., Kinney, S. E., Hardy, R. W., Hahn, J. F., & Luders, H. (1987b). Acoustic (loudspeaker) facial EMG monitoring: II. Use of evoked EMG activity during acoustic neuroma resection. *Archives of Otolaryngology—Head and Neck Surgery, 97,* 541–551.

Radke, R. A., Erwin, C. W. (1988). Intraoperative monitoring of auditory and brain-stem function. *Neurology Clinics of North America, 6,* 899–915.

Radke, R. A., Erwin, C. W., & Wilkins, R. H. (1989). Intraoperative brainstem auditory evoked potentials: Significant decrease in postoperative morbidity. *Neurology, 39,* 187–191.

Rice, D. H., & Cone-Wesson, B. (1991). Intraoperative recurrent laryngeal nerve monitoring. *Archives of Otolaryngology—Head and Neck Surgery, 105,* 372–375.

Richmond, I. L., & Mahla, M. (1985). Use of antidromic recording to monitor facial nerve function intraoperatively. *Neurosurgery, 16,* 458–462.

Roland, P. S., & Meyerhoff, W. L. (1994). Intraoperative electrophysiological monitoring of the facial nerve: Is it standard of practice? *American Journal of Otolaryngology, 15,* 267–270.

Ruben, R. J., Hudson, W., & Chiong, A. (1963). Anatomical and physiological effects of chronic section of the eighth nerve in cat. *Acta Otolaryngologica, 55,* 473–484.

Sabin, H. I., Prasher, D., Bentivoglio, P., & Symon, L. (1987). Preservation of cochlear potentials in a deaf patient fifteen months after excision of an acoustic neuroma. *Scandinavian Audiology, 16,* 109–111.

Schramm, J., Mosrusch, T., Fahlbusch, R., & Hochstetter, A. (1988). Detailed analysis of intraoperative changes monitoring brainstem acoustic evoked potentials. *Neurosurgery, 22,* 694–702.

Schwaber, M. K., & Hall, J. W. III. (1990). A simplified approach for transtympanic electrocochleography. *American Journal of Otology, 11,* 260–265.

Schwartz, D. M., Gennarelli, T. A., Young, M., Fedder, S. L., & Schwinn, D. (1989). Intraoperative monitoring of brainstem auditory evoked potentials following emergency evacuation of a cerebellar vascular malformation. *Journal of Clinical Monitoring, 5,* 116–118.

Schwender, D., Kaiser, A., Klasing, S., Peter, K., & Poppel, E. (1994). Midlatency auditory evoked potentials and explicit and implicit memory in patients undergoing cardiac surgery. *Anesthesiology, 80,* 493–501.

Sekiya, T., & Møller, A. R. (1987a). Avulsion rupture of the internal auditory artery during operations in the cerebellopontine angle: a study in monkeys. *Neurosurgery, 21,* 631–637.

Sekiya, T., & Møller, A. R. (1987b). Cochlear nerve injuries caused by cerebellopontine angle manipulations. An electrophysiological and morphological study in dogs. *Journal of Neurosurgery, 67,* 244–249.

Selesnick, S. H., Carew, J. F., Victor, J. D., Heise, C. W., & Levine, J. (1996). Predictive value of facial nerve electrophysiologic stimulation thresholds in cerebellopontine-angle surgery. *Laryngoscope, 106,* 633–638.

Silverstein, H., McDaniel, A. B., & Norrell, H. (1985a). Hearing preservation after acoustic neuroma surgery using intraoperative direct eighth cranial nerve monitoring. *American Journal of Otology (Supplement),* 99–106.

Silverstein, H., McDaniel, A., Norrell, H., & Haberkamp, T. (1986). Hearing preservation after acoustic neuroma surgery with intraoperative direct eighth cranial nerve monitoring: Part II. A classification of results. *Archives of Otolaryngology—Head and Neck Surgery, 95,* 285–291.

Silverstein, H., McDaniel, A., Wazen, J., & Norrell, H. (1985b). Retrolabyrinthine vestibular neurectomy with simultaneous monitoring of eighth nerve and brain stem auditory evoked potentials. *Archives of Otolaryngology—Head and Neck Surgery, 93,* 736–742.

Silverstein, H., Smouha, E. E., & Jones, R. (1988a). Routine identification of the facial nerve using electrical stimulation during otological and neurotological surgery. *Laryngoscope, 98,* 726–730.

Silverstein, H., Smouha, E. E., & Jones, R. (1988b). Routine intraoperative facial nerve monitoring during otologic surgery. *American Journal of Otology, 9,* 269–275.

Sindou, M., Fobe, J. L., Ciriano, D., Fischer, C. (1992). Hearing prognosis and intraoperative guidance of brainstem auditory evoked potential in microvascular decompression. *Laryngoscope, 102,* 678–682.

Slavit, D. H., Harner, S. G., Harper, C. M., Jr., & Beatty, C. W. (1991). Auditory monitoring during acoustic neuroma removal. *Archives of Otolaryngology—Head and Neck Surgery, 117,* 1153–1157.

Stanton, S. G., Cashman, M. Z., Harrison, R. V., Nedzelski, J. M., & Rowed, D. W. (1989). Cochlear nerve action potentials during cerebellopontine angle surgery: Relationship of latency, amplitude, and threshold measurements to hearing. *Ear and Hearing, 10,* 23–28.

Symon, L., Sabin, H. I., Bentivoglio, P., Cheesman, A. D., Prasher, D., & Barratt, H. (1988). Intraoperative monitoring of the electrocochleogram and the preservation of hearing during acoustic neuroma excision. *Acta Neurochirurgica (Supplement), 42,* 27–30.

Tator, C. H., & Nedzelski, J. M. (1985). Preservation of hearing in patients undergoing excision of acoustic neuromas and other cerebellopontine angle tumors. *Journal of Neurosurgery, 63,* 168–174.

Telian, S., Kileny, P. R., Niparko, J. K., Kemink, J. L., & Graham, M. D. (1989). Normal auditory brainstem response in patients with acoustic neuroma. *Laryngoscope, 99,* 10–14.

Telischi, F. F., Widick, M. P., Lonsbury-Martin, B. L., & McCoy, M. J. (1995). Monitoring cochlear function intraoperatively using distortion product otoacoustic emissions. *American Journal of Otology, 16,* 597–608.

Uziel, A., Benezech, J., & Frerebeau, P. (1993). Intraoperative facial nerve monitoring in posterior fossa acoustic neuroma surgery. *Archives of Otolaryngology—Head and Neck Surgery, 108,* 126–134.

Wade, P. J., & House, W. (1984). Hearing preservation in patients with acoustic neuromas via the middle fossa approach. *Archives of Otolaryngology—Head and Neck Surgery, 92,* 184–193.

Waring, M. D. (1992). Electrically evoked auditory brainstem response monitoring of auditory brainstem implant integrity during facial nerve tumor surgery. *Laryngoscope, 102,* 1293–1295.

Yingling, C. D. (1994). Intraoperative monitoring of cranial nerves in skull base surgery. In R. K. Jackler & D. E. Brackmann (Eds.), *Neurotology* (pp. 967–1002). St. Louis: Mosby.

Yokoyama, T., Uemura, K., & Ryu, H. (1991). Facial nerve monitoring by monopolar low constant current stimulation during ascoustic neurinoma surgery. *Surgical Neurology, 36,* 12–18.

York, D. H., Chabot, R. J., & Gaines, R. W. (1987). Response variability of somatosensory evoked potentials during scoliosis surgery. *Spine, 12,* 874–876.

CHAPTER 10

PEDIATRIC AUDIOLOGIC ASSESSMENT

JUDITH S. GRAVEL
LINDA J. HOOD

DEVELOPING AN APPROACH TO PEDIATRIC ASSESSMENT

Technology, as well as the demand for quality and cost-effective health care delivery, will only continue to advance in the twenty-first century. These factors will influence not only the test procedures available but also the numbers of individuals who will require services. We should expect that the demand for efficient, high-quality, and cost-effective pediatric audiologic services will only increase in future years, driven by advances in medical care, as well as by public health care policy. With innovative new approaches to evaluation increasingly available, there will be new procedures vying for our consideration. Clinicians will need to go beyond their ability to technically perform certain behavioral and physiologic test procedures: They will need to justify the inclusion of each procedure in their test armamentarium. Inclusion will be determined on outcomes-based evidence, test efficiency, and economics.

Consider, for example, the current activity focused on newborn hearing screening. As the number of programs screening hearing in neonates grows, there will be an increased need to comprehensively assess the hearing of very young infants who have been identified by such screening initiatives as being at risk for hearing loss. Parents and health care providers will demand that audiologic assessments be timely, appropriate, and comprehensive. Interven-tion providers will want details of the infant's hearing loss quickly so that individualized habilitation strategies can be initiated as soon after diagnosis as possible. Primary health care providers and specialists will need data that will assist them in determining the etiology of the hearing loss and the medical follow-up and further evaluations that may be required. Payers will want evidence that audiologists conducting the assessment provided only necessary and reliable services that could be demonstrated to positively influence the child's outcome.

The goal of the current chapter is to address pediatric audiologic assessment in view of what we believe to be both best current and future practice. We begin this chapter with a discussion of the important tenets of pediatric audiologic assessment. Our general approach is to retain those principles and procedures that have served us well, to consider others in new ways, and to abandon some that cannot be demonstrated to contribute reliable and unique information to the diagnostic process.

Family and Team Involvement

A complete assessment of a child's hearing should include information from others who are closely associated with the child. As the degree of diagnostic difficulty increases, the input from these individuals is particularly important. Observations of the child's behavioral responses to sound, characterization of the child's abilities and social responsiveness, and specific knowledge of the child's communication competence are all pertinent to the audiologic assessment. Parents, care providers, teachers, and therapists can provide valuable insights. Individuals who observe the child daily can help clarify audiologic indicators that considered alone could be perplexing. Moreover, when the audiologist has a good relationship with these individuals, longer-term management and follow-up plans are more likely to be followed.

Acknowledgments: We wish to acknowledge the contributions of several individuals who have assisted in the development and refinement of the clinical techniques in use at the Rose F. Kennedy Center, Albert Einstein College of Medicine, and the Kresge Hearing Research Laboratory. They include: Martha Anne Ellis and Wei Wei Lee of the Kennedy Center's Auditory Behavioral Laboratory; Charles Berlin, Director of Kresge Hearing Research Laboratory; and the Audiology Clinical Service, Jill Bordelon, Leah Goforth-Barter, Annette Hurley, Patti St. John, and Diane Wilensky. Judith Gravel is supported by a NIH NIDCD Center Grant. Research studies at Kresge Laboratory leading to development of some of the physiologic techniques described have been supported by NIH NIDCD, Kam's Fund for Hearing Research, and the Louisiana Lions Eye Foundation.

Test Battery Approach and the Cross-Check Principle

The need for a test-battery approach and the use of confirmatory tests in pediatric assessment cannot be over-emphasized. The "cross-check principle" has served our profession well over the years, evolving out of the classic 1976 paper of the same name by Jerger and Hayes. The principle states that the results of any single audiometric test cannot be considered valid without independent verification from another test. At the time of the Jerger and Hayes paper, new technologies (such as tympanometry, middle ear muscle assessment, and auditory evoked potentials) were becoming available in clinical settings. For the first time, audiologists had physiologic tests that could be used to corroborate behavioral findings. While technology has added to the pediatric tests available today, still no one measure can be used alone for the assessment of hearing in children. Thus, adherence to the "cross-check principle" in pediatric clinical practice remains a fundamental tenet of our field.

The selection of procedures included in the pediatric test battery must be predicated on a thorough knowledge of the advantages and limitations of each test procedure and how it should be applied specifically to infants and children. Moreover, the information contributed by any one test should add some unique information to the assessment process. Today, with more procedures available, our challenge is to differentially select and administer only those tests that have been demonstrated to be appropriate, efficient, reliable, and effective in delineating the auditory status of infants and children.

Delineating Peripheral Sensitivity

Interventions (such as medical, surgical, or amplification) proceed most efficiently and effectively when the child's hearing sensitivity has been completely delineated. Moreover, today's pediatric prescriptive hearing aid fitting procedures require frequency-specific, individual-ear threshold data for optimal fitting of amplification devices (Seewald, Moodie, Sinclair, & Cornelisse, 1996). Knowledge of the hearing sensitivity of each ear, including the type, degree, and configuration of any existing hearing loss should be the goal of the audiologic assessment. Currently, behavioral and physiologic techniques that are ear- and frequency-specific are available to achieve this purpose. The sections of this chapter that follow will review those procedures. It is critical that audiologists evaluating children be prepared to administer and interpret such procedures, or have referral resources available that can provide such data in a timely manner if their own facilities cannot (Bess, Chase, Gravel, Seewald, Stelmachowicz, Tharpe, & Hedley-Williams, 1996).

Assessing Global Auditory Function

Some clinicians consider physiologic test results to be sufficient for audiologic assessment purposes. However, the pediatric audiologic assessment is not complete unless the audiologist has information regarding the child's global hearing abilities. Said differently, it is important to determine how the child is using his or her hearing for the purpose of communication acquisition. Such results are useful in monitoring and management planning. Thus, physiologic threshold measures alone are insufficient and the pediatric audiologic assessment is incomplete unless it includes measures of behavioral auditory function. However, neither should management decisions be delayed until reliable behavioral threshold tests have been completed. When the cross-check of physiologic results with developmentally appropriate behavioral measures of hearing status are in accord, intervention should proceed without delay.

Formulating Management Strategies

Management decisions must be individualized, appropriate, and evidence-based. Information obtained during the pediatric audiologic assessment is often critical to the formulation and evaluation of appropriate intervention. Realistic goals for the short and long term can be established and the achievement of those objectives can be documented during the audiologic evaluation. This information can help in demonstrating to clinicians, therapists, educators, and parents the effect of specific auditory interventions.

We believe it is important that evidence-based decision making be part of the formulation of management strategies. To clarify, treatments of various types are available for children with auditory disabilities. Some of these interventions are supported by research and their efficacy is undisputed. Some interventions, however, are not evidence-based, yet such therapies will be sought out by concerned parents based on anecdotal information they obtain from others as well as through the media. The recommendations or support voiced for specific auditory management procedures by audiologists should be scientifically based and evidence of the efficacy of the intervention for children should be available.

ASSESSMENT METHODS

Factors Impacting Assessment

Some of the most critical factors influencing the pediatric audiologic assessment are the age, developmental level, and neuromaturation of the child being evaluated. Age and developmental level influence the choice of behavioral test methodology, as well as the interpretation of physiologic tests. Normative values to which an individual child's responses are compared are critical for the accurate interpretation of procedures, when they are used as measures of sensitivity, auditory function, and neurological integrity. The interpretation of behavioral and physiologic test procedures must be based on a knowledge of the typical responses displayed by infants and children who are developing normally.

When audiologic test procedures (in particular, those that evaluate auditory function such as speech measures) involve language either for instruction, stimuli, or response, then the linguistic level of the child must be fully appreciated. Expressive and receptive language competency can influence test results and should always be considered in test interpretation. The child's attention to the task as well as his or her motivation to respond are known to influence results. We would suggest that the child's attention and motivation during the test be monitored. As will be discussed in this chapter, there are techniques that allow these factors to be quantified.

Otitis media (OM), or inflammation of the middle ear space, is a fairly ubiquitous condition of early childhood. Nearly every child has at least one episode in the first three years of life. OM with effusion (OME) is the presence of fluid within the middle ear space that results in some degree of fluctuant but temporary conductive hearing loss (Gravel & Nozza, 1997). Because OME can confound both behavioral and physiologic test interpretation, and since the condition is so common in young children, middle ear status must always be considered when interpreting the results of the audiologic assessment.

Finally, many children with hearing loss have other developmental disabilities that complicate their assessment and management. The interpretation of both behavioral and physiologic tests is influenced by children who have concomitant medical, neurological, cognitive, behavioral, and visual disabilities. In the sections that follow, special mention will be made of assessment considerations for children who have developmental disabilities. However, this chapter will not provide details regarding the assessment of infants and children within these special populations.

Behavioral Test Methods

Behavioral testing has been criticized for being a potentially unreliable and invalid means of determining a young child's auditory status (Berlin & Hood, 1993). This has been attributed to faulty response-conditioning techniques and lax criteria (see below) (Berlin & Hood, 1993). However, when practiced with cognizance of potential pitfalls and time constraints, and employing protocols and procedures that have been demonstrated to increase the reliability and validity of the method, behavioral audiometry can be an efficient and cost-effective test method for clinical use (Diefendorf & Gravel, 1996). Considering the importance of using a test-battery and cross-check approach to pediatric

audiologic assessment (Jerger & Hayes, 1976), behavioral audiometry becomes a useful tool for identification, assessment, and management of infants and children with hearing loss (e.g., Diefendorf & Gravel, 1996; Merer & Gravel, 1997; Roush & Gravel, 1994).

Thus, behavioral assessment is useful for two purposes. While these objectives are not mutually exclusive, they are decidedly different. When used for audiometric purposes, behavioral methodologies should provide a means for quantifying hearing sensitivity, that is, determining frequency-specific thresholds across the speech range (minimally, 500 through 4000 Hz). When used for functional purposes, the auditory assessment is used to qualitatively examine the child's auditory behaviors, determining whether they are typical for age. It is useful for counseling and intervention planning to determine whether the child has developmentally appropriate auditory behaviors such as accurate sound-source localization and selective listening abilities.

Pediatric behavioral tests can be considered according to two general categories: those that examine overt, unconditioned responses to sound to estimate auditory sensitivity and/or auditory function and those that use operant conditioning procedures to achieve similar purposes. Figure 10.1 displays these two general categories of behavioral approaches used in pediatric audiometry as well as the specific procedures.

Conditioned Response Procedures

Visual Reinforcement Audiometry. By the time an infant has reached a chronological/developmental age of 5 to 6 months, an operant conditioning paradigm becomes a viable approach to behavioral audiometry. Increases or decreases in an operant behavior are the result of changes that occur because of the behavior to the organism's environment (Diefendorf & Gravel, 1996). In an operant discrimination (yes-no) procedure, the stimulus is used to cue the infant that a response behavior will result in positive reinforcement. If the reinforcer is sufficiently powerful, the response will be continued over repeated presentations of the stimulus. As demonstrated by Moore and his colleagues (Moore, Thompson, & Thompson, 1975; Moore, Wilson, & Thompson, 1977), test signals that are useful for audiometric purposes have limited reinforcing properties. Consequently, a positive reinforcer having high interest value (appealing to the infant) is used to reinforce the response behavior. Therefore, the stimulus (of little intrinsic interest) cues the availability of reinforcement (Diefendorf & Gravel, 1996).

Visual Reinforcement Audiometry (VRA) was a term first used by Liden and Kankkunen (1969). However, it was the report of Suzuki and Ogiba in 1960 on the conditioned orientation response (COR) that is the basis of the clinical procedure known today as VRA. The seminal

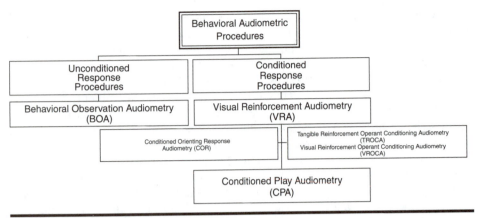

FIGURE 10.1   Two general categories of behavioral audiometric procedures used in pediatric assessment. Specific test procedures are displayed under each general behavioral approach (unconditioned and conditioned response procedures).

studies of Moore, Thompson, Wilson, and their colleagues and students at the University of Washington, Seattle serve as the foundation for the clinical application of operant audiometric response procedures (Diefendorf & Gravel, 1996). In these and subsequent studies, VRA has been demonstrated to be a valid and reliable test procedure for use in the audiometric assessment of infants and young children beginning at 5 to 6 months of age through 2 years of age (e.g., Widen, 1993). Indeed, the VRA procedure is appropriate for use with children who, because of developmental disabilities, function at the same levels. In VRA, a head turn response cued by an auditory stimulus is reinforced visually through the activation and illumination of a three-dimensional animated toy. Highly complex visual reinforcers are critical for maintaining response behaviors over repeated trials (Moore et al., 1975).

Clinical VRA.   Figure 10.2 presents the configuration of the test suite most commonly used for VRA. The audiologist is located outside the test suite. The infant, parent, and a second examiner are located within the test suite. The infant is seated comfortably on her or his parent's lap. The infant's attention is brought to the midline position by the examiner seated to one side (a) or directly in front (b) of the baby. An appealing toy is manipulated by the examiner in front of the infant as a distractor. The examiner's role is to maintain the infant's attention at midline and return the infant to this position once a response is made. The toy used for this purpose should be appealing, but not be so attractive as to overly occupy the infant. Conversely, if the examiner and toy are not sufficiently interesting, the likelihood of false alarms (the infant making noncontingent head turns in the direction of the reinforcer) will be high.

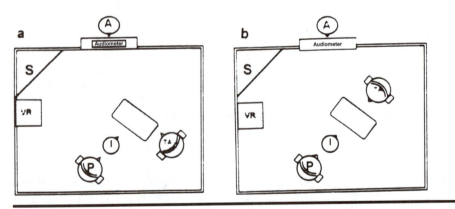

FIGURE 10.2   Configurations of the test suite arrangements commonly used for Visual Reinforcement Audiometry (VRA). See text for detailed explanations. A = audiologist; S = loudspeaker; VR = visual reinforcer display; I = infant; P = parent; TA = test assistant. (Adapted from J. S. Gravel, 1997, Behavioral audiologic assessment. In A. Lalwani & K. Grundfast [Eds.], *Pediatric Otology and Neurology.* Philadelphia: J. B. Lippincott)

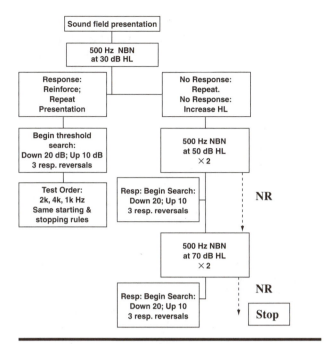

FIGURE 10.3   A suggested Visual Reinforcement Audiometry (VRA) clinical test protocol. This figure shows the approach used to teach the infant the VRA task and obtain air-conducted sound-field thresholds.

In classical VRA, the response is shaped (conditioned) during a training phase that occurs before threshold acquisition commences. A supra-threshold level stimulus is paired with the availability of the reinforcement until after several pairings, the infant demonstrates operant responding—that is, responds contingently upon the presentation of the test stimulus. Successful completion of the training phase is the achievement of a predetermined criterion: a proportion of correct (contingent) responses. The problem with this classic approach for clinical purposes is that the true hearing status often is not known. Consequently, the stimulus intensity used during the training phase may not be above the threshold of an infant referred with suspicion of hearing loss. Therefore, the possibility exists that the stimulus selected to shape the response behavior might be inaudible. In this case, reinforcement would be delivered randomly, and the baby might never learn the response contingency. Responses obtained would therefore be unreliable. The worst-case scenario would be that by chance alone, an infant with severely impaired hearing could provide behavioral responses that suggested that hearing was normal or near-normal (e.g., Berlin & Hood, 1993).

Thus, for clinical audiometry, a traditional period of classic conditioning (pairing the stimulus presentation with reinforcement) is not recommended *unless* there is information available (from physiologic assessments) that the discriminative stimulus is well above the infant's hearing threshold. Rather, for daily practice, the head-turn response

is shaped according a protocol that both optimizes the likelihood of obtaining an orientation response (Thompson & Folsom, 1984) and optimizes test efficiency (e.g., Eilers, Miskiel, Özdamar, Urbano, & Widen, 1991; Eilers, Widen, Urbano, Hudson, & Gonzales, 1991; Primus, 1992; Tharpe & Ashmead, 1993; Widen, 1993).

Thresholds obtained with the VRA procedure for infants 6 to 12 months of age have been shown to be within 10 to 15 dB of those obtained from older children and adults (Gravel & Wallace, 1998; Nozza & Wilson, 1984). Moreover, VRA thresholds are similar across the age span (6 months to 24 months) and show good reliability when compared to thresholds obtained in the same child at older ages (Diefendorf, 1988).

Clinical VRA Protocol.   Figures 10.3 and 10.4 depict a recommended clinical VRA protocol. A stimulus is delivered through a loudspeaker with the visual reinforcer (VR) immediately adjacent (Primus, 1992). The loudspeaker and VR are positioned approximately 90 degrees to one side of

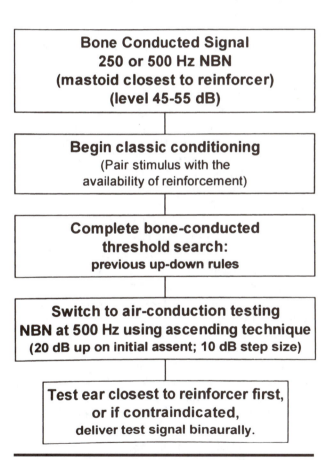

FIGURE 10.4   The approach used when the infant fails to respond to the sound-field training phase. Bone-conducted signals are used to shape the head-turn response prior to obtaining air-conduction thresholds. See text for complete explanation.

the infant. A 500 Hz narrow band of noise is presented at 30 dB HL (Thompson & Folsom, 1984). If the infant turns (orients) towards the sound source, the behavior is reinforced. If no orientation response occurs, no reinforcement is delivered. The same stimulus is delivered a second time. If the infant responds, the behavior is reinforced and the threshold search begins (the baby twice orienting toward the signal).

If the infant fails to respond to both presentations, the intensity level of the stimulus is raised by 20 dB and the procedure is repeated. As described previously, the reinforcement rules are the same: An orienting response from the infant results in reinforcement; no response, no reinforcement. Two reinforced head turns at this level are followed by the initiation of threshold acquisition. If the infant fails to respond to the 500 Hz narrowband noise at 50 dB HL, the stimulus level is raised to 70 dB and the sequence is repeated. As before, an orientation towards the loudspeaker is reinforced and two responses allow the threshold search to begin. If the infant fails to orient to the signal at 70 dB HL, sound field air-conduction presentations are discontinued. (See below for sequence on classic conditioning using the bone oscillator.)

As suggested above, the actual audiometric threshold search begins as soon as two head turns to a test signal at one intensity level have been obtained. On the third trial, the test intensity is lowered by 20 dB; step size remains 20 dB until the infant fails to respond (the first miss). Subsequently, the test signal intensity is raised and then lowered using a conventional staircase (up-down) procedure with a step size of 10 dB. (Reinforcement schedule and stopping rules are described below). Once threshold has been obtained at 500 Hz, 2000 Hz is usually tested next using the same test strategy. Thereafter, sound-field thresholds are established at 4000 and 1000 Hz.

Once sound-field thresholds have been obtained, ear-specific responses are sought. The preferable transducers are insert earphones. Inserts are useful for a number of reasons, including their comfort, light weight, stability, increased interaural attenuation compared to conventional supra-aural earphone/headset assemblies, and reduced risk of ear-canal collapse. However, the majority of typically developing infants can be assessed using conventional earphones (Gravel & Traquina, 1992). Ear- and frequency-specific audiometric information is critical to the medical and audiologic follow-up process. This is particularly true for the prescriptive fitting of amplification devices. Insert earphones should be used for threshold assessment when hearing aid selection is the next step in the management process. Individual real-ear-to-coupler difference (RECD) values may then be applied to provide a better estimate of threshold for use in determining prescriptive hearing aid gain and output targets (Seewald et al., 1996). A test protocol similar to that described above is used. Unless contraindicated, the test stimulus is delivered to the ear

closest to the VR, taking advantage of the probability that the infant will lateralize the sound. When the second ear is tested, if a head turn is made in the direction opposite to the VR location, the reinforcer display is activated regardless. This usually attracts the infant's attention (if not, the parent turns the infant's head towards the VR). Usually subsequent responses are made with a head turn towards the reinforcer. It is important to remember that VRA is not assessing the infant's ability to lateralize or localize a signal. Rather, the head turn (in one direction only) is a convenient and developmentally appropriate behavioral response indicator that can be easily brought under operant control (contrast this with the discussion of COR audiometry that follows).

Following air-conduction testing, bone-conduction thresholds are obtained. A pediatric headband with a foam cushion beneath is used. Generally, the bone oscillator is placed on the mastoid closest to the VR. Unmasked bone-conduction responses are obtained if threshold elevations are evident. Masked thresholds may be obtained; the use of an insert earphone is particularly helpful. The baby is reinforced only for correct responses in the presence of masking noise. The masker is introduced using an ascending method. The infant may respond initially to the masker but will usually cease doing so when he or she is not reinforced for the response.

When infants do not respond to the 70 dB HL stimuli in sound field, classical conditioning is initiated using the bone oscillator placed on the mastoid closest to the VR (Figure 10.4). A 55 dB HL 500 Hz narrowband noise, or 250 Hz narrowband noise at 45 dB HL, is presented and the VR is activated. Thus, the stimulus (in this case, vibrotactile) is paired with the availability of reinforcement. An infant with severe or profound hearing loss with no other developmental disabilities will show contingent behavioral responses as long as the stimulus is salient (can be felt, even if not heard). Responses are obtained in this manner; earphone presentations follow with starting levels dependent upon the bone-conduction responses and any other information that is available (physiologic tests). If the infant or young child fails to display conditioned responding, then other developmental disabilities or immaturities are suspected. We have found it possible to assess hearing in infants with severe and profound degrees of cochlear hearing loss using this protocol (Gravel, 1992, 1997).

Test Rules. Initiating and completing VRA testing is predicated on a body of literature that supports the decisions (test rules) that clinicians adopt during assessment. Some, such as the starting intensity and stimuli, have been discussed previously. Others (stopping rules, reinforcement schedule, acceptable false alarm rate) will be covered in this section. In the practice of pediatric behavioral audiometry it is reassuring to know that the clinical science of our profession supports the decisions we make in the practical application of test procedures.

Primus and Thompson (1985) found no effect of a 100% reinforcement schedule (reinforcement for every correct response) compared to intermittent reinforcement (less than 100% reinforcement schedule for correct responses) on either response habituation or on the total number of responses obtained from 2-year-olds. Therefore, a 100% reinforcement schedule is used initially in VRA. Since Primus and Thompson's data suggest that withholding reinforcement should not affect the level of stimulus control, reinforcement should not be provided if the clinician is at all uncertain about the validity of a response (Diefendorf & Gravel, 1996). Intermittent reinforcement is preferable to a 100% reinforcement schedule that might inadvertently reinforce an incorrect (false-alarm) responses. Reinforcing incorrect responses is confusing to the infant and increases the false alarm rate (turning when no stimulus is present). Collectively, these circumstances negatively influence threshold acquisition (Berlin & Hood, 1993; Diefendorf & Gravel, 1996).

Throughout testing, it is important to present two types of trials: signal trials that contain a test stimulus and control trials that do not. As discussed previously, VR is provided only for correct responses that occur during signal trials (usually a fixed time period encompassing the stimulus as well as a response period immediately following). It is equally important to quantify response behaviors during control-trial intervals. A head-turn during a control interval (a false alarm) should never be reinforced (see above). However, keeping track of the false-alarm rate provides important information regarding whether the infant is under stimulus control (task oriented: Eilers, Miskiel, et al., 1991). High false alarm rates (over 50%) require the clinician to consider that the test results may be inaccurate. Changing the reinforcement schedule or reinstituting the shaping phase of testing may be necessary. In addition, false alarms may be reduced by increasing the novelty of the distracting toy (Gravel, 1989). Eilers, Miskiel, and colleagues (1991) suggest that a false-alarm rate of 30% to 40% is acceptable and adopting such a rate as acceptable does not compromise the accuracy of thresholds for clinical purposes.

Testing at one frequency may be ceased once the infant has exhibited between 3 and 4 response reversals after the first miss (stopping rule: Eilers, Miskiel, et al., 1991; Eilers, Widen, et al., 1991). Eilers and her colleagues found that 6 versus 3 response reversals before discontinuing the threshold search has minimal effect on threshold. Indeed, beyond 4 response reversals, their computer simulations found little improvement in accuracy of thresholds. Thus, there is no need to waste valuable responses when the data obtained are not substantially better because of it. Moreover, the length of testing can be shortened appreciably by adopting the 3- or 4-reversal criterion. The number of test trials needed to obtain threshold was halved by a 4-reversal versus 6-reversal stopping criterion. Thus, a test session may be made more efficient, thereby, optimizing the probability of obtaining thresholds at multiple test frequencies during one test session.

For manual VRA, test schedules may be easily developed using predetermined values (percentages) of signal and control test intervals (Gravel, 1992). By maintaining a record of the infant's responses during signal and control intervals, the audiologist can quantify the amount of stimulus control observed during testing.

The use of computer-assisted test procedures increases the efficiency of VRA testing. Only one examiner is used for assessment. Figure 10.5A depicts the test suite arrangement. The audiologist communicates with the computer via a hand switch, signaling when the baby is ready for a trial and whether a response was made during the trial interval. When the infant makes a correct response, the computer delivers reinforcement. The computer initiates the threshold search, presents the up-down staircase according to the predetermined rules, maintains a trial-by-trial record of performance, presents control trials to monitor the false-alarm rate, and terminates the test once the stopping criterion has been achieved. A light on the hand switch or test box indicates that a trial is occurring; the audiologist (wearing ear plugs or listening to masking noise) is unaware of whether the trial contains a signal or is a control interval. Thus, observer bias is greatly reduced and the reliability of the infant's thresholds may be quantified.

Bernstein and Gravel (1990) described a computer-assisted procedure that interleaved three test frequencies (500, 2000, and 4000 Hz), maintaining a record of correct responses ("hits") and false alarms. In addition, the algorithm incorporated higher-intensity probe trials that were randomly interspersed during the threshold search as a means of monitoring the infant's attention and motivation throughout the procedure.

A commercially available system known as Intelligent VRA (IVRA: Intelligent Hearing Systems, Miami FL) has an option for a traditional single frequency up-down threshold search procedure. Additionally, a four-frequency (500, 1000, 2000, and 4000 Hz) interleaving procedure incorporates an algorithm that quickly restricts trials to the intensity region around threshold, thus making efficient use of the infant's response behaviors (Optimized Hearing Test Algorithm, OHTA; Eilers, Widen, et al., 1991). Finally, IVRA has a hearing screening option known as the Classification of Audiograms by Sequential Testing (CAST) procedure. Bayesian mathematical theory is used to predict which one of 9 patterns is most similar to the audiogram configuration. CAST has been shown to be useful for the hearing screening of children 6 months to 60 months of age (Merer & Gravel, 1997; Widen, 1990). Control trials and probe trials are used in all of the algorithms available on the IVRA system.

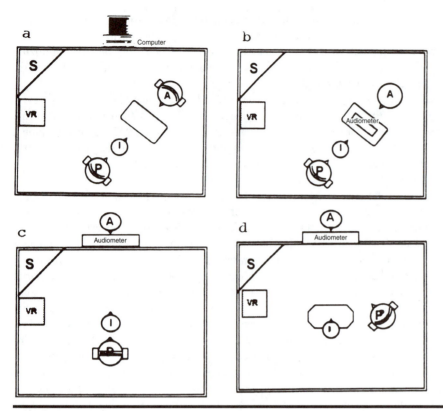

FIGURE 10.5 Additional configurations of the test suite arrangements commonly used for Visual Reinforcement Audiometry (VRA). See text for detailed explanations. A = audiologist; S = loudspeaker; VR = visual reinforcer display; I = infant; P = parent; TA = test assistant. (Adapted from J. S. Gravel, 1997, Behavioral audiologic assessment. In A. Lalwani & K. Grundfast [Eds.], *Pediatric Otology and Neurology*. Philadelphia: J. B. Lippincott)

Figure 10.5B, C, and D presents other test suite arrangements that are used for VRA. Note that these arrangements use only one examiner for testing. In many settings this is preferable as other audiologists and/or support personnel may not be available or are being used for other purposes. Moreover, many clinicians feel that they have better control of the test situation when they alone are controlling the test situation. Note that for traditional test purposes, the audiologist may be located inside or outside of the test suite. When located within the test booth, the audiologist controls all aspects of the test procedure, including stimulus presentation, delivery of reinforcement, and maintaining the infant in the midline position (Gravel, 1989, 1992, 1994, 1997). When the audiologist is outside in the control room, it is useful to seat the infant in a high chair and use the parent to manipulate the distractor toys.

The problem with all of these arrangements is the increased probability of observer/examiner bias influencing the test results. Potential biases may be reduced by having the parent use ear plugs or listen to a masker (such as music) during the test session so that she or he is unaware of the test signals. Similarly, if two examiners are used for VRA, the examiner in the test suite with the baby should be unaware of whether a trial is a signal or control interval. Consequently, ear plugs or the use of a masker are necessary for the test assistant. When only one person is involved in testing, the potential for observer bias is similar to that during audiometry with older children or adults. The same precautions regarding stimulus timing, presentation patterns, and accidental cueing must be undertaken. The use of a stimulus-response record form (as discussed previously) is strongly advised.

Conditioned Orienting Response (COR). VRA and COR audiometry are often used interchangeably. While both procedures reinforce correct responses, the two procedures are different and the terms cannot be used synonymously. The test suite arrangement for COR is depicted in Figure 10.6. Note that two loudspeakers and two separate VRs are positioned to either side of the infant. This is a different arrangement than the single loudspeaker and one VR display used in VRA. As its name implies, COR audiometry

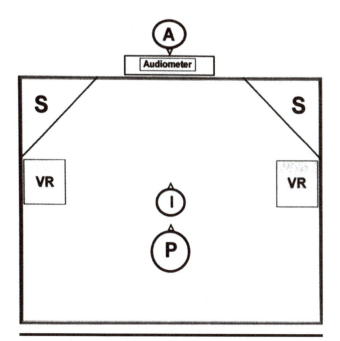

FIGURE 10.6 Test suite arrangement typically used for Conditioned Orienting Response (COR) audiometry. See text for detailed explanation. A = audiologist; S = loudspeaker; VR = visual reinforcer display; I = infant; P = parent; T = test assistant. (From J. S. Gravel, 1997, Behavioral audiologic assessment. In A. Lalwani & K. Grundfast [Eds.], *Pediatric Otology and Neurology*. Philadelphia: J. B. Lippincott)

requires the infant to orient (look) towards the source of the test signal. Test signals are presented from either loudspeaker. The child's responses are judged "correct" only when the head turn is made toward the side (right or left) corresponding to the signal source. When used as a functional indicator of localization ability, the COR procedure can provide useful information. However, for audiometric purposes (ear- and frequency-specific threshold data), the technique has limitations. COR is most often used for sound-field assessment, yet when hearing test results are reported, it is often implied that a head turn towards the right speaker indicates a response from the right ear while a head turn to the left indicates a response attributable to the left ear. Sound-field measures, however, are not sufficient to ensure that ear-specificity has been achieved. An infant with asymmetrical hearing thresholds will likely provide a non-specific sound-field audiometric profile. Moreover, when the infant is required to make two decisions before responding (detection and correct orientation), thresholds may be poorer than when the head turn is only a response indicator (as is the case in the VRA procedure) (Diefendorf & Gravel, 1996; Wilson & Thompson, 1984). Thus, the two test methods are fundamentally different and clinicians should

specify precisely which specific method (VRA or COR) was used to obtain the reported audiometric results.

Play Audiometry. Audiometric assessment of preschoolers and young children is facilitated through use of conditioned response procedures. Indeed, the traditional conditioned play audiometry (CPA) procedure uses reinforcement of correct response behaviors for threshold acquisition (Wilson & Thompson, 1984). Similar to the operant head-turn procedure described previously, play audiometry (including visual/tangible reinforcement operant audiometry, VROCA/ TROCA) uses positive reinforcement to support the response behavior. In the case of VROCA/TROCA, the reinforcer is either an illuminated mechanical toy (VROCA) or tangible (TROCA) treat (food, small toy). In addition, conditioned play procedures have benefited from traditional "play" response indicators (i.e., block drop, ring stack) being "rewarding." The child's responses are supported by a pleasurable activity. However, as with VRA, true conditioned play audiometry should use a reinforcer (illuminated toy; changing computer screen display) that is separate from the response to support repeated response behaviors (Diefendorf & Gravel, 1996). Undoubtedly with the advent of computer-assisted procedures, more manufacturers/ developers of clinical hardware/software will provide as options conditioned behavioral response methodology that will be readily used for the audiometric assessment of young children.

Once children have reached an age of approximately 6 years, the response indicators (behaviors) used are similar to adults, that is, hand-raise or button-push responses. While the response is the same as used for adults, the need to maintain attention and motivation during testing is an issue. Children with developmental disabilities or those with attention deficits may benefit from response and reinforcement paradigms that are used with younger children. Thus, reinforcement or tangible rewards are sometimes useful in audiometric testing of the older child with developmental disabilities. Finally, it is cautioned that simply because children's behavioral responses during audiometry may be similar to that of adults, their performance on some procedures (for example, speech audiometry; see below) will not be adult-like.

Unconditioned Response Methods

Behavioral Observation Audiometry. Northern and Downs have detailed the use of behavioral observation procedures for audiometric purposes in their classic *Auditory Response Index* (Northern & Downs, 1973, 1983, 1991). The *Index* is predicated on observations that healthy newborns, infants, and young children display overt responses to sound that follow a developmental continuum. Indeed, the audiometric procedure known as Behavioral Observation

Audiometry (BOA) has been highly influenced by the work of Marion Downs, beginning in the 1960s and 1970s. In turn, Downs was influenced by methods (the *Distraction Test*) developed in Great Britain, particularly those of Lord and Lady Ewing and Kevin Murphy (Northern & Downs, 1991). The BOA procedure has been used for hearing screening as well as audiometric assessment for more than 25 years, and many consider the procedure the "mainstay" of pediatric audiometry.

Limitations of BOA. Studies done at the University of Washington have demonstrated that the use of unconditioned behavioral response procedures for audiologic assessment can be problematic. In their now-classic studies, Moore, Thompson, and Thompson (1975) and Moore, Wilson, and Thompson (1977) demonstrated that the bandwidth as well as the intensity level of the test stimulus were critical factors influencing the probability of eliciting a behavioral response from a young infant. Moderate to moderately high levels of broadband, complex auditory signals were more likely to elicit an observable response from infants than were less intense and less complex stimuli (e.g., narrow bands of noise or FM tones). With increasing age, the variability was lower, but the effects of signal type and intensity were still present.

While responses to broadband signals such as speech and white noise provide a global estimate of hearing sensitivity, they are insufficient for audiometric purposes and particularly for the fitting of hearing aids. The novelty of even an initially interesting complex sound usually dissipates rapidly, and a "new" (novel) stimulus must be introduced to reinstate response behaviors. Responses that habituate quickly make threshold assessment difficult. The intrinsic appeal of frequency-specific test signals (such as pure tones) is low (Moore, Thompson, & Thompson, 1975). Thus, the signals important for delineating a child's audiometric profile are the stimuli least likely to elicit a response. Moreover, if reliable responses are more likely to occur to signals at higher intensity levels, it is difficult to determine whether an infant has normal hearing or is experiencing some elevation of hearing threshold. Therefore, differentiating normal hearing from mild to moderate degrees of hearing loss is difficult. Finally, behavioral observations are often biased since observers who know when test signals are presented are often used in BOA. Regardless of the number of observers (one, two, or more), if examiners are aware of when a test signal is presented, the possibility of test bias cannot be overlooked. At a minimum, the observer in the test booth with the child, as well as the parent, should be unaware of the presentation of the test signal. As recommended in VRA, this can be accomplished through the use of noise masking (Diefendorf & Gravel, 1996).

Application of the **Auditory Response Index.** Many audiologists routinely use the *Auditory Response Index* for audiological assessment of infants. Specifically, a baby's overt responses (in dB HL) to stimuli (speech, warble tone, noise makers) are compared to the *Index* values, which are tabled according to age. This is used to determine whether an infant exhibits "normal" or "abnormal" hearing sensitivity "for age." As discussed, for numerous reasons the use of unconditioned response procedures is not a sufficiently reliable method for audiometric assessment of infants and is likely not to provide accurate and reliable hearing thresholds.

However, when used as an indicator of auditory development, the *Auditory Response Index* has clinical value in the evaluation of the maturity of the young child's auditory responses (Northern & Downs, 1991). Observations of auditory responses are particularly beneficial once it has been verified by physiologic methods that the infant or child has normal hearing sensitivity. These can be helpful in the comprehensive assessment of children with developmental disabilities and in the formulation of appropriate habilitation goals (Gans & Flexer, 1983). For example, consider a child of 18 months chronological age with suspected cognitive delays but known normal peripheral hearing sensitivity (by physiologic tests—see sections that follow). If the child demonstrates unconditioned behavioral responses to sound that are typical of an infant 4 to 5 months of age, the child's auditory maturation significantly lags behind that expected for his or her chronological age. Thus, for this child, intervention (and indeed, communication) approaches might be focused toward strategies that would promote auditory skill development with the *Auditory Response Index* continuum serving as a guide.

Speech Audiometry

Speech audiometry has been used in the pediatric audiologic assessment for a variety of purposes. For example, speech audiometry is useful in cross-checking other test results, in determining the development of aural language acquisition, and in the validation of hearing aid fitting. Indeed, using speech as a stimulus has obvious face validity if our goal is the comprehensive assessment of hearing. As a stimulus, speech has been found to be particularly useful with infants and young children because it has inherently high interest value and a complex spectrum.

However, speech audiometry has limitations for use with the pediatric population. Unfortunately, the lack of frequency-specificity often limits its usefulness in accurately delineating the configuration of any existing hearing loss. Moreover, when speech is used to quantify the development of speech recognition abilities, the young child's receptive and expressive language skills may compromise the validity of the outcome measure. Thus, it is important to recognize the clinical uses and limitations of speech audiometry in the test battery. Test selection and interpretation should be based on available normative criteria for the pediatric population.

Stimuli used in speech audiometry may vary from phonemes in isolation, to words (monosyllables, spondees, trochees), short phrases, and sentences. Speech may be presented in quiet or competitive noise, to both ears or to one alone. The child's task might be detection or discrimination (simple yes-no wherein the child is required to detect the presence-absence of sound or indicate whether a pair of speech tokens are the same or different; responses: head turn, hand-raise, button push, block drop, verbal yes-no, etc.). Or, the child may be asked to recognize or identify a speech stimulus by repeating the token or indicating the picture or object representing the speech item.

For speech recognition testing, performance can be influenced by the child's lexicon, receptive and expressive language ability, own speech clarity (articulation), and auditory memory (Jerger, 1984). Moreover, performance on the test is influenced by presentation level. A single intensity level (e.g., the "most comfortable" listening level), an adaptive approach (to determine a *speech reception threshold* or *speech recognition threshold*, SRT, or message-to-competition ratio), or a performance-intensity (P-I) function may be developed at levels spanning just above threshold to just below discomfort.

Performance on speech recognition tests is often expressed as a percent-correct score. In some cases, incorrect responses are recorded and a phoneme analysis is completed, or a confusion matrix is developed. The message set used may be "open" (unrestricted) or "closed" (restricted number of items from which to select the correct response). Restrictions on the message set influence the steepness of the slope of the performance-intensity function (Jerger, 1984). Closed message sets increase the probability of chance performance and influence the determination of true test-retest differences.

Below are some examples of speech tests that we have found useful with the pediatric population. The tests have been organized to reflect their use in assessing the detection, discrimination, or recognition of speech (Erber, 1982). (For a comprehensive table that delineates most of the pediatric speech audiometry materials currently available, refer to Appendix 1 of Bess et al., 1996). For a complete discussion of speech audiometry, see Chapter 2 by Wilson and Strouse in this text.

Speech Detection Tests. For speech detection tests, stimuli such as the child's name, CV syllables ("bye-bye," "oh-oh"), short phrases ("look here baby"), or an individual

speech sound (/s/, /sh/) are delivered (usually using monitored live voice presentations) through a loudspeaker, earphone, or bone oscillator. Using an ascending presentation method and beginning below the presumed threshold of hearing, the intensity at which the child's response first occurs is taken as the minimal response level (unconditioned response procedure) for speech. A speech detection threshold (SDT) is obtained when an up-down adaptive test procedure is used. A limitation of the SDT is that, depending upon the speech stimuli used, the threshold may not be frequency specific. The SDT often reflects the best regions of hearing sensitivity in the low- or high-frequency range. When used as a speech detection task, the child is required to merely detect a signal in quiet. Thus, the task lends itself well to conditioned response procedures, making it useful with young infants, children with developmental disabilities, or those with severe and profound degrees of hearing loss.

The *Six-Sound Test* (Ling, 1989) is useful in the evaluation of children because the six phonemes (/ah/, /oo/, /ee/, /m/, /sh/, and /s/) of the test span the speech spectrum from low to high frequency regions. With infants, the test is adaptable for use in a VRA paradigm. Often the older child is taught the behavioral response (e.g., play task or hand-raise) using visual plus auditory input. Then, by removing the visual cues (hiding the lips), the test is completed in the auditory-alone condition. The *Six-Sound Test* is also useful as a simple and practical tool for parents, teachers, or therapists who need to monitor the child's unaided or aided hearing at home or in school.

Speech Discrimination Tests. The *Minimal Pairs Test* (Robbins, Renshaw, Miyamoto, Osberger, & Pope, 1988) is a discrimination test often used in the assessment of children with severe and profound hearing loss, pre- and post-cochlear implantation. The child is not required to identify the words (monosyllables). Rather, the child indicates whether the items of a stimulus pair are the same or different. The test is useful for children of about 5 years of age and older and is limited by whether the child has the concept of "same-different."

Speech Recognition/Intelligibility Tests. Materials used for estimating a child's speech recognition abilities are numerous. Surprisingly, many audiologists do not routinely perform speech audiometry with children, due to the time involved and the limitations of available materials. Yet information useful to the evaluation, monitoring, and intervention process can be obtained from carefully selected speech recognition measures. Some speech intelligibility measures that are used with children were developed for use with adults (for example, the *Northwestern University Test*

No. 6 [NU-6] or the *Central Institute for the Deaf W-22* [CID W-22] lists). Interestingly, the *Phonetically Balanced Kindergarten* (PBK-50s: Haskins, 1949) test, while developed from items known to be within the vocabulary of kindergarten-aged children, was standardized on adult listeners.

The *Word Intelligibility by Picture Identification* (WIPI) test represented an important milestone in pediatric speech audiometry. Children with hearing loss were used in the test's development and the format employed was a colorful picture-point, 6-item closed-set response task. Moreover, because foil items were selected to differ by only one phoneme (as much as was possible), incorrect responses may be examined for consonant confusions. The WIPI can be completed in the auditory alone, visual alone, or combined (auditory plus vision) mode. This is useful for examining the contributions of each sensory input channel and their combination, for use in long-term follow-up, educational, and habilitational recommendations (Ross & Lerman, 1970). The WIPI was standardized on and recommended for use with children from 5 to 6 years of age with mild and moderate hearing loss, and children from 6 to 7 years of age with severe degrees of hearing loss (Ross & Lerman, 1970).

Sanderson-Leepa and Rintelmann (1976) examined the NU-6, PBK-50, and the WIPI in children with normal hearing who ranged in age from 3½ years to 11½ years. Age of the child was found to significantly influence performance on the measures. The most difficult test was the NU-6, followed by the PBK-50s and the WIPI. In fact, Sanderson-Leepa and Rintelmann (1976) recommended that the WIPI be used with children aged 3½ years over use of the PBK-50s. The PBK-50s and the WIPI were found appropriate for use with children age 5½ years, and the NU-6 was more difficult (lower scores, more variability) than the PBK-50s in children aged 7½ to 11½ years of age.

Another important speech measure specifically developed for children is the *Pediatric Speech Intelligibility* (PSI; Jerger, Lewis, Hawkins, & Jerger, 1980) test. The test incorporates two types of measures: performance-intensity (PI) functions and message-to-competition ratio (MCR) functions. PI functions in competition and MCR functions for ipsilateral and contralateral competing messages are useful in examining peripheral and central auditory processing in children. The Pediatric Speech Intelligibility test items are selected closed-sets of words (monosyllables) and sentences actually generated by children 3 to 6 years of age. The test has been shown to be useful in differentiating among children with various auditory versus nonauditory central nervous system dysfunctions (Jerger, 1987). The test is appropriate for children 3 to 10 years of age and can be used with children having mild to moderate hearing loss (Bess at al., 1996). Characteristics

of the PSI have been extensively evaluated making it an extremely useful procedure to use with children (Jerger & Jerger, 1982).

The *Bamford-Kowal-Bench Sentence Lists for Children* (BKB; Bench, Kowal, & Bamford, 1979) sentence materials were developed for older children 8 to 15 years of age with mild to moderate hearing loss. The BKB sentences were constructed to reflect typical language usage of children, thus incorporating vocabulary, grammar, and sentence length appropriate for a pediatric population (Bench et al., 1979). The response required is sentence repetition; the message set is open, and key words are scored.

Recently, a modification of the adult *Hearing-In-Noise Test* (HINT; Nilsson, Soli, & Sullivan, 1994); the *Hearing-In-Noise Test for Children* (HINT-C; Nilsson, Soli, & Gelnett, 1996) has been introduced. The test examines binaural speech understanding and is useful for children 6 to 12 years of age. The sentence items (based on the BKB Sentences) selected for the HINT-C could be repeated accurately in quiet by 5- to 6-year-olds with normal hearing. The reception threshold for sentences (RTS) is determined adaptively with the speech and speech-spectrum-shaped noise presented from 0 degrees azimuth, and with the noise at 90 degrees and 270 degrees relative to the speech signal (0 degrees). Age-correction factors are applied to adult normative data in interpreting the results from children.

PHYSIOLOGIC TECHNIQUES

Physiologic measures take on particular importance when evaluating the integrity of the auditory system in infants and children. While physiologic techniques cannot measure the "moment of hearing," they have proven useful in determining the mechanical and neural integrity of the auditory system, which are critical factors for normal hearing.

Newborn infants and some toddlers and children cannot provide reliable behavioral responses to auditory stimuli. In these cases, use of physiologic measures is critical. Even when reliable behavioral responses are obtained, physiologic measures can provide additional important information. Thus, using physiologic measures either as the primary measure or as a cross-check with other tests is particularly valuable in these populations.

Several objective physiologic techniques are available to the clinician to determine the functional integrity of the auditory system from the middle ear to the cortex. The most commonly used measures include middle ear immittance and middle ear muscle reflexes, otoacoustic emissions, and auditory evoked potentials. Additional measurement and interpretation details related to a number of these measures as they apply to pediatric populations are discussed in other chapters of this text.

Immittance and Middle Ear Muscle Reflexes

Middle ear measurements of immittance and the middle ear muscle reflex (MEMR) provide important information about the integrity of the middle ear system and the neural reflex arc through the lower brainstem pathways that carry information to elicit contraction of the stapedius muscle. These measures are considered an integral part of the basic hearing evaluation in audiologic practice and are particularly important in infants and children due to the higher incidence of middle ear problems in these groups.

Middle ear tests are effective in testing for middle ear pathology, testing for the presence or absence of middle ear muscle reflexes, and evaluating facial nerve function. It is essential to keep in mind exactly what is being measured and to understand both the advantages and limits of each component of the middle ear test battery in order to make appropriate interpretation of the results. Immittance measures the mechanical properties of the auditory path from the external ear to the stapedial footplate. Since flexible external ear tissues and partly formed or immature canal walls can give spurious results, care must be taken when completing these measures in infants. However, this does not mean that these measures should not be used. If normal tympanograms and MEMRs are obtained, then it is highly likely that there are no middle ear pathologies and that the infant does not have a severe hearing loss. In contrast, a normal-appearing tympanogram with absent MEMRs may suggest a severe or profound hearing loss but may also be misleading due to flexible ear canal geometry that could simulate a normal tympanogram when using a 220 Hz tone. Therefore, a normal-appearing tympanogram and absent reflexes in young babies should be interpreted with care, while a normal tympanogram and MEMRs is most likely indicative of normal middle ear function.

Middle ear tests are best used in conjunction with the auditory brainstem response (ABR) and/or a full audiologic test battery. They provide a useful cross-check for other clinical measures of the middle ear, cochlea, and lower brainstem pathways. When using middle ear measures in sedated infants or children, immittance and MEMRs should be completed before beginning the ABR, since positive pressure in the middle ear may build up over time in infants or children who snore or breath heavily during sedated sleep. Obviously, if pressure does deviate from normal over the period of time needed to complete the ABR, then the validity of the middle ear measures will be compromised. Experience has shown that MEMRs can be measured in most sedated infants and children without awakening them.

When no MEMR responses are obtained, testing for the presence of nonacoustic reflexes should be completed. It is erroneous to think that absence of a stapedius reflex response due to physical absence of the middle ear muscles themselves is common. Nonacoustic reflexes can be elicited by a puff of air to the eyelid or a gentle rub of a wisp of cotton in the anterior tragal region. If there is contraction of the middle ear muscles to nonacoustic stimulation but no contraction to acoustic stimulation, this is not a normal variation and should be further evaluated.

Patterns among middle ear measurements and other test results can provide important insights into auditory function. For example, it is highly unlikely that a child who has no response behaviorally to sound is physiologically deaf if MEMRs are present at levels between 70 and 80 dB HL. Conversely, a child who appears to give behavioral responses in normal hearing or mild hearing loss ranges and has normal tympanograms but no MEMRs is still highly suspect for a severe hearing loss. The exception to this possibility would be in young infants, as noted above, and this result may also be seen in patients with auditory neuropathy, which will be discussed below. It should also be remembered that normal MEMRs are often obtained in patients with mild or moderate cochlear losses, so normal middle ear reflex responses cannot rule out hearing losses in this range. Refer to Chapters 4 and 5 for a detailed discussion of immittance and middle ear muscle reflex measurements.

Evoked Otoacoustic Emissions

Evoked otoacoustic emissions (EOAEs) have several clinical applications when evaluating newborns, infants, and children. Types of evoked otoacoustic emissions that are used extensively for clinical purposes are click-evoked otoacoustic emissions and distortion product emissions. EOAEs are widely used in screening programs to rule out hearing loss in newborn infants, and EOAEs and ABR are considered standard methods for this purpose by most audiologists. EOAEs are growing in importance as part of the clinical test battery and as a cross-check to behavioral tests, middle ear measures, and evoked potential results.

Otoacoustic emissions are particularly robust in infants who are free of external and/or middle ear pathology (Kemp, Ryan, & Bray, 1990; Lafreniere, Smurzynski, Jung, Leonard, & Kim, 1993). This characteristic makes EOAEs particularly useful in this population and, even though infants are often physiologically "noisier" than adults, the higher amplitude of the EOAEs allows their acquisition while maintaining acceptable signal-to-noise relationships. EOAE amplitude increases from newborn to ages of from 1 to 9 months, while decreases in amplitude have been observed in children aged 4 to 13 years with an average amplitude for click EOAEs of 15 dB SPL in that age range (Norton & Widen, 1990; Widen, 1997).

Otoacoustic emissions are expected to be present in ears that have hearing sensitivity that is better than approximately 30 to 40 dB HL with an absence of any external or middle ear pathologies. Thus, OAEs can be used as a screening measure to determine whether a hearing loss may be present. Because physical characteristics of the external and middle ears can influence the amplitude of emissions, actual hearing sensitivity cannot be readily predicted. Emissions have been shown to fluctuate with cochlear hearing loss, to provide information about the configuration of hearing loss, and they are used in monitoring the effects of ototoxic medications. Otoacoustic emissions also have particular value, when used in conjunction with the auditory brainstem response, in identifying patients with auditory neuropathy. The ease of recording emissions, their generally robust nature, and their reliability contribute to their value as a clinical test. For detailed discussion of otoacoustic emissions see Chapter 6.

Auditory Evoked Potentials

An important clinical application of auditory evoked potentials is as an objective technique to learn about auditory function. Indeed, Hallowell Davis' pioneering work with cortical potentials was, in part, directed toward the development of a technique to assess auditory function without the need for patient participation. Evoked potentials from the cochlea to the cortex have been studied as possible methods to assess hearing.

If the goal of hearing testing is to determine peripheral hearing sensitivity, then measurement of responses directly from the cochlea would seem ideal. Electrocochleography (ECochG) proved a very useful technique in the 1960s and 1970s. However, the somewhat invasive nature of transtympanic or eardrum recording sites limited its widespread clinical application for this purpose. Cortical responses and middle latency responses proved useful but required that the patient be awake, cooperative, and alert during testing, limiting applications in infants and children, the population most needing an objective "hearing test" method. The relative ease of recording the ABR and its resistance to the effects of sleep and sedation facilitated its widespread use in hearing assessment, particularly in infants and children.

Estimating Auditory Sensitivity with Auditory Evoked Potentials.
While auditory evoked potentials (AEPs) have proven useful in estimating hearing sensitivity, it is important to remember that the ABR is NOT a test of hearing! The ABR and other evoked potentials test neural synchrony, that is, the ability of the central nervous system to respond to external stimulation in a synchronous manner. This synchronous neural response results from the firing of a large group of neurons at the same time. When the central nervous system is functioning normally, we can use these evoked potentials to record neural responses to stimuli presented at various intensity levels. Thus, we can find the lowest intensity level where a neural response is present

and relate that to a threshold for hearing. ABRs can be obtained at intensities close to behavioral thresholds if a sufficient number of responses are averaged to adequately reduce the background physiologic noise (Elberling & Don, 1987). In routine clinical procedures where fewer averages are used, responses can generally be obtained near, but not at, behavioral thresholds.

When to Use Auditory Evoked Potentials to Estimate Auditory Function.
Auditory evoked potentials are best utilized when the clinician desires a noninvasive, safe approach to assessment of auditory function in infants and children who cannot provide reliable responses to behavioral audiometry procedures. AEPs are especially useful when one wishes to know the sensitivity of each cochlea separately, to compare responses by air and bone conduction with or without masking, and to estimate auditory function in low and high frequencies. Since AEPs are a test of the neural system, insight into the integrity of the neural pathways can also be obtained. AEPs should not be used in lieu of a behavioral audiogram in patients who can provide reliable behavioral responses and an ultimate goal in all children should be to obtain behavioral responses. In young infants and children with developmental disabilities, behavioral thresholds may be obtained at a later time, but appropriate management can begin based on AEP results.

Test Protocols and Procedures.
A comprehensive ABR test protocol includes responses to (1) air-conducted clicks to assess the higher frequency range, primarily 2000 to 4000 Hz; (2) low-frequency (generally 500 Hz) tonebursts to assess the lower frequency range; and (3) bone-conducted clicks to distinguish between conductive and sensorineural hearing losses. Outlined below are procedures used at Kresge Laboratory and its associated clinics.

Estimates of auditory function can be obtained from ABRs by progressively decreasing the intensity of the stimulus until no response is discernible. Because Wave V remains at lower intensities, the approach often used is to begin well above the anticipated threshold (based on history or other clinical information) and then decrease intensity by 20 dB steps while following the progressive increase in Wave V latency. Recommended test parameters are provided in Figure 10.7.

We encourage use of two-channel, four-electrode recordings with electrodes placed at the vertex, medial side of each earlobe, and a ground at the forehead. In infants, recording electrodes may be placed at the high forehead and mastoid areas. In addition, when testing infants, lowering the low-frequency filter setting from 100 Hz to 30 Hz will often enhance the amplitude of infant ABRs (Sininger, 1995; Spivak, 1993).

Type of Test Target	ABR Air conduction (higher frequencies)	ABR Air conduction (lower frequencies)	ABR Bone conduction
Time Window	15 msec	20 msec	20 msec
Number Sweeps	1500 or Fsp	1500–2000	1500
Stimulus	100 μsec pulse	500 Hz toneburst	100 μsec pulse
Polarity	Condensation and Rarefaction	Condensation	Alternating
Rate	27.7/sec	39.1/sec	27.7/sec
Filters	100–3000 Hz	30 1500 Hz	100–3000 Hz
Transducer	Insert earphones	Insert earphones	Bone oscillator

FIGURE 10.7 Recommended test parameters for the Auditory Brainstem Response (ABR). See text for explanation.

ABR to Air-Conducted Clicks. Responses to air-conducted clicks are recorded for each ear individually. There are several methods that can be used to obtain the necessary information. We generally obtain a response from each ear using 75 dB nHL 100 μsec clicks in order to determine the latencies of Waves I, III, and V to assess neural function. In patients older than 18 months, adult normative data can be used in interpretation. In infants, we expect increased absolute and interwave latencies and use the normative data provided by Zimmerman, Morgan, and Dubno (1987). If no response is obtained at 75 dB nHL, then the click level is increased to the limits of the equipment to attempt to obtain a response.

We also obtain responses using both condensation and rarefaction clicks at a high intensity and compare the responses obtained with each polarity. This is helpful in distinguishing the cochlear microphonic response (which will reverse in phase as the stimulus does) from Wave I of the ABR (which will not show a phase reversal). Recently, we have observed a series of patients in our practice who, at high intensities, seem to show repeatable waves that turn out not to be an ABR, but a cochlear response instead (Berlin, Bordelon, St. John, Wilensky, Hurley, Kluka, & Hood, 1997). In these patients the "waves" represent a cochlear, not brainstem, response and a neural disorder should be suspected.

Following acquisition of responses at 75 dB nHL, the intensity of the click is decreased in 20 dB steps until no response is obtained. If the patient is quiet and we predict that sufficient time will be available to complete all parts of the test battery, then the click level is increased 10 dB to determine the presence of a response at an intermediary level. For example, if responses are obtained at 75, 55, and 35 dB nHL, but no response is observed at 15 dB nHL, then stimuli are presented at 25 dB nHL. At higher intensities, where responses are readily seen over the noise, fewer than 1000 averages may be sufficient. Closer to threshold, more than 2000 averages may be necessary.

Each of these responses is obtained twice, unless an Fsp or other signal-to-noise estimation is used, to judge replicability and assist in determination of threshold. Latency of the response increases and amplitude decreases, quite predictably, with decreases in stimulus intensity. We generally obtain responses to click stimuli in infants and young children who have normal hearing and are quiet at 15 to 25 dB nHL. An example of an intensity series for an infant obtained using air-conducted clicks is shown in Figure 10.8.

Modifications to Improve Test Efficiency. There are several modifications that can be used to improve test efficiency by decreasing test time. Some instruments have the capability to estimate signal-to-noise levels using the Fsp statistic, which may necessitate fewer averages, reduce the need to replicate the response, and provide an objective estimate of response presence (Sininger, 1993). Another method uses very high stimulus rates (on the order of 500 to 1000 stimuli per second) with randomized presentation sequences known as maximum length sequences (e.g., Picton, Champagne, & Kellett, 1992). Different sequences can be

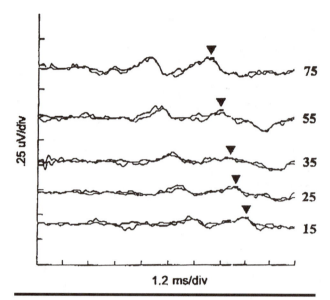

FIGURE 10.8 Example of an Auditory Brainstem Response (ABR) intensity series for an infant obtained using air-conducted clicks.

presented to each ear, which allows testing of both ears simultaneously. When coupled with fast presentation rates, this procedure greatly decreases overall test time. We find both of these techniques useful in our practice.

Two other methods that can be used with any evoked potential system are a binaural-monaural combination of presentation and use of faster stimulus rates. Jerger, Oliver, and Stach (1985) recommended using binaural stimuli at high and low intensities to estimate response threshold. With that information, one knows that at least one ear has a normal synchrony. Then, each ear can be tested individually by presenting stimuli at about 10 dB above the lowest level where the binaural response was obtained. The purpose of this procedure is to reduce the number of averages necessary by focusing in on threshold quickly.

Picton (1978) recommended the use of faster stimulus rates when in the threshold-seeking mode of testing, on the order of 50 to 70 clicks per second to reduce test time. While Wave V latency is prolonged, the amplitude is not reduced as much as for earlier components, making acquisition of responses near threshold possible.

ABR to Bone-Conducted Clicks.   When responses to auditory stimuli are seen at normal threshold levels, there is no need to obtain bone-conducted responses, as would be the practice in conventional audiometry. However, when either click or 500 Hz toneburst responses are not present at expected normal levels, then ABRs should be completed using bone-conducted clicks.

The test parameters used are the same as those for air-conducted clicks except for the use of alternating polarity (see Figure 10.7). The reason for use of alternating polarity with bone-conducted stimuli is the large electrical artifact emitted from the bone oscillator. Oscillator placement can be either at the forehead or mastoid. We use mastoid placement in infants since stimuli from the bone oscillator are conducted across the scalp less efficiently in infants than in adults (Yang, Stuart, Mencher, Mencher, & Vincer, 1993).

The spectrum of bone-conducted clicks is somewhat different than that of air-conducted clicks due to differences in the frequency responses of the two transducers. More importantly, the dynamic range is different, as is true in audiometry. The dynamic range of the bone-conducted stimulus rarely exceeds 45 to 55 dB, and the relationship between the output of the oscillator and the "dial reading" varies with different instruments. Thus, it is important to determine what the dial reading means and how this relates to the oscillator output. To obtain the ABR, bone-conducted stimuli are presented beginning at the highest output level and then decreasing in 20 dB steps as for air conduction. Responses are first obtained without masking, and then, if response thresholds are better than those obtained by air-conduction and/or there is an asymmetry between ears, masking with broadband noise is used.

Since the output in bone conduction is limited, the responses obtained by bone conduction will rarely show the familiar five-wave complex seen at high intensities in standard air-conduction ABRs. Responses will resemble those obtained with air-conducted clicks in the threshold to 50 dB range. Since we are only interested in determining threshold of the response, Wave V is the only component necessary to assess.

Frequency-Specific ABRs Using 500 Hz Stimuli.   ABRs obtained with click stimuli primarily provide information about hearing sensitivity in the 2000 to 4000 Hz range (e.g., Jerger, Hayes, & Jordan, 1980). Patients who have responses to clicks at normal levels may still have a low-frequency hearing loss. Patients who have elevated or no responses to clicks may have anything from normal hearing to a severe hearing loss in the low frequencies. Thus, click information alone is not sufficient to understand auditory function across the frequency range or to fit amplification. Acquisition of responses to low-frequency stimuli is necessary. We have found eliciting the ABR with a 500 Hz toneburst stimulus very effective.

For 500 Hz toneburst ABRs, we change the filters to 30–1500 Hz to accommodate lower-frequency physiologic activity (see Figure 10.7). Tonebursts with 4 millisecond (2 cycles) rise and fall times, Hanning or Blackman envelopes, and either condensation or rarefaction polarity are used (but not alternating). The time window is extended to 20 or 25 milliseconds, since these responses have longer latencies than responses to clicks. Stimuli are presented at a rate near 40 per second (e.g., 39.1 per second) to each ear individually, beginning at 75 dB nHL and then decreasing in 20 dB steps until no response is obtained.

When interpreting the responses obtained to 500 Hz tonebursts, we look for a single replicable peak that represents Wave V of the ABR. An example of an ABR intensity series obtained from an infant using a 500 Hz toneburst is shown in Figure 10.9. The other components of the ABR (e.g., Waves I and III) generally are not seen with these low-frequency stimuli. The latencies obtained range from 8 to 10 msec for high-intensity stimuli to 14 to 16 msec nearer threshold (Gorga, Kaminski, Beauchaine, & Jesteadt, 1988). In infants, these latencies will be even longer. In our experience, ABRs to 500 Hz tonebursts obtained from normal-hearing infants and children using the test parameters shown here are generally between 25 and 35 nHL (above behavioral threshold) (e.g., Hood & Berlin, 1986).

Stapells, Gravel, and Martin (1995) report a mean ABR threshold of 23.6 dB nHL for 500 Hz tones in notched noise in infants and children with normal hearing. A mean difference of 8.6 dB between ABR and behavioral thresholds was found for both normal hearing and hearing impaired groups at 500 Hz.

General Cautions and Considerations.   As with any test, there are a number of factors to keep in mind in making appropriate application and in correctly interpreting test results. Some of the many factors to consider when using auditory evoked potentials are the following:

1. Measuring auditory evoked potentials requires an intact neural system. Thus, abnormalities that can affect the neural system must be considered in interpretation of test results. For example, in the presence of hydrocephalus the ABR can be obliterated despite normal peripheral hearing (Kraus, Özdamar, Heydemann, Stein, & Reed, 1984). We and others have also seen infants and adults who have an apparent auditory neuropathy where the ABR is absent even though otoacoustic emissions are normal (e.g., Berlin, Hood, Cecola, Jackson, & Szabo, 1993; Starr, Picton, Sininger, Hood, & Berlin, 1996). Thus, it is important to obtain otoacoustic emissions in patients who fail to show an ABR at any intensity. Presence of an ABR at high intensities but not to lower intensity stimuli is consistent with a peripheral hearing loss. Absence of an ABR to high and low intensities may mean either a peripheral hearing loss or a neural disorder. Otoacoustic emissions are useful in distinguishing these two groups and we therefore always obtain otoacoustic emissions in patients who fail to show an ABR response.

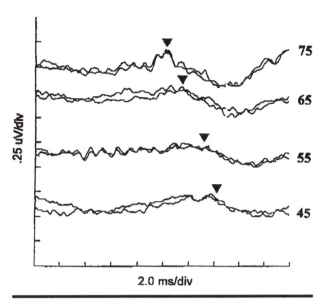

FIGURE 10.9   Example of an Auditory Brainstem Response (ABR) intensity series obtained from an infant using air-conducted 500 Hz tone bursts.

2. Use of insert earphones avoids the possibility of collapsing ear canals, a common problem in infants. These earphones are also more comfortable, which may enhance the patient's state of relaxation or sleep. These thresholds are also more useful in the hearing aid fitting process.

3. An evoked potential test battery should include tympanograms and middle ear muscle reflexes as well as otoacoustic emissions. If the child, as in the case of infants over about 4 months of age and young children, is sedated, then it is important to obtain middle ear and OAE measures before doing the ABR. During sedated deep sleep, positive pressure may build up in the middle ears that will compromise the results of middle ear measures and otoacoustic emissions.

4. Finally, it is always important to remember that the ABR and other auditory evoked potentials are not hearing tests. In those patients who do not demonstrate good neural synchrony, other means of estimating auditory function must be sought. In addition, passing an ABR as an infant does not preclude the possibility of acquired or later onset hereditary hearing loss. Thus, in reporting test results, we always inform parents and referral sources of the importance of monitoring a child's speech and language development and observing their responses to their auditory environment. Should a child fail to develop speech and language, parents are advised to seek appropriate evaluation and management.

In summary, auditory evoked potentials, when used and interpreted properly, provide a powerful method of obtaining reliable estimates of auditory sensitivity in infants, young children, and other individuals who cannot participate in behavioral testing or provide reliable behavioral responses. Auditory evoked potentials also provide an important physiologic cross-check of behavioral test results.

Examining Auditory Pathway Integrity

Auditory evoked potentials are useful in the evaluation of neural integrity in children who present with suspected auditory processing problems. Determining the presence or absence of functional abnormalities in the neural pathways can be used to support observed behavioral difficulties with auditory tasks. To accomplish this, a combination of ABR, middle latency responses (MLR), and cortical potentials can be used.

When ABR testing is completed, even though the overall purpose of the testing may be to obtain information about hearing sensitivity, replicable responses should be obtained at an intensity level that allows identification of Waves I, III, and V in order to evaluate absolute and interwave latencies and assess responses from a neural standpoint. While immaturity of the neural pathways must be considered in patients below 12 to 18 months of age, the clinician should look for presence of response components and general similarities between responses obtained from each ear.

Middle latency responses and cortical potentials are affected by sleep and sedation, are susceptible to muscle activity, and have a longer neuromaturational time course than the ABR. The MLR has been used in objective determination of hearing thresholds, assessment of auditory pathway function, localization of lesions, and assessment of cochlear implant function. While these potentials may be more difficult to record reliably in young children, researchers and clinicians have developed various techniques to distract or involve children according to the requirements of the protocol.

Responses that reflect ability to distinguish between stimuli appear promising in evaluating and understanding various aspects of auditory perception in children. Cortical potentials such as the P300 response and mismatch negativity (MMN) are "event-related potentials" that occur when the brain makes a decision about whether one stimulus differs from another. For these responses, two different stimuli are presented randomly with one of the stimuli occurring only rarely. The patient's task in recording the P300 response is to count the number of "different" or rarely occurring stimuli. Mismatch negativity responses are recorded without participation of the patient, other than remaining quiet, and thus may be particularly useful in pediatric populations. MMNs have been recorded reliably in school-aged children and appear to be a promising technique in understanding various auditory perception abilities in children, assessing the effectiveness of cochlear implants, and

monitoring the effectiveness of intervention programs (Kraus, McGee, Carrell, & Sharma, 1995).

Combining ABRs and OAEs to Identify Patients with Auditory Neuropathy

Recently, patients have been described who demonstrate normal otoacoustic emissions and absent or grossly abnormal ABRs, having what has been termed an auditory neuropathy (Berlin et al., 1993; Starr et al., 1996). The normal otoacoustic emissions suggest normal outer hair cell function, while the abnormal ABRs are consistent with a neural disorder. Some of these patients demonstrate timing problems (Starr, McPherson, Patterson, Don, Luxford, Shannon, Sininger, Tonokawa, & Waring, 1991), which is suggestive of a neural synchrony problem. Possible sites of the disorder may involve the inner hair cells, the synaptic juncture between the inner hair cells and the cochlear branch of the vestibulocochlear (VIIIth) nerve, or the nerve itself; it is not yet known precisely which structures may be involved. Auditory neuropathies most likely have several etiologies, and cases of unilateral auditory neuropathy also have been reported.

These patients are readily identifiable clinically and of particular interest to pediatric evaluation is the fact that a number of infants and young children have been identified with auditory neuropathy (Berlin et al., 1997; Stein, Tremblay, Pasternak, Banerjee, Lindemann, & Kraus, 1996). These patients may show ABRs that seem to have repeatable responses. However, on close examination, it is found that the latency of the responses does not increase with decreasing intensity, as should occur with neural responses. When polarity of the stimulus (i.e., changing from condensation to rarefaction clicks) is reversed, the recorded responses also reverse, which is characteristic of a cochlear response rather than an ABR.

Audiologic characteristics of patients with auditory neuropathy are normal otoacoustic emissions, abnormal ABRs, absent MEMRs to acoustic stimuli, abnormal masking level differences, and poor word recognition. Pure-tone configurations vary widely from the normal to severe hearing level ranges.

Management strategies in older children and adults include use of FM devices to deliver as clear a signal as possible and strategies to maximize use of visual information. Patients generally have not found amplification helpful, which is expected in view of their normal otoacoustic emissions, and we do not recommend use of hearing aids for our auditory neuropathy patients. In infants and young children, we encourage the use of Cued Speech or other methods that introduce visual information that follows the structure of English (Berlin et al., 1997). As these children are followed over time, it is possible that some of them may "outgrow" their neuropathy

Example of Pediatric Protocol

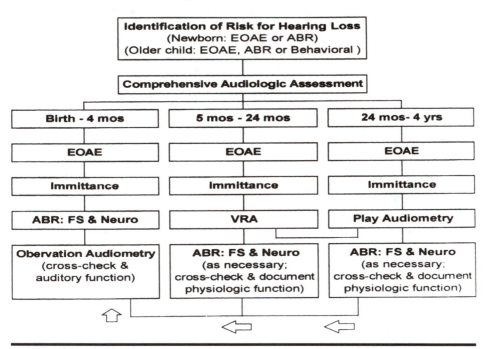

FIGURE 10.10   Pediatric audiometric assessment protocols based on a test battery approach and the cross-check principle (Jerger & Hayes, 1976). Protocols are depicted for three general age/developmental levels (birth to 4 months, 5 months to 24 months, and 24 months to 4 years). EOAE = Evoked otoacoustic emission; ABR = Auditory Brainstem Response; FS = Frequency specific; Neuro = neurologic; VRA = Visual Reinforcement Audiometry.

and later be able to use auditory information in a normal manner. We have observed improvement in auditory function in some patients, while auditory function in others has deteriorated over time. While the probability of such changes is simply not known at the present time, management for all children with auditory neuropathy should focus on facilitating development of language and communication skills.

CONCLUSION

In summary, a test battery approach and the cross-check principle should be adopted in the comprehensive audiologic assessment of infants and children. Behavioral and physiologic tests have important roles in the pediatric test armamentarium. The strengths and limitations of test procedures must be considered in their application to the pediatric population, particularly with children who have developmental deficits. Figure 10.10 presents such an approach for the pediatric population.

Current technology and techniques now allow the pediatric audiologist the opportunity to apply efficient, reliable, and valid test procedures for the audiometric evaluation of a population that can be challenging and often present

assessment dilemmas. As recommended by the Pediatric Working Group (Bess et al., 1996), if the test procedures described in this chapter are not available to the clinician responsible for evaluating the hearing of an infant or young child, it is the clinician's responsibility to identify other facilities who can complete the procedures. Children should be referred for the assessment(s) in a timely manner. This approach will ensure that accurate and comprehensive assessments will be available to infants and children at risk for hearing loss and that intervention will be begun based on the best audiologic data possible.

REFERENCES

Bench, J., Kowal, A., & Bamford, J. (1979). The BKB (Bamford-Kowal-Bench) sentence lists for partially hearing children. *British Journal of Audiology, 13,* 108–112.

Berlin, C. I., Bordelon, J., St. John, P., Wilensky, D., Hurley, A., Kluka, E., & Hood, L. J. (1997). Reversing click polarity may uncover auditory neuropathy in children. *Ear and Hearing,* in press.

Berlin, C., & Hood, L. (1993). Pseudo central hearing loss: A confusion of central for peripheral hearing loss caused by faulty conditioning techniques and lax criteria. *Seminars in Hearing, 14,* 215–223.

Berlin, C. I., Hood, L. J., Cecola, R. P., Jackson, D. F., & Szabo, P. (1993). Does Type I afferent neuron dysfunction reveal itself through lack of efferent suppression? *Hearing Research, 65,* 40–50.

Bernstein, R. S., & Gravel, J. S. (1990). A method for determining hearing sensitivity in infants: The Interweaving Staircase Procedure (ISP). *Journal of the American Academy of Audiology, 1,* 138–145.

Bernstein, R. S., & Gravel, J. S. (1992). Neonatal orienting as a measure of hearing. In F. H. Bess & J. W. Hall (Eds.), *Screening Children for Auditory Function* (pp. 181–190). Nashville, TN: Bill Wilkerson Press.

Bess, F. H., Chase, P. A., Gravel, J. S., Seewald, R. C., Stelmachowicz, P. A., Tharpe, A. M., & Hedley-Williams, A. (1996). Amplification for infants and children with hearing loss. (Pediatric Working Group of the Conference on Amplification for Children with Auditory Deficits). *American Journal of Audiology, 5,* 53–68.

Diefendorf, A. O. (1988). Behavioral evaluation of hearing-impaired children. In F. Bess (Ed.), *Hearing Impairment in Children* (pp. 133–151). Parkton, MD: York Press.

Diefendorf, A. O., & Gravel, J. S. (1996). Behavioral observation and visual reinforcement audiometry. In S. Gerber (Ed.), *Handbook of Pediatric Audiology* (pp. 55–83). Washington DC: Gallaudet University Press.

Eilers, R. E., Miskiel, E., Özdamar, Ö., Urbano, R., & Widen, J. (1991). Optimization of automated hearing test algorithms: Simulations using an infant response model. *Ear and Hearing, 12,* 191–198.

Eilers, R. E., Widen, J. E., Urbano, R., Hudson, T. M., & Gonzales, L. (1991). Optimization of automated hearing test algorithms: A comparison of data from simulations and young children. *Ear and Hearing, 12,* 199–204.

Elberling, C., & Don, M. (1987). Threshold characteristics of the human auditory brain stem response. *Journal of the Acoustical Society of America, 81,* 115–121.

Erber, N. P. (1982). *Auditory Training.* Washington DC: Alexander Graham Bell Association for the Deaf.

Gans, D. P., & Flexer, C. (1983). Auditory response behavior of severely handicapped children. *Journal of Audiologic Research, 23,* 137–148.

Gorga, M. P., Kaminski, J. R., Beauchaine, K. A., & Jesteadt, W. (1988). Auditory brainstem responses to tone bursts in normally hearing subjects. *Journal of Speech and Hearing Research, 31,* 87–97.

Gravel, J. S. (1989). Behavioral assessment of auditory function. *Seminars in Hearing, 10,* 216–228.

Gravel, J. S. (1992). Audiologic assessment of infants and toddlers. *ASHA Monographs-Report 21,* 55–62.

Gravel, J. S. (1994) Auditory assessment of infants. *Seminars in Hearing, 15*(2), 100–113.

Gravel, J. S. (1997). Behavioral audiologic testing. In A. Lalwani & K. Grundfast (Eds.), *Pediatric Otology and Neurotology* (pp. 103–111). Philadelphia: J. B. Lippincott.

Gravel, J. S., & Nozza, R. J. (1997). Hearing loss among children with otitis media with effusion. In J. Roberts, I. Wallace, & F. Henderson (Eds.), *Otitis Media in Young Children: Medical, Developmental and Educational Considerations* (pp. 63–92). Baltimore: Brookes.

Gravel, J. S., & Traquina, D. M. (1992). Experience with the audiologic assessment of infants and toddlers. *International Journal of Pediatric Otorhinolaryngology, 23,* 59–71.

Gravel, J. S., & Wallace, I. F. (1998). Audiologic management of otitis media. In F. Bess (Ed.), *Children with Hearing Loss: Contemporary Trends* (pp. 215–230). Nashville: Vanderbilt Bill Wilkerson Center Press.

Haskins, H. A. (1949). A phonetically balanced test of speech discrimination in children. Master's thesis, Northwestern University, Evanston, IL

Hood, L. J., & Berlin, C. I. (1986). *Auditory Evoked Potentials.* Austin, Texas: Pro-Ed.

Jerger, J., & Hayes, D. (1976). The cross-check principle in pediatric audiometry. *Archives of Otolaryngology, 102,* 614–620.

Jerger, J., Hayes, D., & Jordan, C. (1980). Clinical experience with auditory brainstem response audiometry in pediatric assessment. *Ear and Hearing, 1,* 19–25.

Jerger, J., Oliver, T., & Stach, B. (1985). Auditory brainstem response testing strategies. In J. T. Jacobson (Ed.), *The Auditory Brainstem Response.* San Diego: College-Hill Press.

Jerger, S. (1984). Speech audiometry. In J. Jerger (Ed.), *Pediatric Audiology* (pp. 71–93). San Diego, CA: College Hill Press.

Jerger, S. (1987). Validation of the Pediatric Speech Intelligibility test in children with central nervous system lesions. *Audiology, 26,* 298–311.

Jerger, S., & Jerger, J. (1982). Pediatric Speech Intelligibility test: Performance-intensity characteristics. *Ear and Hearing, 3,* 325–334.

Jerger, S., Lewis, S., Hawkins, J., & Jerger, J. (1980). Pediatric Speech Intelligibility test. I. Generation of test materials. *International Journal of Pediatric Otorhinolaryngology, 2,* 217–230.

Kemp, D. T., Ryan, S., & Bray, P. (1990). A guide to the effective use of otoacoustic emissions. *Ear and Hearing, 11,* 93– 105.

Kraus, N., Özdamar, Ö., Heydemann, P. T., Stein, L., & Reed, N. (1984). Auditory brainstem responses in hydrocephalic patients. *Electroencephalography and Clinical Neurophysiology, 59,* 310–317.

Kraus, N., McGee, T., Carrell, T. D., & Sharma, A. (1995). Neurophysiologic bases of speech discrimination. *Ear and Hearing, 16,* 19–37.

Lafreniere, O., Smurzynski, J., Jung, M. D., Leonard, G., & Kim, D. O. (1993). Otoacoustic emissions in full-term newborns at risk for hearing loss. *Laryngoscope, 103,* 1334–1341.

Liden, G., & Kankkunen, A. (1969). Visual reinforcement audiometry. *Acta Otolaryngologica, 67,* 281–292.

Ling, D. (1989). *Foundations of Spoken Language for Hearing Impaired Children.* Washington, DC: Alexander Graham Bell Association for the Deaf.

Merer, D. M., & Gravel, J. S. (1997). Screening infants and children for hearing loss: An examination of the CAST procedure. *Journal of the American Academy of Audiology, 8,* 233–242.

Moore, J. M., Thompson, G., & Thompson, M. (1975). Auditory localization of infants as a function of reinforcement conditions. *Journal of Speech and Hearing Disorders, 40,* 29–34.

Moore, J. M., Wilson, W. R., & Thompson, G. (1977). Visual reinforcement of head turn responses in infants under 12 months of age. *Journal of Speech and Hearing Disorders, 42,* 328–334.

Nilsson, M. J., Soli, S. D., & Gelnett, D. J. (1996). *Development of the Hearing In Noise Test for Children (HINT-C)* (pp. 1–9). Los Angeles: House Ear Institute.

Nilsson, M. J., Soli, S. D., & Sullivan, J. (1994). Development of a hearing in noise test for the measurement of speech reception threshold. *Journal of the Acoustical Society of America, 95,* 1085–1099.

Northern, J. L., & Downs, M. P. (1978, 1984, 1991). *Hearing in Children.* Baltimore: Williams & Wilkins.

Norton, S. J., & Widen, J. E. (1990). Evoked otoacoustic emissions in normal-hearing infants and children: Emerging data and issues. *Ear and Hearing, 11,* 121–127.

Nozza, R. J., & Wilson, W. R. (1984). Masked and unmasked pure-tone thresholds of infants and adults: Development of auditory frequency selectivity and sensitivity. *Journal of Speech and Hearing Research, 27,* 613–622.

Picton, T. W. (1978). The strategy of evoked potential audiometry. In S. E. Gerber & G. T. Mencher (Eds), *Early Diagnosis of Hearing Loss* (pp. 279–307). New York: Grune and Stratton.

Picton, T. W., Champagne, S. C., & Kellett, A. J. C. (1992). Human auditory evoked potentials recorded using maximum length sequences. *Electroencephalography and Clinical Neurophysiology, 84,* 90–100.

Primus, M. (1992). The role of localization in visual reinforcement audiometry. *Journal of Speech and Hearing Research, 35,* 1137–1141.

Primus, M. A., & Thompson, G. (1985). Response strength of young children in operant audiometry. *Journal of Speech and Hearing Research, 28,* 539–547.

Robbins, A. M., Renshaw, J. J., Miyamoto, R. T., Osberger, M. J., & Pope, M. L. (1988). *Minimal Pairs Test.* Indianapolis: Indiana University School of Medicine.

Ross, M., & Lerman, J. (1970). A picture identification test for hearing-impaired children. *Journal of Speech and Hearing Research, 13,* 44–53.

Roush, J., & Gravel, J. S. (1994). Acoustic amplification and sensory devices for infants and toddlers. In J. Roush & N. Matkin (Eds.), *Infants and Toddlers with Hearing Loss: Family Centered Assessment and Intervention* (pp. 65–79). Baltimore, MD: York Press.

Sanderson-Leepa, M. E., & Rintelmann, W. F. (1976). Articulation functions and test-retest performance of normal-hearing children on three speech discrimination tests: WIPI, PBK-50, and NU Auditory Test No. 6. *Journal of Speech and Hearing Disorders, 41,* 503–519.

Seewald, R. C., Moodie, K. S., Sinclair, S. T., & Cornelisse, L. E. (1996). Traditional and theoretical approaches to selecting amplification for infants and young children. In F. Bess, J. Gravel, & A. M. Tharpe (Eds.), *Amplification for Children with Auditory Deficits* (pp. 161–192). Nashville: Bill Wilkerson Press.

Sininger, Y. S. (1993). Auditory brain stem response for objective measures of hearing. *Ear and Hearing, 14,* 23–30.

Sininger, Y. S. (1995). Filtering and spectral characteristics of average auditory brain-stem response and background noise in infants. *Journal of the Acoustical Society of America, 98,* 2048–2055.

Spivak, L. (1993). Spectral composition of infant auditory brain-stem responses: Implications for filtering. *Audiology, 32,* 185–194.

Stapells, D. R., Gravel, J. S., & Martin, B. A. (1995). Thresholds for auditory brain stem responses to tones in notched noise from infants and young children with normal hearing and sensorineural hearing loss. *Ear and Hearing, 16,* 361–371.

Starr, A., McPherson, D., Patterson, J., Don, M., Luxford, W., Shannon, R., Sininger, Y., Tonokawa, L., & Waring, M. (1991). Absence of both auditory evoked potentials and auditory percepts dependent on timing cues. *Brain, 114,* 1157–1180.

Starr, A., Picton, T. W., Sininger, Y., Hood, L. J., & Berlin, C. I. (1996). Auditory neuropathy. *Brain, 119,* 741–753.

Stein, L., Tremblay, K., Pasternak, J., Banerjee, S., Lindemann, K., & Kraus, N. (1996). Brainstem abnormalities in neonates with normal otoacoustic emissions. *Seminars in Hearing, 17,* 197–213.

Suzuki, T., & Ogiba, Y. (1960). A technique of pure-tone audiometry for children under three years of age: Conditioned orientation reflex (COR) audiometry. *Revue De Laryngologie, Otologie, Rhinologie, 81,* 33–45.

Tharpe, A. M., & Ashmead, D. H. (1993). Computer simulation technique for assessing pediatric auditory test protocols. *Journal of the American Academy of Audiology, 4,* 80–90.

Thompson, G., & Folsom, R. C. (1984). A comparison of two conditioning procedures in the use of visual reinforcement audiometry (VRA). *Journal of Speech and Hearing Disorders, 49,* 241–245.

Thompson, G., & Weber, B. A. (1974). Responses of infants and young children to behavior observation audiometry (BOA). *Journal of Speech and Hearing Disorders, 39,* 140–147.

Thompson, G., Wilson, W. R., & Moore, J. M. (1979). Application of visual reinforcement audiometry (VRA) to low-functioning children. *Journal of Speech and Hearing Disorders, 44,* 80–90.

Thompson, M., & Thompson, G. (1972). Response of infants and young children as a function of auditory stimuli and test method. *Journal of Speech and Hearing Research, 15,* 699–707.

Widen, J. E. (1990). Behavioral screening of high-risk infants using visual reinforcement audiometry. *Seminars in Hearing, 11*(4), 342–356.

Widen, J. E. (1993). Adding objectivity to infant behavioral audiometry. *Ear and Hearing, 14,* 49–57.

Widen, J. E. (1997). Evoked otoacoustic emissions in evaluating children. In M. S. Robinette & T. J. Glattke (Eds.), *Otoacoustic Emissions: Clinical Applications* (pp. 271–306). New York: Thieme.

Wilson, W. R., & Thompson, G. (1984). Behavioral audiometry. In J. Jerger (Ed.), *Pediatric Audiology* (pp. 1–44). San Diego, CA: College Hill Press.

Yang, E., Stuart, A., Mencher, G. T., Mencher, L. S., & Vincer, M. J. (1993). Auditory brain stem responses to air- and bone-conducted clicks in the audiologic assessment of at-risk infants. *Ear and Hearing, 14,* 175–182.

Zimmerman, M. C., Morgan, D. E., & Dubno, J. R. (1987). Auditory brain stem evoked response characteristics in developing infants. *Annals of Otology, Rhinology and Laryngology, 96,* 291–299.

GLOSSARY

Auditory brainstem response (ABR) An auditory evoked potential that represents neural activity from the VIIIth cranial nerve and auditory pathways of the brainstem.

Auditory evoked potentials (AEPs) Electrophysiologic responses representing neural responses of auditory pathways from the VIIIth cranial nerve to the cortex.

Cross-check principle A principle in audiometry that states that the results of any single audiometric test cannot be considered valid without independent verification from another test.

Distortion product otoacoustic emissions (DPOAEs) Used clinically, otoacoustic emissions that represent the cubic distortion product (2f1-f2) occurring from simultaneous presentation of combinations of two pure tones (f1 and f2).

Evoked otoacoustic emissions (EOAEs) Otoacoustic emissions that occur in response to acoustic stimulation.

Immittance A term representing energy flow through the middle ear including admittance, compliance, conductance, impedance, reactance, resistance, and susceptance.

Late cortical responses Long-latency auditory evoked potentials that may include the vertex response (N1-P2), P300, mismatch negativity (MMN), and other responses from the auditory pathways of the cortex.

Middle ear muscle reflexes (MEMRs) Reflexive contraction of the stapedius and tensor tympani muscles of the middle ear in response to loud sound.

Middle latency response (MLR) An auditory evoked potential representing neural activity from, at least in part, auditory radiations from the thalamus to the cortex and the primary auditory cortex.

Mismatch negativity (MMN) A late auditory evoked potential occurring in the 100 to 200 millisecond latency range that represents neural activity obtained by utilizing combinations of auditory stimuli presented in an oddball paradigm.

Otoacoustic emissions (OAEs) Low-level sounds emitted by the normal cochlea.

P300 response A late auditory evoked potential occurring in the 300 millisecond latency range that represents neural activity obtained by utilizing combinations of auditory stimuli presented in an oddball paradigm.

Tympanogram A graph of middle ear immittance as a function of the amount of air pressure delivered to the ear canal.

CHAPTER 11

NEWBORN HEARING SCREENING

BRUCE A. WEBER
ALLAN DIEFENDORF

In audiology texts written just a few years ago the reader will find a very straightforward discussion of newborn hearing screening. They describe how an audiologist takes a clinical auditory brainstem response (ABR) testing unit into the neonatal intensive care unit (NICU) to screen all babies who have been determined to be at high risk for hearing loss. Indeed, at that time there were some differences in protocol between hospital screening programs, but, for the most part, these minor differences related to such factors as the rate of stimulus presentation or placement of the recording electrodes. Newborn hearing screening programs tended to be very similar because there was a broad consensus regarding how such programs should be carried out.

In recent years this situation has changed markedly. There are now strikingly different points of view regarding newborn hearing screening, and, as a result, screening programs now differ widely. Several factors have led to these differences. First, an automated ABR screener has been introduced that permits nurses and nonprofessionals to perform the screening test. Second, the clinical application of evoked otoacoustic emissions (EOAEs) has provided an alternative technique to rival the auditory brainstem response (ABR) as the procedure of choice. Third, there has been a greater expression of the view that *all*, not just high-risk, babies should receive hearing screening prior to hospital discharge.

As a result of these factors, a screening program today may be quite different from the traditional program widely advocated less than ten years ago. Now, instead of an audiologist performing the nursery hearing screening, it may be a nurse, technician, or volunteer who carries out the testing. Instead of using flexible, and more expensive, clinical ABR test equipment, the examiner now may use a dedicated automated ABR screener, or EOAE test unit. Instead of confining screening to babies who are at high risk for hearing loss, all newborns in the hospital may be included in the screening program. There are also early identification programs that elect to perform the screening after the baby has been discharged from the hospital.

Given this current diversity of approaches to early identification of hearing loss, it should not be surprising that there are strong and, in some instances, heatedly opposing points of views. This chapter will attempt to address the major aspects of newborn hearing screening with special attention given to areas where changes have occurred in recent years. The aim of this chapter is not to provide the reader with a blueprint for the initiation of a hearing screening program because we do not believe that a single design is best for all screening environments. The information presented here, however, should assist the reader in appreciating the importance of early identification of hearing loss and the factors that must be considered before a screening program can be initiated.

IMPACT OF CONGENITAL HEARING LOSS

Children with congenital hearing loss may not have immediate access to language and thus may differ from their normal hearing peers in their language development and in their facility with communication. The effect of hearing loss on the development of speech and language skills is both varied and complex. Though children with hearing loss represent a heterogeneous population, the more severe the hearing loss and the earlier the onset, the greater the effects on developmental processes.

No dispute exists as to whether congenital and early onset childhood hearing loss can impose burdens on the affected child, on the family, and on society. There is the widely held view that early identification of hearing loss and immediate intervention for children with a hearing loss increases the likelihood of optimizing children's potential in receptive and expressive language, literacy (reading and writing), academic achievement, and emotional/social development.

Children with hearing loss run the risk of failing to learn language at the normal time or rate because the learning of language is primarily an auditory event. Thus, deficits in communication function interfere with the educational process during the early years and in all the school years that follow. A barrier to the child's progress that is second in importance only to oral language is failure to learn to read. Practically all of the information not presented to a child in the form of oral language will reach the child in printed form. The development of good reading skills depends on the development of good language skills. The two cannot be separated and under optimal conditions should be sequentially learned. As a general rule, children with severe hearing loss do not exhibit sufficient knowledge of language to ensure a basis for the normal development of reading skills and subsequent writing skills.

Children with hearing loss may demonstrate reduced performance in those academic subjects that are language based and/or dependent on the ability to learn new information through reading. Even mathematics performance is affected, although to a lesser extent than other subjects. One measure of educational problems of children with hearing loss is the proportion who have repeated grades in school. Davis and colleagues (Davis, Elfenbein, Schum, & Bentler, 1986) surveyed 376 children enrolled in itinerant teaching programs and reported 27.5% had repeated a grade. The range was from first to eleventh, but failure of the fourth, fifth, and sixth grades was most common.

Difficulties in communication and frequently associated poor academic performance may lead to lowered self-esteem and to social isolation in children with hearing loss. Since they are frequently the only students with hearing loss in the schools, it is not unusual for them to feel isolated, not fitting into either the deaf or the hearing world. Davis (1988) has hypothesized that much of the social isolation experienced by these children comes about because they are so much like children with normal hearing without being enough like them. The end result of social isolation and reduced self-esteem occurs when a child feels rejected by those children with whom daily interactions are necessary.

Hearing impairment also imposes a significant economic burden. Relatively few deaf persons are employed in professional, technical, and managerial positions. The lifetime economic cost of congenital deafness is estimated to currently exceed one million dollars. Other less tangible costs borne by affected individuals and by their families derive from emotional stress, breakdowns in family communication, and isolation from peers and educational systems.

NATIONAL PERSPECTIVE ON EARLY IDENTIFICATION OF HEARING LOSS

Several efforts have directed attention to the issue of identification of hearing loss in infants. In 1988, C. Everett Koop, then Surgeon General of the United States, issued a challenge that by the year 2000, 90% of all children with significant hearing loss should be identified by 12 months of age. At about the same time, the U.S. Department of Health and Human Services was involved in a national initiative for health promotion and disease prevention. By 1990, a coalition of 300 national organizations and state and territorial health departments had designed the *Healthy People 2000* initiative. At that time the age of identification was estimated to be between 24 and 30 months. As part of the initiative related to hearing, a goal was established to reduce the average age at which children with significant hearing impairment are identified to no more than 12 months by the year 2000. The document also stated:

> The future of a child born with a significant hearing impairment depends to a very large degree on early identification (i.e., audiological diagnosis before 12 months of age) followed by immediate and appropriate intervention. If hearing-impaired children are not identified early, it is difficult, if not impossible, for many of them to acquire the fundamental language, social, and cognitive skills that provide the foundation for later schooling and success in society. When early identification and intervention occurs, hearing-impaired children make dramatic progress, are more successful in school, and become more productive members of society. The earlier intervention and habilitation begins, the more dramatic the benefits. (U.S. Department of Health and Human Services, 1990, p. 464).

Achievement of the *Healthy People 2000* goal is dependent upon finding better ways to identify hearing impairment in young children. Toward that end, in 1993 the Expert Panel of the National Institutes of Health (NIH) Consensus Development Conference on Early Identification of Hearing Impairment in Infants and Young Children recommended that *all* newborns (both high and low risk) be screened for hearing loss prior to discharge from the newborn nursery. Additionally, the Panel emphasized that comprehensive intervention and management for those infants identified with hearing loss must be an integral part of a universal screening program. Moreover, in the past several years the National Institute on Deafness and Other Communicative Disorders (NIDCD) as well as the Bureau of Maternal and Child Health (MCH) of the federal government has assigned high priority to funding research projects that address issues related to early identification of hearing loss in infants.

In 1994 the National Joint Committee on Infant Hearing (JCIH) endorsed the goal of *universal detection* of infants with hearing loss as early as possible. The JCIH further stated that *all* infants with hearing loss should be identified before 3 months of age and receive intervention by 6 months of age. Moreover, when hearing loss is identified, evaluation and early intervention should be provided in accordance with the Individuals with Disabilities Education Act (IDEA). Since 1986, this federal legislation has existed for early and appropriate services to all infants with disabilities and their families through IDEA (U.S. Report 99-860, 1986).

EPIDEMIOLOGIC PERSPECTIVE ON EARLY IDENTIFICATION OF HEARING LOSS

The process of early detection of hearing loss should facilitate early intervention; yet, without careful planning the process can lead to development or delivery of unwarranted services that are neither efficient or cost-effective. Hence, in today's sociopolitical context of increasing costs and declining allocations for human services, an epidemiological approach to justifying early detection of hearing loss is essential.

For a disorder to warrant screening, several criteria must be met:

1. The ramifications of not detecting the disorder must have significant consequences in terms of death, impairment, or suffering.
2. The screening method (procedure and tools) must be sensitive and reliable.
3. Treatment for the disorder must be accessible, efficacious, and readily complied with.
4. The benefit(s) of early detection and treatment must outweigh any harms and justify the costs.
5. There must be a professional discipline able to carry out the vision, mission, and supervision of early detection programs.

Consequences of an Undetected Hearing Loss

No dispute exists regarding the potential consequences of a childhood sensorineural hearing loss. As indicated earlier in this chapter, the impact of congenital hearing loss on primary language (spoken language) and secondary language (reading and writing) is significant. Moreover, the subsequent effects on academic achievement, social development, and family dynamics have been well documented for thirty years (Bess, 1985; Davis, 1990; de Villiers, 1992; Karchmer, 1991; Quigley & Thomure, 1968).

Available Screening Tools

Over the years a number of different behavioral and electrophysiological techniques have been used to screen the hearing of newborns. Of these various approaches, two physiologic measures (auditory brainstem response [ABR] and otoacoustic emissions [OAE]) have been shown to be most effective. These techniques will be discussed in some detail later in the chapter.

Available Treatment

It is improper to screen for a disorder without certainty that facilities for appropriate follow-up of individuals who fail and their families are both available and accessible. Access to services for infants and young children with hearing loss and their families has been enhanced as a result of federal and state legislative actions. Public Laws 102-119 and 94-142 provide guidelines for Individualized Family Service Plans (IFSPs) and Individualized Educational Plans (IEPs) respectively. To facilitate follow-up and access, amendments to the federal Education of the Handicapped Act (PL 102-119) provide for statewide, comprehensive, coordinated multidisciplinary, interagency programs of early intervention services for all handicapped children and their families in order to meet the infant's or young child's developmental needs.

Cost versus Benefit

Evidence is mounting that demonstrates the efficacy of treatment for children with hearing loss. Studies involving children who are deaf and hard of hearing show that intervention during the crucial period from birth to $2\frac{1}{2}$ or 3 years of age results in greater linguistic and academic gains than intervention after $2\frac{1}{2}$ or 3 years. That is, when comparisons are made between "early" intervention (prior to about 30 months of age) and "late" intervention (after about 30 months of age), results typically show greater progress for the children receiving "early" intervention on a variety of outcome variables (Glover, Watkins, Pittman, Johnson, & Barringer, 1994). In one of the most thorough longitudinal studies of language and communication skills of children with hearing loss, Levitt, McGarr, and Geffner (1987) reported that, of the many variables examined, age at which special education began showed the largest effect on the development of language and communication skills. Those children who received early intervention showed significantly higher speech and language scores that continued to be evident more than ten years later. In a more recent study, Yoshinaga-Itano (1995) reported findings of early identification and early intervention for young children with varying degrees of hearing loss. Her data indicate that early identification of hearing loss, particularly at birth, not only minimizes the deleterious effect upon communication development, but can prevent delays in development from ever occurring.

Qualified Professionals

Audiology represents the professional discipline able to accept the challenge of universal detection of infants with hearing loss. Accepting this clinical challenge requires audiologists to determine efficient and cost-effective ways to screen the anticipated 4 million babies born in the United States each year, follow all screening failures, and secure appropriate intervention services for those children identified. As the stewards of newborn hearing screening programs, audiology can ensure the quality and value of these programs to infants and their families.

Hearing loss meets all the requirements necessary to warrant screening to permit early identification. Arguing the concept of newborn hearing screening is one thing; the actual implementation is another. It is no small task.

CHARACTERISTICS OF HEARING LOSS TODAY

When all factors are considered, the prevalence of a handicapping hearing loss has been estimated to be as high as six babies for every 1000 live births (Northern & Hayes, 1994). Very little is known about the prevalence of mild to moderate hearing loss in newborns (Mauk & Behrens, 1993).

The characteristics of hearing impairment in children are changing significantly. That is, the etiology of childhood hearing impairment in the 1990s (e.g., persistent pulmonary hypertension; intraventricular hemorrhage) are different from those in the 1970s (e.g., maternal rubella, Rh incompatibility) and the 1980s (e.g., hemophilus influenza type B meningitis). Not only has there been a change in the causes of infant hearing loss, there also has been an apparent shift from the severe-to-profound hearing loss categories to the milder forms of hearing impairment.

With the continued improvement in modern day neonatal intensive care units, there has been a marked increase in the survival rate of premature, high-risk infants including very-low-birth-weight (VLBW) neonates and other severely compromised newborns. In fact, the perinatal and neonatal mortality rates for VLBW babies have shown an accelerated decline since the mid 1970s (Shenai, 1992). Although the prevalence of neurodevelopmental handicaps among VLBW survivors also appears to be decreasing with evolving neonatal intensive care, VLBW infants remain about three times as likely as normal newborn infants to have an adverse neuro-developmental outcome, and the risk increases with decreasing birth weight. For example, these youngsters are at increased risk for respiratory insufficiency from hyaline membrane disease, increased susceptibility to broncho-pulmonary dysplasia (BPD), periventricular-intraventricular hemorrhage, perinatal asphyxia, and hyperbilirubinemia, to name several. In addition, more than 5.5% of these NICU survivors exhibit handicaps characterized by cerebral palsy, hearing loss, mental retardation, or retinopathy of prematurity (Shenai, 1992). Immaturity is a common denominator among several studies examining the neonatal risk factors for sensorineural hearing loss (Halpern, Hosford-Dunn, & Malachowski, 1987; Salamy, Eldridge, & Tooley, 1989). These findings suggest that with decreasing gestational age of patients in the NICU, a concomitant increase in the incidence of sensorineural hearing loss can be expected to occur.

Changes in the makeup of sensorineural hearing loss have occurred due to the incidence of both etiology and severity of hearing loss. Several factors have contributed to this development: (1) advances in knowledge and treatment of various neonatal diseases; (2) the use of inoculations for many infectious diseases that once produced severe to profound sensorineural hearing loss (e.g., hemophilus influenza type B vaccine for meningitis); (3) better understanding of the deleterious effects of many ototoxic drugs; (4) improved medical management with phototherapy or exchange transfusion for neonates with hyperbilirubinemia; and (5) greater accessibility of medical care. The changing characteristics of hearing impairment in neonates and infants will undoubtedly present challenges to individuals responsible for early detection programs.

CURRENT AGE OF DETECTION OF HEARING LOSS

In 1982 and again in 1990, the Joint Committee on Infant Hearing (JCIH) advocated infant hearing screening optimally by three months of age, but no later than six months of age. It further recommended that, whenever possible, the diagnostic process should be completed and habilitation begun by the age of six months. In 1994, the JCIH strengthened its position by advocating detection *before three months* of age. Although the Joint Committee recognized that it is not always possible to meet these guidelines, the recommendation does represent an ideal endorsed and sought by audiologists, physicians, educators, and others concerned with the habilitation of deaf and hard-of-hearing children. Actual practice, however, falls well short of this goal.

Numerous studies have reported the actual ages of identification of hearing loss occur substantially later than six months of age. Stein, Clark, and Kraus (1983) and Stein, Jabaley, Spitz, Stoakley, and McGee (1990), examined ages of identification of hearing loss for graduates of a well-baby nursery (WBN) and neonatal intensive care unit (NICU). For babies from the NICU, the median age of diagnosis was 12.6 and 13.0 months in the 1983 and 1990 studies, respectively. This was significantly earlier than for the WBN graduates, for whom the median ages of diagnosis were 16.5 months and 16.0 months in the 1983 and 1990 studies respectively. Elssman, Matkin, and Sabo (1987) examined questionnaires completed by parents of 159 hearing-impaired children. They found the average age of identification to be 19 months. Surprisingly, results indicated that there was minimal difference in age of identification between babies with no known risk history and those who were at high risk. Children with a moderate degree of hearing impairment and no known risk factors had the highest age of identification (43 months). The situation may even be worse for children with mild hearing losses who are frequently not identified until 5 to 6 years of age (Mauk & Behrens, 1993). It is clear that the goal of the JCIH (identification before three months of age) is far from being met.

WHEN TO SCREEN

Hearing screening in infants is a process driven by the program goals, clinical setting, and the characteristics of the population being served. Thus, it is of utmost importance to establish clearly the intent of any hearing screening program. At a minimum, the following steps should be included in planning a screening program:

1. Define the purpose of the program and set program goals.
2. Choose the test(s) or procedure(s) to be used in screening.
3. Determine the population to be screened.
4. Arrange for diagnostic follow-up.
5. Arrange for treatment/intervention.
6. Select and train program personnel.
7. Monitor the outcome(s) of the screening program (i.e., programmatic assessment and validation), including assurance of linkage from patient assessment to patient benefit.

If the decision has been made to initiate an early identification program, there are some strong reasons for conducting the screening within the newborn nursery prior to the babies' discharge:

1. During the first few days of life newborns spend a large portion of their day in quiet sleep that is ideal for hearing screening. The extent of quiet periods reduces as they grow older.
2. A visit to the nursery allows a check on the status of a number of babies. Selection of a baby for screening can be made on such factors as anticipated discharge date, sleep state, and other pending procedures. Even if one baby is not ready for screening, often there is another baby who can be screened. As a result, several babies can routinely be tested during a single visit. Outpatient testing is seldom as efficient.
3. If follow-up is needed, this can be integrated into the baby's discharge summary and overall medical management.
4. Screening in the newborn nursery eliminates the program's dependence on a caregiver to return the infant to the clinic for testing as an outpatient.

There are, however, also some disadvantages with performing hearing screening directly within the newborn nursery:

1. A potential problem is the routinely high noise levels found in the nursery. It should be noted, however, that a noise attenuating double-walled polyethylene acoustic isolette is now commercially available. This isolette, specially designed for newborn hearing screening, reduces the level of lower frequencies (500 Hz and 1000 Hz) about 20 dB and attenuates higher frequencies (2000 Hz–8000 Hz) approximately 30 dB.
2. Shortly after birth babies commonly have vernix in the ear canals, and it is not uncommon for otitis media to be present.
3. For premature babies health status and immaturity can influence test results.
4. The length of hospital stay for well babies is now very short and this poses logistical problems to insure that screening is performed prior to discharge.
5. Some hearing impairments have a delayed onset or are progressive and these will be missed when hearing is screened in the newborn nursery.

PRINCIPLES OF SCREENING

It makes little sense to undertake newborn hearing screening if available techniques are not effective in sorting normal hearing babies from those who have impaired hearing. A number of factors contribute to a test protocol's degree of effectiveness. It is not the intent of this chapter to discuss this issue in depth, but a brief discussion of the principles of screening seems appropriate to assist us in evaluating alternative screening strategies and techniques. The interested reader can find more information elsewhere (Turner, 1991, 1992a, 1992b).

The selection of a screening test must be made on the basis of demonstrated performance, not on its practical advantages (Weber & Jacobson, 1994). A screening technique may be attractive for a variety of reasons (e.g., cost, brevity, or ease of operation), but unless it can be shown to effectively separate normal-hearing from hearing-impaired babies, it is not worthy of adoption. In evaluating a technique, two questions must be asked. First, if a baby has a hearing impairment, what is the probability that he or she will fail the screening test? Second, if a baby's hearing is normal, what is the probability that the screening test will be passed?

The simplest way to display answers to these questions is in the form of a 2 × 2 table that compares screening test outcome with the actual presence and absence of a hearing loss. Such a matrix is shown in Table 11.1. It can be seen

TABLE 11.1 Screening test outcomes.

	HEARING STATUS	
	Hearing Loss	*Normal Hearing*
Failed Screening	**True Positive**	**False Positive**
Passed Screening	**False Negative**	**True Negative**

that for any individual screening test there are four possible outcomes. Desirable outcomes occur when a baby with a hearing loss fails the screening test (true positive) or a normal-hearing baby passes the test (true negative). Undesirable outcomes occur when a hearing-impaired baby passes the screening (false negative) or a normal-hearing baby fails the screening test (false positive).

It is obvious that the ideal hearing screening test would fail all hearing-impaired babies and would pass all normal-hearing babies. Unfortunately, no technique can reasonably be expected to perform at this level. It is possible, however, to determine how close it comes to this ideal. Table 11.2 gives an example of expected screening results if a 4% prevalence of hearing loss is assumed. In this hypothetical group of 5000 babies, 660 babies failed the test and 4340 passed. Of the 660 failures, 180 were subsequently found to have a hearing loss. Of the 4340 passes, 20 were later found to have a hearing loss. Thus, there were 180 true positives and 4320 true negatives, but there were also 20 false negatives and 480 false positives.

This information can be used to determine the probabilities of the screening outcomes that will occur if the same technique is used in the future. The probability that a hearing-impaired baby will fail the test is referred to as the test's *sensitivity*. It is calculated dividing the number of true positives by the sum of the number of true positives and the number of false negatives. In the example in Table 11.2, dividing 180 by 200 (180 + 20) yields a test sensitivity of 90%. *Specificity* is the probability that a normal-hearing baby will pass the screening test. It is calculated by dividing the number of true negatives by the sum of the number of true negatives and the number of false positives. In our example the specificity of the test is 90% as determined by dividing 4320 by 4800 (4320 + 480).

The positive predictive value of a test is one more important description of its performance. It indicates what percentage of the individuals who fail a screening test actually have the impairment being screened. The positive predictive value of the test equals the number of true positives divided by the total number of babies who failed the test. In the example in Table 11.2 the positive predictive value is obtained by dividing 180 by 660 (180 + 480) for a positive

predictive value of 27.3%. This is very important information because it tells us that, in our example, only a little over one-fourth of the babies who fail the screening test actually have a hearing loss.

It is obvious that high sensitivity and high specificity is desirable in a screening test. A number of factors influence sensitivity and specificity. Assuming a 30 dB screening level in the above example, the values would change if the pass-fail cutoff is either made more stringent (e.g., 20 dB) or less stringent (e.g., 40 dB). When the screening level is made more stringent, more babies will fail the test, which will increase the likelihood that a hearing-impaired baby will fail the test. As a result, sensitivity will go up. However, more normal-hearing babies will also fail the test, so specificity will go down. Using a less stringent screening level will have just the opposite effect. It can be seen that selecting a specific screening protocol results in a tradeoff between optimum sensitivity and optimum specificity.

The performance of a hearing screening test is also influenced by such factors as the presence of a hearing loss due to transient middle ear pathology. The hearing screening test may accurately detect conductive hearing loss in the nursery, only to have the middle ear problem resolved by the time the baby is retested. Thus, the baby will be classified as a false positive outcome.

ALTERNATIVE SCREENING TECHNIQUES

The JCIH position statement did not indicate a preferred screening technique. Rather, it recommended that each program review the alternatives and select the one that is most appropriate for its specific care practice (JCIH, 1994). It is worthwhile, therefore, to examine the relative strengths and weakness of the primary screening techniques.

Conventional Auditory Brainstem Response Screening

The ABR, or the Brainstem Auditory Evoked Response (BAER), as it is commonly referred to in the pediatric and neonatology literature, has been utilized in newborn hearing screening for over twenty years. A train of from 2000 to 4000 abrupt click stimuli are presented to the baby at rates around 30/sec. Following each stimulus presentation an averaging computer records the electrophysiologic activity from recording electrodes on the baby's scalp. Individual responses are summated by the computer and a composite final response reflects the synchronous neural firings within the auditory nerve and brainstem. The nature of the response and the recording technique is discussed in much greater detail in Chapter 7.

As a measure for hearing screening, the ABR has several strengths: (1) the response is very stable and not influenced by the baby's sleep level; (2) it can be recorded from

TABLE 11.2 Example of screening test results on 5000 babies with a high prevalence (4%) of hearing loss.

	HEARING STATUS		
	Hearing Loss	Normal Hearing	Total
Failed Screening	180	480	660
Passed Screening	20	4320	4340
Total	200	4800	5000

babies as young as 28 weeks conceptual age; (3) the ABR can be detected in the presence of minor conductive ear problems; (4) if no response is detected at the screening level (often 30–35 dB nHL), the stimulus level can be raised to probe for threshold; (5) it is possible to use bone-conducted click stimuli to assist in differentiating between conductive and sensorineural impairments (Hooks & Weber, 1984; Stuart, Yang, & Green, 1994) and, with special software, stimulus presentation rates up to several hundred clicks per second are possible (Weber & Roush, 1993); 6) the response can be detected even in a relatively noisy environment such as the NICU. Hyde, Riko, and Malazia (1990), using conventional ABR in a large sample of infants, established a sensitivity rate for sensorineural hearing loss of 98% with specificity of 96%.

Because of its unique combination of strengths, conventional ABR testing has been widely viewed as the method of choice for the electrophysiologic testing of not only newborns, but infants and other difficult-to-test children as well (Jacobson & Jacobson, 1996). Conventional ABR screening, however, is not without its limitations: (1) The test equipment is expensive; (2) the examiner must have a high level of expertise in order to appropriately administer the test and interpret the test results; (3) recording electrodes must be attached to the baby's scalp, so the procedure is quite time consuming; (4) responses can be influenced by the baby's neurological status; (5) the acoustic click routinely used in newborn hearing screening has its energy in the 2000 Hz to 4000 Hz range, so a response provides no information about hearing status for lower frequencies.

Automated ABR Testing

The most common automated ABR screener, the ALGO-2 screener, advances evoked potential technology by using automation and objective data analysis to simplify the task of ABR infant hearing screening while rigorously maintaining accurate, consistent, and effective performance.

One of the ALGO-2 key features is a method of *response detection* frequently referred to as a *weighted-binary template-matching algorithm*. After the examiner has positioned recording sensors on the baby's scalp, the ALGO-2 is activated and the unit automatically presents 35 dBHL click stimuli whenever electrode impedance, ambient noise level, and movement artifacts are within acceptable limits. As the stimuli are presented, the ALGO-2 is comparing the infant's accumulated response in computer memory with an internal template of the typical neonatal ABR. When the likelihood of a response (likelihood ratio) reaches a predetermined criterion level, the test stimuli automatically cease and a display panel indicates that the baby has passed the screening test. A baby cannot pass until the likelihood ratio reaches 160, which is the point where the probability of response exceeds 0.99997. To account for variation in

the latency of ABR component Wave V for premature and full-term infants, the ALGO-2 shifts the template ±1.5 msec in 0.25 msec steps, testing for detection for each latency shift, to find the best fit of the template.

The low false-negative rate reflects the design's emphasis on not passing a deaf baby. Yet, to avoid false-positive identifications, the number of sweeps needed to refer a baby is set extremely high (15,000). If the likelihood of a response does not meet the stringent criteria for a pass at the end of 15,000 trials, testing automatically is halted and the display panel indicates that the infant should be referred for further testing.

An alternative automated ABR hearing screener (Smart-EP) has recently been introduced. Rather than comparing a baby's response to a predetermined template as the ALGO-2 does, this unit records two separate responses and compares their agreement through cross-correlation analysis (Özdamar, Delgado, Eilers, & Urbano, 1994). Multiple time windows are used to locate the region of maximum correlation and this agreement is defined as a response if it exceeds a preset response criterion. The Smart EP system has multiple built-in protocols and is capable of automatically obtaining addition pairs of records at different stimulus intensities. The combination of automatic response detection and stimulus manipulation provides the examiner with an estimate of the patient's threshold

Two major advantages of an automated ABR screening are: (1) a sophisticated examiner is not required, and (2) objective data are collected under controlled conditions with stringent criteria for a pass. This means that the same statistical criterion is applied to *every* test while examiner and interpretation bias is eliminated. A comparison of automated ABR hearing screening with conventional ABR hearing screening reveals a test sensitivity of 100% and test specificity of 96% to 98% (Hall, Kileny, Ruth, & Kripal, 1987; Herrmann, Thornton, & Joseph, 1995; Jacobson, Jacobson, & Spahr, 1990).

Over the past three years, different screening programs utilizing different personnel have reported strikingly similar results (Diefendorf, Reitz, Cox, & Hussain, 1996; Northern & Marlowe, 1995; Stewart, 1995). Thus, the ability to utilize various personnel minimizes personnel cost and increases cost effectiveness.

An automated ABR screener is relatively inexpensive compared to the cost of diagnostic ABR test units, but this cost savings creates some limitations: (1) It is not possible to probe for threshold if the baby does not pass the screening test; (2) in poor recording conditions it is not possible to alter recording parameters, such as stimulus rate or filter settings, to improve the quality of response; (3) bone-conduction stimuli cannot be used. It also should be noted that disposable ear cushions and electrodes cost about $10/baby, which is of significance when attempts are made to keep test cost as low as possible.

Evoked Otoacoustic Emission (EOAE) Testing

This is the most recent alternative to ABR hearing screening. The principles of EOAE testing are discussed in Chapter 6 and only its application to newborn screening will be covered here.

Transient evoked otacoustic emissions (TEOAEs) from neonates have been studied and discussed for a number of years (e.g., Johnsen, Bagli, & Elberling, 1983). However, unlike the ABR, which has been used in newborn screening for over twenty years, the clinical application of TEOAEs with this group is more recent (Bonfils, Uziel, & Narcy, 1989; Bray & Kemp, 1987; Stevens, Webb, Hutchinson, Connell, Smith, & Buffin, 1990). Because most of the earlier studies and applications occurred in Europe, the United States trailed many other countries in the use of TEOAEs in newborn screening. Within the United States the first large-scale investigation of EOAEs in the newborn nursery was conducted in the large federally funded Rhode Island Hearing Assessment Project (White, Vohr, & Behrens, 1993). In this investigation 1850 babies were screened (16.4% were from the NICU) and the clinical utility of TEOAEs as a screening tool was demonstrated. Follow-up studies of infants screened by TEOAEs suggest that this technique can identify infants with hearing loss of approximately 30 dB HL and greater (Kennedy, Kimm, Dees, Evans, Hunter, Lenton, & Thornton, 1991). When TEOAE screening results were compared to ABR results obtained three months after the babies due date, sensitivity and specificity were 93% and 84% respectively (Stevens, Webb, Hutchinson, Connell, Smith, & Buffin, 1989).

Use of TEOAEs as the screening tool has several advantages: (1) It does not require attachment of recording electrodes and is thus less time consuming. Stevens and colleagues (1989) found that emissions testing was nearly twice as fast as ABR screening. (2) TEOAE screening can be performed by technicians or volunteers, though a professional is needed to "read" the tracings to determine if a baby passed the screening. (3) Because the EOAE originates from the hair cells of the inner ear, it is not affected by babies' neurological status.

Screening with TEOAEs also has its disadvantages and limitations: (1) Because the technique utilizes a sound (the emission) as the response, it is obvious that ambient noise levels in the test environment are critical. Babies from some noisy nurseries may need to be removed to a quieter location. As noted above, a sound attenuating isolette is now commercially available. (2) Emissions cannot be recorded if the baby's ear canal is blocked with debris or if the baby has middle ear effusion. Because this is common in very young babies, it can result in very high failure rate in babies tested less than 48 hours after birth. Chang, Vohr, Norton, and Lakes (1993) found that EOAE pass rate improved from 76% to 91% after the newborns' ear canals were cleared of vernix caseosa and debris. It is known that neonatal TEOAE responses improve over the first 24 to 48 hours of life, and there is speculation that this improvement in the EOAE relates to the clearing of fluid from the newborn's middle ear (Kok, Van Zanten, Brocaar, & Wallenburg, 1993). (3) Presence of an emission is evidence of grossly normal hair cell function. If the emission is absent, however, the stimulus parameters cannot be manipulated to provide more information about the baby's cochlear status. (4) The specificity of TOAE screening is lower than that of the ABR, resulting in a higher overreferral rate. This shortcoming, however, may be reduced when consensus is reached regarding OAE pass-fail criteria.

After reviewing the relative strengths and weaknesses of ABR and TEOAE newborn screening, the 1993 NIH Consensus Development Panel recommended emission testing as the initial screening procedure, followed by an auditory brainstem response test for all infants who fail the evoked emissions test. This recommendation was initially met with some surprise and dismay because of the limited research data that were available at that time. There was also the belief by some that the case for automated ABR screening was not given sufficient airing. Since the 1993 report, numerous scientific reports have appeared and major federally funded research is currently underway. Based on the information available today, conventional ABR, automated ABR, and emissions testing are all viable screening techniques and have their strong proponents. The unique characteristics of the individual screening program will determine which technique is best suited for its purposes.

It should be noted that the above discussion of otoacoustic emissions referred exclusively to transient emissions produced by click stimuli. There is also a newer EOAE technique that uses pairs of tones to elicit distortion product evoked otoacoustic emissions (DPOAEs). This technique also has been shown to be applicable to newborn screening and gives comparable information (Bergman, Gorga, Neely, Kaminski, Beauchaine, & Peters, 1995). However, there are still a number of procedural issues to be resolved with the DPOAE, so its clinical position is not as well established. Data available to date suggests that it possesses all the strengths and weaknesses mentioned above for the TEOAE.

SELECTING THE BABIES TO BE SCREENED

At the core of any screening program is its scope, that is, which individuals should be screened and which do not warrant screening? Professional leadership in this area has been provided largely by the Joint Committee on Infant Hearing (JCIH), first established in the late 1960s. The JCIH derives its influence from the fact that is it multidisciplinary, drawing its membership from the American Speech-Language-Hearing Association, the American Academy of Otolaryngology—Head and Neck Surgery, the American

Academy of Pediatrics, the American Academy of Audiology, the Council on Education of the Deaf, and the Directors of Speech and Hearing Programs in State Health and Welfare Agencies.

Initially, in 1969, the JCIH did not recommend mass hearing screening for all newborns. The JCIH instead endorsed the concept of a high-risk register (HRR) for *selecting* infants who should receive hearing assessment. Five factors were identified in 1972 as placing an infant at increased risk for hearing loss (see Table 11.3). The JCIH revised and expanded the high-risk criteria in 1982 and more recently in 1990 to include the ten risk factors shown in Table 11.3. The TORCH mentioned in the table is an acronym for the major infections that may be acquired in utero: T—taxoplasmosis; O—other, including syphilis; R—rubella; C—cytomegalovirus; and H—herpes simplex.

In 1983, Stein, Clark and Kraus reported that nearly one-third of hearing-impaired infants residing in a well-baby nursery would not have been detected through the 1982 HRR. Pappas (1983), found that only 46% of infants would have been identified using the 1982 HRR. That is, 54% of the infants were not suspected of being at risk for hearing loss based on the 1982 criteria and thus were not referred for hearing evaluation during the neonatal period. Elssmann and colleagues (1987) also reported that of the infants with congenital hearing impairment in their study, only 48% had high-risk factors for hearing loss. Mauk, White, Mortensen, and Behrens (1991) reported results drawn from a birth certificate–based high-risk register. They found that only 50% of the children with sensorineural hearing losses exhibited any of the risk criteria recommended by the JCIH in 1982. Consequently, despite the use of the HRR in different applications (hospital-based and birth certificate–based), there is general agreement that the HRR identifies only about 50% of infants with sensorineural hearing loss. The 1994 JCIH Position Statement acknowledged that failure to identify the remaining 50% of children with hearing loss results in diagnosis and intervention at an unacceptably late age.

TABLE 11.3   Risk factors for hearing deficit.

1972	1.	Family history
	2.	Hyperbilirubinemia requiring exchange
	3.	Congenital infections (TORCH)
	4.	Craniofacial anomalies (defects)
	5.	Birth weight < 1500 grams
1982	6.	Bacterial meningitis
	7.	Asphyxia
		Apgar score < 3 at 5 minutes
1990	8.	Ototoxic medication > 5 days
	9.	Mechanical ventilation > 10 days
	10.	Syndromes that include hearing loss

TABLE 11.4   JCIH 1994 indicators for use with neonates (birth–28 days) when universal screening is not available.

1. Family history of hereditary childhood sensorineural hearing loss.
2. In utero infection, such as cytomegalovirus, rubella, syphilis, herpes, and toxoplasmosis.
3. Craniofacial anomalies, including those with morphological abnormalities of the pinna and ear canal.
4. Birth weight less than 1500 grams (3.3 lbs).
5. Hyperbilirubinemia at a serum level requiring exchange transfusion.
6. Ototoxic medications including but not limited to the aminoglycosides used in multiple courses or in combination with loop diuretics.
7. Bacterial meningitis.
8. Apgar scores of 0–4 at one minute or 0–6 at five minutes.
9. Mechanical ventilation lasting 5 days or longer.
10. Stigmata or other findings associated with a syndrome known to include a sensorineural and/or a conductive hearing loss.

Thus, the 1994 JCIH Position Statement addressed the need to identify *all* infants with hearing loss, not just those who manifest one of the risk factors. The 1994 Position Statement (ASHA, 1994) endorses the goal of universal detection of infants with hearing loss as early as possible, but still maintains a role for the high risk indicators. That is, when universal screening for hearing loss is not achievable, the 10 neonatal (birth through age 28 days) indicators (updated from 1990, and presented in Table 11.4) should be utilized to select neonates who should receive hearing assessment. Additionally, the JCIH recognized that certain health conditions may develop with infants (age 29 days through 2 years) that require rescreening. Therefore, infant indicators are identified (Table 11.5) that define, at minimum, infants for whom necessary follow-up of hearing

TABLE 11.5   JCIH 1994 indicators for use with infants (29 days–2 years) when certain health conditions develop that may require screening.

1. Parent/caregiver concern regarding hearing, speech, language, and/or developmental delay.
2. Bacterial meningitis and other infections associated with sensorineural hearing loss.
3. Head trauma associated with loss of consciousness or skull fracture.
4. Stigmata or other findings associated with a syndrome known to include a sensorineural and/or conductive hearing loss.
5. Ototoxic medications including but not limited to chemotherapeutic agents or aminoglycosides used in multiple courses or in combination with loop diuretics.
6. Recurrent or persistent otitis media with effusion for at least 3 months.

status is essential. Lastly, the JCIH recognized that some neonates and infants may pass initial hearing screening, but may have indicators (Table 11.6) that would require periodic monitoring of hearing to detect delayed-onset sensorineural and/or conductive hearing loss.

Kile (1993) recently observed that much is still not known about the relationship between accepted risk indicators and hearing impairment. Therefore, follow-up information is needed to determine if the 1994 indicators are more sensitive to hearing loss and result in detecting more than 50% of children ultimately identified with hearing loss. Neonatal hearing screening programs that rely on the HRR as the first filter for screening *all* newborns in need of further assessment likely will fall short of the objective of identifying *all* infants with hearing loss before 3 months of age. An effective way to comply with the JCIH 1994 goals is to implement valid, reliable, and cost-effective testing that can be used to screen newborns from both well-baby nurseries and intensive care nurseries before hospital discharge. Yet, high risk indicators *maintain an important role* in ongoing audiologic surveillance, parent awareness, and primary-care vigilance.

The panel at the 1993 National Institutes of Health Consensus Development Conference on Early Identification of Hearing Impairment concluded that all infants admitted to the neonatal intensive care unit should be screened for hearing prior to discharge. The panel further concluded that universal screening should be implemented for *all*

TABLE 11.6 JCIH 1994 indicators for infants (29 days–3 years) who require periodic monitoring of hearing.

Some newborns and infants may pass initial hearing screening but will require periodic monitoring of hearing to detect delayed onset sensorineural and/or conductive hearing loss. Infants with these indicators require hearing evaluation at least every 6 months until age 3 years and at appropriate intervals thereafter.

Indicators associated with delayed onset sensorineural hearing loss include:

1. Family history of hereditary childhood hearing loss.
2. In utero infection, such as cytomegalovirus, rubella, syphilis, herpes, or toxoplasmosis.
3. Neurofibromatosis Type II and neurodegenerative disorders.
4. Persistent pulmonary hypertension in the newborn period.

Indicators associated with conductive hearing loss include:

1. Recurrent or persistent otitis media with effusion.
2. Anatomic deformities and other disorders that affect eustachian tube function.
3. Neurodegenerative disorders.

---

infants within the first three months of life. The Joint Committee on Infant Hearing also has supported this concept of universal detection.

Not all have embraced implementation of universal hearing screening. Bess and Paradise (1994) challenged the long-held belief that even a mild hearing loss can influence early development and that the impact of a hearing loss can be reduced if it is detected early and management initiated as soon thereafter as possible. They pointed out that there are limited research data to support this assumption and without more information, under more carefully controlled conditions, universal hearing screening cannot be justified. Others have acknowledged that carefully controlled investigations are lacking, but they argue that this is largely due to the difficulties involved in carrying out tightly controlled longitudinal studies (Carney, 1996). The 1994 Bess and Paradise article resulted in a large outpouring of letters, largely in heated opposition to their views. Most argued strongly and passionately that screening should not be restricted just because there is a shortage of well-controlled investigations. They contended that adequate information already is available to support early intervention and the cost of delayed management exceeds the cost of early screening. More recently, many have acknowledged that the Bess and Paradise article served a valuable function because it caused individuals to reexamine the scientific basis of some of their clinical assumptions.

Whatever one's personal viewpoint on universal hearing screening, the fact remains that currently only 3% to 5% of newborns in the United States are screened for hearing loss (Mauk & Behrens, 1993). Thus, universal hearing screening is still a long way from implementation.

DISORDER PREVALENCE AND SCREENING TEST PERFORMANCE

There is a less obvious change that occurs when the scope of screening is increased: the influence of the prevalence of the disorder being screened on the performance of the screening test. As was discussed in an earlier section, no screening test is perfect, so some normal babies will fail the screening and some hearing impaired babies will pass. The example shown in Table 11.2 was based on the assumption that a hearing loss occurs in 4% in the target population. This prevalence value is close to what would be expected in a group of high-risk newborns.

The rarer the condition, the lower is the positive predictive value of a screening test. That is, the less is the likelihood that a screening failure actually means that the baby has the disorder. If the target population of a hearing screening program is composed of well babies, the overall prevalence of hearing loss will be about 0.2%, which is much less than the approximately 4% found in the high risk population. How this affects the positive predictive value of the screening test is shown in Table 11.7. As in Table

TABLE 11.7   Example of screening test outcomes on 5000 babies with a low prevalence (0.2%) of hearing loss.

	HEARING STATUS		
	Hearing Loss	Normal Hearing	Total
Failed Screening	9	499	508
Passed Screening	1	4491	4492
Total	10	4990	5000

11.2, the sensitivity and specificity of the screening test are assumed to be 90%. Note, however, the differences between Table 11.2 and Table 11.7 in the ratio between the number of babies who failed the screening and the number of hearing losses identified. In Table 11.2, 660 babies failed the screening, of whom 180 had a hearing loss for a predictive value of 27.3%. In contrast, in Table 11.7, where the prevalence is closer to that of the well-baby population, the positive predictive value drops to 1.8% because only 9 of the 508 babies who failed the screening test actually had a hearing loss. In this example, over 98% of the babies who failed the screening test have normal hearing.

All babies who fail a screening test obviously require follow-up testing. When the prevalence of hearing loss is low, a high proportion of the retesting (98% in our last example) will be performed on normal-hearing babies. This adds to the overall costs involved in identifying each hearing-impaired baby (Berlin, 1996). Very successful universal hearing screening programs exist (e.g., Marlowe, 1993) and their number has increased from three in 1991 to 120 in 1995 (Robinette & White, 1997), so the problems involved are far from insurmountable.

FINANCIAL CONSIDERATIONS

There is a finite amount of health care dollars and, as a result, there is increasing pressure to use the limited financial resources wisely. In the current health care climate, test procedures and treatments are undergoing close unemotional scrutiny. Increasingly, practitioners are being held accountable for the cost/benefits of their clinical activities. Devoting more resources to one area that is essential drains resources from other areas. Often compromises must be made because there must be a solid balance between performance and cost. One cannot advocate adoption of a screening program without first considering the financial factors involved.

Personnel Costs

A major component of the costs of newborn screening relates to the personnel. Traditionally, the audiologist has performed the hearing screening. This is highly desirable because he or she can interact effectively with the physicians,

nursery staff, and parents. Use of audiologists also should ensure a high level of professionalism, quality control, and continuity. The use of professionals, of course, affects the cost of conducting the screening program, and this is likely to be reflected in the fee charged for each test. Given the current health care maintenance atmosphere, cost is a primary consideration and the use of audiologists for newborn screening may be becoming prohibitively expensive. A related consideration is the inadequate number of audiologists available to carry out widespread screening, particularly if scope of screening is expanded to include all of the estimated 4 million live births each year (Jacobson & Jacobson, 1996).

An alternative to screening by an audiologist is the use of a trained technician. This has been used widely with X-ray and EEG procedures for years. The clear advantage is reduced cost, but not all newborn screening programs can keep such an individual busy on a full-time basis. Unless there are alternative duties for the technician, the financial advantage may be lost when there are no babies to be screened. Since demand for screening is highly variable, a part-time employee is satisfactory only if the work schedule is very flexible. At present, the definition of a hearing screening technician is vague because there are no established technician training programs or recognized credentialing mechanism. This raises liability issues when hearing screening is performed by unlicensed personnel.

The use of volunteers is obviously the least expensive personnel option. This includes semi-volunteers (i.e., students). Successful use of volunteers has been reported in programs utilizing automated ABR (Marlowe, 1993). In her program, after a 20-hour orientation, the volunteers devote 3 to 4 hours a week so the team is available for screening 365 days of the year. Turnover of personnel and the need for frequent training sessions can be a concern, though Marlowe reports that the average length of volunteer service is about five years. Johnson, Maxon, White, and Vohr (1993) agree that volunteers provide very useful services, but have found that paid employees are necessary to insure continuity and insure appropriate follow-through. If volunteers are utilized for some duties within a screening program, audiologists will still be required to supervise the program to insure that quality remains high. As mentioned for technicians, when sub-professionals are used, liability issues need to be a significant concern (Marlowe, 1996).

If universal hearing screening is to become a reality, sub-professionals will have to be utilized in newborn screening because there are not a sufficient number of audiologists.

Other Costs

Obviously, there are other costs besides those related to the personnel involved. Test equipment is expensive. Items such as clerical supplies and postage also must be viewed as part of the costs of conducting a hearing screening program.

There always are indirect costs associated with any work-place setting (space, heat, lights, water, etc.) that must be considered.

It should be remembered that the true cost of detection of a hearing loss must include costs related to post-screening testing for all babies who fail the initial screening. Looking at only the cost of the initial test does not give an adequate picture of the process. A more expensive screening test actually may be less costly overall if it minimizes the number of babies who need to be retested. The proper way to assess the cost of a screening program is to calculate the cost per detection of a hearing impaired baby. Maxon, White, Behrens, and Vohr (1995) described the costs involved in conducting a large-scale universal TEOAE screening program. They calculated a cost of $26 for every baby screened and $4378 for every baby identified with a significant sensorineural hearing loss. In his modeling of screening program costs, Turner (1991) described ABR screening costs at $60 per infant and the cost for each hearing-impaired infant identified at $5500. Markowitz (1990) presented screening costs ranging from $4 per test to $75 per test and cost per identification ranging from $2000 to over $3000. These values are examples. As discussed elsewhere in this chapter, a number of factors influence an individual program's actual costs required to identify a hearing impaired infant.

Benefits to Society

It has been argued that the costs to society for newborn screening will be more than offset by a reduction in needed special education and by a corresponding increase in productivity and taxable income these individuals will provide. Available data suggest that individuals who are deaf or hard-of-hearing in the United States earn up to 30% less than the general population resulting in income *loss* of $79 billion annually (Northern & Downs, 1991; Schein & Delk, 1974). Deaf and hard-of-hearing individuals who had normal hearing *until* 3 years of age, however, earn 5% more than those born deaf or hard-of-hearing (Schein & Delk, 1974). Detection at birth and immediate intervention for the congenitally deaf should result in some approximation of language skills similar to those with onset of hearing loss at age 3. In fact, Yoshinaga-Itano (1995) suggested that early identification of hearing loss, particularly at birth, not only minimizes the deleterious effect upon communication development, but can prevent delays in development from ever occurring. Therefore, if early detection and early intervention *prevent* delays from occurring, the estimated cost to society from deafness and hearing impairments stated above ($79 billion per year) might be reduced by 5% through neonatal detection and early intervention, that is, up to $3.9 billion per year. Unfortunately, though a strong case can be made that society does gain through early hearing

programs, this fact may not convince an individual hospital administration that a screening program should operate at a financial deficit for the overall good of the country.

The Changing Fee-for-Service Model

It is important to note that the classic fee-for-service model is undergoing a dramatic change as health services move toward managed care. Approximately 80% of infants admitted to newborn nurseries are now in some form of fixed-fee payment plan such as an HMO or Medicaid. This means that for these patients the hospital receives a given amount of reimbursement rather than an amount for each service provided. Thus, for such patients there is the same level of reimbursement regardless of whether hearing screening was performed during the baby's hospital stay. When hospital administration evaluates the cost effectiveness of a program, it looks at the actual amount of revenue the program produces. It is more difficult to justify the cost effectiveness of a program when the submitted charges do not result in additional income to the hospital.

The best way to resolve the reimbursement issue would be through a national or state legislative mandate that would provide tax money to ensure adequate reimbursement for newborn screening. An attempt to mandate newborn screening at the national level was first made in 1991 and again in 1998. Rep. James Walsh (R-NY) introduced a bill entitled the Hearing Loss Testing Act. Passage of this resolution would have required inclusion of hearing screening in all health plans and insurance policies that cover newborns. There also was provision in this bill to provide for screening of newborns not covered by private insurance or Medicaid. At the time of this writing, this bill still remains in committee in hopes that additional support will develop in the future (Marlowe, 1996). The current climate regarding health care reform, however, causes one to be pessimistic about any significant changes in the near future. On a brighter note, Barringer and Mauk (1997) found that 73% of parents would be willing to use their own money to pay for newborn screening if the cost was around $30.

LEGAL/ETHICAL CONSIDERATIONS

After reading the earlier sections of this chapter, it should be clear that nearly every aspect of newborn hearing screening has undergone significant changes in recent years. These changes, in turn, impact what is viewed as the standard of care in this area. That is, it tends to define the level of care that is appropriate given current level of knowledge and technology. There are legal and ethical implications if a hospital fails to provide its patients accepted standard of care. Because of the many changes in the area of newborn hearing screening, the issue of current standard of care needs to be addressed.

Implications of Care Standards

The publication of guidelines and position statements advocating universal detection of hearing loss, along with the availability of technology that makes these guidelines feasible in newborn nurseries, constitute a formidable logical argument for the existence of a new standard of care level (Marlowe, 1996). Additionally, the fact that 20 states currently have legislatively mandated newborn hearing screening statutes makes it difficult to argue that a hospital is exempt from a care standard just because it happens to practice in a state without a mandate.

Delaying recognition and implementation of emerging standards of care until they are mandated can be construed as ignoring the standard, thereby increasing the risk of legal consequences. When there is a failure to acknowledge and conform to a standard of care, thereby causing injury that can be measured in costs and monetary damages, negligence may be proven.

The legal responsibility ultimately lies in the courts. If the parents of a hearing-impaired child with a preventable condition (e.g., the loss of the ability to develop language, with all of its implications) became aware that an eminent panel of experts convened by a government body (1993 NIH Consensus Development Conference) had addressed the problem and had published a solution, there could be legal ramifications for the hospital, attending physicians, as well as for the audiologists involved. This would apply to hospitals without screening programs and also to hospitals where babies are discharged before screening can take place.

Because there currently is no clear statement of standard of care, it is open to various interpretations and may have to be decided on a case by case basis if legal actions are taken (Marlowe, 1996).

Implications of the Use of Unlicensed Personnel

As discussed in a previous section, there are strong arguments for using sub-professional personnel to carry out newborn screening. The NIH (1993) consensus statement supports the use of sub-professionals for some aspects of infant screening if they are trained and supervised by an audiologist. This viewpoint likely was influenced by the fact that 4 million babies are born each year and the number of audiologists is inadequate even if all were assigned to this task alone. Thus, there must be a mechanism for support personnel. These personnel have to be carefully selected, carefully trained, and carefully supervised. There also needs to be some flexibility for those hospitals who find cross-training an attractive option.

Each state may have specific policies through its state licensure laws that define the qualifications of the practitioner and scope of audiology practice, and these should be understood thoroughly before sub-professionals are utilized.

Two examples illustrate this point. In the state of Illinois volunteers may not screen hearing. The Illinois licensing laws prohibit anyone who is not licensed, or exempt from the license (e.g., physicians, school nurses who have passed a course given by the Department of Health, and specially trained technicians doing only industrial testing), from performing evaluation services. Evaluation services are defined as the application of nonmedical methods and procedures for the identification, measurement, testing, and appraisal of hearing or vestibular function. The Illinois law has been interpreted to mean that identification (screening) is to be treated no differently than diagnostic testing. In the state of Ohio, the newborn hearing screening mandate calls for the completion of a checklist of risk factors on each baby and defines this process as screening. Any additional procedure (ABR, automated ABR, or OAE) is considered an assessment and, as such, only may performed by audiologists and licensed aids. Qualifications for licensure as an aid are strictly defined and audiologists are limited to supervising two support personnel. Exceptions to this policy to allow volunteer support staff, for example, must be made by application to the state and cannot be assumed to be allowed. These two examples illustrate the importance of linkage between program development and the widely differing state licensure laws throughout the fifty states.

Implications of False Positives

In Table 11.7 an example was shown in which the test sensitivity and specificity were 90%, but the positive predictive value of the test was less than 2% because of the low prevalence of hearing loss in the target population. In this realistic example, 98% of the babies who failed the screening had normal hearing and thus were false positive outcomes. False positive identifications can overload any service delivery system. The expense of otherwise unnecessary testing is significant, particularly if the overreferral rate is high as in the above example. In addition to the financial consequences is the potential for emotional stress that parents may feel if their baby does not pass the screening. The diagnostic process is often a period of extreme anxiety for most family members awaiting news that confirms or negates the presence of a hearing loss. Parents must deal with their own anxiety and try to deal with misunderstandings that can affect the entire family unit. Several reports (Sorenson, Levy, Mangione, & Sepe, 1984; Tluczek, Mischler, Farrell, et al., 1992) document the extent to which parental anxiety concerning false-positive identifications may persist as an important problem long after the diagnosis in question has been dismissed. This potential for long-term emotional impact is the basis for what has been referred to as "vulnerable child" syndrome. That is, parents treat their children as if they are easily susceptible to accidents or medical problems, resulting in overprotective behavior.

On a positive note, Abdala de Uzcategui and Yoshinaga-Itano (1997) studied parents' emotional responses resulting from their children's hearing screening tests and subsequent referrals. Although the sample was small, and the results represent short-term status, parents generally did not report negative emotional responses. In fact, parents generally reported positive emotions: 81% felt informed, 62% felt comforted, 59% felt encouraged, and 68% felt satisfied with the process.

Even if only a small minority of parents experience emotional stress when their baby does not pass the hearing screening, the potential psycho-social impact may be adverse. Therefore, whenever a baby is referred for additional testing, the audiologist should provide information and support for the family. In instances where follow-up testing indicates that the baby was a false positive the audiologist again must be prepared to provide face-to-face counseling to help family members address their emotional needs.

Implications of Babies Who Are Missed

The problems created by a false positive outcome pale when compared to the impact of a false negative outcome. When a hearing-impaired baby passes the hearing screening, he or she may actually have been harmed by the process. If developmental problems occur, parents and professionals incorrectly may assume that hearing loss has been ruled out as a contributing factor. Infants with hearing loss who incorrectly are discharged from hearing loss detection programs are at significant risk for late identification. Many of these children will not have their hearing loss confirmed until three to five years post-discharge, depending on the nature and degree of their hearing impairment. The lost time for intervention during the crucial years of speech and language development, the impact of late identification on family adjustment, and the potential legal ramifications, all represent significant consequences of false negative outcomes. Most false positive outcomes can be detected on follow-up testing. Because no such testing will occur for false negative babies, it emphasizes that screening test protocols should be designed to keep false negatives to an absolute minimum.

Because there are no systematic screening programs in most communities for children between birth and kindergarten, the burden of early detection and referral for these children falls upon the shoulders of others, including the primary care physician. Yet, it is relatively uncommon for hearing loss to be suspected by the child's physician. Shah, Chandler, and Dale (1978) found that the child's hearing loss was first suspected by the parents in over 75% of the cases, whereas the possibility of a hearing loss was raised by the child's physician in only 7.5% of the sample studied.

Moreover, selected studies have reported delays of 7.1 months (Elssmann et al., 1987), 11.5 months (Shah et al., 1978), and 24 months (Boison, 1987) between parental suspicion of hearing loss and physician referral for audiologic assessment. As would be expected, the greater the degree of hearing loss and the older the age of the child, the more parents notice that their children do not exhibit developmentally appropriate, auditory-related behaviors. In short, physicians should heed parents' intuition that something is wrong, and they should refer to a center specializing in the evaluation of pediatric communicative disorders when parental/caregiver concerns are raised.

Physicians play a key role in timely recognition and referral of children with hearing loss during the period from birth to kindergarten if attention is focused on determining those children who are manifesting significant early delays in speech and language development. Information on developmental milestones for hearing and communication must be provided to all parents upon discharge from a hospital and/or at the time of well-baby check-ups. Increased parent awareness is an inexpensive approach to increase the likelihood of detecting an infant with hearing loss who has been missed in a neonatal hearing screening program.

FOLLOW-UP

It is improper to screen for a disorder without certainty that accessible services exist to provide appropriate follow-up to babies and their families. It is easy for the audiologist to lose sight of the real purpose of a newborn hearing screening program. With pressures to demonstrate the program's effectiveness, there is the tendency to focus attention on maximizing the number of babies who are screened with the view that the more babies that are tested the better is the program. The real test of a screening program, however, is not in how many screenings were performed, but in how those screenings resulted in prompt identification and appropriate management of a hearing-impaired infant. The most important aspect of a newborn screening program really begins when attention is directed toward the subgroup of babies who failed the screening and who now must be viewed as being at particularly high risk for hearing loss. What happens to these babies is the true yardstick for measuring the effectiveness of an early identification program. It is essential that all these babies receive follow-up testing to either confirm or rule out a hearing impairment. This is a difficult goal to achieve.

Parental Compliance

Because hearing loss is not a visible impairment, it is easy for parents to deny or ignore the possibility of a problem. As a result, even the most aggressive efforts to insure follow-up testing may end up with less than satisfactory results. In a summary report on twenty years of NICU screening, Galambos, Wilson, and Silva (1994) found that only about half of the babies who failed the initial screening returned for follow-up testing. Shimizu and colleagues (Shimizu, Walters, Proctor, Kennedy, Allen, & Markowitz, 1990) put forth considerable effort to increase the likelihood that babies would return for outpatient follow-up testing. These efforts included free evaluations, free parking, transportation when needed, and frequent contact by telephone and letter. Despite these efforts, 26% of the babies who failed the newborn screening did not return for their follow-up testing. College-educated mothers were twice as likely to return their infants for testing than were mothers with a ninth-grade education. Noncompliance also is higher in the poor, non-English speaking, single parents, and individuals with transportation problems.

Maximizing Follow-up

In spite of the difficulties involved, it is essential that every reasonable effort be made to maximize parental compliance. This would include: (1) coordinating multiple medical center appointments for the same day, making scheduling easier for the parent, particularly those with transportation problems; (2) whenever possible, counseling the family prior to baby's discharge, emphasizing the importance of additional testing; (3) sending a follow-up letter explaining the nature and significance of the hearing screening test results; (4) sending a letter to the primary-care physician, social worker, or local health department (primary-care provider) enlisting their support in facilitating follow-up testing (Diefendorf & Weber, 1994).

An alternative approach is to attempt follow-up testing on screening failures before the babies leave the hospital. Because as high as 80% of the babies will pass the second test (Maxon et al., 1995), this approach significantly reduces the number of babies who must return as outpatients. However, because initial screening usually is conducted very close to discharge (to take advantage of increased maturation and improved health status), there often is insufficient time to perform a second test before the baby leaves the hospital.

Aside from the logistical problems involved in retesting screening failures prior to hospital discharge, there are some advantages in waiting several weeks before the second test is performed. These advantages include increased maturity, better overall health status, and resolution of debris in the ear canals or transient middle ear problems. Of course, testing in an audiology clinic provides a much quieter test environment. The technique that is used for the initial hearing screening may not be the best technique for follow-up testing. The clinical ABR is the most appropriate procedure for the second level testing because of the ability to vary stimulus intensity to provide information about degree of hearing loss.

Management of Hearing Loss

Getting the baby back for retesting is one concern; the next is what to do if a hearing loss is confirmed on follow-up testing. It can be argued logically that early screening without this testing leading to early intervention defeats the whole intent of an early identification program. Identifying that a baby has a hearing impairment by itself is of little value and may actually produce negative consequences, such as stress on the family, if prompt management is not initiated. The time between initial screening failure and intervention should be the interval needed to adequately confirm that the infant has a hearing impairment. Obviously, this time interval should be as short as possible. It is appropriate, therefore, to think of the goal of newborn screening as permitting earlier initiation of management than would have occurred if screening had not been performed. If this does not occur, the program has failed regardless of the number of babies who were screened. The merit of a hearing screening program, therefore, should not be judged by the number of babies screened, but by the number of babies identified and by the age when their management began.

When hearing loss is confirmed, early intervention services should be provided in accordance with the Individuals with Disabilities Education Act (IDEA), Part C Public Law 102-119 (formerly PL 99-457). A multidisciplinary evaluation will be completed to determine eligibility and to assist in developing an individualized family service plan (IFSP) to describe the early intervention program. The process for developing the IFSP consists of the gathering, sharing, and exchange of information between families and staff to enable families to make informed choices about the early intervention services they want for their children and themselves. Because specific services and eligibility requirements are not uniform from state to state, potential service users and service providers should contact their state Part C service coordinator either through the Department of Health and Human Services or the Department of Education.

The multidisciplinary evaluation and assessment of an infant identified with hearing loss should be performed by a team of professionals working in conjunction with the parent/caregiver. Since there are many cultural styles, values, and family structures in American society, it is necessary to ask who are the important players in a family's life? Family/professional collaboration and partnerships are the keys to family-centered early intervention and to successful implementation of the IFSP process. In turn, the team will develop a program of early intervention services based on the child's unique strengths and needs, and consistent with the family's resources, priorities, and concerns related to enhancing the child's development.

Elements of an early intervention program for children with hearing loss and their families should include the following:

1. Family support and information regarding hearing loss and the range of available communication and educational intervention options. The ultimate goal in working with parents is to help them grow to independent function in dealing with their child's changing status from infancy to adulthood.
2. Implementation of learning environments and services designed with attention to the family's preference. It is important for parents to begin taking control of the decision-making process regarding their children from the outset. This philosophy helps promote services that are family-centered.
3. Intervention that promotes the child in all developmental areas with particular attention to language acquisition and communication skills
4. Services that provide ongoing monitoring of the child's overall health status, audiologic needs, and development of communication skills.
5. Curriculum planning that integrates and coordinates multidisciplinary personnel and resources so that intended outcomes of the IFSP are achieved. Importantly, service coordination models and practices should reflect the implicit and explicit intent of the IFSP.

Periodic Monitoring

Concern for hearing loss should not stop at birth. It must be recognized that limiting hearing screening to the neonatal period will result in a large number of children with hearing loss escaping early detection. Some newborns and infants may pass initial hearing screening but require periodic monitoring of hearing to detect delayed-onset sensorineural and/or conductive hearing loss. For infants identified with JCIH 1994 indicators associated with delayed-onset hearing loss (refer to Tables 11.3 and 11.4), ongoing monitoring and evaluation will be necessary. Infants with these indicators require hearing evaluation *at least* every six months until age 3 years, and at appropriate intervals thereafter.

Different studies have examined premature, high-risk infants relative to general early growth and development, and educational sequelae (Rubin, Rosenblatt, & Barlow, 1973; Kenworthy, Bess, Stahman, & Lindstrom, 1987). In general, these studies have reported that many high-risk infants exhibit delays in several areas of child development.

The development in communication appears to present no exception. The prevalence of communicative disorders in this sub-population of children is well in excess of the prevalence noted for normal babies. Moreover, with the increasing numbers of premature infants who survive, there likely will be a commensurate increase in infants with communication complications.

There may be a growing number of high-risk children who exhibit some degree of mild, high-frequency hearing impairment (Kenworthy et al., 1987). Detailed audiologic evaluation on a periodic basis is required to better isolate the source of hearing impairment (conductive, sensorineural, mixed) in these children. In addition, many of these children will manifest significant lags in speech/language development. Therefore, it would appear justified to include routine, periodic screening of hearing, speech/language, and psycho-educational abilities of these children at various age levels as part of a comprehensive management strategy.

CONCLUSIONS

No aspect of audiology is more important than the early identification and prompt management of the infants with hearing impairments. Because hearing loss impairs both receptive and expressive speech and language development, it strikes at the very foundation of child development. In spite of the numerous obstacles involved, every hospital should address how it can best insure that its newborns will be screened for hearing loss. In addition to establishing a screening protocol, a follow-up network must be developed to track all infants who fail the initial screen, as well as selected infants who pass the screening. This follow-up is required in order to ensure that all infants with hearing impairment are identified and managed with a minimum of delay. Financial planning for such a system must be given the same importance as for the hearing screening itself.

REFERENCES

Abdala de Uzcategui, C., & Yoshinaga-Itano, C. (1997). Parent's reactions to newborn hearing screening. *Audiology Today, 9,* 24–27.

American Speech-Language-Hearing Association. (1994, December). Joint Committee on Infant Hearing 1994 Position Statement. *Asha, 36,* 38–41.

Barringer, D. G., & Mauk, G. W. (1997). Survey of parents' perceptions regarding hospital-based newborn hearing screening. *Audiology Today, 9,* 18–19.

Bergman, B. M., Gorga, M. P., Neely, S. T., Kaminski, J. R., Beauchaine, K. L., & Peters, J. (1995). Preliminary descriptions of transient-evoked and distortion-product otoacoustic emissions from graduates of an intensive care nursery. *Journal of the American Academy of Audiology, 6,* 150–152.

Berlin, C. I. (1996). Role of infant hearing screening in health care. *Seminars in Hearing, 17,* 115–124.

Bess, F. H. (1985) The minimally hearing impaired child. *Ear and Hearing, 6,* 43–47.

Bess, F. H., & Paradise, J. L. (1994). Universal screening for infant hearing impairment: Not simple, not risk-free, not necessarily beneficial, and not presently justified. *Pediatrics, 98,* 330–334.

Boison, K. B. (1987). Diagnosis of deafness: A study of family responses and needs. *International Journal of Rehabilitation Research, 10,* 220–224.

Bonfils, P., Uziel, A., & Narcy, P. (1989). The properties of spontaneous and evoked acoustic emissions in neonates and children: A preliminary report. *Archives of Otorhinolaryngology, 246,* 249–251.

Bray, P., & Kemp, D. (1987). An advanced cochlear echo technique suitable for infant screening. *British Journal of Audiology, 21,* 191–204.

Carney, A. E. (1996). Early intervention and management of the infant with hearing loss: What's science got to do with it? *Seminars in Hearing, 17,* 185–195.

Chang, K. W., Vohr, B. R., Norton, S. J., & Lakes, M. D. (1993). External and middle ear status related to evoked otoacoustic emissions in neonates. *Archives of Otolaryngology—Head and Neck Surgery, 119,* 276–282.

Davis, J. M. (1988). Management of the school age child: A psychosocial perspective. In F. H. Bess (Ed.), *Hearing Impairment in Children* (pp. 401–416). Parkton, MD: York Press.

Davis, J. (Ed.) (1990). *Our Forgotten Children: Hard of Hearing Pupils in the Schools.* Washington, DC: U.S. Department of Education, 1–2.

Davis, J. M., Elfenbein, J., Schum, D., & Bentler, R. A. (1986). Effects of mild and moderate hearing impairment on language, educational, and psychosocial behavior of children. *Journal of Speech and Hearing Disorders, 51,* 53–62.

de Villiers, P. A. (1992). Educational implications of deafness: Language and literacy. In R. D. Eavey & J. O. Klein (Eds.), *Hearing Loss in Childhood: A Primer* (pp. 127–135). Report of the 102nd Ross Conference on Pediatric Research. Columbus, OH: Ross Laboratories.

Diefendorf, A. O., Reitz, P. S., Cox, J., & Hussain, D. Z. (1996). *A Comparison between Automated ABR and Transient Evoked Otoacoustic Emissions in a Special Care Nursery.* Paper presented at Operating a Successful Universal Newborn Hearing Screening Program, Park City, UT.

Diefendorf, A. O., & Weber, B. A. (1994). Identification of hearing loss: Programmatic and procedural considerations. In J. Roush & M. D. Matkin (Eds.), *Infants and Toddlers with Hearing Loss* (43–64). Baltimore: York Press.

Elssman, S. F., Matkin, N. D., & Sabo, M. P. (1987). Early identification of congenital sensorineural hearing impairment. *Hearing Journal, 9,* 13–17.

Galambos, R., Wilson, M., & Silva, P. (1994). Identifying hearing loss in the intensive care nursery: A 20-year summary. *Journal of the American Academy of Audiology, 5,* 151–162.

Glover, B., Watkins, S., Pittman, P., Johnson, D., & Barringer, D. (1994). SKI-HI home intervention for families with infants, toddlers, and preschool children who are deaf or hard of hearing. *Infant-Toddler Intervention: The Transdisciplinary Journal, 4,* 319–332.

Hall, J. W., Kileny, P. R., Ruth, R. A., & Kripal, J. (1987). Newborn auditory screening with Algo-1 vs. conventional auditory brainstem. Paper presented at the American Speech-Language-Hearing Association Convention, New Orleans, LA.

Halpern, J., Hosford-Dunn, H., & Malachowski, N. (1987). Four factors that accurately predict hearing loss in "high-risk" neonates. *Ear and Hearing, 8,* 21–25.

Herrmann, B. S., Thornton, A. R., & Joseph, J. M. (1995). Automated infant hearing screening using the ABR: Development and validation. *American Journal of Audiology, 4,* 6–14.

Hooks, R. G., & Weber, B. A. (1984). Auditory brain stem responses of premature infants to bone-conducted stimuli: A feasibility study. *Ear and Hearing, 5,* 42–45.

Hyde, M. L., Riko, K., & Malazia, K. (1990). Audiometric accuracy of the click ABR in infants at risk for hearing loss. *Journal of the American Academy of Audiology, 1,* 59–66.

Jacobson, J. T., & Jacobson, C. A. (1996). Current technology in newborn universal hearing detection. *Seminars in Hearing, 17,* 125–138.

Jacobson, J. T., Jacobson, C. A., & Spahr, R. C. (1990). Automated and conventional ABR screening techniques in high-risk infants. *Journal of the American Academy of Audiology, 1,* 187–195.

Johnsen, N. J., Bagli, P., & Elberling, C. (1983). Evoked otoacoustic emissions from the human ear. III. Findings in neonates. *Scandinavian Audiology, 12,* 17–24.

Johnson, M. J., Maxon, A. B., White, K. R., & Vohr, B. R. (1993). Operating a hospital-based universal newborn hearing screening program using transient evoked otoacoustic emissions. *Seminars in Hearing, 14,* 46–56.

Joint Committee on Infant Hearing (JCIH). (1982). 1982 position statement. *Asha, 24,* 1017–1018.

Joint Committee on Infant Hearing (JCIH). (1991). 1990 position statement. *Asha, 33,* 3–6.

Joint Committee on Infant Hearing (JCIH). (1994). 1994 position statement. *Audiology Today, 6,* 6–9.

Karchmer, M. A. (1991). *1990 Stanford Achievement Test Norms for Hearing Impaired Students.* Washington: Gallaudet University, Office of Demographic Studies.

Kennedy, C. R., Kimm, L., Dees, D. C., Evans, P. I. P., Hunter, M., Lenton, S., & Thornton, R. D. (1991). Otoacoustic emissions and auditory brainstem responses in the newborn. *Archives of Disease in Childhood, 66,* 1124–1129.

Kenworthy, O. T., Bess, F. H., Stahman, M. T., & Lindstrom, D. P. (1987). Hearing, speech, and language outcomes in infants with extreme immaturity. *The American Journal of Otology, 8,* 419–425.

Kile, J. E. (1993). Identification of hearing impairment in children: A 25-year review. *Infant-Toddler Intervention: The Transdisciplinary Journal, 4,* 299–318.

Kok, M. R., van Zanten, G. A., Brocaar, M. P., & Wallenburg, H. C. S. (1993). Click evoked otacoustic emissions in 1036 ears of healthy newborns. *Audiology, 32,* 213–224.

Levitt, H., McGarr, N. S., & Geffner, D. (1987). Development of language and communication skills in hearing-impaired children. In H. Levitt, N. S. McGarr, & D. Geffner (Eds.), *Development of Language and Communication Skills in Hearing-Impaired Children* (ASHA Monograph No 26, pp. 1–8). Rockville, MD: American Speech-Language-Hearing Association.

Markowitz, R. K. (1990). Cost-effectiveness comparisons of hearing screening in the neonatal intensive care unit. *Seminars in Hearing, 11,* 161–166.

Marlowe, J. A. (1993). Screening all newborns for hearing in a community hospital. *American Journal of Audiology, 2,* 22–25.

Marlowe, J. A. (1996). Legal and risk management issues in newborn hearing screening. *Seminars in Hearing, 17,* 153–164.

Mauk, G. W., & Behrens, T. R. (1993). Historical, political, and technological context associated with early identification of hearing loss. *Seminars in Hearing, 14,* 1–17.

Mauk, G. W., White, K. R., Mortensen, L. B., & Behrens, T. R. (1991). The effectiveness of screening programs based on high-risk characteristics in early identification of hearing impairment. *Ear and Hearing, 12,* 312–319.

Maxon, A. B., White, K. R., Behrens, T. R., & Vohr, B. R. (1995). Referral rates and cost efficiency in a universal newborn hearing screening program using transient evoked otoacoustic emissions. *American Journal of Audiology, 6,* 271–277.

NIH Consensus Statement. (1993). *Early Identification of Hearing Impairment in Infants and Young Children, 11,* 1–24.

Northern, J. L., & Downs, M. P. (1991). *Hearing in Children* (4th ed., pp. 1–31). Baltimore; Williams and Wilkins.

Northern, J. L., & Hayes, D. (1994). Universal screening for infant hearing impairment: Necessary, beneficial, and justifiable. *Audiology Today, 6,* 10–13.

Northern, J. L., & Marlowe, J. A. (1995). Hearing screening using the ALGO-2. Paper presented at the National Symposium on Hearing in Infants, Vail, CO.

Özdamar, Ö., Delgado, R. E., Eilers, R. E., & Urbano, R. C., (1994). Automated electrophysiologic hearing testing using a threshold seeking algorithm. *Journal of the American Academy of Audiology, 5,* 77–88.

Pappas, D. G. (1983). A study of the high-risk registry for sensorineural hearing impairment. *Archives of Otolaryngology—Head and Neck Surgery, 91,* 41–44.

Quigley, S. P., & Thomure, F. E. (1968). *Some Effects of Hearing Impairment on School Performance.* Springfield, IL: Illinois Office of Education.

Robinette, M., & White, K., (1997). Top ten reasons universal newborn hearing screening should be standard of care in the US. *Audiology Today, 9,* 21–23.

Rubin, R., Rosenblatt, C., & Barlow, B. (1973). Psychological and educational sequelae of prematurity. *Pediatrics, 52,* 532.

Salamy, A., Eldridge, L., & Tooley, W. H. (1989). Neonatal status and hearing loss in high risk infants. *Journal of Pediatrics, 114,* 847–852.

Schein, J. D., & Delk, M. T. (1974). *The Deaf Population of the United States.* Silver Springs, MD: National Association of the Deaf.

Shah, C., Chandler, D., & Dale, R. (1978). Delay in referral of children with impaired hearing. *Volta Review, 80,* 207.

Shenai, J. P. (1992). Changing demographics of infants in the neonatal intensive care unit: Impact on auditory function. In F. H. Bess & J. W. Hall (Eds.), *Screening Children for Auditory Function* (pp. 31–36). Nashville, TN: Bill Wilkerson Center Press.

Shimizu, H., Walters, R. J., Proctor, L. R., Kennedy, D. W., Allen, M. C., & Markowitz, R. K. (1990). Identification of hearing impairment in the neonatal intensive care population: Outcome of a five-year project at the Johns Hopkins Hospital. *Seminars in Hearing, 11,* 150–160.

Sorenson, J. R., Levy, H. L., Mangione, T. W., & Sepe, S. J. (1984). Parental response to repeat testing of infants with "false-positive" results in a newborn screening program. *Pediatrics, 73,* 183–187.

Stein, L., Clark, S., & Kraus, N. (1983). The hearing-impaired infant: Patterns of identification and habilitation. *Ear and Hearing, 4,* 232–236.

Stein, L. K., Jabaley, T., Spitz, R., Stoakley, D., & McGee, T. (1990). The hearing-impaired infant: Patterns of identification and habilitation revisited. *Ear and Hearing, 11,* 201–205.

Stevens, J. C., Webb, H. D., Hutchinson, J. Connell, J., Smith, M. F., & Buffin, J. T. (1989). Click evoked otoacoustic emissions compared with brainstem electric response. *Archives of Disease in Childhood, 64,* 1105–1111.

Stevens, J. C., Webb, H. D., Hutchinson, J., Connell, J., Smith, M. F., & Buffin, J. T. (1990). Click evoked otoacoustic emissions in neonatal screening. *Ear and Hearing, 11,* 128–133.

Stewart, D. L. (1995). *Hearing Screening at Baptist Memorial Hospital, Memphis, TN.* Paper presented at Universal Infant Hearing Screening National Seminar; November, Nashville, TN.

Stuart, A., Yang, E. Y., & Green, W. B., (1994). Neonatal auditory brainstem response thresholds to air- and bone-conducted clicks: 0 to 96 hours postpartum. *Journal of the American Academy of Audiology, 5,* 163–172.

Tluczek, A., Mischler, E. H., Farrell, P. M., et al. (1992). Parents' knowledge of neonatal screening and response to false-positive cystic fibrosis testing. *Journal Developmental Behavioral Pediatrics, 13,* 181–186.

Turner, R. G. (1991). Modeling the cost and performance of early identification protocols. *Journal of the American Academy of Audiology, 2,* 195–205.

Turner, R. G. (1992a). Comparison of four hearing screening protocols. *Journal of the American Academy of Audiology, 3,* 200–207.

Turner, R. G. (1992b). Factors that determine the cost and performance of early identification protocols. *Journal of the American Academy of Audiology, 3,* 233–241.

U.S. Department of Health and Human Services, Public Health Service. (1990). *Healthy People 2000: National Health Promotion and Disease Prevention Objectives.* Washington, DC: U.S. Government Printing Office.

United States House of Representatives 99th Congress, 2nd session. (1986). Report 99-860. *Report Accompanying the Education of the Handicapped Act Amendment of 1986.* Washington, DC: U.S. Government Printing Office.

Weber, B. A., & Jacobson, C. (1994). Newborn hearing screening. In J. Jacobson (Ed.), *Principles and Applications in Auditory Evoked Potentials* (pp. 357–383). Boston: Allyn & Bacon.

Weber, B. A., & Roush, P. A. (1993). Application of maximum length sequence analysis to auditory brainstem response testing of premature newborns. *Journal of the American Academy of Audiology, 4,* 157–172.

White, K. R., Vohr, B. R., & Behrens, T. R., (1993). Universal newborn hearing screening using transient evoked otoacoustic emissions: Results of the Rhode Island hearing assessment project. *Seminars in Hearing, 14,* 18–29.

Yoshinaga-Itano, C. (1995). Universal hearing screening for infants: Simple, risk-free, beneficial and justified. *Audiology Today, 7,* 13.

CHAPTER 12

AUDIOLOGIC ASSESSMENT
OF THE ELDERLY

FRED H. BESS
ANDREA HEDLEY-WILLIAMS
MICHAEL J. LICHTENSTEIN

The number of individuals over 65 years of age in the United States is growing steadily and is expected to approach 21 million (Garstecki, 1996). This continual increase in longevity is due in part to the general population's awareness of the benefits of a healthy lifestyle (i.e., exercise and eating habits), as well as to the success in controlling infectious diseases and managing chronic illnesses. Hence, a critical need has developed for the health professions to meet the long-term health care needs of the elderly population. One of these health care needs is rehabilitation of hearing impairment.

Sensorineural hearing loss is a frequent by-product of the aging process. Hearing impairment ranks as one of the three most prevalent chronic conditions, following only arthritis and hypertension. Prevalence studies indicate that the number of individuals 75 years of age with audiologically measurable hearing loss is approximately 4 million. Seven million individuals over 75 years of age are hearing impaired (Garstecki & Erler, 1995). The number of hearing-impaired individuals in middle and later life is considerable. In addition, as shown in Table 12.1, the hearing loss progresses with each succeeding decade (Harford & Dodds, 1982).

The magnitude of the problem is demonstrated clearly in Table 12.2. This table illustrates the results from three different studies in terms of the percentage of hearing-impaired persons for a given age range and sex. The studies include the Health Examination Survey (HES; 1960–62), the Wilkins Study (which conducted a home interview survey on some 31,000 individuals in 1947), and the Health Interview Survey (conducted in the United States on 134,000 people from 44,000 households in 1971). All three studies show a significant increase in the prevalence of hearing impairment with increasing age. It also is noted that the prevalence rates are different for each study. This

is mostly due to methodological differences. Interview surveys typically underestimate the prevalence of hearing impairment, especially for those over 55 years of age. Finally, there appears to be a slight trend for males to exhibit a greater prevalence of hearing loss in the different age ranges than females.

Hearing loss among older persons is associated with reduced communication function. It is reportedly associated with the psychologic features of withdrawal (Weinstein, 1985), negativism (Alpiner, 1978), isolation (Weinstein, 1985), depressive symptoms (Herbst, 1983; Mulrow, Aguilar, Endicott, Tuley, Velez, Charlip, et al., 1990a), frustration (Weinstein, 1985), anxiety and loneliness (Bess, Lichtenstein, Logan, Burger, & Nelson, 1989; Hull, 1980; Maurer & Rupp, 1979), and poor social and emotional well-being (Mulrow et al., 1990a). In addition, hearing impairment has been associated with the functional problems of poor general health, reduced mobility, and reduced interpersonal communications (Herbst, 1983; Bess et al., 1989).

This chapter is concerned with the audiologic findings associated with aging. Toward this end, the chapter covers the pathological changes in the auditory system associated with aging, the early identification of hearing loss in the elderly, and the audiometric findings commonly found in the aged.

ANATOMIC AND PHYSIOLOGIC EFFECTS OF AGING ON THE AUDITORY SYSTEM

Presbycusis (from the Greek *presbys*, old, and *akouein*, to hear) is defined in the strictest sense as hearing loss assessed in an individual in the fifth decade or older due to age-related changes alone, possibly with a genetic basis. *Socioacusis* defines hearing loss associated with exogenous and endogenous sources, including nonoccupational noise exposure, faulty diet, heavy metals, solvents, industrial reagents, pollutants, and tobacco. *Nosoacusis* relates to hearing loss from diseases with otoacoustic effects such as vascular disease, systemic disease, neoplastic problems, inflammations,

Acknowledgment: The authors gratefully acknowledge Shelia Lewis, who typed the manuscript, and Mark Hedrick, who provided assistance with several sections of this chapter. Preparation of this chapter was supported in part by the Retirement Research Foundation.

TABLE 12.1 Mean right-ear pure-tone air conduction threshold levels (in dB HL) for three groups of adults.

Frequency (Hz)	60–69 YEARS (N = 135) Mean (SD)	70–79 YEARS (N = 264) Mean (SD)	80+ YEARS (N = 142) Mean (SD)
250	28.9 (15.0)	31.2 (10.2)	36.1 (15.1)
500	28.6 (16.5)	32.5 (14.6)	38.5 (16.0)
1000	26.9 (18.0)	32.4 (16.8)	41.3 (18.1)
2000	31.0 (22.0)	39.1 (19.6)	50.0 (18.2)
4000	44.5 (22.0)	50.1 (21.8)	63.4 (15.7)
8000	58.2 (21.0)	67.7 (18.3)	80.2 (14.0)

Harford & Dodds (1982)

concussive damage, nutrition, ototoxic drugs, and hyperlipidemia (Mills, 1996). Occupational and nonoccupational noise is perhaps the most common factor that causes cochlear damage and thus complicates the study of presbycusis.

The ISO 1999 "Acoustics: Determination of Occupational Noise Exposure and Estimation of Noise-Induced Hearing Impairment" has compiled data representing pure aging effects—these data are depicted in Figure 12.1. Hearing loss begins in the measured frequency range by approximately age 30 and increases steadily. Interestingly, elderly populations living in quiet rural regions—for example, the Mabaan tribe in an undeveloped part of Africa exhibit significantly less hearing loss for both males and females ages 60 through 90 than do similar groups from highly industrialized communities (Rosen, Bergman, Plester, El-Mofty, & Salti, 1962). This work certainly supports the effects of socioacusis and nosoacusis in age-related hearing loss but does not explain presbycusis. Recent work in age-related changes of the cochlea, taken from animal models, in particular that of Mongolian gerbils, afford the opportunity to study age related changes in the cochlea without the concurrent effects of socioacusis and nosoacousis as well as

the effects of occupational noise exposure. Such research supports age-related hearing loss independent of socioacusis and nosoacusis.

The traditional framework for defining cochlear pathology and presbycusis was originated by Schuknecht (1955, 1964, 1974). Histological evidence, case history data, and audiological measurements were combined and correlated to delineate four specific types of presbycusis. They include: (1) *sensory degeneration* of hair cells and supporting cells at the base of the cochlea with subsequent cochlear fiber degeneration. This type of presbycusis produces an abrupt high-frequency sensorineural hearing loss. (2) *Strial* or *metabolic degeneration* of the stria vascularis, resulting in changes in cochlear electrical potentials and possible effects upon energy production in the organ of Corti. Strial presbycusis produces a flat audiometric configuration usually accompanied by very good speech recognition. (3) *Neural loss of cochlear neurons*, resulting in problems of transmission information coding. Neural presbycusis results in poorer speech recognition than expected from the audiometric data. Although Schuknecht (1974) urged that more histopathological evidence for central auditory nervous system (CANS) degeneration would be useful, he presented no direct evidence for CANS involvement. He stated, however, that individuals with neural presbycusis tend to have diffuse CANS degeneration including motor control problems, memory loss, and intellectual deterioration. (4) *Mechanical* or *cochlear conductive* hypothetical type of presbycusis resulting from alterations to cochlear mechanics produced by mass/stiffness changes or spiral ligament atrophy. Cochlear conductive presbycusis supposedly would produce a straight-line audiometric loss with descending bone-conduction thresholds; speech recognition is inversely related to the steepness of the audiometric configuration.

According to Schuknecht (1974), one or more of these different types of presbycusis can occur in a given individual, thus complicating the relationship between audiometric

TABLE 12.2 Percentage of people reported as hearing-impaired in three different studies (Health Examination Survey, 1960–62, <HES>; Wilkins, 1947, <WIL>; Health Interview Survey, 1971, <HIS>).

AGE GROUP (YEARS)	MALE HES	MALE WIL	MALE HIS	FEMALE HES	FEMALE WIL	FEMALE HIS	BOTH SEXES HES	BOTH SEXES WIL	BOTH SEXES HIS
18–24	1.2	1.2	—	0.4	0.9	—	0.8	1.0	—
25–34	1.4	1.8	5.1	1.3	1.5	3.4	1.3	1.6	4.2
35–44	3.7	2.1	—	2.2	2.9	—	2.9	2.5	—
45–54	4.1	4.9	14.0	4.6	4.6	9.0	4.3	4.7	11.4
55–64	10.6	6.2	—	10.1	6.4	—	10.3	6.4	—
65–74	30.5	12.4	28.0	26.2	12.1	19.0	28.2	12.2	23.1
74–79	48.7	28.0	44.0	47.4	25.0	36.0	48.0	26.0	39.8

Adapted from Davis (1983)

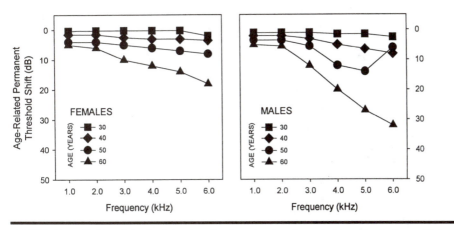

FIGURE 12.1 Epidemiologic data showing hearing levels and chronological age. Data are from an international standard, ISO 1999. Data represents a sample that was highly screened in an effort to eliminate the potential influence of the effects of exposure to noise. (From J. H. Mills, "Presbycusis," in J. J. Ballenger & J. B. Snow, Eds., *Otorhinolaryngology—Head and Neck Surgery*, 15th ed., pp. 1133–1141, 1996. Redrawn with permission from Willliams & Wilkins, Baltimore.)

configuration and histological correlates. In fact, Suga and Lindsay (1976) could not specify correlations between audiometric configuration and site of cochlear involvement; they stated that neural ganglion cell degeneration was the most common finding.

In addition to the Schuknecht data, there are other forms of presbycusic pathophysiology reported in the literature. For example, Nadol (1979) mentioned loss of several outer hair cell afferent synapses, although light microscopy showed presence of outer hair cells and normal myelinated fibers. Thus, normal light microscopy exams of the cochlea do not guarantee the presence of functional hair cell fibers' synapses. Similar studies of age-related changes in the cochleas of mongolian gerbils also show significant outer hair cell deterioration with aging (Tarnowski, Schmiedt, Hellstrom, Lee, & Adams, 1991).

Hawkins and Johnsson (1985) noted two additional types of peripheral presbycusis, *hyperstotic* and *vascular.* It has been suggested that with age, the internal auditory meatus can show hyperstosis (abnormal growth of bony tissue). This new growth could then compress the eighth nerve and internal auditory artery, causing dysfunction/degeneration of the eighth nerve fibers and inner ear tissue. Analysis of a series of human temporal bones showed substantial devascularization involving the capillaries and arterioles of the inner ear, particularly in the regions of the spiral lamina and lateral wall (Schulte & Schmiedt, 1992).

There is a considerable body of evidence to suggest cochlear degeneration in elderly patients with hearing loss (Tarnowski et al., 1991). Structural changes in the auditory nerve and along the central pathways at the brainstem and temporal lobe level resulting in central auditory nervous system dysfunction are also associated with aging (Corso,

1977; Fisch, 1972; Hansen & Reske-Neilsen, 1979; Krmpotic-Nemic, 1971; Schuknecht, 1974). The resulting effect is one of phonemic regression where measured speech intelligibility is poorer than expected from pure tone audiometry. Retrocochlear cell degeneration is associated with slowly progressing high-frequency hearing loss with poorer than expected word understanding. This is known as *central presbycusis* (Hinchcliffe, 1962; Schuknecht, 1955). Stach, Spretnjak, and Jerger (1990) reported a prevalence of central presbycusis of 17% in individuals ages 50 to 54 compared to 90 to 95% in those age 80 and older. Humes, Christopherson, and Cokely (1991), however, demonstrated that prevalence is not so high when one controls for peripheral hearing loss. The loss of cells may also be related to loss of synchrony in the central auditory pathways. Such a loss can be detected electrophysiologically by the decreased phase coherence of the middle latency response (MLR) in elderly adults exhibiting central auditory processing disorders (CAPD). Audiometrically measured CAPD in the elderly appear independent of peripheral sensitivity loss (Jerger, Jerger, Oliver, & Pirozzolo, 1993), but the decreased speed of information processing prevalent in this aged population can greatly affect speech perception performance. In addition, when CAPD and non-CAPD subjects were matched on the relevant variables of age, hearing loss, and intellectual ability, there were no significant group differences on the cognitive measures (Jerger et al., 1993). It appears, then, that CAPD can exist independently of cognitive deficit in this aged population. Figure 12.2 illustrates the various types of presbycusis described in the literature and their associated sites of pathologic changes.

An ever-increasing segment of the elderly population is stricken by a disease process known as Alzheimer's.

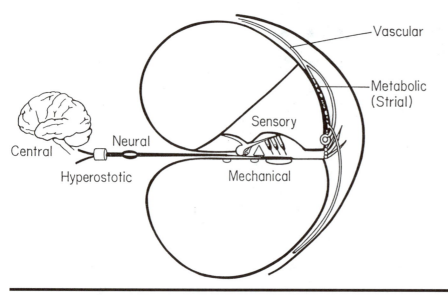

FIGURE 12.2   Cross-section of the human cochlea to illustrate the types of presbycusis and the accompanying sites of pathological change. (Redrawn with permission from "Otopathological changes associated with presbycusis," by J. E. Hawkins & L. G. Johnsson, 1985, *Seminars in Hearing, 6,* 115–134.)

Individuals with Alzheimer's disease exhibit pathological changes in the basal forebrain and midbrain that result in decreased thinking and memory abilities (Esiri, Pearson, & Powell, 1986; Hyman, Maskey, Van Hoesen, & Damasio, 1988; Lewis, Campbell, Terry, & Morrison, 1987; Selkoe, 1992). Auditory processing, which involves learning and memory, is also inhibited by this disease process (Musiek & Hoffman, 1990; Sherif, Gottfries, Alafuzoff, & Ireland, 1992). When matched for hearing sensitivity, age and gender, electrophysiological test results indicate no difference in cochlear function in individuals with Alzheimer's disease (Bess & Strouse, 1996; Strouse, DeChicchis, & Bess, 1996). It appears that primarily higher level auditory functions are affected by this disease process. One study by Kurylo and colleagues (Kurylo, Corkin, Allard, Zatorre, & Browden, 1993) showed significantly poorer performance on localization tasks by Alzheimer's patients than for elderly controls. Most studies in auditory evoked potentials show deficits in the late auditory evoked responses, in particular, the P300. In many patients with Alzheimer's disease, the P300 has increased latency and decreased amplitude (Onofrj, Ghilardi, Fulgente, Nobilio, Bazzano, Ferracco, & Malatesta, 1990; Syndulko, Hansch, Cohen, Pearce, Goldberg, et al., 1982). Increased latency in the P300 is believed to correlate systematically with increased cognition dysfunction and poorer auditory attention (Polich, Ladish, & Bloom, 1990).

IDENTIFICATION AND EVALUATION OF THE ELDERLY HEARING IMPAIRED

Early Identification

Early identification and intervention is considered an important rehabilitative strategy for the elderly hearing impaired. Indeed, there is some evidence to suggest, albeit indirect, that the earlier the hearing loss is identified and hearing aid rehabilitation ensues, the greater the potential for hearing aid success (Davis, 1983; Solomon, 1986). The following review highlights some of the more important issues concerned with screening the elderly population.

Principles of Screening.   Screening for a chronic condition involves the examination of asymptomatic persons to determine if they are likely or unlikely to have the target disorder of interest (Morrison, 1985). Once a screening test is positive, the individual must be further evaluated to determine the presence or absence of the condition. Hearing impairment in the aged is a prototypic disorder for screening: It is a common, progressive, easily detected disorder, for which the belief is held that early identification and rehabilitation will ameliorate its consequences.

To judge the effectiveness of a screening program, seven questions must be answered (Cadman, Chambers, Feldman, & Sackett, 1984). This provides a framework for assessment and future investigation. The questions are:

1. *Has the effectiveness of the program been demonstrated in a randomized trial?* Yes. Mulrow and colleagues (1990a) randomly assigned 194 elderly patients to either a hearing aid or to a waiting list. Following a 4-month trial period, hearing aids were found to be associated with significant improvements in social and emotional function and communication.

2. *Are efficacious treatments available?* Yes. Hearing aids, though not curative, provide the amplification necessary to overcome the hearing deficit. Overall efficacy, however, must be judged by the aged subjects' use of and satisfaction with the aid. Increasingly, outcome measures are being incorporated as a part of the hearing aid fitting process to quantify such hearing aid benefit.

3. *Does the burden of suffering warrant screening?* Yes. As noted earlier, hearing impairment consistently and strongly is associated with functional deficits and impairments beyond just the ability to communicate. Depending on the definition used, hearing impairment affects 30% of persons over 65 years of age. Moreover, hearing impairment is associated with depression and dementia (Herbst & Humphrey, 1980; Mulrow et al., 1990a; Weinstein & Amsell, 1986).

4. *Is there a good screening test?* Yes. Traditional physical diagnostic tests such as the finger rub and whispered voice have been validated and are diagnostically useful (Uhlmann, Rees, Psaty, & Duckert, 1989). The use of other instruments, a hand-held audioscope, and a self-administered questionnaire, the Hearing Handicap Inventory for the Elderly—screening version (HHIE-S) have also been validated (Lichtenstein, Bess, & Logan, 1988b).

5. *Does the program reach those who could benefit?* Possibly. Most older persons will see a primary care physician on an annual or biannual basis. Screening tests could be administered in the physician's office. The ability of a screening program to reach other aged subjects (homebound, institutionalized, or those who do not see physicians) remains to be demonstrated.

6. *Can the health care system cope with the program?* Unknown. If hearing aid rehabilitation results in reduced functional disability and improved quality of life, as demonstrated in studies by Bess and colleagues (1989) and Mulrow and colleagues (1990a), there will be increased pressure to provide and pay for these services. However, with the onset of managed care, insurance coverage of services not directly related to illness is increasingly difficult. Resource analyses as well as studies indicating increased Quality of Life Years (QALY) are needed before public policy can be changed to cover the large segment of the aging population that would be eligible for rehabilitation.

7. *Do persons with positive screenings comply with advice and interventions?* Unknown. In one study, 59% of persons complied with further hearing assessment with pure tone audiometry, regardless of the outcome of a screening test (Lichtenstein, Bess, & Logan, 1988a). This figure may be higher if only persons with a positive screen are referred for evaluation.

These questions are applicable for any screening program, not just one involving hearing impairment. Although progress is being made to investigate these problems, hearing function should be assessed in aged persons as part of a standard physical examination with the primary care physician.

Description of Screening Instruments

Principles of Diagnostic Test Performance. When a patient presents to a caregiver with a complaint, the clinician's first task is to make a diagnosis. This involves a process where information is obtained that is both valid (true) and reliable (the same result is obtained when the information is obtained on more than one occasion). A diagnostic test is any information that may be used to sort out the patient's problem. The primary care provider should be familiar with how useful the testing methods are in ruling in or out a particular diagnosis. This section covers some principles of how to assess the usefulness of two diagnostic tests for detecting hearing impairment in the aged.

Figure 12.3 sets the stage for understanding the diagnostic process. For any problem in a population, we wish to be able to distinguish those persons *with* the characteristic (A + B) from those *without* the characteristic (C + D).

The usefulness of a diagnostic test must be evaluated against an independent standard, the results of which everyone agrees determine the presence or absence of the characteristic. For example, in evaluation for hearing impairment, pure tone audiometry is the gold standard for evaluating screening tests.

When the diagnostic test is compared against the independent standards, the following 2 × 2 table is generated:

| | | Independent Gold Standard CHARACTERISTIC | | |
		Present	Absent	Total
Diagnostic Test	Positive	A	C	A + C
	Negative	B	D	B + D
	Total	A + B	C + D	A + B + C + D

From this table and Figure 12.3 the following proportions may be calculated.

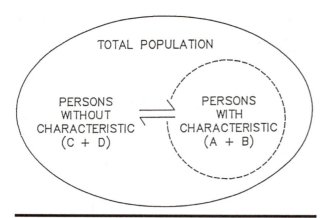

FIGURE 12.3   Schematic diagram for understanding diagnostic tests. The affected subset with the target disorder (A + B) is part of a larger population (A + B + C + D). A good screening test should distinguish between those with the target disorder (A + B) from those without the target disorder (C + D).

- **Prevalence** = A + B/A + B + C + D: The proportion of persons in the population with the characteristic.
- **Pretest Probability:** Another use for prevalence, this represents the a priori probability that the characteristic is present. For example, the prevalence of hearing impairment in aged women is about 30%. When an older woman walks into the office, she has a 30% chance of being hearing impaired, and this is true before any diagnostic tests are performed on her.
- **Sensitivity** = A/A + B: The proportion of persons *with* the characteristic correctly identified by the test. Sensitivity is affected by severity of the characteristic (the more advanced the condition, the higher the sensitivity).
- **Specificity** = D/C + D: The proportion of persons *without* the characteristic correctly identified by the test.
- **Positive Predictive Value** = A/A + C: The proportion of persons with positive tests who have the characteristic. The post-test probability that, given a positive test, the characteristic is present. Positive predictive values are dependent on sensitivity, specificity, and prevalence.
- **Negative Predictive Value** = D/B + D: The proportion of persons with negative tests who do not have the characteristic. The post-test probability that, given a negative test, the characteristic is absent. Negative predictive values also are dependent on sensitivity, specificity, and prevalence.
- **Test Accuracy** = A + D/A + B + C + D: The proportion of persons, with or without the characteristic, correctly identified by the test. In screening, the most valuable tests are those that have the highest accuracy (i.e., they minimize false-positive and false-negative results).

Principles of Screening Instruments

Pure Tone Measures.   The Welch-Allyn Audioscope is a hand-held instrument that delivers a 20, 30, or 40 dB hearing level (HL) tone at 500, 1000, 2000, and 4000 Hz (see Figure 12.4). To use the audioscope the largest ear speculum needed to achieve a seal within the external auditory canal is selected. The tympanic membrane is then visualized—if obstructed by cerumen, the impaction must be removed before testing. Then the tonal sequence is initiated, with the subject indicating whether he or she heard the tone by raising a finger.

The audioscope has been validated in the elderly against pure tone audiometry (Lichtenstein et al., 1988a) using the definition for hearing impairment proposed by Ventry and Weinstein (1983): The subjects were considered hearing impaired if they had a 40 dB loss at 1000 or 2000 Hz in each ear or at both 1000 and 2000 Hz in one ear. Subjects were tested in physicians' offices and in a hearing center.

The sensitivities and specificities of the audioscope by signal frequency and site of testing are shown in Table 12.3. The prevalence of having a 40 dB deficit by audiogram increases from 14% to 16% for 500 Hz to 63% to 69% for 4000 Hz. In general, the sensitivity of the audioscope

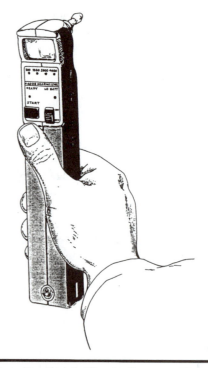

FIGURE 12.4   The Welch-Allyn Audioscope. (Reprinted with permission from "Validation of screening tools for identifying hearing-impaired elderly in primary care," by M. J. Lichtenstein, F. H. Bess, & S. A. Logan, 1988a, *Journal of the American Medical Association, 259,* 2876. Copyright 1988, American Medical Association.)

TABLE 12.3 Sensitivity and specificity of audioscope by signal frequency and test site.

SIGNAL FREQUENCY (Hz)	FAILURE TO HEAR (%)	PHYSICIANS' OFFICE			HEARING CENTER		
		N	Sens (%)	Spec (%)	N	Sens (%)	Spec (%)
Right Ear							
500	13.7	175	79	76	172	92	93
1000	18.3	175	91	69	172	97	85
2000	31.4	175	87	88	172	79	96
4000	63.0	173	89	78	172	89	91
Left Ear							
500	16.1	174	79	77	172	89	94
1000	16.7	174	93	70	172	97	87
2000	32.8	174	88	89	171	88	93
4000	69.0	171	83	72	170	87	87

was essentially the same and the specificity markedly better at each frequency in the hearing center than in the physicians' offices.

Between-occasion and between-observer agreement for the audioscope results were tested using the kappa statistic, which is a measure of the observed agreement not due to chance (Sackett, Haynes, & Tugwell, 1985). The between-location agreement of audioscope results are listed in Table 12.4 by frequency and ear. The kappa values ranged from .41 for the left ear at 500 Hz to .74 for the left ear at 2000 Hz.

The performance of the audioscope against the audiogram definition of hearing impairment is shown in Table 12.5. Using this definition, the prevalence of hearing impairment was 30%. The sensitivity of the audioscope in the physician's office and the hearing center was identical, 94%.

The specificity of the audioscope was significantly lower in the physician's offices compared to the hearing center

(72% vs. 90%). The lower specificity in the physicians' offices probably arises from higher ambient background noise levels in these settings. Thus, the audioscope is a sensitive, repeatable test for the detection of elderly hearing impaired. Its moderate specificity in the primary care setting would have the effect of an increase in false-positive identification of hearing impairment.

TABLE 12.4 Between location agreement of audioscope results: Physicians' offices vs. hearing center.

FREQUENCY (Hz)	KAPPA STATISTIC*	
	Right Ear	Left Ear
500	0.50	0.41
1000	0.50	0.51
2000	0.71	0.74
4000	0.65	0.62

*All values are statistically significant at P < 0.0001

TABLE 12.5 Sensitivity and specificity of the audioscope for detecting hearing impairment when compared to the audiogram.*

LOCATION	PREVALENCE OF HEARING IMPAIRMENT (%)	NUMBER OF PERSONS	SENSITIVITY (%)	SPECIFICITY (%)
Physicians' offices	30	174	94	72
Hearing center	30	171	94	90

*Pure tone test at 40 dB HL at 1000 and 2000 Hz in each ear. Hearing impairment defined as either (a) inability to hear tone at one frequency in *each* ear, or (b) inability to hear both frequencies in one ear.

TABLE 12.6 Hearing Handicap Inventory for the Elderly (Screening Version).

Does a hearing problem cause you to feel embarrassed when you meet new people?

Does a hearing problem cause you to feel frustrated when talking to members of your family?

Do you have difficulty hearing when someone speaks in a whisper?

Do you feel handicapped by a hearing problem?

Does a hearing problem cause you difficulty when visiting friends, relatives, or neighbors?

Does a hearing problem cause you to attend religious services less often than you would like?

Does a hearing problem cause you to have arguments with family members?

Does a hearing problem cause you to have difficulty when listening to television or radio?

Do you feel that any difficulty with your hearing limits/hampers your personal or social life?

Does a hearing problem cause you difficulty when in a restaurant with relatives or friends?

Self-Perception Scales. The Hearing Handicap Inventory for the Elderly–Screening Version (HHIE-S) is a self-administered 10-item questionnaire designed to detect emotional and social problems associated with impaired hearing (Table 12.6; Ventry & Weinstein, 1983). Subjects respond to questions about circumstances related to hearing by stating whether the situation presents a problem. A "no" response scores 0, "sometimes" scores 2, and "yes" scores 4. Total HHIE-S scores range from 0 to 40.

Test-retest repeatability for the HHIE-S as determined using Pearson product-moment correlation is .84 (p < .001) indicating a high degree of repeatability.

The performance of the HHIE-S scores against the audiogram definition of hearing impairment is illustrated in Figure 12.5. Sensitivities and specificities were determined for the performance of the audioscope and HHIE-S by examining the distributions of test results in those with and without hearing impairment as defined by the audiogram. The receiver operating curves for the HHIE-S at the physicians' offices and the hearing center are virtually superimposable (Figure 12.5). Using a cutoff of 8, the sensitivity of the HHIE-S was 72% and 76%, and specificity was 77% and 71% in the hearing center and physicians' offices, respectively. Above a score of 24, the specificity of the HHIE-S was 98% in the hearing center and 96% in the physicians' offices. The corresponding sensitivities were 24% and 30%.

The likelihood ratios for different levels of the HHIE-S are given in Table 12.7. In this group the pretest probability of having a hearing impairment was 30%. For those with HHIE-S scores of 0 to 8, the likelihood ratio was 0.36, with a post-test probability of hearing impairment calculated as 13%. For those with scores of 10 to 24, the likelihood ratio was 2.3 with a post-test probability of hearing impairment of 50%; scores of 26 to 40, yielded a likelihood ratio of 12.00 with a post-test probability of 84%. The HHIE-S shows similar likelihood ratios across different definitions of hearing impairment, such as speech frequency pure tone averages, high-frequency pure tone averages, and speech recognition thresholds (all at 25 dB HL in the better ear; Lichtenstein et al., 1988b). Thus, the HHIE-S is a valid repeatable screening test with a robust performance against different definitions of hearing impairment.

Combining the Audioscope and HHIE-S Results. Both the audioscope and HHIE-S are repeatable valid measures of hearing impairment. The audioscope is very sensitive but moderately specific in the physicians' offices. The HHIE-S is moderately sensitive but highly specific at scores greater than 24. The greatest test accuracy in identifying hearing impairment was found when the two tests were combined

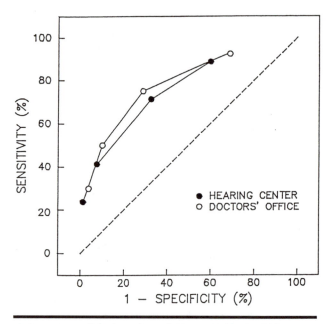

FIGURE 12.5 Receiver operating curves for HHIE-S scores against audiogram measures of hearing impairment. Hearing impairment defined by the criteria of Ventry and Weinstein (see text). From left to right, the four plotted points on each curve indicate the sensitivity and specificity of HHIE-S cut-off points of 24, 16, 8, and 2. (Reprinted with permission from "Validation of screening tools for identifying hearing-impaired elderly in primary care," by M. J. Lichtenstein, F. H. Bess, & S. A. Logan, 1988a, *Journal of the American Medical Association, 259,* 2877. Copyright 1988, American Medical Association.)

TABLE 12.7   Probability of hearing impairment given a Hearing Handicap Inventory for the Elderly (HHIE-S) Score.*

HHIE-S	PRE-TEST PROBABILITY OF HEARING IMPAIRMENT	LIKELIHOOD RATIO (95% CONFIDENCE INTERVAL)	POST-TEST PROBABILITY OF HEARING IMPAIRMENT
0–8	30%	0.36 (0.19–0.68)	13%
10–24	30%	2.30 (1.22–4.32)	50%
26–40	30%	12.00 (2.62–55.00)	84%

*HHIE-S completed at the hearing center. Pure tone test at 40 dB HL at 1000 and 2000 Hz in each ear. Hearing impairment defined as either (a) inability to hear tone at one frequency in *each* ear, or (b) inability to hear both frequencies in one ear.

(Table 12.8). Persons should be considered in need of referral if they fail the audioscope *and* have an HHIE-S score greater than 8 *or* they pass the audioscope *and* have an HHIE-S score greater than 24.

Physical Diagnostic Maneuvers.   Traditional maneuvers for detecting hearing impairment in the elderly also have diagnostic utility (Uhlmann et al., 1989). The performance of a 512 Hz tuning fork, 1024 Hz tuning fork, a finger rub, and whispered voice have been tested against pure tone audiometry in demented and nondemented subjects. In this study ears were considered hearing-impaired if the average loss at 500, 1000, 2000, and 3000 Hz was greater than or equal to 40 dB HL. The results are given in Table 12.9. In demented patients, at set sensitivities, the observed specificities are comparable to those found with the audioscope; however, among nondemented subjects, the specificities are lower. The tests also were found to be repeatable (Table

12.9), but this may depend on the setting in which the tests are performed and differences between observers in administering the tests. Compared to the traditional physical diagnostic tests, the audioscope delivers a standard signal at a standard distance (right at the external auditory canal). The HHIE-S offers the advantage of removing observers from the screening process and relying on self-report. All the studied tests are useful screening tools for hearing impairment; to determine which is optimal (if one is better than the others) would require a direct comparative study performed under field conditions.

MEASURING AUDIOLOGIC CHARACTERISTICS ASSOCIATED WITH AGING

The aging auditory system typically exhibits a loss in threshold sensitivity and a decreased ability to understand

TABLE 12.8   Sensitivity, specificity, and predictive values for diagnostic tests in the diagnosis of hearing-impaired elderly.

TEST	SENSITIVITY (%)	SPECIFICITY (%)	PREDICTIVE VALUES* (%) Positive	Negative	TEST ACCURACY (%)
Audioscope	94	72	60	97	79
HHIE-S Score:					
> 8	76	71	53	88	73
> 24	30	96	75	76	73
Combined: Audioscope Fail *and* HHIE > 8 *or* Audioscope Pass *and* HHIE > 24	75	86	70	89	83

*Predictive values apply at hearing impairment prevalence of 30%.

TABLE 12.9 Sensitivities and specificities of physical examination tests in detecting hearing impairment.

TEST	DISTANCE*	SPEC	DISTANCE*	SPEC	TEST/RETEST RELIABILITY (38 EARS)
	Demented Patients (68 Ears)				
	Sens = 90%		Sens = 80%		
512 Hz tuning fork	40	53%	27	82%	0.66
1024 Hz tuning fork	36	63%	23	95%	0.38
Finger rub	8	85%	3	95%	0.89
Whispered voice	19	78%	14	89%	0.67

TEST	DISTANCE*	SPEC	DISTANCE*	SPEC	TEST/RETEST RELIABILITY (44 EARS)
	Nondemented Patients (68 Ears)				
	Sens = 90%		Sens = 80%		
512 Hz tuning fork	40	56%	34	64%	0.87
1024 Hz tuning fork	45	44%	31	69%	0.58
Finger rub	21	44%	16	49%	0.90
Whispered voice	29	70%	21	82%	0.78

*Distance of test from ear in centimeters.

comfortably loud speech. The audiologic manifestations can reflect the pathological changes occurring within the auditory system. Because one or more types of presbycusis often are present, however, it is sometimes difficult to determine site of lesion from the audiometric data.

Pure-Tone Threshold Measures

The hearing loss among those individuals over the age of 60 years primarily affects the high frequencies, especially those above 1000 Hz. The hearing sensitivity changes that are known to occur as a function of age are shown in Figure 12.6. These data, taken from the Framingham Heart Study (Moscicki, Elkins, Baum, & McNamara, 1985), represent the mean audiometric configurations in the better ear (0.5, 1, 2 kHz) as a function of age for both males and females. The study sample is composed of 935 males and 1358 females. Both males and females age 60 years and older are seen to exhibit hearing loss sensitivity especially in the high-frequency regions (2000–8000 Hz). Furthermore, threshold values for males are poorer than for females. It generally is thought that these differences are due to the occupational noise exposure many males experience throughout their lifetimes (exogenous sources not inherent in socioacusis or nosoacusis).

A problem that consistently has plagued the study of threshold change with age has been the influence of environmental factors (socioacustic agents) that can contaminate the threshold sensitivity data. That is, the influence of high noise levels (particularly inherent to industrialized nations) and other variables known to damage the auditory system.

Although the hearing loss typically is sensorineural, there is some data to suggest that a conductive component can be related to the phenomenon known as presbycusis (Glorig & Davis, 1961; Milne, 1977; Nixon, Glorig, & High, 1962). In general, the air-bone gap is reported to increase with increasing hearing loss. The air-bone gap at the high frequencies, particularly 4000 Hz, has been reported to increase from 10 dB at 50 years of age to 40 dB by 80 years of age (Glorig & Davis, 1961; Marshall, Martinez, & Schlamen, 1983). The cause of the observed conductive component is not clearly understood. Glorig and Davis (1961) suggested that the air-bone gap was due to an age-related increase in the stiffness of the cochlear partition. The conductive loss also may be attributed to the changes that can occur in the middle ear (i.e., stiffness of the ossicular chain and tympanic membrane) as well as decreased soft tissue in the external auditory meatus. Another possible cause of the conductive component may be the tissue reduction in the elderly, which produces changes in the properties of the mastoid. Finally, it is possible that the conductive component in the high-frequency region could be due to ear canal collapse or to the use of an earphone with a hard cushion that has a poor fit to the auricle (Bess & Humes, 1995; Gordon-Salant, 1987).

Speech Recognition Measures

In conjunction with poorer performance on pure tone measures, the speech recognition threshold (SRT) worsens with increasing age. An example of poorer SRT scores with increasing age is shown in Figure 12.7.

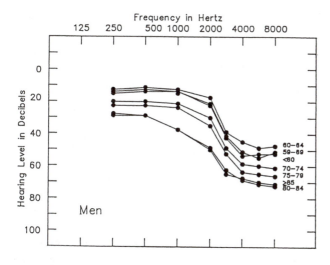

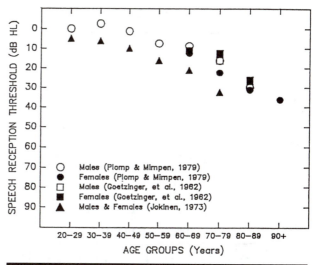

FIGURE 12.7 Speech recognition thresholds (SRTs) as a function of age. Data taken from several studies. (Reprinted with permission from "Basic hearing evaluation," by S. Gordon-Salant, 1987, in H. G. Mueller & V. C. Geoffrey, Eds., *Communication Disorders in Aging*, Figure 4, p. 308. Washington, DC: Gallaudet University Press.)

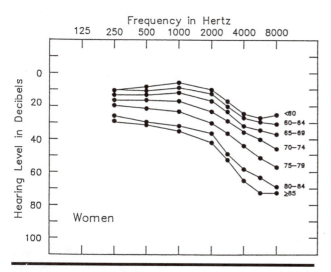

FIGURE 12.6 Mean audiometric thresholds in the better ear for males and females as a function of age. (Redrawn from "Hearing in the elderly: An epidemiologic study of the Framingham heart study cohort," by E. K. Moscicki, E. F. Elkins, H. M. Baum, & P. M. McNamara, 1985, *Ear and Hearing, 6*, 186.)

When speech recognition of comfortably loud speech is assessed in quiet the performance scores of persons matched for equivalent hearing loss are similar across all age groups (Kasden, 1970; Schum, Matthews, & Lee, 1991; Surr, 1977, Townsend & Bess, 1980). Most studies that report poor speech recognition in quiet among the elderly presented the speech material at a fixed intensity level, usually 25 to 40 dB SL. Because the subjects demonstrated high-frequency sensorineural hearing losses, a presentation level of 25 to 40 dB SL often was insufficient

to obtain a maximum speech recognition score. The resulting decrease in speech recognition scores reflected the hearing loss present and not an effect of aging. In fact, Jerger and Hayes (1977) illustrated that PB-max scores in quiet remain relatively stable at 50 through 59 years of age and exhibit only a slight decrease above 59 years. Hence, "an arbitrary presentation level of 95 dB SPL or the use of an adaptive estimate of the PB-max level is preferred" over a fixed presentation level when assessing speech recognition ability in this age population (Gordon-Salant, 1987, p. 309).

The breakdown in speech understanding among the aged appears to be exacerbated even among normal hearers when the listening task is made more difficult through degradation of the speech signal. Dubno, Dirks, and Morgan (1984) found that, regardless of intensity, normal and hearing-impaired listeners over age 65 required more favorable signal-to-babble (S/B) ratios to achieve the same score (50% criterion score) on low predictability items on the Speech Intelligibility in Noise (SPIN) test than did younger subjects with equivalent hearing sensitivity. Figure 12.8 illustrates the S/B ratios required for 50% recognition in four groups of subjects: normal hearing and less than 44 years of age, normal hearing and older than 65 years of age, mild sensorineural hearing loss and less than 44 years of age, and mild sensorineural hearing loss and older than 65 years of age. The more difficult the speech material becomes (high predictability [PH] to low predictability [PL]) the more favorable the S/B ratios must be

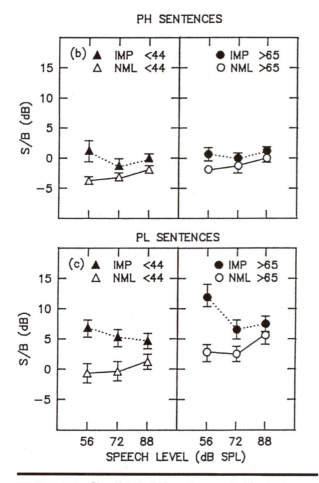

FIGURE 12.8 Signal-to-babble ratios needed for 50% recognition of sentence material (SPIN-PH and PL) in four groups of subjects: young normal (NML) and hearing-impaired (IMP) listeners (left side of the graphs) and older normal (NML) and hearing-impaired (IMP) listeners (right side of the graphs). (Redrawn with permission from "Effects of age and mild hearing loss on speech recognition in noise," by J. R. Dubno, D. D. Dirks, & D. E. Morgan, 1984, *Journal of the Acoustical Society of America, 76,* 87–96. Copyright 1984, Acoustical Society of America.)

for the older subjects, even those with normal pure tone sensitivity, to achieve the same performance of younger ones. These data support the assumption that performance in noise deteriorates with age, with or without increases in threshold sensitivity (Schum et al., 1991). According to Jerger and Hayes (1977), sentence recognition performance decreases systematically with age beginning at 30 to 39 years based on synthetic sentence identification (SSI) scores using an ipsilateral speech competition (message to competition ratio of 0). Sentence recognition performance in competition was much poorer than for monosyllabic materials in quiet for older persons. They attributed this finding to a "central aging effect." Shirinian and Arnst (1982) confirmed these findings but noted greater decline

in speech recognition scores at higher intensity levels. This "rollover" effect has also been reported in subjects with eighth nerve disorders and central auditory dysfunction (Jerger, Neely, & Jerger, 1980).

It appears that the breakdown in speech recognition is even greater when the temporal domain of the speech signal is altered (Bosatra & Russolo, 1982; Jerger, 1973; Konkle, Beasley, & Bess, 1977). Konkle and colleagues examined the effect of time compression on word recognition in four age groups ranging from 54 to 84 years of age. All of the subjects had similar pure tone data and word recognition scores in quiet of 90% or better. The findings from this study are summarized in Figure 12.9. This figure presents the mean word recognition scores for the different age groups at several conditions of time compression and sensation level. It is seen that word recognition decreases with increasing time compression, age, and decreasing sensation level. Konkle and colleagues theorized that this degradation in speech understanding under time-compressed conditions was related to senescent changes in the central auditory mechanism. However, a subsequent study by Otto and McCandless (1982), in which younger and older subjects were more closely matched for high-frequency hearing loss, did not show the same difference in test scores across age groups.

Jerger, Jerger, Oliver, and Pirozzolo (1989) examined the contributions of peripheral, central, and cognitive factors to the speech recognition problems of the elderly population. Following comprehensive audiologic and neuropsychologic evaluations (N = 130), data were analyzed to determine the central auditory and cognitive status of the elderly patients. The prevalence of central auditory processing problems was 50%, whereas the prevalence for cognitive deficits was evident in 41% of the population. The study revealed that speech understanding problems in the aged cannot be totally explained by peripheral hearing loss or cognitive decline and suggested that central deficits are a contributing factor. More specifically, central auditory problems can be evident when there is no cognitive decline and cognitive abnormality can exist independent of central auditory deficits.

Similarly, Cooper and Gates (1991) reported that advancing age accounts for only 15% of the variables influencing the presence of CAPD and may reflect age as a factor for increased risk of developing CAPD rather than the cause of CAPD itself.

When measured, age effects appear task dependent. More complex listening tasks using speech materials presented in less favorable conditions show greater deterioration in test scores for elderly individuals than for younger counterparts.

Loudness Measures

With the onset of sensorineural hearing loss, the sensory-impaired ear may be susceptible to loudness recruitment. Low-input sounds may not be perceived normally by the hearing-impaired ear but high-input sounds are perceived

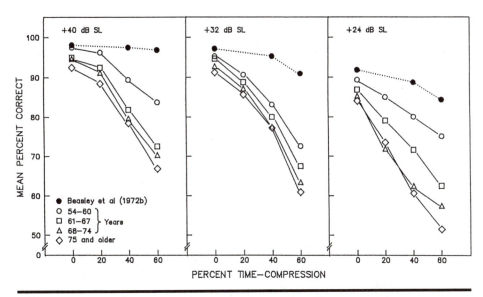

FIGURE 12.9   Mean word recognition scores for the four different age groups as a function of time compression and sensation level. (Redrawn with permission from "Intelligibility of time-altered speech in relation to chronological aging," by D. F. Konkle, D. S. Beasley, & F. H. Bess, 1977, *Journal of Speech and Hearing Research, 20,* 112. © 1977 American Speech-Language-Hearing Association.)

with the same loudness as the normal hearing ear (Sweetow, 1994). As a result, the dynamic range of hearing (range between where sound is perceptible (threshold) and uncomfortable (loudness discomfort level, LDL) is reduced. If amplification is to be provided as a means of rehabilitation for hearing loss present in the older adult, loudness growth measures must be an integral part of the diagnostic assessment protocol. Only by determining both the level of sound necessary to restore audibility as well as the loudness discomfort level can amplification be set to the most comfortable listening range of the listener. Loudness discomfort measures are behavioral tests aimed at eliciting a subjective response from the listener. Currently, there are several methods for obtaining these values. Hawkins and colleagues (Hawkins, Walden, Montgomery, & Prosek, 1987) delineated the levels of loudness shown below.

Levels of Loudness

Painfully loud
Extremely uncomfortable
Uncomfortably loud
Loud but OK
Comfortable, but slightly loud
Comfortable
Comfortable, but slightly soft
Soft
Very soft

Because the instructions given may influence whether an individual accepts or rejects presented stimuli, preset instructions defined by Hawkins are first read to the subject.

The subject then rates pure tone or speech stimuli according to the above categories of loudness.

In the loudness growth by octave band (LGOB) test the nonlinear response of the cochlea from low-level to high-level input is assessed in octave bands and then plotted as a function of perceived loudness versus SPL input (Allen, Hall, & Jeng, 1990).

The Independent Hearing Aid Fitting Forum (IHAFF) proposes a method for assessing loudness growth in a low- and high-frequency band from threshold to perceived uncomfortable loudness. Utilizing the first seven of Hawkins' levels of loudness, the patient rates the audibility of presented pure tones at increasing loudness levels typically at 500Hz and 3000 Hz (IHAFF, 1994).

The goal of all these fitting procedures is to assist in the selection of amplification that provides optimal reception of speech while maintaining normal loudness relationships among environmental sounds (IHAFF, 1994).

Acoustic Immittance Measures

Acoustic immittance at the tympanic membrane is a sensitive and objective diagnostic tool used to identify the presence of fluid behind the tympanic membrane, to evaluate Eustachian tube and facial nerve function, to predict audiometric findings, to determine the nature of the hearing loss, and to assist in the diagnosis of different auditory disorders (Bess & Humes, 1995). In order to interpret immittance test results accurately, the audiologist must recognize the manner in which age may or may not affect the various parameters of acoustic immittance.

Tympanometry and Static Acoustic Immittance. There is limited information available on tympanometric measurements in the elderly population. In a study by Gates and colleagues (Gates, Cooper, Kannel, & Miller, 1990), 95% of ears in this population exhibited pressure between ±100 mmH20, a measurement within normal limits. However, poor Eustachian tube function was measured in a small percentage of older adults (Nerbonne, Schow, & Gosset, 1976). Eustachian tube dysfunction may be reflected in excessive negative pressure on tympanogram findings (Gordon-Salant, 1991). Elderly individuals, then, should be checked for Eustachian tube dysfunction as part of their basic audiologic evaluation.

Static Admittance Values for Older Adults Yield Conflicting Data. When assessing middle ear function, static admittance measures show minimal change as a result of aging (Gordon-Salant, 1987). Static compliance, however, does decline with increasing age (Hall, 1979). But, the static compliance values obtained still fall within accepted normal limits for younger individuals (Gordon-Salant, 1991; Jerger, Jerger & Mauldin, 1972).

Acoustic Reflex. There are a number of studies that have investigated the effect of age on the acoustic reflex. The acoustic reflex is elicited among normal subjects between 80 and 100 dB HL. Of course, the threshold will be elevated for subjects with sensorineural hearing loss. Jerger and co-

workers (Jerger et al., 1972; Jerger, Jerger, Mauldin, & Segal, 1974) reported that the acoustic reflex threshold generally decreases from 96 dB HL to about 84 dB HL in subjects between 3 and 80 years. In support of these data, Osterhammel and Osterhammel (1979) noted that the acoustic reflex declines at approximately 3.5 dB per decade when expressed in sensation level (SL); however, no differences were seen when the data were expressed in terms of hearing level. Quaranta, Cassano, and Amoroso (1980) reported that 55% of their elderly subjects showed absent or abnormal acoustic reflexes for both ipsilateral and contralateral stimulation. Wilson (1981) measured an increase in thresholds, particularly at 4000 Hz, with increasing age. Despite the apparent disagreement among research reports, studies suggest that if age effects exist they are at best minimal for pure tone stimuli below 2000 Hz. Tonal stimuli above 2000 Hz as well as broadband noise do produce statistically significant changes in this age population (Gordon-Salant, 1991; Jerger et al. 1972; Silverman, Silman, & Miller, 1983; Wilson & Margolis, 1991).

Age also influences the acoustic reflex amplitude. Hall (1982) examined individuals ranging in age from 20 to 80 years and reported that the maximum reflex amplitude decreased by about 56% over this age range. The amplitude changes typically are greater for uncrossed reflexes as opposed to crossed reflexes. The uncrossed and crossed acoustic reflex amplitudes for a 1000 Hz signal in three different age groups as a function of signal level are shown in Figure 12.10. At the higher intensity signals the differences in

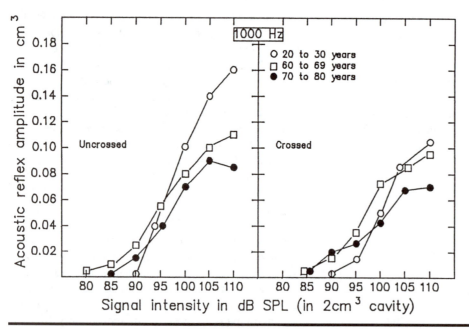

FIGURE 12.10 Crossed and uncrossed acoustic reflex amplitude (1000 Hz signal) in three age groups. (Redrawn with permission from "Acoustic reflex amplitude. II: Effect of age-related auditory dysfunction," by J. Hall, 1982, *Audiology, 21,* 386–399.)

TABLE 12.10   Effect of age on performance on immittance tests.

TEST	EFFECT OF AGE ON PERFORMANCE
Static admittance values	No significant age effect, as static immittance values appear to be within the range considered to be normal for young adults.
Tympanometry	No significant effect, as 95% of ears had pressure between ±100 mm H_2O.[a]
Eustachian tube function tests	Pressure-equalization studies show ventilating inefficiency in a small proportion of older adults.
Acoustic reflex thresholds	No evidence of a systematic age effect for tonal activators below 2000 Hz.[b,c]
	Small age-effect apparent (i.e., elevated reflex levels) when broadband noise is the activator signal.[c]
Acoustic-reflex decay test	No evidence of an age effect on tests of acoustic-reflex decay.[a,c]

[a]Gates et al. (1990).
[b]Gordon-Salant (1991).
[c]Wilson & Margolis (1991).

amplitude become more apparent particularly for uncrossed reflexes. The basis for such age effects is not altogether clear. One possibility is the evidence of age-related dysfunction in the middle ear musculature. Decreased middle ear efficiency would be reflected in reduced capacity for maximal contraction. Another possibility may be related to age changes in the innervation of the stapedius muscle, which of course would diminish the reflex amplitude (Hall, 1979).

At present, there are no data to suggest changes in acoustic reflex decay measures as a result of the aging process. The effect of age on performance on immittance tests is summarized in Table 12.10 using the combined data from these studies (Gates et al., 1990; Gordon-Salant, 1991; Wilson & Margolis, 1991).

Auditory Brainstem Response.   The measurement of auditory brainstem responses (ABR) is considered now an important component of the audiologic test battery. It typically is used in the identification and estimation of hearing impairment of those patients who cannot be tested in a behavioral format (i.e., newborns and infants) or as a special auditory test in neuro-otologic diagnosis. Although the stability and reliability of brainstem responses are considered quite good for the general population, there are a number of extrinsic (i.e., stimulus rate, stimulus intensity, filter setting) and intrinsic (i.e., age, gender, hearing loss) variables that can affect the ABR response. More specific to this discussion, the influence of age and gender on ABR responses has been studied by many investigators and is the subject of some disagreement. For example, Jerger and Hall (1980) reported that latency increased by approximately

0.2 ms over the age range of 25 to 55 years. Furthermore, the Wave V amplitude decreased by about 10% over the same age range. The ABR Wave I-V interval also is reported to increase over the age range of 60 to 86 years, implying that there may be brainstem involvement (Hall, 1990). Rowe (1978) compared the ABR responses for young adults to an older population and found that the elderly group exhibited latency delays on the order of 0.30 ms to 0.50 ms relative to the younger population. According to Thomsen, Terkildsen, and Osterhammel (1978) the Wave V latency increases at approximately 0.10 ms per decade of life. This shift in latency may reflect the hearing loss in higher frequencies seen in this age group. Ottaviani, Maurizi, D'Alatri, and Madori (1991) found no significant differences in the absolute and interwave latencies of older and younger subjects with similar degrees of hearing impairment. According to Jerger and Chmiel (1991), these changes in latency do not affect the use of the ABR for clinical purposes in this age population. Using signal levels of 80 dBnHL, test results obtained are resistant to age effects. However, the ASHA Working Group on Auditory Evoked Potential Measurements (ASHA, 1988) does recommend that the possible effects of the aging process and degree of hearing impairment be considered when the hearing level at 4000 Hz exceeds 50 dBHL in subjects 50 years of age or older. In addition, Schwartz and colleagues (Schwartz, Morris, Spydell, Grim, Schwartz, & Civitello, 1989) emphasized that because elderly individuals tend to be more anxious and noisy, audiologists should maintain an optimal signal-to-noise ratio so that contaminating myogenic activity will not obscure Wave I.

Self-Assessment Scales

An imperfect relationship exists among hearing impairment, hearing disability, and hearing handicap. *Hearing impairment* or *hearing loss* usually denotes a change for the worse in auditory structure or auditory function, outside the range of normal hearing (ASHA, 1981). *Hearing disability* occurs when there is a change in hearing function that causes problems with the perception of speech and environmental sounds (Solomon, 1986). The term *hearing handicap* is used to denote a change in hearing that interferes with performing activities of daily living (Solomon, 1986; Weinstein, 1984). It is possible for a person with mild to moderate loss to experience no disability or handicap; conversely, individuals with marginal hearing loss may perceive themselves as having a significant disability or handicap. Because of the varying response to a hearing impairment, self-assessment techniques have been advocated as a supplement to our pure tone classification schemes (Bess et al., 1989; Schow & Nerbonne, 1982; Ventry & Weinstein, 1983). An understanding of the relationship among hearing impairment, hearing disability, and hearing handicap will offer insight into the impact of hearing impairment in the aged and the rehabilitative needs of this population.

Self-assessment scales and questionnaires allow the audiologist to delve into the patient's and family's perception of their communication difficulties, monitor their progress, and locate their hearing needs outside of the standard audiometric test battery. These tools not only can provide an objective method for evaluating the patient's progress in a rehabilitation paradigm but also provide the professional information for counseling the hearing impaired and his or her "significant others." Moreover, self-assessment scales provide quantifiable measures of perceived benefit by the patient. These scores can serve as a tool for quality assurance assessment of clinical services. If audiological services are to emerge as a reimbursable service under managed care, quantifiable data demonstrating patient benefit is a necessity.

The following review summarizes some of the more common self-assessment scales used for older adults. Some of these scales tap only information regarding the perception of difficulty relating to hearing loss, whereas others delve into the vocational, emotional, and social consequences of hearing loss.

Hearing Handicap Scale. The Hearing Handicap Scale (HHS) Forms A and B (High, Fairbanks, & Glorig, 1964) was the first self-assessment questionnaire developed to evaluate the effectiveness of rehabilitation procedures. The instrument was designed to probe for a person's everyday hearing experiences for persons living in urban environments and focuses primarily on speech communication. Each form contains 20 items and the test takes only about 5 minutes to administer. The questions require only a low level of reading ability. The items are rated on a 5-step continuum from practically always to almost never.

Hearing Measurement Scale. Several years after the introduction of the Hearing Handicap Scale, the Hearing Measurement Scale (HMS) was developed (Noble, 1978, 1979; Noble & Atherly, 1970). This test measures auditory disability for persons with noise-induced sensorineural hearing loss, although it can be used with any hearing impaired adult. It contains 42 scoring items divided into the following seven subcategories: (1) speech-hearing, (2) acuity for nonspeech sounds, (3) localization, (4) emotional response, (5) speech distortion, (6) tinnitus, and (7) personal opinion of hearing loss. Scoring ranges in 5 categories from all of the time to never. The items are weighted to give a measure of disability.

The Denver Scale of Communication Function (DSCF). The Denver Scale of Communication Function (Alpiner, Chevrette, Glascoe, Metz, & Olsen, 1974) was developed to evaluate the client's communication function before and after therapeutic management. There are 25 questions that cover communication in the following areas: family, self, social-vocational, and general communication. Both pre- and post-therapeutic responses are plotted on a grid so that the client can view his or her rehabilitative progress.

The Denver Scale of Communication Function for Senior Citizens Living in Retirement Centers (DSCF-SCLRC). The DSCF-SCLRC (Zarnoch & Alpiner, 1977) is a brief 7-item questionnaire designed specifically for older adults in long-term care and addresses problem areas specific to this population. It is designed to measure pre- and post-rehabilitative performance.

Hearing Performance Inventory (HPI). The Hearing Performance Inventory (Giolas, Owens, Lamb, & Schubert, 1979) asks the client to rate his or her ability to function in problem listening situations. The original inventory contained 158 items and took almost one hour to administer and score. The following areas were probed: understanding speech, signal intensity, response to auditory failure, social aspects of hearing loss, personal and occupational difficulties. In scoring the inventory, the percentage of difficulty was obtained by adding the numerical responses (1 to 5) for all the items answered, dividing by the number of items attempted, and multiplying by 20. The revised HPI (HPI-R) (Lamb, Owens, & Schubert, 1983) has 90 items and takes slightly over half an hour to administer and score. The subsections remain the same. The resulting score can be calculated pre- and post-intervention from amplification as a measure of validating hearing aid performance.

The McCarthy-Alpiner Scale of Hearing Handicap (M-A Scale). The McCarthy-Alpiner Scale of Hearing Handicap (McCarthy & Alpiner, 1980) is a 34-item questionnaire. Form A is for the client to fill out, and Form B is for a family member to use. The only difference in the two forms is a change in the pronoun. The scale was developed to assess the psychological, social, and vocational aspects of hearing loss. The results of the validation study showed a difference in perception between the hearing-impaired person and his or her family. The findings suggest the need to include the family member in the rehabilitation process.

Hearing Handicap Inventory for the Elderly (HHIE).
The Hearing Handicap Inventory for the Elderly (Ventry & Weinstein, 1982) was developed to assess the impact of hearing loss on the emotional and social adjustment of the elderly client. The authors wanted a tool that would assess the handicap imposed by a hearing impairment. The questions were developed to be easy to read and pertinent to the life of an elderly individual. There are 25 items—13 items explore the emotional consequences of hearing loss and 12 items pertain to the social and situational effects. Patients respond to questions regarding their hearing by acknowledging whether the situation presents a problem. A no response scores 0, a sometimes scores 2, and a yes scores 4. Ventry and Weinstein interpreted a score of 18% or greater as suggesting a self-perceived handicap that should lead to further intervention.

Hearing Handicap Inventory for the Elderly—Screening Version (HHIE-S) A 10-item screening version of the HHIE (Ventry & Weinstein, 1983) that assesses the emotional, social/situational and total impact of hearing loss on the older adult. Likelihood of hearing impairment is predicted from the total score: 0–8 = 13%; 10–24 = 50%; 26–40 = 84% probability of hearing impairment (Appendix 12A).

Quantified Denver Scale (QDS) The Quantified Denver Scale (Schow & Nerbonne, 1980) compares the hearing impaired listener's performance to other hearing impaired listeners, providing an estimate of handicap ranging from normal (0–15%) to slight (16–30%) to mild-moderate (31% or greater). There are 25 items divided into four subcategories: family, self, social and general communication.

Hearing Aid Performance Inventory (HAPI) The purpose of the 64-item Hearing Aid Performance Inventory (Walden, Demorest, & Hepler, 1984) is to assess hearing aid benefit based on patient report. The four subsections determine hearing aid benefit in areas typically encountered in daily living: noisy situations, situations involving nonspeech stimuli, situations involving reduced signal information and quiet situations with the speaker in close proximity.

Profile of Hearing Aid Benefit (PHAB) The 66-item Profile of Hearing Aid Benefit questionnaire (Cox & Rivera, 1992) compares unaided and aided performance in speech communication in different listening situations as well as reaction to environmental sounds. There are seven subsections: familiar talkers, ease of communication, reverberation, reduced cues, background noise, aversiveness of sounds, and distortion of sounds. The patient responds on a 7-item continuum from always to never. When unaided and aided scores are calculated together, a score representing hearing aid benefit is obtained. This is useful in measuring reduction of handicap post intervention.

Abbreviated Profile of Hearing Aid Benefit (APHAB)
This shortened version of the PHAB (Cox & Alexander, 1995) reduces the questionnaire to 24 items divided into four 6-item subsections (ease of communication, reverberation, background noise, and aversiveness of sounds). It requires only 10 minutes to administer and yields unaided, aided, and hearing aid benefit scores.

Communication Scale for Older Adults (CSOA) Designed to assess difficult listening situations specific to elderly adults, the 72-item Communication Scale for Older Adults (Kaplan, in review) is divided into two subsections: communication strategies and attitudes. Responses can be scored on a 3-point continuum from almost always to almost never or on a 5-point continuum from always to never.

Self-Assessment of Communication (SAC) and the Significant Other Assessment of Communication (SOAC)
The SAC (Schow & Nerbonne, 1982) is a 10-item self-report questionnaire that assesses (a) primary communication difficulties in different situations, as well as (b) emotional responses to the hearing impairment, and (c) the social consequences or perception of the attitudes of others toward the person's hearing abilities. Response choices range in five categories from almost never to practically always. Total scores on the SAC range from 10 to 50 and a score over 18 constitutes a fail. The Significant Other Assessment of Communication (SOAC) contains the same 10 items as does the SAC with only pronoun changes. It is used to obtain the impressions of a family member or significant other of the client's hearing difficulty (Geier, 1996).

Global Functional Scales: The Sickness Impact Profile (SIP) The scales discussed to this point are all communication-specific because the questions are weighted toward communication difficulties caused by the hearing loss. More recently, attempts have been made to assess the impact of hearing loss on more global measures of function such as functional health status and psychosocial well-being.

Measures of functional health status provide us with insight into the prognosis of a condition, the impact of intervention on general health, and the ramifications of a disease on an individual's life quality (Bess et al., 1989). One measure of functional health status is the Sickness Impact Profile (SIP; Skinner, 1977). The SIP is a 136-statement standardized questionnaire that assesses function in a behavioral context (Bergner, Bobbitt, Carter, & Gilson, 1981; Bergner, Bobbitt, Pollard, Martin, & Gilson, 1976; Gilson, Gilson, Bergner, Bobbitt, Kressel, Pollard, & Vesselago, 1975). The statements are weighted and grouped into 12 subscales: ambulation, mobility, body care/movement, social interaction, communication, alertness, emotional, sleep/rest, eating, work, home management, and recreation/ pastimes. In - addition, there are three main scales: Physical (combining ambulation, mobility, body care/movement), Psychosocial (combining social interaction, communication, alertness, emotional), and Overall (combining all 12 subscales). The higher the SIP score, the greater the perceived functional impairment. The SIP is a valid, reliable tool that has been applied in a number of areas to measure sickness-related dysfunction (Carter, Bobbitt, Bergner, & Gilson, 1976; Pollard, Bobbitt, Bergner, Martin, & Gilson, 1986). As examples, the SIP has been used in studies of end-stage renal disease (Hart & Evans, 1987), survivors of myocardial infarction (Bergner, Hallstrom, Bergner, Eisenberg, & Cobb, 1985), chronic obstructive pulmonary disease (McSweeney, Grant, Heaton, Adams, & Timms, 1982), and rheumatoid arthritis (Deyo & Inui, 1984). In addition, SIP scores have been associated with level of hearing impairment: As hearing worsens in the elderly, SIP scores increase (Bess et al., 1989).

Medical Outcomes Study Short Form Health Survey (MOS SF-36) The MOS SF-36 (Ware, 1993) is a shortened form of the Medical Outcomes Study (MOS) and was designed to monitor patient outcomes in medical and clinical research settings. The questionnaire is divided into 8 subsections ranging from physical functioning, role—physical, bodily pain, mental health, role—emotional, social functioning, vitality, and general health perceptions (McHorney, Ware, & Raczek, 1993). In validation studies, subcategories of physical functioning, general health perception, and role-physical best reflect chronic medical conditions. Mental health and role-emotional best reflect psychiatric problems. Social functioning and bodily pain appear sensitive to both medical and psychiatric problems (McHorney, Ware, Rogers, Raczek, & Lu, 1992). Affect of hearing impairment may best be reflected in the categories of role-emotional, social functioning, and vitality, sensitive to differences in subjective well-being (Ware & Sherbourne, 1992). The MOS SF-36 can be incorporated into the rehabilitative protocol for the elderly adult to assist in monitoring overall effect of hearing impairment and hearing aid/intervention benefit.

FUNCTIONAL IMPACT OF HEARING LOSS IN THE ELDERLY

Investigators who have used communication-specific interview scales to assess the functional impact of hearing loss on older individuals have reported repeatedly that the hearing-impaired elderly experience a wide variety of listening complications (Bess, in press; Schow & Nerbonne, 1982; Ventry & Weinstein, 1982; Weinstein, 1985). An important question, however, is this: Does hearing loss in the elderly produce only a local disturbance in a person's ability to hear and understand speech, or does the impairment produce wider ripple effects that have an impact on some of the more basic areas of human performance? A major study was conducted in Great Britain to examine the social and psychological implications of hearing impairment among adult populations (Herbst, 1983). In part, this study contrasted hearing-impaired with normal-hearing elderly across several different life dimensions including general health, use of welfare services, experience of loneliness, and interactions with friends and family and the experience of hearing impairment. Some of the pertinent findings from this study include the following:

1. Hearing loss appears to be associated with poor general health and is closely linked with such factors as reduced mobility as well as reduction in activities and number of excursions outside the home.
2. Hearing impairment causes a significant reduction in interpersonal interplay and contacts.
3. Hearing impairment appears to be associated with reduced enjoyment of life.
4. Elderly hearing impaired are more likely to be depressed.

In support of Herbst's findings, Bess and colleagues (1989, 1990) analyzed the impact of hearing impairment on individuals over 65 years of age screened in primary care practices. Functional and psychosocial impairment was measured using the Sickness Impact Profile (SIP), a standardized questionnaire for assessing sickness related dysfunction. The findings of this study are summarized in Figure 12.11. These data reflect the average SIP scores for three different dimensions on the functional measure including physical, psychosocial, and an overall score. For the Physical Scale the mean SIP score increased from 3.3 in individuals with no hearing impairment to 18.9 among those with a loss of 41 dB HL or greater in the better ear. The comparable contrast in the Psychosocial Scale are 4.0 and 16.8. For the Overall Scale the contrasts are 5.3 and 17.1, respectively. In addition, Bess and co-workers conducted a step-wise multiple linear regression to adjust for baseline differences in age, race, sex, educational level, number of illnesses, presence of diabetes and ischemic heart disease, number of medications, near visual acuity, and mental status between the hearing-impaired and non-hearing-impaired

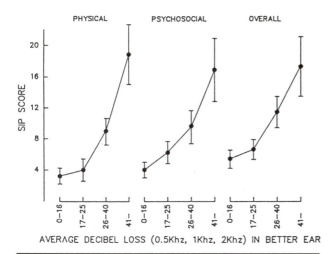

AVERAGE DECIBEL LOSS (0.5Khz, 1Khz, 2Khz) IN BETTER EAR

FIGURE 12.11 Mean physical, psychosocial, and overall Sickness Impact Profile (SIP) scores plotted by level of hearing impairment (average dB loss at 500, 1000, 2000 Hz in the better ear) in 153 elderly subjects. The intervals plotted around the means represent one standard error. (Reprinted with permission from "Hearing impairment as a determinant of function in the elderly," by F. H. Bess, M. J. Lichtenstein, S. A. Logan, M. C. Burger, & E. Nelson, 1989, *Journal of the American Geriatrics Society, 37,* 126.)

elderly. In these multivariate analyses the score of each SIP scale served as the dependent variable. The regression coefficient was reported as a change in SIP score per change in hearing level. After adjustment for confounding variables, higher SIP scores were observed on all three main scales with every 10 dB increase in hearing loss, suggesting strong evidence for a relationship between degree of hearing impairment and functional capacity.

In contrast to the studies by Herbst (1983) and Bess and colleagues (1989), Solomon, Vesterager, and Jagd (1988) reported that life satisfaction, self-perception, and general activity level were not influenced by hearing level.

Several studies have explored the relationship between dementia and deafness. These studies demonstrated that a high percentage of patients with some degree of senile dementia also exhibited significant hearing loss (Herbst, 1983). These studies concluded, however, that hearing loss does not cause dementia, but rather the two conditions coexist among elderly patients. Weinstein and Amsell (1986) reported further that there was a trend among patients with dementia to have more severe hearing losses. Finally, Herbst and Humphrey (1980) showed a significant relationship between depression and hearing impairment. They concluded that "while deafness is not a major cause of depression in old age, it is certainly a contributing factor and one that may be more readily ameliorated than many others" (p. 905).

MANAGEMENT ISSUES IN THE ELDERLY

The primary rehabilitation tool for the elderly hearing-impaired population is amplification. Nevertheless, only 11% of hearing-impaired individuals actually receive hearing aids (Kochkin, 1998). A primary reason for the elderly not receiving amplification is that primary care physicians and "caring others" often fail to recognize hearing impairment. Even if a patient complains of hearing loss, there is only a 52% chance that he or she will be referred for further testing and a 30% chance that he or she will receive a specific recommendation for hearing aids (Kochkin, 1998). In spite of these data, it is estimated that 65% of all hearing aid users are 65 years of age or older (Kochkin, 1992). Most of these individuals are wearing amplification for the first time. Many potential hearing aid patients obtain their initial information regarding amplification from newspaper advertisements, magazines, and friends. Hence, they have already formed an opinion as to the style and type of hearing aid they desire prior to the hearing aid evaluation.

A review of the hearing aid selection process for the elderly hearing-impaired patient is beyond the scope of this chapter. Some issues concerning the specific amplification needs of the elderly, however, are worthy of comment.

When selecting a hearing aid for the elderly patient the audiologist should consider the following areas: (1) the patient's choice of style, (2) vision, (3) ability to manipulate the different types and components of hearing aids, (4) cost, and (5) amplification requirements. It is important to discuss with the elderly hearing-impaired the various hearing aid styles available and which instruments will be most appropriate for a given individual. If a person with a severe hearing loss desires a canal-style hearing aid, the limitations on both aided benefit and physical feasibility of these instruments should be brought to his or her attention.

Another important aspect to consider during the prefitting process with the elderly patient is visual status. Given that visual acuity decreases dramatically with older age, it is worthwhile to obtain information regarding the patient's corrected visual status by using near and far vision eye charts or by simply inquiring about visual status.

In addition to amplification restrictions many older persons have a decreased sense of touch as well as some restricted movement and decreased dexterity. Hence, it is important for the audiologist to determine whether the patient can adjust the controls and change the hearing aid battery on a particular hearing aid style before proceeding with the evaluation.

Although the majority of elderly patients are fitted with in-the-ear style hearing aids, the type and style of hearing aid selected should depend on the patient's ability to operate the aid, not just the degree and configuration of the hearing loss. For persons who cannot manipulate the traditional types of hearing aids, manufacturers have provided audiologists with several options. Simply requesting the hearing aid manufacturer to provide a raised volume control on the in-the-ear instrument may be an option. For some individuals with decreased vision and dexterity, programmable hearing aids using a larger, easier to see and manipulate remote control are a good alternative. In addition, hearing aids with automatic volume control requiring no manual adjustment are an option. One hearing aid company has devised an in-the-ear hearing aid for use with older adults in residential care facilities. This device has an automatic on/off switch when placed in and removed from the case and uses a larger battery, affording six months of use before a change of battery is required.

Finally, the cost of the instrument needs to be weighed against the flexibility for providing the most appropriate electroacoustic response. Because of the degrading effects of distance, noise, and reverberation, optimum speech understanding cannot be achieved in some listening situations with only a hearing aid. Aural rehabilitation classes can help the individual learn about the limitations of hearing loss and hearing aids as well as appropriate ways to compensate through both speaker and listener adjustments to communication strategies (see Appendixes 12B and 12C).

Assistive devices can also offer help through direct sound amplification as well as visual and vibrotactile alerts (Bess & Humes, 1995). The lifestyle of the older individual will help dictate the need for particular assistive devices. If the individual is still employed and active in the community, the needs will be different from the person who is bedridden. For example, if the person is retired, the interest in recreation may take precedence over meetings and conferences. Ross (1986) reported that telephone listening ranks first in importance with hearing-impaired individuals, followed by television and large space listening.

Individuals who rarely leave their homes rely on television as an important source of information. Assistive listening devices are available to enhance listening to television. These devices have either hardwire connections to the television or a remote system such as infrared or FM transmission. In addition, as required by the FCC, due largely to the Americans with Disabilities Act (1992), all television sets 13 inches or larger manufactured after 1992 are now equipped with closed captioning option. The decision as to the appropriate device for improved television listening depends on cost, clarity, and ease of operation.

Assistive devices also can prove to be valuable with use of the telephone. There are many telephone devices available. Some are portable and can attach to any phone. Others replace the existing phone console. Amplified telephones allow the listener to adjust the volume of the incoming speaker. Some also allow for adjustments in the volume, rate, and frequency of the ring and may provide a flashing light as well as auditory ring. Individuals with significant speech understanding problems may benefit from purchasing a telecommunication device for the deaf.

Amplified doorbell ringers that increase the volume of the ring and may couple to a flashing light signal can be hardwired into an existing doorbell or added to a home. The projected flashing light or auditory signal can be received in one or many rooms of the house by a remote or hardwired transmission of the incoming signal.

Churches, synagogues, and public facilities are now using assistive listening devices to enhance speech understanding for the hearing impaired. The FM wireless system, infrared systems, and electromagnetic loops are available for group listening. If the patient's church has a loop system, then the need for a telephone (telecoil) switch on the individual's personal hearing aid(s) may be a necessary option. Again, with the implementation of the Americans with Disabilities Act, group amplification systems in public facilities (such as theaters, movie theaters, and lecture halls) are more readily available. The elderly hearing impaired individual should be instructed in how to request and use these devices. To be effective with dispensing assistive devices it is important to first let older adults describe their specific needs, show them the options that are available, and then guide them in making educated choices.

Finally, many active adults choose to travel by automobile, bus, or plane. An assistive device can enhance communication in the automobile by improving the signal-to-noise ratio reaching the ear. A direct connection from a microphone to a behind the ear hearing aid is efficient; however, because many hearing aid users have in-the-ear models, an inexpensive FM system, such as a pocket talker utilizing an earphone with an adjustable amplified signal for the hearing impaired listener and microphone to direct at the speaker, may be more desirable.

CONCLUSION

It is estimated that one out of every three individuals over the age of 65 exhibits a significant hearing impairment. When one considers the growing number of elderly people in this country, it becomes clear that the audiologist will play an important role in the identification and management of hearing problems with that population. This chapter has focused on the early identification of hearing loss among the elderly population. In addition to the basic audiologic test battery, this chapter has emphasized the value of self-assessment scales. The use of such scales can be of significant benefit in learning more about the patient's communication difficulty, monitoring progress, and objectively assessing the value of amplification. Finally, some brief comments relative to the management issues concerned with elderly hearing impaired patients have been reviewed.

APPENDIX 12A HEARING HANDICAP INVENTORY FOR THE ELDERLY-SCREENING VERSION (HHIE-S)

(Enter: 4 for a "yes" answer; 2 for a "sometimes" answer; 0 for a "no" answer.**)**

1. Does a hearing problem cause you to feel embarrassed when you meet new people? _____
2. Does a hearing problem cause you to feel frustrated when talking to members of your family? _____
3. Do you have difficulty hearing when someone speaks in a whisper? _____
4. Do you feel handicapped by a hearing problem? _____
5. Does a hearing problem cause you difficulty when visiting friends, relatives, or neighbors? _____
6. Does a hearing problem cause you to attend religious services less often than you would like? _____
7. Does a hearing problem cause you to have arguments with family members? _____
8. Does a hearing problem cause you to have difficulty when listening to television or radio? _____
9. Do you feel that any difficulty with your hearing limits/hampers your personal or social life? _____
10. Does a hearing problem cause you difficulty when in a restaurant with relatives or friends? _____

TOTAL _____

Now add the points and see where you fall on the following chart:

HHIE-S Score	Probability of Hearing Impairment %
0–8	13
9–23	48
24 or greater	83

Adapted from Ventry & Weinstein (1983), Lichtenstein, Bess, & Logan (1988b)

APPENDIX 12B COMMUNICATION GUIDELINES FOR PEOPLE WITH HEARING LOSS

1. *Reduce noise and increase light:* Dimly lit and noisy areas can create difficult listening situations even for those with normal hearing. For those with hearing loss such areas can greatly increase the listening difficulties encountered. Whenever possible, if you find yourself in a poorly lit or noisy area, invite your communication partner to an area more appropriate for conversing.
2. *Prepare:* With a little preplanning it is often possible to anticipate difficult listening situations and thereby lessen their impact. As an example, when going out for dinner make reservations for a less busy (noisy) time and tell the host you would like a seat in a well-lit area away from high-traffic areas. Similarly, arriving early to a meeting or lecture will allow you to select a seat that may allow you to hear better.
3. *Inform others of your hearing loss:* When you misunderstand what has been said, do not simply ask for a repetition. Tell the speaker you have a hearing loss and what is helpful to you (i.e., "Please face me when you talk and speak slightly slower and a little louder").
4. *Be attentive:* When hearing is difficult, it is easy to allow the mind to wander. Practice paying close attention to the speaker at all times. Paying close attention can sometimes be exhausting; therefore, arrange for frequent breaks if discussion or meetings are expected to run long.
5. *Watch the speaker:* Although you may have had no formal training in speech reading (lip reading), research has demonstrated that the addition of visual cues to what the ear hears can increase understanding as much as 20%. Always strive for a clear, unobstructed view of the speaker's face. An optimal distance for communication exchange is 3 to 5 feet.
6. *Write things down:* Important instructions, information, or key words such as addresses, telephone numbers, measurements, dollar figures, and so on, should always be written out to avoid confusion.
7. *Be specific how other people can help you understand:* Let others know when you do or do not understand what has been said. Keep in mind that "Huh?" "What?" "Please repeat that" are all ineffective in that they do not tell the speaker what would be helpful. Statements such as "Please raise the volume of your voice," "Please face me when you talk to me," or "I need you to slow down a little" are all much more effective.
8. *Try not to interrupt too often:* How frequently to interrupt calls for a great deal of judgment, but always try to be as unobtrusive as possible. Sometimes a prearranged hand signal for the speaker to slow down, speak up, or to move a hand from in front of the face, and so on, can be useful.
9. *Provide feedback:* Let people know how well they are doing. No one likes to hear only about what is wrong. "Your voice volume and speed are just right; I'm understanding everything you are saying" provides a nice verbal pat on the back as well as important information to the speaker about how best to communicate.
10. *Do not bluff!:* Bluffing robs you of opportunities to practice good communication skills. The risk of not informing others about your hearing loss is an increase in the occurrence of misinterpretations and the possibility of damaged relationships.

11. ***Set realistic goals:*** Be realistic about what you can expect to understand. If you are in a nearly impossible listening situation, it may be best to relax and ride it out. More manageable listening settings will be forthcoming.

12. ***Remember that hearing aids have limitations:*** Often the use of additional assistive listening devices can turn an impossible listening situation into one that is possible.

Boone, M., Clark, J. G., & Trychin, S. (1994). Communication guidelines for people with hearing loss. *Effective Counseling in Audiology: Perspectives and Practice* (pp. 275–276). Englewood Cliffs, NJ: Prentice Hall.

APPENDIX 12C COMMUNICATION GUIDELINES FOR SPEAKING TO PEOPLE WITH HEARING LOSS

1. ***Have their attention first:*** Be sure to get the hard-of-hearing person's attention before you speak. Saying the person's name and waiting for acknowledgment before beginning can greatly decrease your need for repetitions. Similarly, keep in mind that the individual with a hearing loss may not hear the soft sounds of someone entering the room. Calling the person's name as you are approaching or knocking on the door (even if it is open) is a gentle means of alerting the individual that someone is coming.

2. ***Speak face to face:*** The speaker should never speak directly into the ears of someone with a hearing loss, since this, of course, makes it impossible for the listener to make use of visual cues. Research has shown that the addition of visual cues can raise the intelligibility of received speech by approximately 20%.

3. ***Do not put obstacles in front of your face:*** Always speak without anything in your mouth. Pipes, cigarettes, pencils, eyeglass frames, chewing gum, and so on, are distracting to those with hearing loss who may be using visual cues from the speaker's lips.

4. ***Speak clearly and slow down:*** Decrease your speech to slow-normal rate to allow the listener to "catch up." Pausing between sentences can also be helpful.

5. ***Ask if your voice is the right level:*** Do not hesitate to ask the listener if you are speaking at an effective level. Typically it is helpful to speak slightly louder than normal, *but do not shout.* Too much loudness can actually distort the speech signal in an ear with hearing loss.

6. ***Use facial expressions and gestures:*** These will supplement what you are saying. *Facial expressions do not mean overarticulation.* Overarticulation not only distorts the sounds of speech, but also the speaker's face, making the use of visual cues more difficult. Facial expressions and gestures help clarify the message seen on the lips.

7. ***Turn up the lighting:*** To maximize these nonverbal signals, be sure there is adequate lighting on your face. Remember that for the hard of hearing, face-to-face communication is a must, with an optimal distance for communication exchange between 3 to 6 feet.

8. ***Explain the topic:*** Alert the listener with a hearing loss that the subject is shifting when changing topics during group or individual conversations. A statement such as the following can be helpful: "We're talking about last night's Reds' game, Tom."

9. ***Rephrase instead of repeat:*** If the person with a hearing loss does not appear to understand what is being said, try rephrasing the statement rather than simply repeating the misunderstood words. Quite often the same one or two words in the sentence will continue to be missed during each repetition. Rephrasing eliminates many frustrations. This is extremely important, but too often overlooked.

10. ***Turn down the noise:*** Avoid conversation if the television or radio is playing, or if the dishwasher is running, and so on. If you are talking with a person who has a hearing loss, invite that person to move with you to the other side of the room where it might be less noisy.

11. ***Talk to hard-of-hearing people, not about them:*** Too often hearing family members may avoid the need to repeat by talking around the person with a hearing loss. "How is Uncle John doing?" may be directed at Aunt Mary while John is 2 feet away. In such instances, the hard-of-hearing person becomes, at best, a marginal member in any group situation.

12. ***Keep your patience and sense of humor:*** Communication with a hard-of-hearing person can be difficult at times. If you can follow these guidelines and remain patient, positive, and relaxed, you will find the benefits worthwhile. When you become impatient, negative, and tense, communication will become more difficult.

13. ***Ask how to help:*** When in doubt, ask the hard-of-hearing person for suggestions about ways to improve communication.

Boone, M., Clark, J. G. & Trychin, S. (1994). Communication guidelines for speaking to people with hearing loss. *Effective Counseling in Audiology: Perspectives and Practice* (pp. 273–274). Englewood Cliffs, NJ: Prentice Hall.

REFERENCES

Alberti, P., & Kristensen, R. (1970). The clinical application of impedance audiometry. *Laryngoscope, 80,* 735–746.

Allen, J. B., Hall, J. L., & Jeng, P. S. (1990). Loudness growth in ½ octave bands (LGOB)—A procedure for the assessment of loudness. *Journal of the Acoustical Society of America, 88,* 745–753.

Alpiner, J. G. (1978). Rehabilitation of the geriatric client. In J. G. Alpiner (Ed.), *Handbook of Adult Rehabilitative Audiology* (pp. 141–165). Baltimore: Williams & Wilkins.

Alpiner, J. G., Chevrette, W., Glascoe, G., Metz, M., & Olsen, F. (1974). *The Denver Scale of Communication Function.* Unpublished study, University of Denver.

American Speech-Language-Hearing Association. (1981). On the definition of hearing handicap. *Asha, 23,* 293–297.

American Speech-Language-Hearing Association. (1988). *The Short Latency Auditory Evoked Potentials.* ASHA Audiologic Group on Auditory Evoked Potential Measurement.

Bergner, L., Hallstrom, A. P., Bergner, M., Eisenberg, M. S., & Cobb, L. A. (1985). Health status of survivors of cardiac arrest and of myocardial infarction controls. *American Journal of Public Health, 75,* 1321–1323.

Bergner, M., Bobbitt, R. A., Carter, W. B., & Gilson, B. S. (1981). The Sickness Impact Profile: Developments and final revision of a health status measure. *Medical Care, 19,* 787–805.

Bergner, M., Bobbitt, R. A., Pollard W. E., Martin, D. P., & Gilson, B. S. (1976). The Sickness Impact Profile: Validation of a health status measure. *Medical Care, 14,* 57–67.

Bess, F. H. (in press). Hearing impairment in the elderly. *Geriatric Review.*

Bess, F. H., & Humes, L. E. (1995). *Audiology: The Fundamentals.* (2nd ed.) Baltimore: Williams & Wilkins.

Bess, F. H., Lichtenstein, M. J., & Logan, S. A. (1989). Functional impact of hearing loss on the elderly. *ASHA Reports, 19,* 144–149.

Bess, F. H., Lichtenstein, M. J., & Logan, S. A. (1990). Making hearing impairment functionally relevant: Linkages with hearing disability and handicap. *Acta Otolaryngologica, Supplement, 476,* 226–231.

Bess, F. H., Lichtenstein, M. J., Logan, S. A., Burger, M. C., & Nelson, E. C. (1989). Hearing impairment as a determinant of function in the elderly. *Journal of the American Geriatric Society, 37,* 123–128.

Bess, F. H., Logan, S. A., Lichtenstein, M. J., & Hedley, A. (1987). Early identification and referral of hearing-impaired elderly. In M. S. Robinette & C. D. Bauch (Eds.), *Proceedings of a Symposium in Audiology* (pp. 1–27). Rochester, MN: Mayo Clinic/Mayo Foundation.

Bess, F. H., & Strouse, A. L. (1996). Presbycusis. In J. L. Northern (Ed.), *Hearing Disorders* (3rd ed., pp. 199–211). Boston: Allyn & Bacon.

Bess, F. H., & Townsend, T. H. (1977). Word discrimination for listeners with flat sensorineural hearing losses. *Journal of Speech and Hearing Disorders, 42,* 232–237.

Boone, M., Clark, J. G. & Trychin, S. (1994). Communication guidelines for people with hearing loss. *Effective Counseling in Audiology: Perspectives and Practice* (pp. 275–276). Englewood Cliffs, NJ: Prentice Hall.

Bosatra, A., & Russolo, M. (1982). Comparison between central tonal tests and central speech tests in elderly subjects. *Audiology, 21,* 334–341.

Cadman, D., Chambers, L., Feldman, W., & Sackett, D. (1984). Assessing the effectiveness of community screening programs. *Journal of the American Medical Association, 252,* 1580–1585.

Carter, W. B., Bobbitt, R. A., Bergner, M., & Gilson, B. S. (1976). Validation of an internal scaling: The Sickness Impact Profile. *Health Service Research, 74,* 516–528.

Cooper, J. C., & Gates, G. A. (1991). Hearing in the elderly—The Framingham Cohort, 1983–1985: Part II. Prevalence of central auditory processing disorders. *Ear and Hearing, 12*(5), 304–311.

Corso, J. (1977). Auditory perception and communication. In J. E. Birren & K. W. Schaie (Eds.), *Handbook of the Psychology of Aging* (pp. 535–553). New York: Van Nostrand Reinhold.

Cox, R. M., & Alexander, O. C. (1995). The abbreviated profile of hearing aid benefit. *Ear and Hearing, 16,* 176–186.

Cox, R. M., & Rivera, I. M. (1992). Predictability and reliability of hearing aid benefit measured using the PHAB. *Journal of the American Academy of Audiology, 3,* 242–254.

Cranmer, K. (1986). Hearing instrument dispensing. *Hearing Instruments, 6,* 4–14.

Davies, J. W., & Mueller, H. G. (1987). Hearing aid selection. In H. G. Mueller & V. C. Geoffrey (Eds.), *Communication Disorder in Aging: Assessment and Management* (pp. 408–436). Washington, DC: Gallaudet University Press.

Davis, A. (1983). The epidemiology of hearing disorders. In R. Hinchcliffe (Ed.), *Hearing and Balance in the Elderly* (pp. 1–43). Edinburgh: Churchill Livingstone.

Deyo, R. A., & Inui, T. S. (1984). Toward clinical applications of health status measures: Sensitivity of scales to clinically important changes. *Health Service Research, 19,* 275–289.

Dubno, J. R., Dirks, D. D., & Morgan, D. E. (1984). Effects of age and mild hearing loss on speech recognition in noise. *Journal of the Acoustical Society of America, 76,* 87–96.

Esiri, M. M., Pearson, R. C. A., Powell, T. P. S. (1986). The cortex of the primary auditory area in Alzheimer's disease. *Brain Research, 366,* 385–387.

Fein, D. J. (1983). Projections of speech and hearing impairments to 2050. *Asha, 25,* 31.

Feller, A. B. (February, 1981). *Prevalence of Selected Impairments: United States—1977* (DHHS publication No. 81-1562, Vital and Health Statistics, Series 10, No. 134). Washington, DC: National Health Center for Statistics.

Fisch, U. (1972). Degenerative changes of the arterial vessels of the internal auditory meatus during the aging process. *Acta Otolaryngologica, 73,* 259–266.

Garstecki, D. (1996). Older adults: Hearing handicap and hearing aid management. *American Journal of Audiology, 5*(3), 25–33.

Garstecki, D., & Erler, S. (1995). Older women and hearing. *American Journal of Audiology, 4*(2), 41–46.

Gates, G., Cooper, J., Kannel, W., & Miller, N. (1990). Hearing in the elderly: The Framingham Cohort 1983–85, Part I. Basic audiometric test results. *Ear and Hearing, 11,* 247–256.

Geier, K. (1996). *Handbook of Self-Assessment and Verification Measures of Communication Performance.* Columbia, SC: Academy of Dispensing Audiologists.

Gilson, B. S., Gilson, J. S., Bergner, M., Bobbitt, R. A., Kressel, S., Pollard, W. E., & Vesselago, M. (1975). The Sickness Impact Profile: Development of an outcome measure of healthcare. *American Journal of Public Health, 65,* 1304–1310.

Giolas, T. G., Owens, E., Lamb, S. H., & Schubert, E. D. (1979). Hearing Performance Inventory. *Journal of Speech and Hearing Disorders, 44,* 169–195.

Glass, L. E. (1986). Rehabilitation for deaf and hearing-impaired elderly. In S. J. Brody & G. E. Ruff (Eds.), *Aging and Rehabilitation* (pp. 218–237). New York: Springer.

Glorig, A., & Davis, H. (1961). Age, noise and hearing loss. *Annals of Otology, Rhinology, and Laryngology, 60,* 407–516.

Gordon-Salant, S. (1987). Basic hearing evaluation. In H. G. Mueller & V. C. Geoffrey (Eds.), *Communication Disorders in Aging* (pp. 301–333). Washington, DC: Gallaudet University Press.

Gordon-Salant, S. (1991). The audiologic assessment. In D. Ripich (Ed.), *Handbook of Geriatric Communication Disorders* (pp. 367–393). Austin, TX: Pro-Ed.

Hall, J. (1979). Effects of age and sex on static compliance. *Archives of Otolaryngology, 105,* 153–156.

Hall, J. (1982). Acoustic reflex amplitude. I. Effects of age and sex. *Audiology, 21,* 294–309.

Hall, J. (1990). *Handbook of Auditory Evoked Responses.* Boston: College-Hill Press.

Hansen, C., & Reske-Neilsen, E. (1979). Pathological studies in presbycusis: Cochlear and central findings in 12 aged patients. *Archives of Otolaryngology, 105,* 9–12.

Harford, E. R., & Dodds, E. (1982). Hearing status of ambulatory senior citizens. *Ear and Hearing, 3,*105–109.

Hart, L. G., & Evans, R. W. (1987). The functional status of ESRD patients as measured by the Sickness Impact Profile. *Journal of Chronic Diseases, 40,* 117S–130S.

Hawkins, D. B. (1980). Loudness discomfort levels: A clinical procedure for hearing aid evaluations. *Journal of Speech and Hearing Disorders, 45,* 3–15.

Hawkins, D. B., Walden, B., Montgomery, A., & Prosek, R. (1987). Description and validation of an LDL procedure designed to select SSPL90. *Ear and Hearing, 8*(3), 162–169.

Hawkins, J. E., & Johnsson, L. G. (1985). Otopathological changes associated with presbycusis. *Seminars in Hearing, 6,* 115–134.

Herbst, K. R. G. (1983). Psychosocial consequences of disorders of hearing in the elderly. In R. Hinchcliffe (Ed.), *Hearing and Balance in the Elderly* (pp. 174–200). Edinburgh: Churchill Livingstone.

Herbst, K. R. G., & Humphrey, C. (1980). Hearing impairment and mental state in the elderly living at home. *British Medical Journal, 281,* 903–905.

High, W. S., Fairbanks, G., & Glorig, A. (1964). Scale for Self-Assessment of Hearing Handicap. *Journal of Speech and Hearing Disorders, 29,* 215–230.

Hinchcliffe, R. (1962). The anatomical focus of presbycusis. *Journal of Speech and Hearing Disorders, 27,* 301–310.

Hull, R. H. (1980). Aural rehabilitation for the elderly. In R. Schow & M. A. Nerbonne (Eds.), *Introduction to Aural Rehabilitation* (pp. 311–348). Baltimore: University Park Press.

Humes, L., Christopherson, L., & Cokely, M. (1991). Central auditory processing disorders in the elderly: Fact or fiction? In J. Katz, N. Steder, & D. Henderson (Eds.), *Central Auditory Processing: A Transdisciplinary View* (pp. 141–149). St. Louis: Mosby-Year Book.

Humphrey, C., Herbst, K., & Faurgi, S. (1981). Some characteristics of the hearing impaired elderly who do not present themselves for rehabilitation. *British Journal of Audiology, 15,* 25–30.

Hyman, B. T., Maskey, K. P., Van Hoesen, G. W., & Damasio, A. R. (1988). The auditory system in Alzheimer's disease (AD): Hierarchical pattern of pathology. *Neurology, 38*(1), 133.

IHAFF unveils fitting protocol at Jackson Hole Rendezvous. (1994). *The Hearing Review, 9*(1).

International Standards Organization (ISO). (1999). *Acoustics: Determination of Occupational Noise Exposure and Estimation of Noise-Induced Hearing Impairment.*

Jerger, J. (1973). Audiological findings in the aging. *Advances in Otology, Rhinology, and Laryngology, 20,* 115–124.

Jerger, J., & Chmiel, R. (1991). *Effect of Age on Auditory Evoked Potentials.* Paper presented at the Third Annual Convention of the American Academy of Audiology, Denver, CO.

Jerger, J., & Hall, J. (1980). Effects of age and sex on auditory brainstem response. *Archives of Otolaryngology, 106,* 387–391.

Jerger, J., & Hayes, D. (1977). Diagnostic speech audiometry. *Archives of Otolaryngology, 103,* 216–222.

Jerger, J., Jerger, S., & Mauldin, L. (1972). Studies in impedance audiometry. I: Normal and sensorineural ears. *Archives of Otolaryngology, 96,* 513–523.

Jerger, J., Jerger, S., Mauldin, L., & Segal, P. (1974). Studies in impedance audiometry. II: Children less than 6 years old. *Archives of Otolaryngology, 99,* 1–9.

Jerger, J., Jerger, S., Oliver, T., & Pirozzolo, F. (1989). Speech understanding in the elderly. *Ear and Hearing, 10,* 79–89.

Jerger, J., Jerger, S., Oliver, T., & Pirozzolo, F. (1993). Speech understanding in the elderly. In B. R. Alford & S. Jerger (Eds.), *Clinical Audiology: The Jerger Perspective.* San Diego: Singular.

Jerger, J., Neely, J., & Jerger, S. (1980). Speech, impedance and auditory brainstem audiometry in brainstem tumors. *Archives of Otolaryngology, 106,* 218–223.

Johnsson, L. G., & Hawkins, J. E., Jr. (1972). Vascular changes in the human inner ear associated with aging. *Annals of Otology, Rhinology, and Laryngology, 81*(3), 364–376.

Kaplan, H. (in review). Communication scale for older adults. *Journal of the American Academy of Audiology.*

Kasden, S. (1970). Speech discrimination in two age groups matched for hearing loss. *Journal of Auditory Research, 10,* 210–212.

Kochkin, S. (1992). MarkeTrac III: Higher hearing aid sales don't signal better market penetration. *The Hearing Journal, 45*(7), 1–7.

Kochkin, S. (1998). MarkeTrac IV: Correlates of hearing aid purchase intent. *The Hearing Journal, 51*(1), 30–41.

Konkle, D. F., Beasley, D. S., & Bess, F. H. (1977). Intelligibility of time-altered speech in relation to chronological aging. *Journal of Speech and Hearing Research, 20,* 108–115.

Krmpotic-Nemic, J. (1971). A new concept of the pathogenesis of presbycusis. *Archives of Otolaryngology, 93,* 161–166.

Kurylo, D. D., Corkin, S., Allard, T., Zatorre, R. J., & Browden, J. H. (1993). Auditory function in Alzheimer's disease. *Neurology, 43,* 1893–1899.

Lamb, S. H., Owens, E., & Schubert, E. D. (1983). The revised form of the Hearing Performance Inventory. *Ear and Hearing, 4,* 152–159.

Lewis, D. A., Campbell, M. J., Terry, R. D., & Morrison, J. H. (1987). Laminar and regional distributions of neurofibrillary tangles and neuritic plaques in Alzheimer's disease: Augmentative study of visual and auditory cortices. *Journal of Neuroscience, 7*(16), 1799–1808.

Lichtenstein, M. J., Bess, F. H., & Logan, S. L. (1988a). Validation of screening tools for identifying hearing-impaired elderly in primary care. *Journal of the American Medical Association, 259,* 2875–2878.

Lichtenstein, M. J., Bess, F. H., & Logan, S. L. (1988b). Diagnostic performance of the Hearing Handicap Inventory for the Elderly (Screening Version) against differing definitions of hearing loss. *Ear and Hearing, 9,* 209–211.

Marshall, L., Martinez, S. A., & Schlamen, M. E. (1983). Reassessment of high frequency air-bone gaps in older adults. *Acta Otolaryngologica, 109,* 601–606.

Maurer, J. F., & Rupp, R. R. (1979). *Hearing and Aging: Tactics for Intervention.* New York: Grune & Stratton.

McCarthy, P. A., & Alpiner, J. G. (1980). *The McCarthy-Alpiner Scale of Hearing Handicap.* Unpublished manuscript.

McCarthy, P. A., & Alpiner, J. G. (1983). An assessment scale of hearing handicap for use in family counseling. *Journal of the Academy of Rehabilitative Audiology, 16,* 256–270.

McHorney, C. A., Ware, J. E., & Raczek, A. E. (1993). The MOS 36-item short-form health survey (SF-36): II. Psychometric and clinical tests of validity in measuring physical and mental health constructs. *Medical Care, 31*(3), 247–2630.

McHorney, C. A., Ware, J. E., Rogers, W., Raczek, A. E., & Lu, J. F. R. (1992). The validity and relative precision of MOS short- and long-term Health Status scales and Dartmouth COOP charts: Results from the medical outcomes study. *Medical Care, 30*(5) (*Supplement*).

McSweeney, A., Grant, I., Heaton, R. K., Adams, K. M., & Timms, R. M. (1982). Life quality of patients with chronic obstructive pulmonary disease. *Archives of Internal Medicine, 142,* 473–478.

Mills, J. H. (1996). Presbycusis. In J. J. Ballenger & J. B. Snow, Jr. (Eds.), *Otorhinolaryngology—Head and Neck Surgery* (15th ed., pp. 1133–1141). Baltimore: Williams & Wilkins.

Mills, J., Schmiedt, R., & Kulish, L. (1990). Age-related changes in auditory potentials of Mongolian gerbil. *Hearing Research, 46,* 201–210.

Milne, J. M. (1977). The air-bone gap in older people. *British Journal of Audiology, 11,* 1–6.

Morrison, A. S. (1985). Screening in chronic disease. *Monographs in Epidemiology and Biostatistics, 7,* 1–182.

Moscicki, E. K., Elkins, E. F., Baum, H. M., & McNamara, P. M. (1985). Hearing loss in the elderly: An epidemiologic study of the Framingham Heart Study Cohort. *Ear and Hearing, 6,* 184–190.

Moss, A. J., & Parson, V. C. (1986). Current estimates from the National Interview Survey, U.S., 1985. Washington, DC: National Center for Health Statistics. *DHHS Publication (PHS) 86, 1588,* 21–30.

Mulrow, C. D. (1991). Screening for hearing impairment in the elderly. *Hospital Practice,* February, 79–86.

Mulrow, C. D., Aguilar, C., Endicott, J. E., Tuley, M. R., Velez, R., Charlip, W. S., Rhodes, M. C., Hill, J. A., & DeNino, L. A. (1990a). Quality of life changes and hearing impairment: Results of a randomized trial. *American College of Physicians, 113,* 188–194.

Mulrow, C. D., Aguilar, C., Endicott, J. E., Velez, R., Tuley, M. R., Charlip, W. S., & Hill, J. A. (1990b). Association between hearing impairment and the quality of life of elderly individuals. *Journal of the American Geriatric Society, 38,* 45–50.

Mulrow, C. D., & Lichtenstein, M. J. (1991). Screening for hearing impairment in the elderly: Rationale and strategy. *Journal of General Internal Medicine, 6,* 249–258.

Musiek, F. E., & Hoffman, D. W. (1990). An introduction to the functional neurochemistry of the auditory system. *Ear and Hearing, 11,* 395–402.

Nadol, J. (1979). Electron microscopic findings in presbycusic degeneration of the basal turn of the human cochlea. *Otolaryngology—Head and Neck Surgery, 87,* 818–836.

Nerbonne, M., Schow, R., & Gosset, F. (1976). *Prevalence of Conductive Pathology in a Nursing Home Population* (Laboratory Research Reports). Pocatello: Idaho State University, Department of Speech Pathology and Audiology.

Nixon, J., Glorig, A., & High, W. (1962). Changes in air and bone conduction thresholds as a function of age. *Journal of Laryngology and Otology, 74,* 288–299.

Noble, W. G. (1978). *Test Manual for the Hearing Measurement Scale.* Armidele, NSW, Australia: University of New England.

Noble, W. G. (1979). The Hearing Instrument Scale as a paper-pencil form: Preliminary results. *Journal of the American Auditory Society, 5,* 95–106.

Noble, W. G., & Atherly, G. R. C. (1970). The hearing measure scale: A questionnaire for the assessment of auditory disability. *Journal of Auditory Research, 10,* 229–250.

Onofrj, M. C., Ghilardi, M. F., Fulgente, T., Nobilio, D., Bazzano, S., Ferracco, F., & Malatesta, G. (1990). Mapping of event-related potentials to auditory and visual odd-ball paradigms. *Electroencephalitis and Clinical Neurophysiology, 41,* 183–201.

Osterhammel, D., & Osterhammel, P. (1979). Age and sex variations for the normal stapedial reflex thresholds and tympanometric compliance values. *Scandinavian Audiology, 8,* 153–158.

Ottaviani, F., Maurizi, M., D'Alatri, A., & Madori, G. (1991). Auditory brainstem response in the aged. *Acta Otolaryngologica,* (*Supplement,* Stockholm), *476,* 110–114.

Otto, W., & McCandless, G. (1982). Aging and auditory site of lesion. *Ear and Hearing, 3,* 110–117.

Polich, J., Ladish, C., & Bloom, F. E. (1990). P300 assessment of early Alzheimer's disease. *Electroencephalitis and Clinical Neurophysiology, 77,* 179–189.

Pollard, W. E., Bobbitt, R. A., Bergner, M., Martin, D. P., & Gilson, B. S. (1986). The Sickness Impact Profile: Reliability of a health status measure. *Medical Care, 14,* 146–155.

Prevalence of selective impairments—1977. Hyattsville, MD: *U.S. Department of Health and Human Services,* DHHS Publication No. (PHS) 81–1562.

Projections of the population of the United States: 1982–2050 (Advance Report). (1982). Washington, DC: *U.S. Bureau of the Census,* 9–21.

Quaranta, A., Cassano, P. & Amoroso, C. (1980). Presbyacousie et reflexmetrie stapedienne. *Audiology, 19,* 310–315.

Rosen, S., Bergman, M., Plester, D., El-Mofty, A., & Salti, M. (1962). Presbycusis: Study of a relatively noise free population in the Sudan. *Annals of Otology, Rhinology, and Laryngology, 71,* 727–743.

Ross, M. (1986). Thoughts on ALDS. *Hearing Instruments, 87,* 16–21.

Rowe, M. (1978). Normal variability of the brain-stem auditory evoked response in young and old adult subjects. *Electroencephalography and Clinical Neurophysiology, 44,* 459–470.

Sackett, D. L., Haynes, R. B., & Tugwell, P. (1985). *Clinical Epidemiology: A Basic Science for Clinical Medicine.* Boston/Toronto: Little, Brown.

Saunders, J. C., Dean, S. P., & Schneider, M. E. (1985). The anatomical consequences of acoustic energy: A review and tutorial. *Journal of the Acoustical Society of America, 78,* 833–860.

Schow, R. L., & Nerbonne, M. A. (1980). Hearing handicap and Denver scales: Applications, categories, interpretation. *Journal of the Academy of Rehabilitative Audiology, 13,* 66–77.

Schow, R. L., & Nerbonne, M. A. (1982). Communication screening profile: Use with elderly clients. *Ear and Hearing, 3,* 135–147.

Schuknecht, H. F. (1955). Presbycusis. *Laryngoscope, 65,* 407–419.

Schuknecht, H. F. (1964). Further observations on the pathology of presbycusis. *Archives of Otolaryngology, 80,* 369–382.

Schuknecht, H. F. (1974). *Pathology of the Ear.* Cambridge, MA: Harvard University Press.

Schulte, B., & Schmiedt, R. (1992). Lateral wall Na K-ATPase and cholocochlear potentials decline with age in quiet-reared gerbils. *Hearing Research, 61,* 35–46.

Schum, D., Matthews, L., & Lee, F. (1991). Actual and predicted word-recognition performance of elderly hearing-impaired listeners. *Journal of Speech and Hearing Research, 34,* 636–642.

Schwartz, D. M., Morris, M. D., Spydell, J. D., Grim, M. A., Schwartz, J. A., & Civitello, B. A. (1989). *The Brainstem Auditory Evoked Response (BAER) in Patients with High Frequency Cochlear Hearing Loss: New Perspectives on an Old Clinical Problem.* Manuscript submitted for publication.

Selkoe, D. S. (1992). Aging brain, aging mind. *Scientific Americas,* September, 135–142.

Sherif, F., Gottfries, C. G., Alafuzoff, I., & Ireland, L. (1992). Brain gamma-aminotransferase (GABA-T) and monamine orxidase (MAD) in patients with Alzheimer's disease. *Journal of Neural Transmission,* (P-D Sect.), 4, 227–240.

Shirinian, M., & Arnst, D. (1982). Patterns in performance-intensity functions for phonetically balanced word lists and synthetic sentences in aged listeners. *Archives of Otolaryngology, 108,* 15–20.

Silverman, C. A., Silman, S., & Miller, M. H. (1983). The acoustic reflex threshold in aging ears. *Journal of the Acoustical Society of America, 73,* 248–255.

Skinner, A. (1977). *Sickness Impact Profile (SIP).* Baltimore: Johns Hopkins University.

Solomon, G. (1986, November). Hearing problems in the elderly. *Danish Medical Bulletin, Special Supplement Series, 3,* 1–22.

Solomon, G., Vesterager, V., & Jagd, J. (1988). Age-related difficulties: I. Hearing impairment, disability, and handicap—a controlled study. *Audiology, 27,* 164–178.

Stach, B., Spretnjak, M., & Jerger, J. (1990). The prevalence of central presbycusis in clinical populations. *Journal of the American Academy of Audiology, 1,* 109–115.

Strouse, A. L., DeChicchis, A. R., & Bess, F. H. (1996). Changes in hearing with aging. In R. Lubinski & J. Higginbotham (Eds.), *Communication Technologies for the Elderly: Hearing, Speech, and Vision* (pp. 103–128). San Diego: Singular Publishing.

Suga, F., & Lindsay, J. R. (1976). Histopathological observations of presbycusis. *Annals of Otology, Rhinology and Laryngology, 85,* 169–184.

Surr, R. K. (1977). Effect of age on clinical hearing and evaluation results. *Journal of the American Audiology Society, 3,* 1–5.

Sweetow, R. (1994). Fitting strategies for noise-induced hearing loss. In M. Valente (Ed.), *Strategies for Detecting and Verifying Hearing Aid Fittings* (pp. 156–162). New York: Thieme Medical Publishers.

Syndulko, K., Hansch, E. L., Cohen, S. N., Pearce, J. W., Goldberg, Z., Montan, B., Tourtellotte, W. W., & Potrin, A. R. (1982). Long latency event-related potentials in normal aging and dementia. In J. Courjin, F. Mauguiere, M. Revol (Eds.), *Clinical Applications of Evoked Potentials* (pp. 279–285). New York: Raven Press.

Tarnowski, B., Schmeidt, R., Hellstrom, L, Lee, F., & Adams, J. (1991). Age related changes in cochleas of mongolian gerbils. *Hearing Research, 54*:123–124.

Thomsen, J., Terkildsen, K., & Osterhammel, P. (1978). Auditory brainstem responses in patients with acoustic neuromes. *Scandinavian Audiology, 7,* 179–183.

Townsend, T. H., & Bess, F. H. (1980). Effects of age and sensorineural hearing loss on word recognition. *Scandinavian Audiology, 9,* 245–248.

Uhlmann, R. F., Larson, E. B., & Koepsell, T. D. (1986). Hearing impairment and cognitive decline in senile dementia of the Alzheimer's type. *Journal of the American Geriatric Society, 34,* 207–210.

Uhlmann, R. F., Rees, T. S., Psaty, B. M., & Duckert, L. G. (1989). Validity and reliability of auditory screening tests in demented and non-demented older adults. *Journal of General Internal Medicine, 4,* 90–96.

Ventry, I. M., & Weinstein, B. (1982). The Hearing Handicap Inventory for the Elderly: A new tool. *Ear and Hearing, 3,* 128–134.

Ventry, I. M., & Weinstein, B. (1983). Identification of elderly people with hearing problems. *Asha, 25,* 37–42.

Walden, B. E., Demorest, M. E., & Hepler, E. L. (1984). Self-report approach to assessment benefit derived from amplification. *Journal of Speech and Hearing Research, 27,* 49–56.

Ware, J. E. (1993). *SF-36 Health Survey: Manual and Interpretation Guide.* Boston: The Medical Outcomes Trust.

Ware, J. E., & Sherbourne, C. D. (1992). The MOS 36 item short form health survey (SF-36). *Medical Care, 3016,* 473–483.

Weinstein, B. E. (1984). A review of hearing handicap scales. *Audiology, 9,* 91–109.

Weinstein, B. E. (1985). *Hearing Problems in the Elderly: Identification and Management.* New York: The Brookdale Institute on Aging and Adult Human Development, Columbia University.

Weinstein, B. E. (1994). Presbycusis. In J. Katz (Ed.) *Handbook of Clinical Audiology* (4th ed., pp. 568–584). Baltimore: Williams and Wilkins.

Weinstein, B. E., & Amsell, L. (1986). Hearing loss and senile dementia in the institutionalized elderly. *Clinical Gerontologist, 4,* 3–15.

Wilson, R. (1981). The effects of aging on the magnitude of the acoustic reflex. *Journal of Speech and Hearing Research, 24,* 406–414.

Wilson, R., & Margolis, R. (1991). Acoustic reflex measurements. In W. Rintelmann (Ed.), *Hearing Assessment* (2nd ed., pp. 247–319). Austin, TX: Pro-Ed.

Zarnoch, J., & Alpiner, J. (1977). *Denver Scale of Communication Function for Senior Citizens Living in Retirement Centers.* Unpublished study, University of Denver.

CHAPTER 13

BEHAVIORAL ASSESSMENT OF THE CENTRAL AUDITORY NERVOUS SYSTEM

JANE A. BARAN
FRANK E. MUSIEK

The central auditory nervous system (CANS) is a complex system of neural pathways that can be affected by a number of developmental and pathological conditions. Because of this complexity within the CANS neural pathways, assessment of the central auditory system presents a unique challenge, and the audiologist involved in central auditory assessments must possess in-depth knowledge of the CANS and how pathological conditions are likely to affect its function. This chapter provides an overview of the research and clinical developments that have led to the current practice patterns within the field of central auditory assessment. The central auditory pathways, as well as the terms *central auditory processing* and *central auditory processing disorder*, are defined and detailed information is provided for the central auditory tests that are currently used in the behavioral assessment of the CANS. Examples of the more popular versions of many of these tests can be found on the compact auditory disc that accompanies this text. Finally, considerations for test selection, administration, and interpretation are discussed and case studies are highlighted.

HISTORICAL PERSPECTIVE

The beginning of central auditory testing can be traced back to the 1950s when Bocca and his colleagues (Bocca, Calearo, & Cassinari, 1954; Bocca, Calearo, Cassinari, & Migliavacca, 1955) first used a monaural distorted speech test to assess central auditory function in patients with CANS lesions. These Italian physicians recognized that peripheral auditory tests, such as pure tone and speech recognition tests, were not sensitive to the auditory difficulties that were being reported by many of their patients with compromise of the CANS. Specifically, they noted that patients with temporal lobe lesions complained of subjective differences in both the quality and clarity of the sounds perceived in the ear contralateral to the compromised hemisphere in spite of normal peripheral auditory findings. In an attempt to identify a test that would document the existence of these difficulties, these investigators developed a low-pass filtered speech test and administered

it to 18 patients with confirmed temporal lobe lesions. Their results revealed asymmetrical performance in their patients, with depressed scores being noted in the ear contralateral to the damaged hemisphere. Since the time of the introduction of the low-pass filtered speech test, a number of other monaural low redundancy or distorted speech tests have been introduced. These have included band-pass filtered speech, compressed speech, speech recognition in noise, performance-intensity functions, and interrupted speech tests.

Binaural interaction tests, also referred to as binaural integration tests, were first used to assess CANS function in subjects with brain pathology in the late 1950s. Sanchez-Longo and colleagues (Sanchez-Longo & Forster, 1958; Sanchez-Longo, Forster, & Auth, 1957) demonstrated impaired sound localization ability in the auditory field contralateral to temporal lobe lesions in a group of brain-damaged adults. Subsequently, Pinheiro and Tobin (1969, 1971) found that patients with temporal or parietal lobe lesions typically demonstrated abnormal interaural intensity differences (IIDs), whereas patients with frontal or occipital lobe lesions showed normal IIDs. Although it is believed that the critical neural events involved in the processing of the IIDs occur at the brainstem level, the perception of the location of the sound appears to be a cortical function (Pickles, 1985). Other binaural interaction tasks, which were reported as being particularly sensitive to brainstem pathology, appeared in the late 1950s and early 1960s. These included binaural fusion, rapidly alternating speech perception, and masking level differences.

In the early 1960s, Kimura (1961a, 1961b) introduced a dichotic speech test in which digit triads were presented simultaneously to both ears of a group of patients with unilateral temporal lobe lesions. Kimura noted depressed recognition scores for the contralateral ears of her subjects when the stimuli were presented in a competing or dichotic condition. However, if the stimuli were presented in a non-competing condition, no deficits were noted unless the left or dominant hemisphere for speech and language was affected. In this case, depressed scores were typically noted for both ears.

Based upon these findings and some earlier physiological evidence provided by Rosenzweig (1951), Kimura (1961a, 1961b) developed a model that could be used to explain the function of the CANS in the perception of dichotically presented stimuli. In situations where only monaural input is provided to the auditory system, either pathway (ipsilateral or contralateral) is capable of initiating the appropriate neural response. In dichotic situations, however, the weaker ipsilateral pathways are believed to be suppressed and the stronger or privileged contralateral pathways take precedent. Thus, if one hemisphere is compromised in a patient, one would expect reduced performance in the contralateral ear whenever the test stimuli are presented in a competing dichotic manner. In addition, ipsilateral deficits are expected if the left, or dominant, hemisphere for speech and language is affected. Although other theories have been advanced in an attempt to explain dichotic speech perception (Sidtis, 1982; Speaks, Gray, Miller, & Rubens, 1975), Kimura's model remains the most popular. Since the introduction of dichotic digits, several other dichotic speech tests have been introduced. These have included dichotic words, competing or dichotic sentences, and dichotic CVs (consonants-vowels).

In the early to mid 1960s, several researchers began to use temporal ordering or sequencing tasks in the assessment of CANS disorders (Milner, 1962; Milner, Kimura, & Taylor, 1965; Shankweiler, 1966). Results of these early investigations showed that subjects with temporal lobe lesions demonstrated deficits in the perception of tonal sequences.

In the early 1970s, Swisher and Hirsh (1972) used a test paradigm in which they presented two tones of different pitches and with various onset time differences to either the same or to opposite ears of their subjects. Their subjects consisted of two groups of normal control subjects (young and old adults) and three groups of adults with brain injuries. The subjects were asked to indicate the order of the two tones. The authors found that subjects with left hemisphere damage and fluent aphasia required the longest intervals to order stimuli, particularly if the stimuli were presented to the same ear. Subjects with right hemisphere damage and no aphasia required smaller time intervals (approximating those for normal subjects) to make temporal order judgments if the two stimuli were presented to the same ear. These subjects did, however, show greater deficits than the normal subjects when the tonal stimuli were presented to opposite ears.

Lackner and Teuber (1973) presented dichotic clicks that varied in terms of their onsets to the two ears of subjects with cortical involvement. They found that subjects with cortical damage required a longer silent interval between the clicks in order to perceive separation than did subjects with right hemisphere damage.

More recently, Efron and his associates (Efron, 1985; Efron & Crandall, 1983; Efron, Crandall, Koss, Divenyi, & Yund, 1983; Efron, Dennis, & Yund, 1977; Efron, Yund, Nichols, & Crandall, 1985) have conducted a series of experiments with nonspeech auditory signals that demonstrated contralateral ear deficits in individuals with temporal lobe lesions for a variety of auditory tasks (e.g., gap detection, sound lateralization, and temporal ordering tasks). These researchers found consistent contralateral ear effects not only in subjects with posterior temporal lobe involvement, but also in subjects with anterior temporal lobe resections that reportedly involved sections of the temporal lobe previously believed to have no role in auditory processing. Based upon some of their early findings, Efron and Crandall (1983) suggested the existence of a contralaterally organized efferent pathway in each temporal lobe that when activated significantly enhances one's ability to perceive auditory stimuli on the contralateral side of auditory space. It is interesting to note that Seltzer and Pandya (1978) had previously discovered such an efferent multisynaptic pathway in the rhesus monkey.

One of the first temporal patterning tests used in behavioral assessment of the CANS was an intensity pattern sequences test (Pinheiro & Ptacek, 1971; Ptacek & Pinheiro, 1971). This test consisted of 120 sequences of three tone bursts. The tone bursts were of two different intensity levels and the sequences were constructed in such a manner that in each sequence two of the tones were of the same intensity and one was of a different intensity. Given these test parameters six test sequences were generated (*soft-soft-loud, soft-loud-soft, soft-loud-loud, loud-loud-soft, loud-soft-loud,* and *loud-soft-soft*). The patient was asked to verbally describe the sequences perceived.

Perhaps the most popular temporal patterning test used today is the frequency pattern sequences test developed by Pinheiro (1976, 1977). This test is composed of 120 test sequences, with each test sequence containing three tone bursts. In each sequence, two of the three tone bursts are of the same frequency, whereas the third tone is of a different frequency. Typically the patient is asked to describe verbally each sequence heard and a percent correct identification score is derived for each ear. Patients with lesions of either hemisphere or of the interhemispheric pathways have difficulty describing the monaurally presented sequences (Musiek, Kibbe, & Baran, 1984; Musiek & Pinheiro, 1986, 1987; Musiek, Pinheiro, & Wilson, 1980; Pinheiro, 1976; Pinheiro, Weidner, Suren, & Gaydos, 1977). It is interesting to note that some of these same investigators have shown that if split-brain patients are asked to "hum" the sequences they can do so with close to 100% accuracy in spite of the fact that they typically cannot describe the sequences (Musiek, Baran, & Pinheiro, 1994; Musiek, Kibbe, & Baran, 1984; Musiek, Pinheiro, & Wilson, 1980). These results suggest that some processing of the stimuli occurs in both hemispheres and that the auditory interhemispheric connections must be intact if a verbal report of the test sequences is required.

More recently, Divenyi and Robinson (1989) demonstrated the involvement of the left hemisphere in the processing of spectral, as well as temporal, information. These investigators administered seven nonlinguistic auditory tests to three subject groups, including (1) 11 aphasic subjects with left cerebrovascular accidents (CVAs), (2) 4 nonaphasic subjects with right CVAs, and (3) 11 normal control subjects. Their seven auditory tests included frequency discrimination, gap detection, gap discrimination, temporal order discrimination, detection of tones in noise with and without frequency uncertainty, and a tone-by-narrowband masking test to establish frequency selectivity contours. These researchers noted the expected deficits in certain temporal processing functions (e.g., temporal order discrimination) in the left CVA group, but also found that spectral processing functions were affected in this same group of subjects. Based upon their specific findings, these authors suggested that left hemisphere lesions are likely to result in some deficits in the spectral analysis of separate auditory events, but that the major impact will be evident in the subject's ability to readjust the spectral focus of listening.

When Divenyi and Robinson compared the test results for their right-CVA and left-CVA subjects, significant differences were noted for four of the seven tests administered. All of them were pitch-related. For the most part the differences could be attributed to the highly abnormal performance of the right-CVA group as compared to the left-CVA group. Based on these findings the authors proposed the existence of a bilateral cortical representation for most, if not all, of the auditory functions studied. They did, however, acknowledge the prominence of the right hemisphere in the processing of spectral information.

Finally, these researchers found that in their aphasic patients there was an orderly deterioration in test performance on four of the seven auditory tests as the level of linguistic comprehension (as measured by a variety of language tests) decreased, and that as a group, nonfluent aphasics did better than fluent aphasics on six of the seven tests administered. Acknowledging the limitations of their study in terms of subject numbers, these researchers suggested that there is some evidence in their data to suggest that a generic auditory comprehension dysfunction may either parallel, or underlie, the linguistic auditory comprehension dysfunctions often associated with aphasia, as well as the fluency of aphasia.

The foregoing comments provide a cursory discussion of the development of the field of CANS assessment involving behavioral assessment tools. This review hopefully has placed the development of the field in perspective for the reader. Additional information regarding the development of CANS testing can be found in Musiek and Baran (1987). Later in this chapter more in-depth information on the behavioral tests that are currently employed in CANS assessments is provided and some of the important variables that affect one's selection of the tests to be administered and their interpretation are discussed.

DEFINING THE CENTRAL AUDITORY NERVOUS SYSTEM

The importance and popularity of clinical evaluation of the CANS have increased steadily since the 1970s. This is due in large part to recent advances in our understanding of the structure and function of the CANS and the proliferation of new behavioral tests to assess CANS functioning. At the present time the field of audiology possesses both the technology and the knowledge that should enable audiologists to meet the demanding challenge of assessing the auditory status of neurologically involved patients. However, the full clinical value of central auditory testing may not be realized if the audiologist does not possess detailed knowledge of the central auditory system. Before anyone becomes involved in the assessment of central auditory function, that individual should have a thorough understanding of the anatomy and physiology of the CANS.

Because of space limitations, the neuroanatomy and neurophysiology of the CANS will not be discussed in detail within the context of this chapter. A basic overview of the system is provided and the reader requiring additional details is encouraged to seek out other sources for more detailed information about the CANS (Chermak & Musiek, 1997; Musiek, 1986a, 1986b; Musiek & Baran, 1986; Musiek et al., 1994; Pickles, 1988).

The ascending pathways of the CANS originate at the cochlear nucleus complex, which is located at the posterior-lateral aspect of the pontomedullary junction (Figure 13.1). The other nuclei in the ascending auditory pathways of the brainstem include the superior olivary complex (caudal-most pons), the nuclei of the lateral lemniscus (mid pons), the inferior colliculus (mid brain), and the medial geniculate complex (caudal-posterior thalamus). The projections from the medial geniculate take several subcortical routes to the cortex. Currently, the details of these are not well known; however, there are at least two main fiber groups that project to Heschl's gyrus in the superior temporal lobe and to the insula. In addition to the superior temporal lobe and the insula, the posterior-inferior frontal lobe and the inferior parietal lobe have areas that are responsive to acoustic stimulation. Throughout the CANS there are many points where several of the ascending auditory fibers cross over and course contralaterally, thereby increasing

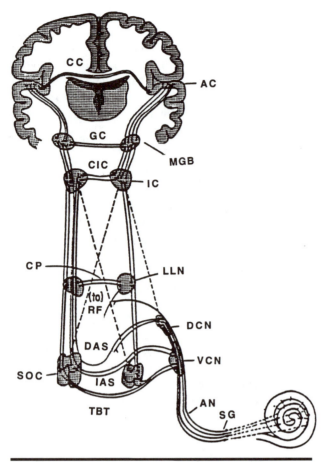

FIGURE 13.1 The main auditory fiber pathways and nuclei in the central auditory nervous system. Key: SG: spiral ganglion; AN: auditory nerve; VCN: ventral cochlear nucleus; DCN: dorsal cochlear nucleus; TBT: trapezoid body tract; IAS: intermediate acoustic stria; DAS: dorsal acoustic stria; SOC: superior olivary complex; RF: reticular formation; LLN: lateral lemniscus nuclei; CP: commissure of Probst; IC: inferior colliculus; MGB: medial geniculate body; CIC: commissure of the inferior colliculus; GC: Gudden's commissure; AC: auditory cortex; CC: corpus callosum.

the intrinsic redundancy of the CANS. The first major crossover occurs at the level of the superior olivary complex. It is for this reason that lesions above this level rarely result in significant losses in terms of threshold sensitivity or speech recognition abilities.

The corpus callosum, which connects the two halves of the brain, also contains auditory fibers that serve to connect the auditory portions of the two hemispheres. Some early primate work by Pandya and colleagues (Pandya, Karol, & Heilbornn, 1971), together with some recent studies of central auditory function in partial split-brain patients (Baran, Musiek, & Reeves, 1986; Musiek et al., 1994; Musiek, Kibbe, & Baran, 1984), have shown that the

interhemispheric auditory fibers are located in the posterior half of the corpus callosum.

The final portion of the auditory system includes the descending efferent auditory pathways that course caudally from the cortical regions to the cochleas. The descending pathways travel both ipsilaterally and contralaterally, taking an anatomical course that is similar to that of the ascending fibers. Their function, however, is very different from the ascending sensory fibers. Because the central auditory pathways represent the largest portion of the auditory system, it is important that the audiologist possesses knowledge not only about the structure and function of the CANS, but also about how lesions and/or pathology in these areas can affect overall auditory functioning.

DEFINING CENTRAL AUDITORY PROCESSING AND CENTRAL AUDITORY PROCESSING DISORDERS

With the development of central auditory testing and the attempts to assess CANS functioning using a variety of behavioral as well as electrophysiological tests came many attempts to define the term *central auditory processing*. For years a definition of this term has eluded the profession and considerable debate has ensued as to its definition as well as to what constitutes a central auditory processing disorder (CAPD). Questions were raised as to whether central auditory processing disorders represented a unique clinical entity or whether they were simply manifestations of other disorders (e.g., language processing disorders, attention disorders, etc.).

In 1993, the American Speech-Language-Hearing Association convened a task force to develop a consensus statement on the topic of central auditory processing. One result of the deliberations of this task force was the development of a definition of central auditory processes.

Central auditory processes are the auditory system mechanisms and processes responsible for the following behavioral phenomena: sound localization and lateralization; auditory discrimination; auditory pattern recognition; temporal aspects of audition, including temporal resolution, temporal masking, temporal integration, and temporal ordering; auditory performance with competing signals; and auditory performance with degraded acoustic signals (ASHA, 1996, p. 41).

The report further qualifies this definition by indicating that these mechanisms are presumed to apply to both nonverbal and verbal signals and that many neurocognitive mechanisms and processes are involved in auditory processing tasks. Some of these are specifically dedicated to processing of acoustic signals, while others are not necessarily unique to the processing of auditory information (e.g., attentional processes and long-term language representations). In the latter case, the term *central auditory processes* refers to the engagement of these mechanisms and processes in the activity of acoustic signal processing.

Having defined the term central auditory processes, the task force went on to develop a definition of a central auditory processing disorder (CAPD).

A **central auditory processing disorder** is an observed deficiency in one or more of the above-listed behaviors. For some persons, a CAPD is presumed to result from the dysfunction of processes and mechanisms dedicated to audition; for others, a CAPD may stem from some more general dysfunction, such as an attention deficit or neural timing deficit, that affects performance across modalities. It is also possible for CAPD to reflect coexisting dysfunctions of both types (ASHA, 1996, p. 41).

Significant in this definition is the recognition that CAPDs can result from dysfunction of the processes that are dedicated to audition, as well from more global deficits (e.g., language deficits, memory deficits, and attention deficits) that are likely to cut across a variety of sensory systems. The only constraint is that in the latter case, the deficits must impact negatively on the processing of auditory information. This should not be construed to mean that there is no value in attempting to tease out the specific auditory perceptual or cognitive deficits that form the basis of a CAPD as these are likely to have direct implications for the management of the individual with the diagnosis of CAPD. Rather the definition recognizes that an auditory-specific processing deficit can coexist with a more global processing deficit, and it lays aside the need to determine which type of deficit underlies the other in those individuals who demonstrate both bottom-up (i.e., auditory-perceptual) and top-down processing (global or higher order) deficits. Additional discussion of this topic can be found in Chermak and Musiek (1997) and McFarland and Cacace (1995).

BINAURAL INTERACTION TESTS

Binaural interaction or integration tests encompass those CANS tests that require the interaction of both ears in order to effect closure for dichotic speech signals that are separated by time, frequency, or intensity factors between the two ears. These tests were designed to assess the ability of the CANS to take disparate information presented to the two ears and to unify this disparate and typically unrecognizable information into one perceptual event. This unification is believed to occur in the brainstem. Thus, these tests are presumed to be sensitive to brainstem pathology. They can, however, also be affected by cerebral lesions.

Rapidly Alternating Speech Perception

Rapidly alternating speech perception (RASP) tests require the integration of segments of speech stimuli delivered alternately between the two ears over time. The best known test in this category is the RASP test developed by Willeford (1976). In this test, segments of sentences are presented to the patient's two ears in an alternating fashion. The alternation rate is 300 msec and a presentation level of 40 dB SL re: pure tone average is recommended. The ear that receives the first 300 msec of each sentence is designated as the lead channel and 10 sentences are presented. Then the lead channel is switched to the opposite ear and 10 additional sentences are presented. However, testing experience has revealed that this procedure may be unnecessary because there is interaction between the two ears. If an abnormality exists in the pathways being assessed by this test, an abnormal score should result, regardless of which ear receives the first segment of the stimulus. Therefore, a single score is all that is required and may in fact constitute a more accurate representation of the function of the CANS being assessed by this particular behavioral test.

The results of various investigations suggest that the number of alternations per second does not make a difference in the performance of normal listeners over a wide range of alternation rates (Bocca & Calearo, 1963; Lynn & Gilroy, 1977). Bocca and Calearo (1963) employed alternating segments of running speech ranging from 20 to 500 msec in duration without any disruption in intelligibility. Lynn and Gilroy (1977) and Willeford (1976) selected 300 msec for their work with RASP. However, it is not known at this time what alternation rate would reveal minimum degrees of brainstem involvement because changes in alternation rates have not been systematically investigated in this population of patients.

There is some question as to whether the RASP test is sensitive to other than grossly abnormal brainstem function. Only 6 of 47 subjects tested by Lynn and Gilroy (1977) had clearly positive test results. Musiek (1983c), using the Willeford version of the test, reported that 5 of 10 subjects with brainstem involvement demonstrated abnormal performance. Lynn and Gilroy (1977) found that for the most part subjects with cortical and interhemispheric involvement performed normally on their RASP test. They did, however, note that some patients with diffuse central lesions demonstrated abnormal performance.

Binaural Fusion

There have been several variations of the binaural fusion test (BF). These tests involve the presentation of bandpass filtered speech to the two ears. Generally, the stimuli for these tests are passed through two bandpass filters. Typically, a low bandpass filtered speech stimulus is delivered to one ear and a high bandpass filtered stimulus is delivered to the opposite ear. In some versions of this test, the ear receiving the bandpass segments is alternated so that one is able to derive a score for two test conditions; that is, a score is obtained when the low bandpass segment is presented to the right ear and a second score is derived when the left ear receives the low bandpass information. In addition, many researchers and clinicians derive a diotic test score. In this test condition, both bandpass segments are presented to both ears simultaneously. Research findings have shown that the bandpass segments are not highly intelligible when presented monaurally, whereas recognition tends to be quite high when both segments are presented simultaneously either to the same ear or to opposite ears.

Matzker (1959) used a binaural fusion test with over 1700 patients. His test consisted of 41 two-syllable words that were phonetically balanced. The test stimuli were bandpass filtered into a low band (500–800 Hz) and a high band (1815–2500 Hz), and vowel recognition rather than word recognition was used as the criterion for correctness. The test was given three times to each subject. The first and third presentations were filtered bands, whereas the second presentation was diotic in nature and did not require fusion. Matzker reported that several patients with brainstem lesions had difficulty with the resynthesis of the two bands, whereas patients with cortical lesions tended to perform normally on this test.

Linden (1964) used an adaptation of the Matzker test for resynthesis. In this case, test stimuli consisted of nine Swedish spondaic word lists of 15 items each. The test stimuli were bandpass filtered similarly to those of Matzker, except that the filtering was somewhat more restrictive, especially in the high-frequency band. In addition, rather than scoring for vowel recognition, Linden used word recognition scores. He also tested at several sensation levels, because he found that performance improved in normal subjects with increases in sensation level (SL); for example, from 35% at 25 dB SL to 89% at 40 dB SL. His findings were reported to be negative for the most part, suggesting that the BF test was not sensitive to brainstem lesions. However, Tobin (1985) suggested that if the test results were reinterpreted, 4 of Linden's 18 subjects may have shown some evidence of brainstem involvement.

Smith and Resnick (1972) chose to use phonetically balanced monosyllabic words for their study of BF. They believed that the lower redundancy of the signal would tax the system further, but this fact would limit application of the test to those individuals with at least fair discrimination ability. These researchers used two resynthesis tasks and a diotic task for their test. The two resynthesis scores were compared to the diotic score. If the scores were similar, the results were considered to be normal. If, however, the dichotic score was significantly higher than either resynthesis score, the results were considered to be positive for brainstem pathology. The authors presented four cases with brainstem pathology. In all four cases the test results were positive.

One of the more popular binaural fusion tests today is the one that is part of Willeford's (1976) test battery. Test stimuli consist of filtered words that were bandpass filtered at 500 to 700 Hz and from 1900 to 2100 Hz with slopes of 36 dB per octave. Presentation levels are 30 dB SL re: the pure tone threshold at 500 Hz for the low band and 30 dB SL re: the pure tone threshold at 2000 Hz for the high band. Abnormal test results have been found in 3 of 10 subjects with brainstem lesions by Musiek (1983c) and for a single patient with a gunshot wound to the right pons by Pinheiro, Jacobson, and Boller (1982). Lynn and Gilroy (1975) reported abnormal findings for patients with brainstem lesions, whereas subjects with cerebral lesions tended to perform normally. These results, however, suggest that the BF test is only moderately sensitive, at best, to brainstem lesions.

Masking Level Differences

The test protocol for obtaining masking level differences (MLDs) involves the presentation of either a pulsed tone, typically a 500 Hz tone, or spondee words to both ears at the same time that a masking noise is being delivered binaurally. The patient normally is tested under two conditions. In the homophasic condition, both the speech or the pulsed tone and the masking noise are presented to both ears in-phase. In the second, or antiphasic condition, one of the signals is presented 180° out-of-phase between the two ears, whereas the other is held in-phase (Hirsh, 1948; Licklider, 1948).

When administering the MLD test, consideration should be given to several variables. Townsend and Goldstein (1972) found that in the antiphasic conditions the amount of release from masking decreased as the sensation level for the presentation of the signals increased. Pengelly, Mueller, and Hill (1982) noted that there was no difference in the size of the MLD when either a broadband or narrowband masker was used in normal subjects. However, in a group of subjects with high-frequency hearing losses, the narrowband masker produced significantly larger MLDs for a 500 Hz signal. Finally, the size of the MLD also appears to be affected by the duration of the masker. Green (1966) and McFadden (1966) showed that a continuous masker tended to produce larger MLDs than did maskers that were gated to follow the duty cycle of the signal. For further information about these considerations, the reader is referred to Durlach and Colburn (1978) and Tobin (1985).

In the first comprehensive clinical investigation of MLDs, Olsen, Noffsinger, and Carhart (1976) found a greater release from masking could be demonstrated in both normal and impaired subjects if the $S_\pi N_0$, as opposed to the $S_0 N_\pi$ antiphasic condition was used. This is the condition in which the masking noise is delivered to the two ears in-phase (N_0), whereas the pure tone or speech signals are delivered out-of-phase (S_π). Similar results were reported in a subsequent investigation by Pengelly and colleagues (1982).

In 1981 Lynn, Gilroy, Taylor, and Leiser reported test results for 26 patients with either brainstem or cortical lesions. Their results showed that patients with low brainstem involvement demonstrated little or no release from masking (i.e., abnormal test results), whereas patients with lesions higher in the CANS tended to perform similarly to a group of normal control subjects. More recently, Noffsinger, Martinez, and Schafer (1982) demonstrated a close correspondence between MLD and ABR results. These investigators found that patients with abnormalities of Waves I, II, or III of the ABR yielded small or absent MLDs, whereas patients with abnormalities of Waves IV or V demonstrated normal MLDs.

Other Binaural Interaction Tests

In the late 1950s Sanchez-Longo and colleagues (Sanchez-Longo & Forster, 1958; Sanchez-Longo et al., 1957) demonstrated impairment of the sound localization ability in the auditory field contralateral to the temporal lobe lesion in a group of brain-damaged subjects. These results suggest that the auditory cortex might have a role in forming the concept of auditory space. A subsequent investigation (Pinheiro & Tobin, 1971) using an Interaural Intensity Difference (IID) test paradigm revealed that subjects with central lesion required a larger IID in the ear ipsilateral to the site of lesion than did normal ears or ears with sensorineural hearing losses, whereas the contralateral ear required only an IID of about 4 dB for lateralization. Pinheiro and Tobin also noted that patients with abnormal IIDs showed neurological signs of temporal and/or parietal lobe involvement, whereas patients with occipital or frontal lobe lesions tended to demonstrate normal IIDs. These results suggest that the perception of the location of sound is a cortical function, even though the critical processing for the IID presumably occurs at the brainstem level (Pickles, 1985). For additional information regarding sound localization and lateralization tasks the reader is directed to Tobin (1985).

TEMPORAL PATTERNING TESTS

In the 1960s and 1970s several researchers began to use temporal patterning or sequencing tasks in an attempt to study the relationship between temporal ordering skills and CANS pathology. Unfortunately, few of these early research test protocols have gained widespread clinical use in spite of the fact that they appeared to be quite sensitive to CANS compromise.

Early Temporal Sequencing Tasks

In 1962, Milner reported that patients with temporal lobe lesions performed poorly when presented with two sequences of three to five tones and asked to identify which tone in the second series was different than the series of tones in the first sequence. He also noted that patients with right temporal lobectomies made more errors than did subjects with left temporal lobectomies. Similar findings have been reported for other patients with temporal lobectomies for binaurally presented bird songs (Milner et al., 1965) and dichotic melodies (Shankweiler, 1966).

Swisher and Hirsh (1972) studied the ability of subjects with cerebral damage to temporally order two tones. For this investigation they used a test paradigm in which they presented two tones of different pitches and with various onset time differences. The two tones were presented either to the same ear or to opposite ears, and the subjects were asked to indicate the order of the two tones. Participants consisted of young adults, older control subjects, and three groups of brain-damaged subjects, including left brain damage with fluent aphasia, left brain damage with nonfluent aphasia, and right brain damage with no aphasia. Fluent aphasics required the longest intervals to order stimuli, particularly if the two stimuli were presented to the same ear. In subjects with right hemisphere damage the differences required to make temporal order judgments between the two stimuli presented were smaller and approximated those demonstrated by the control subjects. They did, however, show greater deficits when the tonal stimuli were presented to opposite ears.

Lackner and Teuber (1973) presented dichotic clicks to the two ears that varied in terms of their onsets. Their subjects included 24 veterans with left hemisphere damage and 19 with right hemisphere damage. They found that subjects with left hemisphere damage required a longer silent interval between the stimuli in order to perceive separation.

A number of additional studies in the 1970s revealed temporal ordering deficits for patients with cerebral lesions (Belmont & Handler, 1971; Carmon & Nachson, 1971; DeRenzi, Faglioni, & Villa, 1977; Karaseva, 1972; Lhermitte, Chain, Escourolle, Ducarne, Pillou, & Chedru, 1971). Lhermitte and colleagues (1971) found that patients with bilateral temporal lobe damage could recognize frequency and intensity differences, but they could not discriminate between two different temporal sequences. Karaseva (1972) found that patients with unilateral damage to the auditory projection areas of the temporal lobe were impaired in the discrimination of rhythmic patterns of clicks in the ear contralateral to the lesions. Contralateral deficits also were reported by Belmont and Handler (1971) for hemiplegics who were asked to indicate the order of stimulation between the two ears when they were stimulated with 500 Hz tones of 200 msec duration separated by delays of 20, 50, or 80 msec. DeRenzi and colleagues (1977) reported deficits in the ability of a group of brain-damaged subjects to use a verbal memory code to recall serial order information. Finally, Carmon and Nachson (1971) noted that patients with left hemisphere damage were severely impaired in their ability to point to the locations in correct order for a sequence of three to five bimodal stimuli (consisting of lights and tones) presented in a temporal order, while patients with right hemisphere lesions performed as well as normal subjects.

As mentioned previously, Efron and associates (Efron, 1985; Efron & Crandall, 1983; Efron et al., 1983; Efron et al., 1977; Efron et al., 1985) have conducted a series of experiments with nonspeech auditory signals and have demonstrated contralateral ear deficits in individuals with temporal lobe lesions for a variety of auditory tasks (e.g., gap detection, sound lateralization, temporal ordering tasks). These authors noted consistent contralateral ear effects in subjects with either posterior temporal lobe involvement or anterior temporal lobe resections. The latter findings were remarkable in that previous to these findings, it was believed that the anterior temporal lobe did not play a role in auditory processing. It is also interesting to note that Efron and Crandall (1983) have postulated the existence of a contralaterally organized efferent pathway that is located within each temporal lobe and that, when activated, significantly enhances our ability to perceive auditory stimuli on the contralateral side of auditory space.

More recently, Blaettner, Scherg, and Von Cramon (1989) introduced a new psychoacoustic pattern discrimination test. For this test, sequences of noise bursts or click trains are presented dichotically at suprathreshold levels, and the subject is asked to discriminate monaural changes in either the intensity or click pattern. The subject simply indicates his or her response by pressing a button whenever a monaural change is noted. This test was administered to 62 patients with unilateral cerebrovascular accidents. Results indicated that abnormal test results correlated highly (76%) with presence of a cerebral lesion and that isolated lesions of the acoustic radiations and/or of the auditory association areas were sufficient to cause an abnormality on this test. As with most behavioral tests, contralateral ear deficits were most prominent. In addition, these researchers found no evidence of ear dominance in normal subjects on this test, nor was the size of the laterality effect on this test larger in either the right or left hemisphere lesion groups. It is therefore likely that this test taps a low level of auditory processing at which hemispheric specialization has not yet taken over. This is an important feature because ear dominance may be confounded with lesion effects. A second advantage of this test is that it can be used to assess auditory function in patients who may be incapable of responding verbally.

Frequency Pattern Sequences

One of the more popular temporal patterning tasks used today is the frequency pattern sequences test developed by Pinheiro (1976). It is composed of 120 test sequences, with each sequence containing three tone bursts. In each sequence two of the tone bursts are of the same frequency, whereas the third tone burst is of a different frequency. The tone bursts used in the sequences include a low-frequency tone (880 Hz) and a high-frequency tone (1122 Hz) and have a 10 msec rise-fall time. The total duration of each tone burst is 150 msec and there is an interstimulus interval of 200 msec between successive tones in the sequences. Given these parameters, six different sequences can be generated (i.e., *high-high-low, high-low-high, high-low-low, low-low-high, low-high-low,* and *low-high-high*). The sequences are typically presented at 50 dB SL re: speech recognition threshold (SRT) and the patient is asked to verbally describe each sequence heard. Percent correct identification scores are derived for each ear. If patients are unable to describe the sequences, they may either hum or manually indicate the sequence heard.

Patients with compromise of the auditory areas of either hemisphere or of the interhemispheric pathways have difficulty describing the monaurally presented test sequences (Musiek et al., 1994; Musiek, Kibbe, & Baran, 1984, Musiek & Pinheiro, 1986, 1987; Musiek et al., 1980; Pinheiro, 1976, Pinheiro & Musiek, 1985; Pinheiro et al., 1977). However, patients who have undergone posterior commissurotomies are often able to hum the sequences with close to 100% accuracy (Musiek, Kibbe, & Baran, 1984). These results suggest that some processing of the stimuli occurs in both hemispheres and that the auditory interhemispheric connections must be intact for normal performance if a verbal response is required. For these reasons, performance is most often found to be bilaterally normal or bilaterally depressed. Given these expected findings (i.e., virtually no ear differences), many audiologists have begun to derive a single binaural score either in the sound field or diotically under headphones.

Musiek and Pinheiro (1987) used frequency pattern sequences to assess CANS function in three groups of patients with different pathologies (cerebral, brainstem, cochlear). Their results revealed that the frequency pattern sequences test is highly sensitive to cerebral lesions (83%), but not as sensitive to brainstem lesions (45%). A total of 12% of the subjects with cochlear hearing loss performed abnormally on this test.

Auditory Duration Patterns

This test is similar to the frequency pattern sequences test in that it also involves the presentation of sequences containing three tone bursts and the patient is asked to verbally describe the sequences heard. On this test, however, the frequency of the tones is maintained at 1000 Hz and the duration of the tones is varied (250 msec and 500 msec). In each sequence two of the three tones have the same duration, whereas the third tone is of a different duration. The interstimulus interval is maintained at 300 msec between successive tones in the sequences and the rise-fall time is maintained at 10 msec. Given these parameters, a total of six sequences are possible (*long-long-short, long-short-long, long-short-short, short-short-long, short-long-short,* and *short-long-long*). The sequences are typically presented at 50 dB SL re: SRT and percent correct identification scores are derived for each ear individually. However, as was the case with frequency patterns, many audiologists may elect to derive a single binaural score.

Musiek, Baran, and Pinheiro (1990) administered this test to three groups of subjects including 50 individuals with normal hearing, 24 subjects with cochlear hearing loss, and 21 individuals with CANS lesions. Their results revealed that the test was highly sensitive to cerebral lesions (86%) with most of the subjects with cochlear hearing loss (92%) showing normal performance. In addition, these researchers reported that 12 of their neurologically involved subjects had received both frequency pattern and auditory duration pattern tests. It is interesting to note that 5 of these 12 subjects performed normally on the frequency pattern sequences test and abnormally on the auditory duration patterns test. These results suggest that these two tests may be assessing different underlying processes even though on the surface they appear to have similar test constructions and parameters. It therefore may be of value to use both tests to assess central auditory function whenever cerebral involvement is suspected.

Other Temporal Patterning Tests

Pinheiro and Ptacek initially utilized temporal sequences of tones that varied in terms of their intensity features (Pinheiro & Ptacek, 1971; Ptacek & Pinheiro, 1971). As mentioned previously, these consisted of tone sequences containing loud and soft tones in a parallel construction to that described above for frequency and duration pattern tests. To date this test has not enjoyed the popularity that the frequency pattern sequences and auditory duration patterns tests have, and most of the research conducted on this test has been limited to subjects without CANS compromise. More recently, Tallal and her colleagues have used a gap detection procedure to test temporal processing abilities in a number of clinical populations. A review of this work can be found in Tallal, Miller, and Fitch (1993) and Tallal and colleagues (Tallal, Miller, Bedi, Byma, Wang, et al., 1996). Until 1997, however, this test was not available commercially. With its commercial release, it is anticipated that this test will be subjected to considerable clinical testing.

MONAURAL LOW-REDUNDANCY SPEECH TESTS

Monaural low-redundancy speech tests have been used extensively in the assessment of subjects with CANS pathology. The stimuli for these tests typically are degraded by electroacoustically or digitally modifying the frequency, temporal, or intensity characteristics of the undistorted signal.

Filtered Speech

Bocca and his colleagues (Bocca et al., 1954; Bocca et al., 1955) first used a low-pass filtered speech test to assess CANS functioning in patients with cerebral tumors affecting the temporal lobe. Their results revealed reduced performance in the contralateral ear for the majority of patients tested. Since the time of these early investigations, several other investigators have used low-pass and bandpass filtered speech tasks to assess CANS function in individuals with intracranial lesions or pathology (Baran et al., 1986; Bocca, 1958; Calearo & Antonelli, 1968; Gilroy & Lynn, 1974; Hodgson, 1967; Jerger, 1960a, 1960b, 1964; Korsan-Bengtsen, 1973; Lynn, Benitez, Eisenbrey, Gilroy, & Wilner, 1972; Lynn & Gilroy, 1971, 1972, 1975, 1976, 1977; Musiek et al., 1994; Musiek & Geurkink, 1982, Musiek et al., 1984; Musiek, Wilson, & Pinheiro, 1979). These studies varied greatly in terms of the test stimuli employed and the frequency cutoff and filter cutoff characteristics used. In general, the results of these studies revealed contralateral deficits in subjects with temporal lobe lesions (Bocca, 1958; Hodgson, 1967; Jerger, 1960a, 1960b, 1964; Korsan-Bengtsen, 1973; Lynn & Gilroy, 1972, 1977; Musiek et al., 1994) and essentially normal results with no obvious differences in subjects with involvement of the interhemispheric pathways (Baran et al., 1986; Gilroy & Lynn, 1974; Lynn et al., 1972; Lynn & Gilroy, 1971, 1972, 1975, 1977; Musiek et al., 1994; Musiek et al., 1984; Musiek et al., 1979). In subjects with brainstem lesions, no consistent pattern of performance has been noted (Calearo & Antonelli, 1968; Lynn & Gilroy, 1977; Musiek & Geurkink, 1982). Contralateral ear deficits have been reported for some subjects, whereas ipsilateral deficits, bilateral deficits, or normal results were noted for other subjects. It appears that factors, such as the level and size of the lesion, as well as whether it is an extra- or intra-axial lesion, may determine laterality effects of brainstem lesions (Musiek & Geurkink, 1982).

Lynn and Gilroy (1977), in an attempt to determine the sensitivity and specificity of low-pass filtered speech, studied 34 patients with temporal lobe lesions and 27 patients with parietal lobe lesions. Seventy-four percent of the temporal lobe patients demonstrated the expected contralateral ear deficits on this test, whereas 74% of the parietal lobe patients demonstrated normal performance.

The most widely used filtered speech test today is the low-pass filtered speech test of Willeford's (1976) central auditory processing test battery. The test consists of two 50-item lists of the Michigan consonant-nucleus-consonant (CNC) words that were selected because they were highly intelligible to adults even when filtered. The stimuli were low-pass filtered with a cutoff frequency of 500 Hz and an 18 dB per octave rejection rate. Stimuli are presented monaurally at 50 dB relative to the pure tone average. Patients are asked to repeat the stimuli perceived, and a percent correct identification score is derived for each ear.

Based on the foregoing test results, it appears that low-pass filtered speech is moderately sensitive to the presence of CANS lesions. The results suggest that filtered speech tests can be useful in documenting the presence of a central lesion, however, they are not useful in locating the specific location of the lesion.

Compressed Speech

An accelerated speech test was first used by some Italian researchers (Bocca, 1958; Calearo & Lazzaroni, 1957). These investigators employed a procedure by which they accelerated sentence stimuli, distorting both the time and frequency characteristics of the test stimuli. They found reduced performance in the ear contralateral to lesions in the auditory cortex, whereas diffuse lesions tended to show reduced performance in both ears. Similar results were reported in a number of other investigations (de Quiros, 1964; Korsan-Bengtsen, 1973; Quaranta & Cervellera, 1977).

To date, four different methods of accelerating and/or compressing the speech stimuli have been used. These have included (1) having the speaker accelerate his or her speech rate, (2) accelerating the recorded signal via a faster playback rate, (3) removing segments of the signals electromechanically, and (4) computer manipulation and/or generation of time-compressed speech materials. A detailed discussion of the first three procedures can be found in Beasley and Maki (1976) and the last in Wilson, Preece, Salomon, Sperry, and Bornstein (1994).

Beasley and his colleagues (Beasley, Forman, & Rintelmann, 1972; Beasley, Schwimmer, & Rintelmann, 1972) generated tapes of compressed speech stimuli (NU-6 word lists) at several different compression ratios using the method of electromechanical time compression introduced by Fairbanks, Everitt, and Jaeger (1954). These investigators studied the intelligibility of NU-6 word lists as a function of both compression rate (at 0% and from 30 to 70% in 10% increments) and sensation level (8 to 40 dB in 8 dB steps) and provided extensive normative data for their compressed speech test. Their results showed a gradual reduction in the speech recognition scores of normal adults

as the compression rate was increased to 70%. At this point a substantial reduction in performance was noted. As sensation level increased, word recognition scores increased in a curvilinear fashion up to 32 dB SL. Recently, Letowski and Poch (1995) showed that not only is the compression ratio an important factor to consider when evaluating the difficulty and clinical usefulness of compressed speech tasks, but that discard interval is also a factor needing consideration.

Kurdziel, Noffsinger, and Olsen (1976) used 0%, 40% and 60% compressed NU-6 word lists in the evaluation of 31 patients with brain lesions (15 had diffuse lesions and 16 had undergone anterior temporal lobe surgery). Reduced performance was noted in the contralateral ear of the patients with diffuse lesions, especially at the 60% compression rate, whereas patients with discrete lesions (anterior temporal lobe surgery) demonstrated essentially equivalent performance for both ears, with recognition scores at 60% compression being only slightly reduced compared to recognition scores at 0% compression. Similar results were reported in an earlier study by Rintelmann, Beasley, and Lynn (1974).

In a large study of Vietnam veterans with discrete cerebral lesions, Mueller, Beck, and Sedge (1987) found that performance was poorest for a group of subjects with lesions in Heschl's gyrus, whereas performance in patients with lesions outside the primary auditory area was relatively good. These authors point out, however, that the mean differences in performance of their pathological subjects (regardless of the location of their lesions) and their controls were small. Also, they failed to note obvious contralateral effects in their subjects. Based upon these results, these authors have suggested that the compressed speech test may be relatively sensitive to identifying patients with diffuse lesions, but that the test may be relatively insensitive to discrete lesions.

Baran and colleagues (Baran, Verkest, Gollegly, Kibble-Michael, Rintelmann, & Musiek, 1985) found that compressed speech is a moderately sensitive test for intracranial lesions involving the temporal lobe. In approximately two-thirds of subjects with confirmed lesions, performance was found to be reduced in one or both ears. The more typical pattern was for reduced performance in the contralateral ear.

A review of the literature failed to reveal any investigations that have employed compressed speech with patients having brainstem lesions. However, two earlier investigations used accelerated speech with this population. In one investigation, reduced performance was noted in one ear for 13 of 14 subjects (Calearo & Antonelli, 1968). In a subsequent study, Quaranta and Cervellera (1977) reported that none of their 9 subjects with brainstem lesions showed reduced performance.

Speech-in-Noise

A third method of reducing the redundancy of speech stimuli has involved the addition of an ipsilateral competing noise. Most commonly, either white noise or speech spectrum noise is employed and signal-to-noise ratios (S/Ns) of 0 to +10 dB are most commonly encountered. Stimuli are typically presented at 40 dB SL re: SRT.

As early as 1959, Sinha found reduced performance on a speech-in-noise test for contralateral ears in individuals with cortical lesions. Subsequent investigations have revealed abnormal findings for the ipsilateral ear of a patient with an extra-axial brainstem lesion (Dayal, Tarantino, & Swisher, 1966), in one or both ears of patients with intra-axial brainstem lesions (Morales-Garcia & Poole, 1972; Noffsinger, Olsen, Carhart, Hart, & Sahgal, 1972), and for contralateral ears in patients with temporal lobe disorders (Heilman, Hammer, & Wilder, 1973; Morales-Garcia & Poole, 1972).

In their 1972 investigation, Morales-Garcia and Poole used S/Ns of 0 and +5 dB in 32 patients with different types of intracranial lesions. They found that 14 of 15 patients with brainstem lesions had abnormal scores, with mean scores falling 20% below normal for both S/Ns. However, no clear pattern of performance emerged as to laterality effects or to the level of the lesions. In addition, they noted that all 10 of their patients with temporal lobe lesions showed depressed contralateral ear scores for at least one of the S/Ns with normal results in the ipsilateral ear, whereas none of their 7 patients with lesions outside the temporal lobe demonstrated a significant contralateral ear deficit.

Olsen, Noffsinger, and Kurdziel (1975) used NU-6 word lists and an ipsilateral white noise (0 dB S/N). These investigators derived not only absolute scores, but also difference scores. Based upon their normative data, they determined that difference scores of greater than 40% were significant. Significant mean ear differences were noted for Ménière's patients (41%, N = 24), eighth nerve patients (47%, N = 21), and temporal lobe patients (43%, N = 24). For temporal lobe patients, all abnormal scores were noted in the contralateral ear. However, inspection of the data for this group revealed that in spite of the significant mean ear difference, more than half of the temporal lobe subjects scored within normal limits of variability. Because of the large range of scores and similar findings for different pathology groups, these investigators concluded that speech-in-noise testing may have some usefulness in detecting CANS disorders, but not in specifying the site of lesion.

Synthetic Sentence Identification with Ipsilateral Competing Message

The synthetic sentence identification with ipsilateral competing message test (SSI-ICM) is composed of 10 third-order approximations of English sentences that are presented along with a competing message consisting of continuous discourse (Jerger & Jerger, 1974). The 10 sentences were originally designed to minimize the subject's reliance on linguistic skills, and they have been carefully controlled for both informational content and length. The sentences are presented to the test ear in the presence of a competing message, and the subject is asked to point to 1 of 10 printed sentences that corresponds to the stimulus presented. The test can be presented in two ways: (a) by varying the message-to-competition ratio, or (b) by keeping the signal-to-competition ratio constant (usually 0 dB) and presenting the sentences at several intensity levels from high to low. If the latter procedure is used in subjects with brainstem involvement, word recognition performance typically decreases as intensity is increased.

The incidence of SSI-ICM abnormality in populations with brainstem involvement is relatively impressive. Jerger and Jerger (1974) reported that 11 of 11 patients with intra-axial brainstem lesions had scores in one or both ears that fell below the normal criteria. In another study of patients with brainstem involvement, an average deficit of 40% was noted for the contralateral ear to the lesioned side of the brainstem (Jerger & Jerger, 1975). Reports using a modification of the SSI-ICM showed that 7 of 13 (Stephens & Thornton, 1976) and 8 of 12 patients (Antonelli, Bellotto, & Grandori, 1987) with brainstem lesions had abnormal results on this test.

The majority of the central tests that appear to be particularly sensitive to brainstem lesions are sensitive to lesions in the low to mid brainstem. For the most part they are likely to miss lesions in the rostral-most portion of the brainstem. The SSI-ICM appears to be sensitive to both rostral and caudal lesions, though it may also be affected, but to a lesser degree, by cerebral involvement (Jerger & Jerger, 1974, 1975).

Other Monaural Low-Redundancy Speech Tests

In addition to the tests discussed above, other investigations have used interrupted speech, expanded speech, and low-sensation level speech tests to study CANS function in pathological cases. These tests have received limited use clinically and therefore will not be discussed here. Also, performance-intensity functions have been used to assess CANS function in patients with low brainstem pathology (Jerger, 1973; Jerger & Jerger, 1971). Although this test is frequently not classified under this category, abnormal results have been reported for some individuals with brainstem lesions and the test may have some utility in identifying CANS compromise. The reader who is interested in any of these tests should see Rintelmann (1985).

DICHOTIC SPEECH TESTS

As mentioned previously, Kimura (1961a, 1961b) typically is credited with the introduction of dichotic speech tests into the field of central auditory assessment. Since that time, several variations of the dichotic digits test, as well as several other dichotic speech tests, have been introduced. For the most part, these tests have been shown to be particularly sensitive to cortical pathology and compromise of the interhemispheric neural pathways, though abnormal results also have been reported for subjects with brainstem involvement.

Dichotic Digits

In the early 1960s Kimura (1961a, 1961b) administered a dichotic digits test in which dichotic triads were presented simultaneously to each ear to a group of patients with unilateral temporal lobe lesions. She found impaired digit recognition in the contralateral ear when the stimuli were presented in a dichotic paradigm, whereas no deficits were noted in either ear if the stimuli were presented in a noncompeting condition—that is, unless the left or dominant hemisphere was affected. In this case, bilaterally depressed scores typically were noted.

More recently, Musiek (1983a) introduced a revised version of the dichotic digits test. The version differs from Kimura's original test in that two rather than three digits are presented simultaneously to each ear and a percent correct score is derived for each ear. Test stimuli are usually presented at 50 dB SL re: SRT. This new version of the test takes only 4 minutes to administer and is easily scored. This ease of scoring results in reduced variability among examiners.

There have been several other variations of the dichotic digits test. These have included having the subject report all test stimuli perceived in one ear first, followed by those perceived in the second ear, or having the subject add the numbers heard in each ear and report a total figure for each ear. Also there has been some work with dichotic words. A review of these procedures can be found in Musiek and Pinheiro (1985).

Test results have shown that the dichotic digits test is fairly sensitive to brainstem and cortical lesions. Musiek (1983a) reported that 17 of 21 patients with intracranial lesions (9 brainstem, 12 hemispheric) showed abnormal performance in either one or both ears on the dichotic digits test. In addition, abnormal test results have been demonstrated for several individuals with complete and/or posterior sections of the corpus callosum (Musiek, Kibbe, & Baran, 1984). Other researchers have found contralateral ear deficits with right temporal lobe lesions and bilaterally depressed scores with left temporal lobe lesions (Mueller, Sedge, & Salazar, 1985; Sedge, Mueller, & Dillon, 1982).

In a large study of Vietnam veterans mentioned previously, Mueller and colleagues (1987) reported that the performance of subjects with cortical damage outside of the temporal lobe of either hemisphere on a dichotic digits test did not differ from that of a group of control subjects. However, if right posterior temporal lobe damage was present, a small decrease in mean right ear performance was noted (3.4%) relative to the mean right ear performance of the control subjects, whereas a larger left ear deficit was noted (i.e., a decrease of 9% compared to the mean score for the control subjects). In patients with injury to the left posterior temporal lobe, greater deficits were noted for both ears when compared to the control group; however, no obvious ear differences were noted in that the mean score for the right ear was 15% lower than that for the normal subjects and the left ear score was 16.3% lower. Sparks, Goodglass, and Nichel (1970) reported contralateral ear deficits with right hemisphere damage. They suggested that the ipsilateral deficits were noted because the lesions were deep and affected the callosal fibers from the right hemisphere. Therefore, the test results were similar to those expected with right hemisphere lesions. To date there have been only a few investigations that have studied the dichotic digits performance of individuals with brainstem lesion. Results revealed that 3 of 13 patients (Stephens & Thornton, 1976) and 7 of 10 subjects (Musiek & Geurkink, 1982) showed abnormal performance on a dichotic digits test.

Results of a comparative study that investigated the relative sensitivity of three dichotic speech tests (dichotic digits, competing sentences, and staggered spondaic words) in the assessment of CANS disorders in 12 subjects with brainstem involvement and 18 with cortical lesions showed that the dichotic digits test yielded slightly more abnormal findings for both groups than did either one of the two remaining tests (Musiek, 1983b). Given the moderately high sensitivity of this test to brainstem, cortical, and interhemispheric lesions, its ease of administration, and its relatively short administration time, this particular test would constitute a good screening tool for CANS disorders. Abnormal findings should alert the audiologist to the need to conduct additional central auditory testing.

Staggered Spondaic Words

Approximately one year after Kimura's introduction of the dichotic speech paradigm into the field of central auditory assessment, Katz (1962) introduced a unique modification of this psychophysical procedure. His Staggered Spondaic Word (SSW) test is among the best known and most frequently used dichotic speech tests in use today. The test stimuli consist of 40 pairs of spondee words that are presented with a staggered onset. In order to achieve the staggered onsets, the first half of one test item is presented in a noncompeting condition, followed by a competing condition in which the second half of the first spondee and the first half of the second spondee are presented in a competing dichotic manner. Finally, the second half of the second spondee is presented in a noncompeting condition. The test stimuli are alternated between the two channels of the audiometer so that the ear receiving the first spondee constantly changes back and forth between the two ears. The procedures for scoring the test are quite complicated and are not used universally. The reader is directed to Brunt (1978) for details regarding test administration and scoring procedures. Many audiologists frequently use the SSW in their neuroaudiological assessments of the CANS. However, when administering this test, many audiologists will present the test stimuli at 50 dB SL re: SRT and derive percent correct identification scores for the right and left ears under the competing conditions only.

Several studies by Katz and associates (Katz, 1962, 1968, 1970, 1977; Katz, Basil, & Smith, 1963; Katz & Pack, 1975) have demonstrated a close correspondence between SSW test results and site of CANS damage. The results of these investigations have shown moderately to severely depressed SSW scores (i.e., competing condition) for the contralateral ear in individuals with cortical lesions involving the primary auditory reception areas of either hemisphere, whereas subjects with lesions outside the primary auditory reception areas have shown only mildly depressed contralateral deficits or normal test results. Lynn and Gilroy (1977) also demonstrated depressed scores for 5 patients with anterior temporal lobe lesions and 5 patients with posterior temporal lobe lesions. They noted that patients with posterior lesions tended to demonstrate more severely depressed scores than did those patients with anterior temporal lobe lesions.

Other investigators also demonstrated abnormal test results in patients with both right and left hemisphere lesions (Lynn & Gilroy, 1975; McClellen, Wertz, & Collins, 1973). However, these researchers noted primarily contralateral deficits if the lesion affected the right hemisphere, and smaller ear differences if the lesion affected the left hemisphere. These findings are consistent with those of Mueller and colleagues (1987), who noted a significant contralateral ear effect in their subjects with right posterior temporal lobe involvement. In this group of subjects mean performance was depressed 10% relative to that of a group of control subjects, whereas mean ipsilateral performance was found to be similar to that of the control subjects. When damage was located in the left posterior temporal lobe, scores were found to be bilaterally depressed when compared to control subjects, that is, 8.8% for the right ear and 8.9% for the left ear.

Results of several investigations for subjects with brainstem lesions have shown mixed results. Jerger and Jerger (1975) studied 10 patients with intra-axial brainstem lesions and 10 control subjects. These investigators found

the pathological group demonstrated mean scores that were 44% and 16% poorer than those of the control subjects for contralateral and ipsilateral ears, respectively. Stephens and Thornton (1976) reported that 6 of 14 subjects demonstrated abnormal test results, whereas Musiek and Geurkink (1982) reported that approximately 60% of their brainstem subjects demonstrated abnormal test results. Other investigators (Pinheiro et al., 1982; Rintelmann & Lynn, 1983) reported abnormal results for a small number of brainstem lesions.

Dichotic CVs

In the early 1970s Berlin and his co-workers (Berlin, Cullen, Hughes, et al., 1975; Berlin, Lowe-Bell, Jannetta, & Kline, 1972) introduced another dichotic speech test, dichotic CVs, into the CANS assessment area. In this test, dichotic CV stimuli are presented to the two ears dichotically while the onsets of the two stimuli are varied. The test stimuli consist of the following CVs: *ba, da, ga, pa, ta,* and *ka.* In one part of the test, the alignments of the two stimuli are close to simultaneous, whereas in other instances the onsets of the second or lagging stimuli are delayed by a specific length of time relative to the onsets of the leading stimuli. Onset lags of 15, 30, 60, and 90 msec are used. In the earlier investigation, Berlin and colleagues (1972) found that normal subjects obtained better scores if the onsets of the lagging CVs were delayed by 30 to 90 msec. A similar improvement in performance, however, was not noted for 4 patients who had undergone temporal lobectomies.

In a subsequent study, Berlin, Cullen, Hughes, and co-workers (1975) administered the dichotic CV test to 3 temporal lobectomy patients and 4 hemispherectomy patients. They found that in both groups, weak ear (i.e., ear contralateral to lesion) performance declined to near chance levels following surgery, whereas strong ear performance (i.e., ear ipsilateral to lesion) performance improved. They reported, however, a significant difference in the amount of improvement noted for the strong ear performance of the two groups. In the lobectomy group a small improvement was noted, but the scores did not begin to approach 100%, whereas in the hemispherectomy group performance rose to nearly 100%. The authors suggested that the differences could be accounted for on the basis of a competition for neural substrate that was still present in the lobectomy group, but that was effectively eliminated in the hemispherectomy group.

Zurif and Ramier (1972) administered dichotic CVs to 20 patients with left hemisphere damage and 20 with right hemisphere damage and noted right brain-damaged subjects showed contralateral ear deficits, whereas left brain-damaged subjects tended to show similar scores for both ears. Speaks and colleagues (1975) demonstrated that 10 of 10 subjects with CANS pathology showed depressed contralateral ear scores, whereas Olsen (1977) found that 31 of 40 patients with temporal lobectomies had depressed scores for one or both ears. In Mueller, Beck, and Sedge's 1987 investigation of CANS results in Vietnam veterans, a substantial reduction in mean performance was noted for the left ear (23.6%) in subjects with right temporal lobe involvement, whereas the mean right ear score did not differ substantially from that of the control group. In subjects with left temporal lobe involvement a similar, but less pronounced, contralateral ear effect (17.7%) was noted. In addition, a small ipsilateral effect (7.2%) was observed.

Limited research has been reported for patients with brainstem involvement. Berlin, Cullen, Berlin, Tobey, and Mouney (1975) demonstrated almost complete suppression of the CVs presented to the left ear of a patient with a lesion in the area of the right medial geniculate body, whereas right ear results were normal.

Synthetic Sentence Identification with Contralateral Competing Message

The Synthetic Sentence Identification with Contralateral Competing Message (SSI-CCM) test is identical to the SSI-ICM test described previously, except that in this case, the sentences and the competing messages are presented to opposite ears rather than the same ear (Jerger & Jerger, 1974, 1975). These investigators found that individuals with brainstem lesions generally performed within normal limits on the SSI-CCM version of this test, whereas they tended to show depressed scores in the ear contralateral to the lesion on the SSI-ICM test. On the other hand, patients with temporal lobe lesions typically demonstrated depressed SSI-CCM scores in the contralateral ear. Similar findings have been reported for other patients with temporal lobe disorders by Keith (1977) and Jerger and Jerger (1981).

In 1983 Fifer, Jerger, Berlin, Tobey, and Campell introduced a modification of the SSI-CCM test. This modification of the SSI-CCM, referred to as the Dichotic Sentence Identification (DSI) test, uses the original sentences of the SSI-CCM test, but rather than presenting the sentences to one ear and a competing discourse message the opposite ear, the sentences were paired and presented dichotically. This particular test was designed in the hope of developing a dichotic speech test that would be minimally affected by peripheral hearing loss. To date, there have been only a few investigations that have studied the sensitivity of the DSI to CANS lesions. In their original article, Fifer and his co-workers reported that 5 of 6 subjects with CANS lesions demonstrated abnormal results on one ear, whereas the sixth subject showed bilateral deficits. Mueller and colleagues (1987) reported test results for 90 subjects with cerebral lesions. Of these subjects 22 had damage to the right or left posterior temporal lobe, whereas the remainder

of the subjects had damage to structures outside the primary auditory areas. Their results showed that this test yielded sensitivity and specificity ratings that were comparable to those obtained with other dichotic speech tests, namely, dichotic digits, staggered spondaic words, and dichotic CVs. This finding, in light of earlier evidence that the test may be relatively resistant to the effects of peripheral hearing loss, suggests that the DSI would be a useful dichotic speech test to incorporate in a CANS test battery, particularly if one is assessing individuals with a peripheral hearing impairment. However, more research is needed to support this contention.

Competing Sentences

In the late 1960s Willeford, along with some of his graduate students, developed a competing sentences test that is one of the most popular tests of this particular type used in clinics today. The test is composed of 25 sentence pairs that average six to seven words in length. The sentences are presented dichotically with the target sentences presented at 35 dB SL (re: SRT) and the competing sentences presented at 50 dB SL (re: SRT). The patient is instructed to repeat the target sentences and to ignore the competing sentences. A total of 10 target sentences are typically presented to each ear, with the remaining 5 sentence pairs used for training or other purposes. One of the major problems with this particular test is that the guidelines for scoring are not well specified in the literature. This leaves open the door for considerable variability in test scores among different testers.

For the most part this test has been used in the assessment of children with auditory processing disorders; however, there have been some investigations that have looked at the performance of individuals with CANS disorders on this test (Lynn & Gilroy, 1972, 1975, 1977; Musiek, 1983a, 1983b, Musiek & Geurkink, 1982; Pinheiro, Jacobson, & Boller, 1982; Rintelmann & Lynn, 1983). These studies have shown that approximately one-half of the subjects studied with brainstem lesions showed abnormal performance in the ear ipsilateral to the lesion. For subjects with temporal lobe lesions, contralateral deficits were noted for individuals with posterior temporal lobe lesions whereas for the most part no deficits were noted in subjects with anterior temporal lobe lesions. As mentioned earlier, Musiek (1983b) reported that the competing sentences test was the least sensitive of three dichotic speech tests administered to subjects with intracranial lesions. Similar findings were reported by Lynn and Gilroy (1972, 1975, 1977) when comparing the staggered spondaic and competing sentences tests.

A recent procedural variation on the traditional competing sentences test was introduced by Bergman, Hirsch, Solzi, and Mankowitz (1987). In their test, referred to as the Threshold-of-Interference Test, these researchers determined the sensation level at which competing sentences interfered with the subject's ability to repeat target sentences. Their test stimuli included Hebrew sentences that were all three words in length. Target sentences were typically presented at 25 dB relative to the threshold of intelligibility for the sentences, and the level of competing sentences was increased from threshold level until the subject could no longer repeat the target sentences. The inability of the subject to attend to and repeat the primary message when the level of the competing message was at, or within, 5 dB of the competing message ear's threshold was labeled "complete suppression," whereas "partial suppression" was defined as a disabling competing message of 30 to 35 dB SL. These investigators administered the test to 27 subjects with CANS involvement and found that 10 of 17 subjects with right hemisphere damage showed complete left ear suppression, whereas 4 of 10 subjects with left hemisphere damage showed left ear suppression. Two additional subjects with right hemisphere damage showed partial suppression of left ear targets and one demonstrated mildly depressed scores for both ears with the larger deficit noted in the contralateral left ear. As with the other dichotic tests, contralateral deficits were noted with right hemisphere damage. However, in 4 of 10 cases with left hemisphere damage, ipsilateral left ear deficits were noted. An inspection of the CT scans for these four patients revealed involvement of the callosal fibers traveling from the right side for at least three out of four of these patients. The authors suggested that this test is useful in exposing strong hemispheric suppression, particularly in case of right hemisphere damage.

Dichotic Rhymes

The dichotic rhyme test was developed by Wexler and Haiwes in 1983. The stimuli for this test consist of monosyllabic word pairs that begin with one of the stop consonants and differ only in the initial consonantal element (e.g., *pig* and *dig*). The stimuli were digitized and computer sliced so that the nondistinct portions of both words were identical (i.e., the medial vowel and the final consonant). The spectral and temporal characteristics of these words are such that when presented in a dichotic manner the stimuli tend to become fused perceptually and typically only one word is perceived by the patient. A total of 15 word pairs have been pseudo-randomized to generate a list of 30 test items with the items being counterbalanced so that each item of each pair is presented to each ear only once during the administration of the test. The stimuli are presented at 50 dB SL re: SRT and a percentage correct score is derived for each ear. Since only one word is perceived in most cases, normal performance is expected at approximately 50% correct identification for each ear. There is,

however, a slight right ear advantage on this test and therefore different norms are used to determine whether a patient's responses are within normal limits for the right and left ears. In addition, the number of double wrongs and an ear difference score can be calculated and these can be compared to norms.

Musiek and his co-workers have used this test with a number of patients and have reported abnormal test results for patients with a variety of cortical lesions (Musiek et al., 1994) as well as for patients who have undergone posterior or complete commissurotomies (Musiek, Kurdziel-Schwan, Kibbe, Gollegly, Baran, & Rintelmann, 1989).

Other Dichotic Speech Tests

In addition to the dichotic speech tests described above, tests such as the Northwestern University Test No. 2 and the Northwestern University Test No. 20 have been used in the assessment of CANS pathology. In both cases, the monosyllabic test stimuli are presented to one ear while a competing message is delivered to the opposite ear. Because these tests have received limited attention in CANS assessment, they will not be reviewed in detail here. Additional information can be found in Musiek and Pinheiro (1985).

NEUROAUDIOLOGICAL FINDINGS IN SPECIAL CLINICAL POPULATIONS

Split-Brain Patients

In the late 1960s, two articles appeared in the literature that reported depressed left ear scores on dichotic speech tests for patients who had undergone complete surgical sections of the corpus callosum (Milner, Taylor, & Sperry, 1968; Sparks & Geschwind, 1968). Since that time similar findings have been reported for a number of additional patients with either complete or posterior sections of the corpus callosum (Gazzaniga, Risse, Springer, Clark, & Wilson, 1975; Musiek et al., 1994; Musiek & Kibbe, 1985; Musiek, Kibbe, & Baran, 1984; Musiek, Reeves, & Baran, 1985; Musiek & Wilson, 1979; Musiek et al., 1979; Springer & Gazzaniga, 1975; Springer, Sidtis, Wilson, & Gazzaniga, 1978). Unfortunately, in many of these investigations no preoperative data were provided. Therefore, it is difficult for the reader to determine if the deficits noted following surgery were related to surgical sectioning of the corpus callosum or to some preexisting hemispheric involvement.

Here at our clinic we have been able to assess the preoperative and postoperative performance of several patients who have had posterior and/or complete commissurotomies (Musiek & Kibbe, 1985; Musiek et al., 1994; Musiek et al., 1984; Musiek, Reeves, & Baran, 1985; Musiek &

Wilson, 1979; Musiek et al., 1979), as well as a number of subjects whose surgical sections were limited to the anterior position of the corpus callosum (Baran et al., 1986). Our results have shown that patients with posterior and/or complete commissurotomies (1) perform normally on a monaural low-redundancy speech test (LPFS), (2) demonstrate left ear deficits on dichotic speech tests (SSW and DD), and (3) show bilateral deficits on a monaural temporal patterning task (FPS). On the other hand, we found that sectioning of the anterior half of the corpus callosum does not result in similar postsurgical deficits. Figure 13.2

displays the test results for four of our subjects with complete commissurotomies and eight subjects with anterior sections of the corpus callosum.

The differences noted between the test results of these two groups of subjects can be explained on an anatomical basis. Given our test results, as well as some the results of some earlier work with primates (Pandya et al., 1971), it appears that the auditory interhemispheric fibers lie in the posterior portion of the corpus callosum. Thus, surgical sectioning of this part of the corpus callosum should result in the deficits observed above, given that the necessary

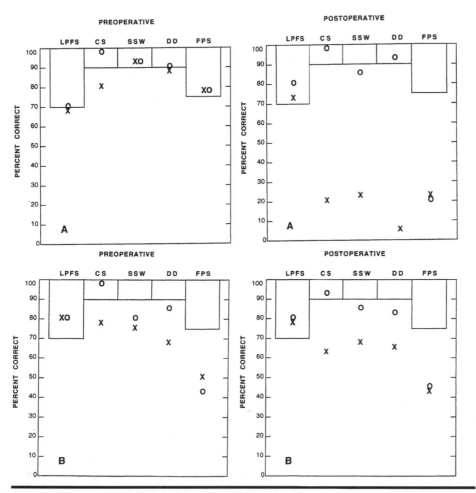

FIGURE 13.2   Panel A: Mean preoperative and postoperative scores for four patients with complete sections of the corpus callosum on five central auditory tests (LPFS: Low-Pass Filtered Speech; CS: Competing Sentences; SSW: Staggered Spondaic Words; DD: Dichotic Digits; FPS: Frequency Pattern Sequences). Data are presented for the right (O) and left (X) ears. The boxes at the top of each panel represent the range of normal performance. (Adapted with permission from "Neurological results from split-brain patients," by F. E. Musiek, K. Kibbe, & J. A. Baran, 1984, *Seminars in Hearing, 5*, 219–229. Copyright by Thieme Medical Publishers, New York.) Panel B: Mean preoperative and postoperative scores for eight patients with anterior sections of the corpus callosum. Specifications are the same as described for Panel A. (Adapted with permission from "Central auditory function following anterior sectioning of the corpus callosum," by J. A. Baran, F. E. Musiek, & A. G. Reeves, 1986, *Ear and Hearing, 7*, 359–362. Copyright by Williams & Wilkins, Baltimore.)

interhemispheric transfer of auditory information would be prevented. The left ear deficits noted on the dichotic speech tests occur because the stronger contralateral pathways from the left ear to the right hemisphere are rendered ineffective by sectioning of the corpus callosum, whereas at the same time the ipsilateral pathways are being suppressed because of the dichotic nature of the task. The bilateral deficits noted on the frequency pattern sequences test occur because sectioning of the posterior portion of the corpus callosum prohibits the necessary interaction of the two hemispheres. Both hemispheres are involved in the processing of tonal sequences (right hemisphere), which require verbal labeling (left hemisphere). No deficits are noted on the monaural low-redundancy speech test because the ipsilateral left ear to left hemisphere pathway is not suppressed during monaural stimulation, and the contralateral right ear to left hemisphere pathway is not affected by the surgical procedure.

The observation of similar test profiles in other pathological subjects could assist in the identification of the site of dysfunction in individuals with CANS lesion that may be affecting the interhemispheric pathways. For example, Damasio and Damasio (1979) reported severe left ear deficits in a group of patients with lesions near the lateral wall of the lateral ventricle at the level of the trigone. These authors concluded that the interhemispheric pathways diverge from the geniculocortical pathways by traveling posteriorly and rostrally to wrap around the lateral ventricle and join the corpus callosum in its posterior position. These results suggest that the interhemispheric fibers may be compromised in at least some hemispheric lesions. Additional evidence of such callosal compromise with hemispheric involvement can be found in an earlier article by Sparks and colleagues (1970). If you recall, these authors noted ipsilateral ear deficits for a dichotic digits test in a number of patients with left hemisphere damage. It was suggested that the deficits were the result of deep left hemisphere lesions that affected the callosal fibers crossing from the right hemisphere.

Ruebens and his associates (Ruebens, Froehling, Slater, & Anderson, 1985) demonstrated severe left ear deficits on dichotic listening tasks in a group of patients with multiple sclerosis. These investigators suggested that the left ear deficits were the result of demyelination of the interhemispheric fibers of the corpus callosum and supported this contention with CT scans demonstrating this callosal abnormality.

Essentially any type of cerebral lesion can compromise the interhemispheric auditory fibers. If only the white matter is involved, the neuroaudiological profile should be similar to that of the split-brain patient. However, if a left hemisphere lesion affects both the gray (cortex) and white (corpus callosum) matter, a slightly different picture emerges. In the latter case, dichotic scores should be abnormal for both ears. This bilateral deficit results from involvement of the left auditory cortex, which causes the classic right ear deficit and the presence of the corpus callosum pathology, which disrupts the transfer of auditory information from the right to the left hemisphere, causing a left ear deficit. Monaural low-redundancy tasks, such as filtered speech, reveal only a contralateral right ear deficit. This occurs because this task does not require interhemispheric transfer of neural information for verbal report of left ear stimuli because the ipsilateral pathways are not suppressed. Temporal patterning test results would reveal bilateral abnormalities because the necessary interhemispheric processing described above cannot be accomplished.

Cases of Central Auditory Deafness

Although cases of central deafness are extremely rare, they can provide a valuable insight into central auditory function and its clinical correlates. Central auditory deafness occurs when the auditory areas in both hemispheres are severely compromised. This type of bihemispheric compromise usually is caused by vascular lesions affecting the middle cerebral artery or one of its main branches. Though these patients do not respond behaviorally to sound, results of tests such as acoustic reflexes and ABRs usually are normal, suggesting normal peripheral auditory function.

In the late 1960s and early 1970s, Jerger and his associates (Jerger, Lovering, & Wertz, 1972; Jerger, Weikers, Sharbrough, & Jerger, 1969) presented audiological test results for two subjects with tandem bilateral temporal lobe lesions. Both of these subjects demonstrated transient aphasia, but no hearing loss after an initial left-sided episode, and a severe hearing loss after a subsequent right-sided episode. In both cases, the hearing losses reportedly recovered within three months of the second episode; however, both subjects continued to demonstrate a marked inability to recognize words or sentences even under ideal listening conditions. Moreover, these investigators noted that if any type of distortion was introduced, recognition declined to near 0%.

Graham, Greenwood, and Lecky (1980) reported similar findings for a third patient who became completely deaf after bilateral temporal lobe embolisms. In addition, these authors provided a comprehensive review of the data presented in twelve earlier case reports. The common symptom noted in all these cases was an auditory agnosia for speech, that is, the patients were unable to comprehend the spoken words even though many of the subjects recognized the stimuli as speech.

Michel, Peronnet, and Schott (1980) reported a case of a 40-year-old male subject with bilateral temporoparietal lobe lesions who had central auditory deficits with aphasic disturbances. Their patient demonstrated deficits for speech recognition tasks, but he could read and write normally. In addition, they found absent late auditory evoked potentials bilaterally.

More recently, Musiek and colleagues (1994) have reported on 3 additional patients and Hood, Berlin, and Allen (1994) have presented 1 additional patient who have demonstrated similar auditory agnosias coincident with bihemispheric compromise of the temporal lobes. In each of these patients, normal ABR and abnormal middle latency and/or late auditory evoked potentials were noted.

The review of the literature demonstrates the critical role that the central auditory mechanism plays in simple, as well as complex, hearing tasks. It also highlights the fact that deficits in audition to any degree can have a central as well as a peripheral origin. Therefore, the audiologist must be alert to the possibility that what may appear to be an apparent peripheral hearing loss may in fact be the audiological manifestation of a central involvement.

Children with Learning Disabilities

Central auditory testing of the child with learning disabilities (LD) began to gain momentum in the early to mid-1970s. Prior to this time, clinical attention primarily was focused on the use of central auditory tests in the assessment of neurologically impaired adults. A great deal of the motivation for testing children came about as the result of the development of a test battery by Willeford (1976), which was specifically designed to assess central auditory processing abilities in young children. Here, rather than attempting to document the presence or absence of a lesion, the tests were used to assess the functional integrity of the CANS in an attempt to tease out deficits that could explain any difficulties the child was having in terms of his or her academic, communicative, and/or social skills. In essence, the goal of central auditory testing with the LD child was to employ tests that would stress the auditory mechanisms at various levels of the CANS in order to identify weaknesses in the system (i.e., by demonstrating age/performance deficits) that could account for the child's problems. It is now commonly accepted that large numbers of children have subtle auditory deficits in spite of normal neurological test results. Therefore, the number of referrals for central auditory assessments has been steadily increasing since the mid 1970s.

As alluded to above, much of the research concerning auditory processing skills of children with language or learning disabilities documented the children's auditory processing deficits in comparison to adult performance. Recently, however, a number of investigations have attempted to examine the natural course of auditory processing skill development for children who are normally developing, and then to compare the performance of children with language or learning disabilities to that of their normally developing peers. Cranford, Morgan, Scudder, and Moore

(1993) asked normally developing children between the ages of 6 and 12 years to report the perceived location of a stationary fused auditory image and to track the apparent movement of a moving fused auditory image. Movement of the fused auditory image was simulated by presenting clicks from each of two matched loudspeakers positioned on opposite sides of the listener and incrementally varying the delays between the pairs of clicks presented. These researchers found that although the children performed similarly to a group of adult subjects tested previously (Moore, Cranford, & Rahn, 1990) on the stationary fused image task, a significant age-related trend was noted on the moving fused auditory image task. On this task, the younger subjects demonstrated poorer tracking abilities than did the older children, who performed similarly to the adults on this task. These findings implicate the presence of significant changes in binaural auditory processing abilities as the normal child matures.

In a subsequent investigation, Visto, Cranford, and Scudder (1996) compared the performance of children with specific language impairment (SLI) on the moving fused image task to that of two groups of normally developing children (i.e., a group of children matched to the SLI group on the basis of chronological age and a second group of children matched to the SLI group on the basis of language age). The results of this investigation revealed that the performance of the SLI group was similar to that of the language-age matched children (i.e., younger children) suggesting that the SLI subjects were delayed in their ability to use binaural acoustic information in a dynamic ongoing fashion. The authors suggest that the processing required for the moving fused auditory image task may be similar to that involved in the ongoing processing of rapid changes in the spectral and temporal components of speech, particularly when one considers the similarity in performance between the SLI group and the younger normally developing children who were matched to the SLI group on the basis of language-age as opposed to chronological age.

Nozza, Wagner, and Crandell (1988) investigated the amount of binaural release from masking for a speech sound (*ba*) in three groups of subjects (infants, preschoolers, and adults). Masking level differences were derived under the S_0N_0 and $S_\pi N_0$ conditions and the results indicated significant differences between the infants and adults, whereas the performance of the preschoolers was not significantly different from that of the adult subjects. In a subsequent investigation by Hall and Grose (1990), MLDs were derived using a pulsed tone (500 Hz) in the presence of two different bandpass noise conditions (300 Hz wide and 40 Hz wide) in children between the ages of 3.9 to 9.5 years. Results showed that the MLD in the 300 Hz wide masking noise condition increased in size up until the age of 5 to 6 years, whereas the MLD for the 40 Hz wide maskers for 5- to 6-year-old children continued to fall below adult values.

The results of these investigations suggest that developmental changes in binaural analysis of acoustic information occurs postnatally as the child matures. The authors suggest that although it is possible that the small MLDs noted in children may be related to imprecise coding of the acoustic information within the auditory periphery, it is more likely that the basis for the small MLDs lie in inefficient central auditory processes responsible for the extraction of the interaural acoustic information.

Hall and Grose (1993) conducted a second investigation that studied the effect of otitis media on MLDs and ABRs. Their subjects included children with a history of otitis media with effusion (OME) and a group of children with no known history of OME. Both groups of children had normal peripheral hearing at the time of the testing. Their results demonstrated that children with a history of OME demonstrated significantly reduced MLDs and prolonged ABR Waves III and V and I–III and III–V interwave intervals. The results of these studies suggest that the reduction noted in the MLD in children having histories of OME may be related to abnormal brainstem processing.

Along similar lines of investigation, Grose, Hall, and Gibbs (1993) investigated the development of temporal resolution as a function of frequency region using a modified masking period pattern or comodulation masking release (CMR) paradigm. Their CMR paradigm permitted age-dependent comparisons of temporal resolution both within channel (monotic) as well as across channel (dichotic). The authors found that temporal resolution improves with age and approaches adult levels of performance for high frequencies at approximately 6 years of age, whereas for low frequencies the improvement with age continues beyond 10 years of age. A subsequent investigation revealed that children with OME are likely to have reduced monotic CMRs and that these are likely to remain reduced for several months after hearing has returned to normal levels, whereas no effects of OME were noted for the dichotic CMRs (Hall & Grose, 1994). The authors suggest that the present findings may suggest a deficit in these children in terms of their ability to segregate an auditory signal from a competing noise, and as such may represent the basis of the speech intelligibility in noise deficits often experienced by children with CAPD.

Many of the tests detailed in this chapter have also been used with children. Research on monotic low-redundancy tests has included low-pass filtered speech (Farrer & Keith, 1981; Martin & Clark, 1977; Musiek et al., 1994; Musiek & Geurkink, 1980; Musiek, Geurkink, & Keitel, 1982; Musiek, Gollegly, & Baran, 1984; White, 1977; Willeford, 1976, 1977a, 1977b, 1980; Willeford & Billger, 1978), compressed speech (Beasley, Maki, & Orchik, 1976; Bornstein & Musiek, 1992; Freeman & Beasley, 1976; Manning, Johnston, & Beasley, 1977; Musiek et al., 1994; Orchik & Oelschlaeger, 1977; Willeford, 1980), speech-in-

noise (Cohen, 1980; Gravel & Stapells, 1993; McCroskey & Kasten, 1980; Papso & Blood, 1989; Rupp, 1983; Willeford & Billger, 1978), and synthetic sentence identification with ipsilateral competing message (Decker & Nelson, 1981; Jerger, 1980; Orchik & Burgess, 1977). Collectively, the results of these investigations have demonstrated (1) that performance on monaural low-redundancy speech tests tends to improve with age, suggesting that these skills are maturational; (2) that there is little difference between the right and left ears on these tests; and (3) that there is considerable variability in performance at each age level. Given these considerations, scores are typically considered abnormal only if the scores are severely depressed in one or both ears compared to age-appropriate norms, or if there is a marked asymmetry between the scores of the two ears.

Dichotic speech tests administered to this population have included dichotic digits (Bakker, Hoefkens, & Van der Vlugt, 1979; Hiscock & Kinsbourne, 1980; Koomar & Cermak, 1981; Kraft, 1984; Musiek et al., 1994; Musiek et al., 1984; Musiek & Geurkink, 1980; Musiek et al., 1982; Newell & Rugel, 1981; Pettit & Helms, 1979; Sommers & Taylor, 1972; Witelson & Rabinovitch, 1972), staggered spondaic words (Berrick, Shubow, Schultz, Freed, Fournier, & Hughes, 1984; Dempsey, 1977; Musiek et al., 1994; Musiek & Geurkink, 1980; Musiek et al., 1982; Musiek et al., 1984; Pinheiro, 1977; Protti, 1983; Riccio, Hynd, Cohen, & Molt, 1996; Sweitzer, 1977; White, 1977; Young, 1983), competing sentences (Dempsey, 1977, 1983; McCroskey & Kasten, 1980; Musiek & Geurkink, 1980; Musiek et al., 1994; Musiek et al., 1984; Musiek et al., 1982; Pinheiro, 1977; Protti, 1983; Protti & Young, 1980; Welsh, Welsh, & Healy, 1980; White, 1977; Willeford, 1977a, 1977b, 1978, 1980; Willeford & Billger, 1978; Young, 1983), dichotic CVs (Berlin, Hughes, Lowe-Bell, & Berlin, 1973; Dermody, Katsch, & Mackie, 1983; Harris, Keith, & Novak, 1983; Hynd, Cohen, & Obrzut, 1983; Hynd & Obrzut, 1977; Koomar & Cermak, 1981; Mirabile, Porter, Hughes, & Berlin, 1978; Roeser, Millay, & Morrow, 1983; Tobey, Cullen, & Rampp, 1979), and the synthetic sentence identification with contralateral competing message test (Jerger, 1980; Orchik & Burgess, 1977). The results of these investigations have demonstrated an obvious right ear advantage on these tests in young children and that performance on these tests tends to improve with age. However, generally more dramatic improvements are noted in the left ear, because even at early ages right ear performance tends to be high. For the most part, test results with LD children have demonstrated depressed left ear scores compared to age-appropriate norms, whereas right ear scores tend to be normal.

Frequency pattern sequences have also been used with children in order to assess pattern perception and temporal sequencing abilities. Pinheiro (1977) demonstrated depressed scores in dyslexic children when she compared their performance to that of normal children on this task. Similar findings have been reported by Musiek and his colleagues (1982, 1984, 1994).

Finally, binaural fusion and rapidly alternating speech tests have been used to assess the binaural integration abilities of young children (Davis & McCroskey, 1980; Musiek & Geurkink, 1980; Musiek et al., 1982; Palva & Jokinen, 1975; Pinheiro, 1977; Plakke, Orchik, & Beasley, 1981; Roush & Tait, 1984; Welsh et al., 1980; Welsh, Welsh, Healy, & Cooper, 1982; White, 1977; Willeford & Billger, 1978; Willeford & Burleigh, 1985). Results have shown that some children demonstrate difficulties on both tests with the BF test having a higher hit rate than the RASP test. Of the tests mentioned thus far, the RASP appears to be the least sensitive.

A consideration of the research on normally developing children suggests that CANS functioning has a relatively long course of maturation with development of functions mediated at the lower centers of the auditory system reaching adult stages of development at an earlier age than those mediated at higher centers within the CANS (Cranford et al., 1993; Grose et al., 1993; Hall & Grose, 1990; Musiek et al., 1984). It is interesting to note that normally developing children tend to achieve adult levels of performance on virtually all of the various tests discussed in this chapter by the age of 10 to 11 years. This appears to be the same age at which myelination of the CANS reaches adult stages of development (Yakovlev & LeCours, 1967), providing evidence that neural and behavioral maturation are codependent processes.

The research on children with CAPD has suggested that the auditory deficits noted in these children may be related to at least three different causes. Musiek and colleagues (1984) suggested that in a large number of children referred for testing, the etiology may be related to delays in the neuromaturational development of the CANS. Other investigators have implicated static neurological involvement (Musiek, Gollegly, & Ross, 1985), whereas others point out that the deficits may be related to actual CANS lesions, similar to those noted in adults (Jerger, 1987; Jerger, Johnson, & Loiselle, 1988; Musiek et al., 1985). In addition, researchers have suggested that the central auditory processing disorders observed in children may be differentiated on an auditory-specific perceptual and/or linguistic basis (Jerger et al., 1988).

It is important to note that when testing children it is essential that a variety of tests be used. In many of the studies mentioned above where more than one test was administered, a given child may have performed abnormally on one test and normally on a second test. It is, therefore, important that the audiologist who is attempting to assess children selects tests that assess different processes. It is also important that he or she take into consideration the age appropriateness of the tests to be used and how sensitive the tests may be for a given age group.

Adults with Obscure Auditory Dysfunction

At the present time audiologists are beginning to see an increasing number of adults presenting with significant auditory complaints (e.g., difficulty hearing in noise) but with apparently normal peripheral hearing. In the past these individuals were frequently dismissed as being overly anxious, but currently evidence exists that in many of these individuals the bases for these hearing difficulties may lie in CANS dysfunction. Although there does not appear to be a unitary cause for these auditory difficulties, the evidence suggests CANS dysfunction may be the underlying cause in many of these adults (Baran & Musiek, 1994). The central auditory deficits experienced by these adults can be related to a number of etiological factors that affect the CANS, such as frank neurological compromise, subtle cerebral morphological abnormalities, and normal aging processes. There are, however, other etiological bases for the hearing difficulties reported in this population that must also be considered. These include (1) subtle subclinical compromise of the peripheral hearing mechanism, (2) cognitive deficits, (3) psychological/emotional problems, (4) language differences, and (5) changes in acoustic environment.

In 1989 Saunders and Haggard coined the term *obscure auditory dysfunction (OAD)* to refer to the auditory difficulties experienced by some individuals with normal audiograms while avoiding specific pathophysiological connotations. It is clear from the evidence available that the underlying bases of the problems in this group of individuals are numerous and varied (Baran & Musiek, 1994; Saunders & Haggard, 1989). In some of these individuals clear pathophysiological bases can be established. In others, the deficits may be more difficult to link to a specific underlying etiological basis. However, in any case presenting with auditory complaints and normal audiograms, involvement of the CANS must be questioned if other etiological bases for the auditory problems cannot be ruled out.

The Elderly

The assessment of CANS functioning in the elderly patient presents the audiologist with a unique challenge. This challenge is related to the fact that there are various sites of aging effects in the elderly clients that can complicate the CANS assessment of the elderly patient. For example, Schnuknecht (1964, 1974) identified four distinct types of presbycusis. These include (1) sensory presbycusis, related to atrophy of the Organ of Corti and degeneration of the hair cells beginning at the basal end of the cochlea and moving toward the apex; (2) neural presbycusis, related to loss of neurons in the auditory pathways and the eighth nerve; (3) stria vascularis atrophy or metabolic presbycusis, related to the degeneration of the stria vascularis in the apical turn of the cochlea; and (4) inner ear conductive-type presbycusis, which probably is related to an increase in the stiffness of the supporting structures of the cochlear duct. These various pathologies manifest themselves in different audiometric configurations, and often more than one may coexist at the same time. Matters are complicated further by the fact that although binaural hearing thresholds may appear similar, both ears may not have the same capacity at suprathreshold levels. Recruitment and problems related to temporal factors may be present. Therefore, one must be aware of the potential confounding effects of peripheral hearing loss on the central tests being used.

With the elderly patient the audiologist may not only be dealing with a cochlear hearing loss but also with a central disability that is not related to a frank neurological lesion. In many presbycusic losses, the central auditory structures, as well as the peripheral mechanisms, are affected by the aging process. Senile changes in the CANS have been reported for both brainstem and cortical structures (Brody, 1955; Kirikae, Sato, & Shitara, 1964; Smith & Sethi, 1975). In the older patient, central auditory function may be depressed by a general loss of neurons throughout the CANS. Blood flow may be reduced by fatty deposits in the arteries supplying the brain. There may be age-related changes in the cerebral metabolism that do not affect peripheral hearing. Glucose metabolism and oxygen consumption decrease with aging. The problem that faces the audiologist is how to account for these differences and their effects on CANS function, which appear to be primarily physiological and not chronological. Therefore, establishing norms by chronological age will not necessarily solve the problem.

There have been a number of attempts to study the CANS function in the geriatric population. Investigations of elderly patients with no known central lesions demonstrated higher percentages of abnormal findings on low-pass filtered speech (Bergman, 1980; Bocca, 1958; Divenyi & Haupt, 1997a; Kirikae et al., 1964), time-compressed or accelerated speech (Calearo & Lazzaroni, 1957; Divenyi & Haupt, 1997a; Konkle, Beasley, & Bess, 1977; Letowski & Poch, 1995, 1996; Schmitt, 1983; Sticht & Gray, 1969), speech-in-noise (Divenyi & Haupt, 1997a; Schum & Matthews, 1992), staggered spondaic words (Divenyi & Haupt, 1997a), synthetic or dichotic sentence identification (Divenyi & Haupt, 1997a; Jerger, Chmiel, Allen, & Wilson, 1994; Jerger & Hayes, 1977; Noffsinger, Martinez, & Andrews, 1996), dichotic nonsense syllables (Dermody, 1976; Kurdziel & Noffsinger, 1977; Noffsinger

et al., 1996), dichotic digits (Divenyi & Haupt, 1997a; Noffsinger et al., 1996), masking level differences (Findlay & Schuchman, 1976; Tillman, Carhart, & Nicholls, 1973), and interrupted speech (Antonelli, 1970; Bergman, 1971; Bocca, 1958; Kirikae et al., 1964).

The foregoing test results implicate a reduction in the efficiency with which the aging CANS processes difficult auditory stimuli. Although these investigations appear to document CANS compromise, the question of the extent of CANS compromise in the geriatric population remains an issue of much debate and controversy. Several investigators have argued that the depressed performance of elderly subjects on these tests is likely to be due to the presence of peripheral hearing loss and cognitive deficits that are common in the geriatric population, and therefore not necessarily due to CANS compromise.

Recently several investigators have attempted to identify the factors that could explain the speech comprehension deficits often experienced by the geriatric patient (Divenyi & Haupt, 1997a, 1997b; Humes & Christopherson, 1991; Humes, Coughlin, & Talley, 1996; Humes, Watson, Christensen, Cokely, Halling, & Lee, 1994; Jerger & Chmiel, 1997; van Rooij & Plomp, 1990). Although there were a number of differences among these studies, three factors consistently emerged from these data that could be used to account for the deficits observed in the elderly subjects tested in these investigations: (1) speech audibility, (2) general speech understanding ability, and (3) speech understanding ability in noise. Other factors also emerged in these studies. These included frequency analysis, spatial and temporal processing, and dichotic competition. It should be noted, however, that not all of the investigations referenced above included tests that would assess each of these areas. Therefore, the fact that these latter factors are not listed above should not be interpreted as suggesting that these factors are not significant contributors to the auditory problems experienced by elderly patients. In fact, dichotic competition emerged as a primary factor in three investigations that included dichotic test measures (Humes et al., 1996; Humes et al., 1994; Jerger & Chmiel, 1997) and temporal processing emerged as a primary factor in two investigations that included such tests (Divenyi & Haupt, 1997b; Humes et al., 1996). Moreover, it is interesting to note that in two of these investigations (Humes et al., 1994; Jerger & Chmiel, 1997), the dichotic speech test performance of the two ears was analyzed separately in the factor analysis undertaken, and in both investigations the auditory processing abilities of the ears emerged as separate factors. These results are consistent with earlier behavioral and electrophysiological findings that suggested that ear differences (which may exist but are typically quite small in young adults) tend to increase with age and in some individuals may become quite pronounced (Jerger, Alford,

Lew, Rivera, & Chmiel, 1995; Jerger et al., 1994). Jerger and his colleagues (1995) have attributed these findings to an age-related progressive deterioration in corpus callosum functioning, which results in a systematic decline in the efficiency of interhemispheric transfer. Although this is not likely to be the only site of deterioration of function in the CANS of the elderly patient, it is likely to be a significant site of senile changes and the basis of some of the speech comprehension difficulties of older patients.

The evidence provided above suggests that reduced capacity or efficacy of function is present throughout the CANS from the brainstem to the cortex and the interhemispheric pathways, and that many of these degenerative changes may occur in some individuals as early as the sixth decade of life. Given these findings, it would appear to be prudent for the audiologist to assess not only the peripheral, but also the central, auditory function of the elderly patient who presents with auditory comprehension difficulties as the elucidation of the extent of CANS compromise may lead to differential decisions regarding management strategies (Musiek & Baran, 1996).

Cases of Binaural Interference

Most audiologists have encountered at one time or another that patient who appears to be a good candidate for binaural hearing aids based upon audiometric and personal data, but who when fitted with amplification does not perform up to expectations. It is possible that in these patients some type of CANS compromise or involvement may be the limiting factor and this possibility warrants further investigation.

Recently, Jerger, Silman, Lew, and Chmiel (1993) presented four cases where evidence of binaural interference (i.e., condition where binaural performance is actually poorer than monaural performance) was provided. In three of the cases, aided binaural speech recognition scores were compared to the aided monaural speech recognition scores, and in each case, the binaural score was found to be noticeably depressed relative to the "better" monaural score. In addition, middle latency responses (MLRs) were derived for both monaural and binaural stimulus presentation conditions in two of these three patients as well as in a fourth patient. In each case, the MLRs derived from one ear revealed better waveform morphology (i.e., the waveforms replicated and the Pa and Na responses could be identified), whereas the responses obtained from the poorer ear were either absent or not well-defined. Interestingly, in all three cases the binaurally derived response lacked the definition of the "better" monaural response. The typical expectation for each of these two tests would have been for the binaural performance to be either improved compared to the better monaural response because of binaural summation effects, or at least equal to the performance of the better ear. Although the exact mechanisms underlying this type of binaural interference have not been elucidated, it is likely that the interference is centrally mediated as the effects are evident only under conditions of binaural stimulation. Additional research needs to be conducted in order to evaluate the extent of this type of central auditory system compromise and to determine which tests should be used to document the presence of this type of disorder. It may no longer be wise to assume that binaural fittings are preferable for most, if not all, hearing aid users. Candidacy for binaural fittings could be better documented if central auditory screenings or assessments were included as part of the hearing aid selection and fitting procedures. For additional information on the utilization of central auditory assessments as part of hearing aid selection and fitting protocols, as well as a discussion of additional case studies with CANS compromise the reader is referred to Musiek and Baran (1996).

Case Illustrations

The first case (Figure 13.3) involves a 69-year-old woman with a left-sided brainstem tumor. The lesion was positioned at the lateral aspect of the low to mid pons. Though this patient did have a mild-to-moderate sensorineural hearing loss, it was bilaterally symmetrical. The results of three dichotic speech tests (staggered spondaic words, dichotic digits, and competing sentences) revealed markedly depressed left ear scores, although all dichotic speech test results were depressed bilaterally. Given that the audiogram was bilaterally symmetrical, the marked difference between the two ears on these central tests would not be expected unless there was central involvement. Frequency pattern test results were normal bilaterally. These findings are consistent with what was mentioned in the text; that is, frequency patterns are not highly sensitive to brainstem lesions and are often not affected by mild to moderate hearing loss.

The second case (Figure 13.4) is one demonstrating the classical contralateral ear effect. This teenage boy had a large lesion involving the left thalamus and medial segments of the left hemisphere. Involvement of the auditory radiations from the medical geniculate was highly probable. In this case and all subsequent cases, peripheral auditory function was normal. Severe right ear deficits are noted for the two dichotic speech tests (staggered spondaic words and competing sentences). Also, a right ear deficit is noted on the monaural low redundancy speech test (low-pass filtered speech). Frequency pattern sequences test results show bilateral deficits even though only one hemisphere is compromised. This bilaterally depressed score is common with this test in that it is believed both hemispheres must be intact to perform normally on this test (see text for further explanation).

a

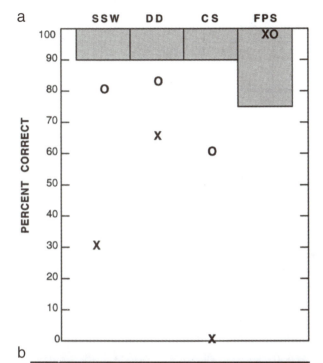

b

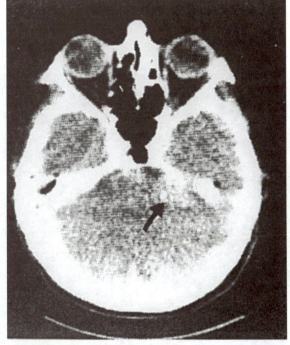

FIGURE 13.3 (A) Central auditory test results for a 69-year-old woman with a mild-to-moderate bilaterally symmetrical sensorineural hearing loss and a left-sided brainstem tumor. Data are presented for four central auditory tests (SSW: Staggered Spondaic Words; DD: Dichotic Digits; CS: Competing Sentences; FPS: Frequency Pattern Sequences) for the right (O) and left (X) ears. The shaded area represents the range of normal performance. (B) CT scan for the patient described in Panel A, documenting the presence of a left-sided brainstem tumor located at the lateral aspect of the low to mid pons.

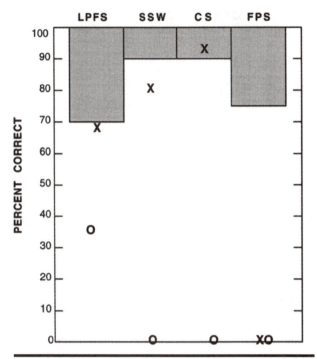

FIGURE 13.4 Central auditory test results for a teenage boy with normal peripheral auditory test results and a large lesion involving the left thalamus and medial segments of the left hemisphere. Data are presented for four auditory tests (LPFS: Low-Pass Filtered Speech; SSW: Staggered Spondaic Words; DD: CS: Competing Sentences; FPS: Frequency Pattern Sequences) for the right (O) and left (X) ears. The shaded area represents the range of normal performance.

The third case (Figure 13.5) is a woman in her mid-forties with a mid, right temporal lobe involvement. Again, a contralateral ear effect is noted for compressed speech and dichotic digits, and though the left ear is worse than the right on frequency patterns, both ears are below normal.

The fourth case (Figure 13.6) is another example of the contralateral ear effect. This case involves a 56-year-old woman with a right hemisphere stroke primarily affecting the temporoparietal region. Test results are depressed for the contralateral left ear for two dichotic speech tests (dichotic rhymes and digits). In addition, frequency pattern sequences test scores were severely depressed for both ears.

The fifth case (Figure 13.7) is a 50-year-old male with a stroke affecting the left temporoparietal area. Test results are depressed for the contralateral right ear on the low-pass filtered speech test and the dichotic rhyme test and for both ears on the dichotic digits test. Frequency pattern sequences test results are normal for both ears.

The sixth case (Figure 13.8) portrays the test results for a young woman with bilateral involvement of both temporal lobes. Note that all central auditory tests (dichotic digits,

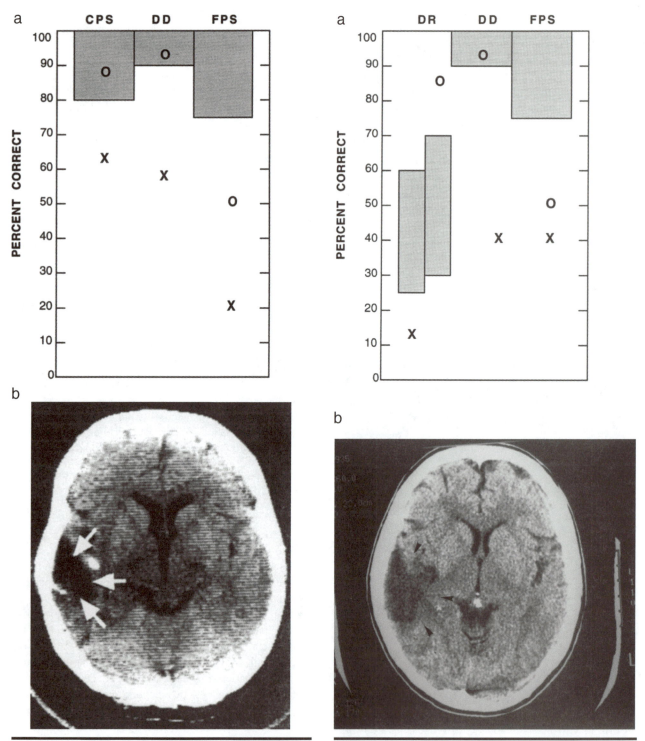

FIGURE 13.5 (A) Central auditory test results for a woman in her mid-forties with normal peripheral auditory test results and a right temporal lobe resection secondary to a tumor. Data are presented for three central auditory tests (CPS: Compressed Speech; DD: Dichotic Digits; FPS: Frequency Pattern Sequences) for the right (O) and left (X) ears. The shaded area represents the range of normal performance. (B) CT scan documenting the right hemisphere involvement for the patient described in (A).

FIGURE 13.6 (A) Central auditory test results for a 56-year-old woman with normal peripheral auditory test results and a right cerebrovascular accident (CVA) affecting the temporoparietal region. Data are presented for three central auditory tests (DR: Dichotic Rhymes; DD: Dichotic Digits; FPS: Frequency Pattern Sequences) for the right (O) and left (X) ears. The shaded area represents the range of normal performance. (B) CAT scan documenting the right hemisphere involvement for the patient described in (A).

a

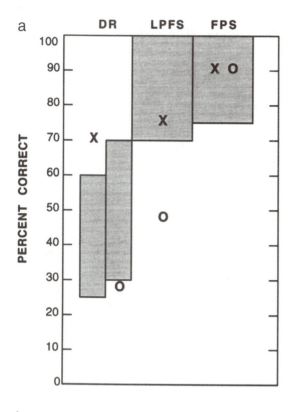

b

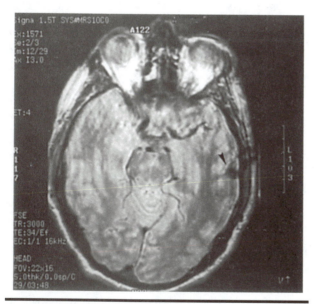

FIGURE 13.7 (A) Central auditory test results for a 50-year-old man with normal peripheral auditory test results and a left cerebrovascular accident (CVA) affecting the temporoparietal region. Data are presented for three central auditory tests (DR: Dichotic Rhymes; LPFS: Low-Pass Filtered Speech; FPS: Frequency Pattern Sequences) for the right (O) and left (X) ears. The shaded area represents the range of normal performance. (B) MRI scan documenting the left hemisphere involvement for the patient described in (A).

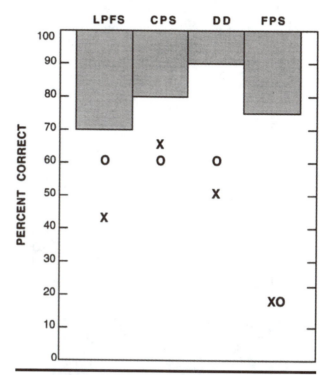

FIGURE 13.8 Central auditory test results for a young woman with normal peripheral auditory test results and bilateral temporal lobe epilepsy and slight cortical atrophy. Data are presented for four central auditory tests (LPFS: Low-Pass Filtered Speech; DD: Dichotic Digits; CPS: Compressed Speech; FPS: Frequency Pattern Sequences) for the right (O) and left (X) ears. The shaded area represents the range of normal performance.

compressed speech, low-pass filtered speech, and frequency pattern sequences) revealed bilaterally reduced scores heralding the consideration of bilateral hemispheric problems.

The final case (Figure 13.9) involves a teenage boy with a large lesion involving the cortex in the left hemisphere and the interhemispheric fibers. It is evident that all dichotic speech tests and frequency patterns demonstrate bilateral deficits, whereas only low-pass filtered speech results show the contralateral ear effect. The dichotic tests are bilaterally depressed because, as explained in the text, these tests require intact callosal fibers as well as an intact cortex. Filtered speech responses do not require an intact corpus callosum and therefore reflect only the compromise of the left cortex by a contralateral (right) ear deficit.

The foregoing illustrative cases attest to the fact that behavioral central auditory tests can be useful in the identification of CANS pathology, but they may not be particularly useful in the identification of the exact location of a lesion. At the present time there is no evidence establishing a direct relationship between CANS test results and site of CANS pathology. Therefore, the audiologist must proceed cautiously when attempting to interpret CANS test results.

a

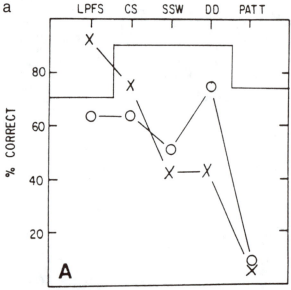

b

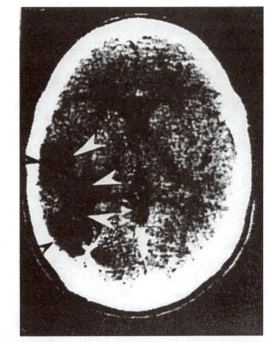

FIGURE 13.9 (A) Central auditory test results for a teenage boy with normal peripheral hearing and a large left temporoparietal tumor involving the auditory cortex and corpus callosum. Data are presented for five central auditory tests (LPFS: Low-Pass Filtered Speech; CS: Competing Sentences; SSW: Staggered Spondaic Words; DD: Dichotic Digits; FPS: Frequency Pattern Sequences) for the right (O) and left (X) ears. The solid line cutting across the upper portion of this figure delineates the lower limits of normal adult performance. (B) CT scan documenting the location of the lesion described in (A). (Reprinted with permission from "Central auditory assessment: Thirty years of challenge and change," by F. E. Musiek & J. A. Baran, 1987, *Ear and Hearing, 8,* 22S-35S. Copyright by Williams & Wilkins, Baltimore.)

CONSIDERATIONS IN TEST SELECTION

There are a number of factors that should be considered when selecting a central auditory test or tests for administration. These factors include both test variables and factors related to the individual being tested.

Sensitivity and Specificity

The goal of central auditory assessment is the accurate identification of those patients having auditory processing disorders and the appropriate exclusion of those individuals without central auditory processing disorders as not having this disorder. There are several measures that are related to these goals, but two measures in particular are central to our discussion of this topic (i.e., test sensitivity and specificity). *Sensitivity*, or hit rate (HR), refers the percentage of patients with a given condition or pathology that the test accurately identifies as having the condition or pathology (Eq. 13.1). For example, if a test is specifically designed to identify brainstem dysfunction, then the sensitivity measure provides an indication as to how many patients with CANS compromise at the level of the brainstem performed abnormally on this test. A second measure that is important to consider when selecting a test or tests to be used for assessing central auditory function is its specificity or correct rejection rate (CR). *Specificity* refers to the percentage of individuals without the condition or pathology for which the test was designed who performed normally or at least differently from the designated population on the test (Eq. 13.2).

$$HR = tp/dp \qquad (13.1)$$
$$CR = tn/np \qquad (13.2)$$

where HR = Hit Rate, tp = number of true positives, dp = number of diseased patients, CR = Correct Rejection Rate, tn = number of true negatives, and np = nondiseased subjects.

The best choices for clinical assessments would be those tests that are high on both measures. For most tests, however, there is a trade-off between the two measures. For example, it is possible to select a cut-off criterion that is sufficiently lax so that any patient with the condition, pathology, or disorder would fall below the criterion; however, as the criterion is relaxed the number of individuals without the designated condition, pathology, or disorder is likely to increase. Clinically, the audiologist may be faced with the decision as to what type of error is more acceptable. Is it more desirable to identify as many patients as possible with a given pathology, recognizing that a number of individuals without the condition will be falsely identified (i.e., false positives)? Or would it be preferable to limit the number of "false alarms" and accept the fact that a number of patients with a given condition will not be identified (i.e., false negatives)? Obviously, these can be important decisions that require careful consideration of a number of factors, including the morbidity rates associated with the condition, the financial and emotional cost of overreferral, and so forth.

This chapter has provided a review of the behavioral tests that have been used to assess CANS function in patients (or probably more appropriately, subjects) with known CANS function. One of the problems that persists in the field of central auditory assessment is proliferation of central tests that are being used to assess central auditory function, many of which have not been subjected to rigorous psychometric testing. Most of the data reported in the various investigations reviewed in this chapter were obtained from the administration of tests designed for research purposes. These studies provide some information about the sensitivity or hit rates of the tests, but frequently there is no information provided regarding the specificity of the test or tests used in the investigations.

Although sensitivity data is not available for all of these tests, a review of the literature can lead one to some informed decisions regarding the potential sensitivity of these tests or categories of tests to lesions at various sites along the CANS. Table 13.1 provides predictions offered by Baran and Musiek (1995) based upon their review of the literature and their personal experience.

Recently, there has been an increased interest in applying clinical decision analysis to determine test efficiency. For example, Hurley and Musiek (1997) retrospectively evaluated the clinical effectiveness of two of the central auditory tests discussed in this chapter (dichotic digits, auditory duration patterns) for assessing CANS dysfunction in subjects with intracranial lesions. Their results revealed that both tests were quite high on both sensitivity and specificity measures, whereas a third measure (P300s) did not fare as well. As more of the behavioral and electrophysiological tests used in clinical assessments of the CANS are subjected to these types of analysis, audiologists will be in a better position to make informed decisions regarding the selection of a given test or tests for a given patient. A detailed review of clinical decision analysis is beyond the scope of this chapter. The reader interested in this topic should refer to Chapter 15 of this text.

Test Availability and Quality of Stimulus Recordings

One of the major problems in the field of central auditory processing at the present time is the inability to easily compare test results across investigations or clinical settings. This is due in large part to the differences that exist in stimulus parameters and test protocols for tests that share the same title, the limited availability of several of these tests on a commercial basis, the less than ideal quality of stimulus reproduction on many of the recordings that do exist, and the susceptibility of audiotapes to deterioration with age and continued use. A recent development in the field of central auditory assessment that should address many of these issues and concerns is the introduction of a compact auditory disc (*Tonal and Speech Materials for Auditory Perceptual Assessment, Disc 1.0*). This disc contains a variety of behavioral tests that have been developed

TABLE 13.1   Expected test results for behavioral tests administered to patients with lesions occurring at various sites along the central auditory nervous system.

TEST CLASSIFICATION	LOW BRAINSTEM	HIGH BRAINSTEM	AUDITORY CORTEX	INTERHEMISPHERIC PATHWAYS
Phase Tests (e.g., MLD)	Binaural deficit* (3)	Little or no deficit (3)	Little or no deficit (3)	Little or no deficit (3)
Binaural Interaction Tests	Binaural deficit* (2)	Little or no deficit (3)	Little or no deficit (3)	Little or no deficit (3)
Monaural Low-Redundancy Speech Tests	Ipsilateral ear deficit (2)	Contralateral ear deficit (2) Bilateral deficits (2) Ipsilateral ear deficit (1)	Contralateral ear deficit (3)	No deficit (3)
Dichotic Speech Tests	Ipsilateral ear deficit (2)	Contralateral ear deficit (2) Bilateral deficits (2) Ipsilateral ear deficit (2)	Contralateral ear deficit (3) Bilateral deficits (1)	Contralateral ear deficit (3)
Temporal Patterning Tests	Ipsilateral ear deficit (1)	Contralateral ear deficit (1) Bilateral deficits (1) Ipsilateral ear deficit (1)	Bilateral deficits (3)	Bilateral deficits (3)

Source: Adapted with permission from "Central auditory processing disorders in children and adults," by J. A. Baran and F. E. Musiek. In L. G. Wall (Ed.), *Hearing for the Speech-Language Pathologist and Health Care Professional*, 1995. Copyright by Butterworth-Heinemann Medical Publishers, Boston.

Key: (3) high probability of occurrence, (2) moderate probability of occurrence, (1) low probability of occurrence.

*Binaural is used in this context since both ears are receiving segments of the stimulus and only one score is derived.

with careful attention to stimulus generation and development of test protocols (Noffsinger, Wilson, & Musiek, 1994). Each of the tests on the disc has been subjected to extensive psychometric testing at nine different test sites around the United States. Table 13.2 provides a listing of each of the central auditory tests available on the disc and classifies each test according to the classification system used in this chapter. Also provided in the table are the test parameters for each test and the number of subjects included in the normative studies. For additional information on any of these tests, the reader is referred to the references accompanying each of the tests listed on the table. Some of the data from the initial psychometric investigations on some of the speech tests is also available in Chapter 2 of this text. Although there is limited information regarding the efficiency of these specific tests with clinical populations to date, it is anticipated that the tests on the disc will compare favorably with data obtained using the comparable tests from earlier audio recorded versions of many of these tests.

Influence of Peripheral Hearing Loss

Obviously the best situation for defining a central auditory processing disorder is to have a patient with normal peripheral hearing. Although this situation does occur in many cases, in many other cases, it does not and one has to either bypass central auditory testing or in some way account for the potential confounding effects of the peripheral hearing loss. Fortunately, careful selection of the central tests to be administered and interpretation of test results can lead to the accurate diagnosis of a central auditory processing deficit in an individual with a peripheral hearing loss.

There have been a number of investigations that have studied the effects of peripheral hearing loss on central auditory test performance. These studies have shown that the presence of a peripheral hearing loss can affect the results of many of the tests mentioned in this chapter including filtered speech, time-compressed speech, speech-in-noise, rapidly alternating speech perception, binaural fusion, masking level differences, dichotic sentences, dichotic CVs, dichotic digits, staggered spondaic words, frequency pattern sequences, and auditory duration patterns (Divenyi & Haupt, 1997b; Fifer et al., 1983; Grimes, Mueller, & Williams, 1984; Humes et al., 1996; Kurdziel et al., 1976; Miltenberger, Dawson, & Raica, 1978; Musiek et al., 1990; Musiek, Gollegly, Kibbe, & Verkest-Lenz, 1991; Musiek & Pinheiro, 1987; Noffsinger, 1982; Olsen et al., 1976; Orchik & Burgess, 1977; Roeser, Johns, & Price, 1976; Speaks, Niccum, & Van Tasell, 1985). However, in spite of the fact that virtually all central tests can be affected by the presence of a peripheral hearing loss, some of the tests discussed in this chapter appear to be less affected than others. For example, some investigators have found that the dichotic digits test (Musiek et al., 1991; Speaks et al., 1985) and the dichotic sentence identification test (Fifer et al., 1983) are relatively more resistant to the effects of mild to moderate peripheral hearing loss than other speech perception tests. Also, both frequency patterns and auditory duration patterns have been found to be quite resistant to the potentially confounding effects of peripheral hearing loss (Musiek et al., 1990; Musiek & Pinheiro, 1987). More recently, Humes and colleagues (1996) investigated the effects of peripheral hearing loss and aging in a group of elderly subjects on ten of the fifteen central auditory tests contained on the compact auditory disc referenced above. Their results indicated that five of the tests were negatively affected by the presence of peripheral hearing loss in this population (dichotic digits, dichotic sentence identification, filtered NU-6 words, 45% time-compressed speech, and 65% time compressed speech), whereas five other tests (two dichotic CVs tests, a binaural fusion task, frequency pattern sequences, and auditory duration patterns) were found to be relatively unaffected by the presence of a peripheral hearing impairment in this population.

Although it is fair to say that peripheral hearing loss can affect virtually any of the central tests, the administration of central auditory tests to a patient with a mild-to-moderate peripheral hearing loss should not be avoided as the coexistence of a central hearing loss with a peripheral hearing loss can have profound implications for the diagnosis and management of the patient with hearing loss.

The presence or absence of a coexisting CAPD in a patient with a peripheral hearing impairment can be established in a number of circumstances, including (1) if hearing loss is present and the central auditory test results fall within the normal range, then the presence of CANS compromise can be ruled out; (2) if hearing loss is present but bilaterally symmetrical and the central auditory test results are clearly asymmetrical, then the presence of a CAPD is implicated; and (3) if a hearing loss is present and it is unilateral or asymmetrical and the central auditory test results reveal "poorer" performance for the better ear, then CANS compromise is likely. In each of these three clinical profiles, the presence or absence of a CAPD can be made with a fair degree of confidence. Fortunately, many patients will fit into one of these three situations and decisions regarding management of these individuals can proceed in an informed manner. There are, however, some patients who will not fit into any of these situations. In these cases, a determination of the status of the CANS and the presence or absence of a coexisting CAPD disorder is difficult, if not impossible to make and management of these patients will have to take place without the benefit of this knowledge.

TABLE 13.2 A list of the auditory perceptual tests contained on the *Tonal and Speech Materials for Auditory Perceptual Assessment, Disc 1.0*. A brief summary of test parameters is provided for each entry along with the number of subjects in the normative data pool and a reference for additional test description.

TEST	CLASSIFICATION	STIMULI	LEVEL	SUBJECTS	REFERENCE
Masking level difference	binaural interaction/ phase test	10 spondee words in 2000 msec gated noise[a]	65 and 85 dB SPL noise level	60 per noise level	Wilson, Zizz, & Sperry (1994)
Dichotic nonsense syllables (simultaneous onset)	dichotic speech test	consonant-vowel combinations (*pa, ta, ka, ba, da, ga*)	50, 60, 70 dB HL	40 per level	Noffsinger, Martinez, & Wilson (1994)
Dichotic nonsense syllables (staggered onset)	dichotic speech test	same as above, but w/ a 90 msec difference in onsets of the CVs	50, 60, 70 dB HL	40 per level	Noffsinger, Martinez, & Wilson (1994)
Dichotic monosyllabic digits	dichotic speech test	digits from 1 to 10, excluding the number 7	50, 60, 70 dB HL	40 per level	Noffsinger, Martinez, & Wilson (1994)
Dichotic synthetic sentences	dichotic speech test	3rd order approximations of English sentences	50, 60, 70 dB HL	40 per level	Noffsinger, Martinez, & Wilson (1994)
Alternated CVC segments[c]	binaural interaction	monosyllabic words segmented into consonant & vowel segments	0, 6, 12, 18, 24, & 30 dB HL	20 per level	Wilson (1994)
Consonant segments[c]	monaural low redundancy	consonant segments	40, 50, 60 dB HL	20 per level	Wilson (1994)
Vowel segments[c]	monaural low redundancy	vowel segments	20, 30, 40 dB HL	20 per level	Wilson (1994)
Binaural NU#6 low and high-pass filtered[d]	binaural interaction	low-pass and high-pass filtered monosyllabic words	0, 6, 12, 18 24, & 30 dB HL	20 per level	Bornstein, Wilson, & Cambron (1994)
NU#6 low-pass filtered[d]	monaural low redundancy	low-pass filtered monosyllabic words	15, 25, 35, 45, 55, & 65 dB HL	20 per level[b]	Bornstein et al. (1994)
NU#6 high-pass filtered[d]	monaural low redundancy	high-pass filtered monosyllabic words	15, 25, 35, 45, 55, & 65 dB HL	20 per level[b]	Bornstein et al. (1994)
NU#6 time compressed	monaural low redundancy	45% time compressed monosyllabic words	5, 15, 25, 35, 45, & 55 dB HL	20 per level[b]	Wilson, Preece, et al. (1994)
NU#6 time compressed w/ reverberation	monaural low redundancy	same as above, but with 0.3 dB reverberation added	same as above	20 per level[b]	Wilson, Preece, et al. (1994)
NU#6 time compressed	monaural low redundancy	65% time compressed monosyllabic words	10, 20, 30, 40, 50, & 60 dB HL	20 per level[b]	Wilson, Preece, et al. (1994)
NU#6 time compressed w/ reverberation	monaural low redundancy	same as above, but with 0.3 dB reverberation added	same as above	20 per level[b]	Wilson, Preece, et al. (1994)
Dichotic chords (simultaneous onset)	dichotic nonspeech test	two three-tone complexes (1 to each ear) & four diotic chords[e]	50, 60, & 70 dB HL	30 per level	Noffsinger, Martinez, Friedrich, & Wilson (1994)

(continued)

TABLE 13.2 Continued

TEST	CLASSIFICATION	STIMULI	LEVEL	SUBJECTS	REFERENCE
Dichotic chords (staggered onset)	dichotic nonspeech test	same as above, but w/ a 90 msec difference in onsets of the chords[e]	50, 60, & 70 dB HL	30 per level	Noffsinger, Martinez, et al. (1994)
Frequency patterns	temporal patterning	three-tone sequences[f]	20 & 50 dB HL	60 per level	Musiek (1994)
Duration patterns	temporal patterning	three-tone sequences[g]	20 & 50 dB HL	60 per level	Musiek (1994)

Source: Adapted with permission from "Speech perception test materials for central auditory processing assessment," by J. A. Baran. In L. Lucks Mendel and J. L. Danhauer (Eds.), *Audiologic Evaluation and Management and Speech Perception Assessment,* 1997. Copyright 1997 by Singular Publishing Group, Inc., San Diego, CA.

[a]Four spondee stimuli are recorded at 16 signal-to-noise ratios varying in 2 dB increments between 0 and –30 dB. Thresholds are established with the spondees and noise in-phase between the ears and with the spondees 180° out-of-phase between the two ears and the noise in-phase. Thresholds are calculated using the Spearman-Karber method (Wilson & Margolis, 1983).

[b]An additional forty subjects were tested at the highest presentation level reported.

[c]The consonant and vowel segments used in the monaural low redundancy tests are the same segmental stimuli used in the alternated CVC segments test.

[d]The low-pass and high-pass stimuli used in the monaural low redundancy tests are the same filtered stimuli used in the binaural NU#6 low and high-pass filtered speech test.

[e]Two chords are presented dichotically followed by the diotic presentation of four chords. The listener's task is to pick the two chords out of the four presented diotically that were perceived under the dichotic presentation. Six different tonal complexes serve as stimuli in this test.

[f]Stimuli consist of tone sequences composed of high (1122 Hz) and low (880 Hz) tones presented in a series of three 150 msec tones. In each stimulus, one of the tones differs in frequency from the other two tones (e.g., HHL, HLL, HLH, LLH, LHH, LHL).

[g]Stimuli consist of tone sequences composed of long (500 msec) and short (250 msec) tones presented in a series of three 1000 Hz tones. In each stimulus one of the tones in the series differs from the other two by being longer of shorter (e.g., LLS, LSS, LSL, SSL, SLL, SLS).

Age, Linguistic, and Cognitive Factors

There are a number of patient variables in addition to presence of a peripheral hearing loss that should be considered whenever one is preparing to administer a central auditory test battery to an individual. Foremost among these variables are the patient's age and his or her linguistic and cognitive capabilities. As mentioned in the discussion on assessment of children who may have central auditory processing disorders, most of the tests that are currently available for clinical use were originally designed to be used in assessing adults with frank neurological involvement. Only later were these tests used to assess CANS function in children who were regarded as learning or language disabled. Since the available evidence suggests that the CANS does not mature until the age of 10 to 11 years (Yakovlev & Lecours, 1967), it is important to select those tests for which age-appropriate norms are available. Tests should be scrutinized to ensure that the items used in the tests are within the child's expected receptive vocabulary and that the child is capable of providing the type of response required by the test.

A number of tests have been designed for use with children, and these tests should be given serious consideration when selecting tests for young children. Four of the tests described earlier in this chapter (rapidly alternating speech perception, binaural fusion, low-pass filtered speech, and competing sentences) are tests included in a battery of tests developed by Willeford (1976) for the express purpose of assessing children with learning problems and have undergone considerable normative study for use with children. There are a number of other tests that have been specifically designed for children that should be given consideration. These include the *Pediatric Speech Intelligibility Test* (Jerger & Jerger, 1984), the *SCAN: A Screening Test for Auditory Processing Disorders* (Keith, 1986), the *SCAN-A: A Screening Test for Adolescents and Adults* (Keith, 1994), the *Selective Auditory Attention Test* (Cherry, 1980), the *Flowers-Costello Test of Central Auditory Abilities* (Flowers, Costello, & Small, 1970), and the *Goldman-Fristoe-Woodcock Auditory Skills Battery* (Goldman, Fristoe, & Woodcock, 1974).

On the other end of the age continuum is the elderly patient who may have significant cognitive deficits and motor disabilities (in addition to peripheral hearing loss) that may limit the applicability of some of the tests discussed in this chapter. Efforts should made to select those tests that are less likely to be affected by general cognitive decline and/or limited motor capabilities if an elderly patient presents with either of these types of disability.

Need for a Test Battery

Few behavioral tests can differentiate brainstem from cerebral lesions when used in isolation. As mentioned earlier, MLDs are primarily a test of caudal brainstem function and are not influenced by lesions of the cortex (Lynn et al., 1981). In addition, the SSI-ICM is reported to be more affected by brainstem than cerebral lesions (Jerger & Jerger, 1974, 1975). Therefore, for patients with good hearing sensitivity and poor scores on either of these two tests the inference is brainstem involvement. Unfortunately, few other behavioral tests offer such clear brainstem/cerebral differentiation. This is due to the fact that the CANS is highly redundant and complex. Therefore, the use of a test battery in the assessment of CANS function is not only prudent, but necessary. Different tests assess different processes. Thus, the utilization of a number of tests is the key to identification of dysfunction in a highly redundant system. Although this chapter has focused on behavioral tests of CANS function, the audiologist engaged in assessment of individuals with potential CANS compromise is encouraged to consider inclusion of one or more of the various electrophysiological tests (auditory brainstem response [ABR], middle late response [MLR], late auditory evoked response [LAER], and auditory cognitive [P3] potential) discussed elsewhere in this text (Chapters 7 and 8) in a given assessment battery as these may help to elucidate the site of lesion or compromise.

The audiologist has a number of tests from which to choose when designing a test battery for a specific patient. It is neither feasible, nor advisable, for an audiologist to administer all tests to all patients, or even the same test battery to all patients. Therefore, the audiologist must be capable of selecting those particular tests (behavioral and/or electrophysiological) that will be most likely to provide documentation of dysfunction in a given patient. Background information, both medical and audiological, may provide insight as to whether a given patient is likely to have a brainstem or cerebral lesion. If this insight is gained, then one can bias his or her battery. If a cerebral lesion is expected or needs to be ruled out, a temporal patterning task (e.g., auditory duration patterns), a dichotic speech test (e.g., dichotic digits), MLR or LAER, and possibly a monaural low-redundancy test (e.g., compressed speech) can be used. If a brainstem lesion is suspected, MLDs and SSI-ICM should be included (also ABR and acoustic reflexes). If the audiologist is unsure of which way to bias the test selection, it is wise for him or her to use some tests from each category.

CONCLUDING REMARKS

There have been a number of significant developments in the field of central auditory assessment since the first central test was administered to patients with CANS compromise in the early 1950s. Our understanding of the neuroanatomy and neurophysiology of the CANS has grown substantially since the time of these early references to the use of central auditory tests in the assessment of the CANS. We are beginning to see some consensus among researchers and clinicians as to what constitutes a central

auditory processing disorder and which test protocols and procedures should be used to assess potential CANS lesions. The recent introduction of a compact disc is expected to further advance the field of central auditory assessment. The fifteen tests contained on the disc have already been subjected to extensive psychometric testing with adults. Similar testing, however, is needed with children and special clinical populations. Additional research is needed to determine the effects of peripheral hearing loss on all central tests and to elucidate what tests are most appropriate for which populations.

REFERENCES

Antonelli, A. (1970). Sensitized speech tests in aged people. In C. Rojskjaer (Ed.), *Speech Audiometry* (pp. 66–77). (2nd Danavox Symposium). Odennse, Denmark: Danavox Foundation.

Antonelli, A., Bellotto, R., & Grandori, F. (1987). Audiologic diagnosis of central versus VIII nerve and cochlear impairment. *Audiology, 26,* 209–226.

American Speech-Language-Hearing Association. (1996). Central auditory processing: Current status and implications for clinical practice. *American Journal of Audiology, 5,* 41–54.

Bakker, D. J., Hoefkens, M., & Van der Vlugt, H. (1979). Hemispheric specialization in children as reflected in the longitudinal development of ear asymmetry. *Cortex, 15,* 619–625.

Baran, J. A. (1997). Speech perception test materials for central auditory processing assessment. In L. Lucks Mendel & J. L. Danhauer (Eds.), *Audiologic Evaluation and Management and Speech Perception Assessment* (pp. 147–168). San Diego: Singular Publishing Group.

Baran, J. A., & Musiek, F. E. (1994). Evaluation of the adult with hearing complaints and normal audiograms. *Audiology Today, 6* (5), 9–11.

Baran, J. A., & Musiek, F. E. (1995). Central auditory processing disorders in children and adults. In L. G. Wall (Ed.), *Hearing for the Speech-Language Pathologist and Health Care Professional* (pp. 415–440). Boston: Butterworth-Heinemann.

Baran, J. A., Musiek, F. E., & Reeves, A. G. (1986). Central auditory function following anterior sectioning of corpus callosum. *Ear and Hearing, 7,* 359–362.

Baran, J. A., Verkest, S., Gollegly, K., Kibble-Michal, K., Rintelmann, W. F., & Musiek, F. E. (1985). *Use of Time-Compressed Speech in the Assessment of Central Nervous System Disorders.* Paper presented to the American Acoustical Society, Nashville.

Beasley, D. S., Forman, B., & Rintelmann, W. F. (1972). Perception of time-compressed CNC monosyllables by normal listeners. *Journal of Auditory Research, 12,* 71–75.

Beasley, D. S., & Maki, J. (1976). Time-and frequency-altered speech. In N. Lass (Ed.), *Contemporary Issues in Experimental Phonetics* (pp. 419–458). New York: Academic Press.

Beasley, D. S., Maki, J., & Orchik, D. (1976). Children's perception of time-compressed speech using two measures of speech discrimination. *Journal of Speech and Hearing Disorders, 41,* 216–225.

Beasley, D. S., Schwimmer, S., & Rintelmann, W. F. (1972). Intelligibility of time-compressed CNC monosyllables. *Journal of Speech and Hearing Research, 15*, 340–350.

Belmont, I., & Handler, A. (1971). Delayed information processing and judgment of temporal order following cerebral damage. *Journal of Nervous and Mental Disease, 152*, 353–361.

Bergman, M. (1971). Hearing and aging: Implications of recent research findings. *Audiology, 10*, 164–171.

Bergman, M. (1980). *Aging and the Perception of Speech*. Baltimore: University Park Press.

Bergman, M., Hirsch, S., Solzi, P., & Mankowitz, Z. (1987). The Threshold-of-Interference Test: A new test of interhemispheric suppression in brain injury. *Ear and Hearing, 8*, 147–150.

Berlin, C. I., Cullen, J., Berlin, H., Tobey, E., & Mouney, D. (1975, November). *Dichotic Listening in a Patient with a Presumed Lesion in the Region of the Medial Geniculate Bodies*. Paper presented at the 90th Meeting of the Acoustical Society of America, San Francisco.

Berlin, C. I., Cullen, J. K., Hughes, L. F., Berlin, J. L., Lowe-Bell, S. S., & Thompson, C. L. (1975). Dichotic processing of speech: Acoustic and phonetic variables. In M. D. Sullivan (Ed.), *Central Auditory Processing Disorders* (pp. 36–46). Proceedings of a Conference at the University of Nebraska Medical Center, Omaha.

Berlin, C. I., Hughes, L. F., Lowe-Bell, S. S., & Berlin, H. L. (1973). Dichotic right ear advantage in children 5–13. *Cortex, 9*, 394–402.

Berlin, C. I., Lowe-Bell, S. S., Jannetta, P. J., & Kline, D. G. (1972). Central auditory deficits after temporal lobectomy. *Archives of Otolaryngology, 96*, 4–10.

Berrick, J. M., Shubow, G. F., Schultz, M. C., Freed, H., Fournier, S. R., & Hughes, J. P. (1984). Auditory processing tests for children: Normative and clinical results on the SSW with children. *Journal of Speech and Hearing Disorders, 49*, 318–325.

Blaettner, U., Scherg, M., & Von Cramon, D. (1989). Diagnosis of unilateral telecephalic hearing disorders: Evaluation of a simple psychoacoustic pattern discrimination test. *Brain, 112*, 177–195.

Bocca, E. (1958). Clinical aspects of cortical deafness. *Laryngoscope, 68*, 301–309.

Bocca, E., & Calearo, C. (1963). Central hearing processes. In J. Jerger (Ed.), *Modern Developments in Audiology* (pp. 337–370). New York: Academic Press.

Bocca, E., Calearo, C., & Cassinari, V. (1954). A new method for testing hearing in temporal lobe tumors. *Acta Otolaryngologica, 42*, 289–304.

Bocca, E., Calearo, C., Cassinari, V., & Migliavacca, F. (1955). Testing "cortical" hearing in temporal lobe tumors. *Acta Otolaryngologica, 42*, 289–304.

Bornstein, S. P., & Musiek, F. E. (1992). Recognition of distorted speech in children with and without learning disabilities. *Journal of the American Academy of Audiology, 3*, 22–32.

Bornstein, S. P., Wilson, R. H., & Cambron, N. K. (1994). Low- and high-pass filtered Northwestern University Auditory Test No. 6 for monaural and binaural evaluation. *Journal of the American Academy of Audiology, 5*, 259–264.

Brody, H. (1955). Organization of cerebral cortex: III. A study of aging in human cerebral cortex. *Journal of Comparative Neurology, 102*, 511–536.

Brunt, M. A. (1978). The staggered spondaic word test. In J. Katz (Ed.), *Handbook of Clinical Audiology* (pp. 334–356). Baltimore: Williams & Wilkins.

Calearo, C., & Antonelli, A. R. (1968). Audiometric findings in brainstem lesions. *Acta Otolaryngologica, 66*, 305–319.

Calearo, C., & Lazzaroni, A. (1957). A speech intelligibility in relation to the speed of the message. *Laryngoscope, 67*, 410–419.

Carmon, A., & Nachshon, I. (1971). Effect of unilateral brain damage on perception of temporal order. *Cortex, 7*, 410–418.

Chermak, G. D., & Musiek, F. E. (1997). *Central Auditory Processing Disorders: New Perspectives*. San Diego: Singular Publishing Group.

Cherry, R. (1980). *Selective Auditory Attention Test (SAAT)*. St. Louis: Auditec.

Cohen, R. L. (1980). Auditory skills and the communicative process. *Seminars in Speech, Language and Hearing, 1*, 197–116.

Cranford, J. L., Morgan, M., Scudder, R., & Moore, C. (1993). Tracing of "moving" fused auditory images by children. *Journal of Speech and Hearing Research, 36*, 424–430.

Damasio, H., & Damasio, A. (1979). Paradoxic ear extinction in dichotic listening: Possible anatomic significance. *Neurology, 29*, 644–653.

Davis, S., & McCroskey, R. I. (1980). Auditory fusion in children. *Child Development, 51*, 75–80.

Dayal, V. S., Tarantino, L., & Swisher, L. P. (1966). Neurootologic studies in multiple sclerosis. *Laryngoscope, 76*, 1798–1809.

Decker, T. N., & Nelson, P. W. (1981). Maturation effects on the synthetic sentence identification-ipsilateral competing message. *Ear and Hearing, 2*, 165–169.

Dempsey, C. (1977). Some thoughts concerning alternate explanations of central auditory test results. In R. W. Keith (Ed.), *Central Auditory Dysfunction* (pp. 293–318). New York: Grune & Stratton.

Dempsey, C. (1983). Selecting tests of auditory function in children. In E. Z. Lasky & J. Katz (Eds.), *Central Auditory Processing Disorders* (pp. 203–222). Baltimore: University Park Press.

de Quiros, J. (1964). Accelerated speech audiometry, an examination of test results. (Translated by J. Tonndorf). *Transactions of the Beltone Institute of Hearing Research, 17*, 48.

DeRenzi, E., Faglioni, P., & Villa, P. (1977). Sequential memory for figures in brain-damaged patients. *Neuropsychologia, 15*, 43–49.

Dermody, P. (1976, April). *Auditory Processing Factors in Dichotic Listening*. Paper presented at the 91st meeting of the Acoustical Society of America, Washington, DC.

Dermody, P., Katsch, R., & Mackie, K. (1983). Auditory processing limitations in low verbal children: Evidence from a two-response dichotic listening task. *Ear and Hearing, 4*, 272–277.

Divenyi, P. L., & Haupt, R. M. (1997a). Audiological correlates of speech understanding in elderly listeners with mild-to-moderate hearing loss. I: Age and lateral asymmetry effects. *Ear and Hearing, 18,* 42–61.

Divenyi, P. L., & Haupt, R. M. (1997b). Audiological correlates of speech understanding in elderly listeners with mild-to-moderate hearing loss. III: Factor representation. *Ear and Hearing, 18,* 189–201.

Divenyi, P. L., & Robinson, A. J. (1989). Nonlinguistic auditory capabilities in aphasia. *Brain and Language, 37,* 290–326.

Durlach, N. I., & Colburn, H. S. (1978). Binaural phenomena. In E. C. Carterette & M. P. Friedman (Eds.), *Handbook of Perception* (Vol. 4, pp. 365–466). New York: Academic Press.

Efron, R. (1985). The central auditory system and issues related to hemispheric specialization. In M. L. Pinheiro & F. E. Musiek (Eds.), *Assessment of Central Auditory Dysfunction: Foundations and Clinical Correlates* (pp. 143–154). Baltimore: Williams & Wilkins.

Efron, R., & Crandall, P. H. (1983). Central auditory processing: Effects of anterior temporal lobectomy. *Brain and Language, 19,* 237–253.

Efron, R., Crandall, P. H., Koss, D., Divenyi, P. L., & Yund, E. W. (1983). Central auditory processing: III. The "Cocktail Party" effect and anterior temporal lobectomy. *Brain and Language, 19,* 254–263.

Efron, R., Dennis, M., & Yund, E. W. (1977). The perception of dichotic chords by hemispherectomized subjects. *Brain and Language, 4,* 537–549.

Efron, R., Yund, E. W., Nichols, D., & Crandall, P. H. (1985). An ear asymmetry for gap detection following anterior temporal lobectomy. *Neuropsychologia, 23,* 43–50.

Fairbanks, G., Everitt, W., & Jaeger, R. (1954). Methods for time or frequency compression-expansion of speech. *Trans IRE-PGA, AU-2,* 7–12.

Farrer, S. M., & Keith, R. W. (1981). Filtered word testing in the assessment of children's central auditory abilities. *Ear and Hearing, 2,* 267–269.

Fifer, R. C., Jerger, J. F., Berlin, C. I., Tobey, E., & Campbell, J. (1983). Development of a dichotic sentence identification test for hearing impaired adults. *Ear and Hearing, 4,* 300–305.

Findlay, R. C., & Schuchman, G. I. (1976). Masking level differences for speech: Effects of ear dominance and age. *Audiology, 15,* 232–241.

Flowers, A., Costello, M., & Small, V. (1970). *The Flowers-Costello Test of Central Auditory Abilities.* Dearborn: MI: Perceptual Learning Systems.

Freeman, B., & Beasley, D. (1976, November). *Performance of Reading-Impaired and Normal Reading Children on Time-Compressed Monosyllabic and Sentential Stimuli.* Paper presented to the American Speech-Language-Hearing Association, Houston.

Gazzaniga, M. S., Risse, G., Springer, S., Clark, E., & Wilson, D. H. (1975). Psychological and neurological consequences of partial and complete commissurotomy. *Neurology, 25,* 10–15.

Gilroy, J., & Lynn, G. E. (1974). Reversibility of abnormal auditory findings in cerebral hemisphere lesions. *Journal of Neurological Sciences, 21,* 117–131.

Goldman, R., Fristoe, M., & Woodcock, R. (1974). *Goldman-Fristoe-Woodcock Auditory Skills Test Battery.* Circle Press, MN: American Guidance Service.

Graham, J., Greenwood, R., & Lecky, B. (1980). Cortical deafness: A case report and review of the literature. *Journal of Neurological Sciences, 48,* 35–49.

Gravel, J. S., & Stapells, D. R. (1993). Behavioral, electrophysiologic and otoacoustic measures from a child with auditory processing dysfunction. *Journal of the American Academy of Audiology, 4,* 412–419.

Green, D. M. (1966). Interaural phase effects in the masking of signals of different durations. *Journal of the Acoustical Society of America, 39,* 720–724.

Grimes, A. M., Mueller, H. G., & Williams, D. L. (1984). Clinical considerations in the use of time-compressed speech. *Ear and Hearing, 5,* 114–117.

Grose, J. H., Hall, J. W., & Gibbs, C. (1993). Temporal analysis in children. *Journal of Speech, Language and Hearing Research, 36,* 351–356.

Hall, J. W., & Grose, J. H. (1990). The masking level difference in children. *Journal of the American Academy of Audiology, 1,* 81–88.

Hall, J. W., & Grose, J. H. (1993). The effects of otitis media with effusion on the masking level difference and the auditory brainstem response. *Journal of Speech and Hearing Research, 36,* 210–217.

Hall, J. W., & Grose, J. H. (1994). The effects of otitis media with effusion on comodulation masking release in children. *Journal of Speech and Hearing Research, 37,* 1441–1449.

Harris, V. L., Keith, R. W., & Novak, K. K. (1983). Relationship between two dichotic listening tests and the token test for children. *Ear and Hearing, 4,* 278–282.

Heilman, K. M., Hammer, L. C., & Wilder, B. J. (1973). An audiometric defect in temporal lobe dysfunction. *Neurology, 23,* 384–386.

Hirsh, I. J. (1948). The influence of interaural phase on interaural summation and inhibition. *Journal of the Acoustical Society of America, 20,* 536–544.

Hiscock, M., & Kinsbourne, M. (1980). Asymmetries of selective listening and attention switching in children. *Developmental Psychology, 16,* 70–82.

Hodgson, W. (1967). Audiological report of a patient with left hemispherectomy. *Journal of Speech and Hearing Disorders, 32,* 39–45.

Hood, L. J., Berlin, C. I., & Allen, P. (1994). Cortical deafness: A longitudinal study. *Journal of the American Academy of Audiology, 5,* 330–342.

Humes, L. E., & Christopherson, L. (1991). Speech identification difficulties of hearing-impaired persons: The contributions of auditory processing deficits. *Journal of Speech and Hearing Research, 34,* 686–693.

Humes, L. E., Coughlin, M., & Talley, L. (1996). Evaluation of the use of a new compact disc for auditory perceptual assessment in the elderly. *Journal of the American Academy of Audiology, 7,* 419–427.

Humes, L. E., Watson, B., Christensen, L., Cokely, C., Halling, D., & Lee, L. (1994). Factors associated with individual differences in clinical measures of speech recognition among the elderly. *Journal of Speech and Hearing Research, 37,* 465–474.

Hurley, R. E., & Musiek, F. E. (1997). Effectiveness of three central auditory processing (CAP) tests in identifying cerebral lesions. *Journal of the American Academy of Audiology, 8,* 257–262.

Hynd, G. W., Cohen, M., & Obrzut, J. E. (1983). Dichotic consonant vowel (CV) testing in the diagnosis of learning disabilities in children. *Ear and Hearing, 4,* 283–286.

Hynd, G. W., & Obrzut, J. E. (1977). Effects of grade level and sex on the magnitude of the dichotic ear advantage. *Neuropsychologia, 15,* 669–692.

Jerger, J. (1960a). Audiological manifestations of lesions in the auditory nervous system. *Laryngoscope, 70,* 417–425.

Jerger, J. (1960b). Observations on auditory behavior in lesions of the central auditory pathways. *Archives of Otolaryngology, 71,* 797–806.

Jerger, J. (1964). Auditory tests for disorders of the central auditory mechanism. In B. R. Alford & W. S. Fields (Eds.), *Neurological Aspects of Auditory and Vestibular Disorders* (pp. 77–86). Springfield, IL: Charles C. Thomas.

Jerger, J. (1973). Diagnostic audiometry. In J. Jerger (Ed.), *Modern Developments in Audiology* (pp. 75–115). New York: Academic Press.

Jerger, J., Alford, B., Lew, H., Rivera, V., & Chmiel, R. (1995). Dichotic listening, event-related potentials, and interhemispheric transfer in the elderly. *Ear and Hearing, 16,* 482–498.

Jerger, J., & Chmiel, R. (1997). Factor analytic structure of auditory impairment in elderly persons. *Journal of the American Academy of Audiology, 8,* 269–276.

Jerger, J., Chmiel, R., Allen, J., & Wilson, A. (1994). Effects of age and gender on Dichotic Sentence Identification. *Ear and Hearing, 15,* 274–286.

Jerger, J., & Hayes, D. (1977). Diagnostic speech audiometry. *Archives of Otolaryngology, 103,* 216–222.

Jerger, J., & Jerger, S. (1971). Diagnostic significance of PB word functions. *Archives of Otolaryngology, 93,* 573–580.

Jerger, J. F., & Jerger, S. W. (1974). Auditory findings in brainstem disorders. *Archives of Otolaryngology, 99,* 342–349.

Jerger, J. F., & Jerger, S. W. (1975). Clinical validity of central auditory tests. *Scandinavian Audiology, 4,* 147–163.

Jerger, J., & Jerger, S. (1981). *Auditory disorders: A manual for clinical evaluation.* Boston: Little & Brown.

Jerger, J., Lovering, L., & Wertz, M. (1972). Auditory disorder following bilateral temporal lobe insult: Report of a case. *Journal of Speech and Hearing Disorders, 37,* 532–535.

Jerger, J., Silman, S., Lew, H., & Chmiel, R. (1993). Case studies in binaural interference: Converging data from behavioral and electrophysiologic measures. *Journal of the American Academy of Audiology, 4,* 122–131.

Jerger, J., Weikers, N. J., Sharbrough, F. W., & Jerger, S. (1969). Bilateral lesions of the temporal lobe: A case study. *Acta Otolaryngologica, 258* (Suppl.), 1–57.

Jerger, S. (1980). Evaluation of central auditory function in children. In R. W. Keith (Ed.), *Central Auditory and Language Disorders in Children* (pp. 30–60). Houston: College-Hill Press.

Jerger, S. (1987). Validation of the pediatric speech intelligibility test in children with central nervous system lesions. *Audiology, 26,* 298–311.

Jerger, S., & Jerger, J. (1984). *The Pediatric Speech Intelligibility Test (PSI).* St. Louis: Auditec.

Jerger, S., Johnson, K., & Loiselle, L. (1988). Pediatric central auditory dysfunction: Comparison of children with confirmed lesions versus suspected processing disorders. *American Journal of Otology, 9* (Suppl.) 63–71.

Karaseva, T. A. (1972). The role of the temporal lobe in human auditory perception. *Neuropsychologia, 10,* 227–231.

Katz, J. (1962). The use of staggered spondaic words for assessing the integrity of the central auditory system. *Journal of Auditory Research, 2,* 327–337.

Katz, J. (1968). The SSW test: An interim report. *Journal of Speech and Hearing Disorders, 33,* 132–146.

Katz, J. (1970). Audiologic diagnosis: Cochlea to cortex. *Menorah Medical Journal, 1,* 25–38.

Katz, J. (1977). The Staggered Spondaic Word test. In R. W. Keith (Ed.), *Central Auditory Dysfunction* (pp. 103–128). New York: Grune & Stratton.

Katz, J., Basil, R. A., & Smith, J. M. (1963). A staggered spondaic word test for detecting central auditory lesions. *Annals of Otology, Rhinology and Laryngology, 72,* 906–917.

Katz, J., & Pack, G. (1975). New developments in differential diagnosis using the SSW test. In M. D. Sullivan (Ed.), *Central Auditory Processing Disorders* (pp. 84–107). Proceedings of a Conference at the University of Nebraska Medical Center, Omaha.

Keith, R. W. (1977). Synthetic sentence identification test. In R. W. Keith (Ed.), *Central Auditory Dysfunction* (pp. 73–102). New York: Grune & Stratton.

Keith, R. W. (1986). *SCAN: A Screening Test for Auditory Processing Disorders.* San Antonio: The Psychological Corporation.

Keith, R. W. (1994). *SCAN-A: Test of Auditory Processing in Adolescents and Adults.* San Antonio: The Psychological Corporation.

Kimura, D. (1961a). Cerebral dominance and the perception of verbal stimuli. *Canadian Journal of Psychology, 15,* 166–171.

Kimura, D. (1961b). Some effects of temporal lobe damage on auditory perception. *Canadian Journal of Psychology, 15,* 157–165.

Kirikae, I., Sato, T., & Shitara, T. (1964). A study of hearing in advanced age. *Laryngoscope, 74,* 205–220.

Konkle, D. F., Beasley, D. S., & Bess, F. (1977). Intelligibility of time-altered speech in relation to chronological aging. *Journal of Speech and Hearing Research, 20,* 108–115.

Koomar, J. A., & Cermak, S. A. (1981). Reliability of dichotic listening using two stimulus formats with normal and learning-disabled children. *American Journal of Occupational Therapy, 35,* 456–463.

Korsan-Bengtsen, M. (1973). Distorted speech audiometry: A methodological and clinical study. *Acta Otolaryngologica* (Stockholm), *310* (Suppl.), 7–75.

Kraft, R. H. (1984). Lateral specialization and verbal/spatial ability in preschool children: Age, sex, and familial handedness differences. *Neuropsychologia, 22*, 319–335.

Kurdziel, S., & Noffsinger, D. (1977, November). *Unusual Time-Staggering Effects via Dichotic Listening with Aged Subjects*. Paper presented at the annual meeting of the American Speech and Hearing Association, Chicago.

Kurdziel, S., Noffsinger, D., & Olsen, W. (1976). Performance by cortical lesion patients on 40% and 60% time-compressed materials. *Journal of American Audiological Society, 2*, 3–7.

Lackner, J., & Teuber, H. L. (1973). Alterations in auditory fusion thresholds after cerebral injury in man. *Neuropsychologia, 11*, 409–415.

Letowski, T., & Poch, N. (1995). Understanding of time-compressed speech by older adults: Effects of discard interval. *Journal of the American Academy of Audiology, 6*, 433–439.

Letowski, T., & Poch, N. (1996). Comprehension of time-compressed speech: Effects of age and speech complexity. *Journal of the American Academy of Audiology, 7*, 447–457.

Lhermitte, F., Chain, F., Escourolle, R., Ducarne, B., Pillou, B., & Chedru, G. (1971). Etude des troubles perceptifs auditifs dans les lesions temporales bilaterales.[Study of the auditory perceptual problems in bilateral temporal lobe lesions]. *Revue Neurologique, 124*, 329–351.

Licklider, J. C. R. (1948). The influence of interaural phase relationships upon the masking of speech by white noise. *Journal of the Acoustical Society of America, 20*, 150–159.

Linden, A. (1964). Distorted speech and binaural speech resynthesis tests. *Acta Otolaryngologica* (Stockholm), *58*, 32–48.

Lynn, G. E., Benitez, J. T., Eisenbrey, A. B., Gilroy, J., & Wilner, H. I. (1972). Neuroaudiological correlates in cerebral hemisphere lesions: Temporal and parietal lobe tumors. *Audiology: Journal of Auditory Communication, 11*, 115–134.

Lynn, G. E., & Gilroy, J. (1971). Auditory manifestations of lesions of the corpus callosum. *Asha, 13*, 566.

Lynn, G. E., & Gilroy, J. (1972). Neuro-audiological abnormalities in patients with temporal lobe tumors. *Journal of Neurological Sciences, 17*, 167–184.

Lynn, G. E., & Gilroy, J. (1975). Effects of brain lesions on the perception of monotic and dichotic speech stimuli. In M. D. Sullivan (Ed.), *Central Auditory Processing Disorders* (pp. 47–83). Proceeding of a Conference at the University of Nebraska, Omaha.

Lynn, G. E., & Gilroy, J. (1976). Central aspects of audition. In J. Northern (Ed.), *Hearing Disorders* (pp. 102–116). Boston: Little & Brown.

Lynn, G. E., & Gilroy, J. (1977). Evaluation of central auditory dysfunction in patients with neurological disorders. In R. W. Keith (Ed.), *Central Auditory Dysfunction* (pp. 177–221). New York: Grune & Stratton.

Lynn, G. E., Gilroy, J., Taylor, P. C., & Leiser, R. P. (1981). Binaural masking-level differences in neurological disorders. *Archives of Otolaryngology, 107*, 357–362.

Manning, W. H., Johnston, K. L., & Beasley, D. S. (1977). The performance of children with auditory perceptual disorders on a time-compressed speech discrimination measure. *Journal of Speech and Hearing Disorders, 42*, 77–84.

Martin, F., & Clark, J. (1977). Audiologic detection of auditory processing disorders in children. *Journal of the American Audiological Society, 3*, 140–146.

Matzker, J. (1959). Two methods for the assessment of central auditory functions in cases of brain disease. *Annals of Otology, Rhinology and Laryngology, 68*, 1155–1197.

McClellen, M., Wertz, R., & Collins, M. (1983, November). *The Effects of Interhemispheric Lesions on Central Auditory Behavior*. Paper presented at the annual meeting of the American Speech-Language-Hearing Association, Detroit.

McCroskey, R., & Kasten, R. (1980). Assessment of central auditory processing. In R. Rupp & K. Stockdell (Eds.), *Speech Protocols in Audiology* (pp. 339–390). New York: Grune & Stratton.

McFadden, D. (1966). Masking-level differences with continuous and with burst masking noise. *Journal of the Acoustical Society of America, 40*, 1414–1419.

McFarland, D. J., & Cacace, A. T. (1995). Modality specificity as a criterion for diagnosing central auditory processing disorders. *American Journal of Audiology: A Journal of Clinical Practice, 4*, 36–48.

Michel, F., Peronnet, F., & Schott, B. (1980). A case of cortical deafness: Clinical and electrophysiological data. *Brain and Language, 10*, 367–377.

Milner, B. (1962). Laterality effects in audition. In V. B. Mountcastle (Ed.). *Interhemispheric Relations and Cerebral Dominance* (pp. 117–195). Baltimore: John Hopkins Press.

Milner, B., Kimura, D., & Taylor, L. B. (1965, April). *Nonverbal Auditory Learning after Frontal or Temporal Lobectomy in Man*. Paper presented at a meeting of the Eastern Psychological Association, Boston, Massachusetts.

Milner, B., Taylor, S., & Sperry, R. (1968). Lateralized suppression of dichotically presented digits after commissural section in man. *Science, 161*, 184–185.

Miltenberger, G., Dawson, G., & Raica, A. (1978). Central auditory testing with peripheral hearing loss. *Archives of Otolaryngology, 104*, 11–15.

Mirabile, P. J., Porter, R. J., Hughes, L. F., & Berlin, C. I. (1978). Dichotic lag effect in children 7–15. *Developmental Psychobiology, 14*, 277–285.

Moore, C. A., Cranford, J. L., & Rahn, A. E. (1990). Tracking of a "moving" fused auditory image under conditions that elicit the precedence effect. *Journal of Speech and Hearing Research, 33*, 141–148.

Morales-Garcia, C., & Poole, J. O. (1972). Masked speech audiometry in central deafness. *Acta Otolaryngologica, 74*, 307–316.

Mueller, H. G., Beck, W. G., & Sedge, R. K. (1987). Comparison of the efficiency of cortical level speech tests. *Seminars in Hearing, 8*, 279–298.

Mueller, H. G., Sedge, R. K., & Salazar, A. M. (1985). Auditory assessment of neural trauma. In M. Miner & K. Wagner (Eds.), *Neural Trauma: Treatment, Monitoring and Rehabilitation Issues* (pp. 155–158). Boston: Butterworth.

Musiek, F. E. (1983a). Assessment of central auditory dysfunction: The dichotic digit test revisited. *Ear and Hearing, 4*, 79–83.

Musiek, F. E. (1983b). Assessment of three dichotic speech tests on subjects with intracranial lesions. *Ear and Hearing, 4*, 318–323.

Musiek, F. E. (1983c). The evaluation of brainstem disorders using ABR and central auditory tests. *Monographs in Contemporary Audiology*, *4*, 1–24.

Musiek, F. E. (1986a). Neuroanatomy, neurophysiology, and central auditory assessment. Part II: The cerebrum. *Ear and Hearing*, *7*, 283–294.

Musiek, F. E. (1986b). Neuroanatomy, neurophysiology, and central auditory assessment. Part III: Corpus callosum and efferent pathways. *Ear and Hearing*, *7*, 349–358.

Musiek, F. E. (1994). Frequency (pitch) and duration pattern tests. *Journal of the American Academy of Audiology*, *5*, 265–268.

Musiek, F. E., & Baran, J. A. (1986). Neuroanatomy, neurophysiology, and central auditory assessment. Part I: Brainstem. *Ear and Hearing*, *7*, 207–219.

Musiek, F. E., & Baran, J. A. (1987). Central auditory assessment: Thirty years of challenge and change. *Ear and Hearing*, *8*, 22S–35S.

Musiek, F. E., & Baran, J. A. (1996). Amplification and the central auditory nervous system. In M. Valente (Ed.), *Hearing Aids: Standards, Options, and Limitations* (pp. 407–438). New York: Thieme Medical Publishers.

Musiek, F. E., Baran, J. A., & Pinheiro, M. L. (1990). Duration pattern recognition in normal subjects and in patients with cerebral and cochlear lesions. *Audiology*, *29*, 304–313.

Musiek, F. E., Baran, J. A., & Pinheiro, M. L. (1994). *Neuroaudiology: Case Studies*. San Diego: Singular Publishing Group, Inc.

Musiek, F. E., & Geurkink, N. A. (1980). Auditory perceptual problems in children: Considerations for the otolaryngologist and audiologist. *Laryngoscope*, *90*, 962–971.

Musiek, F. E., & Geurkink, N. A. (1982). Auditory brainstem response and central auditory test findings for patients with brainstem lesions: A preliminary report. *Laryngoscope*, *92*, 891–900.

Musiek, F. E., Geurkink, N. A., & Keitel, S. (1982). Test battery assessment of auditory perceptual dysfunction in children. *Laryngoscope*, *92*, 251–257.

Musiek, F. E., Gollegly, K. M., & Baran, J. A. (1984). Myelination of the corpus callosum in learning disabled children: Theoretical and clinical correlates. *Seminars in Hearing*, *5*, 231–242.

Musiek, F. E., Gollegly, K. M., Kibbe, K., & Verkest-Lenz, S. (1991). Proposed screening test for central auditory disorders: Follow-up on the dichotic digits test. *American Journal of Otolaryngology*, *12*, 109–113.

Musiek, F. E., Gollegly, K. M., & Ross, M. K. (1985). Profiles of types of central auditory processing disorders in children with learning disabilities. *Journal of Childhood Communication Disorders*, *9*, 43–61.

Musiek, F. E., & Kibbe, K. (1985). An overview of audiological test results in patients with commissurotomy. In A. G. Reeves (Ed.), *Epilepsy and the Corpus Callosum* (pp. 393–399). New York: Plenum Press.

Musiek, F. E., Kibbe, K., & Baran, J. A. (1984). Neuroaudiological results from split-brain patients. *Seminars in Hearing*, *5*, 219–229.

Musiek, F. E., Kurdziel-Schwan, S., Kibbe, K., Gollegly, K. M., Baran, J. A., & Rintelmann, W. F. (1989). The dichotic rhyme test: Results in split brain patients. *Ear and Hearing*, *10*, 33–39.

Musiek, F. E., & Pinheiro, M. L. (1985). Dichotic speech tests in the detection of central auditory dysfunction. In M. L. Pinheiro & F. E. Musiek (Eds.), *Assessment of Central Auditory Dysfunction: Foundations and Clinical Correlates* (pp. 201–218). Baltimore: Williams & Wilkins.

Musiek, F. E., & Pinheiro, M. L. (1986). Effect of peripheral and central auditory lesions on auditory pattern perception. *Journal of the Acoustical Society of America*, *79*, 548.

Musiek, F. E., & Pinheiro, M. L. (1987). Frequency patterns in cochlear, brainstem, and cerebral lesions. *Audiology*, *26*, 79–88.

Musiek, F. E., Pinheiro, M. L., & Wilson, D. H. (1980). Auditory pattern perception in "split-brain" patients. *Archives of Otolaryngology*, *106*, 610–612.

Musiek, F. E., Reeves, A. G., & Baran, J. A. (1985). Release from central auditory competition in the split-brain patient. *Neurology*, *35*, 983–987.

Musiek, F. E., & Wilson, D. H. (1979). SSW and dichotic digit results pre- and post-commissurotomy: A case report. *Journal of Speech and Hearing Disorders*, *44*, 528–533.

Musiek, F. E., Wilson, D. H., & Pinheiro, M. L. (1979). Audiological manifestations in split-brain patients. *Journal of the American Audiological Society*, *5*, 25–29.

Newell, D., & Rugel, R. P. (1981). Hemispheric specialization in normal and disabled readers. *Journal of Learning Disabilities*, *14*, 296–297.

Noffsinger, D. (1982). Clinical applications of selected binaural effects. *Scandinavian Audiology*, *15* (Suppl.), 157–165.

Noffsinger, D., Martinez, C. D., & Andrews, M. (1996). Dichotic listening to speech: VA-CD data from elderly subjects. *Journal of the American Academy of Audiology*, *7*, 49–56.

Noffsinger, D., Martinez, C. D., Friedrich, B. W., & Wilson, R. H. (1994). Dichotic listening to musical chords: Background and preliminary data. *Journal of the American Academy of Audiology*, *5*, 243–247.

Noffsinger, D., Martinez, C. D., & Schaefer, A. (1982). Auditory brainstem responses and masking level differences from persons with brainstem lesions. *Scandinavian Audiology*, *15*, 81–93.

Noffsinger, D., Martinez, C. D., & Wilson, R. H. (1994). Dichotic listening to speech: Background and preliminary data for digits, sentences, and nonsense syllables. *Journal of the American Academy of Audiology*, *5*, 248–254.

Noffsinger, D., Olsen, W. O., Carhart, R., Hart, C. W., & Sahgal, V. (1972). Auditory and vestibular aberrations in multiple sclerosis. *Acta Otolaryngologica*, *303* (Suppl.), 1–63.

Noffsinger D., Wilson, R. H., & Musiek, F. E. (1994). Department of Veterans Affairs compact disc (VA-CD) recording of auditory perceptual assessment: Background and introduction. *Journal of the American Academy of Audiology*, *5*, 231–235.

Nozza, R. J., Wagner, E. F., & Crandell, M. A. (1988). Binaural release for masking for speech sounds in infants, preschoolers, and adults. *Journal of Speech and Hearing Research*, *31*, 212–218.

Olsen, W. O. (1977, November). *Performance of Temporal Lobectomy Patients with Dichotic CV Test Materials*. Paper presented to the American Speech and Hearing Association, Chicago.

Olsen, W. O., Noffsinger, D., & Carhart, R. (1976). Masking level differences encountered in clinical populations. *Audiology*, *15*, 287–301.

Olsen, W. O., Noffsinger, D., & Kurdziel, S. (1975). Speech discrimination in noise by patients with peripheral and central lesions. *Acta Otolaryngologica*, *80*, 375–382.

Orchik, D., & Burgess, T. (1977). Synthetic sentence identification as a function of the age of the listener. *Journal of the American Auditory Society*, *3*, 42–26.

Orchik, D., & Oelschlaeger, M. (1977). Time-compressed speech discrimination in children and its relationship to articulation. *Journal of the American Audiological Society*, *3*, 37–41.

Palva, A., & Jokinen, K. (1975). Unfiltered and filtered speech audiometry in children with normal hearing. *Acta Otolaryngologica*, *80*, 383–388.

Pandya, D., Karol, E., & Heilbornn, D. (1971). The topographical distribution of interhemispheric projections in the corpus callosum of the Rhesus monkey. *Brain Research*, *32*, 31–43.

Papso, C. F., & Blood, I. M. (1989). Word recognition skills of children and adults in background noise. *Ear and Hearing*, *10*, 235–236.

Pengelly, M., Mueller, H. G., & Hill, B. (1982, November). *Masking Level Difference: Effects of High Frequency Hearing Loss and Masking Stimuli*. Paper presented to the American Speech-Language-Hearing Association, Toronto.

Pettit, J. M., & Helms, S. (1979). Hemispheric language dominance of language-disordered, articulation-disordered, and normal children. *Journal of Learning Disabilities*, *12*, 12–17.

Pickles, J. O. (1985). Physiology of the cerebral auditory system. In M. L. Pinheiro & F. E. Musiek (Eds.), *Assessment of Central Auditory Dysfunction: Foundations and Clinical Correlates* (pp. 67–86). Baltimore: Williams and Wilkins.

Pickles, J. O. (1988). *An Introduction to the Physiology of Hearing* (2nd ed.). New York: Academic Press.

Pinheiro, M. L. (1976). Auditory pattern reversal in auditory perception in patients with left and right hemisphere lesions. *Ohio Journal of Speech and Hearing*, *12*, 9–20.

Pinheiro, M. L. (1977). Tests of central auditory function in children with learning disabilities. In R. W. Keith (Ed.), *Central Auditory Dysfunction* (pp. 223–256). New York: Grune & Stratton.

Pinheiro, M. L, Jacobson, G. P., & Boller, F. (1982). Auditory dysfunction following a gunshot wound of the pons. *Journal of Speech and Hearing Disorders*, *47*, 296–300.

Pinheiro, M. L., & Musiek, F. E. (1985). Sequencing and temporal ordering in the auditory system. In M. L. Pinheiro & F. E. Musiek (Eds.), *Assessment of Central Auditory Dysfunction: Foundations and Clinical Correlates* (pp. 219–238). Baltimore: Williams & Wilkins.

Pinheiro, M. L., & Ptacek, P. H. (1971). Reversals in the perception of noise and tone patterns. *Journal of the Acoustical Society of America*, *49*, 1778–1782.

Pinheiro, M. L., & Tobin, H. (1969). Interaural intensity difference for intercranial lateralization. *Journal of the Acoustical Society of America*, *46*, 1482–1487.

Pinheiro, M. L., & Tobin, H. (1971). The interaural intensity difference as a diagnostic indicator. *Acta Otolaryngologica* (Stockholm), *71*, 326–328.

Pinheiro, M. L., Weidner, W. E., Suren, S. M., & Gaydos, M. L. (1977, October). *Sequencing of Pitch Patterns with Competing Music and Competing Discourse by Patients with Right and Left Hemisphere Lesions*. Paper presented at the meeting of the Academy of Aphasia, Montreal.

Plakke, B. L., Orchik, D. J., & Beasley, D. S. (1981). Children's performance on a binaural fusion task. *Journal of Speech and Hearing Research*, *24*, 520–535.

Ptacek, P. H., & Pinheiro, M. L. (1971). Pattern reversal in auditory perception. *Journal of the Acoustical Society of America*, *49*, 493–498.

Protti, E. (1983). Brainstem auditory pathways and auditory processing disorders: Diagnostic implications of subjective and objective tests. In E. Z. Lasky & J. Katz (Eds.), *Central Auditory Processing Disorders* (pp. 117–140). Baltimore: University Park Press.

Protti, E., & Young, M. (1980). The evaluation of a child with auditory perceptual deficiencies: An interdisciplinary approach. *Seminars in Speech, Language and Hearing*, *1*, 167–180.

Quaranta, A., & Cervellera, G. (1977). Masking level differences in central nervous system diseases. *Archives of Otolaryngology*, *103*, 483–484.

Riccio, C. A., Hynd, G. W., Cohen, M. J., & Molt, L. (1996). The Staggered Spondaic Word Test: Performance of children with attention-deficit hyperactivity disorder. *Journal of the American Academy of Audiology*, *5*, 55–62.

Rintelmann, W. F. (1985). Monaural speech tests in the detection of central auditory disorders. In M. L. Pinheiro & F. E. Musiek (Eds.), *Assessment of Central Auditory Dysfunction: Foundations and Clinical Correlates* (pp. 173–200). Baltimore: Williams & Wilkins.

Rintelmann, W. F., Beasley, D., & Lynn, G. E. (1974, April). *Time-Compressed CNC Monosyllables: Case Findings in Central Auditory Disorders*. Paper presented to the Michigan Speech and Hearing Association, Detroit.

Rintelmann, W. F., & Lynn, G. E. (1983). Speech stimuli for assessment of central auditory disorders. In D. Konkle & W. F. Rintelmann (Eds.), *Principles of Speech Audiometry* (pp. 231–284). Baltimore: University Park Press.

Roeser, R., Johns, D., & Price, L. (1976). Dichotic listening in adults with sensorineural hearing loss. *Journal of the American Audiological Society*, *2*, 19–25.

Roeser, R. J., Millay, K. K., & Morrow, J. M. (1983). Dichotic consonant-vowel (CV) perception in normal and learning-impaired children. *Ear and Hearing*, *4*, 293–299.

Rosenzweig, M. (1951). Representation of the two ears at the auditory cortex. *American Journal of Physiology*, *165*, 147–158.

Roush, J., & Tait, C. A. (1984). Binaural fusion, masking level differences, and auditory brain stem responses in children with language-learning disabilities. *Ear and Hearing*, *5*, 37–41.

Ruebens, A., Froehling, B., Slater, G., & Anderson, D. (1985). Left ear suppression on verbal dichotic tests in patients with multiple sclerosis. *Annals of Neurology*, *18*, 459–463.

Rupp, R. R. (1983). Establishing norms for speech-in-noise skills for children. *Hearing Journal, 36,* 16–19.

Sanchez-Longo, L. P., & Forster, F. M. (1958). Clinical significance of impairment of sound localization. *Neurology, 8,* 1191–1225.

Sanchez-Longo, L. P., Forster, F. M., & Auth, T. L. (1957). A clinical test for sound localization and its applications. *Neurology, 7,* 653–655.

Saunders, G. H., & Haggard, M. P. (1989). The clinical assessment of obscure auditory dysfunction. *Ear and Hearing, 10,* 200–208.

Schmitt, J. F. (1983). The effects of time compression and time expansion on passage comprehension by elderly listeners. *Journal of Speech and Hearing Research, 26,* 373–377.

Schuknecht, H. F. (1964). Further observations on the pathology of presbycusis. *Archives of Otolaryngology, 80,* 369–382.

Schuknecht, H. F. (1974). *Pathology of the Ear.* Cambridge, MA: Harvard University Press.

Schum, D. J., & Matthews, L. J. (1992). SPIN test performance of elderly hearing-impaired listeners. *Journal of the American Academy of Audiology, 3,* 303–307.

Sedge, R. K., Mueller, H. G., & Dillon, J. D. (1982, November). *Dichotic Digit and CV Results for Individuals with Head Injuries.* Paper presented at the annual meeting of the American Speech-Language-Hearing Association, Toronto.

Seltzer, B., & Pandya, D. N. (1978). Afferent cortical connections and architectonics of the superior temporal sulcus and surrounding cortex in the Rhesus monkey. *Brain Research, 149,* 1–24.

Shankweiler, D. (1966). Effects of temporal lobe damage on perception of dichotically presented melodies. *Journal of Comparative and Physiological Psychology, 62,* 115–119.

Sidtis, J. (1982). Predicting brain organization from dichotic listening performance: Cortical and subcortical functional asymmetries contribute to perceptual asymmetries. *Brain and Language, 17,* 287–300.

Sinha, S. O. (1959). The role of the temporal lobe in hearing. Unpublished master's thesis, McGill University, Montreal, Quebec.

Smith, B. B., & Resnick, D. M. (1972). An auditory test for assessing brain stem integrity: Preliminary report. *Laryngoscope, 82,* 414–424.

Smith, B. H., & Sethi, P. H. (1975). Aging and the nervous system. *Geriatrics, 30,* 109–115.

Sommers, R. K., & Taylor, M. L. (1972). Cerebral speech dominance in language-disordered and normal children. *Cortex, 4,* 3–16.

Sparks, R., & Geschwind, N. (1968). Dichotic listening in man after section of the neocortical commissures. *Cortex, 4,* 3–16.

Sparks, R., Goodglass, H., & Nichel, B. (1970). Ipsilateral versus contralateral extinction in dichotic listening resulting from hemisphere lesions. *Cortex, 6,* 249–260.

Speaks, C., Gray, T., Miller, J., & Rubens, A. (1975). Central auditory deficits and temporal lobe lesions. *Journal of Speech and Hearing Disorders, 40,* 192–205.

Speaks, C., Niccum, N., & Van Tasell, D. (1985). Effects of stimulus material on the dichotic listening performance of patients with sensorineural hearing loss. *Journal of Speech and Hearing Research, 18,* 16–25.

Springer, S. P., & Gazzaniga, M. S. (1975). Dichotic testing of partial and complete split-brain patients. *Neuropsychologia, 13,* 341–346.

Springer, S. P., Sidtis, J., Wilson, D. H., & Gazzaniga, M. S. (1978). Left ear performance in dichotic listening following commissurotomy. *Neuropsychologia, 16,* 305–312.

Stephens, S., & Thornton, A. (1976). Subjective and electrophysiologic tests in brainstem lesions. *Archives of Otolaryngology, 102,* 608–613.

Sticht, T. G., & Gray, B. B. (1969). The intelligibility of time-compressed words as a function of age and hearing loss. *Journal of Speech and Hearing Disorders, 12,* 443–448.

Sweitzer, R. (1977). Team evaluation of auditory perceptually-handicapped children. In R. W. Keith (Ed.), *Central Auditory Dysfunction* (pp. 341–360). New York: Grune & Stratton.

Swisher, L., & Hirsh, I. J. (1972). Brain damage and the ordering of two temporally successive stimuli. *Neuropsychologia, 10,* 137–152.

Tallal, P., Miller, S., Bedi, G., Byma, G., Wang, X., Nagarajan, S. S., Schreiner, C., Jenkins, W. M., & Merzenich, M. H. (1996). Language comprehension in language-learning impaired children improved with acoustically modified speech, *Science, 271,* 81–84.

Tallal, P., Miller, S., & Fitch, R. (1993). Neurobiological basis of speech: A case for the preeminence of temporal processing. In P. Tallal, A. Galaburda, R. Llinas, & C. von Euler (Eds.), *Temporal Information Processing in the Nervous System* (pp. 27–37). New York: New York Academy of Sciences.

Tillman, T. N., Carhart, R., & Nicholls, S. (1973). Release from multiple maskers in elderly persons. *Journal of Speech and Hearing Research, 16,* 152–160.

Tobey, E. A., Cullen, J. K., & Rampp, D. L. (1979). Effects of stimulus-onset asynchrony on the dichotic performance of children with auditory-processing disorders. *Journal of Speech and Hearing Research, 22,* 197–211.

Tobin, H. (1985). Binaural interaction tasks. In M. L. Pinheiro & F. E. Musiek (Eds.), *Assessment of Central Auditory Dysfunction: Foundations and Clinical Correlates* (pp. 155–172). Baltimore: Williams & Wilkins.

Townsend, T. H., & Goldstein, D. P. (1972). Supra-threshold binaural unmasking. *Journal of the Acoustical Society of America, 51,* 621–624.

van Rooij, J., & Plomp, R. (1990). Auditive and cognitive factors in speech perception by elderly listeners. II: Multivariate analyses. *Journal of the Acoustical Society of America, 88,* 2611–2624.

Visto, J. C., Cranford, J. L., & Scudder, R. (1996). Dynamic temporal processing of nonspeech acoustic information by children with specific language impairment. *Journal of Speech and Hearing Disorders, 39,* 510–517.

Welsh, L. W., Welsh, J. J., & Healy, M. (1980). Central auditory testing and dyslexia. *Laryngoscope, 90,* 972–984.

Welsh, L. W., Welsh, J. J., Healy, M., & Cooper, B. (1982). Cortical, subcortical, and brainstem dysfunction: A correlation in dyslexic children. *Annals of Otology, Rhinology and Laryngology, 91,* 310–315.

Wexler, B., & Halwes, T. (1983). Increasing the power of dichotic methods: The fused rhymed words test. *Neuropsychologia, 21,* 59–66.

White, E. (1977). Children's performance on the SSW test and Willeford Battery: Interim clinical report. In R. W. Keith (Ed.), *Central Auditory Dysfunction* (pp. 319–340). New York: Grune & Stratton.

Willeford, J. (1976). Differential diagnosis of central auditory dysfunction. In L. Bradford (Ed.), *Audiology: An Audio Journal for Continuing Education* (Vol. 2). New York: Grune & Stratton.

Willeford, J. (1977a). Assessing central auditory behavior in children: A test battery approach. In R. W. Keith (Ed.), *Central Auditory Dysfunction* (pp. 43–72). New York: Grune & Stratton.

Willeford, J. (1977b). Evaluation of central auditory disorders in learning disabled children. In L. Bradford (Ed.), *Learning Disabilities: An Audio Journal for Continuing Education* (Vol. 1). New York: Grune & Stratton.

Willeford, J. (1978). Sentence tests of central auditory function. In J. Katz (Ed.), *Handbook of Clinical Audiology* (2nd ed., pp. 252–261). Baltimore: Williams & Wilkins.

Willeford, J. (1980). Central auditory behaviors in learning disabled children. *Seminars in Speech, Language and Hearing, 1,* 127–140.

Willeford, J. A., & Billger, J. A. (1978). Auditory perception in children with learning disabilities. In J. Katz (Ed.), *Handbook of Clinical Audiology* (2nd ed.) (pp. 410–425). Baltimore: Williams & Wilkins.

Willeford, J. A., & Burleigh, J. M. (1985). *Handbook of Central Auditory Processing Disorders in Children*. New York: Grune & Stratton.

Wilson, R. H. (1994). Word recognition with segmented-alternated CVC words: Compact disc trials. *Journal of the American Academy of Audiology, 5,* 255–258.

Wilson, R. H., & Margolis, R. H. (1983). Measurement of auditory thresholds for speech stimuli. In D. F. Konkle & W. F. Rintelmann (Eds.), *Principles of Speech Audiometry* (pp. 79–126). Baltimore: University Park Press.

Wilson, R. H., Preece, J. P., Salomon, D. L., Sperry, J. L., & Bornstein, S. P. (1994). Effects of time compression plus reverberation on the intelligibility of Northwestern Auditory Test No. 6. *Journal of the American Academy of Audiology, 5,* 269–277.

Wilson, R. H., Zizz, C. A., & Sperry, J. L. (1994). Masking-level difference for spondaic words in 2000-msec bursts of broadband noise. *Journal of the American Academy of Audiology, 5,* 236–242.

Witelson, D. R., & Rabinovitch, M. S. (1972). Hemispheric speech lateralization in children with auditory-linguistic deficits. *Cortex, 8,* 412–424.

Yakovlev, P. I., & Lecours, A. R. (1967). Myelogenetic cycles of regional maturation of the brain. In A. Minkiniwski (Ed.), *Regional Development of the Brain in Early Life* (pp. 3–70). Oxford: Blackwell Press.

Young, M. (1983). Neuroscience, pragmatic competence, and auditory processing. In E. Z. Lasky & J. Katz (Eds.), *Central Auditory Processing Disorders* (pp. 141–162). Baltimore: University Park Press.

Zurif, E. B., & Ramier, A. M. (1972). Some effects of unilateral brain damage on the perception of dichotically presented phoneme sequences and digits. *Neuropsychologia, 10,* 103–110.

CHAPTER 14

PSEUDOHYPACUSIS

WILLIAM F. RINTELMANN
SABINA A. SCHWAN

Most children and adults who are examined by an audiologist or an otologist for a complaint of hearing loss have bona fide disorders of the auditory mechanism that typically require some type of medical treatment, including surgery, and/or audiological management, that is, the need for a hearing aid. The preceding chapters have dealt with various aspects of the assessment of hearing based on the assumption that the patient seen by the clinician has an organic disorder that can account for the behavioral symptoms and auditory test results observed. The focus of this chapter, however, is on the child or adult who exhibits a hearing loss in some fashion, but where there is no physical (organic) basis for the hearing disorder displayed.

In this chapter we will consider the problems of terminology, incidence/prevalence, etiological factors, emotional and psychosocial characteristics, and behavioral manifestations related to the disorder in both children and adults. The primary focus of the chapter concerns the detection and assessment of pseudohypacusis via both conventional and special audiologic tests. These include both behavioral and electrophysiological measures for assessing auditory function. Finally, some discussion is concerned with the management of the problem, especially related to children.

TERMINOLOGY

There is no universally accepted term to describe a hearing loss that cannot be attributed to an organic defect. The terms *nonorganic*, *functional*, and *pseudohypacusis* are commonly used descriptors of this problem without specifically implying whether the origin of this problem is on a conscious or unconscious basis. If the individual (child or adult) purposely is exhibiting symptoms of impaired hearing, the problem often is labeled *malingering*, *feigning*, or is sometimes called *simulated hearing loss*. If, however, the origin of the problem is on an unconscious level, the disorder is termed *hysterical*, *psychogenic*, or *conversion* hearing loss or deafness. These latter terms imply that the patient has a severe emotional disorder resulting from psychological conflict or need (Chodoff & Lyons, 1958; Wolf, Birger, Shoshan, & Kronenberg, 1993). Denying the ability to hear on an unconscious level serves as a "defense mechanism" to avoid resolving the primary emotional conflict.

Some early writers (i.e., Fournier, 1958; Portmann & Portmann, 1961) have stressed the importance of distinguishing between psychogenic deafness and malingering; however, there seems to be general agreement (i.e., Hopkinson, 1973; Kinstler, 1971; Martin, 1994) that it is not the role of audiologists to attempt to determine whether a nonorganic hearing loss is on a conscious or unconscious basis. In fact, there simply are no tests within the audiologist's armamentarium to help make such a distinction.

Goldstein (1966) questioned the validity of psychogenic hearing loss as a clinical entity. He proposed certain criteria that he felt must be met to satisfy the definition of psychogenic hearing loss. Specifically, he felt it is necessary to demonstrate that the patient responds to weaker sounds during electrophysiologic audiometry or under hypnosis than via behavioral audiometry. Also, he stated that the patient's auditory behavior should be consistent between the test situation and his or her daily life activities. Finally, Goldstein argued that a diagnosis of psychogenic deafness can be made only if better auditory sensitivity is displayed behaviorally under all circumstances following successful psychiatric or psychologic therapy or after spontaneous remission of the emotional problem. In short, Goldstein concluded that all cases of nonorganic hearing loss are aware of their simulation, and hence are malingering. He added, however, that feigning probably has a psychogenic basis even when the motive may be related to potential monetary gain.

Hopkinson (1967) and Ventry (1968) disagreed with Goldstein's criteria for "validating" psychogenic hearing loss. Also, Ventry (1968) objected to Goldstein's thesis that such a clinical entity does not exist, and he reported on a case of a veteran with a unilateral psychogenic loss. More recently, while acknowledging that conversion hearing loss is very rarely encountered and difficult to distinguish from malingering, Wolf and colleagues (1993) reported on two adult cases of conversion deafness resulting from different traumatic experiences. Also, Spraggs, Burton, and Graham (1994) reported on 5 patients who were identified as pseudohypacusic via electrophysiological methods (electrocochleography, auditory brainstem response, and cortical evoked response audiometry) while undergoing assessment for cochlear implants. All 5 patients were referred for psychological counseling and none were candidates for cochlear implants. Thus, there is some disagreement among experts on whether malingering can be distinguished from psychogenic hearing loss or even if the latter entity exists. More importantly, however, some clinicians, including these writers, contend that audiologists need not be concerned with this question, but rather, should focus on accurately assessing the organic status of the patient's hearing so that appropriate referral and management can be initiated. This topic is considered later in this chapter.

The use of labels like "malingering," "feigning," and "simulation" imply that the patient is willfully lying, and hence, is dishonest. Such terms, therefore, simply should not be used. If an audiologist has occasion to give "medicolegal" testimony, he or she may state that the patient's test results are discrepant or inconsistent without labeling the patient as a "malingerer." Furthermore, such reports should include as accurate an estimate as possible about the patient's organic hearing threshold level.

The terms "nonorganic," "functional," and "pseudohypacusis" encompass both malingering and psychogenic hearing loss; therefore, use of one of these generic terms is preferable since they avoid the issue of deciding whether the professed hearing loss is on a conscious or unconscious basis. Some writers (i.e., Martin, 1972) prefer the term "nonorganic" because it is immediately clear that the only inference made concerns the organic status of the hearing mechanism. On the other hand, advocates of the term "functional" (Hopkinson, 1973; Ventry & Chaiklin, 1962) point out that the term nonorganic does not provide for the possibility that an actual organic disorder simply has escaped audiologic or otologic identification. Those who prefer the term "functional" stress that in medicine, a functional disease is one in which the organ is not functioning appropriately even though the organ shows no evidence of structural alteration or pathology.

The term "pseudohypoacusis" also has several proponents. This word was modified by Carhart (1961) from "pseudo neural hypacusis" employed by Brockman and Hoversten (1960) and was subsequently used by Rintelmann and Harford (1963). Goldstein (1966) too preferred the use of this term, but slightly shortened to "pseudohypacusis." The abovementioned writers advocated use of this term because it clearly signifies the condition of a false (pseudo) less than normal auditory sensitivity (hypoacusis or hypacusis). In recent years, the term pseudohypacusis has gained in popularity as evidenced by its use by writers who previously preferred the terms nonorganic or functional (e.g., Martin, 1994). The term "pseudohypacusis" will be used primarily for the remainder of this chapter.

It also should be mentioned that some patients may exhibit an "exaggerated overlay" to an actual organic defect. Such cases also must be considered as pseudohypacusic in that they present the same basic problem of auditory assessment to the audiologist and the otologist.

INCIDENCE/PREVALENCE AND ETIOLOGICAL FACTORS

Both "incidence" and "prevalence" are terms used to describe the frequency of occurrence of a particular condition or disorder, but they are not synonymous terms. "Incidence is the number of new occurrences of a condition in a population within a specified time period [whereas] prevalence refers to the total number of cases in a population at, or during, a specified period of time" (Moscicki, 1984, p. 39). The only definitive statement that can be made concerning the incidence or prevalence of pseudohypacusis is that it is highly variable depending upon the population being examined (Altschuler, 1982; Barrs, Althoff, Krueger, & Olsson, 1994; Coles & Mason, 1984; Rickards & De Vidi, 1995; Sulkowski, Sliwinska-Kowalska, Kowalska, & Bazydlo-Golinska, 1994). Further, incidence and prevalence are closely linked to potential causative factors. Hence, these two topics will be discussed together.

A review of the literature on this topic strongly suggests that the highest prevalence figures have been reported in those special populations of adults in which *decibels of hearing loss could be translated into dollars of compensation*. For example, Johnson, Work, and McCoy (1956) reported that the prevalence of nonorganic problems among veterans examined for service-connected hearing loss increased from 10 to 15% to nearly 50% in the ten-year period following World War II. This tremendous increase in pseudohypacusic cases was attributed to essentially three factors: (1) changing the method of compensation from a single lump-sum award to a monthly payment, (2) use of crude hearing tests (i.e., conversation voice) as a basis for verifying the hearing loss, and (3) inadequate counseling when the hearing loss was initially discovered. In contrast, a prevalence figure for the total 1978 patient population of the Walter Reed Hospital, Audiology and Speech Center was reported as 48 pseudohypacusic cases, or 1.74%, from a total of 2765 patients (D. Schwartz, personal communication, January, 1979). Ten years later, in 1988, the prevalence of pseudohypacusis among active duty and retired military personnel who received audiologic evaluations at the Walter Reed Hospital was 1.4% (32 of 2329 persons tested). In contrast, the prevalence of pseudohypacusis during the late 1980s on Army posts among basic trainees and soldiers in combat arms units was *estimated* to be approximately 4 to 5% (R. Atack, personal communication, January, 1989). However, although records typically are not kept concerning the prevalence of pseudohypacusis in the veterans population, the clinical impression of the audiologist queried at one Michigan VA

Audiology center is that there has been a substantial reduction in the number of pseudohypacusic cases in the past three decades, 1968–1997 (G. Peters, personal communication, April, 1997). One reason given for the reduced prevalence of pseudohypacusis since the 1980s in the military and veterans populations is that longitudinal audiologic records are kept for most military personnel; hence, the existence of such detailed "hearing health histories" makes it difficult to suddenly simulate a hearing loss.

Furthermore, undoubtedly, the increased sophistication of "modern audiology" in terms of instrumentation, available tests, and training and experience of personnel has contributed substantially to a significant reduction in the prevalence of this problem during the past three decades.

Another concern is the prevalence of pseudohypacusis among some industrial workers who are exposed to high noise levels. Since the enactment of the Occupational Safety and Health Act of 1970 there has been an increasing awareness by the general public concerning the deleterious effects of prolonged exposure to high noise levels. Although this is a legitimate societal concern, the possibility of industrial workers receiving compensation for job-connected hearing loss clearly provides some individuals with the motivation for either feigning a hearing loss or attempting to exaggerate the degree of a bona fide hearing loss (Armbruster, 1982; Coles & Mason, 1984). To illustrate, Barelli and Ruder (1970) obtained data on 162 medico-legal cases and reported that 24% of the 116 workers who had applied for compensation were found to have a nonorganic hearing loss. In another study, Gosztonyi, Vassallo, and Sataloff (1971) reported on the reliability of manual and self-recording audiometric tests of 100 employees in a heavy industry. They found reliable audiometric results from all of the 50 salaried (office) personnel, whereas unreliable and hence invalid audiograms were obtained from 17 (34%) of the hourly (shop) workers. Commenting on the unreliable audiometric results, Gosztonyi and colleagues stated, "15 were later found to be compensation cases. The unreliable audiograms were deliberate and could be called malingering. In certain instances we also found that workers in relatively quiet departments of the plant were being influenced to complain of hearing loss and file for compensation" (1971, p. 117). Harris (1979) discussed the problem of nonorganic hearing loss in industry and described how to identify the potential "malingerer" both before and during audiometric testing. He suggested methods of documenting invalid hearing tests among industrial workers and stressed the importance of early detection for immediate resolution of the problem. Hence, the potential motivation for pseudohypacusis based on the opportunity for a monetary award may be a serious problem in industrial hearing conservation programs. Conversely, in a more recent study of 246 workers who underwent otologic and audiologic testing as part of a worker's compensation claim

for noise-induced work-related hearing loss, only 9% demonstrated pseudohypacusis, indicating that the incidence of pseudohypacusis in this particular population was fairly low (Barrs et. al., 1994).

Estimates of the prevalence of pseudohypacusis in the general adult population are substantially less than in the two special populations (veterans and industrial workers) briefly discussed above. Although most of these prevalence figures are based on somewhat vague estimates, nevertheless, one can obtain a general notion of the magnitude of the problem. For example, Kinstler (1971) reported on a brief survey made in one large western city. He stated that in two otologic groups with large diagnostic caseloads and sizable surgical practices both groups reported a prevalence of under 2%. Kinstler also stated that one otolaryngologist surveyed had many patients who were involved in medico-legal litigation related to traumatic or noise-induced hearing loss. Estimates of pseudohypacusis among these patients was between 5 and 10%. As Kinstler pointed out, the number of functional loss cases will vary in relationship to the proportion of medico-legal cases in the otologists' practice.

Although there is a dearth of prevalence data on adult pseudohypacusis seen in audiology clinics, a survey conducted in 1951 of 30 audiology centers in the United States reported that the percentage of pseudohypacusic civilians "was 0 in 16 of the centers, less than 5 in 11 of the centers, and 5 or more in only 3 of the centers" (Zwislocki, 1963, cited by Hopkinson, 1973, p. 178). Based on the present writers' experience both in university, hospital-based, and private audiology practices over a period of several years, a prevalence figure of less than 2% in the general adult population (excluding large concentrations of medico-legal cases) appears to be a reasonable estimate for the late 1990s.

The prevalence of pseudohypacusis among children also is difficult to ascertain, again, because there are few solid data upon which to base an accurate estimate. Most of the reports involving children simply state the number of cases seen without relating these numbers to the total patient population for a given period of time. A few early reports, however, provide some limited clues regarding prevalence figures. The 1951 survey of 30 audiology centers mentioned above (Zwislocki, 1963, cited by Hopkinson, 1973) also attempted to determine the prevalence of pseudohypacusis in children. A negligible percentage was reported by 22 centers with 6 centers stating less than 5% and only 2 centers reporting more than 5%. Specific prevalence figures collected by Campanelli (1963) for one audiology center revealed that during a twelve-month period 41 school children, or 1.7%, from a total caseload of 2300 demonstrated significant "simulated" hearing losses. This sample of children ranged in age from 6 to 17 years, with a mean age of 10.9 years. These children were referred by audiologists and school nurses from school hearing screening programs.

Clearly, the prevalence of pseudohypacusis among both children and adults in the typical patient population seen for audiologic and otologic evaluation is not nearly as great as it is among those special populations in which there is an opportunity to receive direct compensation for a job-related hearing loss. It should be noted, however, that no recent prevalence figures have been reported in the literature for pseudohypacusis in either children or adult populations.

Accidents, not necessarily related to job performance, also can be causative factors resulting in pseudohypacusis. For example, if a patient is sent for a hearing evaluation by his (her) attorney because the client (patient) is involved in a suit over an automobile accident in which he (she) allegedly received a traumatic hearing loss, the audiologist should at least consider the possibility of pseudohypacusis. One of us (W. F. R.) recalls a case in which the patient, claiming a severe bilateral hearing loss as a consequence of an auto accident, arrived at our hearing clinic wearing binaural hearing aids. Subsequently, the battery of audiological tests administered to this patient demonstrated normal hearing in both ears.

Motivation or possible etiological factors among children exhibiting pseudohypacusis, too, are based on the possibility of a "reward," in a sense. Contrary to the adult pseudohypacusic where the sought after gain is often monetary, the reward for children may be for various psychological purposes. Based on several reports in the literature (Barr, 1963; Berger, 1965; Brockman & Hoversten, 1960; Dixon & Newby, 1959; Lehrer, Hirschenfang, Miller, & Radpour, 1964; McCanna & De Lapa, 1981; Rintelmann & Harford, 1963), one of the more common causes among school-age children for exhibiting pseudohypacusis is that a hearing loss serves as an acceptable reason for both parents and teachers to account for poor academic performance. Often such children have failed school hearing screening tests and have a history of middle ear disorders, which initially provide the excuse for poor performance in school. After the middle ear problem has been resolved, and if the academic performance does not improve, some children resort to simulating a hearing loss, probably in an effort to continue to have an excuse for their less than satisfactory school performance. A few children even exhibited nonorganic visual problems in addition to pseudohypacusis (Berger, 1965; Dixon & Newby, 1959; Lumio, Jauhiainen, & Gelhar, 1969; Rintelmann & Harford, 1963).

Another possible factor that can contribute to the display of pseudohypacusis in children, according to several investigators including those mentioned above, is the child's need to gain attention. This can be expressed in various ways, such as aggressive behavior at school, strong sibling rivalry at home, or other forms of manifesting social conflict (Aplin & Rowson, 1986; Lumio et al., 1969). Broad (1980) also reported that another cause of pseudohypacusis in children involves a poor self-image.

A typical pattern for the onset of pseudohypacusis in children found by Rintelmann and Harford (1963) is that the child often initially fails a hearing screening test in school. Such failure may be due to an actual hearing loss, or some children with normal hearing may fail a screening test for various reasons (i.e., poor acoustic environment, audiometers improperly calibrated, etc.) The child may next fail a second screening or pure-tone threshold test and subsequently be referred for an otological examination. The child may then be referred to an audiologist, sometimes with the suspicion of pseudohypacusis, but also sometimes for a hearing aid evaluation. Often, by the time the child arrives for a examination at an audiology center, he (she) has exhibited a hearing loss on two or three tests in a period of a few weeks or months. Thus, the pattern has been established for the child to demonstrate a hearing loss in the test situation. Further, if the child has already recognized that a hearing loss may provide certain benefits (i.e., an excuse for poor academic performance), he (she) may be quite committed to continuing to show a hearing loss.

Thus, it appears that pseudohypacusis in both adults and children can be attributed to some form of gain that may be derived from the hearing loss. The motivating factor for pseudohypacusis in adults often can be directly related to potential monetary gain resulting from the hearing loss. Among children the causative factors usually are less obvious, but typically can be traced to some form of psychological gain (i.e., providing a reason [excuse] for poor school achievement), or serving as a means for getting attention and affection.

It is important that the detection and assessment of pseudohypacusis be accomplished, if possible, before the adult or child becomes strongly committed to exhibiting a hearing loss. For children especially, it is critical to identify incorrect responses to hearing tests before the child has the chance to recognize that a hearing loss may provide various types of secondary gains such as those discussed above.

EMOTIONAL AND PSYCHOSOCIAL CHARACTERISTICS

Whether pseudohypacusis is displayed on a conscious or an unconscious basis, clearly in either case the child or adult is exhibiting behavior that deviates to some extent from "normal." In the preceding discussion, it was pointed out that the causative factors can be almost always related to some form of monetary or psychological gain. Pseudohypacusic children may use their alleged hearing loss to gain attention, to excuse poor school performance, or to provide a means of expressing hostility at home or in other social environments. By the very nature of the problem of pseudohypacusis, adults too are exhibiting deviant social behavior. One may then ask: "Are there certain emotional problems or personality characteristics that may be associated with pseudohypacusis?"

Some investigators have reported that pseudohypacusic children often have serious emotional problems (Aplin & Rowson, 1986; Barr, 1963; Berk & Feldman, 1958; Broad, 1980; Brooks & Geoghegan, 1992; Dixon & Newby, 1959). Lehrer and colleagues (1964) conducted extensive psychological evaluations on 10 pseudohypacusic children ranging in age from 11 to 16 years and found that all of the children revealed significant emotional problems that were considered to be associated with pseudohypacusis. The emotional problems typical of these children were: feelings of insecurity and inadequacy resulting in a strong need for attention and approval, hostility towards parents or siblings, and a display of anxious behavior. Each of the children in this study received psychotherapy and the authors reported "a uniformly excellent response to these therapy sessions which were largely supportive in nature" (1964, p. 68). Other studies also suggest that supportive therapy may be all that is necessary in dealing with pseudohypacusic children (Andaz, Heyworth, & Rowe, 1995; Bowdler & Rogers, 1989; Veniar & Salston, 1983). On the other hand, some young children who display inconsistent behavior on audiological tests do not appear to have such emotional problems. These children often are below the age of 8 years or so, and based on our experience should probably simply be called "difficult-to-test" rather than pseudohypacusic.

Many writers have discussed the personality traits and the emotional and social characteristics of adult pseudohypacusics, particularly among the military and veteran populations of World War II. Truex (1946), Knapp (1948), and Johnson and colleagues (1956), among others, mentioned anxiety, depression, and hypochondriasis as common problems. Gleason (1958) compared the psychological profiles of patients showing inconsistent audiological test results with those displaying consistent audiological behavior in a sample of 278 military patients. He found that 30% of the total sample showed inconsistency during audiological testing and that of this subgroup 86% demonstrated a nonorganic overlay to a true hearing loss. Compared to the group of patients who gave consistent test results, the pseudohypacusic group

> showed poorer intellectual performance, a greater degree of psychiatric and psychosomatic complaints, and deviant social behavior.... The group is seen to be heterogeneous and composed of three psychological subclasses. The largest element demonstrates emotional immaturity, instability, and an inadequate response to social demands. The next largest group is a neurotic population high in anxiety and feelings of inferiority and lacking in self-confidence. (Gleason, 1958, p. 46)

Cases in the third group, described as "small," were found to be normal psychologically.

Trier and Levy (1965) compared the social and psychological characteristics of pseudohypacusic veterans with a control group having organic hearing disorders. The pseudohypacusics, compared to the control subjects, revealed a lower socioeconomic status based on lower reported incomes, were somewhat limited in intellectual functioning, and showed poorer emotional stability. The latter was demonstrated on measures of gross emotional disturbance and in preoccupation with and exploitation of physical symptoms. Further, based on interviews with patients, the authors felt that veterans with functional hearing loss probably lack confidence in their ability to meet the needs of everyday life. Such feelings of general inadequacy can include having doubts about their capabilities of providing financially for themselves and their families. Hence, the possibility of obtaining monthly compensation provides the motivation for exaggerating a hearing loss. Trier and Levy concluded: "Because social values are generally opposed to the exaggeration of physical symptoms for gain, this behavior is likely to result in a loss of self-esteem" (1965, p. 255).

In a retrospective study, Gold, Hunsaker, and Haseman (1991) looked at pseudohypacusis as a possible marker for poor general adaptation in a military environment. Military personnel who had exhibited pseudohypacusis were compared to a normal control group concerning age, rank, and military status. Results of this investigation demonstrated a significant difference between the two groups in the rate of premature separation from the military. Results further suggested that pseudohypacusis in a new military recruit may be a strong indicator that the recruit should be separated prematurely from active duty in the military. It may be cost effective for these military recruits to be separated from duty as soon as the diagnosis of pseudohypacusis is made.

A comparable psychosocial profile study has not been reported to date to our knowledge for an adult civilian population. Undoubtedly, this is because the cooperation needed from patients (subjects) to gather such data would be difficult to achieve in most civilian settings. Research of this nature is needed in large industrial settings in which workers are filing compensation claims for job-related noise-induced hearing loss.

Few studies have reported on long-term outcome of patients exhibiting pseudohypacusis; however, Brooks and Geoghegan (1992) attempted to do so. They identified patients who had been diagnosed as pseudohypacusic as much as 27 years previously. Efforts were made to determine if the nonorganic hearing loss exhibited in these patients originally had any long-term effects. Of the 27 patients who were reviewed, it was determined that 1 was established as a "malingerer," 5 exhibited speech problems,

1 may have been dyslexic, and 5 had undergone psychiatric care. The authors suggested that pseudohypacusis may indicate underlying problems that deserve detailed investigation and follow-up.

Finally, one group that is often not thought to exhibit pseudohypacusis are those undergoing medical and audiological evaluation for cochlear implantation. Spraggs and colleagues (1994) found that 5 of 600 patients undergoing cochlear implant assessment in England exhibited pseudohypacusis. Four of these patients were adults and 1 was 17 years of age. This underscores the need to consider the possibility of pseudohypacusis in all patient populations.

BEHAVIORAL MANIFESTATIONS

While the audiologist is obtaining a case history, the patient may display certain behavioral characteristics that could alert the clinician to the possibility of pseudohypacusis. These "behavioral clues" have been described frequently in the literature (Altschuler, 1982; Brockman & Hoversten, 1960; Fournier, 1958; Gibbons, 1962; Harris, 1979; Hopkinson, 1973; Johnson et al., 1956; Kinstler, 1971; Martin, 1994; McCanna & DeLapa, 1981; Nilo & Saunders, 1976). Children frequently will respond to the clinician's informal conversation at levels substantially below what one would predict from their voluntary pure-tone thresholds (Berger, 1965; Campanelli, 1963; Lehrer et al., 1964). Yet, as soon as formal testing begins, they have difficulty hearing. This naive behavior seldom is displayed by adults with "confirmed" pseudohypacusis. Features often exhibited, however, by both children and adult pseudohypacusics are normal voice quality, loudness, and pitch with good speech articulation, while their voluntary pure-tone thresholds usually show severe to profound hearing loss. This too represents naive behavior, since persons with long-standing severe hearing loss typically have defective speech and voice characteristics. The reader should be cautioned, however, that an individual may have a bona fide severe bilateral hearing loss of recent or sudden onset, and hence, have reasonably good speech and voice quality when examined.

Several other behavioral signs may raise the suspicion of pseudohypacusis. The patient may explain his or her ability to follow conversation by claiming excellent lip reading skills and he or she may continue to follow conversation while the examiner's head is turned or the lighting in the room is dimmed. Other pseudohypacusics may behave in an opposite fashion, that is, they may display excessive effort to watch the clinician's mouth, cup their hand over their ear while leaning toward the speaker, and talk in an abnormally loud voice. In general, some pseudohypacusics go through excessive contortions in an effort to impress the clinician with how much trouble they have hearing.

Further clues about the possibility of pseudohypacusis may be obtained from the patient's responses to case history information. Elaborate details may be given about the onset and symptoms of the professed hearing loss, which, when taken in toto, simply do not fit any known set of symptoms that tend to define a particular type of organic disorder. Also, such patients may go into great detail (more than someone with an organic loss) about how their hearing loss is totally handicapping.

Inappropriate statements and actions regarding hearing aid use can provide additional clues to the clinician. These include: exaggerated claims of benefit from amplification; professing daily use of the hearing aid, yet showing lack of familiarity with the aid's operation; and unrealistic statements about battery life and cost.

Other behavioral clues may be gained while administering the battery of audiological tests. Given appropriately calibrated equipment, a cooperative patient, and careful testing procedures, one may expect both proper agreement between tests and good test-retest reliability (Armbruster, 1982). Thus, inconsistent responses that exceed expected test-retest reliability (i.e., about 10 dB for pure-tone thresholds) should raise the suspicion of the possibility of pseudohypacusis. To account for such discrepancies, the patient may claim frequently during testing that he or she is confused between the test tones and the ringing in his or her ears.

Chaiklin and Ventry (1965) pointed out the value of attending to both false positive and false negative responses in the clinical setting. The latter type of response occurs when the subject (patient) fails to respond to signals presented at or slightly above his or her threshold. False negative responses are considered to be characteristic of pseudohypacusis. By the same token, false positive responses occur when the subject responds either when the signal is absent or when the stimulus is presented below thresholds. False positive responses are typical of highly motivated patients with bona fide hearing loss. Chaiklin and Ventry (1965) reported that 86% of their adult subjects with true hearing loss exhibited false positive responses, whereas only 22% of their adult sample with functional hearing loss displayed such responses.

Finally, a word of caution is in order concerning the possibility of overinterpreting the abovementioned kinds of behavioral manifestations. Most patients seen in an audiology center, including those with job-related noise-induced hearing loss, have true organic hearing disorders. While the clinician should remain alert to the possibility of pseudohypacusis, drawing such a conclusion without substantial test battery data clearly is not in the best interest of the patient, and hence, is a serious clinical error. Behavioral clues can be useful in helping the audiologist to make a decision about which tests to give, but such clues should never be used to arrive at an assessment of hearing. The remainder of this chapter deals mostly with those audiological tests that have proven useful in the detection and assessment of pseudohypacusis.

CONVENTIONAL AUDIOLOGIC TESTS

The audiologic tests discussed in this section include both routine and so-called "special" tests that typically are administered to patients having organic disorders of the auditory system. Hence, these are not "special tests" for pseudohypacusis per se and herein is their primary value. Most audiologists who have infrequent opportunity to test patients suspected of pseudohypacusis do not have the facility necessary to properly administer those tests specifically designed for assessing pseudohypacusis (i.e., the Doerfler-Stewart test) without considerable practice. Thus, the fact that pseudohypacusis can be identified and assessed by unique behavior on auditory tests that are commonly employed in a typical audiology center makes these conventional tests especially useful for assessing pseudohypacusis (Rintelmann & Harford, 1963; Rintelmann & Schwan, 1991; Rintelmann, Schwan, & Blakley, 1991). Such auditory measures include pure-tone audiometry, speech audiometry, acoustic immittance, auditory brainstem response, and transient evoked otoacoustic emissions.

Pure-Tone Audiometry

One of the most distinguishing characteristics of pseudohypacusis is inconsistency in responses, or poor reliability, on auditory tests including pure-tone threshold measures (Chaiklin & Ventry, 1963). As stated earlier, a skilled clinician testing a cooperative patient with calibrated equipment in a proper acoustic environment should obtain test-retest agreement of pure-tone thresholds within ±10 dB. If differences of 15 dB or more are obtained, especially within the same test session, suspicion of pseudohypacusis is in order. A simple technique for measuring consistency of pure-tone threshold responses was described by Harris (1958). He suggested using alternately ascending and descending tone presentations in order to increase the difficulty of maintaining a falsely elevated threshold. Although this method is very effective with some pseudohypacusics, others can successfully give consistent responses at suprathreshold levels. In fact, several investigators have reported that some pseudohypacusics demonstrate good test-retest reliability on threshold tests (Berger, 1965; Campanelli, 1963; Lehrer et al., 1964; Shepherd, 1965).

Nilo and Saunders (1976) reported a "modified conventional approach" where the patient is told a discrepancy in pure-tone test results exists. The patient is not placed on the defensive, instead the inconsistencies are blamed on such things as directions may have been misunderstood or the patient may have been nervous. An ascending technique in 2 to 2½ dB steps is then utilized with the patient being pressured to respond. The investigators found that with most cases this modified approach gave reliable test results.

Another simple modification of a conventional technique for measuring pure-tone thresholds that has been advocated for use with children is the "Yes-No" method (Frank, 1976; Miller, Fox & Chan, 1968). Pure-tone thresholds are obtained with the modified ascending technique (Carhart & Jerger, 1959), but the child is asked to say "yes" when he or she hears a tone and "no" when he or she does not. The critical aspect of this procedure is that the child must give an immediate "no" response as soon as the tone is presented. This technique is not applicable to adults since they understand the fallacy of being asked to say "no" to a tone below an admitted threshold. Some children, however, apparently do not recognize the faulty logic of this technique. As a consequence, the "Yes-No" method has been successfully employed to establish organic thresholds in pseudohypacusic children (Frank, 1976; Miller et al., 1968).

Other modifications of pure-tone audiometry also have been employed such as the Variable Intensity Pulse Count Method (VIPCM) described by Ross (1964) as a modification of a procedure used earlier by Dixon and Newby (1959). Using a conventional pure-tone audiometer, a variable number of tone pulses are presented above the child's admitted threshold until accurate responses are obtained several times. Next, the variable intensity of the tones includes presentation levels both above and 10 to 15 dB below the admitted threshold. This process is continued, with the number and intensity of tones randomly varied, until the lowest Hearing Level is found that will elicit three successive responses. Ross found good agreement between the VIPCM pure-tone thresholds and the SRTs of pseudohypacusic children. He pointed out that a critical feature of the VIPCM is to instruct the child that he or she will receive a test of counting ability, thereby diverting attention away from the hearing test per se. Obviously, successful use of this test is dependent upon the child's ability to count to at least 4 or 5.

For individuals exhibiting a unilateral hearing loss, the absence of a shadow curve due to cross-over of the signal to the non-test (normal) ear when masking is not used can be considered as strong evidence for the identification of pseudohypacusis. This is especially true for bone-conduction whereby the interaural attenuation, or cross-over of the pure-tone stimulus from the test to the non-test ear, is about 0 to 5 dB. For air-conduction thresholds the cross-over or shadow curve response for the test ear should occur somewhere between 35 and 65 dB, depending upon frequency, above the threshold of the non-test ear. Hence, when masking is not used, once the signal exceeds the interaural attenuation between ears, the tone will be perceived. If a patient actually has a "dead" ear (no response by air or bone conduction) and a normal ear, the shadow curve audiogram for the poor ear when tested without masking would show a moderate conductive loss with essentially normal bone conduction. Thus, if the patient does not respond, this is a clear indication of pseudohypacusis. For further discussion of interaural attenuation and clinical masking, refer to Chapter 3.

The shape of the audiometric configuration has been suggested by some as providing an additional clue for the detection of pseudohypacusis. Doerfler (1951) reported that the "saucer" audiogram usually found between 50 and 90 dB (re audiometric zero) was present in 80% of those patients with functional hearing losses. He attributed this to the notion that a normal listener simulating a hearing loss probably uses a reference level based on comfortable loudness and that the typical saucer audiogram corresponds to the 60 dB equal loudness contour. Johnson and colleagues (1956) noted that the phenomenon of recruitment will cause the saucer audiogram to be modified for persons with a functional overlay on a high-frequency loss. A functional hearing loss level will vary also with the configuration of a true organic hearing loss. Gelfand and Silman (1985) found that the size of the functional overlay would be the same for all frequencies if hearing were normal or if there were only a mild loss. However, the magnitude of the functional overlay decreased in organic hearing losses as severity of the loss increased.

Other writers (i.e., Aplin & Kane, 1985; Coles & Mason, 1984; Fournier, 1958) have characterized the audiometric pattern as a relatively "flat" loss across frequencies. On the other hand, Ventry and Chaiklin (1965) reported that saucer audiograms were found in only 8% of their pseudohypacusic patients and also were obtained from some cases of true organic loss. Hence, they concluded that the saucer-shaped audiogram has little utility in identifying pseudohypacusis. Finally, it should be noted that saucer or relatively flat audiometric configurations often occur with various types of conductive and sensorineural defects such as otosclerosis and Ménière's syndrome.

Speech Audiometry

In routine audiologic assessments a basic measure of intertest reliability is the comparison between the speech recognition threshold (SRT) and the pure-tone average of 500, 1000, and 2000 Hz or the two best of these three frequencies. Several investigators have studied the relationship between pure-tone and speech thresholds (i.e., Aplin & Kane, 1985; Carhart & Porter, 1971; Siegenthaler & Strand, 1964). Refer to Chapter 2 by Wilson for a detailed discussion of this topic. In general, given properly calibrated equipment, careful testing with appropriate threshold procedures, and a cooperative patient, the agreement between the SRT and the appropriate (two or three frequency) pure-tone average (PTA) should be within ±6–8 dB. If the SRT-PTA differs by as much as 12 dB or more with lower (better) SRTs, this outcome should raise the suspicion of

pseudohypacusis. This SRT-PTA discrepancy in cases of pseudohypacusis was probably first recognized by Carhart (1952), and subsequently has been reported by several investigators (Brockman & Hoversten, 1960; Chaiklin, Ventry, Barrett, & Skalbeck, 1959; Dixon & Newby, 1959; Fournier, 1958). Concerning the efficiency of the SRT-PTA discrepancy for detecting pseudohypacusis, Rintelmann and Harford (1963) found that in a sample of 10 pseudohypacusic children all of the children had SRTs that were substantially better than their PTAs.

Regarding adult pseudohypacusis, Ventry and Chaiklin (1965) evaluated the efficiency of five audiometric measures commonly employed to identify such patients. They reported that the SRT-PTA relationship was the most efficient measure and correctly identified 70% of a sample of 47 subjects. Combined with the pure-tone test-retest agreement, these two measures resulted in 85% correct identifications. Later, Conn, Ventry, and Woods (1972) obtained pure-tone thresholds via an ascending technique and speech thresholds via both ascending and descending methods from adult normal listeners asked to simulate a hearing loss. They found that the SRT-PTA difference was enhanced (made larger) by using the ascending technique as opposed to the descending technique for measuring the SRT. Hence, they recommended that when pseudohypacusis is suspected SRTs should be obtained with an ascending technique. Schlauch, Arnce, Olson, Sanchez, and Doyle (1996) suggested that clinicians employ an ascending technique to measure SRTs and a descending technique to measure pure-tone thresholds in a pseudohypacusic population. This results in a maximum SRT-PTA difference and is recommended as a screening test for pseudohypacusis.

Several writers (i.e., Juers, 1966; Kinstler, 1971) have attempted to explain why SRTs typically demonstrate better hearing than PTAs in cases of pseudohypacusis. For some children the explanation simply may be that they regard the pure-tone test to be the "real" test of their hearing and that when the more common speech signals are presented, they respond as they would in normal conversation. On the other hand, since a large SRT-PTA difference also is found often for the more sophisticated adult pseudohypacusic, another reason must be found to account for this discrepancy. A plausible explanation is that the perceived loudness of spondee words is substantially greater than for pure tones for two reasons. First, the acoustic energy of speech is "broad spectrum" (see Chapter 2), whereas the perceived acoustic energy of a pure tone is that of the fundamental frequency even though some harmonic energy may be present. Secondly, spondaic words that are used for measuring SRT contain strong vowel components, and hence have an emphasis upon low-frequency energy. Since the perceived growth in loudness is greater in the low-frequency region compared to the mid frequencies, this too contributes to the listener's perception of speech stimuli being louder than pure tones. Whatever the reason to account for the SRT-PTA differences found in pseudohypacusis, the fact remains that this audiometric discrepancy is probably the best audiometric clue for alerting the clinician to suspect pseudohypacusis.

Measurement of speech or word recognition (earlier termed speech discrimination) is another routinely used audiologic test that has proved useful in identifying pseudohypacusis. If word recognition scores are obtained immediately after measuring SRTs, it is recommended that such tests be given at a low sensation level (SL) re the SRT (Olsen & Matkin, 1978; Rintelmann & Harford, 1963). Often pseudohypacusics will respond to items on a word recognition test at levels fairly close to their admitted SRT especially if the SRT is substantially above their true organic speech threshold. In fact, Rintelmann and Harford (1963) found that for some pseudohypacusic children high word recognition scores were obtained at Hearing Levels (re audiometric zero) substantially lower (better) than the admitted PTA. Hence, two important qualitative clues for detecting pseudohypacusis can be obtained via word recognition testing. First, it is obviously not possible to obtain high scores at Hearing Levels below admitted PTAs; and secondly, high word recognition scores usually are obtained at SLs of +24 dB or higher depending upon the specific test employed and the type of auditory pathology. See Chapter 2 for further discussion of this topic.

Additional clues for identifying pseudohypacusis can be obtained from analyzing the types of responses given both to SRT and word recognition tests. Writers frequently have noted that the types of errors made by pseudohypacusics are different from those made by persons with true organic hearing loss (Fournier, 1958; Johnson et al., 1956). Often pseudohypacusics will repeat only the first half or second half of the spondee word during SRT testing. Also, they may fail to respond to some words after having repeated several spondees at weaker Hearing Levels. Chaiklin and Ventry (1965) did a quantitative analysis of such errors made by pseudohypacusics and based on their findings constructed a spondee error index (SERI). Applying their SERI to a sample of 20 pseudohypacusics, they reported correct identification in 85% of the subjects. Campbell (1965) analyzed the types of errors made on word recognition tests and constructed an index of "pseudo-discrimination loss" for use with a recorded version of the CID W-22 test. He reported good agreement between the ratings from his index and the independent judgments of three clinical audiologists.

In spite of the encouraging findings of the two studies briefly mentioned above, these methods have received little attention clinically. Lack of interest in such techniques undoubtedly is due to the fact that after the audiologist has taken the time to complete the analysis of the patient's responses, one still has nothing more than qualitative evidence concerning pseudohypacusis. In other words, testing techniques that require substantial time and effort for both administration and interpretation should provide some quantitative information about the patient's true organic level of hearing.

SPECIAL BEHAVIORAL AUDIOLOGIC TESTS

Time-Honored Historic Tests

Beginning in the late 1940s and continuing through the decade of the 1970s, several "special tests" were employed for the identification and assessment of pseudohypacusis. Some of these tests were developed specifically for the problem of pseudohypacusis (i.e., the Doerfler-Stewart, the Lombard, Pure-tone and Speech Delayed Auditory Feedback, and the Falconer Lipreading test). Other tests (i.e., automatic or Bekesy audiometry and the Sensorineural Acuity Level or SAL) were developed and employed to assess "bona fide hearing loss"; however, these latter tests also were found to be useful for the assessment of pseudohypacusis. In fact, Bekesy audiometry, named after the scientist who first described the instrument (Bekesy, 1947), was still used in some clinical settings during the early to middle 1980s.

Reports in the literature concerning the sensitivity (hit rate or true positive) of the abovementioned tests range from sparse (Doerfler-Stewart and Lombard) to fairly extensive (Bekesy audiometry and Delayed Auditory Feedback). For a detailed discussion, including references regarding the abovementioned historically important tests, see Rintelmann and Schwan (1991).

Although the abovementioned tests comprised an important part of our clinical audiology armamentarium for approximately 35 years, they fell into disuse over ten years ago for at least three reasons:

1. They were replaced by newer more sensitive electrophysiologic measures with higher hit rates; that is, a larger percentage of pseudohypacusic cases can be assessed with the newer electrophysiologic tests (i.e., auditory brainstem response, etc.).
2. Most of the older behavioral tests provide primarily qualitative information versus quantitative information, that is, the test can identify pseudohypacusis but does not give a close estimate of the patient's organic hearing threshold levels (i.e., Bekesy type tracings).
3. Those tests designed specifically for pseudohypacusis (i.e., Doerfler-Stewart, Delayed Auditory Feedback, etc.) were so infrequently used that most audiologists lacked sufficient experience to appropriately administer and interpret them.

For reasons stated above, all but one of the time-honored behavioral pseudohypacusic tests have fallen into disuse.

The Pure-Tone and Speech Stenger test remains popular as a screening test even though it too has shortcomings similar to those stated above regarding the other historic behavioral tests. We will now discuss the Stenger test.

Pure-Tone and Speech Stenger Tests

The Stenger test is based on the principle that a tone presented simultaneously to two ears is perceived only in the ear that receives the greater intensity. Hence, this test is most appropriate for persons exhibiting unilateral pseudohypacusis, but it can be used also for testing pseudohypacusics manifesting an asymmetrical bilateral hearing loss if the admitted threshold difference between ears is at least 40 dB.

The Stenger test, originally administered with a pair of matched tuning forks, was one of the first tests developed specifically for the identification of pseudohypacusis (Stenger, 1907). Since the initial description of this test, various procedures for administering it have been proposed. Concerning appropriate instrumentation, a two-channel audiometer should be used to provide separate attenuation to each earphone and whereby the output from a single audio oscillator can be delivered to both earphones. This latter requirement is especially important since no two oscillators in commercial audiometers will produce the exact frequency set on the frequency dial (see Chapter 17). In other words, if a different pure-tone source (oscillator) is used for each earphone, the patient may perceive either a slightly different frequency in each ear or a beating phenomenon. To avoid this problem, the speech Stenger can be employed by presenting the same spondee words to each earphone, but at different intensities.

Although several writers have described a test procedure for the Stenger test, there currently is no standardized method for giving this test (Fournier, 1958; Kinstler, 1971; Watson & Tolan, 1949). When using the Stenger as a screening test, Martin (1994) has recommended introducing the desired pure tone to the better ear at a level of 10 dB above threshold and simultaneously at 10 dB below the admitted threshold of the "poorer" ear. If the patient responds to the tone, this suggests that he perceived it via his better ear, and hence, the loss in the poorer ear is "real." Such an outcome is called a *negative Stenger*. On the other hand, if the patient does not respond, this implies that the tone was heard in the professed poorer ear. Hence, such a result is a *positive Stenger*. In this case, the pure tone is lateralized to the ear receiving the louder signal (poorer ear) and the patient is unaware of the presence of the weaker signal in the better ear. The principle of the Stenger screening test can be applied to a procedure for estimating actual thresholds. Again, begin by presenting the pure tone to the good ear at 10 dB SL while simultaneously giving the tone to the bad ear at 0 dB Hearing Level. The patient should respond.

Next, increase the signal level in the bad ear by 5 dB while keeping the level in the good ear constant. Continue raising the level in the bad ear in 5 dB steps until the patient fails to respond. When this "Stenger effect" occurs, the tone has lateralized to the bad ear, which suggests that the signal to the bad ear is approximately at a 15 dB SL or higher. Recall, the tone is still being delivered to the good ear at a 10 dB SL. According to Martin (1994), this procedure for determining the minimum contralateral interference level should provide a reasonable estimate of the organic threshold of the claimed bad ear. The speech Stenger test can be administered by using essentially this same procedure.

Concerning the clinical efficiency of the Stenger test, the findings reported in the literature vary from less than 50% to 100% correct identification. Ventry and Chaiklin (1965) reported that the Stenger test was appropriate for only 55% of their veteran patients and that correct identification of pseudohypacusis was obtained with only 43% of the cases. These findings are in close agreement with those of Hattler and Schuchman (1971), who reported that this test was applicable with 57% of their patients and that it showed only 48% correct identification of pseudohypacusis. In contrast to the above findings, Kinstler, Phelan, and Lavender (1972) reported 83% correct identification for adult pseudohypacusic patients with the pure-tone Stenger and 75% successful detection with the speech Stenger test. Peck and Ross (1970) administered the pure-tone Stenger by ascending and descending modes to 35 normal-hearing young adults who were told to feign a total unilateral loss. Both methods of signal presentation were found to be 100% efficient in detecting unilateral pseudohypacusis. Monro and Martin (1977) also found the pure-tone Stenger, using the screening technique, to be 100% effective in detecting feigning unilateral hearing loss in a group of young adult normal listeners. However, Martin and Shipp (1982) found that with sophistication and practice the efficiency was reduced for both the pure-tone and speech Stenger tests in providing threshold estimates for young adult normal-hearing subjects who were instructed to feign a unilateral hearing loss.

The most likely explanation for the conflicting findings concerning the efficiency of the Stenger test relates to the amount of asymmetry between ears. The importance of this fact was recognized in each of the above cited studies. For example, Ventry and Chaiklin (1965) noted that both the pure-tone and speech Stenger tests were most efficient when the patients exhibited an interaural difference greater than 40 dB. They found very few positive results with smaller differences between ears. Hence, it appears that in order for the Stenger test to be successfully employed, either via pure-tone or speech, there must be a large interaural discrepancy in the patient's admitted thresholds.

The last historic test to be discussed is the Sensorineural Acuity Level Test. Although this test too has fallen into disuse, it remains an excellent measure for assessing pseudohypacusis.

Sensorineural Acuity Level (SAL) Test

The Sensorineural Acuity Level (SAL) test developed by Jerger and Tillman (1960) as a method for measuring the extent of sensorineural hearing loss was received initially with enthusiasm by audiologists as a means for circumventing some of the problems encountered in measuring bone-conduction thresholds. The SAL test is based upon the principle that a known level of white noise presented via a bone-conduction vibrator placed at the center of the forehead will produce a smaller threshold shift for a person with a sensorineural hearing loss than for someone with normal hearing or with a conductive loss. The difference between the threshold shifts for a normal ear and for an ear with pathology is the amount of the sensorineural hearing loss. Subsequent research (Tillman, 1963) revealed that the SAL test, like bone-conduction, also was plagued with problems. Two major limitations in its employment have been the occlusion effect and spread of masking. (For further discussion see Chapters 1 and 3.) While the above mentioned problems tend to restrict the clinical usefulness of the SAL test, Rintelmann and Harford (1963) found it quite effective for the detection and assessment of pseudohypacusis among children. They found that the SAL thresholds demonstrated substantially better hearing than the pure-tone thresholds for all 10 children tested. Such findings can be explained by the fact that since a pseudohypacusic individual does not have the "built-in attenuation" provided by a cochlear lesion, the bone-conducted threshold shift produced by the noise is similar to that for a normal ear or one with a conductive loss. Thus, if the pseudohypacusic person does not exhibit a conductive loss (which is usually the case), the differences between the air-conduction and SAL thresholds not only help to confirm the suspicion of pseudohypacusis, but also provides some evidence that the patient's thresholds are at least as good as the SAL results indicate.

The SAL test has the same advantage as the Doerfler-Stewart test for assessing pseudohypacusis; that is, the masking noise disrupts the figurative "yardstick" against which sounds (pure tone or speech) are gauged. Although the SAL test was developed originally by Jerger and Tillman (1960) for use with pure tones, a few investigators have adapted this technique for use with speech stimuli. Bragg (1962) employed spondee words to obtain SRT-SAL scores and found close agreement among measures of bone-conduction, pure-tone SAL, and the SRT-SAL in subjects with sensorineural hearing loss. Bailey and Martin (1963) reported that speech SAL using spondees showed a closer relationship to post-operative SRTs than either bone-conduction or pure-tone SAL thresholds in patients with otosclerosis. Rintelmann and Johnson (1970), using spondees, compared speech SAL scores both under earphones and in a sound-field to pure tone SAL scores in three groups of subjects: normal listeners, "plugged" normals, and individuals with sensorineural hearing loss. They found good agreement between the earphone speech SAL score and the 500, 1000, and 2000 Hz average of the pure-tone SAL test. Also, the differences between sound-field and earphone speech SAL scores were consistent with expected minimum audible field-minimum audible pressure differences (i.e., 8.7 dB better via sound-field for the sensorineural group). More recently, Hurley and Mather (1988) reported on the potential clinical use of the SAL test by studying two groups of subjects with feigned hearing loss. Their data demonstrated that this test is useful in prediction of audiometric threshold to within 10 dB.

A word of caution is in order for the reader who may wish to consider using either the pure-tone or speech SAL test for assessing pseudohypacusis. Like any other auditory test, one must first know the normative value of the particular signal being used. Hence, clinicians must establish their own normative data based on the equipment being used. For further discussion of the SAL test, see Chapters 1 and 3.

ELECTROPHYSIOLOGICAL AND OTHER DIRECT MEASURES

In this section the following measures will be discussed: electrodermal audiometry, acoustic reflex, electrocochleography, otoacoustic emissions, auditory brainstem response, and middle and long latency potentials. At the outset it should be emphasized that each of these measures has proven to be useful in assessing the integrity of some portion of the auditory system; however, none of these methods directly measures a person's ability to hear. A major distinction between these procedures and the behavioral methods for assessing auditory function discussed above is that the so-called direct (objective) measures do not necessitate active participation from the patient in the test procedure, but simply require passive cooperation. In a sense, calling these procedures (i.e., auditory brainstem response) objective is somewhat of a misnomer, in that the test results still must be interpreted by the clinician or investigator. Nevertheless, these procedures are called objective (by some) because the patient's role is passive and the particular electrophysiologic response is measured and usually recorded by an instrument.

Electrodermal Audiometry

About fifty years ago, experimental psychologists employed the technique of psychogalvanic skin response (PGSR) as a procedure for measuring autonomic nervous system activity associated with affective or emotional states. In the 1940s the first concentrated efforts were made to use PGSR or GSR for the clinical evaluation of hearing (Bordley & Hardy, 1949; Doerfler, 1948; Knapp & Gold, 1950; Michels & Randt, 1947). Much of the impetus for the application of PGSR, later termed electrodermal audiometry (EDA), to the measurement of hearing thresholds (especially in children) came from the extensive work by Bordley, Hardy, and associates at Johns Hopkins University from the late 1940s through the early 1950s.

The EDA procedure is based on a conditioning paradigm in which the conditioned stimulus (pure-tone) is presented accompanied by the unconditioned stimulus (mild electric shock). Initially, the shock produces a reduction in skin resistance to a low-voltage electric current. These resistance changes are amplified and graphically recorded. After the subject has been conditioned to the pure-tone stimulus, a threshold measurement procedure is begun. A variety of methods have been advocated for measuring pure-tone thresholds. Close agreement has been found, approximately ±5 dB, between EDA and voluntary thresholds (Burk, 1958; Doerfler & McClure, 1954). Also, procedures have been reported for measuring EDA speech thresholds with classical conditioning (Ruhm & Carhart, 1958; Ruhm & Menzel, 1959) and with instrumental avoidance conditioning (Hopkinson, Katz, & Schill, 1960). A comparison of the two conditioning methods for obtaining EDA SRTs in normal listeners was conducted by Katz and Connelly (1964). They found that instrumental avoidance was superior to classical conditioning in that acquisition of conditioning was more rapid and extinction was slower.

The primary application of EDA has been for obtaining pure-tone thresholds on patients suspected of pseudohypacusis in Veterans Administration audiology programs. As stated earlier in this chapter, an important motivating factor among veterans for exhibiting pseudohypacusis has been the compensation claims connected with service-related hearing loss. Hence, during the late 1950s through the middle 1960s, EDA was used as a routine test in VA audiology centers with veterans seeking pensions for service-connected hearing loss. With the sharp reduction in the incidence of pseudohypacusis among veterans and military personnel since the late 1960s, the use of EDA with these populations has diminished greatly. However, Stankiewicz, Fankhauser, and Strom (1981) stated that EDA is very useful in a clinical setting and advocate its use in nonorganic hearing loss cases.

It may seem somewhat paradoxical that during the past several years there has been substantial reduction in the clinical application of EDA, while at the same time investigators have reported impressive results with this technique for obtaining pure-tone thresholds among pseudohypacusic subjects who could be successfully conditioned. But, herein lies a major limitation of EDA. For example, Citron

and Reddell (1976) found that among 86 patients seen for medico-legal audiologic evaluation 25 could not be conditioned; however, 88% of those who were tested by EDA demonstrated close agreement (within ±5 dB) with their voluntary thresholds.

In addition to the problem of not being able to condition some patients for EDA testing, there are other reasons to account for the disuse of this technique. The use of an unpleasant electric shock as an integral part of EDA has long been sufficiently disturbing to many audiologists that they simply will not employ this test. Also, within the past several years legal questions have been raised about the use of shock with EDA; and finally, federal regulations and safety standards (i.e., Underwriters Laboratories) concerning maximum allowable current in instruments used with humans may simply prohibit altogether EDA testing in its present form. Thus, the future role of EDA, which had its beginning in the 1940s with the "birth of audiology," simply may be to mark a part of the history of hearing assessment.

Acoustic Reflex

Acoustic immittance measures (tympanometry, static compliance, and acoustic reflex) have been well established for many years as a routine part of the audiological evaluation (see Chapters 4 and 5). Although the primary application of acoustic immittance (impedance) tests is for the evaluation of organic hearing disorders, it has been recognized for many years that the measurement of middle ear muscle reflex thresholds could be usefully employed in the detection of pseudohypacusis (Gelfand, 1994; Jepsen, 1953; Lamb & Peterson, 1967; Sanders, 1975; Thomsen, 1955).

In persons with normal hearing the acoustic reflex usually is elicited with contralateral stimulation at sensation levels ranging from 70 to 95 dB; the reflex is absent in most cases of conductive pathology; for individuals with cochlear lesions the reflex may be obtained at sensation levels ranging from 15 to 60 dB. Hence, as Wilber (1976) has pointed out, there can be dramatic variability in the precise sensation level that will elicit the acoustic reflex from the patient with cochlear pathology. As a consequence, it is difficult to detect pseudohypacusis based on acoustic reflex thresholds unless reflexes are elicited at sensation levels of 10 dB or lower re the patient's alleged pure-tone thresholds. The classic example, however, is the patient who exhibits either a unilateral or bilateral profound hearing loss with acoustic reflex thresholds present at Hearing Levels better than the admitted voluntary thresholds. Such a result is not possible physiologically, and hence is strong support for the detection of pseudohypacusis. By the same token, the absence of acoustic reflexes taken as a single measure do not confirm a diagnosis of sensorineural hearing loss.

Acoustic reflex measurements also have been used for estimating thresholds. Jerger, Burney, Mauldin, and Crump (1974) refined and evaluated the procedure of Niemeyer and Sesterhenn (1974) in which acoustic reflex thresholds for pure tones are compared to those elicited by broadband white noise and low- and high-frequency filtered white noise. This procedure, termed SPAR (sensitivity prediction from the acoustic reflex), was intended to provide an estimate of the amount of hearing loss as well as an approximation of the audiometric configuration. If this test had proven to be clinically successful, it could have served an important function in the assessment of pseudohypacusis. Unfortunately, however, subsequent studies (i.e., Jerger, Hayes, Anthony, & Mauldin, 1978) have demonstrated that there are some serious limitations to the employment of the SPAR procedure.

It has been suggested by some (i.e., Wilber, 1976) that the very nature of impedance measures, including tympanometry and acoustic reflex, may serve to deter an individual from exhibiting pseudohypacusis, especially if these tests are administered at the outset of the audiological evaluation. As stated by Wilber, if the unsophisticated patient is made aware by the clinician "that every time the sound occurs there is a needle deflection [of the impedance unit] and, thus, he may infer that we are able to 'see' whether he hears or not" (1976, p. 212). Hence, some clinicians feel that the impedance testing atmosphere per se may discourage the potential pseudohypacusic.

Electrocochleography

Electrocochleography (ECochG) is a procedure for measuring and recording the evoked electrical activity that originates within the cochlea and the auditory branch of the VIIIth cranial nerve in response to auditory stimuli. Although there are three distinct electrical potentials that could be measured and analyzed, the most commonly recorded potential in ECochG is the compound VIIIth nerve action potential, which represents the sum of the synchronous discharges of a number of single unit auditory nerve fibers. Refer to Chapter 7 for a discussion of ECochG.

This procedure, like any electrophysiologic method, can provide important information about the integrity of some portion of the auditory system, but like ABR, it is not a direct measure of hearing per se. While the use of ECochG for many years was essentially a laboratory procedure, more recently it is receiving increasing clinical use for a variety of applications (see Chapter 7).

ECochG also can be applied to patients suspected of pseudohypacusis, especially since two noninvasive electrode recording techniques (extratympanic and ear canal) recently have proven to be clinically feasible (see Chapter 7). However, to date we are aware of only one reported application of ECochG to the assessment of pseudohypacusis (Spraggs et al., 1994). These authors reported that since 1982 over 600 patients have been assessed for possible cochlear implants and in this population 5 were identified as pseudohypacusic. In 4 of these 5 cases ECochG was used to verify a nonorganic hearing loss. It is probable that measuring otoacoustic emissions (presented next) will replace ECochG in the test battery for pseudohypacusis.

Otoacoustic Emissions

Transient evoked otoacoustic emissions (TEOAE) recently have been added to the audiologist's test repertoire and they are proving to be important in the assessment of pseudohypacusis (Durrant, Kesterson, & Kamerer, 1997; Kvaerner, Engdahl, Aursnes, Arnesen, & Mair, 1996; Musiek, Bornstein, & Rintelmann, 1995; Robinette, 1992). Otoacoustic emissions offer the audiologist a noninvasive, objective opportunity to measure preneural cochlear function. Otoacoustic emissions are subaudible sounds resulting from an active response from the cochlea (probably the outer hair cells) to various types of acoustic signals. As a screening test, otoacoustic emissions provide information about a wide range of frequencies, and thus have proven to be invaluable for assessing normal cochlear function. Presence of a TEOAE suggests that hearing sensitivity is most likely better than 30 dB HL. See Figure 14.1D in Case Studies below for an example of otoacoustic emission results and also Figure 6.8 in Chapter 6.

The audiologist does need to be aware of the fact that abnormal pure-tone thresholds could result from a lesion of the auditory nerve or pathways of the brainstem as well as from pseudohypacusis. If the cochlea is normal, an evoked otoacoustic emission will be present. However, if the patient presents with voluntary abnormal thresholds, but with a normal evoked otoacoustic emission, the possibility of a retrocochlear lesion as well as pseudohypacusis must be considered. Refer to Chapter 6 for detailed discussion of otoacoustic emissions.

Auditory Brainstem Response, Middle and Long Latency Potentials

Measurement and recording of the evoked electrical activity that originates within the brainstem and higher auditory pathways including the auditory cortex as a consequence of auditory stimulation has received the focus of attention of many auditory physiologists and other investigators since the 1930s. The difficulty in distinguishing evoked electrical potentials resulting from auditory stimulation from the random bioelectric potentials of background noise, however, delayed the clinical application of auditory brainstem response (ABR) audiometry until the development of small signal averaging computers in the 1960s. After these small summing computers became available, many investigators provided evidence to support the clinical application of ABR as a method for determining pure-tone thresholds of patients unable or unwilling to respond appropriately to conventional test procedures (Alberti, 1970; Beagley, 1973; Beagley & Knight, 1968; Hyde, Alberti, Matsumoto, & Li, 1986; McCandless, 1967; McCandless & Best, 1964; McCandless & Lentz, 1968; Sanders & Lazenby, 1983; Shaia & Albright, 1980; Sohmer, Feinmesser, Bauberger-Tell, & Edelstein, 1977). Some of these investigators have reported that ABR thresholds agree within 10 dB of voluntary pure-tone thresholds. Others, however, have cautioned that close agreement between ABR and voluntary thresholds is not always found (Rose, Keating, Hedgecock, Miller, & Schreurs, 1972).

Briefly, it should be noted that auditory brainstem responses are distinguished from higher central auditory system responses on the basis of their latencies from the onset of the auditory signal. The "early" or "short" latency responses (1 to 10 msec) are attributed to VIIIth nerve and brainstem activity, the "middle" (10 to 50 msec) to brainstem/primary cortical projection, whereas the "late" (50 to 300 msec) and "very late" (300 msec and longer) responses are considered to represent higher central auditory nervous system activity (see Chapters 7 and 8).

There clearly is some evidence to support the use of ABR in the assessment of pseudohypacusis (Barrs et al., 1994; Musiek et al., 1995; Sanders & Lazenby, 1983; Sulkowski et al., 1994). Also, during a two-year period (1987 and 1988) we utilized ABR for threshold estimation with 8 pseudohypacusic patients in our own hospital-based audiology clinical setting. In every case we were able to demonstrate that auditory evoked responses were elicited at substantially lower (better) Hearing Levels than voluntary pure-tone thresholds. See Figure 14.2 from Case Two and also Figure 14.1B from Case One.

Interest in both laboratory and clinical activities concerning ABR (reminiscent of impedance studies nearly three decades earlier) has resulted in the use of ABR for the assessment of pseudohypacusis.

Also, middle and long latency auditory evoked responses have received limited application to date in the assessment of pseudohypacusis. Several authors (i.e. Barrs et al., 1994; Hall, 1992; Musiek et al., 1995; Sulkowski et al., 1994) have pointed out that while both the ABR and the middle latency response (MLR) are recordable close to behavioral threshold, the click-evoked ABR is restricted to providing information about the frequency range from 1000 to 4000 Hz, whereas the MLR with tone-burst stimuli can provide frequency-specific threshold estimates. See Case One, Figure 14.1C.

According to some authors, including Musiek and colleagues (1995), perhaps the most accurate but least used electrophysiologic measure for assessing thresholds in pseudohypacusic cases is the slow cortical potential. This test too can provide frequency-specific information close to behavioral threshold. While the literature is sparse about applying this measure to pseudohypacusis, Spraggs and colleagues (1994), cited earlier, used this measure with 4 of the 5 pseudohypacusic patients identified during cochlear implant evaluation. In each case the cortical evoked response test produced thresholds demonstrating that these patients were not suitable candidates for cochlear implants.

The primary limitation of each of the electrophysiologic tests briefly discussed above (ABR, MLR, and slow cortical response) is that they are all fairly time-consuming. Nevertheless, each of these measures can provide reasonably accurate threshold information.

CASE STUDIES

Two pseudohypacusic cases are presented below in which the results of several of the tests described in this chapter are illustrated.

Case One

Case one was a 31-year-old woman with a congenital, profound sensorineural hearing loss in the right ear. Serial audiograms from a referral center indicated a fluctuating hearing loss in the left ear. Multiple blood tests taken at the referral center were within normal limits with the exception of elevated cholesterol levels. She was given steroid therapy (prednisone) with no improvement in her hearing. She was then referred to Dartmouth Hitchcock Medical Center for further evaluation. Figure 14.1A shows her voluntary audiogram. Initially, there was good agreement between the PTA and SRT in the left ear, consistent with a severe hearing loss (77 dB HL vs 70 dB HL, respectively). However, it was highly suspicious that her speech recognition score at a +5 sensation level was 96%. A diagnostic ABR performed at that time indicated a questionable sensorineural hearing loss, although site-of-lesion results did not indicate VIIIth nerve or low brainstem involvement. Due to the diagnosis of hypercholesterolemia, the patient was encouraged to begin a low sodium and cholesterol diet. Figure 14.1B, which displays the ABR completed approximately three months later (with the patient still complaining of hearing loss), shows a large repeatable Wave V at 30 dB nHL. In light of these findings, electrophysiologic measurements were expanded to include the MLR. In this patient, all components of the MLR (Na, Pa, Nb, Pb) were present and repeatable at normal latencies at 30 dB nHL (Figure 14.1C). The TEOAEs were then obtained. Figure 14.1D shows that emissions were present from slightly above 500 Hz through 4000 Hz. The absence

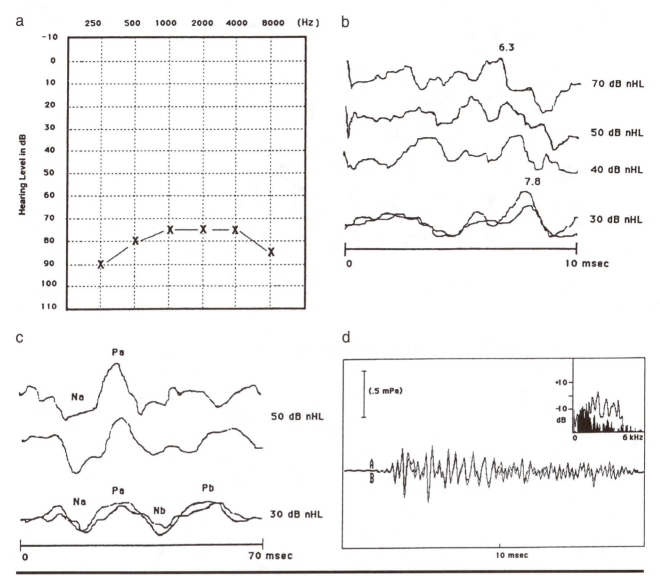

FIGURE 14.1 Case One. (A) Audiogram. There was no response at equipment limits for the right ear. (B) The ABR tracing from the left ear. Top and bottom traces have wave V latencies marked. (C) The MLR for the left ear. Negative and positive waveforms of the MLR are marked. (D) The TEOAE obtained from the left ear. (From F. E. Musiek, S. P. Bornstein, & W. F. Rintelmann. "Transient evoked otoacoustic emissions and pseudo-hypoacusis," *Journal of the American Academy of Audiology, 6*(4), 293–301, July 1995. Reprinted by permission of the American Academy of Audiology.)

of a response at 500 Hz was likely due to excessive noise rather than to lack of an emission at that frequency. The overall echo level of 10.4 dB SPL and the reproducibility value of 85 percent are consistent with normal hearing sensitivity (Musiek, Bornstein, & Rintelmann, 1995).

Case Two

This case presents audiologic test results of a 26-year-old woman that demonstrate bilateral pseudohypacusis (Figure 14.2). Voluntary pure tone thresholds were at a severe

Hearing Level for the right ear and profound (no response to tonal stimuli) for the left ear. The SRT for the right ear was substantially better than pure tone results. Acoustic reflexes were present bilaterally at levels at or below admitted pure tone thresholds. ABR results demonstrated an appropriate latency-intensity function for Wave V down to the normal hearing range for the right ear and down to the level of borderline normal or a mild loss for the left ear. Comparison of ABR results with those of behavioral tests clearly demonstrated test findings consistent with pseudohypacusis.

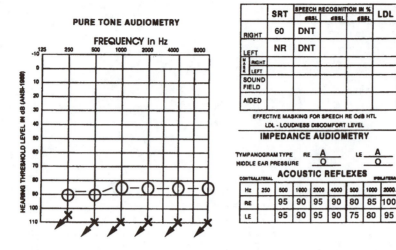

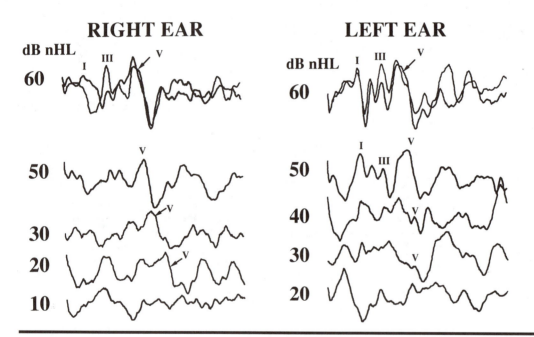

FIGURE 14.2 Case Two: Test results of a 26-year-old woman that demonstrate bilateral pseudohypacusis.

TEST BATTERY PROTOCOL
AND PATIENT MANAGEMENT

If the audiologist has some notion in advance that a patient may attempt to exhibit pseudohypacusis, the order and methods of test administration can be structured appropriately. The pseudohypacusic patient usually responds to threshold tasks at suprathreshold levels; therefore, as mentioned previously, the patient must employ some judgment of loudness as his or her gauge for admitting or denying awareness of the signal because he or she actually will be hearing it all the time. For this reason at the outset of the testing session, the clinician should avoid presenting any auditory signals, pure-tone or speech, at high Hearing Levels. Thus, an ascending technique should be used to establish first SRTs and then pure-tone thresholds in order to obtain the best initial estimate possible of the patient's true organic threshold levels. Recall that in obtaining pure-tone thresholds from children, modified techniques (i.e., the Yes-No method) can be utilized. If a large discrepancy is found between the SRTs and the pure-tone average thresholds (exceeding 10 dB), typically with better (more sensitive) thresholds for speech, the next test administered should be one that will verify the suspicion of pseudohypacusis and hopefully also provide some quantitative estimate of the patient's hearing ability. The clinician may choose any one of several tests depending upon whether the patient is displaying a unilateral or bilateral loss. For a unilateral loss, the speech Stenger would be a good choice, or for either a unilateral or bilateral loss, the pure-tone speech SAL test would be appropriate.

Speech recognition scores should be obtained, preferably at low sensation levels re the SRT (i.e., 10 dB). Acoustic reflexes should be measured, especially if pure-tone thresholds show a profound hearing loss, and tympanometry should be obtained if air-bone gaps are found. Other audiological measures comprising the test battery for pseudohypacusis should include one or more of the electrophysiological measures (i.e., ABR, TEOAE, etc.). Employment of such tests, obviously, would depend upon both the availability of the instrumentation and the experience of the clinician. We prefer to use ABR as the final test with all pseudohypacusic patients because it usually gives the best estimate of the patient's true organic Hearing Level within the frequency range from approximately 1000 to 4000 Hz. However, if one wishes to obtain frequency-specific thresholds, MLR or the slow cortical potential can be measured.

Concerning employment of audiological tests for the detection and assessment of pseudohypacusis, the results of a survey by Martin and Sides (1985) indicated that 99% of the audiologists who responded (227 of 230) did have occasion to use various tests for assessing pseudohypacusis. The Stenger, employed by 88% of the respondents, and acoustic immittance measures, used by 87%, were by far the most popular tests. Also, 34% of the respondents employed ABR for testing pseudohypacusis. Conventional Bekesy audiometry was employed by 20% of the audiologists. The reported frequency of usage of other tests was as follows: the Lombard by 24%, Doerfler-Stewart by 15%, DAF by 9%, EDA by 1%, and "other" tests by 10% of the respondents. More recent surveys by Martin and Morris (1989) and Martin, Armstrong, and Champlin (1994) suggest that the most commonly employed special audiologic test for assessing pseudohypacusis remains the Stenger (89%), whereas acoustic immittance measures showed decreased usage from 79% in 1989 to 51% in 1994. However, ABR gained in usage to 58% in 1994.

We are not aware of any new surveys beyond those cited above, but it is our clinical impression that audiologists continue to use the tests as mentioned above with the addition of otoacoustic emissions.

Concerning patient management during the testing session, as soon as inconsistent results are observed, the clinician should attempt to provide the patient (child or adult) with a graceful way out. It is much easier for the audiologist to provide an adult or child with a way out during initial testing by simply saying something like "I probably didn't explain at first exactly what you should listen to or when you should signal me, but now you seem to understand and you will do much better." On the other hand, if the adult or child has persisted in displaying inappropriate responses for several test sessions, it is difficult for the patient to change his or her test behavior without considerable embarrassment.

A caution is in order concerning the clinician's attitude toward the patient. Since testing pseudohypacusics can be frustrating even for the clinician experienced in evaluating such patients, one must keep in mind that the purpose of the examination is to evaluate (as well as possible) the patient's hearing and not to make value judgments about his or her motivation. This principle applies equally whether testing a 6-year-old child or a mature adult. Further, the audiologist must recognize that he or she is not involved in a game of "matching wits" with the patient. The audiologist must maintain an objective clinical attitude with all patients, including pseudohypacusics.

Concerning transmitting the results of an audiological evaluation on an adult pseudohypacusic, in most cases this is accomplished via a written report to the referral source, (i.e., an otolaryngologist, attorney, etc.). The only information that usually should be conveyed directly to the patient is that the test results are inconclusive due to certain kinds of inconsistent responses that were found during testing. The amount and type of information, however, and the manner in which it is conveyed obviously varies according to several factors. The counseling ability and experience of the clinician are of paramount importance for this phase of the audiological evaluation.

When testing children, the audiologist may have the responsibility of counseling the parents, providing a written report to the school system, family pediatrician, otolaryngologist, and so on. Again, this depends on the referral source. If the test results demonstrate that the child has normal hearing, this information should be presented to the parents in such a way that the child does not get blamed for simulating a hearing loss. This can be done by explaining to the parents that children vary greatly in the way in which they respond to formal hearing tests. In other words, statements should be made to play down the significance of the child's behavior on hearing tests. At the same time it should be made clear that the child has normal hearing and that he or she should be treated accordingly. The teacher, too, should be informed of the status of the child's hearing and that he or she does not need preferential seating in the classroom. The most important notion to convey to both the parents and teacher is that the child should not be confronted with his or her "deception" of a hearing loss.

Also, as indicated earlier in this chapter, some pseudohypacusic children and adults may benefit from a referral to a psychologist or psychiatrist. Such a referral usually should be made by the primary physician who is treating the patient, but if the audiologist has occasion to make a referral to a psychologist or psychiatrist, the discussion of this referral should be treated in a straightforward fashion in the same manner in which any referral (i.e., to an otolaryngologist) is handled. Finally, it cannot be overemphasized that proper audiological management of pseudohypacusic patients requires experience and skill not only in testing but also in counseling.

CONCLUSION

Although pseudohypacusis can be identified fairly readily by most audiologists, the problem of determining the patient's true organic hearing ability is a much more difficult task. Several standard tests that are used routinely in audiological evaluations can be employed successfully for the detection of pseudohypacusis. However, measures that provide quantitative information about the organic status of the patient's auditory system (i.e., various electrophysiologic tests) typically require special equipment and/or some special training or experience on the part of the clinician. Finally, proper audiological evaluation and management of such patients require appropriate clinical experience based on a thorough knowledge and understanding of the problem of pseudohypacusis.

REFERENCES

Alberti, P. (1970). New tools for old tricks. *Annals of Otology, Rhinology and Laryngology, 79,* 900–907.

Altshuler, M. W. (1982). Qualitative indicators of non-organicity: Informal observations and evaluation. In M. B. Kramer & J. M. Armbruster (Eds.), *Forensic Audiology* (pp. 59–68). Baltimore: University Park Press.

Andaz, C., Heyworth, T., & Rowe, S. (1995). Nonorganic hearing loss in children—a 2-year study. *Journal of Oto-Rhino-Laryngology and Its Related Specialties, 57,* 33–35.

Aplin, D. Y., & Kane, J. M. (1985). Variables affecting pure tone and speech audiometry in experimentally simulated hearing loss. *British Journal of Audiology, 19,* 219–228.

Aplin, D. Y., & Rowson, V. J. (1986). Personality and functional hearing loss in children. *British Journal of Clinical Psychology, 25,* 313–314.

Armbruster, J. M. (1982). Indices of exaggerated hearing loss from conventional audiological procedures. In M. B. Kramer & J. M. Armbruster (Eds.), *Forensic Audiology* (pp. 69–95). Baltimore: University Park Press.

Bailey, H. A. T., Jr., & Martin, F. N. (1963). A method for predicting postoperative SRT. *Archives of Otolaryngology, 77,* 177–180.

Barelli, P. A., & Ruder, L. (1970). Medico-legal evaluation of hearing problems. *Eye, Ear, Nose, and Throat Monthly, 49,* 398–405.

Barr, B. (1963). Psychogenic deafness in school children. *International Audiology, 2,* 125–128.

Barrs, D. M., Althoff, L. K., Krueger, W. W., & Olsson, J. E. (1994). Work-related, noise-induced hearing loss: Evaluation including evoked potential audiometry. *Otolaryngology Head & Neck Surgery, 110,* 177–184.

Beagley, H. A. (1973). The role of electro-physiological tests in the diagnosis of non-organic hearing loss. *Audiology, 12,* 470–480.

Beagley, H. A., & Knight, J. J. (1968). The evaluation of suspected non-organic hearing loss. *Journal of Laryngology and Otology, 82,* 693–705.

Bekesy, G. v. (1947). A new audiometer. *Acta Otolaryngologica, 35,* 411–422.

Berger, K. (1965). Nonorganic hearing loss in children. *Laryngoscope, 75,* 447–457.

Berk, R. L., & Feldman, A. S. (1958). Functional hearing loss in children. *New England Journal of Medicine, 259,* 214–216.

Bordley, J., & Hardy, W. (1949). A study in objective audiometry with the use of a psychogalvanometric response. *Annals of Otology, Rhinology, and Laryngology, 58,* 751–760.

Bowdler, D. A., & Rogers, J. (1989). The management of pseudohypoacusis in school-age children. *Clinical Otolaryngology, 15,* 211–215.

Bragg, V. C. (1962, November). *Measurement or Sensorineural Acuity Level Using Spondee Words.* Presented at the convention of the American Speech and Hearing Association, New York.

Broad, R. D. (1980). Developmental and psychodynamic issues related to cases of childhood functional hearing loss. *Child Psychiatry and Human Development, 11,* 49–58.

Brockman, S. J., & Hoversten, G. H. (1960). Pseudo neural hypacusis in children. *Laryngoscope, 70,* 825–839.

Brooks, D. N., & Geoghegan, P. M. (1992). Non-organic hearing loss in young persons: Transient episode or indicator of deep-seated difficulty. *British Journal of Audiology, 26,* 347–350.

Burk, K. (1958). Traditional and psychogalvanic skin response audiometry. *Journal of Speech and Hearing Research, 1,* 275–278.

Campanelli, P. A. (1963). Simulated hearing losses in school children following identification audiometry. *Journal of Auditory Research, 3,* 91–108.

Campbell, R. (1965). An index of pseudo-discrimination loss. *Journal of Speech and Hearing Research, 8,* 77–84.

Carhart, R. (1952). Speech audiometry in clinical evaluation. *Acta Otolaryngologica, 41,* 18–42.

Carhart, R. (1961). Tests for malingering. *Transactions of the American Academy of Ophthalmology and Otolaryngology, 65,* 437.

Carhart, R., & Jerger, J. F. (1959). Preferred method for clinical determination of pure-tone thresholds. *Journal of Speech and Hearing Disorders, 24,* 330–345.

Carhart, R., & Porter, L. S. (1971). Audiometric configuration and prediction of threshold for spondees. *Journal of Speech and Hearing Research, 14,* 486–495.

Chaiklin, J. B., & Ventry, I. M. (1963). Functional hearing loss. In J. Jerger (Ed.), *Modern Developments in Audiology* (pp. 76–125). New York: Academic Press.

Chaiklin, J. B., & Ventry, I. M. (1965). Patient errors during spondee and pure-tone threshold measurement. *Journal of Auditory Research, 5,* 219–230.

Chaiklin, J. B., Ventry, I. M., Barrett, L. S., & Skalbeck, G. S. (1959). Pure-tone threshold patterns observed in functional hearing loss. *Laryngoscope, 69,* 1165–1179.

Chodoff, P., & Lyons, H. (1958). Hysteria; the hysterical personality and "hysterical" conversion. *American Journal of Psychiatry, 114,* 734–740.

Citron, D. III, & Reddell, R. C. (1976). A comparison of EDR, LOT, Pure-tone DAF, and conventional pure-tone threshold audiometry for medical-legal audiological assessment. *Archives of Otolaryngology, l02,* 204–206.

Coles, R. R., & Mason, S. M. (1984). The results of cortical electric response audiometry in medico-legal investigations. *British Journal of Audiology, 18,* 71–78.

Conn, M., Ventry, I. M., & Woods, R. W. (l972). Pure-tone average and spondee threshold relationships in simulated hearing loss. *Journal of Auditory Research, 12,* 234–239.

Dixon, R. F., & Newby, H. A. (1959). Children with non-organic hearing problems. *Archives of Otolaryngology, 70,* 619–623.

Doerfler, L. G. (1948). Neurophysiological clues to auditory acuity. *Journal of Speech and Hearing Disorders, 13,* 227–232.

Doerfler, L. G. (1951). Psychogenic deafness and its detection. *Annals of Otology, Rhinology, and Laryngology, 60,* 1045–1048.

Doerfler, L. G., & McClure, C. (l954). The measurement of hearing loss in adults by galvanic skin response. *Journal of Speech and Hearing Disorders, 19,* 184–189.

Durrant, J. D., Kesterson, R. K., & Kamerer, D. B. (1997). Evaluation of the nonorganic hearing loss suspect. *American Journal of Otology, 18,* 361–367.

Fournier, J. E. (1958). The detection of auditory malingering. *Translations of the Beltone Institute for Hearing Research, 8.*

Frank, T. (1976). Yes-no test for nonorganic hearing loss. *Archives of Otolaryngology, 102,* 162–165.

Gelfand, S. A. (1994). Acoustic reflex threshold tenth percentiles and functional hearing impairment. *Journal of the American Academy of Audiology, 5,* 10–16.

Gelfand, S. A., & Silman, S. (1985). Functional hearing loss and its relationship to resolved hearing levels. *Ear and Hearing, 6,* 151–158.

Gibbons, E. (1962). Aspects of traumatic and military psychogenic deafness and simulation. *International Audiology, 1,* 151–154.

Gleason, W. J. (1958). Psychological characteristics of the audiologically inconsistent patient. *Archives of Otolaryngology, 68,* 42–46.

Gold, S. R., Hunsaker, D. H., & Haseman, E. M. (1991). Pseudohypacusis in a military population. *Ear, Nose, & Throat Journal, 70,* 710–712.

Goldstein, R. (1966). Pseudohypacusis. *Journal of Speech and Hearing Disorders, 31,* 341–352.

Gosztonyi, R. E., Vassallo, L. A., & Sataloff, J. (1971). Audiometric reliability in industry. *Archives of Environmental Health, 22,* 113–118.

Hall, J. W. III (1992). *Handbook of Auditory Evoked Responses.* Boston: Allyn & Bacon.

Harris, D. A. (1958). A rapid and simple technique for the detection of non-organic hearing loss. *Archives of Otolaryngology, 68,* 758–760.

Harris, D. A. (1979). Detecting non-valid hearing tests in industry. *Journal of Occupational Medicine, 21,* 814–820.

Hattler, K. W., & Schuchman, G. I. (1971). Efficiency of Stenger, Doerfler-Stewart and lengthened LOT-time Bekesy tests. *Acta Otolaryngologica, 72,* 252–267.

Hopkinson, N. T. (1967). Comment on pseudohypoacusis. *Journal of Speech and Hearing Disorders, 32,* 293–294.

Hopkinson, N. T. (1973). Functional hearing loss. In J. Jerger (Ed.), *Modern Developments in Audiology* (pp. 175–210). New York: Academic Press.

Hopkinson, N. T., Katz, J., & Schill, H. (1960). Instrumental avoidance galvanic skin response audiometry. *Journal of Speech and Hearing Disorders, 25,* 349–357.

Hurley, R. M., & Mather, J. (1988, November). *Effectiveness of the SAL Test in Identifying Feigned Hearing Loss.* Poster Session presented at the convention of the American Speech and Hearing Association, Boston.

Hyde, M., Alberti, P., Matsumoto. N., & Li, Y. L. (1986). Auditory evoked potentials in audiometric assessment of compensation and medicolegal patients. *Annals of Otology, Rhinology and Laryngology, 95,* 514–519.

Jepsen, O. (1953). Intratympanic muscle reflexes in psychogenic deafness (impedance measurement). *Acta Otolaryngologica Supplement, 109,* 61–69.

Jerger, J., Burney, P., Mauldin, L., & Crump, B. (1974). Predicting hearing loss from the acoustic reflex. *Journal of Speech and Hearing Disorders, 39,* 11–22.

Jerger, J., Hayes, D., Anthony, L., & Mauldin, L. (1978). Factors influencing prediction of hearing level from the acoustic reflex. In D. Schwartz & F. Bess (Eds.), *Monographs in Contemporary Audiology, 1,* 1–20, Minneapolis: Maico Hearing Instruments.

Jerger, J., & Tillman, T. A. (1960). A new method for the clinical determination of sensorineural acuity level (SAL). *Archives of Otolaryngology, 71,* 948–955.

Johnson, K. O., Work, W. P., & McCoy, G. (1956). Functional deafness. *Annals of Otology, Rhinology, and Laryngology, 65,* 154–170.

Juers, A. (1966). Nonorganic hearing problems. *Laryngoscope, 76,* 1714–1723.

Katz, J., & Connelly, R. (1964). Instrumental avoidance vs. classical conditioning in GSR speech audiometry. *Journal of Auditory Research, 4,* 171–179.

Kinstler, D. B. (1971). Functional hearing Loss. In L. E. Travis (Ed.), *Handbook of Speech Pathology* (pp. 375–398). New York: Appleton-Century-Crofts.

Kinstler, D. B., Phelan, J. G., & Lavender, R. W. (1972). The Stenger and speech Stenger tests in functional hearing loss. *Audiology, 11*, 187–193.

Knapp, P. H. (1948). Emotional aspects of hearing Loss. *Psychosomatic Medicine, 10*, 203–222.

Knapp, P. H., & Gold, B. (1950). The galvanic skin response and diagnosis of hearing disorders. *Psychosomatic Medicine, 12*, 6–22.

Kvaerner, K. J., Engdahl, B., Aursnes, J., Arnesen, A. R., & Mair, I. W. S. (1996). Transient-evoked otoacoustic emissions—Helpful tool in the detection of pseudohypacusis. *Scandinavian Audiology, 25*, 173–177.

Lamb, L. E., & Peterson, J. L. (1967). Middle ear reflex measurements in pseudohypacusis. *Journal of Speech and Hearing Disorders, 32*, 46–51.

Lehrer, N. D., Hirschenfang, S., Miller, M. H., & Radpour, S. (1964). Non-organic hearing problems in adolescents. *Laryngoscope, 74*, 64–70.

Lumio, J. S., Jauhiainen, J,. & Gelhar, K. (1969). Three cases of functional deafness in the same family. *Journal of Laryngology, 83*, 299–304.

Martin, F. N. (1972). Nonorganic hearing loss: An overview and pure tone tests. In J. Katz (Ed.), *Handbook of Clinical Audiology* (pp. 357–373). Baltimore: Williams & Wilkins.

Martin, F. N. (1994). Pseudohypacusis. In J. Katz (Ed.), *Handbook of Clinical Audiology* (pp. 553–567). Baltimore: Williams & Wilkins.

Martin, F. N., Armstrong, T. W., & Champlin, C. A. (1994). A survey of audiological practices in the United States. *American Journal of Audiology, 3*(2), 20–26.

Martin, F. N., & Morris, L. J. (1989). Current audiologic practices in the United States. *The Hearing Journal, 42*, 25–44.

Martin, F. N., & Shipp, D. B. (1982). The effects of sophistication on three threshold tests for subjects with simulated hearing loss. *Ear and Hearing, 3*, 34–36.

McCandless, G. (1967). Clinical application of evoked response audiometry. *Journal of Speech and Hearing Research, 10*, 468–478.

McCandless, G. A., & Best, L. (1964). Evoked responses to auditory stimuli in man using a summing computer. *Journal of Speech and Hearing Research, 7*, 193–202.

McCandless, G. A., & Lentz, W. E. (1968). Evoked response (EEG) audiometry in non-organic hearing loss. *Archives of Otolaryngology, 87*, 123–128.

McCanna, D. L., & De Lapa, G. (1981). A clinical study of 27 children exhibiting functional hearing loss. *Language, Speech and Hearing Services in Schools, 12*, 26–35.

Michels, M. W., & Randt, C. T. (1947). Galvanic skin response in the differential diagnosis of deafness. *Archives of Otolaryngology, 65*, 302–311.

Miller, A. L., Fox, M. S., & Chan, G. (1968). Pure tone assessments as an aid in detecting suspected non-organic hearing disorders in children. *Laryngoscope, 78*, 2170–2176.

Monro, D. A., & Martin, F. N. (1977). Effects of sophistication on four tests for nonorganic hearing loss. *Journal of Speech and Hearing Disorders, 42*, 528–534.

Moscicki, E. K. (1984). The prevalence of "Incidence" is too high. *Asha, 26*(8), 39–40.

Musiek, F. E., Bornstein, S. P., & Rintelmann, W. F. (1995). Transient evoked otoacoustic emissions and pseudohypacusis. *Journal of the American Academy of Audiology, 6*, 293–301.

Niemeyer, W., & Sesterhenn, C. (1974). Calculating the hearing threshold from the stapedius reflex threshold for different sound stimuli. *Audiology, 13*, 421–427.

Nilo, E. R., & Saunders, W. H. (1976). Functional hearing loss. *Laryngoscope, 86*, 501–505.

Olsen, W. O., & Matkin, N. D. (1978). Differential audiology. In D. E. Rose (Ed.), *Audiological Assessment* (pp. 368–419). Englewood Cliffs: Prentice-Hall.

Peck, J. E., & Ross, M. (1970). A comparison of the ascending and the descending modes for administration of the pure-tone Stenger test. *Journal of Auditory Research, 10*, 218–220.

Portmann, M., & Portmann, C. (1961). *Clinical Audiometry.* Springfield, IL: Charles C. Thomas.

Rickards, F. W., & De Vidi, S. (1995). Exaggerated hearing loss in noise induced hearing loss compensation claims in Victoria. *Medical Journal of Australia, 163*, 360–363.

Rintelmann, W. F., & Harford, E. (1963). The detection and assessment of pseudohypoacusis among school-age children. *Journal of Speech and Hearing Disorders, 28*, 141–152.

Rintelmann, W. F., & Johnson, K. R. (1970, November). *Comparison of Pure-Tone versus Speech Sensorineural Acuity Level (SAL) Test.* Presented at the convention of the American Speech and Hearing Association, New York.

Rintelmann, W. F., & Schwan, S. A. (1991). Pseudohypacusis. In W. F. Rintelmann (Ed.), *Hearing Assessment* (2nd ed., pp. 603–652). Austin, TX: Pro-Ed.

Rintelmann, W. F., Schwan, S. A., & Blakley, B. W. (1991). Pseudohypacusis. *Otolaryngologic Clinics of North America, 24*, 381–390.

Robinette, M. S. (1992). Clinical observations with transient evoked otoacoustic emissions with adults. *Seminars in Hearing, 13*, 23–36.

Rose, D. E., Keating, L. W., Hedgecock, L. D., Miller, K. E., & Schreurs, K. K. (1972). A comparison of evoked response audiometry and routine clinical audiometry. *Audiology, 11*, 238–243.

Ross, M. (1964). The variable intensity pulse count method (VIPCM) for the detection and measurement of the pure-tone thresholds of children with functional hearing losses. *Journal of Speech and Hearing Disorders, 29*, 477–482.

Ruhm, H. B., & Carhart, R. (1958). Objective speech audiometry: A new method based on electrodermal response. *Journal of Speech and Hearing Research, 1*, 169–178.

Ruhm, H. B., & Menzel, O. J. (1959). Objective speech audiometry in cases of nonorganic hearing loss. *Archives of Otolaryngology, 69*, 212–219.

Sanders, J. W. (1975). Symposium on sensorineural hearing loss in children: Early detection and intervention. Impedance measurement. *Otolaryngologic Clinics of North America, 8*, 109–124.

Sanders, J. W., & Lazenby, B. B. (1983). Auditory brain stem response measurement in the assessment of pseudohypoacusis. *American Journal of Otology, 4*, 292–299.

Schlauch, R. S., Arnce, K. D., Olson, L. M. Sanchez, S., & Doyle, T. (1996). Identification of pseudohypacusis using speech recognition thresholds. *Ear and Hearing, 17,* 229–236.

Shaia, F. T., & Albright, P. (1980). Clinical use of brainstem evoked response audiometry. *Virginia Medical, 107,* 44–45.

Shepherd, D. C. (1965). Non-organic hearing loss and the consistency of behavioral auditory responses. *Journal of Speech and Hearing Research, 8,* 149–163.

Siegenthaler, B., & Strand, R. (1964). Audiogram-average methods and SRT scores. *Journal of the Acoustical Society of America, 36,* 589–593.

Sohmer, H., Feinmesser, M., Bauberger-Tell, L., & Edelstein, E. (1977). Cochlear, brain stem, and cortical evoked responses in nonorganic hearing loss. *Annals of Otology, Rhinology, and Laryngology, 86,* 227–234.

Spraggs, P. D. R., Burton, M. J., & Graham, J. M. (1994). Nonorganic hearing loss in cochlear implant candidates. *American Journal of Otology, 15,* 652–657.

Stankiewicz, J., Fankhauser, C. E., & Strom, C. G. (1981). Electrodermal audiometry: Renewed acquaintance with an old friend. *Otolaryngology—Head and Neck Surgery, 89,* 671–677.

Stenger, P. (1907). Simulation and dissimulation of ear diseases and their identification. *Deutsche Medizinsche Wochenschrift, 33,* 970–973.

Sulkowski, W., Sliwinska-Kowalska, M., Kowalska, S., & Bazydlo-Golinska, G. (1994). Electric response audiometry and compensational noise-induced hearing loss. *Otolaryngologia Polska, 48,* 370–374.

Thomsen, K. A. (1955). Case of psychogenic deafness demonstrated by measuring impedance. *Acta Otolaryngologica, 45,* 82–85.

Tillman, T. W. (1963). Clinical applicability of the SAL test. *Archives of Otolaryngology, 78,* 20–32.

Trier, T., & Levy, R. (1965). Social and psychological characteristics of veterans with functional hearing loss. *Journal of Auditory Research, 5,* 241–255.

Truex, E. H. (1946). Psychogenic deafness. *Connecticut State Medical Journal, 10,* 907–915.

Veniar, F. A., & Salston, R. S. (1983). An approach to the treatment of pseudohypacusis in children. *American Journal of Diseases of Children, 137,* 34–36.

Ventry, I. M. (1968). A case for psychogenic hearing loss. *Journal of Speech and Hearing Disorders, 33,* 89–92.

Ventry, I. M., & Chaiklin, J. B. (1962). Functional hearing loss: A problem in terminology. *Asha, 4,* 251–254.

Ventry, I. M., & Chaiklin, J. B. (1965). Evaluation of puretone audiogram configurations used in identifying adults with functional hearing loss. *Journal of Auditory Research, 5,* 212–218.

Watson, L. A., & Tolan, T. (1949). *Hearing Tests and Hearing Instruments* (p.597). Baltimore: Williams & Wilkins.

Wilber, L. A. (1976). Acoustic reflex measurement—procedures, interpretations and variables. In A. S. Feldman & L. A. Wilber (Eds.), *Acoustic Impedance and Admittance—The Measurement of Middle Ear Function* (pp. 197–216). Baltimore: Williams & Wilkins.

Wolf, M., Birger, M., Shosan, J. B., & Kronenberg, J. (1993). Conversion deafness. *Annals of Otolaryngology, Rhinology, and Laryngology, 102,* 349–352.

Zwislocki, J. (Ed.). (1963). *Critical Evaluation of Methods of Testing and Measurement of Nonorganic Hearing Impairment.* Report of Working Group 36, NAS-NRC Committee on Hearing, Bioacoustics.

CHAPTER 15

CLINICAL DECISIONS

ROBERT G. TURNER
MARTIN S. ROBINETTE
CHRISTOPHER D. BAUCH

This is a revision of a chapter that originally appeared in *Hearing Assessment* (Rintelmann, 1991). Since the fundamentals of decision making have not changed much, the first part of this chapter is almost identical to the original. What has changed are audiologists' attitude toward, and use of, the traditional audiological test battery for the identification of retrocochlear disease. Use of traditional site-of-lesion tests, such as SISI and Bekesy, continues to decline (Martin, Armstrong, & Champlin, 1994). The original section on the audiological test battery has been removed. There is more emphasis in this chapter on auditory brainstem response and acoustic reflex measures for retrocochlear evaluation. In addition, the section on cost-benefit analysis has been expanded. We hope the reader finds these changes useful.

ESSENTIAL DECISION MAKING

As in life, decision making is an essential and unavoidable component of clinical work. Even refusal to decide often constitutes a significant decision. Whether interpreting a test or selecting a hearing aid, it is this professional, educated decision that the audiologist "sells" to his patient. The success of the profession of audiology depends on the ability of the audiologist to make appropriate decisions.

How do we make decisions? There are three basic steps: (1) gathering of data, (2) processing of data, and (3) cost-benefit analysis. Let me illustrate with a simple example. It is Friday night and I want to take my family to the movies. First I check the newspaper for times and admission cost. This is the gathering of data. Next I calculate the exorbitant cost for six people. This is the processing of data. Finally, I consider the benefit I would receive relative to the cost of attending. This is the cost-benefit analysis. I decide to rent a video and watch a movie at home. This is an intelligent decision.

The first step, gathering of data, is extremely important because the correctness of the decision is a function of the accuracy of the data. Despite its importance, we will not consider this step in detail; the difficulties of data collection are particular to the problem. The other two steps are of interest to us. How do we analyze data; that is, how do

we reduce raw data to useful measures and determine cost-benefit?

There are two basic strategies for analysis and decision making: *analytic/objective* and *intuitive/subjective*. In the analytic/objective technique, the emphasis is on quantifying data, costs, and benefits. Mathematics and logic are applied to the data to produce a quantitative result. A well-defined criterion is applied to the result to determine the decision. The advantage of this approach is that subjectivity and bias are removed from the decision process. In addition, there is little "noise" in the analysis since math and logic are very precise techniques. There are, however, several disadvantages. Some problems are too complex to model and describe. A major problem is the necessity of quantifying all relevant issues. Financial costs are easy to quantify, but how do you assign a number to illness or hearing impairment? Another limitation is the individual's expertise with the tools of quantitative analysis. Not everyone, including audiologists, is facile with calculus, Boolean algebra, or complex number theory. Some problems may be possible to quantify, but impossible to analyze. Thus, the analytic/objective approach works best with simpler problems that are within the technical capabilities of the individual.

The intuitive/subjective approach is less well understood, but frequently employed. The essence of this technique is that the analysis takes place, not in the conscious mind, but in the sub- or super-conscious mind. All of us are familiar with intuition and the ability to make good judgments on the basis of limited data. It just "feels" right. This is clearly the basis for decision making for complex problems in our lives and the only technique available for problems so difficult that they defy quantitative analysis. If the reader doubts the existence of this subconscious analytic ability, consider speech perception. The process of converting acoustic waveforms into linguistic concepts is an extremely difficult problem of analysis. This process cannot be duplicated by machine, yet it is performed effortlessly by the human without conscious thought.

The mechanisms of intuitive decision making are not clear. Perhaps we can access, through our subconscious mind, the "answer" or at least data not available to the conscious mind, in some universal store of knowledge. Another possibility is that the subconscious mind has the ability to evaluate and integrate *qualitative* data, permitting the solution of very complex problems. There is an important disadvantage to the intuitive/subjective approach. The decision process cannot be examined by the conscious mind. This makes the process susceptible to undetected error. Decisions may be based on emotion, prejudice, or bias, not a superior form of analysis. There is no way to determine the basis for the decision. In summary, the intuitive/subjective technique works best on complex problems that resist quantitative analysis.

The issue of analytic versus intuitive decision making has important implications for health care. While both techniques are employed, there is a strong tradition of the intuitive approach, reflecting medicine's history as the healing arts. Many problems are too complex to permit analytic analysis; however, there are issues that, with effort, can be quantitatively analyzed. How often is the statement "This decision was based on twenty years experience!" an excuse to avoid the difficulty of an analytic solution to the problem?

The objective of this chapter is to examine some quantitative techniques of decision making, in particular, those techniques that are relevant to the use of diagnostic tests. While this is a fairly narrow perspective, diagnostic audiology has, historically, played an important role in the development of the profession.

Diagnostic tests are used in many specialties of health care. For audiology, the classic example of diagnostic tests are those developed to distinguish between cochlear and retrocochlear site-of-lesion. In this context, diagnostic means to distinguish between several possible conditions, not necessarily to identify the etiology of a disease. All health care professionals using diagnostic tests face the same problem. How do you appropriately select, administer, and interpret diagnostic tests? This is a basic problem in decision making. Next, we will examine some powerful techniques, called clinical decision analysis, that facilitate our use of diagnostic tests.

CLINICAL DECISION ANALYSIS

Clinical decision analysis (CDA) is a quantitative, systematic approach to clinical decision making. It is concerned with both the processing of data and the cost-benefit analysis. The techniques of CDA are largely derived from the theory of signal detection (TSD). TSD began during World War II as an engineering attempt to extract signals from noise, a prime example being radar. Following the war, psychologists applied TSD to the detection of auditory signals by the human observer.

In the past twenty-five years, CDA has been applied to a variety of clinical disciplines and problems. The primary emphasis has been on the evaluation of the performance of screening and diagnostic tests. TSD was developed to extract signal from noise, that is, to make a decision as to the presence of a signal in noise. The use of a diagnostic test is an analogous problem because most diagnostic tests are not infallible; there is some "noise" in the test result. Most tests will produce a range of scores for a particular type of patient, and, more importantly, there will be an overlap in the scores produced by diseased and non-diseased patients. It is this overlap of test scores for the two patient groups that creates a potential for error. A particular score could, with finite probability, be produced by either patient group.

Consider the following situation. A patient, either diseased or non-diseased, receives a diagnostic test. The outcome of the test is either positive or negative for the disease. The test is fallible and makes errors, reflecting the "noise" in the testing process. There are four possible outcomes of the testing, reflecting the result of the test and the state of the patient. These outcomes are represented by a 2×2 decision matrix (Figure 15.1). If the patient is diseased, a positive test is called a hit and a negative result a miss. If the patient is non-diseased, a positive result is a false alarm and a negative result is a correct rejection. The terminology of hits, false alarms, and so on reflect the historical origin of TSD. Different terminology is frequently used in the clinical literature. A hit is a true positive; a miss is a false negative; a false alarm is a false positive; a correct rejection is a true negative. The traditional terminology will be used in this chapter because it is less confusing and more consistent with the historical origin of TSD.

The four elements of the matrix represent the number of hits, misses, false alarms, and correct rejections when the test is given to a number of patients. The hits and correct

TEST RESULT

		Positive	Negative
PATIENT STATE	Diseased (dp)	Hit (hs)	Miss (ms)
	Non-Diseased (np)	False Alarm (fs)	Correct Rejection (cs)

FIGURE 15.1 Decision matrix for diagnostic tests. dp: number of diseased patients; np: number of non-diseased patients; hs: number of hits; ms: number of misses; fs: number of false alarms; cs: number of correct rejections. Hit rate (HT) = hs/dp; false alarm rate (FA) = fs/np.

rejections are correct decisions, whereas, misses and false alarms are errors that degrade the performance of the test. For example, 10 diseased and 20 non-diseased patients are tested. The test is positive on 7 out of 10 diseased patients and 2 out of 20 non-diseased patients. Thus, there would be 7 hits and 3 misses, 2 false alarms and 18 correct rejections. Note that the number of hits plus misses always equals the number of diseased patients. The number of false alarms plus correct rejections equals the number of non-diseased patients.

MEASURES OF INDIVIDUAL TEST PERFORMANCE

Hit Rate and Friends

Next we will consider measures of diagnostic test performance. These measures are discussed in detail in Turner and Nielsen (1984). The most basic measures of test performance can be calculated from the decision matrix. These are *hit rate (HT), miss rate (MS), false alarm rate (FA)*, and *correct rejection rate (CR)*. Hit rate (also called *true positive rate* and *sensitivity*) is the percentage of diseased patients correctly identified as positive for the disease; miss rate (also called *false negative rate*) is the percentage of diseased patients incorrectly identified as negative. False alarm rate (also called *false positive rate*) is the percentage of non-diseased patients incorrectly called positive; correct rejection rate (also called *true negative rate* and *specificity*) is the percentage of non-diseased patients correctly identified as negative. These measures are calculated by the following equations:

$$HT = \frac{hs}{dp} \qquad (15.1)$$

$$MS = \frac{ms}{dp} \qquad (15.2)$$

$$FA = \frac{fs}{np} \qquad (15.3)$$

$$CR = \frac{cs}{np} \qquad (15.4)$$

where dp = number of diseased patients, np = number of non-diseased patients, hs = number of hits, ms = number of misses, fs = number of false alarms, and cs = number of correct rejections. (See Table 15.1 for abbreviations used in this chapter.) It should be noted that these measures can be expressed as a percentage or the equivalent decimal, that is, 50% = .50. For most calculations in this chapter, the

TABLE 15.1   Abbreviations used in chapter.

HT/FA: Hit rate/false alarm rate of an individual test (%)

HTn/FAn: Hit rate/false alarm rate of test in nth block of protocol (%)

HBn/FBn: Hit rate/false alarm rate of nth block in a protocol (%)

HTp/FAp: Hit rate/false alarm rate of protocol (%)

HTp(m)/FAp(m): Hit rate/false alarm rate of protocol with mid-pos correlation (%)

HTp(z)/FAp(z): Hit rate/false alarm rate of protocol with zero correlation (%)

HTp(+)/FAp(+): Hit rate/false alarm rate of protocol with max-pos correlation (%)

HTs/FAs: Hit rate/false alarm rate of a screening protocol used with a definitive test (%)

Pr[+/D]: Hit rate; probability of a positive test result with a diseased patient (%)

Pr[+/N]: False alarm rate; probability of a positive test result with a non-diseased patient (%)

Pr[D/+]: Posterior probability of being correct with a positive test result (%)

Pr[N/–]: Posterior probability of being correct with a negative test result (%)

EF: Efficiency; percentage of correct test results (%)

d': Measure of test performance; larger d' means better performance (%)

A': Measure of test performance; large A' means better performance (%)

PD: Disease prevalence; percentage of test population with disease

dp: Number of diseased patients

np: Number of non-diseased patients

hs: Number of hits

ms: Number of misses

fs: Number of false alarms

cs: Number of correct rejections

CP: Cost per patient tested ($)

CTI: Cost per tumor identified ($)

STI: Savings per tumor identified ($)

TC: Total cost of administrating a protocol ($)

TM: Tumors missed by protocol (%)

decimal form should be used. While all four measures can be calculated, only two, usually HT and FA need be considered. This is because HT + MS = 100% and FA + CR = 100%; thus, MS and CR can always be determined from HT and FA.

HT and FA are easily calculated from clinical data. For example, 100 diseased (dp) and 200 non-diseased patients (np) are tested. The test is positive for 82 (hs) of

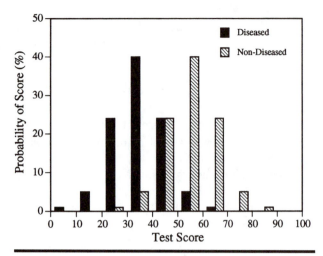

FIGURE 15.2 Probability distribution curves for a theoretical test. One distribution corresponds to test performance for diseased patients, the other for non-diseased patients. Possible test scores are divided into ten intervals: 0–10, 11–20, 21–30, . . . 91–100. The numbers that encompass each cluster of two bars represent the range of the test score. Thus, the bars between "30" and "40" correspond to the score range of 31–40. These two bars give the probability of diseased and non-diseased patients having a test score in the range of 31–40. That probability is 40% for diseased and 5% for non-diseased patients. (Adapted from R. G. Turner & D. W. Nielsen, "Application of clinical decision analysis to audiological tests," *Ear and Hearing, 5,* 125–133, 1984, with permission.)

scores for each population, that is, the number of patients in a group with a score between 0 and 10, 10 and 20, and so on. Next, we divide the number of patients in each score range by the total number of patients in the group to obtain the probability distribution curve (PDC). Essentially, the PDC gives the probability of obtaining a particular score, or range of scores, for each group of patients. PDCs for a theoretical test are shown in Figure 15.2. Note that there are two PDCs, one for diseased patients and one for non-diseased patients. Also note that the two distributions are different; the probability of a particular score is different for the two populations of patients. For example, the probability of a score from 31 to 40 is 40% for diseased patients and 5% for non-diseased patients. Stated another way, 40% of the diseased patients and 5% of the non-diseased patients had scores from 31 to 40.

Because the two PDCs in Figure 15.2 do not completely overlap, we may use this test to distinguish diseased from non-diseased. First, however, we must establish a criterion to determine if a test score is positive or negative for disease. Remember, in the clinic, we do not know the type of patient being tested; that is the purpose of the test. In Figure 15.3 we set the criterion at 50. On average, non-diseased patients have higher scores than diseased patients, therefore, a score greater than 50 is negative and a score less that or equal to 50 is positive for disease. Because there is

the diseased patients and 38 (fs) of the non-diseased patients. HT = 82/100 = .82 = 82%; FA = 38/200 = .19 = 19%. If desired, MS = 100% − HT = 18% and CR = 100% − FA = 81%.

The measures of test performance, HT, FA, MS, and CR, can also be expressed as probabilities. HT is the probability of a positive test result given a diseased patient (Pr[+/D]); FA is the probability of a positive result with a non-diseased patient (Pr[+/N]); MS is the probability of a negative result given a diseased patient (Pr[−/D]), and CR is the probability of a negative result given a non-diseased patient (Pr[−/N]).

Probability Distribution Curve

As shown above, HT and FA can be easily calculated from clinical data, but they are, in fact, determined by the basic properties of the test and the criterion that is selected to determine if the test result is positive or negative. Consider a theoretical test that produces a score from 0 to 100. The test is administered to two groups of patients, one diseased and the other non-diseased. Each group will produce a variety of scores on the test. We could plot a histogram of

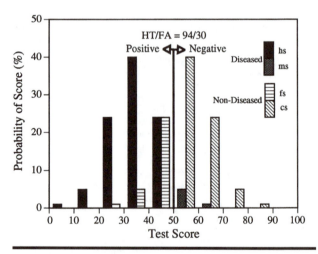

FIGURE 15.3 Establishing criterion to determine test outcome. Test scores below criterion are positive for disease; scores above are negative. The criterion divides the probability distribution curve for diseased patients into hits and misses, the distribution for non-diseased patients into false alarms and correct rejections. Once the criterion is established, the hit rate (HT) and false alarm rate (FA) can be calculated (HT/FA = 94/30%) for the test. (Adapted from R. G. Turner & D. W. Nielsen, "Application of clinical decision analysis to audiological tests," *Ear and Hearing, 5,* 125–133, 1984, with permission.)

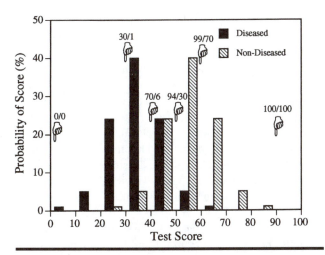

FIGURE 15.4 Effect of criterion on hit rate (HT) and false alarm rate (FA). HT/FA can be varied by changing criterion. Each "hand" indicates a criterion; the corresponding HT/FA is shown above each symbol. (Adapted from R. G. Turner & D. W. Nielsen, "Application of clinical decision analysis to audiological tests," *Ear and Hearing, 5*, 125–133, 1984, with permission.)

some overlap in the two PDCs, the criterion divides the PDCs into four regions corresponding to hits, misses, false alarms, and correct rejections. Below the criterion (<50), the diseased patients constitute the hits and the non-diseased patients the false alarms. Above the criterion, the diseased patients are the misses and the non-diseased patients the correct rejections. HT, FA, MS, and CR can be calculated from the PDCs. For example, HT is the total probability that a diseased patient will have a test score less than or equal to 50. From Figure 15.3, we add all of the probabilities below 50 from the diseased distribution: HT = 1% + 5% + 24% + 40% + 24% = 94%.

We can select any criterion for a test, but different criteria will produce different test performance. HT/FA for various criteria are shown in Figure 15.4 for the PDCs in Figure 15.2. Evident in these calculations are several important results. If criterion is increased (e.g., 50 to 60), there is an increase in HT (94 to 99%) which is good, but there is also an increase in FA (30 to 70%) which is bad. If criterion is reduced (e.g., 50 to 40), the FA will be reduced (30 to 6%), which is good, but so will HT (94 to 70%), which is bad. Thus, we see a fundamental property of diagnostic tests; there is a trade-off between HT and FA when we adjust criterion, that is, you never get something for nothing. Although theoretical PDCs can be defined for which HT will increase without increasing FA, this is unlikely with real tests. This trade-off between HT and FA has important clinical consequences.

Another interesting result occurs with extreme criteria. We could set the criterion at 100 and call all results positive

for disease. This would produce a HT = 100%, a wonderful result. The problem is that FA would also equal 100%. Likewise, with a criterion of 0, all results would be negative for disease. This would produce a FA = 0%, but also a HT = 0%. Thus, criterion can be manipulated to increase HT or decrease FA, but there is the trade-off that limits the value of changing the criterion.

Because any HT or FA can be obtained by adjusting criterion, both HT and FA are needed to evaluate the performance of a test. Yet, the literature is full of studies where a new test is evaluated only with diseased patients. This produces a HT, but no FA because non-diseased patients must be tested to calculate FA. These studies must be interpreted carefully because of the ability to vary HT with criterion.

ROC Curve, d′ and A′

Because HT and FA vary significantly with criterion, how can this important relationship be visualized? The *receiver operating characteristic* (ROC) curve is a plot of HT versus FA for different criteria. The ROC curve can be plotted on linear coordinates or special coordinates called double probability, which are derived from the Gaussian (normal) distribution. The HT/FA data from Figure 15.4 are plotted on linear coordinates in Figure 15.5. The shape of the ROC curve is determined by the PDCs. One special case occurs when the PDCs are Gaussian with equal variance (GEV),

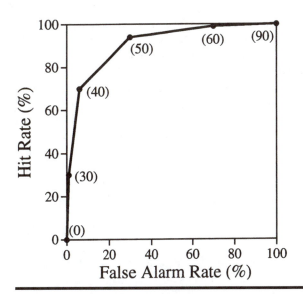

FIGURE 15.5 Receiver operating characteristic (ROC) curve plotted on linear coordinates. The six values calculated from Figure 15.4 are plotted to form the ROC curve. The numbers in parentheses correspond to the criteria used in Figure 15.4 to determine hit rate and false alarm rate.

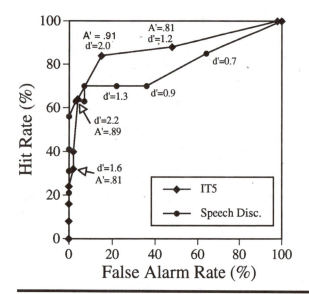

FIGURE 15.6 Receiver operating characteristic curves for speech discrimination (SDS) and ABR interaural wave V latency difference (IT5) plotted on linear coordinates. These curves were derived from probability distribution curves for SDS and IT5 in Figures 8 and 9, Turner and Nielsen (1984). Values of d′ are shown for various points on the ROC curves. Values of A′ are shown for points on the curve for IT5. Note that d′ and A′ can vary with criterion for a particular test. (From R. G. Turner & D. W. Nielsen, "Application of clinical decision analysis to audiological tests," *Ear and Hearing, 5*, 125–133, 1984, with permission.)

as in Figures 15.2, 15.3, and 15.4. On double probability coordinates (not shown), the ROC curve will be a straight line. The ROC curve is not a straight line on linear coordinates (Figure 15.5).

The ability of a test to distinguish patients is related to the amount of overlap of the PDCs. If, in Figure 15.2, the two PDCs completely overlapped, then the test would be useless. For any test score we would have HT = FA, and MS = CR. If there was absolutely no overlap in the PDCs, then the test would be perfect. It would be possible to set the criterion such that HT = 100% and FA = 0%.

A measure of PDC overlap is the parameter d′, which is technically defined for PDCs that are GEV. d′ is the difference of the means of the two PDCs divided by their common standard deviation (the two PDCs have the same variance, therefore, their standard deviation is the same). When the PDCs completely overlap, there is no difference in the means and d′ = 0. The ROC curve corresponds to HT = FA. As the overlap is reduced, d′ increased and the ROC curve moves away from the HT = FA diagonal. On linear coordinates (Figure 15.5), the ROC curve approaches the lines FA = 0% and HT = 100%, that is, the upper left corner.

For many tests, including audiological tests, the PDCs are not GEV. This is illustrated by data for speech discrimination score (SDS) and auditory brainstem response (ABR) interaural Wave V latency difference (IT5). (The PDCs for these two tests are shown in Turner & Nielsen, 1984, Figures 8 and 9.) The ROC curves for these two tests are plotted on linear coordinates (Figure 15.6) and double probability coordinates (Figure 15.7). These ROC curves differ in shape from those for PDCs that are GEV. This is best shown in Figure 15.7 where the straight lines are ROC curves for PDCs that are GEV. The ROC curves for SDS and IT5 deviate significantly from these lines, indicating that they are not GEV.

The parameter d′ is based on the shape of the PDCs, but can also be calculated from HT and FA. Each point on the ROC curve corresponds to a particular value of HT/FA; thus, d′ can be calculated for each point. The easiest way to determine d′ from HT/FA is to use published tables (Swets, 1964). When the PDCs for a test are GEV, there is a single d′ reflecting the amount of overlap of the PDCs. This d′ does not change with criterion. Each point on the ROC curve corresponds to a different HT/FA, but the same d′. That is why in Figure 15.7 each straight line corresponds to a particular value of d′. If the PDCs are not GEV, then d′ will vary with criterion and each point on the ROC curve can have a different d′. This is illustrated in Figure 15.6, where d′ is shown for SDS and IT5.

Another measure of test performance, A′, is calculated from a single point (HT/FA) on the ROC curve (Robinson & Watson, 1972). This measure is independent of the

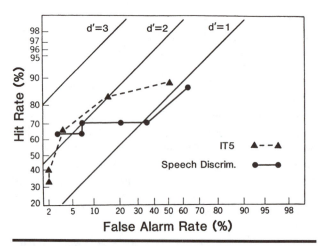

FIGURE 15.7 Receiver operating characteristic curves for SDS and IT5 plotted on double probability coordinates. Same data as in Figure 15.6. Straight lines correspond to constant values of d′. (From R. G. Turner & D. W. Nielsen, "Application of clinical decision analysis to audiological tests," *Ear and Hearing, 5*, 125–133, 1984, with permission.)

shape of the PDCs. A′ is the average of the maximum and minimum possible areas under ROC curves that can be passed through the known point. A′ is an approximation to the area under the actual ROC curve, which is not known. A′ varies from .5 to 1.0 and is given by

$$A' = 0.5 + \frac{(HT - FA) \times (1 + HT - FA)}{4HT \times (1 - FA)} \quad (15.5)$$

where the decimal form of HT and FA are used. The larger the A′, the better the test. A′ can vary with criterion, as in Figure 15.6 where A′ is calculated for several points on the ROC curve for IT5. For further discussions of ROC curves, d′, and A′, see Robinson and Watson, 1972 or Egan, 1975.

Posterior Probabilities and Efficiency

Consider this situation. We are testing a patient in the clinic and the test result is positive. We know the hit rate of the test, but hit rate is the probability of a positive result given a diseased patient. We do not know if the patient is diseased, but we do know the test result. Hit rate tells us little about the accuracy of the test result. What we want is not hit rate, the probability of a positive result given a diseased patient (Pr[+/D]), but the probability that the patient is diseased given a positive test result (Pr[D/+]). This probability is called a *posterior probability*. Another posterior probability is Pr[N/–]; this is the probability of a non-diseased patient given a negative test result. These two posterior probabilities are important because they are the probability of being correct given a particular test result. There are two other posterior probabilities, Pr[D/–] and Pr[N/+], which are the probability of being incorrect given a test result.

Because Pr[D/+] + Pr[N/+] = 100% and Pr[D/–] + Pr[N/–] = 100%, we need calculate only two of the four posterior probabilities. To calculate the posterior probabilities we need HT and FA for the test, plus the *prevalence* (PD) of the disease in the test population. Prevalence is the percentage of the test population that has the disease at the time of testing. Prevalence is often confused with *incidence*, which is the percentage of a population that develop a disease in a specified time period (Moscicki, 1984).

The posterior probabilities are calculated by the following equations. The decimal form of HT, FA, and PD must be used.

$$Pr[D/+] = \frac{1}{1 + \dfrac{(FA)*(1 - PD)}{(HT)*(PD)}} \quad (15.6)$$

$$Pr[N/-] = \frac{1}{1 + \dfrac{(1 - HT)*(PD)}{(1 - FA)*(1 - PD)}} \quad (15.7)$$

The posterior probabilities can also be calculated if we know the number of hits, misses, false alarms, and correct rejections in a particular testing situation. Sometimes, this is an easier strategy than using the equations above.

$$Pr[D/+] = \frac{hs}{hs + fs} \quad (15.8)$$

$$Pr[N/-] = \frac{cs}{cs + ms} \quad (15.9)$$

Stated simply, the probability of being correct with a positive test result is the number of hits divided by the total number of positive test results (hits plus false alarms). Likewise, the probability of being correct with a negative test result is the number of correct rejections divided by the total number of negative results (correct rejections plus misses).

Posterior probabilities are calculated for several audiological tests that are used to identify retrocochlear site-of-lesion (Table 15.2). Consider first Pr[D/+], the probability of being correct with a positive test result. This is calculated for three disease prevalences, PD = 2%, 5%, 50%. Two percent and 5% represent the range of prevalences for retrocochlear disease typically found in clinical practice, similar to the prevalence of hearing loss in a neonatal intensive care nursery. Fifty percent is used to illustrate the effect of prevalence on the posterior probabilities. ABR is considered the best audiological test. With a relatively high prevalence of 5%, the probability of ABR being correct with a positive result is only 31%. With a 2% prevalence, the probability is only 15%. For comparison, consider an excellent theoretical test (ETT) with HT/FA = 99/5%. Even with this test, which is better than any audiological test, the probability of being correct is only 29% for PD = 2% and 51% for PD = 5%. Consider the well-baby nursery; assume a typical prevalence of hearing loss of 0.2% (2 per 1000). Even with the excellent theoretical test, the probability of being correct with a positive result is only 4%. In contrast, when PD = 50% the probability of being correct is >80% for all tests. We see that when prevalence is low, the probability of a positive result being correct is small, even for tests with excellent performance.

It should be clear that the probability of a positive test result being correct is highly dependent on disease prevalence. Thus, anything we can do to increase the prevalence in the test population will improve the probability of being correct. One common technique is to use a screening test. A basic objective of all screening tests is to "fail" most who have the disease while "passing" most who do not. The ultimate result is to significantly increase the prevalence in the population who fail the screening test. Consider this example. We have a population of 1000 with a

TABLE 15.2   Posterior probabilities and efficiency for several audiological tests.[a]

TEST	HT/FA	PR[D/+] 2%	5%	50%	PR[N/−] 5%	50%	EF 5%	50%
ETT	99/5	29	51	95	99+	99	95	97
ABR	95/11	15	31	90	99+	95	89	92
TDT	70/13	10	22	84	98	74	86	79
BEK	49/7	13	27	88	97	65	91	71

[a]All measures in percent. 2%, 5%, 50% indicate disease prevalence. Abbreviations explained in Tables 15.1 and 15.4. ETT: excellent theoretical test.

disease prevalence of 2%. Thus, 20 would have the disease and 980 would not. We use a screening test with a HT = 90% and FA = 10%. We can predict that 18 (20 × 0.9) with disease and 98 (980 × 0.1) without disease would fail the screen. There would be 116 (18 + 98) failures. Since 18 of the 116 would have the disease, the prevalence in this population would be about 16%. Thus, we have increased the prevalence in the test population from 2% to 16% using a screening test.

Another way to increase the prevalence in the test population is to use symptoms for the disease. That is, instead of testing everyone, only test those who display symptoms commonly associated with the disease, for example, unilateral hearing loss. Screening patients by symptom is common practice and is, in fact, equivalent to using a screening test. If we desired, the performance of a particular symptom could be evaluated in terms of hit rate and false alarm rate. An example using symptoms to improve test performance and cost-effectiveness is given at the end of this chapter.

Even with a relatively high prevalence of retrocochlear disease of 5%, the probability of being correct with a positive result is only 20 to 30% for audiological tests. Does this low probability mean the tests are of no value? No, these tests provide some information. Without any tests, the probability of identifying an ear as retrocochlear is PD, the prevalence of disease. For PD = 5%, we would be correct 5% of the time if we arbitrarily call an ear retrocochlear. Using ABR, we would be correct 31% of the time. Thus, our performance is improved from 5% to 31% by using ABR.

Now consider Pr[N/−], the probability of being correct with a negative test result. When prevalence is low (5%), Pr[N/−] is greater than 97% for all tests. If fact, there is little difference between 2% and 5% and, therefore, only 5% is shown in Table 15.2. Only when prevalence is high is there a significant variation in Pr[N/−] with test performance.

It has been claimed in the literature that a positive test result is somehow more meaningful than a negative result. This is an interesting concept considering the calculations in Table 15.2. The posterior probabilities clearly indicate that the probability of being correct with a positive result is much smaller than the probability of being correct with a negative result.

We can interpret the posterior probabilities in a slightly different way. Pr[D/+] = 25% means that the probability of being correct with a positive result is 25%. One out of four positive results will actually be diseased. Stated differently, for every diseased patient identified, there will be three non-diseased patients incorrectly called diseased. Thus, there will be three false alarms for every hit. Because of the low prevalence of retrocochlear disease (2 to 5%), even ABR will produce two to five false alarms for every patient correctly identified. The audiologist should not be discouraged if patients are incorrectly referred for additional testing because of a positive test result. A large number of false alarms are to be expected when prevalence is low. This will be particularly true in the well-baby nursery where the prevalence of hearing loss is a small fraction of a percent.

Several of the posterior probabilities have been given other names, *predictive value* and *information content*, and have been suggested as measures of performance for audiological tests (Jerger, 1983; Jerger & Jerger, 1983). These measures are identical to the posterior probabilities and thus provide the same information.

HT/FA and PD can also be used to calculate efficiency (EF). EF is the percentage of total test results that are correct and is calculated by

$$EF = HT \times PD + (1 - FA) \times (1 - PD) \quad (15.10)$$

The decimal form should be used for HT, FA, and PD. Like the posterior probabilities, efficiency is a function of disease prevalence. When disease prevalence is small, false alarms rate drives efficiency more than hit rate. For example, Bekesy has an efficiency higher than ABR (Table 15.2) for PD = 5%. Even though, ABR has a much higher HT (95 vs. 49%), Bekesy has a lower FA (7% vs. 11%). When prevalence is high, for example, 50%, ABR would have a significantly higher efficiency (92% vs. 71%).

It may seem strange that Bekesy could have a higher efficiency than ABR, but consider this. Assume PD = 5%; if we call all ears negative for retrocochlear then we would be correct 95% of the time. Our efficiency would be 95%; the efficiency with no test would be better than with ABR. The problem is that we would identify no diseased ears. With ABR, efficiency would be 89%; we would make fewer correct decisions, but we would identify most of the diseased ears. Essentially, we would be trading false alarms for misses. We would probably make a subjective cost-benefit decision that misses "cost" more than false alarms.

Comparing Test Performance

Can the measures discussed above be used to determine which test is "best"? The answer to that question depends on the meaning of best. If we mean best in a particular clinic situation, then the answer is usually no. These measures evaluate test performance. The test with the best performance may not be the best test to use because of other issues such as cost of test, morbidity of test, or the availability of necessary equipment. The decision as to the best test is based on a cost-benefit analysis, not simply test performance. The measures described can provide a basis, although somewhat limited, for comparing test performance. It is important, however, to remember the limitations of each performance measure. It is not always possible to rank-order tests on the basis of a single measure of test performance.

Sometimes hit rate and false alarm rate can indicate the test with superior performance. For example, if Test 1 has HT/FA = 85/10% and Test 2 has HT/FA = 75/15%, then Test 1 is better than Test 2 because Test 1 has *both* a higher HT and a lower FA. If, however, Test 2 has HT/FA = 75/5%, then Test 1 has a higher HT and FA; it is no longer obvious which test is superior.

In some situations, the ROC curves for two tests can be compared to determine the superior test. If the ROC curve for one test lies in the ROC space above the curve for a second test, then the first test is superior. The test with the upper curve is superior because for any particular value of FA, the upper test will have a greater HT. If the PDCs for the two tests are not GEV, then the two ROC curves can interweave as for SDS and IT5 in Figure 15.6. Thus, one test will not always lie above the other test and determining the superior test is more difficult. In the case of SDS and IT5, the curve for IT5 is above the curve for SDS for most values of FA. We can reasonably concluded that IT5 is superior to SDS.

For most audiologic tests, the criterion for test interpretation is well defined and, as a result, there is a single value of HT/FA corresponding to the established criterion. This single HT/FA represents one point on the ROC curve.

Seldom is there sufficient published clinical data to construct an entire ROC curve. Thus, when comparing tests we have only single values of HT/FA for each test. A d' can be calculated from a single HT/FA, but is it appropriate to compare tests using d'? If the tests have PDCs that are GEV, then the meaning of d' is clear and all points on the ROC curve have the same d'. The test with the largest d' is superior. If the PDCs are not GEV, then d' can vary with criterion and different points on the ROC curve will have different values of d' (Figure 15.6). In addition, the relation of d' to the shape of the PDC is not clear. When two tests are compared, the test with the larger d' may have the smaller d' if a different criterion was used for either test, as with SDS and IT5. Still, d' can be useful when comparing tests on the basis of single values of d'. When restricted to a particular criterion for each test, which is often the case, the test with the larger d' can be considered to have superior performance.

The posterior probabilities provide extremely useful information about test performance, but can they be used to rank-order tests? When prevalence is low, the posterior probabilities are biased towards tests with low false alarm rates. Consider two tests with HT/FA = 90/20% and 10/2%. With a prevalence of 5%, both tests would have a Pr[RE/+] = 20%, but d' equal to 2.1 and 0.8, respectively. The first test is clearly superior on the basis of d', but both tests have the same posterior probability. The posterior probabilities provide important information, but should not be used to rank-order tests.

APPLICATION TO AUDIOLOGIC TESTS

Cochlear versus Retrocochlear

The techniques of clinical decision analysis can be applied to variety of clinical issues in audiology. We will consider one application in some detail to illustrate the use of the techniques. For many years, a major interest in diagnostic audiology has been the differentiation of cochlear from retrocochlear site-of-lesion. Even though retrocochlear means everything beyond the cochlear, for our purposes we will restrict retrocochlear site-of-lesion to the cerebellopontine angle (CPA) including the VIIIth nerve. We will not consider high brain stem or cortical disease.

The most common tumors of the CPA are acoustic tumors (78%), which are also called acoustic neuromas, neurinomas, neurilemmomas, neurofibromas, or vestibular schwannomas. Other, less frequent, tumors include meningioma, primary cholesteatomas, and glomas body tumors. Acoustic tumors comprise 8 to 10% of all intracranial tumors (Schuknecht, 1974).

In Sweden and Great Britain, statistics indicate about 7 per 1 million (general population) diagnosed cases of acoustic tumor each year (Hirsh & Anderson, 1980).

Applying this statistic to the United States would indicate about 20 new cases per year in a city of 3 million people. The point is that most audiologists will see relatively few patients with acoustic tumors.

The prevalence of retrocochlear disease in a clinic population will be significantly greater than in the general population. Clinic patients are at risk for the disease because of symptoms and case history. In patients suspect for retrocochlear disease, a prevalence as great as 10% (Bauch, Rose, & Harner, 1982) has been reported although 5% is more typical (Hart & Davenport, 1981). The prevalence in a typical clinical situation may be significantly lower than 5%. Referral centers for retrocochlear disease will have a higher prevalence than the general clinic.

The audiologist's role in the detection of retrocochlear disease results from the nature of the symptoms. The initial symptom of an acoustic tumor is auditory about 77% of the time, either hearing loss (69%) or tinnitus (8%). Vestibular problems occur only 3% of the time. The presenting complaint is auditory in 57% of cases and vestibular in 6% (Hart, Gardner, & Howieson, 1983).

Performance of Tests

Many special audiologic, vestibular, and radiologic tests have been developed over the years to assist in identifying retrocochlear lesions. These tests have been used in otoneurologic clinics, sometimes in the "test battery" approach, to evaluate thoroughly patients suspected of having eighth nerve involvement. To use these tests effectively, however, the audiologist must know the performance of these tests.

From an extensive literature review, Turner, Shepard, and Frazer (1984) estimated the relative accuracy of various tests. They calculated hit rates, false alarm rates, receiver operating characteristics, predictive value, and efficiency of a number of tests. Based on their analyses they concluded that the two best audiologic tests for detection of retrocochlear involvement were the auditory brainstem response and the acoustic reflex and reflex decay test. Most of the other audiologic special tests were considerably less accurate in differentiating between cochlear and retrocochlear pathology and consequently have become unnecessary and impractical for otoneurologic assessment. Turner and colleagues further determined that high resolution radiologic tests such as fourth generation CT scans were the most effective in detecting retrocochlear involvement and served as the "gold standard" at that time.

In the past decade magnetic resonance imaging with gadolinium (MRI-G) enhancement has outstripped high resolution CT scanning in its ability to detect even very small tumors (less than 1 cm in size). Hit rate and correct rejection rate of MRI with gadolinium enhancement are at least 99%, according to recent data (Mulkens, Parizel, Martin, Degryse, Van de Heyning, Forton, & De Schepper, 1993).

Table 15.3 describes the test performance of some of the audiologic, vestibular, and radiologic tests that are currently used in assessments to differentiate cochlear and retrocochlear disorders. Also shown are older tests that are seldom used today, but are used in some examples in this chapter. These data represent average performance for these tests based on review of the clinical literature (Turner et al., 1984). Evoked otoacoustic emission (EOAE) tests are not included since they show poor performance in the identification of eight nerve tumors (Robinette & Durrant, 1997). They reported EOAE test results to be diagnostic of retrocochlear pathology for only 18% of 236 surgically confirmed acoustic neuromas. Test abbreviations are defined in Table 15.4.

All of the radiologic tests in Table 15.3 have excellent hit rate and correct rejection rate performance functions, at least 97%, whereas the best non-radiologic test (ABR) has hit rate of 95% and correct rejection rate of 89%. Word recognition, tone decay test and acoustic reflex and decay testing fall well below ABR in overall performance.

Despite the enormous popularity and effectiveness of MRI assessment for patients suspected of having retrocochlear disorders, ABR remains a useful and important measure for many otoneurologic patients. A number of considerations such as cost of the examination, availability or delay for the MRI evaluation, allergic reaction to gadolinium, claustrophobic problems for some patients, and level

TABLE 15.3 Performance of audiological, vestibular, and radiological tests.[a]

TEST	HTa	FAa	d'	A'	PR[D/+]	EF
Older Audiological Tests						
ABLB	59	10	1.5	0.84	23	88
BCL	85	8	2.5	0.94	37	92
BEK	49	7	1.4	0.83	28	91
SDS	45	18	0.8	0.73	11	80
SISI	65	16	1.4	0.83	17	83
Current Audiological Tests						
TDT	70	13	1.6	0.87	22	86
PIPB	74	4	2.4	0.92	48	95
ARC	84	15	2.0	0.91	22	85
ABR	95	11	2.9	0.96	31	89
Vestibular Test						
ENGC	85	33	1.5	0.84	12	68
Radiological Tests						
CTMC	98	2	>4	0.99	75	98
CTGC	97	<1	>4	0.99	90	99
CTHR	98	0	[b]	>0.99	100	>99
MRI-G	>99	<1	>5	>0.99	96	>99

[a]Calculations of posterior probability and efficiency based on an assumed prevalence of retrocochlear disease of 5%. All measures in percent except A' and d'. Abbreviations explained in Tables 15.1 and 15.4. Data from Turner, Frazer & Shepard (1984).
[b]Cannot calculate d' when FAa = 0.

TABLE 15.4 Abbreviations for diagnostic tests.

ABLB: Alternate Binaural Loudness Balance
ABR: Auditory Brain Stem Response
ARC: Immittance—Combined Acoustic Reflex and Decay
BCL: Bekesy Comfortable Loudness
BEK: Bekesy Audiometry
CTMC: CAT with Metrizamide Cisternography
CTGC: CAT with Gas Cisternography
CTHR: High Resolution or 4th Generation CAT
DEF: Definitive Test
ENGC: Electronystagmography—Caloric Response
MRI-G: Magnetic Resonance Imaging with gadolinium-
    DPTA
PIPB: Performance Intensity—Phonetically Balanced
    Speech Discrimination
SDS: Traditional Speech Discrimination
SISI: Short Increment Sensitivity Index
TDT: Tone Decay Test

of suspicion of retrocochlear disease justify the continued use of ABR for some patients. Even though the MRI offers detailed examination of the internal auditory meatus in incredible detail for many patients, the test may not be appropriate or practical for every patient suspected of having a retrocochlear disorder.

Bauch, Olsen, and Pool (1996) evaluated the diagnostic value of ABR in a recent study that included MRI and ABR evaluations of patients suspected to have eighth nerve lesions. They compared results for 75 patients having surgically confirmed eighth nerve tumors (vestibular schwannomas) and 75 nontumor patients whose audiograms were identical or nearly so to the audiograms for tumor patients. That is, audiometric configuration and degree of hearing loss were very similar for the tumor and nontumor groups. Figure 15.8 reports the percentage of abnormal ABR findings for these 75 audiometrically matched pairs of patients. In this figure, hit rate of the various ABR indices is indicated by the percentage of abnormal responses for the eighth nerve tumor patients. False alarm rate of the various indices equals the percentage of abnormal responses for the nontumor patients.

Hit rate was over 90% for two ABR indices, that is, Wave V absolute latency and a combination of abnormal I–V interpeak interval (IPI) *or* abnormal Wave V interaural latency difference (ILD). However, the false alarm rate varied greatly among the indices. Wave V absolute latency measurement had an unacceptably high (37%) false alarm rate. The combination abnormal I–V IPI *or* abnormal Wave V ILD proved to be superior for interpretation of ABR results; ABR hit rate was 92% and the false alarm rate dropped to 12% when this combination was implemented.

Bauch, Olsen, and Pool (1996) also examined the hit rate of ABR testing in identifying retrocochlear lesions as a function of tumor size for these patients. Patients were grouped into small (less than 1 cm), medium (1.1–2.0 cm), and large (greater than 2.0 cm) tumor sizes. The three subgroups were similar in sample size, ranging from 22 to 30 patients in each group (Figure 15.9). Hit rate was 100% for the larger tumors for five different ABR indices (absolute latencies of Waves III and V, I–III IPI, Wave V ILD, and the combination of abnormal I–V IPI or abnormal Wave V ILD). However, hit rate dropped to 93% for the medium size tumors for three different indices (absolute latency of Wave V, Wave V ILD, and the combination of I–V IPI and Wave V ILD, and 82% for two different indices (absolute latency of Wave V and the I–V IPI and Wave V ILD combination) for the patients having the smallest tumors (less than 1 cm).

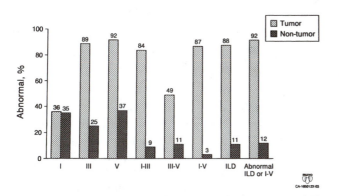

FIGURE 15.8 Percentage of abnormal (delayed or absent) ABR responses for 75 nontumor and 75 tumor patients matched for hearing loss. (From C. D. Bauch, W. O. Olsen, & A. F. Pool, "ABR indices: Sensitivity, specificity, and tumor size," *American Journal of Audiology, 5*(1), 97–104, 1996. Reprinted by permission of the American Speech-Language-Hearing Association.)

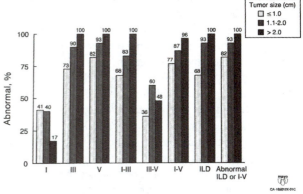

FIGURE 15.9 Percentage of abnormal (delayed or absent) ABR responses for 75 tumor patients as a function of tumor size. (From C. D. Bauch, W. O. Olsen, & A. F. Pool, "ABR indices: Sensitivity, specificity, and tumor size," *American Journal of Audiology, 5*(1), 97–104, 1996. Reprinted by permission of the American Speech-Language-Hearing Association.)

As anticipated, ABR is less sensitive in detecting the smallest of tumors because smaller tumors usually result in less pressure on the eighth nerve. Nevertheless, ABR does offer the neurotologist an excellent option as a screening test at a fraction of the cost of certain imaging tests when the medical suspicion level of eighth nerve tumor is sufficiently low. Further, the ABR may often be used as a baseline for future testing (6 to 12 months) when the neurotologist suggests follow-up studies to assess any progression or change in symptoms and/or hearing status. In these cases the physician must use his or her best judgment in determining which tests to utilize.

TEST PROTOCOLS

Clinical Necessity?

Often, more than one diagnostic test has been developed to identify a particular disease. If any one test is perfect, that is, HT/FA = 100/0%, then only that test is needed. Diagnostic tests, however, seldom have perfect performance. The practice has been to use multiple tests. A combination of individual diagnostic tests is a test protocol. The routine use of test protocols results, to a large degree, from the subjective impression that several tests are better than one test. Are several tests better than one? Before addressing this question we should develop a rationale for combining tests. We cannot evaluate the value of test protocols until we define what we expect to gain from their use.

There are four basic justifications for combining tests into a test protocol: (1) **Super protocol:** A super protocol is a protocol with a hit rate higher *and* a false alarm rate lower than any individual test in the protocol. For example, a protocol consists of two tests with HT/FA = 90/20% and 80/10%. A super test would have HTp > 90% and FAp < 10%, e.g., 95/6%. In this case, protocol performance would be superior, by any measure, to that of the individual tests that form the protocol. (2) **Improved performance**: A protocol may not qualify as a super protocol, but the performance, as indicated by some measure such as d′ or A′, may be better than that of the individual tests. For the example above, we might have HTp/FAp = 90/10%. (3) **Manipulate hit rate or false alarm rate:** We saw earlier that the hit rate and false alarm rate of an individual test varied with criterion. Hit rate could be increased or false alarm rate decreased, but there was always a trade-off. Thus, a desired hit rate or false alarm rate could be obtained, but there was little improvement in the performance of the test. It may be possible to use a protocol to obtain a hit rate higher (or false alarm rate lower) than available with any individual test in the protocol. The higher hit rate (or lower false alarm rate) may be advantageous in a particular clinical situation, even though the performance of the protocol is no better than that of any individual test. For the example above, we might

obtain HTp/FAp = 95/25%. (4) **Screen patients for a definitive test:** Even when tests are available with near perfect performance, such as the definitive radiological tests discussed above, the financial cost, morbidity, and mortality may preclude the use of these tests on every patient. In this case, other tests are needed to screen patients for the definitive test. A protocol consisting of the screening test(s) and a definitive test may be appropriate.

Thus, we see that there are reasonable theoretical justifications for using test protocols. The use of a test protocol, however, raises certain important questions. (1) What tests should be used in the protocol? (2) How should the tests be administered? (3) How is a criterion determined for the protocol? (4) How is protocol performance evaluated? We will now consider some basic issues related to the use of protocols.

Formulation and Use

The test protocol functions much like an individual test and in many ways can be treated as one. The purpose of the protocol is to indicate the state of the patient. The simplest result would be positive or negative for a particular disease, although a protocol may also have more than two outcomes (e.g., positive, negative, uncertain).

There are two basic ways of combining tests into a protocol: *parallel* and *series*. Parallel means that several tests are administered and a decision concerning patient management is made on the basis of multiple test results (Figure 15.10A). When tests are combined in parallel, a criterion is needed to determine if the result of the protocol is positive or negative. The criterion for a protocol differs slightly from the criterion for individual tests. Standard criteria are used to determine if the individual tests are positive or negative. The protocol criterion defines how many individual tests must be positive for the protocol to be positive. For example, five tests are combined in parallel. If all five tests must be positive for the protocol to be positive, then the criterion is "strict." If only one test must be positive, then the criterion is "loose." If two, three, or four tests must be positive, then we have established an "intermediate" criterion.

Tests combined in series are performed sequentially with a decision made after each test (Figure 15.10B). A protocol criterion is not needed for tests combined in series. The protocol is implicit in the design of the series protocol. Tests can be combined in series in two ways: *series-positive* or *series-negative* (Figure 15.11).

With a series-positive protocol, a patient is excluded from additional testing with a negative test result, whereas a positive result means that the patient receives the next test (Figure 15.11A). For a series-positive protocol to be positive, all test results must be positive. Recall that a parallel protocol with a strict criterion required all tests to be

a

Parallel

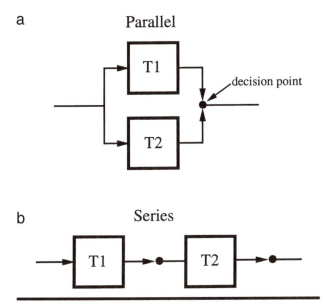

b

Series

FIGURE 15.10   Two techniques for combining tests (T1 and T2) into a protocol. At a decision point (solid dot), a decision is made about future testing or treatment. That decision is based on a single test result for a series protocol and multiple test results for a parallel protocol. (Adapted with permission from R. G. Turner, G. J. Frazer, & N. T. Shepard, "Clinical performance of audiological and related diagnostic tests," *Journal of the American Academy of Audiology, 3*, 233–241, 1984.)

a

Series-Positive

b

Series-Negative

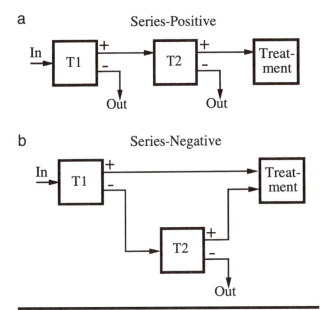

FIGURE 15.11   Two techniques for combining tests (T1 and T2) into a series protocol. "OUT" means that the patient receives no additional testing or treatment. (Adapted with permission from R. G. Turner, G. J. Frazer, & N. T. Shepard, "Clinical performance of audiological and related diagnostic tests," *Journal of the American Academy of Audiology, 3*, 233–241, 1984.)

positive for the protocol to be positive. Thus, a series-positive protocol is analogous to a parallel protocol with a strict criterion. In fact, the performance of a series-positive is identical to the corresponding parallel protocol with a strict criterion. As stated above, the protocol criterion is implicit in the design of a series protocol.

With a series-negative protocol, a positive test result sends the patient for the ultimate treatment (Figure 15.11B). If a test result is negative, the patient receives the next test. For the series-negative protocol to be positive, only one test must be positive. The series-negative protocol is analogous to the parallel protocol with a loose criterion and they have the same performance.

Performance Measures

How can protocol performance be evaluated? The performance measures developed for individual tests can be used with slight modification. Protocol performance can be described in terms of hit rate and false alarm rate. Once this is known, other measures of performance, for example, d′ and efficiency, can be calculated for the protocol.

The most straightforward technique to determine protocol hit rate (HTp) and false alarm rate (FAp) is to calculate them using clinical data. The calculations are similar to those for individual tests. Protocol hit rate is the total

number of protocol hits divided by the total number of diseased patients. False alarm rate is the total number of protocol false alarms divided by the total number of non-diseased patients. The posterior probabilities and efficiency for the protocol are calculated using protocol hit rate, protocol false alarm rate, and disease prevalence.

The calculation of protocol performance is illustrated by a simple example. A test protocol is formed by combining two tests in parallel (Figure 15.12). A population of 10 diseased (dp = 10) and 12 non-diseased (np = 12) patients are tested by the protocol. The prevalence in this

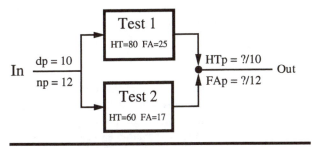

FIGURE 15.12   Simple test protocol for data shown in Table 15.5. (Adapted with permission from R. G. Turner, "Techniques to determine test protocol performance," *Ear and Hearing, 9*, 177–189, 1988.)

TABLE 15.5 Test results for simple protocol in Figure 15.1.[a]

	DISEASED PATIENTS												
PATIENT #	1	2	3	4	5	6	7	8	9	10		*TOTAL*	*HT(%)*
Test 1	+	+		+	+		+	+	+	+		8	80
Test 2		+	+		+		+	+		+		6	60
Protocol													*HTp(%)*
loose	+	+	+	+	+		+	+	+	+		9	90
strict		+			+		+	+		+		5	50

	NON-DISEASED PATIENTS													
PATIENT #	1	2	3	4	5	6	7	8	9	10	11	12	*TOTAL*	*FA(%)*
Test 1				+	+					+			3	25
Test 2		+		+									2	17
Protocol													*FAp(%)*	
loose		+		+	+					+			4	33
strict				+									1	8

[a] Abbreviations explained in Tables 15.1 and 15.4. Adapted from Turner (1988).

test population is PD = dp/(dp + np) = 10/22 = 45%. Test 1 has HT/FA = 80%/25%; Test 2 has HT/FA = 60%/17%. Because the two tests are in parallel, all patients receive both tests. First a loose, then a strict criterion will be considered. Test results are shown in Table 15.5.

With a loose criterion, the protocol is positive if one or both tests are positive. For the diseased patients, 9 show a positive result on one or both tests. Thus, the number of hits for the protocol is 9, as opposed to 8 and 6 for the individual tests. The hit rate for the protocol (HTp) is 9/10 = 90%. For the non-diseased patients, 4 show a positive test result on one or both tests. The number of false alarms for the protocol is 4, compared to 3 and 2 for the individual tests. False alarm rate for the protocol (FAp) is 4/12 = 33%.

The same type of calculations are possible for a strict criterion. For the protocol to be positive, both tests must be positive. For the diseased patients, both tests were positive five times for HTp = 5/10 = 50%. For the non-diseased patients, both test were positive one time for FAp = 1/12 = 8%. Using HTp and FAp, efficiency and the posterior probabilities can be calculated for both a loose and strict criterion.

Test Correlation

When clinical data are available, protocol performance is easily calculated. We shall see later that there has been little clinical evaluation of audiologic protocols. Often, the necessary clinical data are not available to calculate protocol performance. Is there any way to theoretically determine protocol performance? Yes, protocol performance can be predicted if we know (1) the design of the protocol,

(2) the performance (HT/FA) of the individual tests in the protocol, and (3) the correlation between the individual tests. Before proceeding, let us consider what is meant by test correlation.

Test correlation is the tendency of individual tests in a protocol to identify the same patients as positive or negative. If both tests identify the same patients then the tests have maximum-positive (max-pos) correlation. If the two tests identify different patients, then the tests have maximum-negative (max-neg) correlation. The two tests can have zero correlation, in which case the patients identified by Test 1 would not provide any information about the patients identified by Test 2. Test correlation can be anywhere from max-neg to max-pos.

Test correlation has a significant effect on protocol performance. This is best illustrated by an example. Twelve diseased patients are to be tested by two tests. Both Test 1 and Test 2 identify 6 out of 12 patients as positive, HT = 50%. The two tests are combined in parallel with a loose criterion; the protocol is positive if either test is positive. For max-pos correlation, the two tests identify the same 6 patients as positive. Even with a loose criterion, the protocol hit rate is 6/12 = 50%, no better than the individual tests. Next we assume max-neg correlation. In this case, the two tests identify different patients. Thus, all 12 patients are identified by one test or the other. A loose criterion requires only one test to be positive for the protocol to be positive, thus, HTp = 12/12 = 100%. For this simple example, protocol hit rate can vary from 50% to 100% depending on test correlation. In general, protocol hit rate and false alarm rate will vary significantly with test correlation for any protocol criterion.

Limits on Protocol Performance

Do we know test correlation for audiological tests? Data suggest that correlation is mid-positive, that is, between zero and max-pos correlation. Let me emphasize, however, that these data are extremely limited. Later in this chapter, we will develop techniques for predicting protocol performance based on the assumption of mid-pos correlation. First, we will calculate limits on protocol performance that do not require a knowledge of actual test correlation.

We have seen that protocol performance is a function of criterion and test correlation. The extremes of criterion are loose and strict; the extremes of test correlation are max-pos and max-neg. The important point is that protocol performance at the extremes of criterion or correlation define limits on protocol performance. For example, if we calculate protocol hit rate for both a loose and a strict criterion, then hit rate for any intermediate criterion would be between that calculated for loose and strict. Likewise, protocol hit rate for any actual test correlation would lie between that calculated for max-pos and max-neg correlation.

The two extremes of criterion and the two of correlation form four combinations of criterion/correlation: loose/max-pos; loose/max-neg; strict/max-pos; strict/max-neg. If protocol performance is calculated for these four conditions, then these calculated values place limits on actual protocol performance for any criterion or test correlation. We can think of criterion and correlation as axes of a two-dimensional space (Figure 15.13). The four combinations of criterion and correlation define the four corners of a rectangle in that space. Any protocol would define a point in the rectangle based upon the selected criterion of the protocol and actual test correlation. We can calculate limits by calculating protocol hit rate and false alarm rate at the four corners, that is, at the extremes of correlation and criterion.

What follows are the techniques and equations needed to calculate limits on protocol performance. While this information can serve as a useful reference, the reading is somewhat tedious. The more casual reader may want to skip ahead to the next section, "Basic Properties."

Consider a simple protocol of "N" tests combined in parallel (or the equivalent series protocol). The hit rate and false alarm rate of the nth test in the protocol is indicated by HTn/FAn. If we specify a loose criterion and assume max-pos correlation, the protocol performance is given by the following equations:

$$HTp(l/+) = HTx \tag{15.11}$$

$$FAp(l/+) = FAx \tag{15.12}$$

where HTx and FAx are the maximum individual hit rate and false alarm rate of the tests in the protocol. For a strict criterion and max-pos correlation, we have

$$HTp(s/+) = HTm \tag{15.13}$$

$$FAp(s/+) = FAm \tag{15.14}$$

where HTm and FAm are the minimum individual hit rate and false alarm rate of the tests in the protocol.

If we assume max-neg correlation and specify a loose criterion for the protocol, we have

$$HTp(l/-) = MIN\,[\textstyle\sum HTn \text{ or } 100\%] \tag{15.15}$$

$$FAp(l/-) = MIN\,[\textstyle\sum FAn \text{ or } 100\%] \tag{15.16}$$

where $\sum HTn$ and $\sum FAn$ mean the sum of the individual hit rates and false alarm rates, respectively. MIN [A or B] is the smaller of A or B. Finally, for a strict criterion and max-neg correlation the equations are

$$HTp(s/-) = MAX\,[\{\textstyle\sum HTn - 100(N-1)\} \text{ or } 0] \tag{15.17}$$

$$FAp(s/-) = MAX\,[\{\textstyle\sum FAn - 100(N-1)\} \text{ or } 0] \tag{15.18}$$

where MAX [A or B] means the larger of A or B, and 100(N–1) means 100% times one less than the number of individual tests. For convenience, hit rate and false alarm rate are expressed as percent, not decimal, for these calculations.

The derivation of these equations may not be obvious to the reader, nor will it be discussed in detail. The equations

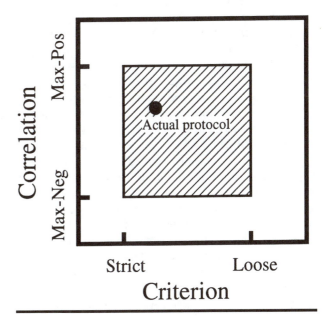

FIGURE 15.13 Space defined by extremes of protocol criterion and test correlation. Any real protocol would lie somewhere in this rectangular space depending on actual test correlation and selected criterion.

(a) Strict   (b) Loose

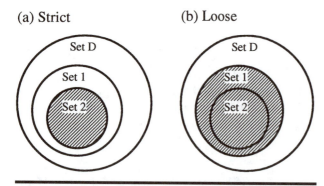

FIGURE 15.14   Set D consists of all diseased patients. Set 1 are all patients identified as positive by Test 1; Set 2 are patients identified as positive by Test 2. For this example, test correlation is maximum-positive. Because of correlation, Set 2 is a subset of Set 1. Test 1 and Test 2 are combined in parallel to form a protocol. The cross-hatched area indicates those patients identified as positive by the protocol (Set P) with a strict (a) and a loose (b) criterion.

are easily determined by using simple set theory. One example will illustrate the strategy. Consider a parallel protocol consisting of Test 1 and Test 2. We assume max-pos correlation. The hit rate of Test 1 (HT1) is 80% and the hit rate of Test 2 (HT2) is 60%. Ten diseased patients are tested by the protocol. These 10 patients can be considered a set, labeled Set D (Figure 15.14). Test 1 will identify 8 of the 10 patients because HT1 = 80%. These 8 patients (Set 1) are a subset of the original 10 (Set D), as shown in Figure 15.14. Test 2 will identify 6 patients (Set 2), which are also a subset of Set D. Because the tests have max-pos correlation, these 6 patients identified by Test 2 are a subset of the 8 identified by Test 1. Thus, Set 2 is a subset of Set 1.

If we choose a strict criterion, then the protocol will be positive only when both tests are positive. The subset of patients identified by the protocol (Set P) will be the intersection of Set 1 and Set 2 (Set P = Set 1 ∩ Set 2). This is true only for the 6 patients identified by *both* tests (Set 2). Thus, the protocol hit rate will equal the smallest hit rate of the individual tests.

If we select a loose criterion, then the protocol will be positive if either test (or both tests) is positive. This corresponds to the union of the two sets (Set P = Set 1 ∪ Set 2). Since Set 2 is a subset of Set 1, the maximum number of positive patients will be those in Set 1. Thus, the protocol hit rate will equal the greatest individual hit rate.

To illustrate the equations developed in this section, we will calculate limits on an example protocol. This protocol is designed to distinguish cochlear from retrocochlear site-of-lesion and consists of the tone decay test (TDT), acoustic reflex-combined (ARC), and auditory brainstem response (ABR) combined in parallel with either a loose or a

strict criterion. These tests have HT/FA of TDT = 70/13%, ARC = 84/15%, and ABR = 95/11%. Limits on performance are shown in Table 15.6. For a particular criterion, note the large variation in protocol hit rate and false alarm rate with test correlation. This variation is, in general, so large that the limits are not usual for evaluating protocol performance. We cannot say from the data in Table 15.6 if this is a "good" or "bad" protocol. These data do, however, reveal some basic properties of test protocols.

Basic Properties

Earlier, we described four theoretical justifications for using a test protocol. The first justification is to create a super protocol. We would like the protocol to have a hit rate higher and a false alarm rate lower than that of any test in the protocol. Again consider the sample protocol of ABR, TDT, and ARC. ABR has the highest individual hit rate, 95%, and the lowest false alarm rate, 11%. Thus, for some criterion, we want the protocol to have HTp > 95% and FAp < 11%. From Table 15.6, it is evident that there is no single combination of criterion and test correlation that produce a HTp > 95% and FAp < 11%. With a loose criterion, the protocol hit rate and false alarm rate can be no lower than the largest individual hit rate (95%) and false alarm rate (15%). Likewise, with a strict criterion, the protocol hit rate and false alarm rate can be no greater that the smallest individual hit rate (70%) and false alarm rate (11%). It is never possible to obtain, for any particular combination of criterion and correlation, a protocol hit rate higher than the highest individual hit rate (95%) *and* a false alarm rate lower than the lowest individual false alarm rate (11%). A basic property of test protocols is that a super protocol is not possible and, therefore, cannot be a justification for using a test protocol.

A second justification for a test protocol is improved performance. Is protocol performance always superior to the performance of the individual tests in the protocol? No, performance is not always improved by combining tests. This can be demonstrated by a simple argument. Consider a

TABLE 15.6   Limits on protocol performance.[a]

	HTp/FAp	
CORRELATION	*Loose*	*Strict*
Max-Positive	95/15	70/11
Max-Negative	100/39	49/0

[a]Protocol consists of ABR, TDT, and ARC combined in parallel. Calculations of protocol hit rate and false alarm rate at the extremes of criterion and correlation define limits on possible protocol performance. Results for loose and strict criteria are indicated. Abbreviations explained in Tables 15.1 and 15.4.

protocol that consists of a definitive test (HT/FA = 100/0%) and a test that is not perfect. If used alone, the definitive test will never make an error. If the second test is combined in any way with the definitive test to form a protocol, the protocol will make some errors because the second test will make errors. Clearly, the performance of the protocol is inferior to the performance of the definitive test alone.

The same point can be made from the data in Table 15.6 for the sample protocol. For max-pos correlation and a loose criterion, HTp/FAp = 95/15%. This is clearly inferior to ABR, which has HT/FA = 95/11%. ABR has the same hit rate, but a lower false alarm rate. Again we see that protocol performance can be inferior to that of the tests in the protocol.

Protocol performance is not always better, but is it ever better than the individual tests? For the example protocol of ABR, ARC, and TDT, we can calculate performance measures d' and A' and compare to that of the individual tests (Table 15.7). Two special test correlations, zero and mid-positive, are also considered. (The techniques for calculating protocol performance with zero and mid-positive correlation will be discussed later in this chapter.) Of the three tests in the example protocol, ABR has the best performance with the highest HT, the lowest FA, and the largest d' and A'. Does the performance of the protocol ever exceed that of ABR? First note that as the hit rate of the protocol increases with a loose criterion, so does the false alarm rate. Likewise, as false alarm rate decreases with a strict criterion, so does hit rate. There is the same general trade-off between hit rate and false alarm rate that is evident for individual tests when criterion is changed. No combination of criterion and correlation produce an A' for the protocol that is better than that for ABR; protocol performance is never as good as that of ABR. Only for zero correlation is d' slightly better for the

protocol than for ABR. For all other correlations, ABR has a larger d'.

Turner (1991a) predicted the performance of four protocols assuming mid-positive correlation. These protocols consisted of a screening audiological protocol combined with a definitive test. He calculated A' and d' for the screening protocols using the predicted values of hit rate and false alarm rate (Table 15.8). We can use these results to determine if screening protocol performance is ever better than individual test performance. Note in Table 15.8 that the first screening protocol, S4, is just ABR; the performance of this protocol is, of course, the same as ABR. Two other protocols, S2 and S4, contain ABR. Is their performance superior to ABR, the best test in the protocol? No, A' and d' for protocols S2 and S4 are less than for ABR. Protocol S3 is of interest because it does not contain ABR. Of the tests in the protocol, PIPB has the largest A' (.92) and d' (2.4). Both A' (.89) and d' (1.9) for the protocol are less than for PIPB. We see that none of the protocols achieved a performance better than that of the best test in the protocol.

What can we conclude about protocol performance? First, it is clear that protocol performance can be inferior to individual test performance. The assumption that performance is always improved by using more tests is incorrect. We evaluated four different audiological protocols and found that, in general, performance was poorer with the protocol. There was, however, one result that suggested improved performance on the basis of d'. It is possible that under some conditions performance might be better than the individual tests. The exact relationship between protocol performance and individual test performance is determined by the design of the protocol and the tests that form the protocol. Some type of theoretical or clinical evaluation is required to demonstrate improved performance with a protocol. This assumption cannot be made *a priori*.

TABLE 15.7 Comparison of individual test performance to protocol performance.[a]

TEST	HT/FA	A'	d'			
ABR	95/11	.96	2.9			
TDT	70/13	.87	1.6			
ARC	84/15	.91	2.0			

	LOOSE			STRICT		
CORRELATION	HTp/FAp	A'	d'	HTp/FAp	A'	d'
Max-Pos	95/15	.95	2.7	70/11	.88	1.8
Mid-Pos	97.4/24.5	.93	2.6	63/5.6	.88	1.9
Zero	99.8/34	.91	3.3	56/0.2	.89	3.0
Max-Neg	100/39	.90	[b]	49/0	.87	[b]

[a] Protocol consists of ABR, TDT, and ARC combined in parallel. Results for loose and strict criteria are indicated. Abbreviations explained in Tables 15.1 and 15.4.
[b] The measure d' cannot be calculated because HTp = 100% or FAp = 0%.

TABLE 15.8 Comparison of individual test performance to screening protocol performance.[a]

TEST	HT/FA	A′	d′
ABR	95/11	.96	2.9
ABLB	59/10	.84	1.5
ARC	84/15	.91	2.0
PIPB	74/4	.92	2.4
SISI	65/16	.83	1.4
TDT	70/13	.87	1.6
SCREENING PROTOCOL	**HTs/FAs**	**A′**	**d′**
S1 ABR	95/11	.96	2.9
S2 ARC + ABR	82/6	.93	2.5
S3 ABLB*ARC*PIPB*SISI*TDT	92/31	.89	1.9
S4 ABLB*ARC*PIPB*SISI*TDT + ABR	89/8	.95	2.6

[a]Screening protocols the same as in Table 15.13. A "+" between tests indicates series-positive; "*" between tests indicates tests in parallel with a loose criterion. The values for HT/FA were taken from Table 15.3; values for HTs/FAs were taken from Table 15.13. Abbreviations are explained in Tables 15.1 and 15.4.

The third justification for a protocol is to manipulate hit rate and false alarm rate. From Table 15.7, it is evident that a protocol can produce hit rates and false alarm rates not available with the individual tests. For any correlation other than max-pos, hit rate can be increased with a loose criterion, and false alarm rate can be reduced with a strict criterion. Even though protocol performance may be no better than the best test, a higher hit rate or a lower false alarm rate may be of clinical value.

The fourth justification for a protocol is to screen for a definitive test. This is a legitimate use of multiple tests and is not affected by protocol properties.

Based on the properties of test protocols, we can state the following conclusions:

1. The super protocol is not possible.
2. Improved diagnostic performance with a protocol is questionable; however, degraded performance is clearly possible.
3. Protocols can be used to manipulate hit rate and false alarm rate. A loose criterion will increase hit rate; a strict criterion will decrease false alarm rate.
4. The legitimate reasons for using a protocol are to manipulate hit rate and false alarm rate or to screen for a definitive test.

PREDICTING PROTOCOL PERFORMANCE

Basic Strategy

Often, appropriate clinical data may not be available for calculating protocol performance, and it may not be practical

to collect the data through clinical studies. Is it possible to theoretically predict protocol performance? Yes, protocol performance can be predicted. The techniques are presented in detail by Turner (1988). We will review the basic strategy and equations that are used. Protocol performance can be predicted given sufficient information. It is necessary to know (1) the design of the protocol, (2) the performance of the individual tests in the protocol, and (3) the correlation between individual tests.

Protocol design is determined by the clinician; therefore, design is always known. Many combinations of tests are possible. For our discussion, protocol construction is initially limited to the basic design shown in Figure 15.15A. This protocol consists of blocks of tests connected in series. The patients begin with the test(s) in Block 1 (In) and proceed through the tests until completed (Out). A block can consist of a single test or several tests combined in parallel. For parallel tests, the criterion is limited to loose or strict. The blocks are combined in either series-positive or series-negative. One possible protocol is shown in Figure 15.15B. Block 1 contains three tests in parallel and Block 3 has two tests in parallel. Block 1 is combined to Block 2 in series-positive. All patients with positive results from Block 1 move to Block 2. The patients with negative results are defined as negative for the protocol and receive no more tests. Block 2 and Block 3 are combined in series-negative. All patients who test negative on Block 2 receive the tests in Block 3. All patients who test positive on Block 2 are defined as positive for the protocol and receive no more tests.

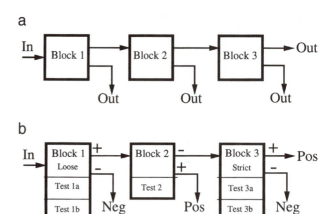

FIGURE 15.15 Basic protocol design. (A) Blocks of tests are connected in series. (B) Within a block, several tests can be combined in parallel with a loose or strict criterion. Blocks may be connected in series-positive or series-negative. (Adapted with permission from R. G. Turner, "Techniques to determine test protocol performance," *Ear and Hearing, 9*, 177–189, 1988.)

TABLE 15.9 Comparison of actual and predicted protocol performance.[a]

	HTp/FAp—LOOSE		HTp/FAp—STRICT	
	Actual	*Predicted*	*Actual*	*Predicted*
ARC*PIPB	90/30	90/34	65/10	60/6
ARC*PIPB*BCL	100/45	92/43	55/0	56/5

[a]Calculations of actual HTp and FAp based on clinical data of Jerger and Jerger (1983). Mid-positive test correlation is assumed for calculating predicted HTp and FAp. Tests are combined in parallel to form protocol. Results are presented for both loose and strict criteria. Abbreviations explained in Tables 15.1 and 15.4. Adapted from Turner (1988).

TABLE 15.10 Comparison of actual and predicted protocol hit rates.[a]

	HTp—LOOSE		HTp—STRICT	
	Actual	*Predicted*	*Actual*	*Predicted*
BEK*SDS	69	68	40	42
BEK*SISI	73	70	48	46
SDS*SISI	76	75	44	45
BEK*SDS*SISI	81	80	38	37

[a]Calculations of actual HTp based on clinical data of Johnson (1977). Mid-positive test correlation is assumed for calculating predicted HTp. Tests are combined in parallel to form protocol. Results are presented for both loose and strict criteria. Abbreviations explained in Tables 15.1 and 15.4. Adapted from Turner (1988).

To determine protocol performance, the HT and FA of the individual tests in the protocol must be known. For audiological tests that distinguish cochlear from retrocochlear site-of-lesion, good estimates of performance are provided by Turner, Shepard, and Frazer (1984). For other tests, the performance measures may not be available.

To calculate protocol performance, it is necessary to know the performance of the individual tests in the protocol; however, this information is not sufficient. It is also necessary to know test correlation. For audiologic tests, very limited data suggest a mid-pos correlation. That is, a test correlation that produces a protocol hit rate and false alarm rate that is halfway between the hit rates and false alarm rates produced by zero test correlation and max-pos correlation. These clinical data (Jerger & Jerger, 1983; Johnson, 1977) are summarized in Tables 15.9 and 15.10. Shown are a comparison of actual protocol hit rates and false alarm rates, calculated from clinical data, as compared to those predicted assuming mid-pos correlation. There is very good agreement between predicted and actual performance indicating an actual test correlation near mid-pos.

What follows in this section are the techniques and equations needed to predict protocol performance. As before, the reader suffering from formula-phobia may wish to skip ahead to the "Example," or to the next topic, "Cost-Benefit Analysis."

Mid-Positive Correlation

Protocol hit rate and false alarm rate for mid-pos correlation [HTp(m)/FAp(m)] is defined to be the average of the protocol hit rates and false alarm rates for zero correlation [HTp(z)/FAp(z)] and max-pos correlation [HTp(+)/FAp(+)]. That is, protocol performance is first calculated assuming zero correlation and then recalculated assuming max-pos correlation. The protocol hit rates for the two correlations are averaged to obtain the protocol hit rate for mid-pos correlation. Protocol false alarm rate

for mid-pos correlation is obtained in a similar way. For mid-pos correlation we have

$$HTp(m) = \frac{HTp(z) + HTp(+)}{2} \qquad (15.19)$$

$$FAp(m) = \frac{FAp(z) + FAp(+)}{2} \qquad (15.20)$$

Protocol hit rates and false alarm rates for max-pos correlation can be calculated using the equations discussed previously for calculating limits on protocol performance (Equations 15.11, 15.12, 15.13, 15.14). To summarize, performance for parallel-strict (or series-positive) is given by **HTp(+) = HTm** and **FAp(+) = FAm** where HTm and FAm are the smallest hit rate and false alarm rate of the individual tests. For parallel-loose (or series-negative) the equations are **HTp(+) = HTx** and **FAp(+) = FAx** where HTx and FAx are the largest hit rate and false alarm rate of the individual tests.

These equations apply when all tests are combined in either parallel or series. Parallel protocols are limited to loose or strict criteria. Series protocols must be entirely series-positive or series-negative.

Zero Correlation

Zero test correlation is a special case of some interest. Not only is performance for zero correlation needed to calculate mid-positive performance, but frequently the assumption is made that tests are independent or uncorrelated. The equations derived for zero correlation have general application.

There are two equations for zero correlation that must be considered. These are for loose and strict criterion with a parallel protocol, or series-positive and series-negative for a series protocol. Recall that the performance of a parallel protocol with a strict criterion is identical to that of a series-positive protocol; thus, they can be considered equivalent when calculating performance. The same is true for parallel-loose and series-negative.

We will first consider the performance of a parallel protocol with strict criterion. Performance is given by

$$HTp(s/z) = \prod_{n=1}^{N} HTn \qquad (15.21)$$

$$FAp(s/z) = \prod_{n=1}^{N} FAn \qquad (15.22)$$

where N = number of individual tests, HTn and FAn are hit rate and false alarm rate of the nth test. The symbol "$\prod$" means the product of the terms. Thus, for three tests in a protocol (N = 3)

$$HTp(z) = HT1*HT2*HT3$$

$$FAp(z) = FA1*FA2*FA3$$

The protocol hit rate and false alarm rate are just the product of the individual tests hit rates and false alarm rates.

Next we consider a parallel protocol with loose criterion. The equations are slightly more complex.

$$HTp(l/z) = HT1 + \sum HTn \times \prod (1 - HTm) \qquad (15.23)$$

$$FAp(l/z) = FA1 + \sum FAn \times \prod (1 - FAm) \qquad (15.24)$$

where N = number of individual tests, HTn and FAn are hit rate and false alarm rate of the nth test, HTm and FAm are hit rate and false alarm rate of the mth test. The symbol "$\sum$" means the sum of the terms. For three tests (N = 3),

$$HTp(z) = HT1 + HT2*(1-HT1) + HT3*(1-HT1)*(1-HT2)$$

$$FAp(z) = FA1 + FAp*(1-FA1) + FA3*(1-FA1)*(1-FA2)$$

Example

The basic techniques for predicting performance will be illustrated by a simple protocol. Complex protocols require some additional techniques that will not be discussed here. Again, the reader is referred to Turner (1988). The protocol consists of three blocks of tests combined in series-positive (Figure 15.16A). The first block contains two tests combined in parallel with a loose criterion. The basic strategy is to determine the hit rate and false alarm rate of each block, and then combine the blocks to determine the performance of the total protocol. Protocol performance will be determined first for zero correlation and then for max-pos correlations. These results will be used to determine performance for mid-pos correlation.

We begin by assuming zero test correlation. The first step is to determine the hit rate and false alarm rate for each block. Block 1 has two tests combined in parallel with a loose criterion. The hit rate and false alarm rate of Block 1 (HB1/FB1) is determined by using Equations 15.23, 15.24.

$$HB1 = HT1a + HT1b*(1–HT1a) = .60 + .76*(1–.60) = .90 = 90\%$$

$$FB1 = FA1a + FA1b*(1–FA1a) = .10 + .22*(1–.10) = .30 = 30\%$$

Block 2 and Block 3 contain just one test each; therefore, the performance of the test in the block is the performance of the block (Figure 15.16B). Now that an equivalent hit rate and false alarm rate has been calculated for each block, the three blocks can be combined using the equation for series-positive (Equations 15.21, 15.22). Recall that series-positive is equivalent to parallel with a strict criterion. The resultant hit rate and false alarm rate are that of the total protocol for zero correlation (HTp(z)/FAp(z)).

$$HTp(z) = HB1*HB2*HB3 = .90*.80*.90 = .65 = 65\%$$

$$FAp(z) = FB1*FB2*FB3 = .30*.20*.16 = .01 = 1\%$$

We can think of reducing the protocol to a single test with a performance equal to that of the protocol (Figure 15.16C).

Next we determine protocol performance for max-pos correlation. Again, the first step is to determine the performance of each block. For max-pos correlation, the performance of Block 1 is given by Equations 15.11, 15.12.

$$HB1 = MAX[HT1a, HT1b] = MAX[60,76] = 76\%$$

$$FB1 = MAX[FA1a, FA1b] = MAX[10, 22] = 22\%$$

As before, the performance of last two blocks equals that of the single test in each block. Protocol performance is determined by calculating the performance of the three blocks combined in series-positive (Equations 15.13, 15.14).

$$HTp(+) = MIN[HB1, HB2, HB3] = MIN[76, 80, 90] = 76\%$$

$$FAp(+) = MIN[FB1, FB2, FB3] = MIN[22, 20, 16] = 16\%$$

The final step is to calculate protocol performance for mid-pos correlation (Equations 15.19, 15.20).

$$HTp(m) = \frac{HTp(z) + HTp(+)}{2} = \frac{65 + 76}{2} = \frac{141}{2} = 71\%$$

$$FAp(m) = \frac{FAp(z) + FAp(+)}{2} = \frac{1+1}{2} = \frac{17}{2} = 8$$

The hit rate of the protocol is 71% and the false alarm rate is 8%, assuming a mid-positive correlation.

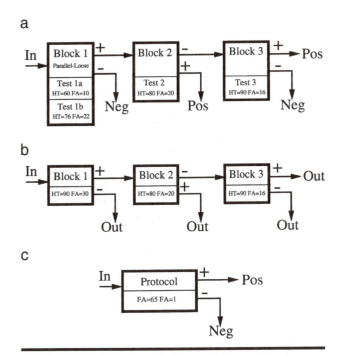

FIGURE 15.16 Basic strategy for predicting protocol performance. (A) Protocol design. (B) First step is to calculate the performance of each block. Protocol can then be represented as an equivalent protocol with one test in each block. (C) The blocks can be combined to calculate protocol performance. Protocol is represented as a single test with equivalent performance.

COST-BENEFIT ANALYSIS

Overview

Cost-benefit analysis is the consideration of factors other than performance when selecting protocols for clinical use. Up to this point, we have been concerned with measures of performance. Cost-benefit analysis is necessary because the protocol with the best performance is not always the appropriate protocol to use. There may be significant financial cost or personal risk to the patient that makes the use of a particular protocol undesirable.

Subjective cost-benefit analysis is common in clinical practice. Ultimately, we must make decisions about patient care; we must decide what tests to administer. In lieu of formal, objective techniques we employ the subjective/intuitive strategy. We may not realize that we have performed a cost-benefit analysis, but we have. Whenever we decide not to use a test because it costs too much, it takes too long, the patients complain, no one uses the information, and so on, we have conducted a cost-benefit analysis. We can avoid the sloppiness and bias of the subjective approach by using a more objective analysis.

The basic strategy of an objective cost-benefit analysis is to quantify the various costs and/or benefits of the protocols. Generally, costs are assigned to errors (misses and false alarms); benefits are assigned to correct decisions (hits and correct rejections). The protocol with the greatest benefits and lowest cost is the one of choice.

While conceptually simple, the cost-benefit analysis can be extremely difficult in practice. Most analyses are based on the number of hits, misses, false alarms, and correct rejections. To determine these numbers, we must know the performance of the protocol and the prevalence of the disease. Unfortunately, this necessary information may not be available from clinical data. The other major problem with cost-benefit analysis is quantifying costs and benefits. The financial cost of a procedure is easy to specify, but how is a number derived for patient suffering or death? Even financial cost can be difficult. For example, data may not be available to determine the long-term financial impact of an undetected disease on patient or society.

All is not lost; even a simple cost-benefit analysis can be useful. We will consider two relatively simple techniques: *cost ratios* and *cost analysis*. Both techniques require a knowledge of hit rate, false alarm rate, and prevalence. Both require calculations of hits and false alarms. Cost ratios require no other information; cost analysis needs the financial cost of administrating each test in the protocol. With both techniques, we avoid the more difficult measures of cost; however, we still need protocol performance. Even that may not be available from clinical data. Fortunately, we have presented techniques in this chapter that can be used to predict protocol performance.

Protocol Performance

Numerous audiologic tests have been developed to identify retrocochlear disease. Turner (1991a) reviewed the performance of many individual tests and combinations of tests to consider performance of the test battery principle. The general strategy has been to combine audiologic (and occasionally vestibular tests) with a definitive radiological test. Although decisions regarding patient treatment are made on the basis of the definitive test, the financial cost, morbidity, and even possible mortality have made it impractical to test every suspect patient with the definitive test. For these reasons other tests must serve as a screening protocol to decide who receives the definitive test.

We will consider several protocols to illustrate the techniques of cost ratios and cost analysis. The protocols will combine a screening protocol with a definitive radiological test. Individuals who test positive on the screening protocol receive the definitive test. For the definitive test, we will use magnetic resonance imaging with gadolinium-DPTA, which has a hit rate approaching 100% and a false alarm rate approaching 0% (Kileny, Telian, & Kemink 1991).

For comparison, the first protocol will consist of MRI-G without a screening protocol. For five protocols, the screening protocol will consist of an individual test: auditory brainstem response (ABR); electronystagmography—caloric response (ENG-C); acoustic reflex and reflex decay—combined (ARC); performance intensity functions for phonetically balanced words (PIPB); and tone decay testing (TDT).

We will consider two additional protocols using ARC and ABR combined with a definitive radiological test. ARC and ABR have the best performance of the audiologic tests in Table 15.3 as measured by d' and A'. For one protocol, ARC and ABR are combined in series-positive. That is, individuals who test positive on ARC are tested by ABR. Those that are positive on ABR are tested with MRI-G. Thus, an individual must test positive on both ARC and ABR to receive MRI-G. For the other protocol, ARC and ABR are combined in series-negative. Individuals who test positive on ARC proceed directly to MRI-G. Those who test negative on ARC are tested by ABR. Those who are positive on ABR receive MRI-G. In this protocol, an individual who tests positive on either ARC or ABR is tested by MRI-G.

First, we must calculate the hit rate and the false alarm rate of the protocols. Note that all individuals identified as positive by the screening protocol (hits and false alarms) will receive the definitive test. The definitive test, having near perfect performance, will correctly identify which individuals were hits on the screening protocol and which were false alarms. The hit rate of the total protocol will, therefore, equal the hit rate of the screening protocol. Individuals not identified in screening remain undetected because they do not receive the definitive test. The false alarm rate

of the total protocol is zero because false alarms from the screening protocol are correctly identified as correct rejections by the definitive test.

Please note that the hit rates and false alarm rates of the screening protocols, not the total protocols, are given in Table 15.11. As stated above, the hit rate of the total protocol equals that of the screening protocol; the false alarm rate of the total protocol equals zero.

The first protocol is just MRI-G. There is no screening protocol; everyone is referred for MRI-G. For screening protocols consisting of one test (P2–P6), hit rate and false alarm rate equal the hit rate and false alarm rate of the individual test. For the two screening protocols that use ARC and ABR (P7, P8), hit rate and false alarm rate are calculated using techniques presented in this chapter, assuming a mid-positive test correlation.

Next we must calculate the number of hits, misses, correct rejections, and false alarms. Olsen (1987) presented a hypothetical sample of 1000 patients having sensorineural hearing loss evaluated because of suspicion of eighth nerve tumors. Hart and Davenport (1981) report 5% as the average prevalence of acoustic tumors in a clinical population suspected for retrocochlear disease. Using a 5% prevalence rate, 50 patients would presumably have eighth nerve lesions and 950 patients would have sensory (cochlear) hearing losses.

Table 15.11 shows the number of the hypothetical 1000 patients identified as hits, misses, correct rejections, and false alarms for the eight screening protocols. The number of hits is simply the screening hit rate (HTs) times the number of patients with eighth nerve lesions (50). The number of false alarms equals the screening false alarm rate (FAs) times the number of patients with sensory hearing loss (950). Misses and correct rejections are calculated from the number of hits and false alarms. Because of the

TABLE 15.11   Performance of eight screening protocols.[a]

| PROTOCOL[b] | HTs | FAs | 50 TUMORS | | 950 COCHLEAR | |
			hs	ms	cs	fs
P1 MRI-G	n/a	n/a	—	—	—	—
P2 ABR + MRI-G	95	11	47	3	846	104
P3 ENG-C + MRI-G	85	33	42	8	637	313
P4 ARC + MRI-G	84	15	42	8	808	142
P5 PIPB + MRI-G	74	4	37	13	912	38
P6 TDT + MRI-G	70	13	35	15	827	123
P7 ARC + ABR + MRI-G	82	6	41	9	893	57
P8 (ARC – ABR) + MRI-G	97	20	48	2	760	190

[a]Screening protocol is everything except MRI-G, the definitive test. Note that Protocol P1 has no screening protocol. The numbers given in table are for screening protocol, not total protocol. Prevalence is assumed to be 5%.

[b]Hit rates and false alarm rates for individual tests are given in Table 15.3. Abbreviations explained in Tables 15.1 and 15.4.

definitive test, the number of hits for the total protocol equals that of the screening protocol. The number of false alarms for the total protocol will equal zero.

Ranking with Cost Ratios

Consider the following situation. We have several possible screening protocols that we wish to combine with a definitive test. We want to evaluate the performance of the screening protocols so as to determine the best protocol for clinical use. Patients who are positive on the screening protocol will receive the definitive test. Patients who test negative will not receive the definitive test and will, in most cases, be lost from the system. Patients who test positive on the screening protocol constitute the hits and false alarms. The definitive test will accurately sort these patients into the two groups. The patients who test negative are the misses and correct rejections. Since these patients do not receive the definitive test, we have no information as to the number in each group.

We would like to calculate the hit rate and the false alarm rate for the screening protocols, but we cannot because we do not have an accurate count of misses and correct rejections. If we had an exact measure of disease prevalence in the test population, then the misses and correct rejections could be calculated from the hits and false alarms. In practice, the exact prevalence will not be known. Is the situation hopeless? No, Dobie (1985) provides a clever technique to rank-order protocols by using only data on patients who test positive (the hits and false alarms) on the screening protocol. This technique requires that (1) a definitive test be used to accurately determine hits and false alarms, and (2) we decide the relative costs of errors, that is, how many false alarms equal one miss.

The technique can be illustrated with this example. Consider three of the screening protocols discussed above that are combined with MRI-G to identify retrocochlear lesion. Protocol 2 is ABR alone, Protocol 7 is ARC combined in series positive with ABR, Protocol 8 is ARC combined in series negative with ABR. We must choose a cost ratio, R; this is the maximum number of false alarms that we will accept for each miss. This decision is the cost-benefit component of this technique and can be somewhat subjective. In this case, we consider a false alarm preferable to a miss because of the danger of an undetected tumor. In other situations, we might consider a miss less costly than a false alarm. We decide to accept up to 5 false alarms for every miss, that is, R = 5.

The relative difference in the cost (CST) of two protocols is given by the following equation:

$$CST(X-Y) = (fsX - fsY) - R*(hsX - hsY) \quad (15.25)$$

where hsX, fsX are the number of hits, false alarms of Protocol X and hsY, fsY are the number of hits, false alarms of Protocol Y. If CST is positive then the cost of Protocol X is greater than the cost of Protocol Y and, therefore, Protocol Y is superior. If CST is negative then Protocol X is superior.

To rank-order our three protocols, we must compute the relative cost of the three pairs of protocols: CST(2–7), CST(2–8), CST(7–8). For this example, assume that 1000 patients were tested with each protocol. With Protocol 2, 151 patients tested positive. MRI-G ultimately demonstrated that the 151 patients consisted of 47 hits and 104 false alarms. Protocol 7 was positive for 98 patients, of which 41 were hits and 57 were false alarms. For Protocol 8, there were 48 hits and 190 false alarms. Calculations of the cost differences are shown in Table 15.12. Note that CST(2–8) and CST(7–8) are both negative indicating that P2 and P7 are both superior to P8. For R = 5, CST(2–7) is positive (+17) indicating that P7 is superior to P2. Thus we could rank-order the three protocols as P7, P2, P8.

These results are somewhat surprising in that ABR was not the best protocol. This is a consequence of R, the cost ratio we selected. What would happen if we permitted 10 false alarms for each miss? The calculations for R = 10 are also shown in Table 15.12. In this case we see that CST(2–7) is negative indicating that P2 (ABR) is superior. The rank-orderings now would be P2, P7, P8. We see that the rank-ordering of the protocols is highly dependent on our selection of R. If R is small, then protocols with low false alarm rates will be favored. If R is large, then protocols with high hit rates are favored.

The primary advantage of this technique is that protocols can be rank-ordered using just hits and false alarms. These numbers are usually more available from clinical data than misses and correct rejections. The technique has, however, several disadvantages. The rank-order is a strong function of the cost ratio we select; the orderings can change significantly with different ratios, as with our example. The selection of the cost ratio can be extremely

TABLE 15.12 Cost ratios of three protocols.[a]

PROTOCOL	HTs/FAs	hs/fs
P2 ABR + MRI-G	95/11	48/105
P7 ARC + ABR + MRI-G	82/6	41/57
P8 (ARC − ABR) + MRI-G	97/20	48/190

RELATIVE COST	R = 5	R = 10
CST(2-7)	+17	−13
CST(2-8)	−81	−76
CST(7-8)	−98	−63

[a]Protocols are the same as in Table 15.12. A "+" between tests indicates series-positive; "(ARC − ABR)" means the two tests are in series-negative. A positive result on either ARC or ABR sends patient for MRI-G. Abbreviations explained in Tables 15.1 and 15.4.

arbitrary and subjective, thus, the resulting rank-order will be equally arbitrary. This technique is only as good as the selection of the cost ratio. The second disadvantage is that these calculations provide a relative ranking, not an absolute measure of the performance of the different protocols. The protocols under consideration may all be terrible, the top-ranked protocol may only be "less bad" than the others. Even with these limitations, this technique is still extremely valuable.

Cost Analysis

Another fairly simple cost-benefit strategy is cost analysis. For this technique, we calculate the financial cost of each protocol. In particular, we determine the average cost for each patient tested and the average cost for each "diseased" patient identified. No attempt is made to assign costs to nonfinancial factors such as morbidity or mortality.

For this example, we will consider the eight protocols in Table 15.11. Financial cost for each protocol is calculated assuming a retrocochlear disease prevalence of 5% and a patient population of 1000. A cost value of 1.0 is assigned to ARC, PIPB, and TDT; a value of 6 is assigned for ABR and ENG-C, because charges for these test generally are about six times higher than for ARC and PIPB; accordingly a value of 30 is assigned to MRI-G. Assuming each unit is worth $50, the ARC, PIPB, and TDT tests are estimated at a cost of $50 each, an ABR or ENG-C at $300 each, and an MRI-G at $1500. While prices may vary by practitioner, region, and over time, it is assumed that these relative value units offer a stable reference point.

Table 15.13 gives the total cost of each protocol, the cost per patient tested, and the cost per patient identified with retrocochlear lesion. Note that for all protocols, with the exception of MRI-G alone (when all 1000 patients receive the MRI-G), the numbers of hits and false alarms on the screening test(s) indicates the number of patients given the definitive test (MRI-G).

In P1, all 1000 patients suspected of a retrocochlear lesion are given the MRI-G without any audiological screening test. It is assumed that all 50 patients with tumors are identified and the total cost is $1,500,000 (i.e., 1000 patients × $1500 per test). The cost per patient tested is, obviously, $1500. Since, in our example, we have 50 patients with tumors, the cost to identify each patient can be found by dividing $1,500,000 by 50 which equals $30,000.

In P2, all 1000 patients are screened by ABR. A total of 151 patients (47 hits and 104 false alarms) receive the MRI-G. The overall cost is $526,500. The relative cost to identify the 47 tumors is $11,202 per identified tumor patient, a savings of $18,798 per tumor patient relative to P1. The limitation however, is that 5% of the tumors were missed.

In P3, only the ENG-C is given to the 1000. A total of 355 patients (42 hits and 313 false alarms) receive the definitive test (MRI-G). The financial cost of this protocol is $832,500, $306,000 higher than the total cost of P2. The high cost of this protocol is attributable to the 33% false alarm rate. More importantly, P3 misses 8 of the true eighth nerve tumor patients in this hypothetical sample.

In P4, the ARC is given all patients. A total of 184 patients receive the MRI-G. This protocol has a hit rate of 42 (the same as the ENG-C) but the relative costs are lower at $331,000 because of the reduced false alarm rate. P4 costs $7881 per identified tumor and is less expensive than P2 (ABR), but misses 5 more tumors than does P2.

The next two screening test protocols have relatively poor hit rates. In P5, the PIPB test is given to all patients, but with a hit rate of 74% identifies only 37 of the 50 tumors. Total costs and costs per identified tumor are low because this test also has the lowest false alarm rate of the audiologic tests (4%), and consequently only 75 patients

TABLE 15.13 Cost analysis of eight protocols.[a]

PROTOCOL[b]	TC($)	CP($)	CTI($)	TM(%)
P1 MRI-G	1,500,000	1,500	30,000	<1
P2 ABR + MRI-G	526,500	526	11,202	5
P3 ENG-C + MRI-G	832,500	832	19,821	15
P4 ARC + MRI-G	331,000	331	7,881	16
P5 PIPB + MRI-G	162,500	162	4,392	26
P6 TDT + MRI-G	287,000	287	8,200	30
P7 ARC + ABR + MRI-G	252,200	252	6,151	18
P8 (ARC − ABR) + MRI-G	651,800	652	13,579	3

[a] Prevalence is assumed to be 5%.

[b] Hit rate and false alarm rate for individual tests are given in Table 15.3. A "+" between tests indicates series-positive; "(ARC − ABR)" means the two tests are in series-negative. A positive result on either ARC or ABR sends patient for MRI-G. TC: total cost; CP: cost per patient tested; CTI: cost per tumor identified; TM: tumors missed by protocol. Other abbreviations explained in Tables 15.1 and 15.4.

receive the MRI-G. With the TDT as the screening test (P6) the hit rate is unacceptable (70%), and the false alarm rate increases to 13%.

Reviewing the data of Table 15.13, it appears that P3 has unacceptable costs and P5 and P6 have unacceptable hit rates as screening tests for retrocochlear lesions. The best alternatives to P1 appear to be P2 and P4 (ABR or ARC). Given this information, it is of interest to combine ABR and ARC. P7 and P8 provide examples of combining these tests in an effort to reduce cost and/or improve hit rate.

In P7, the ARC is combined with ABR in series-positive. This procedure reduces financial cost but the hit rate is also reduced to 82% because ARC and ABR are combined in series and total hit rate can be no better than the hit rate of the poorest test in the series. In this procedure all 1000 patients are screened by ARC; in addition, 184 are also screened by ABR and 98 (41 hits and 57 false alarms) eventually are given the MRI-G. The overall cost of this protocol is $252,200, which is less than one-half the cost of P2, but it also misses more than three times as many of the eighth nerve tumor patients (9 versus 3).

P8 combines ARC and ABR in series-negative. In this procedure all 1000 patients are given the ARC. Those patients testing positive on the ARC are given the MRI-G, patients with negative ARC results are given the ABR, and those with positive ABR findings are evaluated by MRI-G. This series-negative combination yields a higher hit rate (97%) and higher false alarm rate (20%) than either ARC or ABR alone. The total cost, $651,000, is derived from 1000 patients receiving the ARC, 816 receiving the ABR, and 238 having the MRI-G. The cost is slightly higher than P2, but it catches 2% more of the tumor patients.

Cost Analysis—Probability of Eighth Nerve Tumors

One area not addressed by our discussion of CDA is the criteria used to categorize patients as suspect for retrocochlear lesions in the first place. It must be recognized that any patient with an eighth nerve tumor who is seen for an audiologic evaluation but who is not selected for a site-of-lesion protocol is lost to the system as it now functions. This caution serves to reinforce the need for continued evaluation of patient history, initial test selection, test findings, and outcome.

The probability of eighth nerve tumors in patients considered at risk for such lesions will vary depending upon the presenting symptoms. The probability of symptom complexes correlating with the ultimate detection of eighth nerve tumors has been estimated by Welling, Glasscock, Woods, and Jackson (1990). They considered the "classic" symptom group consisting of unilateral asymmetric sensorineural hearing loss, tinnitus, and decreased word recognition as high risk, having >30% probability of being associated with an eighth nerve tumor. Symptoms such as

sudden sensorineural hearing loss or otherwise unexplained persistent unilateral tinnitus were classified as intermediate risk (>5% and <30% probability), and symptoms of isolated vertigo, historically explained unilateral hearing loss, or tinnitus were classified as low risk (<5% probability of an eighth nerve tumor).

Table 15.14 shows the financial implications of using the MRI-G alone as the definitive test, or MRI-G only following a positive ABR result for each of the risk categories (high, intermediate, and low). Hypothetical groups of patients with sensorineural hearing loss are presented, of whom 50 have eighth nerve tumors. Columns in Table 15.14, beginning on the left, show (1) the probability of an eighth nerve tumor (Pt) in the group of patients considered to be of high, intermediate, or low risk; (2) the protocols; (3) the number of patients (N50) required for 50 patients to have an acoustic neuroma, assuming the different probabilities of having a tumor; (4) and (5) the number of hits and false alarms for the screening protocols; (6) the total protocol cost (TC) for all patients tested; (7) the actual cost (CTI) expended to identify each tumor patient; (8) the savings in dollars for each tumor identified, if the ABR test is given to patients suspected to have eighth nerve tumors, and the MRI-G is given only to those patients with positive ABR results.

In our hypothetical sample of patients with a 30% probability of having a tumor, an N of only 165 patients is required to include 50 patients with tumors. Employing the ABR as a screening test results in missing three tumor patients and saving $1982 for each of the 47 patients identified with tumors.

The data for the intermediate risk group (5%) is the same as shown in Tables 15.11 and 15.13 for the MRI-G and ABR + MRI-G protocols. One thousand patients are now needed to include 50 patients with tumors and the costs per identified patient are $30,000 for testing all with MRI-G and $11,202 for the ABR + MRI-G protocol. By using the ABR as a screening test for this intermediate probability group, a savings of $18,797 per patient identified is estimated as compared to giving all 1000 patients the MRI-G.

The value of the screening test protocol is dramatically shown in the low probability risk group shown in this example. Five thousand patients are now needed to include 50 patients with tumors. If an MRI-G were given to each patient, the cost per identified tumor jumps to $150,000. With the ABR as a screening test, the cost per tumor identified is lowered by $99,223. Moreover, the cost of the protocol for all 5000 patients is reduced by $5,113,500 when ABR is used as a screening test.

Decisions regarding referral of patients for MRI-G, without other test results such as ABR, rest on a number of factors. Clearly, the patient's case history, symptoms, as well as his or her anxiety, must be considered in determining

TABLE 15.14 Cost analysis of protocols assuming different probability of tumor.[a]

Pt(%)	PROTOCOL	N50	hs	fs	TC($)	CTI($)	STI($)
30	MRI-G	165	50	0	247,500	4,950	
30	ABR + MRI-G	165	47	13	139,500	2,968	1,982
5	MRI-G	1000	50	0	1,500,000	30,000	
5	ABR + MRI-G	1000	47	104	526,500	11,202	18,797
1	MRI-G	5000	50	0	7,500,000	150,000	
1	ABR + MRI-G	5000	47	544	2,386,500	50,777	99,223

[a]Prevalence is assumed to be 5%.

Hit rate and false alarm rate for protocols are given in Table 15.11. A "+" between tests indicates series-positive. Pt: probability of tumor based on symptoms; N50: number of patients required to yield 50 tumors; TC: total cost; CTI: cost per tumor identified; STI: savings per tumor identified using ABR. Other abbreviations explained in Tables 15.1 and 15.4.

a definitive cause for symptoms. Furthermore, the patient's convenience and access to medical attention in follow-up examinations to assess stability or progression of symptoms or concerns that initiated the evaluation also influence the course taken in the diagnostic protocol.

Nevertheless, the hypothetical data in Tables 15.13 and 15.14 serves to highlight the importance of CDA in an era of medical cost containment coupled with powerful yet expensive diagnostic capabilities. Clearly, the use of clinical decision analysis in audiology opens a new era for defining optimum defensible strategies for identification and differential diagnosis of auditory disorders and a conceptual framework for clinical data analysis.

Some Limitations

This review of clinical decision analysis (CDA) was based primarily on the work of Turner and his colleagues (Turner, 1988; Turner, Frazer, & Shepard, 1984; Turner & Nielsen, 1984; Turner, Shepard, & Frazer, 1984) and is essentially an academic exercise applying several assumptions to data obtained from a literature review. Consequently, some limitations should be addressed before accepting clinical inferences. One critical assumption deals with test correlation. If two tests both identify the same patients, the tests have maximum-positive correlation. If the two tests identify different patients the tests have maximum-negative correlation. Because actual test correlation was not always available, a mid-positive correlation was assumed for the protocols using tests in combination. For example, in P8 of Table 15.11, the use of a mid-positive correlation assumption led to the conclusion that some patients with eighth nerve lesions will be positive for the ARC, but negative for the ABR. Although experience shows that this will happen on occasion (Bauch, Rose, & and Harner 1983; Robinette, Bauch, Olsen, Harner, & Beatty, 1992), the actual correla-

tion between these and other tests has not been validated by clinical studies. Another limitation of CDA as reviewed here is the requirement that test outcomes may only be (+) or (−) for the disorder being identified. Whereas, this assumption may be appropriate for protocols to identify eighth nerve lesions and perhaps for early identification of hearing loss (Jacobson & Jacobson, 1987; Turner, 1991b, 1992a, 1992b), the same assumptions may not suffice for evaluations of central auditory disorders (Musiek, 1991) or for the evaluation of dizzy patients.

REFERENCES

Bauch, C. D., Olsen, W. O., & Pool, A. F. (1996). ABR indices: Sensitivity, specificity, and tumor size. *American Journal of Audiology*, 5(1), 97–104.

Bauch, C. D., Rose, D. E., & Harner, S. G. (1982). Auditory brainstem responses from 255 patients with suspected retrocochlear involvement. *Ear and Hearing, 3*, 83–86.

Bauch, C. D., Rose., D. E., & Harner, S. G. (1983) Auditory brainstem response and acoustic reflex test results for patients with and without tumor matched for hearing loss. *Archives of Otolaryngology, 109*, 522–525.

Dobie, R. A., (1985). The use of relative cost ratios in choosing a diagnostic test. *Ear and Hearing, 6*, 113–116.

Egan, J. P. (1975). *Signal Detection Theory and ROC Analysis.* New York: Academic Press.

Hart, R. G., & Davenport, J. (1981). Diagnosis of acoustic tumors. *Neurosurgery, 9*, 450–463.

Hart, R. G., Gardner, D., & Howieson, J. (1983). Acoustic tumors: Atypical features and recent diagnostic tests. *Neurology, 33*, 211–221.

Hirsh, A., & Anderson, H. (1980). Audiologic test results in 96 patients with tumours affecting the eight nerve. *Acta Otolaryngologica Supplement, 369*, 1–26.

Jacobson, J. T., & Jacobson, C. A. (1987). Principles of decision analysis in high risk infants. *Seminars in Hearing, 8*, 133–141.

Jerger, S. (1983). Decision matrix and information theory analysis in the evaluation of neuro-audiologic tests. *Seminars in Hearing, 4,* 121–132.

Jerger, S., & Jerger, J. (1983). The evaluation of diagnostic audiometric tests. *Audiology, 22,* 144–161.

Johnson, E. W. (1977). Auditory test results in 500 cases of acoustic neuroma. *Archives of Otolaryngology, 103,* 152–158.

Kileny, P. R., Telian, S. A., & Kemink, J. L. (1991). Acoustic neuroma: Diagnosis and management. In J. T. Jacobson, & J. L. Northern (Eds.), *Diagnostic Audiology* (pp. 217–233). Austin, TX: Pro-Ed.

Martin, F. N., Armstrong, T. W., & Champlin, C. A. (1994). A survey of audiological practices in the United States. *American Journal of Audiology, 3*(2), 20–26.

Mulkens, T. H., Parizel, P. M., Martin, J. J., Degryse, H. R., Van de Heyning, P. H., Forton, G. E., & De Schepper, A. M. (1993). Acoustic schwannoma: MR findings in 84 tumors. *American Journal of Radiology, 160,* 395–398.

Moscicki, E. K. (1984). The prevalence of "incidence" is too high. *Asha, 26,* 39–40.

Musiek, F. E. (1991). Auditory evoked responses in site-of-lesion assessment. In W. F. Rintelmann (Ed.), *Hearing Assessment* (2nd ed., pp. 383–427). Austin, TX: Pro-Ed.

Olsen, W. O. (1987). Differential audiology tests. In M. S. Robinette & C. D. Bauch (Eds.), *Proceedings of a Symposium in Audiology.* Rochester, MN: Mayo Clinic.

Rintelmann, W. F. (1991). *Hearing Assessment.* Austin, TX: Pro-Ed.

Robinette, M. S., Bauch, C. D., Olsen, W. O., Harner, S. G., & Beatty, C. W. (1992). Use of TEOAE, ABR, and acoustic reflex measures to assess auditory function in patients with acoustic neuroma. *American Journal of Audiology, 1*(4), 66–72.

Robinette, M. S., & Durrant, J. D. (1997). Contributions of evoked otoacoustic emissions in differential diagnosis. In M.S. Robinette & T. J. Glattke (Eds.), *Otoacoustic Emissions: Clinical Applications* (pp. 205–232). New York: Thieme.

Robinson, D. E., & Watson, C. S. (1972). Psychophysical methods in modern psychoacoustics. In J. V. Tobias (Ed.), *Foundations of Modern Auditory Theory* (pp. 101–131). New York: Academic Press.

Schuknecht, H. (1974). *Pathology of the Ear.* Cambridge, MA: Harvard University Press.

Swets, J. A. (1964). *Signal Detection and Recognition by Human Observers.* New York: John Wiley & Sons.

Turner, R. G. (1988) Techniques to determine test protocol performance. *Ear and Hearing, 9,* 177–189.

Turner, R. G. (1991a). Making clinical decisions. In W. F. Rintelmann (Ed.), *Hearing Assessment* (pp. 679–738). Austin, TX: Pro-Ed.

Turner, R. G. (1991b). Modeling the cost and performance of early identification protocols. *Journal of the American Acedemy of Audiology, 2,* 195–205.

Turner, R. G. (1992a). Comparison of four hearing screening protocols. *Journal of the American Academy of Audiology, 3,* 200–207.

Turner, R. G. (1992b). Factors that determine the cost and performance of early identification protocols. *Journal of the American Academy of Audiology, 3,* 233–241.

Turner, R. G., Frazer, G. J., & Shepard, N. T. (1984). Clinical performance of audiological and related diagnostic tests. *Ear and Hearing, 15,* 187–194.

Turner, R. G., & Nielsen, D. W. (1984). Application of clinical decision analysis to audiological tests. *Ear and Hearing, 5,* 125–133.

Turner, R. G., Shepard, N. T., & Frazer, G. J. (1984). Formulating and evaluating audiological test protocols. *Ear and Hearing, 15,* 321–330.

Welling, D. B., Glasscock, M. E., Woods, C. I., & Jackson, C. G. (1990). Acoustic neuroma: A cost-effective approach. *Otolaryngology—Head and Neck Surgery, 103,*(3) 364–370.

CHAPTER 16

OCCUPATIONAL HEARING LOSS PREVENTION PROGRAMS

THOMAS H. SIMPSON

The National Institute for Occupational Safety and Health (NIOSH) estimates that in 1992, approximately 30 million American workers were exposed to hazardous levels of occupational noise. NIOSH further estimates that the number of exposed workers has increased by over 30% since 1983 (NIOSH, 1998). Traditionally, industrial hearing conservation programs (HCPs) have sought to preserve hearing abilities of workers already demonstrating some degree of occupational hearing loss. This is because federal regulations mandating noise control and hearing protection did not exist until 1969, and specific requirements for "effective" HCPs did not exist prior to 1983 (Federal Register, 1968, 1969a, 1969b, 1974a, 1974b, 1975, 1981, 1983). Consequently, HCPs were often implemented after significant portions of the work force had already been overexposed, and the primary performance goal of these programs was to prevent additional occupationally related hearing loss.

The generation of American workers not fully benefitting from HCPs has either retired or is nearing retirement age. Therefore, the term "hearing conservation" has recently been replaced by "hearing loss prevention," to underscore the notion of "zero tolerance" towards the almost entirely preventable condition of occupational hearing loss (NIOSH, 1998).

Audiologists are uniquely qualified to assume positions of responsibility in occupational hearing loss prevention programs (HLPPs). Professional supervision of audiometric testing programs is necessary to assure reliable and valid data for early identification and intervention. Indifferently implemented hearing testing programs often do little more than document the steady progression of noise-induced hearing loss (Gasaway, 1985).

Audiologists should also acquire knowledge and skills necessary to interact with professionals from other disciplines commonly associated with occupational health and safety. These disciplines include occupational health nurses, physicians, industrial hygienists, safety professionals, and noise control engineers. It is paramount that audiologists be able to serve as effective members of a multidisciplinary team concerned with prevention of occupational hearing loss.

This chapter provides a brief overview of current legal requirements and "best practices" for occupational hearing loss prevention programs (HLPPs). Legal requirements will identify minimum steps necessary to achieve compliance with federal regulations. "Best practices" will identify more proactive approaches thought to lead to truly effective HLPPs.

BACKGROUND

It is beyond the scope of this chapter to review the extensive literature associating noise exposure with hearing loss. Readers are encouraged to consult other sources of information on this well-established link (ACGIH, 1995; Atherley, 1973; Atherley & Martin, 1971; Axlesson, Borchgrevink, Hamernik, Hellstrom, Henderson, & Salvi, 1996; Bohne, Yohman, & Gruner, 1987; Bohne, Zahn, & Bozzay, 1985; Byrne, Henderson, Saunders, Powers, & Farzi, 1988; Ceypek, Kuzniarz, & Lipowczan, 1973; CHABA, 1986; Clark & Bohne, 1986; Clark, Bohne, & Boettcher, 1987; Coles, 1980; Coles, Garinther, Hodge, & Rice, 1968; Coles, Rice, & Martin, 1973; Danielson, Henderson, Gratton, Bianchi, & Salvi, 1991; Eldred, Gannon, & von Gierke, 1955; Fechter, Young, & Carlisle, 1988; von Gierke, Robinson, & Karmy, 1981; Glorig, Ward, & Nixon, 1961; Guberan, Fernandez, Cardinet, & Terrier, 1971; Hamernik, Henderson, Colig, & Salvi, 1981; Helmkamp, Talbott, & Margolis, 1984; Henderson & Hamernik, 1986; Holmgren, Johnsson, Kylin, & Linde, 1971; ISO, 1961; Kryter, Ward, Miller, & Eldredge, 1966; Kuzniarz, Swierczynski, & Lipowczan, 1976; Nilsson, Liden, & Sanden, 1977; Passchier-Vermeer, 1968, 1971, 1973; Price & Kalb, 1991; Robinson, 1968; Sataloff, Vassallo, & Menduke, 1969; U.S. Air Force, 1956; Ward, 1970, 1980, 1986; Ward & Nelson, 1971; Ward & Turner, 1982).

Furthermore, this chapter will not address potential relationships between noise exposure and nonauditory health effects, such as annoyance, hypertension, and anxiety. At this time there is a lack of conclusive evidence associating noise exposure with these conditions (Belli, Sri, Scarficcia, & Sorrentino, 1984; Cohen, 1973, 1976; Delin, 1984; Humes, 1984; Jonsson & Hansson, 1977; Lees &

Roberts, 1979; Malchaire & Mullier, 1979; Manninen & Aro, 1979; Melnick, 1994; Noweir, 1984; Ohrstrom, Martin, & Rylander, 1988; Parvizpoor, 1976; Singh, Rai, Bhatia, & Nayar, 1982; Suter, 1989, 1992b; Talbott, Findlay, Kuller, Lenkner, Matthews, Day, & Ishii, 1990; Talbott, Helmkamp, Matthews, Kuller, Cottington, & Redmond, 1985; Verbeek, van Dijk, & de Vries, 1987; Wilkins & Action, 1982; Wu, Ko, & Chang, 1987). It is furthermore assumed that reduction of noise exposures to protect hearing would secondarily result in benefits for these other potentially deleterious health effects (Melnick, 1994).

Rather, this chapter will focus on basic terminology and concepts underpinning implementation, management, and evaluation of occupational hearing loss prevention programs.

Noise-Induced Hearing Loss—Basic Concepts and Terminology

Prolonged exposure to high levels of noise typically results in sensorineural hearing loss secondary to inner ear damage. Damage may involve cochlear blood supply, sensory cells, nerve cells, and supporting structures within the cochlea. Resulting hearing losses may be temporary or permanent, and these audiometric outcomes have commonly been labeled *temporary threshold shift* (TTS) and *permanent threshold shift* (PTS), respectively. A third type of noise-induced hearing loss is *acoustic trauma*, which is typically associated with brief exposures to very high noise levels often demonstrating abrupt rise times. In general, the mechanisms of noise-induced hearing loss are thought to change with noise exposure levels and noise exposure types. Prolonged exposure to moderate levels of noise is thought to cause vascular changes in the inner ear associated with TTS and PTS, while extreme noise levels are associated with immediate physical trauma to delicate inner ear structures (i.e., acoustic trauma) (Axlesson et al., 1996).

In general, the following concepts relating noise exposure to hearing loss are well-established:

1. Amounts of PTS in humans are generally correlated with exposure levels (in decibels), exposure durations, and temporal/spectral characteristics of the offending noise.
2. For a range of noise exposure levels and durations, there is a "trading relationship" between exposure level and exposure duration. Long durations of modest exposure seem to result in similar amounts of PTS as shorter durations at higher exposure levels.
3. At extremely high exposure levels, no exposure duration may be safe.
4. At very modest exposure levels, unlimited exposure durations may be safe.

5. Intermittent noise exposures seem to be less dangerous than continuous noise exposures, even when the total sound energy (i.e., power or intensity) of the two exposures is quite similar. That is, periods of relative quiet seem to allow for recovery not afforded by more continuous exposures.
6. Impulse noise (e.g., gunfire or an explosion) is particularly hazardous to hearing. Impact noise (such as two pieces of metal banging together) poses similar threats to hearing. The common link between these two types of noise is abrupt onset (i.e., rapid rise time).
7. High-frequency sound (i.e., above 1000 Hz) is generally thought to be more dangerous than low frequency sound (i.e., below 1000 Hz).
8. Both humans and laboratory animals demonstrate wide degrees of individual susceptibility to noise exposure: With similar lifetime noise exposures, employees with "tough" ears will show far less hearing damage than employees with "tender" ears.
9. The audiometric "notching effect" demonstrated at 3, 4, and 6 kHz in audiograms of noise-exposed humans may be related to resonance characteristics of outer and middle ears: Most occupational noise exposures are considered to be broadband in frequency content, and human ears amplify these broadband signals such that audiometric damage in the 3 to 6 kHz frequency range is passed along to the inner ear.
10. Any noise exposure that is capable of inducing TTS in the short term is likely to produce PTS in the long term. That is, temporary threshold shift (TTS) is commonly thought to be a warning sign of permanent threshold shift (PTS). This assumption persists despite evidence that amounts of TTS do not correlate with long-term PTS in humans. That is, some individuals with small amounts of TTS after long term exposure show considerable PTS and vice versa.

Damage Risk Criteria

Damage risk criteria are used by government agencies to set acceptable limits for occupational noise exposure (Melnick, 1994). Considerations in formulating damage risk criteria for occupational hearing loss include:

1. Determination of dose-response relationships between occupational noise exposure and hearing loss. That is, how much noise exposure of what type over how long a duration will result in how much hearing loss?
2. Determination of how much hearing loss is acceptable in what portion of the population over a working lifetime. The term "risk" in damage risk criteria alludes to the high variance in susceptibility to noise in humans. Damage risk criteria must address this issue to determine acceptable limits for occupational exposure.

3. Estimation of how much hearing loss may accrue over a working lifetime from a variety of causes, including (a) occupational noise exposure, (b) aging or presbycusis, (c) nonoccupational noise exposure or sociocusis, and (d) other non-noise related causes of hearing loss, such as hereditary and disease factors sometimes referred to as nosoacusis (Kryter et al., 1966). Damage risk criteria must attempt to parse out the percentage of total hearing loss in a population due specifically to occupational noise exposure versus other potential causation factors.

The International Standards Organization (ISO) has examined these factors comprehensively. Based upon original research by Robinson (1968) and Passchier-Vermeer (1968), ISO released a standard for "assessment of occupational noise exposure for hearing conservation purposes" (ISO, 1971). The standard provides descriptive audiometric summaries from three types of data pools:

1. Industrial workers with known occupational exposures to noise
2. Comparably aged groups demonstrating no significant occupational exposures but who were essentially *unscreened* for sociocusis and nosacusis
3. Other comparably aged groups *highly screened* for sociocusis and nosacusis thought to represent a "purely presbycusic" population

Comparisons of audiometric data among these groups were utilized to estimate percentages of total hearing loss thought to result from occupational noise exposures versus other potential causes of hearing loss such as presbycusis, sociocusis, and nosacusis.

Figure 16.1 was generated from data provided by ISO (1971). The graph depicts median hearing levels at the average of 3, 4, and 6 kHz for males aged 20 to 35 years from the various ISO databases. The dotted line with circles depicts hearing levels for a highly *screened* male population. This group reported no occupational noise exposures, no nonoccupational exposures (i.e., sociocusis), and no significant histories of ear disease or familial hearing loss (i.e., nosacusis). In other words, this line represents median hearing levels thought to accrue purely as a function of aging (i.e., presbycusis) for males between ages 20 and 35.

The dotted line with squares in Figure 16.1 depicts audiometric data from an *unscreened* male population. These are median hearing levels expected in a male population between ages 20 and 35 where some individuals may have experienced recreational noise exposures and/or other threats to hearing such as ear disease. Thus, this line predicts total hearing loss from the combination of presbycusis, sociocusis, and nosacusis.

The solid lines in Figure 16.1 represent hearing levels for males who were occupationally exposed to continuous noise levels of 95 dBA between the ages of 20 and 35. The solid line with circles adds the predicted amount of occupational PTS to a "purely presbycusic" (i.e., screened) population, while the solid line with squares adds the same occupational PTS to a more typical male population whose audiometric data are potentially contaminated by nonoccupational noise and ear disease.

Figure 16.2 was also developed from ISO (1971) data and summarizes median levels of PTS at individual audiometric

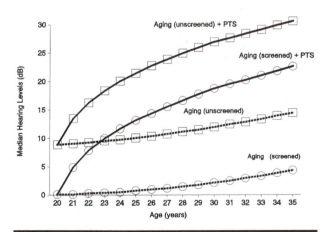

FIGURE 16.1   Median hearing levels (dB) estimated to accrue for males between ages 20 and 35 as a function of aging and permanent threshold shift (PTS) from 95 dBA occupational noise exposures. Screened samples represent estimates for populations with no known nonoccupational noise exposures or ear disease.

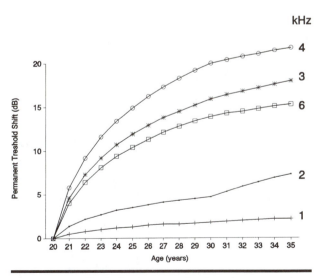

FIGURE 16.2   Single frequency estimates of permanent threshold shift accruing for males between the ages of 20 and 35 experiencing occupational noise exposures of 95 dBA.

frequencies for the same occupationally exposed male population in Figure 16.1. Note that the rate of noise-induced hearing loss is greatest over the first few years of exposure and tends to slow down as hearing loss progresses. Also, note the varying rates of noise-induced hearing loss as a function of audiometric frequency. Clearly, the pace of hearing loss is greatest at 4000 Hz, reflecting the common clinical sign of a "notching" audiometric morphology.

It is important to consider that hearing levels predicting occupational PTS in Figures 16.1 and 16.2 were developed from occupationally exposed, *unprotected* populations. It is nearly impossible to find large populations of workers today who do not wear hearing protection; furthermore, ethical considerations for treatment of human subjects preclude research likely to result in PTS. Therefore, it is likely that the original ISO estimates of the hazardous effects of occupational noise exposure will never be replicated (ISO, 1971, 1990; Johansson, Kylin, & Reopstorff, 1973).

Excess Risk. In 1974, International Standards Organization (ISO), Environmental Protection Agency (EPA) and the National Institute for Occupational Safety and Health (NIOSH), estimated the excess risk of incurring hearing impairment from occupational noise exposure over a forty-year working lifetime (39 Fed. Reg. 43,802, 1974b). The term "excess risk" was used to describe the percentage of occupationally exposed workers suffering impairment after the percent of impaired people from a non-noise-exposed population had been subtracted out. That is, excess risk was taken as the total percent impaired employees minus that percentage of impaired workers who might have become impaired for reasons other than occupational noise exposure.

Estimates of excess risk for hearing impairment from ISO, EPA, and NIOSH are summarized in Figure 16.3. The horizontal axis depicts forty-year lifetime noise exposures (dBA), while the vertical axis gives estimates of excess risk in percent. Each agency defined hearing impairment as hearing levels in excess of 25 dB at the audiometric average of 500, 1000, and 2000 Hz. For a lifetime exposure of 90 dBA, between 21% and 29% excess risk was estimated, while between 0 and 5% excess risk was estimated for lifetime exposures of 80 dBA. These excess risk estimates took on great historical importance in development of damage risk criteria for noise and hearing conservation regulations in the United States.

FEDERAL REGULATIONS

Walsh-Healey and Occupational Safety and Health Acts

The Walsh-Healey Public Contracts Act was passed by Congress in 1935. This act authorized the U.S. Department of Labor to regulate employers doing business with the federal government. In 1969, under authority of the Walsh-Healey Public Contracts Act, the Department of Labor issued the "Walsh-Healey" noise standard, which became the first civilian attempt to regulate noise in the United States. In 1970 the Occupational Safety and Health Act was passed by Congress. This legislation essentially adopted all technical aspects of Walsh-Healey and in addition created the National Institute for Occupational Safety and Health (NIOSH) and the Occupational Safety and Health Administration (OSHA). While NIOSH was charged with a research mission to improve health and safety in the workplace, OSHA was charged with the duties of enacting and enforcing health and safety regulations. Perhaps most importantly, the OSHA Act of 1970 expanded regulatory scope beyond employers with federal contracts to practically all employers in the United States (Suter, 1986).

Both the Walsh-Healey and OSHA Acts introduced the following noise regulations:

1. Maximum permissible exposure levels (PELs) were established for both continuous and impulse/impact noise.
2. If occupational exposures exceeded PELs, employers were required to utilize feasible administrative or engineering noise controls to reduce exposures to within permissible ranges.
3. If noise control efforts failed to sufficiently reduce noise exposures, employers were required to provide

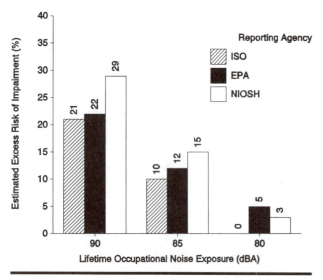

FIGURE 16.3 Estimates of excess risk of hearing impairment attributable to lifetime occupational noise exposures of 80, 85, and 90 dBA from International Standards Organization (ISO), the Environmental Protection Agency (EPA), and the National Institute for Occupational Safety and Health (NIOSH).

and oversee the use of hearing protective devices capable of reducing occupational exposures to within maximum permissible levels.

4. Finally, for all exposures in excess of maximally permissible levels, employers were required to administer "continuing" and "effective" hearing conservation programs (HCPs).

Permissible Exposure Levels. PELs for impulsive or impact noise were established at 140 dB peak sound pressure level. For continuous noise, maximum permissible exposures were characterized by spectral content, exposure duration, and time-weighted-average (TWA) exposure level of the offending noise. Table 16.1 summarizes maximum permissible exposures for continuous noise. The first column in Table 16.1 depicts time-weighted-average (TWA), A-weighted sound levels in decibels (dBA). The second column lists allowable durations for each exposure level, while the third column characterizes total noise exposure accumulations for each combination of exposure level and exposure duration.

Frequency Weighting. Further explanation of terms introduced in Table 16.1 would be helpful at this time. A-weighting refers to a filtering network on sound level meters that attenuates incoming sounds in a manner analogous to the differential frequency sensitivity of the human ear. Figure 16.4 summarizes attenuation factors as a function of octave band center frequencies for A, B, and C filtering networks of a sound level meter. These attenuation

TABLE 16.1. Maximum permissible exposure levels (PELs) of Walsh-Healey (1969) and OSHA (1983) regulations.

TWA dBA	ALLOWABLE DURATION HOURS	ACCUMULATED NOISE DOSE PERCENT
115	0.25	100%
110	0.50	100%
105	1.00	100%
100	2.00	100%
95	4.00	100%
90	8.00	100%
85	16.00	100%

curves correspond to response characteristics of the human ear at 40, 70, and 100 phons, respectively (Earshen, 1986). Phons characterize equal loudness at different frequencies (Stevens, 1936). At moderate loudness levels corresponding to an A-weighting of 40 phons, human ears attenuate significant portions of low-frequency energy. At higher listening levels corresponding to B- and C-weighting at 70 and 100 phons, respectively, human ears have a "flatter" response resulting in progressively less low-frequency attenuation. A-weighting was chosen for measurement of sound exposures for regulatory purposes to strike a reasonable compromise among a number of alternative damage risk criteria that attributed greater risk to human hearing for high frequencies than low frequencies.

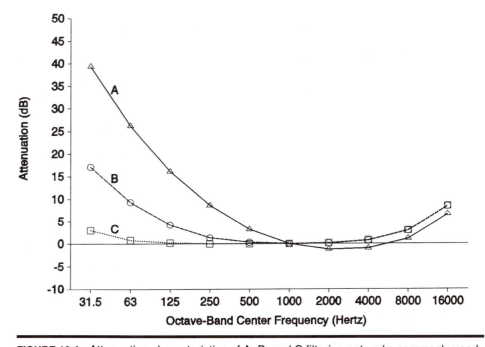

FIGURE 16.4 Attenuation characteristics of A, B, and C filtering networks commonly used in sound measurement.

Time-Weighted-Average. The time-weighted-average (TWA) can be thought of as an average sound level for a specified duration. Most occupational noise exposures are not constant throughout a typical 8-hour work shift. On the contrary, occupational exposure levels may vary highly from moment to moment. The TWA "averages" these fluctuations to an equivalent exposure at a constant level. In Table 16.1, for example, a TWA exposure of 90 dBA is allowed for 8 hours. An actual employee exposure may fluctuate above and below 90 dBA over this period, but the overall 8-hour exposure when "averaged" may not exceed the equivalent of an exposure at a constant level of 90 dBA for this 8-hour period.

Noise Dose. Whereas TWA in Table 16.1 may be considered the average "rate" of exposure accumulation, noise dose (reported in percent) can be thought of as the total amount of accumulated exposure. In a strictly regulatory sense, Table 16.1 tells us that an employee accumulating noise exposure at an average "rate" of 90 dBA for a duration of 8 hours has "bagged the legal limit" (i.e., 100%) of allowable noise exposure for that day. Similarly, an average exposure "rate" of 115 dBA results in the same maximum allowable noise dose (100%) in the very short duration of 0.25 hours or 15 minutes! The concept of noise dose is very useful when communicating the concept of risk to employees. Table 16.1 suggests that exposures of 115 dBA for 15 minutes are equivalent in risk to an 8-hour exposure of 90 dBA.

Doubling Rate or Exchange Rate. A final noteworthy aspect of Table 16.1 is discernable in the mathematical relationships among its three columns. For each 5-decibel increase in TWA, the allowable exposure duration is cut in half while the resultant noise dose remains constant at 100%. This halving of allowable exposure durations for 5 dB increments in exposure levels is referred to as the 5 dB doubling rate or 5 dB exchange rate. These damage risk criteria suggest that risk for noise-induced hearing loss doubles with every 5 dB increase in exposure if exposure duration is held constant.

Hearing Conservation Amendment

Although both Walsh-Healey and OSHA Acts identified the need for employers to administer "continuing" and "effective" HCPs, neither regulation specified the necessary components or characteristics that an "effective" HCP should include. This situation was rectified in 1983 when the hearing conservation amendment became enforceable (OSHA, 1983). The hearing conservation amendment added the following important items to existing federal noise regulations:

1. An "action level" TWA exposure of 85 dBA was introduced to supplement permissible exposure levels (PELs). This 8-hour exposure could be calculated as a total noise dose of 50% (see Table 16.1) and was established as the exposure triggering implementation of an occupational HCP.
2. If employees were exposed to a daily noise dose of 50% or greater, employers were required to:
   a. Establish noise exposure monitoring programs sufficient to identify employee risk
   b. Establish audiometric testing programs to provide early identification of employees at risk for occupational hearing loss
   c. Provide hearing protective devices (HPDs) to employees at no cost to these employees
   d. Provide annual training to employees regarding the effects of noise on hearing and proper use of HPDs
   e. Establish recordkeeping systems for employee audiograms and noise exposures

It is important to remember that major components of the OSHA Act remained unchanged by the hearing conservation amendment. Employers were still required to pursue feasible noise controls and enforce use of HPDs by employees exposed above permissible exposure levels (see Table 16.1).

OCCUPATIONAL HEARING LOSS PREVENTION PROGRAMS

What follows is a discussion of each major component of contemporary occupational hearing loss prevention programs (HLPPs). Each program component will be discussed from two perspectives: (1) achieving minimum compliance with current federal regulations and (2) providing "best practices" for prevention of occupational hearing loss. This approach reflects general consensus among practicing professionals that compliance with federal regulations may not provide sufficient protection to employees exposed to high levels of occupational noise (Abel, Alberti, & Riko, 1978; Berger, 1980, 1981, 1986; Berger, Franks, & Lingren, 1996; Berger & Kieper, 1991; Franks & Berger, 1997; Goff & Blank, 1984; Hachey & Roberts, 1983; Helmkamp, 1986; Hempstock & Hill, 1990; Pekkarinen, 1989).

Historically speaking, federal noise regulations in the United States have generally followed recommendations of the National Institute for Occupational Safety and Health (NIOSH), which is charged with a continuing mission of research to assure that current health and safety regulations are based upon timely empirical data. The hearing conservation amendment of 1983, in fact, was largely based upon formal recommendations of NIOSH in a document entitled "Criteria for a Recommended Standard: Occupational Exposure to Noise" (NIOSH, 1972).

In 1996, NIOSH released draft recommendations for revisions in current federal noise regulations. After a period of public comment, the document was revised by NIOSH to reflect final recommendations toward revision of our current noise regulation. Because it is unknown if OSHA will adopt recommendations of NIOSH, issues relating to *minimum compliance* with federal regulations will reflect contents of the 1983 federal noise rule and hearing conservation amendment (OSHA, 1983). Where appropriate, "best practices" will be based upon the most recent recommendations of NIOSH (1998).

Noise Exposure Monitoring—the Sound Survey

Minimum Compliance. OSHA (1983) requires that noise exposure monitoring be completed if employee TWA exposures are equal to or in excess of 85 dbA or a noise dose of 50%. Practically speaking, the only way to determine if exposures meet OSHA's "action level" is to conduct actual exposure measurements. OSHA suggests that the need to perform exposure monitoring may be indicated by employee complaints about the noise, difficulty in carrying on conversation in the work environment, or indications that employees may be losing their hearing. If exposures are constant throughout the work shift and employees are fairly stationary, OSHA allows the use of area monitoring to estimate employee exposures. That is, general area measurements of noise may be used to represent employee exposures. Representative personal monitoring must be used, however, if exposures are fluctuant and employees move in and out of noisy areas.

In cases where area monitoring is allowable, a single number may be appropriate to estimate employee exposures. When employees are exposed to two or more periods of noise with different levels, OSHA requires that the total daily noise dose be calculated as follows:

$$D = 100(C_1/T_1 + C_2/T_2 + \ldots C_n/T_n)$$

where D indicates noise dose (in percent), C_n indicates calculated exposure duration at a specific noise level, and T_n indicates tabled allowable duration for that specific noise level.

An example calculation is given in Table 16.2. A laborer for a lawn service works approximately 10 hours per day when weather permits. In a typical 10-hour shift, the employee takes 1 hour and 45 minutes for meals, breaks, and clean up, leaving 8 hours and 15 minutes for direct labor. In the morning, the employee operates a lawnmower for 4 hours at an average exposure level of 90 dBA. For this activity the calculated or observed exposure duration

TABLE 16.2. Example calculation of employee noise exposure with two or more significantly different periods of exposure.

ACTIVITY	CALCULATED OBSERVED HOURS C_n	OBSERVED EXPOSURE dBA	TABLED HOURS T_n	C_n/T_n
Operate Lawn Mower	$C_1 = 4$	90	$T_1 = 8$	0.5
Lunch	0.50	0	Infinity	0
Break	0.25	0	Infinity	0
Operate Hedge Trimmer	$C_2 = 4$	85	$T_2 = 16$	0.25
Break	0.50	0	Infinity	0
Operate Leaf Blower	$C_3 = 0.25$	105	$T_3 = 1$	0.25
Clean up	0.50	0	Infinity	0
Totals:	10	$(C_1/T_1 + C_2/T_2 + C_3/T_3) = 1.00$ Dose $= 100 (C_1/T_1 + C_2/T_2 + C_3/T_3) = 100\%$			
		TWA$_8$ = 16.61 × LOG (Dose/100) + 90 = 90 dBA			

(C_1) is 4 hours and the tabled allowable duration (T_1) is 8 hours (from Table 16.1). From our equation above:

$$C_1/T_1 = 4/8 = 0.5.$$

The employee then operates a hedge trimmer for 4 hours at 85 dBA, resulting in a calculated or observed exposure duration (C_2) of 4 hours and a tabled allowable duration (T_2) of 16 hours (again, from Table 16.1). Finally, operation of the leaf blower for 15 minutes at 105 dBA yields a C_3 of 0.25 hours and a T_3 of 1 hour. Substituting these values into our original equation and solving for D (noise dose, in percent), we get:

$$D = 100(C_1/T_1 + C_2/T_2 + \ldots C_n/T_n)$$

$$D = 100(4/8 + 4/16 + 0.25/1)$$

$$D = 100(0.5 + 0.25 + 0.25)$$

$$D = 100(1.0)$$

$$\text{Noise Dose} = 100\%.$$

Thus, our employee in Table 16.2 receives a daily noise dose of 100% from the combination of these activities. OSHA requires that sound levels from 80 to 130 dBA be included in exposure measurements. This requirement has been interpreted such that noise levels falling below 80 dBA may be excluded from the measurement sample. Manufacturers of sound level meters and dosimeters typically include an option to set the threshold or cut-off of a device at 80 dBA to accommodate this strategy. Because no sound levels exceeded 80 dBA during lunch, breaks, and clean up in Table 16.2, these activities were excluded in the overall computation of noise dose. Meter thresholds or cut-offs are generally justified by research supporting the notion that unlimited exposure duration is allowable for some exposure levels (Earshen, 1986).

The bottom row of Table 16.2 provides an additional equation for converting daily noise dose to 8-hour TWA noise exposure (TWA_8) in dBA. Detailed discussion of this equation is beyond the scope of this chapter other than to note that the "+90" term in the equation corresponds to OSHA's permissible exposure level (PEL).

Finally, OSHA requires:

1. Monitoring be performed in a manner sufficient for appropriate selection of HPDs.
2. Monitoring be repeated whenever changes in manufacturing production or processes are suspected of increasing employee exposures.
3. Monitoring equipment to be calibrated according to manufacturers' recommendations.
4. Employees to be allowed to observe monitoring procedures.
5. Employees found to be at or above the "action level" be notified of monitoring results.

6. Employee exposures to be calculated without attenuation factors associated with use of HPDs.
7. That sampling strategies for monitoring programs be designed to include employees in the hearing conservation program.

The requirement that exposure monitoring sampling strategies be inclusive is very important. Problems and pitfalls affecting reliability and validity of noise measurements are well documented (Botsford, 1967; Brogan & Anderson, 1994; Earshen, 1986; Royster, Berger, & Royster, 1986; Shaw, 1985). Therefore, most monitoring programs are conservative, tending to include employees in the HCP when actual exposure estimates may be equivocal.

Best Practice. NIOSH (1998) has recommended that the PEL be reduced from 90 to 85 dBA and also that the doubling rate be reduced from 5 to 3 dB. Table 16.3 summarizes how these PEL and doubling rate changes would affect current damage risk criteria. The first three columns in Table 16.3 repeat current OSHA values for TWA, allowable exposure duration, and accumulated noise dose. These three columns are based on a PEL of 90 and a doubling rate of 5 dB. The last column in Table 16.3 provides recommended exposure levels in dBA commensurate with current OSHA values for allowable duration and noise dose. Note that OSHA currently allows exposure to 115 dBA for a duration of 15 minutes (0.25 hours) while NIOSH recommends that exposures be limited to 100 dBA for the same allowable duration (Suter, 1992a).

Some employers in the United States have already adopted these recommendations of NIOSH (1998). The NIOSH criteria for PEL and doubling rate tend to include more employees in the HCP and also result in more conservative application of HPD programs. Another strategy accomplishes almost the same thing without being so technical. Some employers offer HCP benefits to all employees, not just those whose TWA is 85 dBA or greater.

Audiometric Testing Programs

Minimum Compliance. Employers must establish and maintain audiometric testing programs and make them available to all employees exposed at or above the action level (85 dBA TWA or a dose of 50%). Audiometric testing programs must be under professional supervision of an audiologist, otolaryngologist, or physician. Tests may be performed by technicians certified by the Council for Accreditation in Occupational Hearing Conservation or by technicians demonstrating competence necessary to obtain valid audiograms and properly use an audiometer. Technicians operating microprocessor audiometers need not be certified but must be responsible to an audiologist, otolaryngologist, or physician.

TABLE 16.3 Comparison of effects of 3 versus 5 dB doubling rates on Time-Weighted-Average (TWA) noise exposures of the same duration.

CURRENT OSHA TWA dBA (PEL = 90) (DBL. RATE = 5)	ALLOWABLE DURATION HOURS	ACCUMULATED NOISE DOSE PERCENT	RECOMMENDED NIOSH TWA dBA (PEL = 85) (DBL. RATE = 3)
115	0.25	100%	100
110	0.50	100%	97
105	1.00	100%	94
100	2.00	100%	91
95	4.00	100%	88
90	8.00	100%	85
85	16.00	100%	82

Pure-tone air-conduction thresholds must be obtained at 500, 1000, 2000, 3000, 4000, and 6000 Hz for each ear. Audiometers must meet specifications of, and be maintained in accordance with, American National Standard Specification for Audiometers (ANSI, S3.6-1969). Functional operation of audiometers must be checked on a daily basis. Acoustic calibrations for SPL output, linearity, and tolerances must be performed annually, and exhaustive calibrations must be performed at least every two years. Rooms used for audiometric testing must not demonstrate background sound pressure levels exceeding those in Table 16.4. See Chapter 17 for discussion of audiometer calibration.

Baseline audiograms must be collected on employees within 6 months of an action level exposure. Employers relying on mobile test vans may wait 12 months to collect baselines, but must assure that employees use hearing protection after the first 6 months of exposure. Baseline audiograms must not be contaminated by temporary threshold shift (TTS); therefore, baseline audiograms must be preceded by 14 hours of relative quiet. OSHA allows the use of hearing protection to fulfill this requirement if employees are tested throughout the workshift.

Annual audiograms must be collected on employees remaining at or above action level noise exposures. Annual audiograms are compared to baselines to determine if (1) the annual audiogram is valid, and (2) if a standard threshold shift has taken place. These determinations may be performed by a technician. Standard threshold shift (STS) is defined by OSHA as a change in hearing threshold relative to the baseline audiogram of an average of 10 dB or more at 2000, 3000, and 4000 Hz in either ear. Employers may account for the contribution of presbycusis in the calculation of standard threshold shift.

When test results demonstrate STS, employers may perform a retest within 30 days. If STS is not persistent on the retest audiogram, then the retest audiogram may be substituted for the annual audiogram. If the STS is persistent upon retest, or if a retest audiogram is not completed after the initial STS, employer follow up must include:

1. Written notification to employees within 21 days
2. Employees not using hearing protectors must be fitted with HPDs, trained in their use and care, and required to use them
3. Employees already using HPDs shall be refitted, retrained, and provided with HPDs offering greater attenuation if necessary

Determination of STS may be made by a technician. Problem audiograms, however, must be reviewed by an audiologist, otolaryngologist, or physician. Employees suspected of demonstrating a medical pathology of the ear either caused or aggravated by the use of HPDs must receive appropriate referral at employer expense. Employees suspected of demonstrating medical pathology unrelated to HPD use must be informed of the need for referral, but employers are not held responsible for referral costs.

If the audiologist, otolaryngologist, or physician determines that an annual audiogram demonstrates persistent STS or significant improvement from baseline, this annual

TABLE 16.4 OSHA maximum allowable octave-band sound pressure levels for audiometric test rooms.

OCTAVE BAND CENTER FREQUENCY (Hz)	500	1000	2000	4000	8000
Sound Pressure Level (dB)	40	40	47	57	62

audiogram may become the revised baseline audiogram to which future hearing tests will be compared.

Best Practice.   Many employers offer audiometric testing to all employees, regardless of occupational exposure levels. Although little or no empirical data exist to confirm this, it has been reported that employees demonstrate more positive attitudes towards the HCP when all participate. In these cases, the employees seem to regard the HCP as a health benefit rather than an employer exercise to meet OSHA requirements (Royster & Royster, 1990). Some employers require testing every 6 months when employee exposures are extreme. Requiring more frequent testing for exposures in excess of 100 dBA TWA is fairly common.

Testing all employees allows employers to create a "control group" as part of the audiometric database. Ideally, it would then be possible to match exposed and unexposed employee populations for gender, age, pre-existing hearing loss, and nonoccupational noise exposures. Comparisons between audiometric data from these matched populations should yield highly useful characterizations of HCP performance (Simpson, Steward, & Kaltenbach, 1994).

It is generally accepted that OSHA permissible background noise levels permissible in test environments by OSHA are too high to permit reliable testing at audiometric zero (Morrill, 1986; Morrill & Sterrett, 1981). Therefore, most employers and mobile van consultants strive to meet maximum permissible background sound pressure levels of the American National Standards Organization (ANSI S3.1-1991b).

Although "problem" audiograms must be reviewed by a professional, no criteria are given by OSHA to define problem audiograms. Therefore, audiologists, otolaryngologists, and physicians are tacitly responsible for developing and implementing referral criteria in their programs. Many HCPs, however, do not benefit from direct access to professionals for routine review of audiograms. It has been recommended that HCP professionals develop specific criteria for nonprofessionals to identify cases potentially needing referral for further evaluation.

The Subcommittee on Medical Aspects of Noise of the American Academy of Otolaryngology—Head and Neck Surgery (AAO-HNS, 1983) has provided otologic referral criteria for occupational HCPs. Criteria were developed to guide program directors in determining appropriate referral conditions. Referral criteria may be triggered by case history items, otoscopic findings, or audiometric results.

AAO-HNS recommends referral if an employee reports a history of ear pain; drainage; dizziness; severe persistent tinnitus; sudden, fluctuant, or rapidly progressive hearing loss; or a feeling of fullness or discomfort in one or both ears within the preceding 12 months. Referral is also recommended if otoscopic inspection reveals excessive cerumen accumulation or a foreign body in the ear canal.

AAO-HNS recommends referral if baseline audiograms exhibit (1) average hearing levels at 0.5, 1, 2, and 3 kHz greater than 25 dB in either ear, or (2) a difference in average hearing level between better and poorer ears of more than 15 dB at 0.5, 1, and 2 kHz (low-frequency asymmetry) or more than 30 dB at 3, 4, and 6 kHz (high-frequency asymmetry). For annual or periodic audiograms AAO-HNS recommends referral for declines from baseline in average hearing levels of more than 15 dB at 0.5, 1, and 2 kHz (low-frequency shift) or more than 20 dB at 3, 4, and 6 kHz (high-frequency shift).

AAO-HNS recommends baseline audiograms be designated as first chronologic valid tests for all future comparisons and "revised" baselines be used for OSHA compliance purposes, not for determining referral needs. Also, AAO-HNS suggests that program directors may wish to perform a retest within 90 days to verify shifts before referral action is taken.

Many occupational HCPs adopt procedures and practices of pertinent ANSI standards as they become revised. American National Standard Specification for Audiometers (ANSI, S3.6-1969), for example, has gone through several revisions since promulgation of the hearing conservation amendment of 1983. Keeping HCP practices current with these revised standards assures that programs stay current with changing technology (ANSI, 1978, 1983, 1985, 1986, 1991a, 1991b, 1991c, 1996).

Some programs are examining potential utility of adopting audiometric shift criteria more conservative than OSHA's current definition of STS (Royster, 1992). NIOSH (1998), for example, has proposed single-frequency shifts of 15 dB as a more appropriate "flag" for early intervention than OSHA's three-frequency averaging technique at 2, 3, and 4 kHz. Other programs and consultants are eliminating the practice of age correction when computing STS, as this practice is thought to be less appropriate for individual audiograms than for populations or samples (NIOSH, 1998).

Hearing Protection Programs

Minimum Compliance.   A variety of hearing protective devices (HPDs) must be made available to all employees whose exposures are equal to or in excess of the action level (i.e., 85 TWA or noise dose of 50%). Employers are currently required to enforce use of HPDs by employees whose occupational exposures are in excess of the permissible exposure level (i.e., 90 TWA or noise dose of 100%). Employers are also required to enforce HPD use by employees who have demonstrated STS whose exposures are equal to or in excess of the action level. Furthermore, employers are required to ensure proper initial fitting of HPDs, provide training in their use and care, and supervise their correct use by employees.

At minimum, HPDs must attenuate employee exposures to the PEL (TWA$_8$ of 90 dBA or noise dose of 100%); however, HPDs must attenuate exposures to the action level (TWA$_8$ of 85 dBA or 50% dose) for employees who have demonstrated Standard Threshold Shift (STS). The hearing conservation amendment provides employers four methods to calculate HPD attenuation. The simplest method is provided by the equation:

$$[\text{Protected TWA}_8] = [\text{Exposure TWA}_8] - [\text{NRR}-7],$$

where Protected TWA$_8$ represents the desired level of employee protection, Exposure TWA$_8$ represents an actual employee exposure, and NRR represents the Noise Reduction Rating (in decibels) of a particular HPD. The "–7" term in the above equation is frequently mistakenly identified as a "devaluation" of the NRR because it is subtracted from the NRR. In actuality, this term is a correction factor to account for all inputs to this equation being A-weighted decibels rather than C-weighted decibels, which serve as inputs to the more complicated alternative calculations provided by OSHA.

The Environmental Protection Agency (EPA) requires HPD manufacturers to follow specific protocols to calculate NRR and also requires manufacturers to label all HPDs with the appropriate NRR value. Assuming that an employee has demonstrated a standard threshold shift (STS) and has a TWA$_8$ workplace exposure of 95 dBA, OSHA requires that this employee be protected or attenuated to a TWA$_8$ exposure of 85 dBA. In our example, Protected TWA$_8$ = 85 dBA, and Exposure TWA$_8$ = 95 dBA. If we substitute these values into our original equation and solve for NRR, we can estimate the minimum NRR value that should provide sufficient attenuation for this employee.

Original Equation:
$$[\text{Protected TWA}_8] = [\text{Exposure TWA}_8] - [\text{NRR}-7]$$

Substituting: $85 = 95 - [\text{NRR}-7]$

Solving for NRR: $\text{NRR} - 7 = 95 - 85$

$\text{NRR} - 7 = 10$

$\text{NRR} = 10 + 7$

$\text{NRR} = 17$

In this example, any HPD with a NRR of 17 dB or greater should be sufficient for this employee, according to prescribed OSHA calculations. If another employee with the same exposure (i.e., 95 dBA) did not demonstrate STS, OSHA would require attenuation to only 90 dBA, resulting in a minimum NRR of 12 dB using the same equation.

Best Practice.   Many employers require the use of HPDs at the current action level of 85 dBA. Recall that the National Institute of Occupational Safety and Health (NIOSH) has recently recommended that an 8-hour exposure of 85 dBA become the maximum permissible exposure level (PEL). In short, current regulations compute a noise dose of 50% for a TWA$_8$ of 85 dBA, while NIOSH recommends that the same exposure is equivalent to a noise dose of 100 percent (NIOSH, 1998). Furthermore, a growing body of data supports the notion that a TWA$_8$ of 85 dBA poses sufficient risk to warrant consistent use of HPDs in the workplace (ACGIH, 1995; Axlesson et al., 1996).

Employers who do not require use of HPDs at the action level are faced with a significant administrative problem: How do you force certain employees (i.e., those who have suffered an STS) to wear HPDs in the same exposure environments (i.e., 85 TWA$_8$ to 90 TWA$_8$) where others (i.e., those who have not suffered an STS) are *not* required to wear hearing protectors? Few companies have employee tracking systems sufficient to monitor HPD use in these situations.

Many companies also recognize that current OSHA methods for estimating HPD attenuation are inadequate (NIOSH, 1994). Current EPA-supported laboratory methods for calculating NRR allow manufacturers to use highly motivated test subjects who may be experimentally fit with HPDs by the person supervising the test. These test methods vastly overestimate attenuation achieved in a real-world setting and furthermore are not even statistically predictive of actual attenuations achieved in the field (Berger et al., 1996; Lempert & Edwards, 1983).

Several attempts are currently being undertaken to achieve more realistic estimates of real-world HPD attenuation factors (Berger et al., 1996; Casali & Park, 1991). Unfortunately, the EPA retains statutory authority in this matter, and funding for the EPA Office of Noise Abatement and Control was eliminated during the Reagan administration. Consequently, it is unlikely that regulatory changes will soon be forthcoming. In the interim, NIOSH recommends that NRRs be derated by 25%, 50%, and 70% for earmuffs, formable earplugs, and all other earplugs, respectively (NIOSH, 1998).

Training and Motivation Programs

Minimum Compliance.   Employers are required to institute training programs for all employees exposed to a TWA of 85 dBA or noise dose of 50 percent. Training programs are to be provided on an annual basis for all employees included in the HCP, and these programs must be updated to reflect changes in protective equipment or work processes. Training must include the following topics:

1. The effects of noise on hearing
2. The purpose of HPDs, the advantages, disadvantages of various types, and attenuation of various types, and instructions on selection, fitting, use, and care
3. The purpose of audiometric testing, including an explanation of test procedures

Employers are further required to make copies of the federal noise regulation available to employees and must also post a copy of the federal standard in the workplace. Also, employers must ensure employee participation in the training program and, upon request, make all training materials available to OSHA.

The actual format of training sessions and materials is left to employer discretion. Group training sessions are common, where a group of employees hear a speaker or view a film or slide show. Other training programs consist of little more than an educational pamphlet. Typically, employers document training sessions with attendance records to prove that they have "ensured" employee participation.

Best Practice. Training programs are critical to overall success of the HCP. Employees will not likely be highly motivated to participate when the training program is the same slide show year after year. They will likely be even less responsive to the same pamphlet showing up in their mailboxes every year. Some of the most effective training programs:

1. Eschew group training sessions in favor of individual training at the time of the annual hearing test. Immediate feedback on audiometric outcomes is an important motivator.
2. Involve employees in the formal training sessions. A retiree or older active employee who is wearing binaural hearing aids can go a long way to convince younger employees to protect their hearing.
3. Customize training materials for specific group sessions. A group of employees from the same department may be very interested in the specific noise sources that they have in common, for example.
4. Develop objective measures of training outcomes. Pre- and post-testing of employees may be performed, for example.

Recordkeeping

Minimum Compliance. Employers are required to retain accurate records of employee noise exposure measurements for two years. Audiometric test records must be retained for the duration of employment. Audiometric test records must include:

1. Name and job classification of the employee
2. Audiogram date
3. The examiner's name
4. Date of last audiometer calibration
5. The employee's most recent noise exposure assessment

Records may be accessed by employees and former employees. Employers going out of business are required to

transfer existing records to successor employers, who must maintain these records according to terms of the regulations.

Best Practice. Most employers maintain HCP records indefinitely. It is not unusual, for example, for a company to archive these data for the duration of an employee's life plus fifty years.

But simple record maintenance is not enough. Most successful programs utilize their archival data to track program performance. It is generally accepted that audiometric database analysis is a useful tool for characterizing overall program performance (Royster & Royster, 1990). Successful programs utilize their historical data to track program performance and provide evidence of quality assurance.

Program Evaluation

Minimum Compliance. Current OSHA regulations require "continuing" and "effective" hearing conservation programs but do not specify how to measure effectiveness (OSHA, 1983). Historically, effectiveness has been gauged programmatically: If all components of the HCP were in place, the program was said to be effective (AOMA, 1987; Franks, Davis, & Krieg, 1989, Hetu, 1979). Unfortunately, this regulatory stance has not changed. An OSHA inspection largely consists of determining that all HCP components (i.e., audiometric testing, noise monitoring, training, et cetera) are in place and are being conducted according to federal regulations. Consequently, employers are encouraged to go to great lengths to provide documentation of hearing tests, noise surveys, training sessions, and employee notification letters. They are not necessarily encouraged to examine the efficacy of these programs from the standpoint of quality assurance.

Best Practice. Audiometric database analysis is a growing trend in HCP management. In fact, a number of prescribed analytic protocols are currently available specifically for this purpose (ANSI, 1991c; Byrne & Monk, 1993; Franks et al., 1989; Melnick, 1984; Pell, 1972; Rink, 1989; Royster, 1992; Simpson et al., 1994). Although there is no consensus at this time favoring any single method of audiometric database analysis, NIOSH suggests that the simplest method is to monitor the incidence of standard threshold shift (STS).

Noise Control

Minimum Compliance. Employers have been required since the Walsh-Healey Act (1969) to apply feasible administrative and engineering controls to reduce noise exposures exceeding the maximum PEL (TWA of 90 dBA or noise dose of 100%). Administrative controls may involve rotating employees in and out of excessively noisy jobs to minimize individual exposure durations, while engineering controls involve direct reduction of noise exposure sources.

It is important to understand that hearing protection devices (HPDs) are not considered by OSHA to be a noise control. HPDs and other forms of personal protective equipment such as respirators are considered to be temporary solutions. In fact, all components of the HCP, including audiometric testing, are regarded as interim strategies until hazardous noise exposures can be eliminated (NIOSH, 1995).

Employers are currently allowed to weigh engineering costs against costs of providing effective HCPs in determining economic feasibility of noise controls. Unfortunately, this practice has led to a deemphasis of engineering controls in recent years (OSHA, 1989).

Best Practice.   Progressive employers have already reset their noise control guidelines to take effect at a TWA of 85 dBA. This proactive approach recognizes significant risk to occupational hearing loss below the current maximum PEL of 90 dBA. It is likely that reducing the "trigger" for noise controls from 90 to 85 dBA fosters a higher degree of employee participation in the HCP: Employees are more likely to accept the use of HPDs, for example, if they see an aggressive company program to reduce long-term exposures.

Most aggressive noise control programs have two major components: (1) "buy quiet" policies and (2) active maintenance programs (Brogan & Anderson, 1994; Haag, 1988a, 1988b; NIOSH, 1973, 1975). A widget manufacturer, for example, may need to purchase specialized equipment from third parties to increase efficiency. If these third parties are required to deliver quiet machines, an important first step in noise control has been accomplished. As the machines age, noise is often an expected outcome. Consequently, the widget manufacturer must implement aggressive maintenance programs to keep these machines in good running condition. Many major manufacturers in the United States have developed purchase specifications for new equipment requiring attention to noise control, and proactive machine maintenance programs are becoming far more commonplace.

Worker Compensation

If prevention programs are effective, no employees should suffer from occupational hearing loss. In the United States, noise control and hearing protection have been mandated since 1969 (Federal Register, 1969a, 1969b), and formal HCPs have been required since 1983 (OSHA, 1983); never-theless, occupational hearing loss remains one of our most prevalent work-related illnesses, and employers continue to face rising costs of compensating employees for occupational hearing loss (ASHA, 1992).

The worker compensation system was designed to reduce civil litigation between employees and employers. Employees gave up their right to sue while employers assumed responsibility for work-related injuries and illnesses. At this time, each of the 50 states awards compensation to employees for occupational hearing loss (ASHA, 1992). Some states allow presbycusis to be taken into consideration while others do not. Some states use specific occupational exposure criteria and weigh the use of hearing protective devices in granting financial awards. Some states grant awards for tinnitus, while others do not. Because state compensation systems differ considerably, practitioners are advised to consult more detailed sources for continuous updates on state practices (ASHA, 1992).

Many states use hearing impairment formulae to calculate compensation awards. The formulae yield "percent impairment" scores: Complete impairment is 100 percent, while no impairment is 0 percent. Because the formulae are based upon pure-tone air-conduction thresholds, they do not characterize hearing handicap as well as word discrimination scores or handicap scales (ASHA, 1981; Suter, 1986). But because the pure-tone audiogram is thought to be more reliable, impairment formulae have gained favor as a more "objective" way to compute compensation awards.

Most formulae have the following components:

1. *Frequency averaging.* Ideally, audiometric frequencies are chosen to correlate with ability to discriminate speech. The American Speech-Language-Hearing Association Task Force has proposed the average of 1000, 2000, 3000, and 4000 Hz, for example (ASHA, 1981).

2. *Low fence.* The low fence represents the frequency average where impairment begins. The ASHA Task Force (1981) has recommended a low fence of 25 dB hearing level: When the average of 1–4 kHz exceeds 25 dB, hearing impairment begins.

3. *High fence.* The high fence represents the frequency average for complete or 100% hearing impairment. The ASHA Task Force high fence is 75 dB hearing level (ASHA, 1981).

4. *Rate or slope.* This characterizes increasing impairment in percent per decibel. A low fence of 25 dB (0% impairment) and high fence of 75 dB (100% impairment) creates a range of 50 dB; hence the ASHA Task Force (1981) formula increments hearing impairment at a rate of 2% per dB hearing level for the averaged frequencies.

5. *Better ear weighting.* Individual left and right ear impairments are generally combined to favor the capabilities of the better ear. A better ear weighting of 5 to 1 is common. The formula below illustrates a 5 to 1 better ear weighting:

$$BI = [5(BE) + (PE)]/6$$

where BI represents binaural impairment (in percent), and BE and PE indicate better ear and poorer ear impairments, respectively. In this example, if better and poorer ears demonstrate 20% and 50% impairment, respectively, binaural impairment would be calculated as follows:

$$BI = [5(20\%) + (50\%)]/6$$
$$BI = [100\% + 50\%]/6$$
$$BI = [150\%]/6$$
$$BI = 25\%$$

Unfortunately, some very antiquated impairment formulae are still in use. One commonly used formula employs a low fence of 25 dB and a high fence of 92 dB hearing level for the pure-tone average at 500, 1000, and 2000 Hz (AMA, 1971). The most commonly used formula today was developed by the American Academy of Otolaryngology (AAO, 1979) and employs low and high fences of 25 and 92 dB, respectively, for the pure-tone average at 500, 1000, 2000, and 3000 Hz and better ear weighting of five to one (ASHA, 1992).

As financial awards continue to grow, employers will likely take greater care with HCP implementation and management. But growing financial awards for occupational hearing loss is a two-edged sword: If employers continue to pay out high compensation awards, some may begin to wonder if HCPs are cost effective (Royster & Royster, 1990). Is an ounce of prevention truly worth a pound of cure, or does it take two ounces of prevention? Audiologists need to be actively involved in assuring that properly implemented programs will in fact prevent occupational hearing loss. Our profession needs to develop hearing loss prevention programs, not hearing loss documentation programs.

Research Needs

NIOSH (1998) has identified a number of areas where research is needed to facilitate progress in reduction of occupational hearing loss. These areas include the following:

Noise Control. Research is needed to reduce noise exposures in situations where HPDs are currently thought to be the only solutions. New noise control technologies need to be explored, and existing technologies need to be tested in broader applications.

Impulse Noise. More information is needed to characterize the hazardous aspects of impulse noise (Coles et al., 1968; Pekkarinen, 1987; Starck & Pekkarinen, 1987; Starck, Pekkarinen, & Pyykko, 1988; Sulkowski, Kowalska, & Lipowczan, 1983; Sulkowski & Lipowczan, 1982; Taylor, Lempert, Pelmear, Hemstock, & Kershaw, 1984; Thiery & Meyer-Bisch, 1988). Although existing laboratory and field evidence indicate increased risk for impulse noise, insufficient information exists at this time to formulate valid damage risk criteria for impulse noise.

Nonauditory Effects of Noise. More data are needed to describe potential relationships between noise exposure and nonauditory effects such as hypertension and psychological stress. Little information is known, for example, on how workplace noise may contribute to accidents by interfering with speech communications or ability to hear warning signals.

Ototoxic Chemical Exposures. Some industrial chemicals have shown potential for ototoxicity (Boettcher, Henderson, Gratton, Danielson, & Byrne, 1987; Brown, Brummett, & Fox, 1980; Brown, Brummett, Meikle, & Vernon, 1978; Gannon, Tso, & Chung, 1979; Hamernik & Henderson, 1976; Humes, 1984; Johnson, Juntunen, Nylen, Berg, & Hoglund, 1988; Morata, Dunn, Kretschmer, Lemasters, & Keith, 1993; Rebert, Sorenson, Howd, & Pryor, 1983; Rybak, 1992; Young, Upchurch, Kaufman, & Fechter, 1987). More research is needed to investigate ototoxic risk of these chemicals alone and in combination with noise towards eventual formulation of damage risk criteria.

Noise Monitoring. Formal monitoring protocols incorporating statistical sampling strategies are well established for determining risks for air contaminants (NIOSH, 1977). Little research exists suggesting that similar monitoring strategies are appropriate for assessing risks of noise exposure. Some investigators have suggested that alternative monitoring strategies may be more appropriate (AIHA, 1991; Behar & Plenar, 1984; CSA, 1986; Henry, 1992; Royster et al., 1986; Simpson & Berninger, 1992; Stephenson, 1995). More data are needed to identify strategies for collecting noise exposure data in ways more useful to the ultimate goal of noise control and hazard reduction.

Hearing Protectors. Continued research is needed to develop a laboratory method to estimate attenuations achieved by HPDs used in the field. Furthermore, data are needed in support of a field method to test HPD attenuations in the workplace. Also, research is needed to explore new technologies for development of HPDs affording greater comfort and enhanced communication.

Training and Motivation. Research is needed to develop training and motivation programs that promote employee involvement in health and safety programs. Behavioral survey tools need to be developed to assess worker beliefs, attitudes, and intentions towards the practice of hearing loss prevention (Merry, 1995).

Program Evaluation. Although a number of methods are currently available for evaluating program effectiveness, no single method appears to be superior to the others. Further research and development is needed in this area, and a method that is both accurate and easy to use should be implemented. Audiometric database analysis remains important in this area; however, supplemental methods of program assessment need to be developed that do not rely on audiogram analysis. Survey instruments, for example, should be developed to investigate employee beliefs, intents, and behaviors fostering success in hearing loss prevention programs.

REFERENCES

Abel, S. M., Alberti, P. W., & Riko, K. (1978). User fitting of hearing protectors: Attenuation results. In P. W. Alberti (Ed.), *Personal Hearing Protection in Industry* (pp. 315–322). New York: Raven Press.

American Academy of Otolaryngology (AAO). (1979). Committee on Hearing and Equilibrium and the American Council of Otolaryngology Committee on the Medical Aspects of Noise: Guide for evaluation of hearing handicap. *Journal of the American Medical Association, 241*(19), 2055–2059.

American Academy of Otolaryngology—Head and Neck Surgery (AAO-HNS). (1983). Otologic referral criteria for occupational hearing conservation programs. Washington, DC: Author.

American Conference of Governmental Industrial Hygienists (ACGIH). (1995). *1995–1996 Threshold Limit Values for Chemical Substances and Physical Agents and Biological Exposure Indices.* Cincinnati, OH: Author.

American Industrial Hygiene Association (AIHA). (1991). *A Strategy for Occupational Exposure Assessment.* Akron, OH: Author.

American Medical Association (AMA). (1971). *Guides to the Evaluation of Permanent Impairment.* Chicago: Committee on Rating Mental and Physical Impairment.

American National Standards Institute (ANSI). (1969). *American National Standard Specification for Audiometers.* ANSI S3.6-1969. New York: Author.

American National Standards Institute (ANSI). (1978). *American National Standard Specification for Personal Noise Dosimeters.* ANSI S1.25-1978. New York: Author.

American National Standards Institute (ANSI). (1983). *American National Standard Specification for Sound Level Meters.* ANSI S1.4-1983 (ASA 47). New York: Author.

American National Standards Institute (ANSI). (1985). *American National Standard Specification for Sound Level Meters, Amendment to S1.4-1983.* ANSI S1.4A-1985. New York: Author.

American National Standards Institute (ANSI). (1986). *American National Standard Specification for Octave-Band and Fractional-Octave-Band Analog and Digital Filters.* ANSI S1.11-1986 (ASA 65). New York: Author.

American National Standards Institute (ANSI). (1991a). *American National Standard Specification for Personal Noise Dosimeters.* ANSI 1.25-1991 (ASA 98). New York: Author.

American National Standards Institute (ANSI). (1991b). *American National Standard Maximum Permissible Ambient Noise Levels for Audiometric Test Rooms.* ANSI S3.1-1991 (ASA 99). New York: Author.

American National Standards Institute (ANSI). (1991c). *Draft American National Standard: Evaluating the Effectiveness of Hearing Conservation Programs.* Draft ANSI S12.13-1991. New York: Author.

American National Standards Institute (ANSI). (1996). *American National Standard specification for Audiometers.* ANSI S3.6-1995 (ASA 81). New York: Author.

American Occupational Medicine Association (AOMA). (1987). Guidelines for the conduct of an occupational hearing conservation program. *Journal of Occupational Medicine, 29*(12), 981–982.

American Speech-Language-Hearing Association (ASHA). (1981). American Speech-Language-Hearing Association Task Force on the Definition of Hearing Handicap. On the definition of hearing handicap. *ASHA, 23,* 293–297.

American Speech-Language-Hearing Association (ASHA). (1992). A survey of states' workers compensation practices for occupational hearing loss. *ASHA, 34*(3, Suppl 8), 2–8.

Atherley, G. R. C. (1973). Noise-induced hearing loss: The energy principle for recurrent impact noise and noise exposure close to the recommended limits. *Annals of Occupational Hygiene, 16,* 183–193.

Atherley, G. R. C., & Martin, A. M. (1971). Equivalent-continuous noise level as a measure of injury from impact and impulse noise. *Annals of Occupational Hygiene, 14,* 11–28.

Axlesson, A., Borchgrevink, H., Hamernik, R. P., Hellstrom, P., Henderson, D., & Salvi, R. J. (Eds.). (1996). *Scientific Basis of Noise-Induced Hearing Loss.* New York: Thieme Medical Publishers.

Behar, A., & Plenar, R. (1984). Noise exposure—sampling strategy and risk assessment. *American Industrial Hygiene Association Journal, 45,* 105–109.

Belli, S., Sri, L., Scarficcia, G., & Sorrentino, R. (1984). Arterial hypertension and noise: A cross-sectional study. *American Journal of Industrial Medicine, 6,* 59–65.

Berger, E. H. (1980). E*A*RLog monographs on hearing and hearing protection, *Hearing Protector Performance: How They Work—and—What Goes Wrong in the Real World.* Vol. 5. Indianapolis, IN: Cabot Safety Corporation.

Berger, E. H. (1981). E*A*RLog monographs on hearing and hearing protection: *Motivating Employees to Wear Hearing Protection Devices.* Vol. 7. Indianapolis, IN: Cabot Safety Corporation.

Berger, E. H. (1986). Hearing protection devices. In E. H. Berger, J. C. Morrill, W. D. Ward, & L. H. Royster (Eds.), *Noise and*

Hearing Conservation Manual (pp. 319–382). Akron, OH: American Industrial Hygiene Association.

Berger, E. H., Franks, J. R., & Lingren, F. L. (1996). International review of field studies of hearing protector attenuation. In A. Axlesson, H. Borchgrevink, R. P. Hamernik, P. Hellstrom, D. Henderson, & R. J. Salvi (Eds.), *Scientific Basis of Noise-Induced Hearing Loss* (pp. 361–377). New York: Thieme Medical Publishers.

Berger, E. H., & Kieper, R. W. (1991). *Measurement of the Real-World Attenuation of E*A*R Foam and UltraFit Brand Earplugs on Production Employees*. Indianapolis, IN: Cabot Safety Corporation, Report No. EA-R 91-30/HP.

Boettcher, F., Henderson, D., Gratton, M., Danielson, R., & Byrne, C. (1987). Synergistic interactions of noise and other ototraumatic agents. *Ear and Hearing, 8*, 192–212.

Bohne, B. A., Yohman, L., & Gruner, M. M. (1987). Cochlear damage following interrupted exposure to high-frequency noise. *Hearing Research, 29*, 251–264.

Bohne, B. A., Zahn, S. J.,. & Bozzay, D. G. (1985). Damage to the cochlea following interrupted exposure to low frequency noise. *Annals of Otology, Rhinology and Laryngology, 94*, 122–128.

Botsford, J. H. (1967). Simple method for identifying acceptable noise exposures. *Journal of the Acoustical Society of America, 42*, 810–819.

Brogan, P. A., & Anderson, R. R. (1994). Industrial noise control process. Paper presented at the Annual Meeting of the National Hearing Conservation Association, February 17–19, 1994, Atlanta, GA.

Brown, J., Brummett, R., & Fox, K. (1980). Combined effects of noise and kanamycin. Cochlear pathology and pharmacology. *Archives of Otolaryngology, 106*, 744–750.

Brown, J., Brummett, R., Meikle, M., & Vernon, J. (1978). Combined effects of noise and neomycin: Cochlear changes in the guinea pig. *Acta Otolaryngologica, 86*, 394–400.

Byrne, C., Henderson, D., Saunders, S., Powers, N., & Farzi, F. (1988). Interaction of noise and whole body vibration. In O. Manninen (Ed.), *Recent Advances in Researches on the Combined Effects of Environmental Factors* (pp. 68–79). Tampere, Finland: Py-Paino Oy Printing House.

Byrne, D., & Monk, W. (1993). Evaluating a hearing conservation program: A comparison of the USAEHA method and the ANSI S12.13 method [Abstract]. *Spectrum, 10* (Suppl 1), 19.

Canadian Standards Association (CSA). (1986). *Procedures for the Measurement of Occupational Noise Exposure, A National Standard of Canada*. Toronto, Canada: Author.

Casali, J. G., & Park, M. (1991). Laboratory versus field attenuation of selected hearing protectors. *Sound and Vibration, 25*(10), 26–38.

Ceypek, T. K. J., Kuzniarz, J. J., & Lipowczan, A. (1973). Hearing loss due to impulse noise—A field study. *Proceedings of the International Congress on Noise as a Public Health Problem, Dubrovnik, Yugoslavia*. Washington, DC: U.S. Environmental Protection Agency.

Clark, W. W., & Bohne, B. A. (1986). Cochlear damage: Audiometric correlates? In M. J. Collins, T. Glattke, & L. A. Harker (Eds.), *Sensorineural Hearing Loss: Mechanism, Diagnosis and Treatment*. Iowa City: University of Iowa Press.

Clark, W. W., Bohne, B. A., & Boettcher, F. A. (1987). Effect of periodic rest on hearing loss and cochlear damage following exposure to noise. *Journal of the Acoustical Society of America, 82*, 1253–1264.

Cohen, A. (1973). Extra-auditory effects of occupational noise. Part II: Effects on work performance. *National Safety News, 108*, 68–76.

Cohen, A. (1976). The influence of a company hearing conservation program on extra-auditory problems in workers. *Journal of Safety Research, 8*(4), 146–162.

Coles, R. R. (1980). Effects of impulse noise on hearing—introduction. *Scandinavian Audiology, Supplement 12*, 11–13.

Coles, R. R., Garinther, G. R., Hodge, D.C., & Rice, C. G. (1968). Hazardous exposure to impulse noise. *Journal of the Acoustical Society of America, 43*, 336–346.

Coles, R. R., Rice, C. G., & Martin, A. M. (1973). Noise-induced hearing loss from impulse noise: Present status. In *Proceedings of the International Congress on Noise as a Public Health Problem, Dubrovnik, Yugoslavia, May 13–18, 1973*. Washington, DC: Environmental Protection Agency, EPA Pub No. 550/9-73-008.

Committee on Hearing, Bio-acoustics and Biomechanisms (CHABA). (1986). *Proposed Damage-Risk Criterion for Impulse Noise*. Washington, DC: National Academy of Sciences, National Research Council.

Danielson, R., Henderson, D., Gratton, M. A., Bianchi, L., & Salvi, R. (1991). The importance of "temporal pattern" in traumatic impulse noise exposures. *Journal of the Acoustical Society of America, 90*, 209–218.

Delin, C. (1984). Noisy work and hypertension. *Lancet, 2*, 931.

Earshen, J. J. (1986). Sound measurement: Instrumentation and noise descriptors. In E. H. Berger, W. D. Ward, J. C. Morrill, & L. H. Royster (Eds.), *Noise and Hearing Conservation Manual*. Akron, OH: American Industrial Hygiene Association.

Eldred, K. M., Gannon, W. J., & von Gierke, H. E. (1955). *Criteria for Short Time Exposure of Personnel to High Intensity Jet Aircraft Noise*. Wright-Patterson AFB, OH: U.S. Air Force, WADC Technical Note 55-355.

Fechter, L. D., Young, J. Y., & Carlisle, L. (1988). Potentiation of noise induced threshold shifts and hair cell loss. *Hearing Research, 34*, 39–48.

33 Fed. Reg. 14,258 (1968). Bureau of Labor Standards. Proposed rule making: Occupational noise exposure.

2.34 Fed. Reg. 790 (1969a). Bureau of Labor Standards. Occupational noise exposure.

34 Fed. Reg. 7,948 (1969b). Bureau of Labor Standards. Occupational noise exposure.

39 Fed. Reg. 37,773 (1974a). Occupational Safety and Health Administration. Occupational noise exposure: Proposed requirements and procedures. (Codified at 29 CFR 1910.)

39 Fed. Reg. 43,802 (1974b). U.S. Environmental Protection Agency. Proposed OSHA occupational noise exposure regulation: Request for review and report.

40 Fed. Reg. 12,336 (1975). Occupational Safety and Health Administration: Occupational noise exposure—review and report requested by EPA.

46 Fed. Reg. 4,078 (1981). U.S. Department of Labor. Occupational noise exposure; hearing conservation amendment: Final rule. (Codified at 29 CFR 1910.)

3.48 Fed. Reg. 9,738 (1983). U.S. Department of Labor. Occupational noise exposure; hearing conservation amendment: Final rule. (Codified at 29 CFR 1910.)

Franks, J. R., & Berger, E. H. (1997). Hearing protection—personal protection—overview and philosophy of personal protection. In *ILO Encyclopedia of Occupational Safety and Health*. Geneva, Switzerland: International Labour Organization (in press).

Franks, J. F., Davis, R. R., & Krieg, E. F. (1989). Analysis of a hearing conservation program database: Factors other than workplace noise. *Ear and Hearing, 10*(5), 273–280.

von Gierke, H. E., Robinson, D., & Karmy, S. J. (1981). *Results of the Workshop on Impulse Noise and Auditory Hazard*. Southampton, England: University of Southampton, Institute of Sound and Vibration Research, ISVR Memorandum 618.

Gannon, R. P., Tso, S. S., & Chung, D. Y. (1979). Interaction of kanamycin and noise exposure. *Journal of Laryngology and Otology, 93*, 341–347.

Gasaway, D. C. (1985). Documentation: The weak link in audiometric monitoring programs. *Occupational Health and Safety, 54*(1), 28–33.

Glorig, A., Ward, W. D., & Nixon, J. (1961). Damage risk criteria and noise-induced hearing loss. *Archives of Otolaryngology, 74*, 413–423.

Goff, R. J., & Blank, W. J. (1984). A field of evaluation of muff-type hearing protection devices. *Sound and Vibration, 18*(10), 16–22.

Guberan, E., Fernandez, J., Cardinet, J., & Terrier, G. (1971). Hazardous exposure to industrial impact noise. *Annals of Occupational Hygiene, 14*, 345–350.

Haag, W. M. (1988a). Engineering source controls can reduce worker exposure to noise. *Occupational Health and Safety, 57*(4), 31–33.

Haag, W. M. (1988b). Purchasing power. *Applications of Industrial Hygiene, 3*(9), F22–F23.

Hachey, G. A., & Roberts, J. T. (1983). *Real World Effectiveness of Hearing Protection*. Unpublished paper presented at the American Industrial Hygiene Conference, Philadelphia, PA, May 1983.

Hamernik, R., & Henderson, D. (1976). The potentiation of noise by other ototraumatic agents. In D. Henderson, R. Hamernik, D. Dosanjh, & J. Mills (Eds.), *Effects of Noise on Hearing* (pp. 291–307). New York: Raven Press.

Hamernik, R., Henderson, D., Coling, D., & Salvi, R. (1981). Influence of vibration on asymptotic threshold shift produced by impulse noise. *Audiology, 20*, 259–269.

Helmkamp, J. C. (1986). Why workers do not use hearing protection. *Occupational Health and Safety, 55*(10), 52.

Helmkamp, J. C., Talbott, E. O., & Margolis, H. (1984). Occupational noise exposure and hearing loss characteristics of a blue-collar population. *Journal of Occupational Medicine, 26*, 885–891.

Hempstock, T. I., & Hill, E. (1990). The attenuations of some hearing protectors as used in the workplace. *Annals of Occupational Hygiene, 34*, 453–470.

Henderson, D., & Hamernik, R. (1986). Impulse noise: Critical review. *Journal of the Acoustical Society of America, 80*, 569–584.

Henry, S. D. (1992). *Characterizing TWA Noise Exposures Using Statistical Analysis and Normality*. Unpublished paper presented at the Hearing Conservation Conference, Cincinnati, OH, April 3, 1992.

Hetu, R. (1979). Critical analysis of the effectiveness of secondary prevention of occupational hearing loss. *Journal of Occupational Medicine, 21*, 251–254.

Holmgren, G., Johnsson, L., Kylin, B., & Linde, O. (1971). Noise and hearing of a population of forest workers. In D. W. Robinson (Ed.), *Occupational Hearing Loss*. London and New York: Academic Press.

Humes, L. (1984). Noise-induced hearing loss as influenced by other agents and by some physical characteristics of the individual. *Journal of the Acoustical Society of America, 76*, 1318–1329.

ISO. (1961). *International Organization for Standardization, Acoustics—Draft Proposal for Noise Rating Numbers with Respect to Conservation of Hearing, Speech Communication, and Annoyance*. Geneva, Switzerland: International Organization for Standardization, ISO/TC 43 #219.

ISO. (1971). *International Organization for Standardization, Acoustics—Assessment of Occupational Noise Exposure for Hearing Conservation Purposes*. Geneva, Switzerland: International Organization for Standardization, R-1999.

ISO. (1990). *International Organization for Standardization, Acoustics—Determination of Occupational Noise Exposure and Estimation of Noise-Induced Hearing Impairment*. Geneva, Switzerland: International Organization for Standardization, ISO-1999.

Johansson, B., Kylin, B., & Reopstorff, S. (1973). Evaluation of the hearing damage risk from intermittent noise according to the ISO recommendations. In *Proceedings of the International Congress on Noise as a Public Health Problem*. Washington, DC: U.S. Environmental Protection Agency, EPA Report 550/9-73-008.

Johnson, A., Juntunen, L., Nylen, P., Borg, E., & Hoglund, G. (1988). Effect of interaction between noise and toluene on auditory function in the rat. *Acta Otolaryngologica* (Stockholm), *105*, 56–63.

Jonsson, A., & Hansson, L. (1977). Prolonged exposure to a stressful stimulus (noise) as a cause of raised blood pressure in man. *Lancet, 1*, 86–87.

Kryter, K. D., Ward, W. D., Miller, J. D., & Eldredge, D. H. (1966). Hazardous exposure to intermittent and steady-state noise. *Journal of the Acoustical Society of America, 39*, 451–464.

Kuzniarz, J. J., Swierczynski, Z., & Lipowczan, A. (1976). Impulse noise induced hearing loss in industry and the energy concept: A field study. In *Proceedings of 2nd Conference, Southampton*. London, England: Academic Press.

Lempert, B. L., & Edwards, R. G. (1983). Field investigations of noise reduction afforded by insert-type hearing protectors. *American Industrial Hygiene Association Journal, 44*, 894–902.

Lees, R. E. M., & Roberts, J. H. (1979). Noise-induced hearing loss and blood pressure. *CMA Journal, 120*, 1082–1084.

Malchaire, J. B., & Mullier, M. (1979). Occupational exposure to noise and hypertension: A retrospective study. *Annals of Occupational Hygiene, 22,* 63–66.

Manninen, O., & Aro, S. (1979). Noise-induced hearing loss and blood pressure. *International Archives of Occupational and Environmental Health, 42,* 251–256.

Melnick, W. (1984). Evaluation of industrial hearing conservation programs: A review and analysis. *American Industrial Hygiene Association Journal, 45*(7), 59–67.

Melnick, W. (1994). Industrial hearing conservation. In J. Katz (Ed.), *Handbook of Clinical Audiology* (4th ed., pp. 534–552). Baltimore: Williams & Wilkins.

Merry, C. J. (1995). *Instilling a Safety Culture in the Workplace.* Paper presented at the Hearing Conservation Conference III/XX, Cincinnati, OH, March 22–25, 1995.

Morata, T. C., Dunn, D., Kretschmer, L. W., Lemasters, G. K., & Keith, R. W. (1993). Effects of occupational exposure to organic solvents and noise on hearing. *Scandinavian Journal of Work and Environmental Health, 19*(4), 245–254.

Morrill, J. C. (1986). Hearing measurement. In E. H. Berger, W. D. Ward, J. C. Morrill, & L. H. Royster (Eds.), *Noise and Hearing Conservation Manual.* Akron, OH: American Industrial Hygiene Association.

Morrill, J. C., & Sterrett, M. L. (1981). Quality controls for audiometric testing. *Occupational Health and Safety, 50*(8), 26–33.

National Institute for Occupational Safety and Health (NIOSH). (1972). *Criteria for a Recommended Standard: Occupational Exposure to Noise.* DHEW (NIOSH) Publication No. HSM 73-11001. Cincinnati, OH: U.S. Department of Health, Education, and Welfare.

National Institute for Occupational Safety and Health (NIOSH). (1973). *The Industrial Environment—Its Evaluation and Control.* DHEW (NIOSH), pp. 533–562. Cincinnati, OH: U.S. Department of Health, Education, and Welfare.

National Institute for Occupational Safety and Health (NIOSH). (1975). *Compendium of Materials for Noise Control.* DHEW (NIOSH) Publication No. 75-165. Cincinnati, OH: U.S. Department of Health, Education, and Welfare, Public Health Service, Center for Disease Control, National Institute for Occupational Safety and Health.

National Institute for Occupational Safety and Health (NIOSH). (1977). *Occupational Exposure Sampling Strategy Manual.* DHEW (NIOSH) Publication No. 77-173. Cincinnati, OH: U.S. Department of Health, Education, and Welfare, Public Health Service, Center for Disease Control, National Institute for Occupational Safety and Health.

National Institute for Occupational Safety and Health (NIOSH). (1994). *The NIOSH Compendium of Hearing Protective Devices.* DHHS (NIOSH) Publication No. 95-105. Cincinnati, OH: U.S. Department of Health and Human Services, Public Health Service, Centers for Disease Control and Prevention, National Institute for Occupational Safety and Health.

National Institute for Occupational Safety and Health (NIOSH). (1995). *Preventing Occupational Hearing Loss—A Practical Guide.* DHHS (NIOSH) Publication No. 96-110. Cincinnati, OH: U.S. Department of Health and Human Services, Public Health Service, Centers for Disease Control, National Institute for Occupational Safety and Health.

National Institute for Occupational Safety and Health (NIOSH). (1998). *Occupational Noise Exposure: Revised Criteria for a Recommended Standard.* DHHS (NIOSH) Publication No. 98-126. Cincinnati, OH: U.S. Department of Health and Human Services, Public Health Service, Centers for Disease Control, National Institute for Occupational Safety and Health.

Nilsson, R., Liden, G., & Sanden, A. (1977). Noise exposure and hearing impairment in the shipbuilding industry. *Scandinavian Audiology, 6,* 59–68.

Noweir, M. H. (1984). Noise exposure as related to productivity, disciplinary actions, absenteeism, and accidents among textile workers. *Journal of Safety Research, 15*(4), 163–174.

Occupational Safety and Health Administration (OSHA). (1983). 3.48 Fed. Reg. 9, 738 (1983). U.S. Department of Labor. *Occupational Noise Exposure: Hearing Conservation Amendment: Final Rule.* (Codified at CFR 1910.)

Occupational Safety and Health Administration (OSHA). (1989). *Industrial Hygiene Field Operation Manual.* OSHA Instruction CPL 2.45B. Washington, DC: U.S. Department of Labor.

Ohrstrom, E., Martin, B., Rylander, R. (1988). Noise annoyance with regard to neurophysiological sensitivity, subjective noise sensitivity and personality variables. *Psychological Medicine, 18,* 605–613.

Parvizpoor, D. (1976). Noise exposure and prevalence of high blood pressure among weavers in Iran. *Journal of Occupational Medicine, 18,* 730–731.

Passchier-Vermeer, W. (1968). *Hearing Loss Due to Exposure to Steady-State Broadband Noise.* Delft, Netherlands: Research Institute for Public Health Engineering, Report 35.

Passchier-Vermeer, W. (1971). Steady-state and fluctuating noise: its effect on the hearing of people. In D. W. Robinson (Ed.), *Occupational Hearing Loss.* New York and London: Academic Press.

Passchier-Vermeer, W. (1973). Noise-induced hearing loss from exposure to intermittent and varying noise. In *Proceedings of the International Congress on Noise as a Public Health Problem.* Washington, DC: U.S. Environmental Protection Agency, EPA Report 550/9-73-008.

Pekkarinen, J. (1987). Industrial impulse noise, crest factor and the effects of earmuffs. *American Industrial Hygiene Journal, 48*(10), 861–866.

Pekkarinen, J. (1989). *Exposure to Impulse Noise, Hearing Protection and Combined Risk Factors in the Development of Sensory Neural Hearing Loss.* Kuopio, Finland: University of Kuopio.

Pell, S. (1972). An evaluation of a hearing conservation program. *American Industrial Hygiene Association Journal, 33*(1), 60–70.

Price, G. R., & Kalb, J. T. (1991). Insights into hazards from intense impulses from a mathematical model of the ear. *Journal of the Acoustical Society of America, 90,* 219–227.

Rebert, C. S., Sorenson, S. S., Howd, R. A., & Pryor, G. T. (1983). Toluene-induced hearing loss in rats evidenced by the brainstem auditory-evoked response. *Neurobehavioral Toxicology and Teratology, 5*, 59–62.

Rink, T. (1989). *Clinical Review of Patterns from 300,000 Industrial Audiograms*. Paper presented at the 1989 Industrial Hearing Conservation Conference, April 12–14, 1989, Lexington, KY.

Robinson, D. W. (1968). *The Relationship between Hearing Loss and Noise Exposure*. Teddington, England: National Physical Laboratory, NPL Aero Report Ac 32.

Royster, J. D. (1992). *Evaluation of Different Criteria for Significant Threshold Shift in Occupational Hearing Conservation Programs*. Raleigh, NC: Environmental Noise Consultants, Inc., NTIS No. PB93-159143.

Royster, J. D., & Royster, L. H. (1990). Hearing conservation programs: Practical guidelines for success (pp. 73–75). Chelsea, MI: Lewis Publishers.

Royster, L. H., Berger, E. H., & Royster, J. D. (1986). Noise surveys and data analysis. In E. H. Berger, W. D. Ward, J. C. Morrill, & L. H. Royster (Eds.), *Noise and Hearing Conservation Manual*. Akron, OH: American Industrial Hygiene Association.

Rybak, L. P. (1992). Hearing: The effects of chemicals. *Otolaryngology—Head and Neck Surgery, 106*, 677–686.

Sataloff, J., Vassallo, L., & Menduke, H. (1969). Hearing loss from exposure to interrupted noise. *Archives of Environmental Health, 18*, 972–981.

Shaw, E. A. G. (1985). *Occupational Noise Exposure and Noise-Induced Hearing Loss: Scientific Issues, Technical Arguments and Practical Recommendations*. APS 707. Report prepared for the Special Advisory Committee on the Ontario Noise Regulation. NRCC/CNRC No. 25051. Ottawa, Canada: National Research Council.

Simpson, T. H., & Berninger, S. (1992). *Comparison of Short- and Long-Term Sampling Strategies for Fractional Assessment of Noise Exposure*. Unpublished paper presented at the Hearing Conservation Conference, Cincinnati, OH, April 3, 1992.

Simpson, T. H., Steward, M., & Kaltenbach, J. A. (1994). Early indicators of hearing conservation program performance. *Journal of the American Academy of Audiology, 5*, 300–306.

Singh, A. P., Rai, R. M., Bhatia, M. R., & Nayar, H. S. (1982). Effect of chronic and acute exposure of noise on physiological functions in man. *International Archives of Occupational Environmental Health, 50*, 169–174.

Starck, J., & Pekkarinen, J. (1987). Industrial impulse noise: Crest factor as an additional parameter in exposure measurements. *Applied Acoustics, 20*, .263–274.

Starck, J., Pekkarinen, J., & Pyykko, I. (1988). Impulse noise and hand-arm vibration in relation to sensory neural hearing loss. *Scandinavian Journal of Work and Environmental Health, 14*, 265–271.

Stephenson, M. R. (1995). *Noise Exposure Characterization via Task Based Analysis*. Paper presented at the Hearing Conservation Conference III/XX, Cincinnati, OH, March 22–25, 1995.

Stevens, S. S. (1936). A scale for the measurement of a psychological magnitude: Loudness. *Psychological Review, 43*, 405–416.

Sulkowski, W. J., Kowalska, S., & Lipowczan, A. (1983). Hearing loss in weavers and drop forge hammermen. In T. Rossi (Ed.), *Proceedings of the International Congress on Noise as a Public Health Problem*. Milan, Italy: Centro Ricerche e Studi Amplifon.

Sulkowski, W. J., & Lipowczan, A. (1982). Impulse noise-induced hearing loss in drop forge operators and the energy concept. *Noise Control Engineering, 18*, 24–29.

Suter, A. H. (1986). Hearing conservation. In E. H. Berger, J. C. Morrill, W. D. Ward, & L. H. Royster (Eds.), *Noise and Hearing Conservation Manual* (pp. 1–18). Akron, OH: American Industrial Hygiene Association.

Suter, A. H. (1989). *The Effects of Noise on Performance*. Aberdeen Providing Ground, MD: U.S. Army Human Engineering Laboratory. Technical Memorandum 3-89.

Suter, A. H. (1992a). *The Relationship of the Exchange Rate to Noise-Induced Hearing Loss*. Cincinnati, OH: Alice Suter and Associates, NTIS No. PB93-118610.

Suter, A. H. (1992b). *Communication and Job Performance in Noise: A Review* (pp. 53–78). ASHA Monographs, No. 28. Rockville, Maryland: American Speech-Language-Hearing Association.

Talbott, E., Findlay, R., Kuller, L., Lenkner, L., Matthews, K., Day, R., & Ishii, E. (1990). Noise-induced hearing loss: A possible marker for high blood pressure in older noise-exposed populations. *Journal of Occupational Medicine, 32*, 685–689.

Talbott, E., Helmkamp, J., Matthews, K., Kuller, L., Cottington, E., & Redmond, G. (1985). Occupational noise exposure, noise-induced hearing loss and the epidemiology of high blood pressure. *American Journal of Epidemiology, 121*, 501–514.

Taylor, S. M., Lempert, B., Pelmear, P., Hemstock, L., & Kershaw, J. (1984). Noise levels and hearing thresholds in the drop forging industry. *Journal of the Acoustical Society of America, 76*(3), 807–819.

Thiery, L., & Meyer-Bisch, C. (1988). Hearing loss due to partly impulsive industrial noise exposure at levels between 87 and 90 dB(A). *Journal of the Acoustical Society of America, 84*, 651–659.

U.S. Air Force (1956). *Hazardous Noise Exposure*. Washington, DC: U.S. Air Force, Office of the Surgeon General, AF Regulation 160-3.

Verbeek, J. H. A. M., van Dijk, F. J. H., & de Vries, F. F. (1987). Non-auditory effects of noise in industry: IV. A field study on industrial noise and blood pressure. *International Archives of Occupational and Environmental Health, 59*, 51–54.

Ward, W. D. (1970). Temporary threshold shift and damage risk criteria for intermittent noise exposures. *Journal of the Acoustical Society of America, 48*, 561–574.

Ward, W. D. (1980). Noise-induced hearing loss: Research since 1973. In J. V. Tobias, G. Jansen, W. D. Ward (Eds.), *Proceedings of the Third International Congress on Noise as a Public Health Problem*. Rockville, MD: American Speech-Language Hearing Assoc, ASHA Report 10.

Ward, W. D. (1986). Auditory effects of noise. In E. H. Berger, W. D. Ward, J. C. Morrill, & L. H. Royster (Eds.), *Noise and Hearing Conservation Manual.* Akron, OH: American Industrial Hygiene Association.

Ward, W. D., & Nelson, D. A. (1971). On the equal energy hypothesis relative to damage-risk criteria in the chinchilla. In D. W. Robinson (Ed.), *Occupational Hearing Loss.* London and New York: Academic Press.

Ward, W. D., & Turner, C. W. (1982). The total energy concept as a unifying approach to the prediction of noise trauma and its application to exposure criteria. In R. P. Hamernik, D. Henderson, & R. Salvi (Eds.), *New Perspectives on Noise-Induced Hearing Loss.* New York: Raven Press.

Wilkins, P. A., & Action, W. I. (1982). Noise and accidents—A review. *Annals of Occupational Hygiene, 25,* 249–260.

Wu, T. N., Ko, Y. C., & Chang, P. Y. (1987). Study of noise exposure and high blood pressure in shipyard workers. *American Journal of Industrial Medicine, 12,* 431–438.

Young, S. Y., Upchurch, M. B., Kaufman, M. J., & Fechter, L. D. (1987). Carbon monoxide exposure potentiates high-frequency auditory threshold shifts induced by noise. *Hearing Research, 26,* 37–43.

CHAPTER 17

INSTRUMENTATION AND CALIBRATION

THEODORE J. GLATTKE

The sophistication and flexibility of audiologic instrumentation have undergone unparalleled improvement in recent years due to the development of low-cost, high-speed computers and accessories such as digital sound processing boards. A single computer platform may support a diagnostic audiometer, otoacoustic emission recordings, immittance measurements, hearing aid analysis and programming, and maintenance of clinical records. Recent enhancements of digital storage capabilities will allow audiologists to build libraries of high-quality standardized complex stimulus materials that may be used repeatedly without deterioration of the recording medium. New versions of compact disk (CD) technology have made it possible to increase the storage capacity of the conventional 5-inch CD medium by a factor of 20. Generally called digital video disc (DVD) technology, this development will allow for the creation of standardized evaluation and rehabilitation materials that will include visual as well as auditory components.

Miniature transducers and flexible, calibrated probe microphone assemblies make it possible to capture acoustical signals within the external ear canal to evaluate the performance of hearing aids, and they open the possibility of the development of self-calibrating audiologic instrumentation. Instrumentation used to record electrophysiological responses also has become increasingly adaptable and easy to use while providing more automated features. Many systems are compatible with icon-based computer software that allows the operator to select recording and analysis features from elaborate menus. "Automated" screening for hearing loss through the use of auditory brainstem response (ABR) technology has been shown to produce referrals for follow-up testing that are comparable to those generated by screening techniques in which the pass/fail decision is made by an experienced examiner. Oculomotor behavior can be quantified in terms of velocity and direction of even the most rapid saccades, and recently developed technology precludes the necessity of using electrodes to detect eye motion. As the scope of practice of audiologists has expanded to include the evaluation and rehabilitation of dizzy patients, so has the reliance of clinicians on sophisticated motion translators that can detect and quantify patient sway characteristics.

The technological explosion that has resulted in increased sophistication of instrumentation also has created an increase in the demands that an audiologist faces in terms of maintenance and calibration of clinical tools. The cost of purchase and maintenance of the apparatus needed to perform calibration of bone conduction transducers, insert and supra-aural earphones, loudspeakers, probe microphones, motion translators, and electrophysiological equipment is prohibitive in many settings. Few of us have the knowledge and skills to identify and resolve problems with digital computers and their accessories. We rely increasingly on outside sources to insure that equipment is performing according to its specifications or to the requirements of regulatory agencies and voluntary standards programs. It is important that the clinician who purchases calibration services from another party understands the full scope of calibration requirements.

AMERICAN NATIONAL STANDARDS INSTITUTE

The American National Standards Institute (ANSI) is a voluntary organization that draws its support from manufacturers, professional and scientific organizations, and consumers. The Institute sponsors the development of standards that are of value to government agencies, industry, professional service providers and the general public. ANSI attempts to coordinate its standards with the International Electrotechnical Commission (IEC) and the International Organization for Standardization (ISO). Although the use of standards is entirely voluntary, standards have the impact of law when they are identified in regulations pertaining to clinical practice. It is in the clinician's best interest to insure that the instrumentation that is employed conforms to the applicable standards.

The Acoustical Society of America (ASA) provides the administrative support for standards committees that are identified as S1 (Acoustics), S2 (Mechanical Vibration and Shock), S3 (Bioacoustics), and S12 (Noise). Standards are reviewed every five years. At the time of review, they are reaffirmed, revised, or withdrawn. The current catalog of standards may be obtained by contacting the Standards Secretariat, Acoustical Society of America, 120 Wall Street, 32nd Floor, New York NY 10005-3993. Current instrumentation and procedural standards that may be of particular interest to audiologists include the following:

ANSI S1.1-1994 American National Standard Acoustical Terminology

ANSI S1.4-1983 (R1994) American National Standard Specification for Sound Level Meters

ANSI S1.25-1991 American National Standard Specification for Personal Noise Dosimeters

ANSI S3.1-1991 American National Standard Maximum Permissible Ambient Noise Levels for Audiometric Test Rooms

ANSI S3.2-1989 American National Standard Method for Measuring the Intelligibility of Speech Over Communication Systems

ANSI S3.6-1996 American National Standard Specification for Audiometers

ANSI S3.7-1995 American National Standard Method for Coupler Calibration of Earphones

ANSI S3.13-1987 (R1993) American National Standard Mechanical Coupler for Measurement of Bone Vibrators

ANSI S S3.20-1995 American National Standard Bioacoustical Terminology

ANSI S3.21-1978 (R1992) American National Standard Method for Manual Pure Tone Threshold Audiometry

ANSI S3.25-1989 American National Standard for an Occluded Ear Simulator

ANSI S3.39-1987 American National Standards Specifications for Instruments to Measure Aural Acoustic Impedance and Admittance (Aural Acoustic Immittance)

ANSI S3.43-1992 American National Standard Reference Zero for the Calibration of Pure-Tone Bone-Conduction Audiometers

ANSI S3.44-1996 American National Standards Determination of Occupational Noise Exposure and Estimation of Noise-Induced Hearing Impairment

ANSI S12.2-1995 American National Standard Criteria for Evaluating Room Noise

ANSI S12.6-1984 (R 1990) American National Standard Method for the Measurement of the Real-Ear Attenuation of Hearing Protectors

ANSI S12.18-1994 American National Standard Method for Outdoor Measurement of Sound Pressure Level

Other organizations that produce standards that affect audiological instrumentation include Underwriters Laboratory (UL), which publishes UL544—Standard for Medical and Dental Equipment and UL 2601—Medical Electrical Equipment, Part 1: General Requirements for Safety. The American National Standards Institute and the Association for the Advancement of Medical Instrumentation jointly publish the American National Standard Safe Current Limits for Electromedical Apparatus.

AUDIOMETERS

The basic components of an audiometer include signal and noise sources, provision for accommodation of external signals, a means of controlling the duration and intensity of the signal and a selection of output transducers. These elements are illustrated in Figure 17.1. According to ANSI S 3.6-1996, audiometers are grouped into one of five classes designated by numerals (1, 2, . . . 5) in terms of the facilities that they offer for pure-tone testing and three classes designated by letters (A,B,C) in terms of features that they provide for testing with speech signals. Type 1A is a full-range dual channel instrument and types 4 and 5 are limited-use air-conduction instruments without provision for masking.

Certification that an audiometer meets the current ANSI standard indicates that it meets requirements in the following general areas:

1. Electrical safety
2. Warm-up time
3. Variation in the power supply and environment
4. Generation of unwanted acoustic signals
5. Subject response system
6. Monitoring earphone or loudspeaker system
7. Talk back system

Specific areas that are addressed by the standard include:

1. Tone signal source frequency and sound pressure level ranges, accuracy, and distortion characteristics; signal rise and decay time
2. Speech signal source sound pressure level range, distortion, frequency response, and monitoring capability
3. Properties of masking sounds
4. Resolution, linearity, and accuracy of signal and masker level controls
5. Calibration procedures for supra-aural, circumaural and insert earphones, bone conduction vibrators, and loudspeakers

Tone Signals

The Type 1 audiometer must have the capacity of presenting tones at octave intervals from 125 through 8000 Hz plus 750, 1500, 3000, and 6000 Hz. The latter tones are sometimes called "half octave" frequencies. (A true half octave increase in frequency is equal to $2^{1/2}$ times the starting frequency, or 1.414, and so the actual 1/2 octave points would be 707, 1414, 2828, and 5656 Hz, respectively.) The least stringent requirements are for the type 5 audiometers, with no minimum or a maximum requirements. Frequency accuracy must be within 1% of the stated frequency for type 1 units, 2% for type 2, and 3% for types 3, 4, and 5 units.

The audiometer output is expressed in dB Hearing Level (HL), which, of course, compensates for the fact that

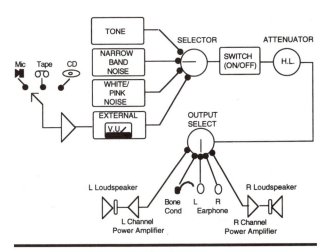

FIGURE 17.1 Schematic of audiometer components in a single channel.

human hearing sensitivity is not equal for all test frequencies. The actual SPL associated with 0 dB HL will vary with the frequency of the stimulus, with the type of earphone that is employed, and with the type of acoustic coupler that links the earphone and measuring microphone. Three types of earphones are described in the standard: supra-aural, circumaural, and insert. The standard calls for the use of an "artificial ear" that is as specified in ANSI 3.7 with the popular Telephonics® style supra-aural earphones. The earphone and cushion are placed on a cavity that is designated as an ANSI 9-A coupler. Under those conditions, the reference pressures for 0 dB HL are as summarized in Table 17.1 for the octave frequencies between 250 and 8000 Hz. The actual SPL value is termed the reference equivalent threshold sound pressure level (RETSPL). The 1996 standard also includes information for calibration of insert receivers. The distal end of the insert receiver is inserted into an occluded ear simulator or into an HA-2 acoustic coupler used to calibrate button-type hearing aid earphone receivers, or the entire eartip is inserted into an HA-1 acoustic coupler and reference SPLs are measured through a conventional calibration microphone system.

TABLE 17.1 Examples of reference equivalent threshold sound pressures for 0 dB HL for standard supra-aural earphones in an ANSI 9-A coupler and for insert earphones in an HA-2 acoustic coupler.

TEST FREQUENCY	250	500	1000	2000	4000	8000 Hz
Reference SPL ANSI 9-A	25.5	11.5	7.0	9.0	9.5	13.0 dB
Reference SPL HA-2	14.0	5.5	0.0	3.0	5.5	0.0 dB

The RETSPL values for insert receivers measured with an HA-2 coupler system also are provided in Table 17.1.

The standard includes an appendix that describes interim or tentative RETSPL values for two types of circumaural earphones that may be employed for extended high-frequency testing. In general, the calibration procedures involve placement of the earphone on a flat-plate adapter that is attached to an IEC "artificial ear" or coupler device.

Bone conduction signals are calibrated through the use of an accelerometer or force transducer system called a mechanical coupler. The standard provides reference force levels for transducer placements on the forehead and on the mastoid. The reference levels are referred to as reference equivalent threshold force levels (RETFL) for bone vibrators. The forehead levels range from 8 to 14 dB higher than the reference force values for the mastoid. All values are provided with the assumption that the nontest ear is masked with a narrowband masker at 40 dB EM (effective masker level) during threshold measurement.

Harmonic Distortion

Harmonic distortion must be measured from the acoustical or mechanical signal, that is to say, from the output of a microphone that is coupled to an earphone in a standard coupler and from the output of a force transducer that is coupled to the bone-conduction vibrator. The maximum distortion is expressed in percentages of the SPL of the test signal. For bone-conducted signals, the total distortion must not exceed 5.5%. This means that the energy in the harmonics must be at least 26 dB below the level of the test signal (dB = 20 log 18). For air-conducted signals, the total energy in the harmonics must be at least 32 dB below the test signal. The level of the second harmonic must be no more than 2% of the level of the intended signal. This is not a very strict criterion. The spectrum pictured in Figure 17.2 illustrates the permissible distortion that would occur under standard test conditions for a signal at 1000 Hz. The signal is presented at 110 dB HL, or 117 dB SPL.

The maximum amplitude of the second harmonic that is allowed is 2% of the intended signal, so the harmonic can emerge at a level that is only 34 dB (dB = 20 log 50) below the intended signal. In this instance the harmonic would be present at 83 dB SPL and not exceed the ANSI standard requirement.

Rise/Fall Time of Tone

When the tone signals are switched on and off, it is imperative that the transition between the two states not be abrupt, so that transient stimulus artifacts can be avoided. A transient artifact produces an audible "click" that can cue the listener about the presence of a sound and lead to a false

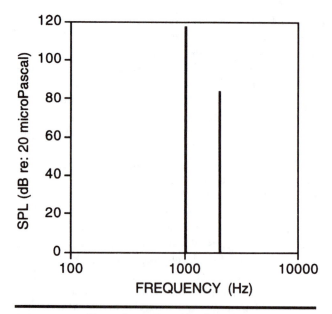

FIGURE 17.2 Example of allowable distortion for a standard test situation. The test signal is 1000 Hz and the second harmonic appears at a level not exceeding 2% of the test signal SPL.

positive response by the listener. The standard specifies that the rise and fall times for the tone must not be less than 20 ms when measured from the point at which the tone is at 10% of its maximum amplitude to the point at which the tone is at 90% of its maximum amplitude. The rise time from 0% to 90% must not exceed 200 ms, and the fall time from 100% to 0% must not exceed 200 ms. When a signal is "off" it must be at least below the 0 dB reference threshold value or 60 dB below the indicated HL dial setting, when the HL dial is set to 60 dB or greater.

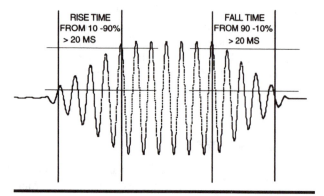

FIGURE 17.3 Example of measurement of rise/fall times for a tonal stimulus.

Attenuator Linearity

The maximum signal strength applied to standard earphones by the audiometer is approximately 1 volt. This will provide an output of about 130 dB SPL for a typical supra-aural earphone and cushion. The voltage applied to the earphone for near 0 dB HL at 1000 Hz is between 1 and 10 μV. The audiometer attenuator system must accommodate this drop in voltage of nearly 1,000,000 to 1 and the audiometer circuitry must not allow the signal to leak around the electrical obstacle posed by the attenuator. The standard requires that the output level of the audiometer always be within 1 dB of the stated value for attenuators marked in 5 dB intervals or 0.3 times the interval of attenuators that are marked in smaller (e.g., 2 dB) intervals. It is very difficult to measure sound pressures near 0 dB HL without specialized equipment that includes narrowband filters or employs other techniques to reduce background noise at frequencies removed from the signal of interest.

Speech Recognition Threshold

The use of the phrase "speech recognition threshold" represents a change from the older terminology of "speech reception threshold" and it is defined as the lowest stimulus level at which the speech signal is recognized 50% of the time. However, speech signals are not used to calibrate the audiometer speech circuit. The standard reference SPL for speech is based on routing a 1000 Hz tone through the external input circuitry and setting the gain of the external tone so that the volume indicator measures a value equivalent to that for the speech material. The reference SPL under those circumstances shall be 12.5 dB greater than the standard for a 1000 Hz pure tone. (See Table 17.1 for examples of SPL values for pure tones delivered via supra-aural and insert earphones.) Therefore, 0 dB HL for speech signals presented via standard supra-aural earphones is 19.5 dB SPL. See Chapter 2 for a discussion of speech audiometry.

Masking

General purpose audiometers routinely provide broad- and narrowband masking sounds. The rationale for the use of narrowband masking is derived from the critical band concept. Briefly, it can be demonstrated that only a narrow band of frequencies near a given pure tone is effective in contributing to the masking of that tone. This narrow band is called the critical band. Audiometers meeting the ANSI specifications for narrow band maskers will produce noise bands that are one-third to one-half octave in width and centered on the frequency of interest. The reading on the HL dial in the case of narrowband masking noise is effective masking or the amount by which the threshold of a normal hearing individual would be shifted in the presence of the noise at the indicated HL value. The appropriate SPL for the narrowband noise masker varies in parallel with the reference threshold values (see Table 17.1) and at 0 dB HL (effective masking) the noise output should be equal to the reference threshold for a signal at the center frequency plus 4 to 8 dB. Refer to Chapter 3 for a discussion of effective masking.

Sound Field Calibration

The standard acknowledges that the environments in which sound field audiometry is conducted may vary considerably. The procedures involved in sound field calibration require that the loudspeakers be placed in the plane of the listener's ears when the listener is seated in the examination room and that measures be obtained for the SPL of frequency modulated (FM) tones at a reference point corresponding to the position of the listener's head. This reference point must be at least one meter from the loudspeaker. Reference equivalent threshold values are related to the angle of incidence of the sound source and they are provided for 45- and 90-degree incidence for monaural threshold testing as well as for 0 degree incidence for both binaural and monaural testing.

Examples of the RETSPLs for sound field measurements are provided in Table 17.2. The sound-field RETSPL values are lower than the coupler measurements (Table 17.1). The differences obtain from the differences between minimum audible pressure (MAP) at the plane of the tympanic membrane, which is estimated by the coupler measurements, and the minimum audible sound field (MAF) surrounding the head. The MAF reference values are influenced by the azimuth, or relative position of the loudspeaker, as indicated in Table 17.2. The azimuth effects are minimum for low-frequency (long wavelength) signals. The complex relationships between azimuth and reference SPL in the higher frequencies are due to resonance and diffraction properties of the head and torso (e.g., Shaw, 1974, Shaw & Vaillancourt, 1985). The requirement that a reference point be one meter from the loudspeaker suggests that it is impossible to create a suitable sound field environment for examination rooms with dimensions that will not permit the listener to be seated at least one meter from the loudspeakers.

Full calibration of the instrument implies that the reference sound pressure levels have been determined for all acoustical transducers and that force measurements have been obtained for the bone conduction vibrator. The person providing the service must have instrumentation that is capable of measuring the rise/fall time of tone bursts, the accuracy of signal frequency and sound pressure level, properties of frequency modulated tones, and distortion. Electrical safety checks specified in the standard include requirements for safe operation of the instrument with power line reversals and in grounded and ungrounded situations. Full calibration of the *test facility* also includes the requirement that background noise levels in the test rooms be compatible with the applicable ANSI standard.

ACOUSTIC IMMITTANCE SYSTEMS

Acoustic immittance measurement systems are described in ANSI S3.39-1987. Four instrument types, designated 1 through 4, are detailed. The full-range instruments are labeled Type 1, and the Type 4 category has no minimum requirement for features. It should be recalled that the principle by which the instruments operate is that the SPL of a standard probe signal measured in the ear canal will vary directly with the impedance, or opposition, that the external, middle, and inner ear components offer to the flow of energy. This impedance measurement will vary inversely with the volume of the external ear canal and so the clinical instruments are designed to produce a measure that is *compensated* for the ear canal volume. The compensation is obtained by comparing the SPL of the probe signal under a condition in which the ear canal is pressurized at a level of +200 decaPascals (daPa) with a measure obtained when the ear canal pressure matches that of the middle ear cavity. Under the former condition, the SPL value is controlled primarily by the ear canal volume and under the latter condition, the SPL value is due to the ear canal volume, and the response of the other peripheral structures.

This is accomplished by delivering the probe signal to the ear through a hermetically sealed apparatus that is inserted into the external auditory canal, adjusting the air pressure and comparing SPL values obtained at various pressures with standard calibrated, values. The resulting readout to the clinician is a *tympanogram* that expresses the change in SPL in impedance units (acoustic ohms), the compliance of an equivalent volume of air (cm^3), or the admittance in acoustic mmhos. The only probe frequency specified in the standard is 226 Hz. At this frequency, the

TABLE 17.2 Examples of reference equivalent threshold sound pressure levels for sound field testing. Examples are provided for three positions of the loudspeaker for monaural testing.

TEST FREQUENCY	250	500	1000	2000	4000 Hz
Binaural	11.0	4.0	2.0	−1.5	−6.5 dB
Monaural 0°	13.0	6.0	4.0	0.5	−4.5 dB
Monaural 45°	12.0	3.0	0.0	−2.5	−8.5 dB
Monaural 90°	11.0	1.5	−1.5	−1.5	−4.0 dB

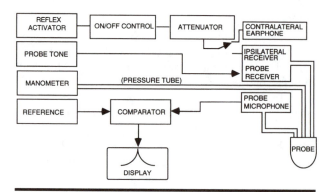

FIGURE 17.4 Components of an acoustic immittance measurement system.

equivalent volume measurement in cm³ is numerically equal to the admittance in acoustic mmhos.

Tone and Noise Generation

As illustrated in Figure 17.4, the typical apparatus consists of an audiometer section and the immittance section. The audiometer section includes tone and noise generators that are used as acoustic reflex activators, a switching apparatus to control the duration of the activator stimulus and an attenuator to control the level of the activator stimulus. The Type 1 instruments must provide tonal stimuli at 500, 1000, 2000, and 4000 Hz. The stimuli may be routed to a receiver that is placed on or in the ear contralateral to the probe, or to the probe for ipsilateral stimulation.

The standards for frequency accuracy, harmonic distortion, attenuator linearity, and rise/fall characteristics of the reflex activating signals are equivalent to those for audiometer circuits. If noise is provided, then it should have a flat spectrum (±5 dB re: the level at 1000 Hz) from 250 through 6000 Hz.

Pressure Manometer

The standard requires that the device have the capacity to control and measure the air pressure in the external ear canal over a range of −600 to +200 decaPascals (daPa) for the full range instruments. The limited range Type 3 device should provide a range of −300 to +100 daPa. The tolerance of the pressure measurement should be 10% in Type 1 and 2 instruments and 15% in the Type 3 instruments. The pressure accuracy must be measured in a 0.5 cm³ test cavity.

Probe Signal

The standard requires a probe signal of 226 Hz. Additional probe frequencies may be supplied for multifrequency tympanometry measurements. For 226 Hz, the probe frequency tolerance is 3% and the probe level must not exceed 90 dB SPL. Harmonic distortion should be less than 5% (harmonics should be at least 26 dB below the level of the probe tone). Calibration of the probe is accomplished by inserting it into three cavities that are supplied by the manufacturer. The standard calls for these cavities to have volumes of 0.5, 2.0 and 5.0 cm³.

Because the presence of an acoustic reflex is detected as a small change of probe SPL, it is critical that the apparatus not misread the presentation of an ipsilateral reflex activating stimulus as that change. The SPL difference associated with acoustic reflex threshold measures is approximately 0.25 dB. The immittance device reduces the possibility of an artifact by employing filter circuitry in the probe microphone circuit to isolate the probe frequency.

Display Dimensions

The configuration of the tympanogram that is displayed by the apparatus will be influenced by the relative dimensions of the vertical and horizontal axes. To reduce the possibility that identical results might be misinterpreted as being different, the standard indicates that the vertical scale, representing acoustic admittance, be segmented so that one division corresponds to 1 acoustic mmho and that the same distance correspond to 300 daPa on the horizontal axis. The standard also recommends that the display employ standard terminology to label the axes. Refer to Chapters 4 and 5 for discussions of tympanometry and acoustic reflexes.

ELECTROPHYSIOLOGICAL MEASUREMENTS

Electrophysiological measurements generally employ large electrodes applied to the surface of the skin to detect electrical events generated in neural or muscle tissue. Recordings that audiologists obtain include

Electromyography (EMG) (recordings of motor potentials)

Electro-oculography (EOG) (recordings of eye potentials) and visual evoked potentials (responses from the visual nervous system)

EOG and electronystagmography (ENG) (recordings of eye motion)

Somatosensory potentials—recorded to study nerve conduction velocity, e.g., during intraoperative monitoring

Auditory evoked potentials, including

Electrocochleography (ECG) (0 to 5 msec after stimulus—recordings of cochlear and auditory nerve events)

Auditory brainstem responses (ABR) (1.5–10 msec after stimulus recordings of auditory nerve, brainstem and mid-brain events)

Middle latency responses (MLR) (10–50 msec after stimulus recordings of cortical electrical activity)

Late evoked potentials (LEP) (>50 msec after stimulus recordings of cortical electrical activity)

The principal standards that exist for electrophysiological recording apparatus pertain to electrical safety for the patient. As mentioned previously, Underwriters Laboratories (UL) publishes UL544—Standard for Medical and Dental Equipment and UL 2601—Medical Electrical Equipment, Part 1: General Requirements for Safety. The American National Standards Institute and the Association for the Advancement of Medical Instrumentation jointly publish the American National Standard Safe Current Limits for Electromedical Apparatus.

The electrophysiological signals that are detected from the surface of the body are complex "graded" events. That is to say, they change in magnitude either as by-products of stimulus characteristics or as the result of changes in subject state. The signals that are detected range from about 0.05 microvolts to nearly 100 microvolts when seen from the surface of the body. To detect the smallest events, an amplifier providing a gain of 1,000,000 or 10,000,000 must be used. The physiological signals range in frequency from very slow phenomena, about 0.25 Hz, to relatively rapid events that contain a broad spectrum.

Apparatus

Although there is no standard that specifies the characteristics of the apparatus or the methods to be employed in electrophysiological records, the apparatus typically includes the following:

1. Electrical contact with the skin through metal or specialized composition material, called an electrode. Intraoperative monitoring may involve invasive electrodes that are placed directly on tissue after surgical exposure.
2. Use of at least three electrical contact points, one called "active" or noninverting, a second called "reference" or inverting, and a third called "common."
3. Specialized, low-noise, high-gain amplifier designed to detect and amplify the difference between the noninverting and inverting electrodes. This differential amplifier is designed to reduce the background electrical noise that is present in most clinic environments.
4. Filters that are employed to emphasize the desired electrical signals and attenuate unwanted signals.
5. Computer-based data collection system that involves an analog-to-digital converter to sample the amplifier output and store the signal in digital form.
6. For evoked potential recordings, the device that will incorporate a stimulus generator and a means of sampling the electrophysiological activity in synchrony with repeated presentations of the stimulus. The repetitive sampling procedure enables the computer to obtain an average of the electrical activity coincident with the stimulus presentation. This process reduces the contribution of nonsynchronized electrical signals to improve the resolution of the desired response.

There are many sources of interference or noise in most clinical environments. The principal sources are illustrated in Figure 17.5. They include radio frequency signals from communications systems and imaging equipment, magnetic fields created by motors that power elevators and air conditioning equipment, and electromagnetic radiation from lights and the transducers used to provide auditory stimulation. In addition, unwanted physiological signals such as EEG, EMG, or ECG can contaminate the recording situation. The effects of the noise are reduced through the use of two techniques: differential amplification and signal averaging.

Differential amplifiers have been employed to improve the signal-to-noise ratio of the desired response for more than 45 years (Tasaki, Davis, & Legouix, 1972). The action of a differential amplifier system is illustrated in schematic form in Figure 17.6. Briefly, the device actually consists of at least three amplifier elements. For routine measurements of small physiological signals, three electrodes are used to make contact with the patient. In ideal recording conditions, one electrode is placed to optimize the detection of the electric potentials that are of interest. This placement often is the vertex, and the lead wire from this electrode is lead to the so-called noninverting input of the differential amplifier. A second electrode is placed at a different site. The placement will, under optimal circumstances, cause the second electrode to detect the same noise as the first electrode. The second electrode is attached to the inverting input of the differential amplifier. A third electrode is placed at a quiet location and serves as a common reference point for the other two electrodes.

The differential amplifier is so called because it amplifies the difference between the two signals at its input. If the noninverting electrode detects the desired response and noise and the inverting electrode detects the same noise as the noninverting electrode, then the output of the amplifier will reduce the noise contribution and leave the desired

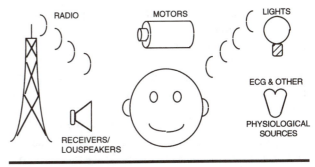

FIGURE 17.5 Examples of sources of competing signals that can compromise electrophysiological recordings.

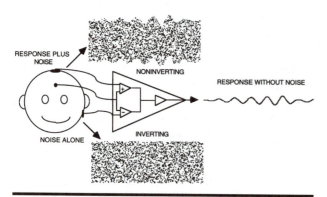

FIGURE 17.6 Schematic illustration of a differential amplifier and the effects of the differential amplifier on signal-to-noise ratio.

response intact. The differential amplifiers are rated in terms of their *common mode rejection* capabilities, usually in dB. Common mode rejection refers to the amount of reduction that the amplifier offers for signals that appear in common at both the inverting and noninverting inputs. A typical common mode rejection value is 60 dB, which means that the noise levels are reduced to 0.001 of their original value if they appear identical at both inputs to the preamplifier system (60 dB = 20 log 1000). In practice, the noninverting and inverting electrodes do not detect identical amounts of noise and they may both detect some of the desired signal. As a result, the differential amplifier is supplemented by a digital averaging system.

Analog-to-Digital Conversion

The first step in the process of obtaining averaged electrophysiological responses is called analog-to-digital conversion. In the most general terms, the A-to-D process involves sampling the signal that is of interest with an appropriate transducer (e.g., microphone or electrodes) amplifying the voltage that is the *analog to the signal of interest* and then representing that voltage on a moment to moment basis in terms of digits that a computer or other storage device can process. Two features of the A-to-D and D-to-A process influence the quality of the result: rate of conversion and resolution of the conversion.

The *rate of conversion* is the number of samples that can be converted in each second. The *resolution* refers to the precision of the conversion process. Said differently, the resolution is expressed by the number of bits used to represent the voltage.

An example of the effect of conversion rate on the fidelity of the signal is illustrated in Figure 17.7A. The signal is a sine wave that has been sampled at a rate equal to 8 times the frequency of the sine wave. Note that the view of the signal that is stored in the computer for later analysis is

a fairly crude representation of the actual signal. There is a rule about sampling rate. The rule says that to detect the presence of some frequency you must sample the signal at a rate equal to at least twice the frequency you are trying to capture. This is termed the *Nyquist frequency*. In the example of Figure 17.7B, the sampling rate is slightly more than twice the frequency of the signal that is being sampled. Note that the actual sine wave is represented very poorly!

If the A-to-D system fails to sample the signal at the Nyquist frequency, false information will be produced in the result. The false information will be the creation of a frequency "alias." The alias will be equal to the difference between the sampling frequency and the highest frequency that is in the signal. In the case of auditory brainstem responses, this means that you would want to sample at about 6000 Hz to capture the most important information (3000 Hz and below). However, as can be seen, the signal is actually poorly represented even when the A-to-D converter is operated at 8 times the actual frequency that is to be captured. In a practical situation involving sound recording, it is common to pass the signal through a low-pass filter, sometimes called an *antialiasing filter*, to help to insure that the signal will not contain high frequencies that might be misread by the analog to digital converter.

The amplitude resolution of the A-to-D converter is determined by the length of the binary number used to represent the moment to moment voltage. A number that is 16 bits in length will allow the incoming signal to be resolved into 2^{16} parts. This is 65,537 parts (including 0). Examples of poor and excellent sampling outcomes are illustrated in Figure 17.7D.

The 16-bit sampling resolution allows you to record/reproduce data with a dynamic range from noise floor to peak of the signal of 96 dB (dB = 20 X log 65,537 to 1, the range that can be counted with 16 bits). Generally, the electrophysiological signals of interest will be buried in background noise, perhaps at 1/1000 or 1/10,000 of the noise levels. You will need to reach down into the noise with the A-to-D converter to find the small signals. To reach down to 0.001 to 0.0001 times the average background noise, you'll need an A-to-D converter with a 60 dB to 80 dB dynamic range. To get a 60 dB range, you will need 10 bits (1024 to 1), 72 dB will require 12 bits (4098 to 1), and 80 dB will require 14 bits (16384 to 1).

Averaging Procedures to Improve Signal-to-Noise Ratio

Once the sampling process has been completed for each presentation of the stimulus, the resulting data is summed and submitted to averaging procedures in the computer memory. The averaging procedures reduce the contribution of unwanted noise while preserving the waveform of responses that are synchronized with repetitive stimulation.

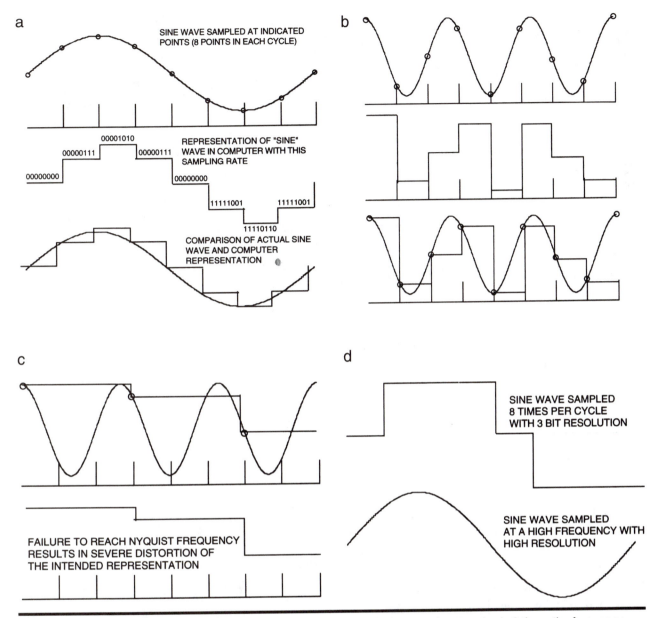

FIGURE 17.7 (A) Example of analog-to-digital conversion pattern when the rate of conversion is 8 times the frequency of the sine wave signal. (B) Example of sampling of a sine wave at a frequency only slightly higher than the Nyquist frequency. (C) Example of the distortion that results when sampling rate does not at least reach the Nyquist frequency. (D) Examples of poor and good amplitude resolution.

The averaging process outcome is simulated in Figure 17.8. Electrical activity that is not synchronized with the stimulus sums to a near zero value when the number of samples is increased. In the illustration at the top of the figure, a small "response" is mixed with random noise that is approximately 10 times greater than the "response." The tracing that is represented is of a single sample of data. When multiple samples are obtained, the amplitude of the nonsynchronized noise is reduced by a factor equal to the square root of the sample size. When two samples are

obtained, the amplitude of the noise is reduced to 71% of the original value ($1/2^{1/2}$). When 10 samples are obtained, as in the next example, the noise is reduced to about 33% of the starting value ($1/10^{1/2}$). When 100 samples are obtained, the noise drops to 10% of the original level.

In most cases, default sampling for auditory brainstem responses involves the collection of 1000 or 2000 samples. This reduces the apparent noise to a level of less than one-thirtieth of its actual level, allowing the small response to emerge from the background noise. Several classes of

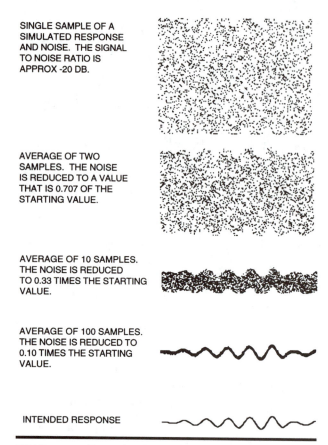

SINGLE SAMPLE OF A SIMULATED RESPONSE AND NOISE. THE SIGNAL TO NOISE RATIO IS APPROX -20 DB.

AVERAGE OF TWO SAMPLES. THE NOISE IS REDUCED TO A VALUE THAT IS 0.707 OF THE STARTING VALUE.

AVERAGE OF 10 SAMPLES. THE NOISE IS REDUCED TO 0.33 TIMES THE STARTING VALUE.

AVERAGE OF 100 SAMPLES. THE NOISE IS REDUCED TO 0.10 TIMES THE STARTING VALUE.

INTENDED RESPONSE

FIGURE 17.8 Example of the effect of repeated sampling on noise reduction.

Figure 17.9, the conventional stimulus is led to the receiver, which is coupled to the sound level meter in the usual way. The AC output of the sound level meter is displayed on an oscilloscope display during the generation of the click stimulus. The SPL reading is ignored, but the peak amplitude of the click is noted in terms of a voltage value on the oscilloscope screen. The pulse is replaced with a continuous tone with a frequency that corresponds to the major peak in the spectrum of the transient stimulus, usually 4 kHz. The continuous tone is adjusted until its amplitude matches the peak amplitude of the click stimulus. At this point the SPL of the tone is read and noted as the stimulus SPL. The behavioral threshold for click stimuli measured in this manner is approximately 35 dB peak equivalent SPL (Glattke, 1983). Most manufacturers of evoked potential equipment specify the stimulus amplitude in terms of *normal Hearing Level* or nHL. This is not a standard amplitude scale, but it is similar to the Hearing Level scale used in audiometers: The 0 dB reference point is the minimum SPL at which listeners with normal pure-tone thresholds can detect the stimulus. There are no standards for distortion, attenuator linearity, masking, or other features of evoked potential equipment. Manufacturers typically recommend that the end user of such equipment obtain "normative" data from a group of listeners who have normal pure tone thresholds prior to attempting to evaluate clinical patients. See Chapters 7, 8, and 9 for discussions of the various electrophysiological measures described above.

evoked potentials have more favorable signal-to-noise ratios and, as a consequence, the number of samples required to extract them from background noise is correspondingly less.

Calibration of the Acoustical Stimuli for Auditory Evoked Potential Testing

There is no standard that applies to the calibration of stimuli used in evoked potential tests. The *stimulus-related potentials,* primarily short-latency neural responses, are most robust when elicited with brief stimuli that have rapid rise/fall times. The clinical examiner must trade imprecision in stimulus frequency composition for the desired stimulus temporal features. It is common to use "clicks" formed by electrical pulses that are 100 μs in duration led to the receiver. The receiver produces a brief acoustical pulse with a leading phase determined by the polarity of the electric signal. The SPL of the stimulus cannot be determined by a conventional sound level meter because the ballistic properties of the meter limit its ability to register a single brief event. It is common to determine the *peak equivalent SPL* following a method outlined by Cullen, Ellis, Berlin, and Lousteau (1972). As illustrated in

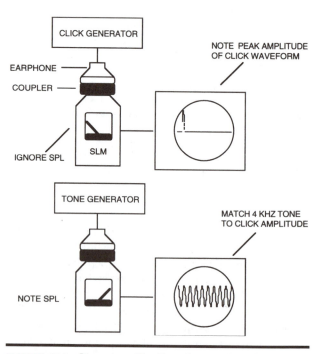

FIGURE 17.9 Steps in calibration of a transient signal to obtain peak equivalent SPL. (After Glattke, 1983)

OTOACOUSTIC EMISSION MEASUREMENTS

Since their discovery twenty years ago, otoacoustic emissions (OAEs) have found widespread application in screening for hearing loss, differential diagnosis, and the identification of individuals with subtle pathology of the auditory system (Robinette & Glattke, 1997). There are no standards, save for electrical safety, that have been developed for the OAE instrumentation that is reaching the marketplace. However, the U.S. Food and Drug Administration has developed regulations that affect the testing features that can be offered by each manufacturer. Several manufacturers offer equipment that is capable of recording spontaneous otoacoustic emissions (SOAEs) and distortion product otoacoustic emissions (DPOAEs). At the present time, only one manufacturer supplies equipment that is capable of recording transient evoked otoacoustic emissions (TEOAEs) and DPOAEs. All of the instrumentation available today has some common features:

1. Personal computer platform
2. Digital sound processing (DSP) components for stimulus generation
3. One or more miniature receivers to produce the acoustic stimulus
4. Miniature microphone to detect signals in the external ear canal
5. Software to produce the stimuli and extract the desired response from background noise

TEOAE recording is virtually identical to recording auditory brainstem responses. The stimulus used to elicit the response is a brief click (or tone burst) presented at about 80 dB peak equivalent SPL at a rate of approximately 50/second. The acoustic signal in the ear canal is sampled coincident with stimulus presentation for approximately 2000 replications of the stimulus and an average response waveform is developed for a 20 msec time period following the stimulus onset. The level of the TEOAE response is about 10 dB SPL in adults, 20 dB SPL in newborns, and it is buried in background noise that is 20 to 40 dB greater than the response amplitude. The TEOAE stimulus and detection probe system consists of a single receiver and microphone, as illustrated in Figure 17.10.

DPOAE responses are obtained for tone bursts formed by delivering two sinusoids to independent receivers. The two signals, f1 and f2, are mixed acoustically in the ear canal. The response of interest is a small signal located at a frequency other than f1 and f2. The response typically is about 50 dB or more below the level of the primary tone bursts. It is imperative that the crosstalk between the two receivers be well below the noise floor of the recording, otherwise contaminated data may be obtained. As Siegel (1995) has noted, some types of probe systems are not free of crosstalk. He urges that manufacturers adopt a uniform

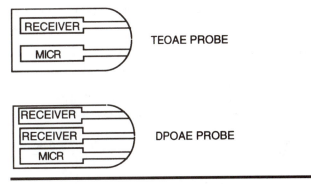

FIGURE 17.10   Otoacoustic emission probe components.

standard for specifying crosstalk. Siegel and Hirohata (1994) also noted that the accuracy of DPOAE measures in the ear canal is highly variable, and that errors may be as large as 20 dB, depending on the position of the measuring device. As the use of OAE measurements expands, the need for standardization in this area will become more acute. See Chapter 6 for more information.

This chapter was not conceived as a guide to the specific steps involved in calibration of acoustical signals or the troubleshooting and repair of equipment. Rather, it was prepared to provide the audiologist with information about the scope of many of the applicable standards and to highlight some areas in which standardization remains elusive. Most clinicians will purchase services related to calibration and maintenance of the equipment that they use in their practice and it is imperative that they be informed consumers of those services. Rapid changes in the technical support of clinical activity can be expected to be delivered with increasing frequency, and it will be increasingly important for audiologists to stay informed of the features and limitations of the instrumentation that is available to them.

REFERENCES

American National Standards Institute (1985). *Safe Current Limits for Electromedical Apparatus*, [ANSI/AAMI ESI-1978 (R1985)]. New York: Author.

American National Standards Institute S1.1-1994. *American National Standard Acoustical Terminology*. New York: Author.

American National Standards Institute S1.4-1983 (R1994). *American National Standard Specification for Sound Level Meters*. New York: Author.

American National Standards Institute S1.25-1991. *American National Standard Specification for Personal Noise Dosimeters*. New York: Author.

American National Standards Institute S3.1-1991. *American National Standard Maximum Permissible Ambient Noise Levels for Audiometric Test Rooms*. New York: Author.

American National Standards Institute S3.2-1989. *American National Standard Method for Measuring the Intelligibility of Speech Over Communication Systems*. New York: Author.

American National Standards Institute S3.6-1996. *American National Standard Specification for Audiometers*. New York: Author.

American National Standards Institute S3.7-1985. *American National Standard Method for Coupler Calibration of Earphones*. New York: Author.

American National Standards Institute S3.13-1987 (R1993). *American National Standard Mechanical Coupler for Measurement of Bone Vibrators*. New York: Author.

American National Standards Institute S3.20-1995. *American National Standard Bioacoustical Terminology*. New York: Author.

American National Standards Institute S3.21-1978. (R1992). *American National Standard Method for Manual Pure Tone Threshold Audiometry*. New York: Author.

American National Standards Institute S3.25-1989. *American National Standard for an Occluded Ear Simulator*. New York: Author.

American National Standards Institute S3.39-1987. *American National Standards Specifications for Instruments to Measure Aural Acoustic Impedance and Admittance (Aural Acoustic Immittance)*. New York: Author.

American National Standards Institute S3.43-1992. *American National Standard Reference Zero for the Calibration of Pure-Tone Bone-Conduction Audiometers*. New York: Author.

American National Standards Institute S3.44-1996. *American National Standards Determination of Occupational Noise Exposure and Estimation of Noise-Induced Hearing Impairment*. New York: Author.

American National Standards Institute S12.2-1995. *American National Standard Criteria for Evaluating Room Noise*. New York: Author.

American National Standards Institute S12.6-1984 (R1990). *American National Standard Method for the Measurement of the Real-Ear Attenuation of Hearing Protectors*. New York: Author.

American National Standards Institute S12.18-1994. *American National Standard Method for Outdoor Measurement of Sound Pressure Level*. New York: Author.

Cullen, J. K., Ellis, M. S., Berlin, C. I., & Lousteau, R. J. (1972). Human acoustic nerve action potential recordings from the tympanic membrane without anesthesia. *Acta Otolaryngologica, 74*, 15–22.

Glattke, T. J. (1983). *Short Latency Auditory Evoked Potentials*. Austin: Pro-Ed.

Robinette, M. S., & Glattke, T. J. (Eds.) (1997). *Otoacoustic Emissions: Clinical Applications*. New York: Thieme.

Shaw, E. A. (1974). Transformation of sound pressure level from the free field to the eardrum in the horizontal plane. *Journal of the Acoustical Society of America, 56*, 1848–1861.

Shaw, E. A., & Vaillancourt, M. M. (1985). Transformation of sound-pressure level from the free field to the eardrum presented in numerical form. *Journal of the Acoustical Society of America, 78*, 1120–1123.

Siegel, J. H. (1995). Cross-talk in otoacoustic emission probes. *Ear and Hearing, 16*, 150–158.

Siegel, J. H., & Hirohata, E. T. (1994). Sound calibration and distortion product otoacoustic emissions at high frequencies. *Hearing Research, 80*, 146–152.

Tasaki, I., Davis, H., & Legouix, J.-P. (1952). The space-time pattern of the cochlear microphonics (guinea pig) as recorded by differential electrodes. *Journal of the Acoustical Society of America, 24*, 502–519.

Underwriters Laboratories (n.d.). UL544—*Standard for Medical and Dental Equipment*. New York: Author.

Underwriters Laboratories (n.d.). UL 2601—*Medical Electrical Equipment, Part 1: General Requirements for Safety*. New York: Author.

A

Aaltonen, O., 247, 252, 253, 254
Abbas, P.J., 209, 215, 289
Abdala de Uzcategui, C., 340
Abe, H., 296
Abel, S.M., 470
Abramson, M., 283
Achim, A., 246
Achor, L.J., 212, 225, 234
Action, W.I., 466
Adachi, M., 107
Adams, J., 349
Adams, K.M., 364
Agbenyega, T., 179
Agranoff, D., 179
Aguilar, C., 347, 351
Ahlstrom, C., 42
Aine, C., 257
Ainslie, P.J., 201
Aittonie, K., 245
Akurekliet, C., 256
Al-Mefty, O., 285
Alafuzoff, I., 350
Alain, C., 246
Alaminos, D., 143
Alarson, J.L., 143
Alberti, P.W., 102, 112, 256, 428, 470
Albright, P., 428
Aleksandrovsky, I.V., 43
Alexander, G.C., 44
Alexander, J., 251
Alexander, L., 171, 174, 177, 179
Alexander, O.C., 363
Alford, B.R., 210, 396
Algazi, A., 253, 260
Alho, K., 247, 252, 253, 254, 259, 260
Allard, T., 350
Allen, J., 51, 395, 396
Allen, J.B., 174, 359
Allen, M.C., 341
Allen, P., 249, 250, 392
Allen, R., 246
Allison, T., 246
Alpiner, J.G., 347, 362, 363
Althoff, L.K., 416, 417, 428
Altshuler, M.W., 416, 420
Alvan, G., 178
Amaddio, M.D., 279
Amadee, R.G., 176
Amadeo, M., 218
Amedofu, G., 179
American Academy of Audiology (AAA), 109, 111
American Academy of Neurology, 280, 299
American Academy of Otolaryngology (AAO), 478
American Academy of Otolaryngology—Head and Neck Surgery (AAO-HNS), 182, 474
American Conference of Governmental Industrial Hygienists (ACGIH), 465, 475
American Encephalographic Society, 290
American Industrial Hygiene Association (AIHA), 478
American Medical Association (AMA), 478
American National Standards Institute (ANSI), 1, 3, 4, 5, 7, 8, 10, 11, 13, 14, 15, 16, 21, 24,
34, 42, 49, 68, 69, 76, 95, 99, 100, 101, 141, 142, *145,* 474, 476, 486, 487, 489
American Occupational Medicine Association (AOMA), 476
American Speech and Hearing Association, 32, 33
American Speech-Language-Hearing Association (ASHA), 4, 7, 8, 15, 32, 33, 105, 108, 109, 111, *197, 199, 203, 204, 212, 213, 214, 215, 216, 218, 220, 221, 224,* 273, 335, 361, 362, 378, 379, 477, 478
American Standards Association, 1, 73, 76
Aminoff, M., 252, 258
Amlie, R.N., 219
Amoroso, C., 360
Amsell, L., 351, 365
Amstutz, L., 259
Anand, V.K., 285
Anari, M., 187
Anch, M., 250
Andaz, C., 419
Anderson, D., 391
Anderson, H., 67, 68, 69, 71, 73, 74, 79, 83, 141, 148, 149, 445
Anderson, L.G., 43
Anderson, R.R., 472, 477
Anderson, S.D., 177
Anderson, C., 249
Andreozzi, M.P., 211, 281
Andrews, M., 395
Andrews, S., 254
Anold, R., 184
Anslie, J., 249
Antablin, J.K., 28, *28,* 43, 54, *54*
Antervo, A., 245, 246
Anthonisen, B., 184
Anthony, L., 145, 427
Antinoro, F., 250
Antonelli, A.R., 383, 384, 385, 395
Aoki, K., 249
Aplin, D.Y., 418, 419, 422
Aponchenko, V., 218
Araki, H., 248
Aran, J.M., 205, 209, 280
Arcos, J.T., 54
Arehart, K.H., 117, 118, *120*
Arehole, S., 256
Arenberg, I.K., 177, 208, 209, 211, 281
Arezzo, J.C., 212, 245, 247
Arick, D.S., 108
Arjona, S.K., 109
Arlinger, S.D., 8
Armbruster, J.M., 417, 420
Armstrong, T.W., 431, 437
Arnce, K.D., 422
Arnesen, A.R., 184, 187, 427
Arnst, D., 358
Aro, S., 466
Aronson, M., 258
Arriaga, M.A., 290
Arslan, E., *197*
Ashmead, D.H., 309
Atherley, G.R.C., 362, 465
Atkins, J.S., 290, 293, 295
Auger, R.G., 286

Augustine, L., 256
Aursnes, J., 187, 427
Auth, T.L., 375, 381
Avery, C., 107, 108
Axlesson, A., 187, 465, 466, 475
Aydogdu, I., 256
Azumi, T., 249

B

Babb, T., 246
Bachman, R., 104, 106, 108, 109, *109*
Backs, R., 257
Bader, C.R., 168
Badier, J., 244
Bagli, P., 334
Bailey, H.A.T. Jr., 425
Bak, C., 245
Bakker, D.J., 393
Balkany, T.J., 117, 169, 177, 178, 179, 230, 235
Ballad, W.J., 201, 217
Balzer, G., 275
Bamford, J.M., 184, 316
Banerjee, S., 322
Barajas, J.J., 143, 246, 251
Baran, J.A., 255, 256, 257, 376, 377, 378, 382, 383, 384, 386, 389, 390, *390,* 393, 394, *394,* 396, *400,* 401, 402, 404
Barber, H.O., 223
Barelli, P.A., 417
Baribeau-Braun, J., 250, 251, 258
Barlow, B., 342
Barnard, S., 210
Barnes, K., 252
Barr, B., 148, 149, 418, 419
Barr, T., 38
Barratt, H., 276, 285
Barrett, L.S., 422
Barringer, D.G., 329, 338
Barrs, D.M., 416, 417, 428
Barthelemy, C., 257
Bartz, W.H., 49
Basil, R.A., 387
Basile, L., 246
Bastien, C., 252
Bastuji, H., 251
Bauberger-Tell, L., 428
Bauch, C.D., 219, 223, 446, 447, 462
Bauer, L., 251
Baum, H.M., 356, *357*
Baumann, S., 245
Bawden, R., 111
Bazydlo-Golinska, G., 416, 428
Bazzano, S., 350
Beagley, H.A., 210, 428
Beardsley, J.V., 217
Beasley, D.S., 47, 358, *359,* 384, 393, 394, 395
Beattie, R.C., 31, 38, 39, 141, 213, 214
Beatty, C.W., 279, 283, 284, 290, 294, 462
Beatty, J., 246
Beauchaine, K.A., 16, 184, 214, 219, 222, 321
Beauchaine, K.L., 104, 106, 107, 334
Beck, D.L., 293
Beck, G., 148
Beck, W.G., 384, 386, 387, 388

G

Gabriel, S., 202
Gafni, M., 212
Gaines, R.W., 280
Galambos, R., 214, 248, 255, 259, 341
Galbraith, G., 257
Gannon, R.P., 478
Gannon, W.J., 465
Gans, D.P., 314
Gantz, B.J., 289
Garber, S.R., 213
Garcia, E., 214
Garcia-Larrea, L., 251
Gardner, D., 446
Gardner, H.J., 41
Gardner, J.C., 212, 232
Garinther, G.R., 465, 478
Garreau, B., 257
Garrido, E., 290
Garstecki, D., 347
Gartner, M., 179
Gasaway, D.C., 465
Gaskill, S.A., 174, 181
Gates, G.A., 107, 108, 109, 358, 360, 361
Gauz, M.T., 16
Gaydos, M.L., 376, 382
Gazzaniga, M.S., 389
Geddes, L.A., 198
Geffner, D., 329
Geier, K., 363
Geisler, C., 243
Geisler, M., 251
Gelfand, S.A., 42, 51, 141, 143, 144, 422, 426
Gelhar, K., 418
Gelnett, D.J., 316
Gengel, R.W., 37
Gennarelli, T.A., 288
Geohegan, P.M., 419
Gerganoff, S., 258
Gerhardt, K.J., 211
Gershon, S., 258
Geschwind, N., 389
Geurkink, N.A., 243, 248, 249, 254, 255, 383, 386, 387, 388, 393, 394
Ghilardi, M.F., 350
Gibbin, K.P., 177, 225
Gibbons, E., 420
Gibbs, C., 393, 394
Gibson, W.P.R., 208, 209, 211, 280, 281
Giebel, A., 184
Giebink, G.S., 107, 108, 112, 121
Giesser, B., 258
Gilmore, C., 44
Gilroy, J., 53, 380, 383, 387, 388, 404
Gilson, B.S., 364
Gilson, J.S., 364
Giolas, T.G., 362
Girod, J., 245
Givens, G., 147, 149
Glascoe, G., 362
Glasscock, M.E., 221, 461
Glattke, T.J., *172,* 173, 494, *494,* 495
Glaze, D., 249
Gleason, W.J., 419
Gleeson, M.J., 290
Glorig, A., 68, 356, 362, 465
Glotzbach, L., 170
Glover, B., 329
Glynn, R.J., 290
Goff, E., 246
Goff, R.J., 470
Goff, W., 246

Gold, B., 426
Gold, S.R., 208, 209, 419
Goldberg, Z., 258, 350
Goldgar, D.E., 222
Goldman, R., 404
Goldstein, B.A., 16, 86
Goldstein, D.P., 15, 380
Goldstein, R., 116, 248, 249, 254, 415, 416
Gollegly, K.M., 49, 221, 245, 254, 384, 389, 394, 402
Golos, E., 236
Gomes, H., 260
Gonzales, L., 309, 311
Goode, R.L., 96
Goodglass, H., 386, 391
Goodhill, V., *133*
Goodin, D., 246, 251, 252, 258
Goodman, J., 256
Goodman, W., 250
Gordon, E., 246
Gordon, M.L., 225
Gordon-Salant, S., 356, 357, *357,* 360, 361
Gorga, M.P., 150, 175, 177, 184, 214, 215, 217, 219, 222, 321, 334
Gosselin, J-Y., 258
Gosset, F., 360
Gosztonyi, R.E., 417
Gottfries, C.G., 350
Gould, H., 254
Govaerts, P.J., 178
Goycoolea, H.G., 102, 103, 104
Grafman, J., 258
Graham, J., 391
Graham, J.M., 415, 420, 427, 428
Graham, J.T., 35, 244
Graham, M., 112
Graham, M.D., 282, 290, 292
Grandori, F., 184, 385
Granseyer, G., 258
Grant, I., 364
Grant, S., 121
Gratton, G., 250
Gratton, M.A., 465, 478
Gravel, J.S., 42, 177, 214, 215, 256, 306, 307, 308, *308,* 309, 310, 311, 312, *312,* 313, *313,* 314, 315, 316, 321, 323, 393
Gravenstein, D., 276, 277, 279, 286
Gray, B.B., 395
Gray, L., 256
Gray, T., 376, 387
Grayson, A., 244, 250
Graziani, L., 245
Green, D.M., 30, 380
Green, D.S., 9, 16
Green, J.D., 290
Green, K.W., 136, *136,* 153, 154, *154*
Green, V., 258
Green, W.B., 333
Greenberg, C.Z., 6, 30
Greenwood, R., 244, 391
Greville, K.A., 234
Griffiths, S.K., 31
Grim, M.A., 361
Grimes, A.M., 402
Grimes, C.T., 15
Grimm, D., 27
Grose, J.H., 392, 393, 394
Grossmann, J., 249
Grote, J.J., 210
Groth, J., 184
Grubb, P.A., 39
Gruber, J., 21

Grundy, B.L., 273, 279
Gruner, M.M., 465
Guberan, E., 465
Guinan, J.J., 135
Gunter, M.B., 31
Gur, R., 256
Gutjahr, P., 178
Gutter, T., 198, 201

H

Haag, W.M., 477
Haas, J., 258
Habener, S.A., 148
Haberkamp, T., 283
Habraken, J.B., 202
Hachey, G.A., 470
Hachikawa, K., 181
Haenel, J.L., 36, 37, *37,* 38
Hagerman, B., 32
Haggard, M.P., 394
Hahn, J.F., 50, 293, 294
Haines, H.L., 35
Haines, S.J., 296
Hake, H.W., 71
Halgren, E., 246, 259
Hall, C., 258
Hall, J.L., 359
Hall, J.W. III, 69, 86, 135, 197, 209, 218, 219, 228, 247, 248, 249, 250, 251, 252, 278, 333, 360, *360,* 361, 392, 393, 394, 428
Hallen, O., 102, 104
Halling, D., 395
Hallstrom, A.P., 364
Halperin, H.R., 35
Halpern, J., 330
Halwes, T., 389
Hamalainen, M., 244, 245, 246, 247
Hamel, G., 215, 254
Hamernik, R.P., 465, 466, 475, 478
Hammer, L.C., 385
Hammerschlag, P.E., 283, 290, 294
Hammond, S.R., 214
Handelsman, L., 258
Handler, A., 381
Handler, S.D., 141, 143, 144
Hanks, W.D., 102
Hanna, T.E., 35
Hansch, E.L., 258, 350
Hansch, M., 258
Hansen, C., 349
Hansen, J., 248
Hanssens, K., 184
Hansson, L., 465
Har'el, Z., 213, 236
Harbert, F., 8
Hardy, R.W., 293, 294
Hardy, W., 426
Harford, E.R., 102, 104, 347, 348, 416, 418, 421, 422, 423, 425
Hari, R., 244, 245, 246, 247
Harner, S.G., 279, 283, 284, 290, 294, 446, 462
Harper, C.M., 279, 283, 284
Harris, D.A., 417, 420, 421
Harris, F.P., 168, 170, 173, 174, 176, 178, 179, 184
Harris, J.D., 11, 35, 48
Harris, R.W., 48
Harris, V.L., 393
Harrison, J., 246
Harrison, R.V., 279
Hart, C.W., 385